VARCAROLIS'S
Canadian Psychiatric Mental Health Nursing
A Clinical Approach | THIRD EDITION

BRIEF CONTENTS

UNIT 1 Foundations in Theory

1. Mental Health and Mental Illness, 2
2. Historical Overview of Psychiatric Mental Health Nursing, 16
3. Overview of Psychiatric Mental Health Nursing Care Within Various Settings, 24
4. Relevant Theories and Therapies for Nursing Practice, 41
5. Understanding Responses to Stress, 59

UNIT 2 Foundations in Practice

6. The Nursing Process and Standards of Care for Psychiatric Mental Health Nursing, 74
7. Ethical Responsibilities and Legal Obligations for Psychiatric Mental Health Nursing Practice, 89
8. Cultural Implications for Psychiatric Mental Health Nursing: A Critical Cultural Perspective, 105

UNIT 3 Biopsychosocial Interventions

9. Therapeutic Relationships, 122
10. Communication and the Clinical Interview, 136
11. Psychotropic Drugs, 153

UNIT 4 Psychobiological Disorders

12. Anxiety and Related Disorders, 180
13. Depressive Disorders, 220
14. Bipolar Disorders, 249
15. Schizophrenia Spectrum and Other Psychotic Disorders, 270
16. Eating and Feeding Disorders, 304
17. Neurocognitive Disorders, 324
18. Psychoactive Substance Use and Treatment, 350
19. Personality Disorders, 390
20. Sleep–Wake Disorders, 413

UNIT 5 Trauma Interventions

21. Crisis and Disaster, 432
22. Suicide and Non-suicidal Self-Injury, 448
23. Anger, Aggression, and Violence, 465
24. Interpersonal Violence: Child, Older Persons, and Intimate Partner Abuse, 481
25. Sexual Assault, 508

UNIT 6 Interventions for Distinct Populations

26. Sexuality and Gender, 524
27. Disorders of Children and Adolescents, 533
28. Psychosocial Needs of the Older Person, 555
29. Recovery, Survivorship, and Public Mental Health Approaches, 572
30. Psychological Needs of Patients With Medical Conditions, 586
31. Care for the Dying and for Those Who Grieve, 594
32. Forensic Psychiatric Nursing, 610

UNIT 7 Advanced Intervention Modalities

33. Therapeutic Groups, 620
34. Family Interventions, 630
35. Integrative and Complementary Therapies, 645

Appendix Standards of Practice, Code of Ethics, Beliefs, and Values, 656
Glossary, 659
Index, 672

VARCAROLIS'S
Canadian Psychiatric Mental Health Nursing
A Clinical Approach | THIRD EDITION

CHERYL L. POLLARD,
RPN, RN, BScN, MN, PhD (Nursing)
Dean
Faculty of Nursing
University of Regina
Regina, Saskatchewan

SONYA L. JAKUBEC,
RN, BHScN, MN, PhD (Nursing)
Professor
Faculty of Health & Community Studies, School of Nursing and Midwifery
Mount Royal University
Calgary, Alberta

US 9th Edition Editor

MARGARET (PEGGY) JORDAN HALTER,
PhD, APRN
Clinical Nurse Specialist
Cleveland Clinic Akron General
Akron, Ohio;
Adjunct Faculty
Ohio State University
Columbus, Ohio

ELSEVIER

Elsevier

VARCAROLIS'S CANADIAN PSYCHIATRIC MENTAL HEALTH NURSING: A CLINICAL APPROACH, THIRD EDITION   ISBN: 9780323778794

Copyright © 2023 by Elsevier Inc. All rights reserved.

Previous editions copyrighted 2019 and 2014 by Elsevier Canada, a Division of Reed Elsevier Canada, Ltd.

Adapted from *Varcarolis' Foundations of Psychiatric-Mental Health Nursing: A Clinical Approach*, 9th Edition, by Margaret Jordan Halter. Copyright © 2022, Elsevier Inc., ISBN: 9780323697071 (paperback). All rights reserved.

No part of this publication may be reproduced or transmitted in any form or by any means, electronic or mechanical, including photocopy, recording, or any information storage and retrieval system, without permission in writing from the publisher. Reproducing passages from this book without such written permission is an infringement of copyright law.

Requests for permission to make copies of any part of the work should be mailed to: College Licensing Officer, access ©, 1 Yonge Street, Suite 1900, Toronto, ON M5E 1E5. Fax: (416) 868-1621. All other inquiries should be directed to the publisher, www.elsevier.com/permissions.

Every reasonable effort has been made to acquire permission for copyrighted material used in this text and to acknowledge all such indebtedness accurately. Any errors and omissions called to the publisher's attention will be corrected in future printings.

Notice

Practitioners and researchers must always rely on their own experience and knowledge in evaluating and using any information, methods, compounds or experiments described herein. Because of rapid advances in the medical sciences, in particular, independent verification of diagnoses and drug dosages should be made. To the fullest extent of the law, no responsibility is assumed by Elsevier, authors, editors or contributors for any injury and/or damage to persons or property as a matter of products liability, negligence or otherwise, or from any use or operation of any methods, products, instructions, or ideas contained in the material herein.

Managing Director, Global Content Partners: Kevonne Holloway
Senior Content Strategist (Acquisitions, Canada): Roberta A. Spinosa-Millman
Content Development Specialist: Theresa Fitzgerald
Publishing Services Manager: Shereen Jameel
Project Manager: Nadhiya Sekar
Design Direction: Brian Salisbury

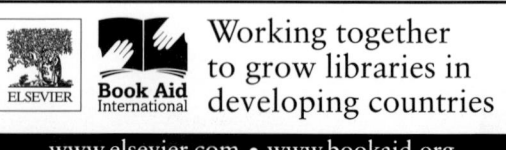

Last digit is the print number: 9 8 7 6 5 4 3 2 1

Walk gently in the lives of others, as not all wounds are visible.
This text is dedicated to those individuals who have courageously shared their lived experience of mental illness with me. It has been through this sharing that caring moments were created and transformational understanding happened.

—Cheryl L. Pollard

For those holding this text, the faculty looking to enliven teaching and practice, and the students seeking to practice in novel ways, this book is yours to inspire us all in our shared responsibility for more compassionate experiences of mental well-being in our daily lives, as well as in our families, communities, workplaces, institutions, and politics. This text is also dedicated to those who have taught me about the power and possibilities of listening, recovery, belonging, and inclusion, in particular to Fran, Elizabeth, Cecile, and all our park inclusion auditors and participants: I am privileged to have worked alongside you all.

—Sonya L. Jakubec

ACKNOWLEDGEMENTS

First, we would like to acknowledge the text from which this book has been adapted. To work from the years of expertise of Elizabeth Varcarolis and Margaret Jordan Halter and their contributors is to stand on the shoulders of giants. Our first edition of this adaptation was developed by a remarkable team and we begin by acknowledging them: our colleague, Mary Haase, who remains an inspiration, and Susan Ray, who is dearly missed. The second edition built upon the foundation of that strong adaptation, and was carefully crafted and edited with outstanding contributors. The second edition also coincided with early implementation of recommendations from the Truth and Reconciliation Commission (TRC) and Canada's adoption of the United Nations Declaration of the Rights of Indigenous Peoples, both serving as significant social and cultural turning points. The power and commitment to changes from these national and international directives is, again, emphasized in this third edition with our use of the terms *Indigenous peoples* and *Indigenous health*, which acknowledge the inherent rights and political views of the diverse groups of people with historical and cultural ties to Canada. These terms are distinct from the term *Aboriginal*, which is a broad term that does not account for the various original peoples in our country. Throughout this third edition, it is important for readers to critically reflect on the terms used to reference the diverse Indigenous populations in Canada. In this textbook we use the term *First Nations, Métis, and Inuit peoples* to replace the term *Aboriginal* unless otherwise specified (for instance, in original source reference material). Mental health nursing practice depends on an informed reading and ability to value the rights of Indigenous peoples to act and claim their identity according to their original names as a form of resistance to the legislated terms that have created inequity and harm over many years. The context and considerations surrounding these terms, as well as racialization and inequities, are discussed in greater depths in Chapter 8, and approaches to culturally safe practice and trauma-informed care are elaborated in this and other chapters. We acknowledge the conditions that shape vulnerabilities, shifting from referring to people as vulnerable, and instead consider the structural vulnerabilities.

Additional changes include updates to all clinical chapters. These changes were based on the most recent evidence available, including Canadian research and statistics, current pharmacological practices, content in a number of contemporary mental health concerns (including substance use and treatment, harm reduction, and gender and sexuality diversity), which provide a current perspective of mental health and mental health practice in Canada.

Our heartfelt appreciation also goes out to the talented group of writers who contributed to both the first and second Canadian editions—and those contributing to this third edition. Your contributions figuratively bind us together in this text, which is a collective source of current knowledge for Canadian practice. We welcome new contributors, Sandra Harrisson, Lisa-Marie Forcier, Eric MacMullin, Gabriel Barrington-Moss, Bonnie Fournier, and Meaghan Thumath, all of whom brought the very latest knowledge and future directions to this edition. Thank you again to returning contributors: Sherri Melrose and Sharon Moore, Martin Davies and Paul Martin Kerr, Richard Csiernik, Melodie B. Hull, and Erin Ziegler. Your clinical and scientific expertise strengthens this text, and your skillful communication makes it all seem easy!

Special thanks go to those authors who significantly revised and adapted chapter content related to culture and equity, in particular, Gwen Campbell McArthur, who, from her experiences as a person of Métis ancestry and a long-time community mental health practitioner, activist, advisor, and researcher, carefully updated the Indigenous mental health section in Chapter 8 in our second edition. We extend this appreciation now to Victoria Smye and Abe Oudshoorn, who have expanded the conversation of culture and psychiatric mental health care in Chapter 8 with a critical equity-informed perspective. Coinciding with the Black Lives Matter and Every Child Matters movements within Canada and striking refugee crises across the globe, Smye and Oudshoorn have put a laser focus on structural vulnerabilities and the community strengths that make mental health and healing possible.

We have indeed sought the expertise of a talented pool of contributors. Their collective knowledge and passion have had a powerful influence on this edition. It has truly been a joy working with each of you. Thanks for the countless hours you spent reading, synthesizing the evidence, writing, and rewriting!

A huge debt of gratitude goes to the many educators and clinicians who reviewed the manuscript and offered valuable suggestions, ideas, opinions, and criticisms. All comments were valued; they helped refine and strengthen the individual chapters, including late production nursing history discoveries from Anne Marie Creamer in New Brunswick.

Throughout this project, a number of people at Elsevier provided superb, and patient, support and encouragement. Sincere thanks go to the Elsevier team: our Senior Content Strategist, Roberta A. Spinosa-Millman, who held the project and us all together with the perfect combination of strong vision, diplomacy, and good humour; Theresa Fitzgerald, our patient, organized, respectful, and always encouraging Content Development Specialist; and the Copy Editing and Production team who have made our work shine.

Finally, we extend a shared thank you to each other as Canadian coeditors, tossing the lead on our work back and forth as needed and keeping the joy and humour in it always; we could ask for no more respectful, clear, and focused companions on this journey.

CONTRIBUTORS

Gabriel Barrington-Moss, RN, MN
Assistant Professor
Chair, Department of Professional Nursing and Allied Health
Faculty of Nursing
MacEwan University
Edmonton, Alberta

Karen Scott Barss, RPN, BHSc, MA
Faculty
Saskatchewan Collaborative Bachelor of Science in Nursing
Saskatchewan Polytechnic
Saskatoon, Saskatchewan

Richard Csiernik, BSc, MSW, PhD
Professor
Social Work
King's University College at Western University
London, Ontario

Martin Davies, BSc, PhD (retired)
Undergraduate Program Coordinator
Faculty of Medicine and Dentistry, Pharmacology
University of Alberta
Edmonton, Alberta

Lisa-Marie Forcier, RN, BSc, BScN (Hons.), MN
Professor
Bridging to University Nursing Program
School of Community and Health Studies
Centennial College
Toronto, Ontario

Bonnie Fournier, RN, BScN, MSc, PhD
Adjunct Professor
Thompson Rivers University
Kamloops, British Columbia

Sandra Harrisson, RN, MSc, PhD
Adjunct Professor
School of Nursing
University of Ottawa
Ottawa, Ontario

Melodie B. Hull, RPN(T), BA, MSc, MEd, PID
Retired Faculty
Nursing
College of the Rockies
Cranbrook, British Columbia
Retired Open Learning Faculty—Nursing & Health
Thompson Rivers University
Kamloops, British Columbia

Paul M. Kerr, BSc, PhD
Associate Professor
Department of Nursing Science
Faculty of Nursing
MacEwan University
Edmonton, Alberta

Eric MacMullin, RN, MScN (Informatics)
Professor
School of Community and Health Studies
Centennial College
Toronto, Ontario

Robert J. Meadus, BN, BVocEd, MSc(N), PhD, RN, CPMHN(C)
Associate Professor
Faculty of Nursing
Memorial University of Newfoundland & Labrador
St. John's, Newfoundland

Sherri Melrose, RN, PhD
Associate Professor
Centre for Nursing and Health Studies
Athabasca University
Athabasca, Alberta

Sharon Moore, BA, RN, R. Psych., MEd, PhD
Professor Emeritus
Faculty of Health Disciplines
Athabasca University
Athabasca, Alberta

Abe Oudshoorn, BScN, PhD
Associate Professor
Arthur Labatt Family School of Nursing
Western University
London, Ontario

Victoria Smye, RN, PhD, FCAN
Director & Associate Professor
Arthur Labatt Family School of Nursing
Western University
London, Ontario

Meaghan Anne Thumath, RN, BSN, MScPH, DLSHTM
Clinical Assistant Professor
School of Nursing
University of British Columbia
Vancouver, British Columbia

Erin Ziegler, BScN, MN, PhD, PHC-NP
Assistant Professor
Daphne Cockwell School of Nursing
Toronto Metropolitan University
Toronto, Ontario

CONTRIBUTORS TO US NINTH EDITION

Leslie A. Briscoe, MSN, RN, PMHCNP
Psychiatric Nurse Practitioner
Louis Stokes Cleveland VA Medical Center
Geriatric Psychiatry: Outpatient and
    Consultation/Liaison Service
Nursing Editorial Advisory Panel
Wolters Kluwer Publishing
Clinical Drug Information/Nursing Division
Hudson, Ohio

Rachel M. Childs, MS, MA, MSSA, PMHNP
Psychiatric Nurse Practitioner
Pediatric Psychiatry
Mary Bridge Children's Hospital
MultiCare Health System
Tacoma, Washington

Carissa R. Enright, MSN, RN, PMHNP BC
Associate Clinical Professor
Texas Women's University
Dallas, Texas

Jodie Flynn, MSN, RN, SANE-A, SANE-P, D-ABMDI
Instructor
Capital University
Columbus, Ohio

Emily Fowler, MSN, APRN, PMHNP-BC
Psychiatric Nurse Practitioner
Native American Community Clinic
Lyn-Lake Psychotherapy and Wellness
Minneapolis, Minnesota

Christina Fratena, MSN, APRN-CNS, BC
Instructor of Nursing
Malone University
Canton, Ohio

Margaret (Peggy) Jordan Halter, PhD, APRN
Clinical Nurse Specialist
Cleveland Clinic Akron General
Akron, Ohio;
Adjunct Faculty
Ohio State University
Columbus, Ohio

Edward A. Herzog, MSN, PMH, APRN-CNS
Faculty Emeritus
College of Nursing
Kent State University
Kent, Ohio

Laura G. Leahy, DrNP, APN, PMH-CNS/FNP, BC
Family Psychiatric Advanced Practice Nurse
APN Solutions, LLC
Sewell, New Jersey

Donna Rolin, PhD, APRN, PMHCNS-BC, PMHNP-BC
Clinical Associate Professor
School of Nursing
University of Texas at Austin
Austin, Texas

Jane Stein-Parbury, BSN, MEd, PhD, FRCNA
Emeritus Professor
Faculty of Health
University of Technology Sydney
Sydney, Australia

Christine A. Tackett, MSN, RN
Associate Professor
Herzing University
Akron, Ohio

Elizabeth M. Varcarolis, RN, MA
Professor Emeritus
Formerly Deputy Chairperson and
    Psychiatric Nursing Coordinator
Department of Nursing
Borough of Manhattan Community College,
    Associate Fellow
Albert Ellis Institute for Rational Emotional
    Behavioral Therapy (REBT)
Former Major, Army Nurse Corps Reserve
New York, New York

REVIEWERS

Lorna Canada-Vanegas Mesa, BScPN, RPN
Instructional Associate
Psychiatric Nursing Department
Faculty of Health Studies
Brandon University
Brandon, Manitoba

Christine Davis, BScN, MEd, MN
Professor
School of Baccalaureate Nursing
St. Lawrence College
Brockville, Ontario

Lori Carre, RN, MN
Professor of Nursing
Faculty of Applied Arts & Health Sciences
Seneca College of Applied Arts & Technologies
Toronto, Ontario

Mary A. Denton, RN(NP), MN, BScN, BSc
Provincial Clinical Placement Coordinator
Practical Nursing Program
Saskatchewan Polytechnic
Saskatoon, Saskatchewan

Arleah D. Johansen, LPN
LPN/Educator/Program Manager
Medical Surgical (LPN)/PN Program
  (Educator and Program Manager)
Nanaimo Regional General Hospital (LPN) and Discovery
  Community College (Educator and Program Manager)
Nanaimo, British Columbia

Colleen MacDonald, RN, BScN, MSN
Professor
School of Health Sciences
  Practical Nursing Program
St. Lawrence College
Cornwall, Ontario

Farhana Madhani, RN, PhD
Assistant Professor
Nursing Department
Brock University
St. Catharines, Ontario

Claudette McDonald, RN, MN
Practical Nursing Faculty
Nova Scotia Community College
Truro, Nova Scotia

Robert J. Meadus, BN, BVocEd, MSc(N), PhD, RN, CPMHN(C)
Associate Professor
Faculty of Nursing
Memorial University of Newfoundland & Labrador
St. John's, Newfoundland

Amanda O'Rae, RN, MPH
Senior Instructor
Faculty of Nursing
University of Calgary
Calgary, Alberta

Bhavik B. Patel, RN, BScN
Professor
Practical Nursing
Loyalist College
Belleville, Ontario

Geraldine M. Smith, RN, MN
Nursing Instructor
Faculty of Health Sciences
University of Lethbridge
Lethbridge, Alberta

Mary J. Thompson, RN, BN, MHS, MPC
Nursing Faculty
Division of Science and Health
Medicine Hat College
Medicine Hat, Alberta

Michelle M. Thompson, RN, BScN, MEd (Counselling)
Part-Time Instructor Post RN BScN
Continuing and Distance Education
St. Francis Xavier University
Antigonish, Nova Scotia

Jacqueline Williamson, RN, BScN, MEd, PhD
Professor
School of Health and Community Services
Durham College
Oshawa, Ontario

Jim Wohlgemuth, RN, MN, CTN-B
Instructor
Nursing Education & Health Studies
Grande Prairie Regional College
Grande Prairie, Alberta

TO THE INSTRUCTOR

The role of the health care provider continues to become more challenging as the impacts of climate change, effects of globalization, realities of competing funding priorities, lack of trained personnel, and the dictates of municipal, provincial and territorial, and federal governments compromise our health care system. We nurses and our patients are from widely diverse historical, cultural, religious, and socioeconomic contexts, bringing together a wide spectrum of knowledge, beliefs, and practices. As a society, we are experiencing the outcome of systemic racism, oppression, and inequities. An in-depth consideration and understanding of these contextual and social experiences are paramount in the administration of responsive and evidence-informed nursing care and are emphasized throughout this third edition.

Emphasizing historical, social, and political concerns, we have made a concentrated effort to align diagnostic terms, where appropriate, with the *Diagnostic and Statistical Manual of Mental Disorders, fifth edition (DSM-5)*. However, note that we have decided to use the term *dementia* when referring to progressive degenerative neurocognitive disorders. Although the term *dementia* was dropped from the *DSM-5*, many current practitioners still frequently use it. Therefore an editorial decision was made to include and use the term to ensure that readers using this text as a basis for clinical practice would be able to understand what is meant when *dementia* is used by more experienced health care providers.

We are living in an age of fast-paced research in neurobiology, genetics, and psychopharmacology that strives to find the most effective evidence-informed approaches for patients and their families, evidence that takes seriously the social organization of everyday life. Legal issues and ethical dilemmas faced by the health care system are magnified accordingly. Given these myriad challenges, knowing how best to teach our students and serve our patients can seem overwhelming. Well researched, with contributions from knowledgeable and experienced nurse educators and interdisciplinary clinical experts with pan-Canadian perspectives, our goal is to bring to you the most current and comprehensive trends and evidence-informed practices in psychiatric mental health nursing.

CONTENT NEW TO THIS EDITION

The following topics are at the forefront of nursing practice and, as such, are considered in detail in this third edition:

- Emphasis on the historical and structural features of Indigenous and refugee mental health concerns, with a focus on cultural safety, equity-informed approaches, and related relational practices including trauma-informed practices (Chapter 8)
- Evidence-informed practices and an emphasis on health promotion, resiliency, and recovery in the clinical chapters (Unit 4) as well as a new chapter on recovery, survivorship, and public mental health approaches (Chapter 29)
- Issues involving opioid withdrawal, harm reduction, and an emphasis on motivational interviewing in substance use disorders, as well as attention to nurses' substance use and support (Chapter 18)
- Disaster preparedness in light of climate change, COVID-19, and other disasters of our times (Chapter 21)
- Neurotransmitter and immune stress responses, stress-inducing events and stress-reducing techniques, self-assessment of nurses' stress levels, and mindfulness (Chapter 5)
- Attention to the language and distinctions of assessment and treatment with suicide and non-suicidal self-injury (Chapter 22)
- Exploration of legislative changes in medically assisted death (MAiD) and wide issues of grief (including ecological grief and grief from historical oppression and trauma) relevant for psychiatric mental health nursing (Chapter 31)
- The important mental health issues concerning gender and sexual diversity, in particular, issues surrounding stigma and discrimination for people from the lesbian, gay, bisexual, transgender, Two Spirited and queer and questioning LGBTQ2 community (Chapter 26)
- Special attention to lifespan mental health assessment, treatment and promotion, and prevention (Chapters 27 and 28)
- Emphasis throughout the text on recovery versus rehabilitation, victimization, social isolation and loneliness, unemployment and poverty, involuntary treatment, incarceration, wellness and recovery action plans, mental health first aid, interventions to promote adherence to treatment, and more
- A recognition of the increased prevalence and implications of sleep disturbances and sleep–wake disorders with a focus on their relationship to psychiatric illness and the nurse's role in assessment and management (Chapter 20)

Refer to the *To the Student* section of this introduction for examples of thoroughly updated familiar features with a fresh perspective, including the new Safety Tips feature boxes in select chapters, How a Nurse Helped Me boxes, Research Highlight boxes, Integrative Therapy boxes, Patient and Family Teaching boxes, Drug Treatment boxes, Considering Culture boxes, Key Points to Remember, Assessment Guidelines, and Vignettes, among others.

ORGANIZATION OF THE TEXT

Chapters are grouped in units to emphasize the clinical perspective and facilitate the location of information. All clinical chapters are organized in a clear, logical, and consistent format with the nursing process as the strong, visible framework. The basic outline for clinical chapters is as follows:

- Clinical Picture: Identifies disorders that fall under the umbrella of the general chapter name. Presents an overview of the disorder(s) and includes *DSM-5* criteria as appropriate.
- Epidemiology: Helps the student to understand the pattern of the problem and characteristics of those who would most likely be affected. This section provides information related to prevalence, lifetime incidence, age of onset, and gender differences.
- Co-Morbidity: Describes the most commonly associated co-morbid conditions. Knowing that co-morbid disorders are often part of the clinical picture of specific disorders helps students and clinicians understand how to better assess and treat their patients.
- Etiology: Provides current views of causation along with formerly held theories. It is based on the biopsychosocial triad and includes biological, psychological, and environmental factors.
- Assessment:
  - General Assessment: Appropriate assessment for a specific disorder, including assessment tools and rating scales. Rating scales, for instance, used to gauge suicide risk, assess anxiety, or assess substance use problems, help to highlight important areas in the assessment. Because the ratings provided by patients are subjective in nature, experienced clinicians use these tools as

a guide when planning care, in addition to their knowledge of their patients.
- Self-Assessment: Discusses topics relevant to the nurse's self-reflection required to enhance self-growth and provide the best possible and most appropriate care to the patient.
- Assessment Guidelines: Provides a summary of specific areas to assess by disorder.
- Diagnosis: *DSM-5* (2013) taxonomy and criteria are discussed in select sections as part of the nursing process.
- Outcomes Identification: *Nursing Interventions Classification (NIC)* for interventions and *Nursing Outcomes Classification (NOC)* for outcomes are introduced in Chapter 1 and used throughout the text where appropriate.
- Planning
- Implementation: Interventions follow Canadian Standards of Psychiatric-Mental Health Nursing (2014, with the release of updated standards set for 2021) set by the Canadian Federation of Mental Health Nurses under the umbrella of the Canadian Nurses Association (CNA). These standards are incorporated throughout the chapters.
- Evaluation

TEACHING AND LEARNING RESOURCES

For Students

Student Resources on Evolve, available at http://evolve.elsevier.com/Canada/Varcarolis/psychiatric/, provide a wealth of valuable learning resources.

The Evolve Resources on the text's inside front cover provides login instructions and access code.

- The **Answers to Critical Thinking** questions provides possible outcomes for the Critical Thinking questions at the end of each chapter.
- The **Answers to Chapter Review** questions provides answers and rationales for the Chapter Review questions at the end of each chapter.
- Critical Reasoning **Case Studies and Nursing Care Plans** provide detailed case studies and care plans for specific psychiatric disorders to supplement those found in the textbook.
- The **Glossary** highlights psychiatric mental health nursing terms with definitions.
- **Review Questions** provided for each chapter will help students prepare for course examinations and for the nursing licensure examination.
- **Pre-Tests and Post-Tests** provide interactive self-assessments for each chapter of the textbook, including instant scoring and feedback at the click of a button.
- **NEW! Next Generation NCLEX®-Style Case Studies** specific to this text.
- **Prepare for Exams:** Test Taking Strategies for psychiatric mental health nursing help prepare you for class tests and the NCLEX® Examination by explaining the various types of exam questions, providing examples and techniques for answering them, and offering general tips for testing success.
- **Key Points** provide a quick reference to reinforce the essential information.
- **DSM-5 Diagnostic Criteria**

For Instructors

Instructor Resources on Evolve, available at http://evolve.elsevier.com/Canada/Varcarolis/psychiatric/, provide a wealth of material to help you make your psychiatric nursing instruction a success. In addition to all of the Student Resources, the following are provided for Faculty:

- **TEACH for Nurses Lesson Plans** focus on the most important content from each chapter and provide innovative strategies for student engagement and learning. These new lesson plans provide teaching strategies that integrate textbook content with activities for pre-class, in-class, online, group, clinical judgement and interprofessional collaboration, all correlated with RN-NGN Clinical Judgement Model and PN Clinical Judgement Skills competencies.
- **PowerPoint Presentations** are organized by chapter, with approximately 650 slides for in-class lectures. These are detailed and include customizable text and image lecture slides to enhance learning in the classroom or in Web-based course modules. If you share them with students, they can use the Notes feature to help them with your lectures.
- **The Test Bank** has more than 1000 test items, complete with correct answers, rationales, the cognitive level of each question, the corresponding step of the nursing process, and appropriate The National Council Licensure Examination (NCLEX-RN® exam) Client Needs labels.
- **ExamView® Test Bank** that features examination format test questions with rationales and answers for all chapters. The robust ExamView® testing application, provided at no cost to faculty, allows instructors to create new tests; edit, add, and delete test questions; sort questions by category, cognitive level, and nursing process step; and administer and grade tests online, with automated scoring and gradebook functionality.
- **NEW! Next Generation NCLEX®-Style Case Studies** for Psychiatric Mental Health Nursing.
- **An Image Collection** provides over 100 full-colour images from the book for instructors to use in lectures.

Sherpath

Sherpath Book-Organized Collections offer digital lessons, mapped chapter-by-chapter to the textbook, so that the reader can conveniently find applicable digital assignment content. Featuring convenient teaching materials that are aligned to the textbook, the lessons are organized by chapter for quick and easy access to invaluable class activities and resources.

Elsevier eBooks

This exciting program is available to faculty who adopt a number of Elsevier texts, including *Varcarolis's Canadian Psychiatric Mental Health Nursing*, third edition. Elsevier eBooks is an integrated electronic study centre consisting of a collection of textbooks made available online. It is carefully designed to "extend" the textbook for an easier and more efficient teaching and learning experience. It includes study aids such as highlighting, e-note taking, and cut-and-paste capabilities. Even more importantly, it allows students and instructors to do a comprehensive search within the specific text or across a number of titles. Please check with your Elsevier Educational Solutions Consultant for more information.

A WORD ON TERMINOLOGY

The authors and contributors of the text recognize and acknowledge the diverse histories of the First Peoples of the lands now referred to as Canada. It is recognized that individual communities identify themselves in various ways; within this text, the term *Indigenous* is used to refer to all First Nations, Inuit, and Métis people within Canada unless there are research findings that are presented uniquely to a population.

Knowledge and language concerning sex, gender, and identity are fluid and continually evolving. The language and terminology presented in this text endeavour to be inclusive of all people and reflect what is, to the best of our knowledge, current at the time of publication. Gender pronouns have been removed whenever possible, using the terms *they* and *them* as acceptable singular references to achieve gender neutrality (see https://en/oxforddictionaries.com/usage/he-or-she-versus-they). Patient profiles in Case Studies, Ethical Dilemmas boxes, and Evidence-Informed Practice: Translating Research into Practice boxes include preferred pronouns and employ initials in place of full names.

Throughout the textbook, when information is specific to the role of the RN, "Registered Nurse" or "RN" has been used; in all other instances, the term *nurse* is used to refer to an RN and/or RPN/LPN, depending on jurisdictional regulations.

"Interprofessional collaboration" is used to refer to any collaboration among health care team members and others (for example, spiritual caregivers).

"Health care provider" can include a physician, nurse practitioner, or an RN for whom the prescribing of medications or treatments is within their scope of practice.

We are grateful to educators who send suggestions and provide feedback, and we hope this third edition helps students learn and appreciate the scope of psychiatric mental health nursing practice.

Cheryl L. Pollard
Sonya L. Jakubec

TO THE STUDENT

Psychiatric mental health nursing challenges us to understand the complexities of human behaviour. In the chapters that follow you will learn about people with psychiatric mental health disorders and how to provide them with quality nursing care and promote their mental health. As you read, keep in mind these special features.

ADDITIONAL LEARNING RESOURCES

Your **1 Evolve Resources** at http://evolve.elsevier.com/Canada/Varcarolis/psychiatric/ offer more helpful study aids, such as additional Case Studies and Nursing Care Plans.

Key Points to Remember listed at the end of each chapter reinforce essential information.

Critical Thinking activities at the end of each chapter are scenario-based critical thinking problems to provide practice in applying what you have learned. **Answer Keys** can be found on the Evolve website.

Multiple-choice **Chapter Review** questions at the end of each chapter help you review the chapter material and study for exams. **Answers** with **rationales** are located on the Evolve website.

READING AND REVIEW TOOLS

2 Objectives and **3 Key Terms and Concepts** introduce the chapter topics and provide a concise overview of the material discussed.

CHAPTER FEATURES

4 How a Nurse Helped Me boxes are patient accounts and narratives that introduce select chapters and invite exploration into the lived experiences of patients and families.

5 Considering Culture boxes reinforce the importance of providing culturally competent care.

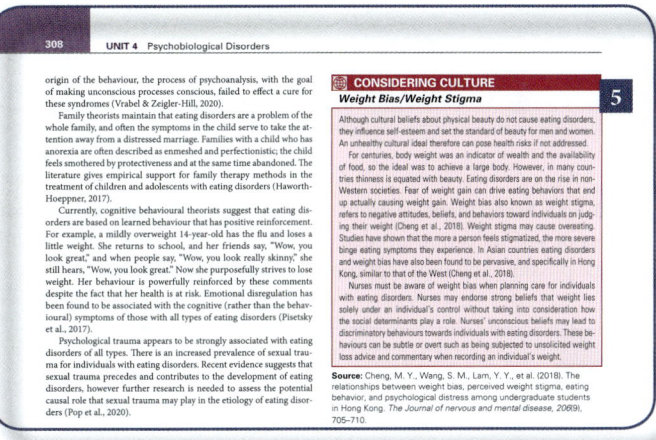

6 Vignettes describe the unique circumstances surrounding individual patients with psychiatric disorders.

7 Assessment Guidelines at the end of each Assessment section in most clinical chapters provide summary points for patient assessment.

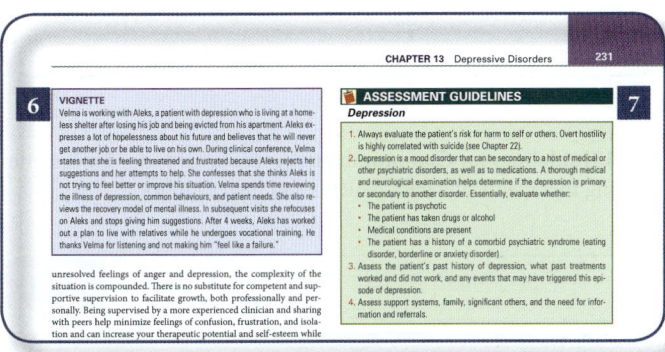

xiii

8 Safety Tip boxes are found in select chapters and shine light on important issues of safety for psychiatric mental health care, patient experiences, and nursing interventions or responses.

9 Research Highlight boxes demonstrate how current research findings affect psychiatric mental health nursing practice and standards of care.

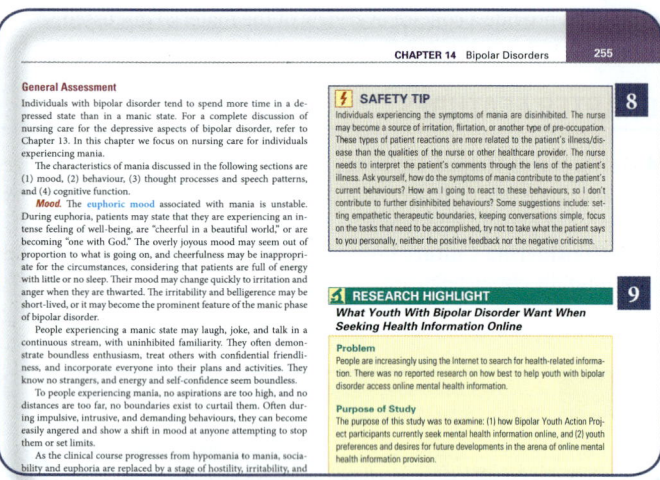

10 Self-Assessment sections discuss topics relevant to a nurse's process of self-reflection needed to enhance self-growth and provide the best possible and most appropriate care to the patient.

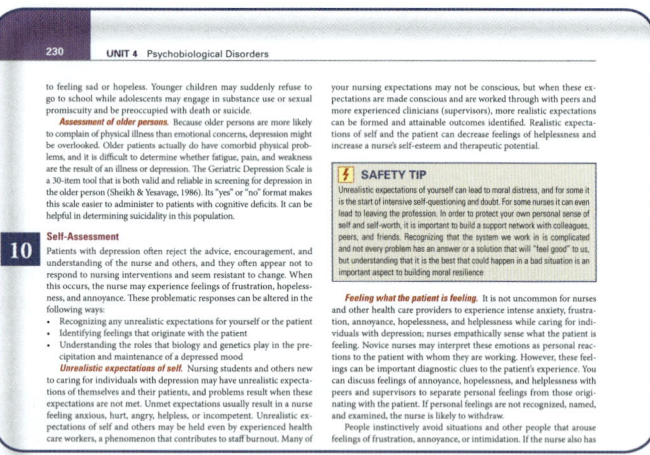

11 Guidelines for Communication boxes provide tips for communicating therapeutically with patients and their families.

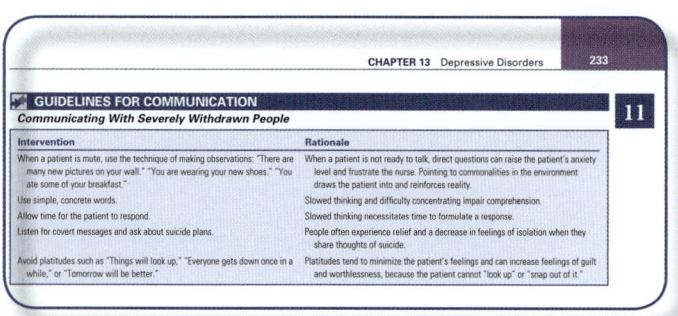

12 Patient and Family Teaching boxes underscore the nurse's role in helping patients and families understand psychiatric disorders, treatments, complications, and medication adverse effects, among other important issues.

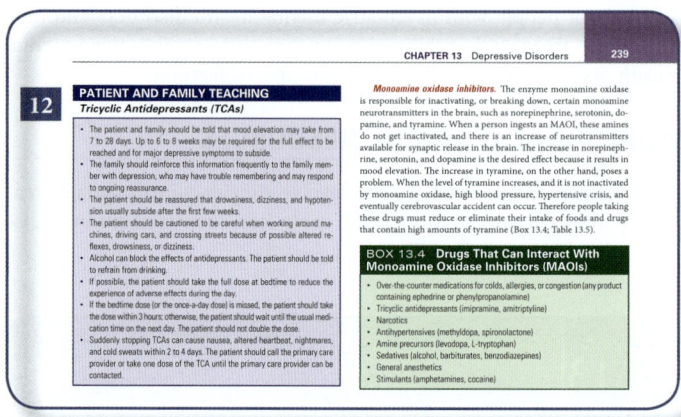

13 Drug Treatment boxes present the latest information on medications used to treat psychiatric disorders.

14 Integrative Therapy boxes discuss significant nursing considerations for complementary and alternative therapies and examine relevant study findings.

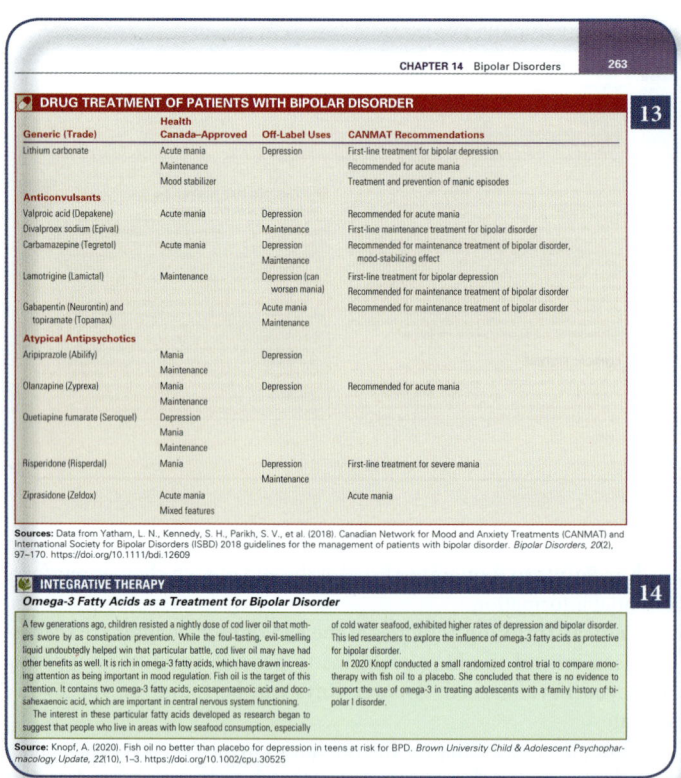

15 *DSM-5* boxes identify the criteria of disorders identified and described in the *Diagnostic and Statistical Manual of Mental Disorders*, fifth edition.

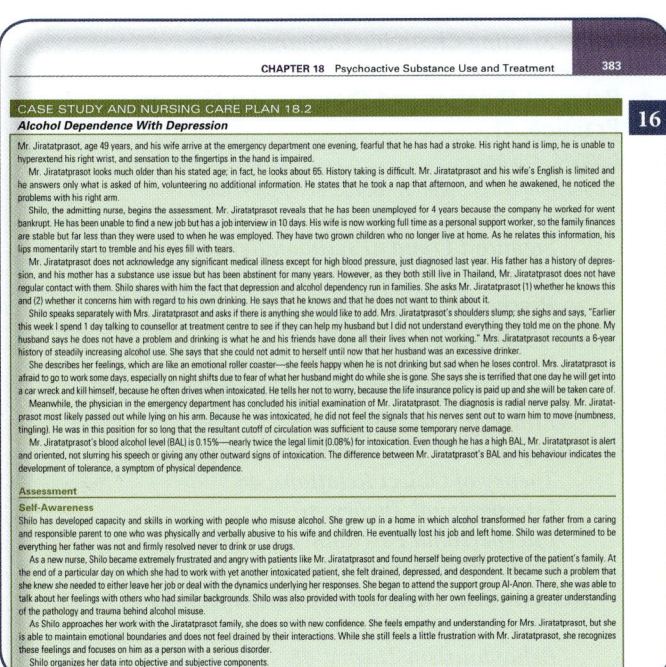

16 Case Studies and Nursing Care Plans present individualized histories of patients with specific psychiatric disorders following the steps of the nursing process. Interventions with rationales and evaluation statements are presented for each patient goal.

Next Generation NCLEX® (NGN)

The National Council for the State Boards of Nursing (NCSBN) is a not-for-profit organization whose members include nursing regulatory bodies. In empowering and supporting nursing regulators in their mandate to protect the public the NCSBN is involved in the development of nursing licensure examinations, such as the NCLEX-RN®. In Canada the NCLEX-RN® was introduced in 2015 and is, as of the writing of this text, the recognized licensure exam required for practising Registered Nurses (RNs) in Canada.

As of 2023, the NCLEX-RN® will be changing in order to ensure that its item types adequately measure clinical judgement, critical thinking, and problem-solving skills on a consistent basis. The NCSBN will also be incorporating into the examination, what they call the Clinical Judgement Measurement Model (CJMM), which is a framework the NCSBN has created to measure a novice nurse's ability to apply clinical judgement in practice.

These changes to the examination come as a result of findings indicating that novice nurses have a much higher than desirable error rate with patients (errors causing patient harm) and, upon NCSBN's investigation, discovering that the overwhelming majority of these errors were caused by failures of clinical judgement.

Clinical judgement has been a foundation underlying nursing education for decades, based on the work of a number of nursing theorists. The theory of clinical judgement that most closely aligns to what NCSBN is basing their CJMM is the work by Christine A. Tanner.

The new version of the NCLEX-RN® is identified loosely as the "Next-Generation NCLEX" or "NGN" and will feature the following:

- Six key skills in the CJMM: recognizing cues, analyzing cues, prioritizing hypotheses, generating solutions, taking actions, and evaluating outcomes.
- Approved item types as of March 2021: multiple response, extended drag and drop, cloze (drop-down), enhanced hot-spot (highlighting), matrix/grid, bow tie, and trend. More question types may be added.
- All new item types are accompanied by mini case studies with comprehensive patient information—some of it relevant to the question, and some of it not.
- Case information may present a single, unchanging moment in time (a "single episode" case study) or multiple moments in time as a patient's condition changes (an "unfolding" case study).
- Single-episode case studies may be accompanied by one to six questions; unfolding case studies are accompanied by six questions.

For more information (and detail) regarding the NCLEX-RN® and changes coming to the exam, visit the NCSBNs websites: https://www.ncsbn.org/11447.htm and https://ncsbn.org/Building_a_Method_for_Writing_Clinical_Judgment_It.pdf.

For further NCLEX-RN® examination preparation resources, see *Elsevier's Canadian Comprehensive Review for the NCLEX-RN Examination*, second edition, ISBN 9780323709385.

Prior to preparing for any nursing licensure examination, please refer to your provincial or territorial nursing regulatory body to determine which licensure examination is required in order for you to practice in your chosen jurisdiction.

CONTENTS

Acknowledgements, vi
Contributors, vii
Contributors to US Ninth Edition, viii
Reviewers, ix
To the Instructor, x
To the Student, xiii

UNIT 1 Foundations in Theory

1 Mental Health and Mental Illness, 2
Sonya L. Jakubec
  Mental Health and Mental Illness, 2
    Two Conceptualizations of Mental Health and Mental Illness, 3
    Contributing Factors, 4
    Perceptions of Mental Health and Mental Illness, 6
    Human Genome Project, 6
    Social Influences on Mental Health Care, 7
    Changing Directions, Changing Lives: The Mental Health Strategy for Canada, 7
  Epidemiology of Mental Disorders, 7
  Classification of Mental Disorders, 9
    The Diagnostic and Statistical Manual, 9
    The ICD-11, 10
  Psychiatric Mental Health Nursing, 10
    What Is Psychiatric Mental Health Nursing?, 10
    Classification of Nursing Diagnoses, Outcomes, and Interventions, 10
    Evidence-Informed Practice, 11
    Levels of Psychiatric Mental Health Clinical Nursing Practice, 11
    Future Challenges and Roles for Psychiatric Mental Health Nurses, 11
  References, 13

2 Historical Overview of Psychiatric Mental Health Nursing, 16
Sandra Harrisson
  Early Mental Illness Care, 16
    Early Canadian Asylums, 17
  Early Psychiatric Treatments, 17
  The Introduction of Nurses to Asylum Care, 18
  Shifts in Control Over Nursing, 18
    Eastern and Atlantic Canada, 19
    Western Canada, 19
  Deinstitutionalization and the Nursing Role in Psychiatric Mental Health Care, 20
  University-Based Nursing Curriculum, 20
  National Organizations for Psychiatric Mental Health Nursing and Canadian Nurses Association Certification, 21
  Advanced-Practice Nursing in Psychiatric Mental Health Care, 21
  The Future of Psychiatric Mental Health Nursing, 21
  References, 22

3 Overview of Psychiatric Mental Health Nursing Care Within Various Settings, 24
Cheryl L. Pollard
  Funding Psychiatric Mental Health Care, 25
  The Continuum of Mental Health Care, 25
    Evolving Venues of Practice, 25
  Psychiatric Mental Health Care Settings, 26
    Community Mental Health Centres, 27
    Mobile Crisis Intervention Teams, 28
    Disaster Response Teams, 28
    Partial Hospitalization Programs, 29
    Inpatient Psychiatric Mental Health Programs, 29
    Assertive Community Treatment, 31
    Ensuring Safety, 31
  Psychiatric Mental Health Nursing: Roles and Responsibilities, 32
  Community Psychiatric Mental Health Nursing, 32
    Biopsychosocial Assessment, 33
    Treatment Goals and Interventions, 34
    Interprofessional Team Member, 35
    Biopsychosocial Care Manager, 35
    Treatment Team, 35
    Nursing Care, 36
  Future Issues, 37
    Barriers to Treatment, 37
    Meeting Changing Demands, 38
  References, 39

4 Relevant Theories and Therapies for Nursing Practice, 41
Cheryl L. Pollard
Originating US chapter by Margaret Jordan Halter
  Psychoanalytic Theories and Therapies, 42
    Sigmund Freud's Psychoanalytic Theory, 42
    Classical Psychoanalysis, 43
    Psychodynamic Therapy, 44
  Developmental Theories, 44
    Cognitive Development, 44
    Stages of Moral Development, 44
    Ethics of Care Theory, 45
  Interpersonal Theories and Therapies, 46
    Theory of Object Relations, 46
    Interpersonal Theory, 46
    Interpersonal Psychotherapy, 46
    Peplau's Theory of Interpersonal Relations, 46
  Behavioural Theories and Therapies, 48
    Classical Conditioning Theory, 48
    Behaviourism Theory, 48
    Operant Conditioning Theory, 48
    Behavioural Therapy, 48
  Cognitive Theories and Therapies, 50
    Rational Emotive Behaviour Therapy, 50
    Cognitive Behavioural Therapy, 50
    Dialectical Behavioural Therapy, 51
  Humanistic Theories, 53
    Abraham Maslow's Humanistic Psychology Theory, 53

Biological Theories and Therapies, 54
    The Advent of Psychopharmacology, 54
    The Biological Model, 54
Additional Therapies, 54
    Milieu Therapy, 54
References, 57

5 Understanding Responses to Stress, 59
Lisa-Marie Forcier
Originating US Chapter by Margaret Jordan Halter, Elizabeth M. Varcarolis

Responses to and Effects of Stress, 59
    Early Stress Response Theories, 59
    Neurotransmitter Stress Responses, 61
    Immune Stress Responses, 61
Mediators of the Stress Response, 62
    Stressors, 62
    Perception, 62
    Personality, 62
    Social Support, 63
    Diet, 63
    Culture, 63
    Spirituality and Religious Beliefs, 63
Nursing Management of Stress Responses, 63
    Measuring Stress, 63
    Adverse Childhood Experiences, 64
    Assessing Coping Styles, 65
    Managing Stress Through Relaxation Techniques, 65
References, 71

UNIT 2 Foundations in Practice

6 The Nursing Process and Standards of Care for Psychiatric Mental Health Nursing, 74
Lisa-Marie Forcier, Eric MacMullin
Originating US chapter by Margaret Jordan Halter, Elizabeth M. Varcarolis

Assessment, 75
    Age Considerations, 76
    Language Barriers, 77
    Psychiatric Mental Health Nursing Assessment, 77
Nursing Diagnosis, 82
Outcomes Identification, 82
Planning, 83
Implementation, 84
    Basic-Level Interventions, 85
    Advanced-Practice Interventions, 85
Evaluation, 85
Documentation, 85
References, 87

7 Ethical Responsibilities and Legal Obligations for Psychiatric Mental Health Nursing Practice, 89
Cheryl L. Pollard

Ethical Concepts, 89
Mental Health Legislation, 93
Establishing Best Practice, 94
    Standards of Practice, 95
    Standards of Care, 95
    Policies and Procedures, 95
    Traditional Practice Knowledge, 95
Guidelines for Ensuring Adherence to Standards of Care, 95
Patients' Rights Under the Law, 95
    Authorization of Treatment, 95
    Autonomy, 96
    Beneficence and Non-maleficence, 97
    Rights Regarding Confidentiality, 98
Civil Obligations and Responsibilities, 99
    Tort Law, 100
References, 103

8 Cultural Implications for Psychiatric Mental Health Nursing: A Critical Cultural Perspective, 105
Victoria Smye, Abe Oudshoorn

Understanding the Landscape of Culture in Mental Health, 105
    Culture, Race, Ethnicity, and the Social Determinants of Health, 105
    Equity-Oriented Health Care (EOHC): Cultural Safety and Trauma- and Violence-Informed Care, 106
    Culture and Our Worldviews, 108
    Critical Thinking: Who Do You Position as Different?, 109
    Culture of Health Care, Mental Illness, Social and Structural Inequity, and Stigma, 110
The Cultural Landscape of Canada, 111
    Indigenous Peoples, Multi-culturalism, and Equity, 111
Mental Health Concerns of Indigenous Peoples, 111
    Historical Trauma, 112
    Suicide, 112
    Interpersonal and Structural Violence, 112
    Substance Use, 113
Mental Health Concerns of Immigrants and Refugees, 113
Barriers and Pathways to Mental Health Care in a Multi-cultural Context, 114
    Guidelines for Clinical Practice: Communication, 114
    Misdiagnosis, 115
References, 116

UNIT 3 Biopsychosocial Interventions

9 Therapeutic Relationships, 122
Cheryl L. Pollard
Originating US chapter by Margaret Jordan Halter, Elizabeth M. Varcarolis

Concepts of the Nurse–Patient Relationship, 123
    Therapeutic Use of Self, 123
    Relationship Boundaries, 124
Values, Beliefs, and Self-Awareness, 126
Peplau's Model of the Nurse–Patient Relationship, 126
    Pre-orientation Phase, 128
    Orientation Phase, 130
    Working Phase, 131
    Termination Phase, 131
What Hinders and What Helps the Nurse–Patient Relationship, 132
Factors that Encourage and Promote Patients' Growth, 133

   Genuineness, 133
   Empathy, 133
   Positive Regard, 133
  References, 135
10 Communication and the Clinical Interview, 136
Erin Ziegler
Originating US chapter by Margaret Jordan Halter, Elizabeth M. Varcarolis
  The Communication Process, 137
  Factors that Affect Communication, 137
   Personal Factors, 137
   Environmental Factors, 137
   Relationship Factors, 137
  Verbal and Non-verbal Communication, 139
   Verbal Communication, 139
   Non-verbal Communication, 139
   Interaction of Verbal and Non-verbal Communication, 139
  Communication Skills for Nurses, 140
   Therapeutic Communication Strategies, 140
   Cultural Considerations, 146
   Assertive Communication, 146
   Evaluation of Communication Skills, 147
  The Clinical Interview, 147
   Preparing for the Interview, 147
   Introductions, 148
   Initiating the Interview, 148
   Tactics to Avoid, 148
   Helpful Guidelines, 148
   Attending Behaviours: The Foundation of Interviewing, 148
   Clinical Supervision, 149
   Process Recordings, 149
  References, 152
11 Psychotropic Drugs, 153
Martin Davies, Paul M. Kerr
  Structure and Function of the Brain, 154
   Functions and Activities of the Brain, 154
   Cellular Composition of the Brain, 156
   Organization of the Brain, 158
   Visualizing the Brain, 160
   Disturbances of Mental Function, 164
  Use of Psychotropic Drugs, 164
   Drugs Used to Treat Anxiety and Insomnia, 165
   Drug Treatment for Depression, 167
   Drug Treatment for Bipolar Disorders, 170
   Drugs Used to Treat Psychosis, 171
   Drug Treatment for Attention-Deficit/Hyperactivity Disorder, 174
   Drug Treatment for Alzheimer's Disease, 174
   Natural Health Products, 174
  References, 176

UNIT 4 Psychobiological Disorders

12 Anxiety and Related Disorders, 180
Cheryl L. Pollard
Originating US chapter by Margaret Jordan Halter
  Anxiety, 181
   Levels of Anxiety, 182
   Defences Against Anxiety, 184
   Clinical Picture, 185
  Anxiety Disorders, 185
   Epidemiology, 190
   Comorbidity, 190
  Somatic Symptom and Related Disorders, 190
   Clinical Picture, 190
   Epidemiology, 193
   Comorbidity, 193
  Obsessive-Compulsive Disorders, 193
   Epidemiology, 194
   Comorbidity, 194
  Trauma- and Stressor-Related Disorders, 196
   Acute Stress Disorder, 196
   Post-Traumatic Stress Disorder, 196
  Dissociative Disorders, 198
   Clinical Picture, 198
   Epidemiology, 199
   Comorbidity, 199
  Etiology of Anxiety-Related Disorders, 199
   Biological Factors, 199
   Psychological Factors, 200
   Environmental Factors, 200
   Sociocultural Factors, 200
  Application of the Nursing Process, 201
   Assessment, 201
   Diagnosis, 205
   Outcomes Identification, 205
   Planning, 205
   Implementation, 207
   Evaluation, 216
  References, 217
13 Depressive Disorders, 220
Cheryl L. Pollard
Originating US chapter by Margaret Jordan Halter
  Clinical Picture, 220
   Disruptive Mood Dysregulation Disorder, 221
   Persistent Depressive Disorder, 222
   Premenstrual Dysphoric Disorder, 222
   Substance/Medication-Induced Depressive Disorder, 222
   Depressive Disorder due to Another Medical Condition, 222
  Epidemiology, 223
   Children and Adolescents, 223
   Older Persons, 223
  Comorbidity, 224
  Etiology, 224
   Biological Factors, 224
   Psychological Factors, 226
  Application of the Nursing Process, 226
   Assessment, 226
  Diagnosis, 231
  Outcomes Identification, 232
   The Recovery Model, 232
  Planning, 232
  Implementation, 232
   Counselling and Communication Techniques, 232
   Health Teaching and Health Promotion, 232
   Promotion of Self-Care Activities, 233
   Milieu Management: Teamwork and Safety, 233

Pharmacological Interventions, 234
Biological Interventions, 241
Evaluation, 243
References, 247

14 Bipolar Disorders, 249
Cheryl L. Pollard
Originating US chapter by Margaret Jordan Halter
Clinical Picture, 249
Bipolar I Disorder, 249
Bipolar II Disorder, 250
Cyclothymic Disorder, 251
Other Bipolar Disorders, 251
Epidemiology, 251
Children and Adolescents, 252
Cyclothymic Disorder, 252
Comorbidity, 252
Bipolar I Disorder, 252
Bipolar II Disorder, 252
Cyclothymic Disorder, 252
Etiology, 252
Biological Factors, 252
Environmental Factors, 253
Psychological Factors, 253
Application of the Nursing Process, 254
Assessment, 254
Nursing Diagnosis, 256
Outcomes Identification, 257
Planning, 258
Implementation, 258
Evaluation, 265
References, 269

15 Schizophrenia Spectrum and Other Psychotic Disorders, 270
Lisa-Marie Forcier, Eric MacMullin
Originating US chapter by Edward A. Herzog
Clinical Picture, 271
Epidemiology, 272
Comorbidity, 272
Etiology, 273
Biological Factors, 273
Psychological, Social, and Environmental Factors, 274
Course of the Disorder, 275
Phases of Schizophrenia, 275
Prognosis, 275
Early Detection, 275
Application of the Nursing Process, 275
Assessment, 275
Diagnosis, 283
Outcomes Identification, 283
Phase I—Acute, 283
Phase II—Stabilization, 283
Phase III—Maintenance, 283
Planning, 283
Phase I—Acute, 283
Phase II—Stabilization and Phase III—Maintenance, 284
Implementation, 284
Phase I—Acute, 284
Phase II—Stabilization and Phase III—Maintenance, 285
Milieu Management, 285
Counselling and Communication Techniques, 285
Health Teaching and Health Promotion, 287
Pharmacological Interventions, 288
Specific Interventions for Paranoia, Catatonia, and Disorganization, 290
Advanced-Practice Interventions, 295
Evaluation, 296
References, 300

16 Eating and Feeding Disorders, 304
Bonnie Fournier
Originating US chapter by Rachel M. Childs, Carissa R. Enright
Clinical Picture, 304
Avoidant/Restrictive Food Intake Disorder, 305
Pica, 305
Rumination Disorder, 305
Epidemiology, 305
Comorbidity, 307
Etiology, 307
Biological Factors, 307
Psychological Factors, 307
Environmental Factors, 308
Anorexia Nervosa, 308
Application of the Nursing Process, 308
Assessment, 308
Diagnosis, 310
Outcomes Identification, 310
Planning, 310
Implementation, 311
Evaluation, 313
Bulimia Nervosa, 313
Application of the Nursing Process, 313
Assessment, 313
Diagnosis, 314
Outcomes Identification, 314
Planning, 315
Implementation, 315
Evaluation, 216
Binge Eating Disorder, 316
References, 322

17 Neurocognitive Disorders, 324
Gabriel Barrington-Moss
Originating US chapter by Jane Stein-Parbury
Delirium, 326
Clinical Picture, 326
Epidemiology, 326
Comorbidity and Etiology, 326
Application of the Nursing Process, 326
Assessment, 326
Diagnosis, 329
Outcomes Identification, 329
Planning, 329
Implementation, 329
Evaluation, 329
Mild and Major Neurocognitive Disorders, 330
Clinical Picture, 332
Epidemiology, 334
Etiology, 334
Application of the Nursing Process, 335
Assessment, 335
Diagnosis, 336

    Outcomes Identification, 336
    Planning, 336
    Implementation, 336
    Evaluation, 344
  References, 348

18 Psychoactive Substance Use and Treatment, 350
Rick Csiernik
  Distinguishing Between an Addiction and a Compulsive Behaviour, 351
    The Process of Addiction Development, 351
    Epidemiology, 352
    Comorbidity, 354
    Etiology, 355
  Application of the Nursing Process, 357
    Assessment, 357
    Helping Patients Change, 369
    Diagnosis, 373
    Outcomes Identification, 373
    Planning, 373
    Implementation, 373
    Substance Misuse Interventions, 374
    Evaluation, 385
  References, 387

19 Personality Disorders, 390
Cheryl L. Pollard
Originating US chapter by Margaret Jordan Halter, Christine A. Tackett
  Clinical Picture, 391
  Epidemiology, 391
  Comorbidity, 392
  Etiology, 392
    Biological Factors, 392
    Psychological Factors, 392
    System Factors, 392
  Cluster A Personality Disorders, 393
    Paranoid Personality Disorder, 393
    Schizoid Personality Disorder, 393
    Schizotypal Personality Disorder, 394
  Cluster B Personality Disorders, 394
    Borderline Personality Disorder, 394
    Anti-social Personality Disorder, 397
    Histrionic Personality Disorder, 398
    Narcissistic Personality Disorder, 399
  Cluster C Personality Disorders, 400
    Avoidant Personality Disorder, 400
    Dependent Personality Disorder, 400
    Obsessive-Compulsive Personality Disorder, 400
  Application of the Nursing Process, 401
    Assessment, 401
    Diagnosis, 402
    Outcomes Identification, 402
    Planning, 402
    Implementation, 402
    Evaluation, 408
  References, 411

20 Sleep–Wake Disorders, 413
Gabriel Barrington-Moss
Originating US chapter by Margaret Jordan Halter
  Sleep, 414
  Consequences of Sleep Loss, 414
  Normal Sleep Cycle, 414
  Regulation of Sleep, 417
  Functions of Sleep, 417
  Sleep Requirements, 417
  Sleep Patterns, 418
  Sleep–Wake Disorders, 418
  Clinical Picture, 418
    Insomnia Disorders, 418
    Hypersomnia Disorders, 419
    Confusional Arousal Disorders, 419
    Kleine–Levin Syndrome, 420
    Sleep–Wake Disorders Related to Breathing, 420
    Circadian Rhythm Sleep Disorder, 420
    Restless Legs Syndrome (Willis-Ekbom Disease), 420
  Epidemiology, 421
  Comorbidity, 421
    Sleep–Wake Disorders and Mental Illness, 421
    Sleep and General Health, 422
  Application of the Nursing Process, 422
    Assessment, 422
    Diagnosis, 424
    Outcomes Identification, 424
    Planning, 424
    Implementation, 425
    Evaluation, 427
  References, 428

Unit 5 Trauma Interventions

21 Crisis and Disaster, 432
Meaghan Thumath
  The Development of Crisis Theory, 433
    Types of Crisis, 434
    Phases of Crisis, 435
  Application of the Nursing Process, 435
    Assessment, 435
    Diagnosis, 437
    Outcomes Identification, 437
    Planning, 439
    Implementation, 439
    Evaluation, 441
  References, 447

22 Suicide and Non-suicidal Self-Injury, 448
Sherri Melrose, Sharon Moore
With contributions by Sonya L. Jakubec
  Epidemiology, 449
    Indigenous Peoples Statistics, 449
    Risk Factors, 450
    Suicide Among Older Persons, 450
  Etiology, 452
    Biological Factors, 452
    Psychosocial Factors, 452
    Societal Considerations, 453
  Application of the Nursing Process, 453
    Assessment, 454
    Implementation, 455
    Evaluation, 459
  Non-suicidal Self-Injury, 459
    Epidemiology, 459
    Comorbidity, 459
    Risk Factors, 459
    Clinical Picture, 459

Assessment, 460
Diagnosis, 460
Outcomes Criteria, 460
Planning, 460
Interventions, 460
Evaluation, 460
References, 461

23 Anger, Aggression, and Violence, 465
Melodie B. Hull
Epidemiology, 467
  Comorbidity, 467
Etiology, 468
  Biological Factors, 468
  Psychological Factors, 468
  Sociocultural Factors, 470
Application of the Nursing Process, 470
  Assessment, 470
  Nursing Diagnosis, 471
  Outcomes, 471
  Planning, 471
  Implementation, 471
  Evaluation, 477
References, 478

24 Interpersonal Violence: Child, Older Persons, and Intimate Partner Abuse, 481
Robert J. Meadus
Originating US chapter by Margaret Jordan Halter
Clinical Picture, 481
  Violence, 482
  Cycle of Violence, 485
Epidemiology, 485
  Child Abuse, 485
  Intimate Partner Violence, 486
  Older Person Abuse, 487
Comorbidity, 487
Etiology, 487
  The Ecological Model of Violence, 487
  Environmental Factors, 487
Application of the Nursing Process: Interpersonal Violence, 489
  Assessment, 489
  Diagnosis, 495
  Outcomes Identification, 496
  Planning, 496
  Implementation, 496
  Evaluation, 502
References, 505

25 Sexual Assault, 508
Erin Ziegler
Originating US chapter by Margaret Jordan Halter, Jodie Flynn
Epidemiology, 509
  Profile of Sexual Perpetrators, 509
Clinical Picture, 509
  Relationships Between Victims and Perpetrators, 509
  Psychological Effects of Sexual Assault, 510
  Rape-Trauma Syndrome, 510
Application of the Nursing Process, 511
  A Trauma-Informed Approach, 511
  Assessment, 512
  Diagnosis, 513
  Outcomes Identification, 515
  Planning, 515
  Implementation, 515
  Evaluation, 519
References, 520

UNIT 6 Interventions for Distinct Populations

26 Sexuality and Gender, 524
Erin Ziegler
Sexuality, 525
Gender, 525
Gender Dysphoria, 526
Gender Incongruence, 526
Clinical Picture, 527
Epidemiology, 527
Nursing Care for Transgender Individuals, 527
Advanced Interventions, 527
  Pharmacological, 527
  Surgical, 527
Application of the Nursing Process, 527
  Assessment, 527
  Planning, 528
  Implementation, 528
Providing Safe and Inclusive Nursing Care, 529
Mental Health Issues in the LGBTQ2 Population, 529
  Clinical Picture, 529
  Depression, 529
  Self-Harm and Suicide, 530
  Substance Use, 530
  Evaluation, 530
References, 531

27 Disorders of Children and Adolescents, 533
Cheryl L. Pollard
Epidemiology, 534
Comorbidity, 534
Risk Factors, 534
Etiology, 535
  Biological Factors, 535
  Environmental Factors, 536
Child and Adolescent Psychiatric Mental Health Nursing, 536
  Assessing Development and Functioning, 537
  General Interventions, 539
Neurodevelopmental Disorders, 542
  Intellectual Disabilities, 542
  Communication Disorders, 542
  Autism Spectrum Disorder, 542
  Attention-Deficit/Hyperactivity Disorder, 543
  Specific Learning Disorder, 544
  Motor Disorders, 544
Application of the Nursing Process, 544
  Assessment, 544
  Diagnosis, 545
  Outcomes Identification, 545
  Implementation, 546
Disruptive, Impulse Control, and Conduct Disorders, 546
  Oppositional Defiant Disorder, 546
  Conduct Disorder, 547
Application of the Nursing Process, 548
  Assessment, 548
  Diagnosis, 548

   Outcomes Identification, 548
   Implementation, 548
  Anxiety Disorders, 550
   Separation Anxiety Disorder, 550
   Generalized Anxiety Disorder, 550
  Application of the Nursing Process, 550
   Assessment, 550
   Diagnosis, 550
   Outcomes Identification, 550
   Implementation, 550
  Other Disorders of Children and Adolescents, 551
   Depressive Disorders and Bipolar and Related Disorders, 551
   Post-Traumatic Stress Disorder, 551
   Feeding and Eating Disorders, 551
  References, 552

28 Psychosocial Needs of the Older Person, 555
Cheryl L. Pollard
Originating US chapter by Margaret Jordan Halter, Leslie A. Briscoe
  Developmental Theories of Aging, 555
  Mental Health Issues Related to Aging, 556
   Late-Life Mental Illness, 556
   Trauma, 558
   Caregiver Burden, 559
   Access to Care, 559
   Ageism, 559
   Ageism and Public Policy, 560
   Ageism and Drug Testing, 560
  Distinguishing Between Psychiatric and Physical Symptoms, 560
   Pain, 560
  Nursing Care of Older Persons, 563
   Assessment Strategies, 564
   Intervention Strategies, 566
   Care Settings, 568
  References, 570

29 Recovery, Survivorship, and Public Mental Health Approaches, 572
Sonya L. Jakubec
  Serious Mental Illness Across the Lifespan, 572
   Older Persons, 572
   Younger Adults, 573
  Development of Serious Mental Illness, 573
  Rehabilitation Versus Recovery: Two Models of Care, 573
  Issues Confronting People With Serious Mental Illness, 574
   Establishing a Meaningful Life, 574
   Comorbid Conditions, 574
   Social Problems, 575
   Economic Challenges, 575
   Treatment Issues, 575
  Resources for People With Serious Mental Illness, 577
   Comprehensive Community Treatment, 577
   Substance Use Treatment, 578
  Evidence-Informed Treatment Approaches, 578
   Assertive Community Treatment, 578
   Cognitive Behavioural Therapy and Meta-cognitive Therapy, 578
   Family Support and Partnerships, 578
   Social Skills Training, 578
   Supportive Psychotherapy and Peer Support, 579
   Vocational Rehabilitation and Related Services, 579
  Other Potentially Beneficial Services or Treatment Approaches, 579
   Consumer-Run Programs, 579
   Wellness and Recovery Action Plans, 579
   Exercise, 579
  Nursing Care of Patients With Serious Mental Illness, 579
   Assessment Strategies, 579
   Intervention Strategies, 579
   Evaluation, 581
  Current Issues, 581
   Population Health and Social Justice Approaches, 581
   Involuntary Treatment, 581
   Criminal Offences and Incarceration, 581
  References, 583

30 Psychological Needs of Patients With Medical Conditions, 586
Cheryl L. Pollard
  Psychological Factors Affecting Medical Conditions, 586
  Psychological Responses to Serious Medical Conditions, 587
   Depression, 587
   Anxiety, 588
   Substance Use, 588
   Grief and Loss, 588
   Denial, 588
   Fear of Dependency, 589
  Human Rights Abuses of Stigmatized Persons With Medical Conditions, 589
  Application of the Nursing Process, 590
   Assessment, 590
   Diagnosis, 591
   Outcomes Identification, 591
   Planning, 591
   Implementation, 591
   Evaluation, 592
  References, 593

31 Care for the Dying and for Those Who Grieve, 594
Sonya L. Jakubec
  Hospice Palliative Care, 594
  Nursing Care at the End of Life, 596
   Hospice Palliative Care Nursing, 596
   The Art, Presence, and Caring of Nursing, 596
   Assessment for Spiritual Issues, 596
   Awareness and Sensitivity of Cultural Contexts, 596
   Palliative Symptom Management, 597
   The Importance of Effective Communication, 597
   Self-Care, 600
  Nursing Care for Those Who Grieve, 601
  Grief Reactions, Bereavement, and Mourning, 601
   Types of Grief, 601
   Theories, 602
   Helping People Cope With Loss, 603
  Current Topics and Future Directions, 604
   Medical Assistance in Dying (MAiD) Legislation, 604
   Palliative Care for Patients With Dementia, 605
   Areas for Future Discovery, 605
  References, 606

32 Forensic Psychiatric Nursing, 610
Lisa-Marie Forcier, Eric MacMullin
- **Forensic Nursing, 611**
  - *Education, 612*
  - *Roles and Functions, 612*
  - *The Forensic Mental Health System in Canada, 613*
- **Forensic Psychiatric Nursing, 613**
  - *Roles and Functions, 613*
- **References, 616**

UNIT 7 Advanced Intervention Modalities

33 Therapeutic Groups, 620
Cheryl L. Pollard
Originating US chapter by Donna Rolin, Emily Fowler
- **Therapeutic Factors Common to All Groups, 620**
- **Planning a Group, 620**
- **Phases of Group Development, 621**
- **Group Member Roles, 621**
- **Group Leadership, 622**
  - *Nurse as Group Leader, 622*
  - *Responsibilities, 622*
  - *Styles of Leadership, 623*
  - *Clinical Supervision, 623*
  - *Group Observation, 624*
  - *Ethical Issues in Group Therapy, 624*
  - *Basic Groups, 625*
  - *Advanced-Practice Nurse or Nurse Therapist, 626*
  - *Dealing With Challenging Member Behaviours, 627*
- **Expected Outcomes, 628**
- **References, 629**

34 Family Interventions, 630
Lisa-Marie Forcier
Originating US chapter by Christina Fratena, Laura G. Leahy
- **Family, 631**
  - *Family Functions, 631*
  - *Families and Mental Illness, 632*
- **Canadian Models of Family Nursing Care and Assessment, 632**
  - *McGill Model of Nursing, 632*
  - *Calgary Family Assessment Model and Calgary Family Intervention Model, 632*
- **Family Therapy, 632**
  - *Issues Associated With Family Therapies, 632*
  - *Family Life Cycle, 633*
  - *Working With the Family, 634*
- **Family Therapy Theory, 635**
  - *The Family as a System, 636*
- **Application of the Nursing Process, 636**
  - *Assessment, 636*
  - *Diagnosis, 639*
  - *Outcomes Identification, 640*
  - *Planning, 640*
  - *Implementation, 640*
  - *Evaluation, 642*
- **References, 643**

35 Integrative and Complementary Therapies, 645
Cheryl L. Pollard
With Contributions From Karen Scott Barss
- **Integrative Health Care in Canada, 645**
  - *Research, 646*
- **Patients and Integrative Care, 646**
  - *Safety, 646*
  - *Efficacy, 647*
- **Integrative Nursing Care, 647**
- **Classification of Integrative Therapies, 647**
  - *Whole Medical Systems, 647*
  - *Mind–Body–Spirit Approaches, 648*
  - *Biologically Based Therapies, 650*
  - *Manipulative Practices, 652*
  - *Energy Therapies, 653*
- **References, 654**

Appendix: Standards of Practice, Code of Ethics, Beliefs, and Values, 656
Glossary, 659
Index, 672

A tailored education experience —

Sherpath book-organized collections

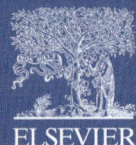

Sherpath book-organized collections offer:

Objective-based, digital lessons, mapped chapter-by-chapter to the textbook, that make it easy to find applicable digital assignment content.

Adaptive quizzing with personalized questions that correlate directly to textbook content.

Teaching materials that align to the text and are organized by chapter for quick and easy access to invaluable class activities and resources.

Elsevier ebooks that provide convenient access to textbook content, even offline.

Sherpath is the digital teaching and learning technology designed specifically for healthcare education.

**VISIT
myevolve.us/sherpath
today to learn more!**

21-CS-0280 TM/AF 6/21

UNIT 1

Foundations in Theory

1. Mental Health and Mental Illness

2. Historical Overview of Psychiatric Mental Health Nursing

3. Overview of Psychiatric Mental Health Nursing Care Within Various Settings

4. Relevant Theories and Therapies for Nursing Practice

5. Understanding Responses to Stress

1

Mental Health and Mental Illness

Sonya L. Jakubec

 http://evolve.elsevier.com/Canada/Varcarolis/psychiatric/

OBJECTIVES

1. Describe the two conceptualizations of mental health and mental illness.
2. Explore the role of resilience in the prevention of and recovery from mental illness and consider your own resilience in response to stress.
3. Identify how culture influences our view of mental illnesses and behaviours associated with them.
4. Define and identify attributes of positive mental health.
5. Discuss the nature/nurture origins of psychiatric disorders.
6. Summarize the social determinants of health in Canada.
7. Explain how findings of epidemiological studies can be used to identify areas for medical and nursing interventions.
8. Identify how the *DSM-5* can influence a clinician to consider a broad range of information before making a diagnosis.
9. Describe the specialty of psychiatric mental health nursing.
10. Compare and contrast a *DSM-5* medical diagnosis with a nursing diagnosis.

KEY TERMS AND CONCEPTS

clinical epidemiology
comorbid condition
Diagnostic and Statistical Manual of Mental Disorders, 5th edition
epidemiology
evidence-informed practice
incidence
mental health
mental illness
Nursing Interventions Classification
Nursing Outcomes Classification
prevalence
resilience
virtual health care

 HOW A NURSE HELPED ME

When a Nurse Becomes a Patient

I am a registered nurse working in the area of mental health. I always prided myself on my ability to give caring and compassionate treatment to all of my patients. Little did I know that one day I would be the patient. I was diagnosed with bipolar disorder when I was 34 years old. For many years, I struggled with devastating depressions and periods of acute mania. I felt stupid, ashamed, and embarrassed about my behaviour during these times. Whenever I needed hospitalization, I begged the ambulance driver to take me to any hospital but the one I worked in. On one occasion, that did not happen, and I was admitted to the unit where I worked as a nurse. I thought I could have died of the deep shame I felt. Judy, the nurse assigned to me, seemed scared and embarrassed to come and speak with me, so I felt uncomfortable when I spoke with her. On about the fourth day of that admission, Brenda, another nurse I knew, was assigned to my care. Brenda started out by telling me that she would be my nurse for the shift and that she would make herself available to me for a one-on-one later in the day. When she came to speak with me, she said, "Let's talk about the elephant in the room, and then we can move into talking about how I can support you in getting well." We talked about my embarrassment and shame. I felt so relieved that she was willing to address my feelings about my mental illness. Over the next several weeks, we had many one-on-one sessions, and I was able to share my story with Brenda. Brenda helped me see that there was hope for my future and that I could learn to live well despite my diagnosis. I would love to say that I got well and stayed well, but actually, I have continued to struggle with my health. I can tell you that Brenda's acknowledgement of my feelings helped me deal with the stigma I felt about my illness. I no longer feel ashamed of having a mental illness.

Because they are frequently mentioned in our daily conversations and in the media, it is likely you routinely hear about people's mood, thinking, emotions, and behaviours. Terms like *depression*, *anxiety*, *psychosis*, *dementia*, *addiction*, *crisis*, and *stress* are used in many different ways. But what does this mean for people who are experiencing distress or problems in their mental health and well-being? How are you to understand and work knowledgeably in this changing and rapidly evolving area of nursing? Certainly, people living with mental illnesses and their families and caregivers experience a range of physical symptoms that result both from the illness itself—and as a consequence of treatment, the social determinants of health—and from the stigma and discrimination that contribute further to distress (Gaebel et al., 2017). Your understanding of the theories of mental health and illness and ongoing self-reflection are important places to begin to establish psychiatric mental health nursing practice that can treat, support, and empower people who suffer unnecessarily from mistreatment, misunderstanding, and social exclusion (da Silva et al., 2020; Ungar, 2018).

MENTAL HEALTH AND MENTAL ILLNESS

The World Health Organization (WHO) maintains that a person cannot be considered healthy without taking into account mental and physical health. The WHO defines mental health as "a state of well-being in which each individual is able to realize his or her own potential, cope with the normal stresses of life, work productively and fruitfully, and make a contribution to the community" (WHO, 2018). Our quality of life and our ability to enjoy life are enhanced by positive mental health and a sense of well-being (Mental Health Commission

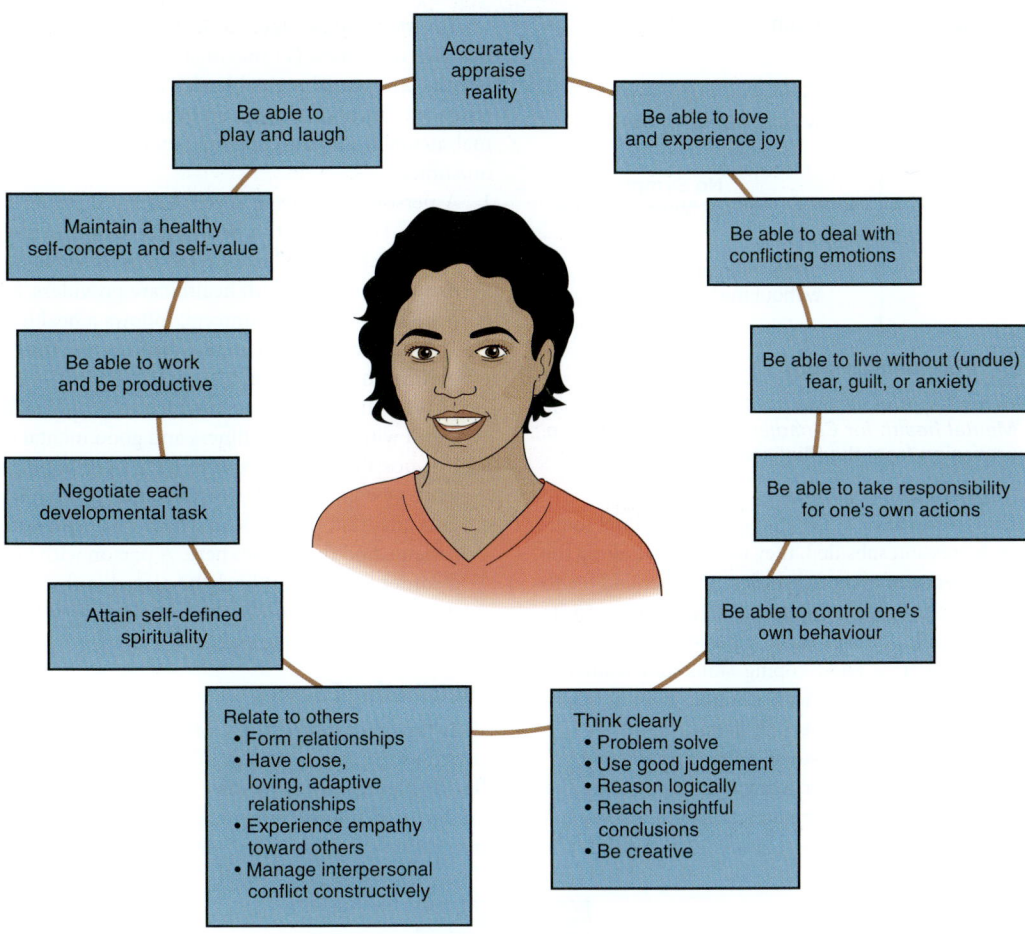

Fig. 1.1 Some attributes of mental health.

of Canada, 2017). Good mental health is associated with better physical health outcomes, improved educational attainment, increased economic participation, and rich social relationships (Alegría et al., 2018; Shim & Compton, 2018). Mental health is described as more than merely the absence of mental disorders or disabilities (WHO, 2018). The Public Health Agency of Canada (2020) also makes the distinction that mental health is not the same as mental illness but asserts that poor mental health can lead to mental and physical illness. Good mental health enables people to feel, think, and act in ways that support the enjoyment of life and ways of coping with the challenges that life brings. The promotion of positive mental health in this way enhances a sense of emotional and spiritual well-being that respects the importance of culture, equity, social justice, interconnections, and personal dignity (Public Health Agency of Canada, 2019). Some of the attributes of positive mental health are presented in Figure 1.1.

Societal and psychiatric definitions of *mental health* are continually evolving. Defining concepts are shaped by the prevailing culture and social values and reflect changes in cultural norms, society's expectations, dominant medical discourse, and corporate and political views. In the past, the term *mental illness* was applied to behaviours considered "strange" or "different," behaviours that occurred infrequently and deviated from an established norm. Such criteria are inadequate because they suggest that mental health requires conformity. But there is a further problem in viewing people whose behaviour is unusual as mentally ill. Such a definition would mean that nonconformists and independent thinkers like Socrates, Mahatma Gandhi, and Canada's suffragettes such as Nellie McClung and Emily Murphy would be considered mentally ill. And although the determination of Viola Desmond, the dedication of Terry Fox, and the artistic abilities of Leonard Cohen are uncommon, virtually none of us would consider the much-admired exceptional behaviours of these Canadian heroes to be signs of mental illness.

It is alterations in cognition, mood, or behaviour coupled with significant distress and impaired functioning that characterize **mental illness** (Public Health Agency of Canada, 2017). *Mental illness* refers to all mental disorders with definable diagnoses. Cognition may be impaired, as in Alzheimer's disease; mood may be affected, as in major depression; behaviour may change, as in schizophrenia; or a combination of the three types of symptoms may be apparent.

Two Conceptualizations of Mental Health and Mental Illness

Published in 1988, *Mental Health for Canadians: Striking a Balance*, commonly called the Epp Report, highlighted the importance of issues related to mental health and mental illness in Canada. It proposed seven guiding principles for the development of public policies to support mental health. Despite the forward thinking of this report, it was not until 2009 that Canada developed a mental health strategy framework (Mental Health Commission of Canada, 2009), with a framework for action established in 2017 (Mental Health Commission of Canada, 2017).

The Epp Report (Epp, 1988) proposed two continua to depict the relationship between mental health and mental disorder. The Mental Disorder Continuum assigns one endpoint as maximal mental disorder and the opposite endpoint as the absence of mental disorder, allowing for a range of impairment and distress. For instance, a person with

Fig. 1.2 Continua from the Epp Report. (Source: Public Health Agency of Canada. (1988). *Mental health for Canadians: striking a balance.* Reproduced with permission from the Minister of Health, 2013.)

a severe clinical depression would be at the endpoint of maximal mental disorder, but as the depression subsided, they would move along the continuum toward the absence of mental disorder. The Mental Health Continuum assigns one pole as optimal mental health and the opposite pole as minimal mental health. On this scale, a person with optimal mental health would demonstrate good coping skills and resilience when faced with stressors, and a person with minimal mental health may decompensate and not be able to cope with stressors.

The interaction between the continua suggested by Epp (Figure 1.2) is interesting and could provide a basis for many research studies. For example, how can nurses support routine physical health assessment for people with schizophrenia?

This depiction of mental health and mental illness allows for four possible outcomes: (1) maximal mental disorder and optimal mental health; (2) optimal mental health and absence of mental disorder; (3) absence of mental disorder and minimal mental health; and (4) minimal mental health and maximal mental disorder. We will look at each outcome:

1. A person may have a severe mental disorder *and* optimal mental health. How could this be possible? Think of the person with a diagnosis of chronic schizophrenia who is stable on their medications, maintains contact with health care providers, has a social network, possibly works or volunteers, follows a healthy diet, and exercises. This person still has a mental disorder, yet they meet the criteria for optimal mental health.
2. This quadrant is the one in which we would all like to be. Imagine a world with no mental illness and good mental health.
3. It is possible for a person to have poor coping skills and no resilience when faced with stressors and yet not have a mental disorder.
4. This quadrant is the one in which we would not like to be, yet many patients find themselves here. A person with borderline personality disorder would most likely be placed in this quadrant.

It is important to note that it is possible to be anywhere along the continua, not just at one end.

Contributing Factors

Many factors can affect the severity and progression of a mental illness, as well as the mental health of a person who does not have a mental illness (Figure 1.3). If possible, these influences need to be evaluated and factored into an individual's plan of care. In fact, the **Diagnostic and Statistical Manual of Mental Disorders, 5th edition (DSM-5)**

Fig. 1.3 Influences that can have an impact on an individual's mental health.

(American Psychiatric Association, 2013), classifies around 350 mental disorders with evidence that suggests that the symptoms and causes of a number of them are influenced by cultural and ethnic factors. The *DSM-5* is discussed in further detail later in this chapter.

Resilience

Researchers, clinicians, and patients are all interested in actively facilitating mental health and reducing mental illness. A characteristic of mental health increasingly being promoted as essential to the recovery process is **resilience**. Canadian researcher Michael Ungar (2018) understands *resilience* as a process and outcome of complex, cultural systems rather than as an individual capacity to overcome adversity. In this way, when exposed to adversity, one's resilience depends on the navigation and negotiation of resources that can support well-being. Ungar's (2018) research emphasizes that resilience depends far more on the quality and interactions of the social and physical ecologies surrounding people than on individual personality traits, cognitions, or talents. Closely associated with the process of *adapting*, resilience helps people face tragedies, loss, trauma, and severe stress. We can see evidence of resilience in the wake of disasters such as the global pandemic that started in 2020 and the civil war in Syria resulting in mass casualties and refugees. Being resilient does not mean being unaffected by stressors; rather, it means that instead of remaining stuck in negative emotions or practices, resilient people and institutions recognize such feelings and negotiate complex personal and societal systems in order to deal with their responses and the responses of others.

Beyond social and environmental understandings of resilience, practically accessing and developing resilience assists people in recovering from painful experiences and difficult events. Resilience is characterized by optimism and a sense of mastery and competence. Research demonstrates that early experiences in emotional regulation and mastering difficult or stressful situations enhance the prefrontal cortex's ability to cope with such situations later (Harrist & Gardner, 2019). You can get an idea of how good you are at regulating your emotions by taking the assessment in Box 1.1. These neurobiological discoveries related to the stress response (refer also to Chapter 5) also shine the light on more upstream measures to prevent distressing and stressful conditions for people. Inequitable, oppressive, discriminatory social structures at the root of distress for people are concerns that require different questions, leading to different solutions and interventions than a view focused on individual biology alone.

BOX 1.1 Assessing Your Resilience

The following questions are intended to provide you with an opportunity to reflect on and perhaps discover your own resilience.
1. What about my life gives me the most meaning?
2. What do others depend on me for?
3. What do I do that others value?
4. What is my philosophy, beliefs about life that guide my day-to-day choices?
5. What do I hope for?
6. How do I respond in difficult times?
7. How have I gotten through difficult times?
8. How do I handle disappointments in life?
9. What is my general outlook in life (optimist, pessimist)?
10. In what ways can I depend on myself?
11. What has changed in my life?
12. What has stayed the same in my life?

As you reflect on your answers, those related to your inner strength, competence, optimism, flexibility, and the ability to cope effectively when faced with adversity are all positively linked to increased levels of resilience.

Mental health recovery. According to the Mental Health Commission of Canada (2015, 2020a), recovery rests on several key concerns: respect for individual contexts and wishes, hope for a better future, dignity and self-determination, collaboration and reflection, and a focus on strengths and personal responsibility. Recovery practices insist that all people are respected for the experience, expertise, and strengths they contribute. Recovery approaches challenge traditional notions of professional power and expertise by helping to break down the conventional notions of expertise that give more weight to professional expertise over lived experience (of patients and families).

VIGNETTE

Elizabeth Anderson lives with schizophrenia. Involvement in a recovery support group has changed her view of her illness, herself, her marriage, and her potential. She has taken the lead role in her own recovery and supports others to do the same through her writing, speaking, and community work. This leadership and her book *Being Mentally Healthy (in spite of a mental illness)* highlight a recipe for recovery and for being mentally healthy while living with a mental illness. According to Elizabeth, the recipe requires six ingredients: "timely intervention; the right medications; supportive people (especially loved ones); a reason to be well; a reason to hope; something important to do, or a higher purpose or calling." Elizabeth describes her life with mental illness in terms of resiliency, and with hope for the future and any number of possibilities, stating: "Yes, I'm doing well and I've got a mental illness."

Learn more about Elizabeth's story here: https://canadianwomen.org/blog/being-mentally-healthy/.

Culture

There is no standard measure for mental health, in part because it is culturally defined and is based on interpretations of effective functioning according to societal norms (WHO, 2018). One approach to differentiating mental health from mental illness is to consider what a particular culture regards as acceptable or unacceptable behaviour. In this view, people with mental illnesses are those who violate social norms and thus threaten (or make anxious) people observing them. For example, there are traditions where people consider suicide to be an act of honour, and others for whom suicide bombing for religious statements or in protest would be considered an act of a holy warrior or martyrs. Contrast these viewpoints with others who would consider any attempt or completed suicide as a feature of mental illness.

Throughout history, people have interpreted health or sickness according to the current and cultural views. A striking example of how cultural change influences the interpretation of mental illness is an old definition of *hysteria*. According to *Webster's Dictionary* (Porter, 1913), hysteria was "a nervous affection, occurring almost exclusively in women, in which the emotional and reflex excitability is exaggerated, and the will power correspondingly diminished, so that the patient loses control over the emotions, becomes the victim of imaginary sensations, and often falls into paroxysm or fits." Treatment for this condition often involved sexual outlets for afflicted women, whose condition was thought to be the result of sexual deprivation. According to some authors, this diagnosis fell into disuse as women gained rights, the family atmosphere became less restrictive, and societal tolerance of sexual practices increased.

Cultures differ not only in their views regarding mental illness but also in the types of behaviour categorized as mental illness. Culture-bound syndromes seem to occur in specific sociocultural contexts, identify local idioms of distress, and are easily recognized by people in those cultures (Stern et al., 2017). For example, one syndrome recognized in parts of Southeast Asia is *running amok*, in which a person (usually a male) runs around engaging in furious, almost indiscriminate violent behaviour. *Pibloktoq*, an uncontrollable desire to tear off one's clothing and expose oneself to severe winter weather, is a recognized psychological disorder in parts of Greenland, Alaska, and the Arctic regions of Canada. In Canada, *anorexia nervosa* (see Chapter 16) is recognized as a psychobiological disorder that entails voluntary starvation. The disorder is well known in Europe, North America, and Australia but unheard of in many other parts of the world.

What is to be made of the fact that certain disorders occur in some cultures but are absent in others? One interpretation is that the conditions necessary for causing a particular disorder occur in some places but are absent in others. Another interpretation is that people learn certain kinds of abnormal behaviour by imitation. However, the fact that some disorders may be culturally determined does not prove that all mental illnesses are determined so. Evidence suggests that schizophrenia (see Chapter 15) and bipolar disorders (see Chapter 14) are found throughout the world. The symptom patterns of schizophrenia have been observed among indigenous Greenlanders and West African villagers as well as in Western culture.

Perceptions of Mental Health and Mental Illness
Mental Illness Versus Physical Illness

People commonly make a distinction between mental illnesses and physical illnesses. It is an odd distinction, considering that *mental* refers to the brain, the most complex and sophisticated part of the body, the organ responsible for the higher thought processes that set us apart from other creatures. Surely the workings of the brain, namely the synaptic connections, the areas of functioning, the spinal innervations and connections, are *physical*. One problem with this distinction is that it implies that psychiatric disorders are "all in the head" and therefore under personal control and indistinguishable from a choice to indulge in bad behaviour. Although some physical disorders, such as a broken arm from skiing or lung cancer from smoking, are blamed on the victim, the majority of physical illnesses are considered to be beyond personal responsibility.

Perhaps the origin of this distinction between mental and physical illness lies in the religious and philosophical tradition of explaining the unexplainable by assigning a mystical or spiritual origin to cognitive processes and emotional activities. Despite many advances in understanding, mental illnesses continue to be viewed differently from illnesses that originate in other parts of the body.

Consider that people with epilepsy were once thought to be possessed by demons, under the attack of gods, or cursed; they were subjected to horrible "cures" and treatments. Today, most people would say that epilepsy is a disorder of the brain and not under one's personal control because epilepsy appears on brain scans as areas of overactivity and excitability. But there are no specific biological tests to diagnose most psychiatric disorders, for example, no blood test to diagnose obsessive-compulsive disorder (OCD). However, researchers are convinced that the root of most mental disorders lies in intercellular abnormalities, and they can now see clear signs of altered brain function in several mental disorders, including schizophrenia, OCD, stress disorders, and depression. Further details about these signs are discussed in Chapter 5 and throughout Unit 4.

Nature Versus Nurture

For students learning about mental illness, one of its most intriguing aspects is its origins. Although for centuries people believed that extremely unusual behaviours were due to demonic forces, in the late 1800s the mental health pendulum swung briefly to a biological focus with the "germ theory of diseases" (Nolan, 1993). Germ theory explained mental illness in the same way other illnesses were being described; that is, they were caused by a specific agent in the environment (Morgan et al., 2020). This perspective led to the segregation and isolation of people who were thought to be "mad," in the same way that those with infections were isolated in order to prevent the infection of others. This theory was abandoned rather quickly because clinicians and researchers could not identify single causative factors for mental illnesses; there was no "mania germ" that could be viewed under a microscope and subsequently treated. Nonetheless, the practices of isolation persisted.

Although biological treatments for mental illness continued to be explored and ultimately dismissed as ineffective, over the next half-century, psychological theories dominated and focused on the science of the mind and behaviour. These theories explained the origin of mental illness as faulty psychological processes that could be corrected by increasing personal insight and understanding. For example, a patient experiencing depression and apathy might be assisted to explore feelings left over from childhood, when his attempts at independence were harshly discouraged by overly protective parents.

This psychological focus was challenged in 1952, when the medication chlorpromazine (Largactil) was found to have a calming effect on agitated, out-of-control patients. Imagine what this discovery must have been like for clinicians who had resorted to every biological treatment imaginable, including wet wraps, insulin shock therapy, and psychosurgery (in which holes were drilled in the head of a patient and probes inserted in the brain), in a futile attempt to change behaviour. Many began to believe that if psychiatric problems respond to medications that alter intercellular components, then the illness must be a disruption of intercellular components to begin with. At this point, the pendulum made steady and sure progress toward a biological explanation of psychiatric problems and disorders.

Currently, the diathesis–stress model, in which diathesis represents biological predisposition and stress represents environmental stress or trauma, is the most accepted explanation for mental illness. This nature-plus-nurture argument asserts that most psychiatric disorders result from a combination of genetic vulnerability and negative environmental stressors. While one person may develop major depressive disorder (MDD) largely as the result of an inherited and biological vulnerability that alters brain chemistry, another person with little vulnerability may develop depression from changes in brain chemistry caused by the insults of a stressful environment. MDD is discussed in Chapter 13.

Human Genome Project

The Human Genome Project was a 13-year project (1990–2003) that was completed on the 50th anniversary of the discovery of the DNA double helix. The project has strengthened some biological and genetic explanations for psychiatric conditions and subsequent therapeutic interventions (Breen et al., 2016). The goals of the project were to:
- Identify the approximately 20 000 to 25 000 genes in human DNA
- Determine the sequences of the 3 billion chemical base pairs that make up human DNA
- Store this information in databases
- Improve tools for data analysis
- Address the ethical, legal, and social issues that may arise from the project.

Although researchers have begun to identify some rare genetic links to mental illness and more common gene–environment interactions (as you will see in the chapters on clinical disorders), it will be some time before we understand the precise contribution of genetics and the environment on mental illness (Bray & O'Donovan, 2018). What we do know is that most psychiatric disorders result from a large, common, and evolutionarily stable collection of genetic variations rather than a single gene. This concept of a common incidence and stable prevalence throughout the population both humanizes these previously stigmatized conditions and instills questions that contribute to misinformation and judgements.

Social Influences on Mental Health Care
Self-Help Movement
In January 1918 the Canadian Mental Health Association (CMHA) was formed by Dr. Clarence M. Hincks and Clifford W. Beers to promote mental health. The CMHA is one of the oldest and most respected voluntary health organizations in Canada (CMHA, 2020). In the latter part of the twentieth century, the CMHA and other organizations and individuals expended tremendous energy on putting the notion of equality, treating people fairly and extinguishing stigmatizing labels, into widespread practice in Canada. In regard to mental illness, decades of institutionalization had created political and social concerns that gave rise to a mental health movement similar to the rights movements for women, people with disabilities, and the LGBTQ2 (lesbian, gay, bisexual, transgender, queer, intersex, and Two-Spirit) population. Groups of people with mental illnesses, or mental health patients, began to advocate for their rights and the rights of others with mental illness and to fight stigma, discrimination, and forced treatment. Practitioners and activists who are concerned for the people in their care, as well as critical and antioppressive approaches to practice, are establishing alternative ways of understanding and addressing the conditions and contexts that organize contemporary psychiatry in Canada and elsewhere (Bull et al., 2018; Burstow, 2015; Menzies et al., 2013).

Decade of the Brain
In 1990, the United States Congress designated the last decade of the past century the "Decade of the Brain." This American initiative stimulated a worldwide growth of neuroscientific research (Leefmann & Hildt, 2017). Among the advances and progress made during the Decade of the Brain were the following:
- Understanding the genetic basis of embryonic and fetal neural development
- Mapping genes involved in neurological illness, including mutations associated with Parkinson's disease, Alzheimer's disease, and epilepsy
- Discovery that the brain uses a relatively small number of neurotransmitters but has a vast assortment of neurotransmitter receptors
- Uncovering the role of cytokines (proteins involved in the immune response) in such brain disorders as depression
- Refinement of neuroimaging techniques, such as positron emission tomography (PET) scans, magnetic resonance imaging (MRI), magnetoencephalography, and event-related electroencephalography (EEG), which have improved our understanding of normal brain functioning as well as areas of difference in pathological states
- Bringing together computer modelling and laboratory research, which resulted in the new discipline of computational neuroscience.

While the Decade of the Brain ended in 2000, the so-called neuroage of expanded scientific exploration of the brain continues to influence society in numerous ways, including biomedical, clinical, political, marketing, and business.

Mental Health for Canadians: Striking a Balance
Mental Health for Canadians: Striking a Balance (Epp, 1988) was one of the first government-generated reports that acknowledged the challenges of the mentally ill population. The purpose of the report was to assist Canadians engaged in developing and reviewing mental health–related policies and programs. Three challenges in mental health were identified: (1) reducing inequities, (2) increasing prevention, and (3) enhancing coping. These challenges continue. For example, the Mental Health Commission of Canada (2012) identified similar challenges, which are reflected in its six strategic directions: (1) promoting mental health across the lifespan; (2) fostering recovery and well-being for people while upholding their rights; (3) providing timely access to treatment and supports; (4) reducing disparities; (5) recognizing the distinct circumstances, rights, and cultures in addressing mental health needs of individuals and communities; and (6) ensuring effective leadership and collaboration across sectors, agencies, and communities.

Changing Directions, Changing Lives: The Mental Health Strategy for Canada
In November 2009, the Mental Health Commission of Canada released a report titled *Toward Recovery & Well-Being: A Framework for a Mental Health Strategy for Canada*. Until this time, Canada did not have a national plan for the development of a mental health strategy. Seven interconnected goals were identified to define what it would take to have a system oriented toward both enabling the recovery of people living with mental health problems and illnesses and fostering the mental health and well-being of everyone living in Canada. This framework was the first phase in the development of a comprehensive Canadian mental health strategy, instrumental in both health reform and social change (Rosen et al., 2010). It put forward the vision and broad goals for the strategy in 2012 and a later action plan in 2017.

The aim of the strategy and action plan is to improve mental health and well-being for all Canadians. The large collaborative teams who have developed the strategy and plan strongly believe that we can create a mental health system that will meet the needs of people of all ages living with mental health problems and illnesses and their families. Implementation of this strategy will help to ensure that people who experience mental health problems and illnesses especially those with the most severe and complex ones, are treated with respect and dignity and enjoy the same rights as all Canadians. Six key strategic directions (Box 1.2) were outlined in the report. Students are encouraged to access the full report to get an understanding of how health care providers, patients, families, and communities can work together to implement the strategies throughout Canada.

The 2017–2022 action plan for this strategy focuses further on four key pillars: leadership and funding, promotion and prevention, access and services, and data and research.

EPIDEMIOLOGY OF MENTAL DISORDERS

Epidemiology, as it applies to psychiatric mental health, is the quantitative study of the distribution of mental disorders in human populations. Once the distribution of mental disorders has been determined quantitatively, epidemiologists can identify high-risk groups and high-risk factors associated with illness onset, duration, and recurrence. The further study of risk factors for mental illness may then lead to important clues about the causes of various mental disorders.

Two different but related words used in epidemiology are *incidence* and *prevalence*. **Incidence** refers to the *number of new cases* of mental disorders in a healthy population within a given period of time; for example, the number of Vancouver adolescents who were diagnosed with MDD between 2010 and 2020. **Prevalence** describes the *total number of cases*, new and existing, in a given population during a specific period of time, regardless of when the subjects became ill; for example,

> **BOX 1.2 Strategic Directions Identified in *Changing Directions, Changing Lives: The Mental Health Strategy for Canada***
>
> **Strategic Direction 1: Promotion and Prevention**
> Promote mental health across the lifespan in homes, schools, and workplaces and prevent mental illness and suicide wherever possible. Reducing the impact of mental health problems and illnesses and improving the mental health of the population require promotion and prevention efforts in everyday settings where the potential impact is greatest.
>
> **Strategic Direction 2: Recovery and Rights**
> Foster recovery and well-being for people of all ages living with mental health problems and illnesses and uphold their rights. The key to recovery is helping people to find the right combination of services, treatments, and supports and eliminating discrimination by removing barriers to full participation in work, education, and community life.
>
> **Strategic Direction 3: Access to Services**
> Provide access to the right combination of services, treatments, and supports, when and where people need them. A full range of services, treatments, and supports includes primary health care, community-based and specialized mental health services, peer support, and supported housing, education, and employment.
>
> **Strategic Direction 4: Disparities and Diversity**
> Reduce disparities in risk factors and access to mental health services and strengthen the response to the needs of diverse communities and Northerners. Mental health should be taken into account when acting to improve overall living conditions and addressing the specific needs of groups such as new Canadians and people in northern and remote communities.
>
> **Strategic Direction 5: First Nations, Inuit, and Métis**
> Work with First Nations, Inuit, and Métis people to address their mental health needs, acknowledging their distinct circumstances, rights, and cultures. By calling for access to a full continuum of culturally safe mental health services, the *Mental Health Strategy for Canada* can contribute to truth, reconciliation, and healing from intergenerational trauma.
>
> **Strategic Direction 6: Leadership and Collaboration**
> Mobilize leadership, improve knowledge, and foster collaboration at all levels. Change will not be possible without a whole-of-government approach to mental health policy, without fostering the leadership roles of people living with mental health problems and illnesses and their families, and without building strong infrastructure to support data collection, research, and human resource development.

Source: Mental Health Commission of Canada. (2012). *Changing directions, changing lives: The mental health strategy for Canada.* https://www.mentalhealthcommission.ca/sites/default/files/MHStrategy_Strategy_ENG.pdf

met the criteria for diagnosed illness meeting the International Classification of Diseases (ICD) from a hospital or other physician visit. Select highlights from the report include:

- "Approximately five million Canadians (or about one in seven people) use health services for a mental illness annually."
- "Women are more likely than men to use health services for a mental illness, especially those between the ages of 25 to 39 years. A combination of genetic, biological, behavioural and sociocultural factors may explain this difference."
- "Almost one in four people aged 80 and over use health services for a mental illness, a trend likely driven by the inclusion of dementias in the International Classification of Diseases under mental disorders."
- "The largest relative increase [of the use of health services for mental illness] occurred among young adolescents (aged 10 to 14)."
- "Boys (under 15 years of age) are more likely to use health services for a mental illness than girls; likely driven by certain disturbance of conduct disorders and attention deficit disorder which are known to occur more frequently among boys."

Many individuals have more than one mental disorder at a time; this state is known as a **comorbid condition**.

Some disorders may have a high incidence but a low prevalence, and vice versa. A disease with a short duration, such as the common cold, tends to have a high incidence (many new cases in a given year) and a low prevalence (not many people suffering from a cold at any given time). Conversely, a chronic disease such as diabetes will have a low incidence because a year (or whatever time increment is used) after diagnosis, the person will be dropped from the list of new cases. Lifetime risk data, or the risk that one will develop a disease in the course of their lifetime, will be higher than both incidence and prevalence. Table 1.1 shows the prevalence of some psychiatric disorders in Canada.

RESEARCH HIGHLIGHT BOX

Mental Health Epidemiology: Differences in Prevalence of Mental Disorders and Suicidality Across Canadian Provinces

> A large Canadian study further examined prevalence data and showed significant differences in the prevalence of mental disorders and suicidality in Canadian provinces. This survey includes a representative sample of Canadians over the age of 15 years in each province. They looked at sociodemographic factors (such as age, sex, income, and marital status) and past-year prevalence of mental disorders and suicidality. A total of 25,113 participants were included in the study. Manitoba had the highest prevalence of any mental disorder (14%). It also had the highest prevalence of major depressive disorder (7%) and alcohol use disorder (4%). Nova Scotia had the highest prevalence of substance use disorders (2.9%). Quebec and Prince Edward Island had the lowest prevalence of any mental disorder (8.5% and 7.7%, respectively). British Columbia and Ontario had the highest prevalence of suicidal planning (1.4% and 1.3%, respectively), and Ontario had the highest prevalence of suicide attempts (0.7%). Differences in provincial prevalence were not related to the sociodemographic factors included in the study. Though the data from the most recent Canadian mental health prevalence surveys are old, these findings point the way to investigate these differences and how they impact the need for mental health services.

Source: Palay, J., Taillieu, T. L., Afifi, T. O., et al. (2019). Prevalence of mental disorders and suicidality in Canadian provinces. *Canadian Journal of Psychiatry. Revue Canadienne de Psychiatrie, 64*(11), 761–769. https://journals.sagepub.com/doi/10.1177/0706743719878987

the number of adolescents who screen positive for MDD in Toronto schools between 2010 and 2020. Each level of investigation supplies information that can be used to improve clinical practice and plan public-health policies.

Report From the Canadian Chronic Disease Surveillance System: Mental Illness in Canada, a report from the Public Health Agency of Canada (2015), describes the major mental illnesses and reports their incidence and prevalence over a 14-year period. The report identified individuals as having used health services for a mental illness if they

TABLE 1.1 Mental Health Profile: Prevalence of Mental Illness and Indicators (Over 12 Months)

Disorder	Prevalence Over 12 Months (%)	Comments
Any mental illnesses (including substance use disorder)	10.1	33.1% (lifetime prevalence)
Schizophrenia or psychosis	1.3	Population aged 15 and over who reported that they have ever been diagnosed by a health professional with schizophrenia or psychosis.
Substance use disorder (alcohol or drug)	4.4	21.6% lifetime prevalence
All mood disorders	7.8 (males 6; females 9.6)	Leading cause of disability in Canada and established economies worldwide
Major depressive episode	4.7	11.3% lifetime prevalence
Bipolar disorder	1.5	2.6% lifetime prevalence
Generalized anxiety disorder	2.6	8.7% lifetime prevalence
		Can begin across life cycle; risk is highest between childhood and middle age
Panic disorder	0.7	Typically develops in adolescence or early adulthood
Obsessive-compulsive disorder (OCD)	1.8	Symptoms begin in childhood or adolescence
Posttraumatic stress disorder (PTSD)	1.7	Current diagnosed condition
Eating disorders	0.4	Current diagnosed condition
Attention deficit disorder	2.6	Current diagnosed condition
Other		
Suicidal behaviour (not classified as a mental disorder but has significant impact on mental well-being, and people with mental illness are at higher risk for suicide)	9.3 per 100 000*	Over 3500 suicides were reported in Canada in 2020. Rates vary by population. The largest population of suicides in Canada are from adults. The suicide rate for Inuit peoples living in Northern Canada is 70 per 100 000 people, significantly higher than the general population.
Suicidal thoughts	3	12% (lifetime)

*Centre for Suicide Prevention. (2021). Suicide stats for Canada, provinces and territories. https://www.suicideinfo.ca/resource/suicide-stats-canada-provinces/

Sources: Palay, J., Taillieu, T. L., Afifi, T. O., et al. (2019). Prevalence of mental disorders and suicidality in Canadian provinces. *Canadian Journal of Psychiatry, 64*(11), 761–769. https://doi.org/10.1177/0706743719878987; Statistics Canada. (2020). *Canadian Community Health Survey, 2019.* https://www150.statcan.gc.ca/n1/daily-quotidien/200806/dq200806a-eng.htm

Clinical epidemiology is a broad field that addresses what happens after people with illnesses are seen by clinical care providers. Using traditional epidemiological methods, studies are conducted in groups that are usually defined by the illness or symptoms or by diagnostic procedures or treatments given to address the illness or symptoms. Clinical epidemiology includes:
- Studies of the natural history of an illness
- Studies of diagnostic screening tests
- Observational and experimental studies of interventions used to treat people with the illness or symptoms.

Results of epidemiological studies are now routinely included in the *Diagnostic and Statistical Manual of Mental Disorders* (discussed below) to describe the frequency of mental disorders. Analysis of such studies can reveal the frequency with which psychological symptoms appear together with physical illness. For example, epidemiological studies demonstrate that depression is a significant risk factor for death in people with cardiovascular disease and for premature death in people with breast cancer.

CLASSIFICATION OF MENTAL DISORDERS

The Diagnostic and Statistical Manual

The first *Diagnostic and Statistical Manual of Mental Disorders* (DSM) was published by the American Psychiatric Association in 1952. Its purpose was to provide clinicians, educators, and researchers with a common framework to understand and communicate about mental disorders. With a common understanding of mental disorders, researchers and clinicians could work together in their attempts to improve care for people with mental illness.

Today, its fifth edition, the *DSM-5*, serves as the official guide for diagnosing psychiatric disorders. Listing more than 350 diagnoses, this authoritative manual was influenced by psychiatrists, psychologists, licensed clinical social workers, licensed counsellors, licensed marriage and family therapists, and advanced-practice psychiatric mental health nurses. Consistent with the purposes of previous editions, the *DSM-5* also serves as a tool for collecting epidemiological statistics about the diagnosis of psychiatric disorders.

A common misconception is that a classification of mental disorders classifies *people*, when actually the *DSM-5* classifies *disorders* people have. For this reason, the *DSM-5* and this textbook avoid the use of expressions such as "a schizophrenic" or "an alcoholic." Viewing the person as a person first and not an illness requires more accurate terms such as "an individual with schizophrenia" or "my patient has major depression."

The *DSM-5* Organizational Structure

The *DSM-5* (American Psychiatric Association, 2013) organizes diagnoses for psychiatric disorders on a developmental hierarchy, meaning that disorders that are usually seen in infancy, childhood, and adolescence are listed in the first chapter and neurodevelopmental disorders and disorders that occur later in life, such as the neurocognitive disorders, are further down the list. Also, within each chapter, specific disorders are listed based on the typical age of onset, from youngest to oldest. Diagnostic groups that are related to one another have been closely situated (for example, schizophrenia spectrum disorders are next to bipolar-related disorders, and feeding and eating disorders are next to elimination disorders).

- Neurodevelopmental disorder
- Schizophrenia spectrum disorder
- Bipolar and related disorders
- Depressive disorders
- Anxiety disorders
- Obsessive-compulsive disorders
- Trauma and stressor disorders
- Dissociative disorders
- Somatic symptom disorders
- Feeding and eating disorders
- Elimination disorders
- Sleep–wake disorders
- Sexual dysfunctions
- Gender dysphoria
- Disruptive, impulse control, and conduct disorders
- Substance and addictive disorders
- Neurocognitive disorders
- Personality disorders
- Paraphilias
- Other disorders

When making a diagnosis based on the *DSM-5*, clinicians and researchers need to consider presenting symptoms and how these symptoms are affecting the patient's life. Assessing the impact that the mental disorder is having on a person's day-to-day functioning requires the Disability Assessment Schedule 2.0, a tool developed by the WHO (https://www.who.int/classifications/icf/whodasii/en/).

The *ICD-11*

The *International Classification of Diseases (ICD)* (WHO, 2020) sets the global health information standard for mortality and morbidity statistics. Clinicians and researchers use this classification system to define diseases, study disease patterns, monitor outcomes, and subsequently allocate resources based on the prevalence of disease. The *ICD* is used globally and has been translated into 43 languages. The 11th edition was published in 2020.

The Canadian Institute for Health Information developed an enhanced version of the previous version, *ICD-10*, referred to as the *ICD-10-CA*. That version extends beyond defining and classifying diseases to describe conditions and situations that are not diseases, including, for example, risk factors to health and psychosocial circumstances. Also, the *ICD-10-CA* better represents the social determinants of health than *ICD-10*. The Canadian Institute for Health Information (2020) continues to assess the implication for implementing *ICD-11* in Canada with the development of support tools and design of further required supplemental resources relative to the Canadian context; until those resources are complete, the *ICD-10-CA* remains the classification system in use in Canada. You can browse the categories of the *ICD-10-CA* here: https://secure.cihi.ca/estore/productSeries.htm?pc=PCC189. And you can view *ICD-11* here: https://icd.who.int/browse11/l-m/en#/http%3a%2f%2fid.who.int%2ficd%2fentity%2f334423054.

PSYCHIATRIC MENTAL HEALTH NURSING

In all clinical settings, nurses work with people who are going through crises, including physical, psychological, mental, and spiritual distress. You will encounter patients who are experiencing feelings of hopelessness, helplessness, anxiety, anger, low self-esteem, or confusion. You will meet people who are withdrawn, suspicious, elated, depressed, hostile, manipulative, suicidal, intoxicated, or withdrawing from a substance. Many of you have already come across people who are going through difficult times in their lives. You may have handled these situations skillfully, but at other times, you may have wished you had additional skills and knowledge. Basic psychosocial nursing concepts will become central to your practice of nursing and increase your competency as a practitioner in all clinical settings. Whatever setting you choose to work in, you will have the opportunity to improve the lives of people who are experiencing mental illness as an additional challenge to their health.

Your experience in the mental health nursing rotation can help you gain insight into yourself and greatly increase your insight into the experiences of others. This part of your nursing education can also give you guidelines for and the opportunity to learn new skills for dealing with a variety of challenging behaviours. The following sections of this chapter present a brief overview of the work of professional psychiatric nurses, their scope of practice, and the challenges and evolving roles in the future health care environment.

What Is Psychiatric Mental Health Nursing?

Psychiatric mental health nurses enrich the health and well-being of Canadians by working with people throughout their lifespan and assisting healthy people who are in crisis or who are experiencing life problems, as well as those with long-term mental illness. Their patients may include people with concurrent disorders (i.e., a mental disorder and a coexisting substance disorder), homeless people and families, people in jail, individuals who have survived abusive situations, and people in crisis. Psychiatric mental health nurses work with individuals, couples, families, and groups in every nursing setting: in hospitals, in patients' homes, in halfway houses, in shelters, in clinics, in storefronts, on the street; virtually everywhere.

Uniquely, Canada has two bodies that provide standards of practice for mental health nursing. In the four western provinces and Yukon, registered psychiatric nurses follow the standards of practice issued by the provincial regulatory bodies with codeveloped *Standards of Psychiatric Nursing Practice* (See 2019 Standards here: https://www.crpnm.mb.ca/wp-content/uploads/2019/10/Standards-of-Psychiatric-Nursing-Practice-FINAL-October-2019.pdf). Registered nurses working in the specialty area of psychiatric mental health nursing follow the standards of practice issued by the Canadian Federation of Mental Health Nurses (CFMHN), an associate group of the Canadian Nurses Association (CNA). The Foundation, through the CNA, developed their 2014 Canadian Standards of Psychiatric-Mental Health Nursing (see https://www.cfmhn.ca/professional-practice/) due for updating in 2021 (Canadian Federation of Mental Health Nurses, 2014).

Classification of Nursing Diagnoses, Outcomes, and Interventions

To provide the most appropriate and scientifically sound care, the psychiatric mental health nurse uses standardized classification systems developed by professional nursing groups. These diagnoses provide a common language to aid in the selection of nursing interventions and ultimately lead to positive outcome achievement. The International Council of Nurses (2017) has a catalogue of 279 nursing diagnoses that are referenced throughout this text and can serve to guide your plan of care with your psychiatric mental health patients. The *Nursing Diagnoses: Definitions and Classification 2018–2020* of the North American Nursing Diagnosis Association International (NANDA-I) (Herdman & Kamitsuru, 2018) also provides 244 standardized diagnoses, more than 40% of which are related to psychosocial and psychiatric nursing care.

DSM-5 and Nursing Diagnoses

A nursing diagnosis is "a clinical judgment about individual, family, or community responses to actual or potential health problems and life processes" (International Nursing Knowledge Association, 2020). A well-defined nursing diagnosis provides the framework for setting priorities and identifying appropriate nursing interventions for dealing with the patient's reaction to the disorder. Those reactions might include confusion, low self-esteem, and impaired ability to function in job or family situations differing from the diagnoses that are made based on the criteria contained within the *DSM-5* that are used to label the patient's disorder.

Nursing Outcomes Classification (NOC)

The *Nursing Outcomes Classification (NOC)* provides "a comprehensive list of standardized outcomes, definitions, and measures to describe client outcomes influenced by nursing practice" (Moorhead et al., 2018). Outcomes are organized into seven domains: functional health, physiological health, psychosocial health, health knowledge and behaviour, perceived health, family health, and community health. The psychosocial health domain, which this text is most concerned with, includes four classes: psychological well-being, psychosocial adaptation, self-control, and social interaction.

Nursing Interventions Classification (NIC)

The *Nursing Interventions Classification (NIC)* is another tool used to standardize, define, and measure nursing care. Butcher and colleagues (2019) define a nursing intervention as "any treatment, based upon clinical judgment and knowledge, that a nurse performs to enhance patient/client outcomes," including direct and indirect care through a series of nursing activities. There are seven domains: basic physiological, complex physiological, behavioural, safety, family, health system, and community. Two domains relate specifically to psychiatric nursing: behavioural, including communication, coping, and education; and safety, covering crisis and risk management.

Evidence-Informed Practice

The nursing diagnosis classification systems mentioned have been researched extensively by nurses across a variety of treatment settings. Along with other best practice guidelines, they form a foundation for the novice or experienced nurse to participate in evidence-informed practice, that is, care based on the collection, interpretation, and integration of valid, important, and applicable patient-reported, clinician-observed, and research-derived evidence (Jakubec & Astle, 2021). In the chapters that follow, you will see examples of the application of nursing diagnoses to specific patients in vignettes and case studies, along with brief descriptions of other relevant research in the Research Highlight boxes, and evidence-informed practice description.

Levels of Psychiatric Mental Health Clinical Nursing Practice

Registered nurses in Canada may choose to work in psychiatric mental health nursing settings without additional certifications. However, many will choose to write the CNA's psychiatric/mental health nursing certification exam for the specialty. Registered psychiatric nurses (in the western provinces and Yukon) write national registration examinations.

Registered nurses and registered psychiatric nurses can further their education at a baccalaureate level or at the graduate level (master's, doctorate) and can become qualified to practise psychiatric mental health nursing at two levels, namely basic and advanced, depending on their educational preparation. Table 1.2 describes basic and advanced psychiatric nursing interventions.

Future Challenges and Roles for Psychiatric Mental Health Nurses

There has been a great demand for psychiatric mental health nurses, and indications suggest this need will increase in the future. Four significant trends that will affect the future of psychiatric mental health nursing in Canada are the aging population, increasing cultural diversity, expanding technology, and an increased awareness of the impact of health determinants on mental illness.

Aging Population

As the population of older adults grows, the prevalence of Alzheimer's disease and other dementias requiring the support of skilled and knowledgeable nurses will increase. Healthier older adults will need more services at home, in retirement communities, or in assisted-living facilities. Long-term care facilities will need to be reimagined with care and ethics

TABLE 1.2 Basic-Level and Advanced-Practice Psychiatric Mental Health Nursing Interventions

Basic-Level Intervention	Description
Coordination of care	Coordinates implementation of the nursing care plan and documents coordination of care
Health teaching and health maintenance	Provides individualized anticipatory guidance to prevent or reduce mental illness or enhance mental health (e.g., community screenings, parenting classes, stress management)
Milieu therapy	Provides, structures, and maintains a safe and therapeutic environment in collaboration with patients, families, and other health care clinicians
Pharmacological, biological, and integrative therapies	Applies current knowledge to assessing patients' responses to medication, provides medication teaching, and communicates observations to other members of the health care team
Advanced-Practice Intervention	**Description**
All of the Above Plus:	
Medication prescription and treatment	Prescribes psychotropic medications, with appropriate use of diagnostic tests; has hospital admitting privileges
Psychotherapy	Provides individual, couple, group, or family therapy using evidence-informed therapeutic frameworks
Consultation	Shares clinical expertise with nurses or those in other disciplines to enhance their treatment of patients or address systems issues

Source: Adapted from American Psychiatric Nurses Association, International Society of Psychiatric-Mental Health Nurses, & American Nurses Association. (2014). *Psychiatric-mental health nursing: Scope and standards of practice—3rd Edition.* Silver Spring, MD: NurseBooks.org.

as a way of combatting competing tensions of clinical versus social care, safety versus risk, regulations versus trust, management versus community control and autonomy, and choice and equity (Armstrong, 2018). For more information on the needs of older adults, refer to Chapters 17, 24, and 28.

Cultural Diversity, Decolonization, and Antiracism

In the early phases of strategic development the Mental Health Commission of Canada identified cultural diversity as a priority for national plans and strategies (Hansson et al., 2010). As explored in greater detail in Chapter 8, the increasing cultural diversity within Canada warrants deeper attention to culturally safe care and concern for the mental health consequences of colonization and racism. The Truth and Reconciliation Commission of Canada's (2015) Calls to Action and the Black Lives Matter movement (Black Lives Matter – Canada, 2020) have emphasized the mental health concerns arising from systematic racism in Canada, and psychiatric mental health nurses are in a key position to bring antiracist practices into patient care and into the organizations where they work (Cénat, 2020).

Expanding Technology

Genetic mapping from the Human Genome Project has resulted in a steady stream of research discoveries concerning genetic markers implicated in a variety of psychiatric illnesses. This information could be helpful in identifying at-risk individuals and in targeting medications specific to certain genetic variants and profiles. However, the legal and ethical implications of responsibly using this technology are staggering and generate questions such as:

- Would you want to know you were at risk for a psychiatric illness like bipolar disorder?
- Who should have access to this information: your primary care provider, your future spouse, a lawyer in a child-custody battle?
- Who will regulate genetic testing centres to protect privacy and prevent 21st-century problems like identity theft and fraud?

Despite these concerns, discoveries and technology provide great promise in the diagnosis and treatment of psychiatric disorders, and nurses will be central as informed educators and caregivers.

Scientific advances through research and technology are certain to shape psychiatric mental health nursing practice. MRI research, in addition to comparing healthy people to people diagnosed with mental illness, is now focusing on the development of preclinical profiles of children and adolescents. The hope of this type of research is to be able to identify people at risk for developing mental illness, thereby allowing earlier interventions to try to decrease impairment.

Virtual health care services provided from a distance are gaining wide acceptance, with many options promoted widely as part of the COVID-19 pandemic response (Mental Health Commission of Canada, 2020b). In the early days of the Internet, patients were cautioned against the questionable wisdom of seeking advice through an unregulated medium. However, the Internet has transformed the way we approach our health care needs. It is used liberally by the young and old alike, with particularly strong associations found in cell/smart phone–based mental health alerts and tools (Berrouiguet et al., 2016). Web-based mental health care has empowered people to advocate for themselves and explore health problems and options related to treatment, supportive care, and mental health promotion (Renfrew et al., 2020).

Telepsychiatry, also known as telemedicine, has evolved over the past 20 years in an attempt to reach the population in rural and remote districts (25% of the Canadian population). In this practice, real-time consultations typically occur in health care facilities using a secured telecommunications connection to enable a psychiatric assessment or consultation. Through the use of telepsychiatry, the mental health needs of a greater range of people in a wider range of locations can be met with timely professional assessments and prescribed interventions (Yellowlees & Shore, 2018).

Inequities and Social Determinants of Health

Discussed earlier as a lens for mental health and illness, psychiatric mental health nurses draw upon the social determinants of health to inform their practice. An ever-increasing body of evidence that addresses what people need to be healthy suggests that spending more on the treatment of illness and disease will not actually improve a person's health. Rather, it is suggested that factors such as income, social status, and education directly affect the physical and mental health of individuals and populations and that more attention should go toward policies directly impacting those factors rather than downstream interventions and therapies (Alegría et al., 2018; Shim & Compton, 2018). Psychiatric mental health nurses will be increasingly required to address patient needs related to disease prevention and health promotion, identified through the assessment of the social determinants of health. Twelve key social determinants of health have been identified and it is not difficult to see how upstream interventions in these areas can prevent mental illness and promote mental health. Each stands alone but is at the same time closely linked to the other determinants of health. The 12 determinants are:

1. Income and social status
2. Employment/working conditions
3. Education and literacy
4. Childhood experiences
5. Physical environments
6. Social supports and coping skills
7. Healthy behaviours
8. Access to health services
9. Biology and genetic endowment
10. Gender
11. Culture
12. Race/Racism.

For more information the context of these health determinants and ways to support the reduction of inequalities related to the determinants, see "Social and Economic Influences on Health" (Public Health Agency of Canada, 2020) at https://www.canada.ca/en/public-health/services/health-promotion/population-health/what-determines-health.html.

KEY POINTS TO REMEMBER

- Resilience is a process and outcome that supports people to navigate stressors and accompanying negative emotions and to negotiate resources in order to deal with the stressor and reactions. This process can be promoted and improved to strengthen supportive environments at individual and broader community and societal levels.
- Mental health and mental illness exist along two distinct but intersecting continua.
- Culture influences behaviour, and symptoms may reflect a person's cultural patterns or beliefs. Symptoms therefore must be understood in terms of a person's cultural background.
- The study of epidemiology can help identify high-risk groups and behaviours, which can lead to a better understanding of the causes of some disorders. Incidence rates provide us with the number of new cases in a given period of time. Prevalence rates help us to identify the proportion of a population experiencing a specific mental disorder at a given time.

- Comorbid conditions are those disorders that occur at the same time as another condition. For example, a person with schizophrenia may also have comorbid diabetes, depression, and hypertension.
- Psychiatric mental health nurses work with a broad population of patients in diverse settings to promote optimal mental health.
- Due to social, cultural, scientific, and political factors, the future holds many challenges and possibilities for the psychiatric mental health nurse.

CRITICAL THINKING

1. Amir, a 19-year-old first-year university student with a grade point average of 3.4, is brought to the emergency department after a suicide attempt. He has been extremely depressed since the death of his girlfriend 5 months previously, when the car he was driving crashed. His parents are devastated. They believe taking one's own life prevents a person from going to heaven. Amir has epilepsy and has had more seizures since the automobile accident. He says he should be punished for his carelessness and does not care what happens to him. Over the past month, he has not been to school or shown up for his part-time job tutoring children in reading.
   a. What might be a possible nursing diagnosis for Amir? Before you plan your care, what are some other factors you would like to assess regarding aspects of Amir's overall health and other influences that can affect his mental health?
   b. Do you think that an antidepressant could help Amir through the grieving process? Why or why not? What additional care do you think Amir needs?
   c. Formulate at least two potential nursing interventions for Amir.
   d. Would the religious beliefs of Amir's parents factor into your plan of care? If so, how?
2. In a small study group, share the experiences you have had with others from unfamiliar cultural, ethnic, religious, or racial backgrounds, and identify two positive learning experiences from these encounters.
3. Consider what it would be like working with a group of healthy women preparing for parenthood versus working with a group of depressed women in a mental health clinic. What do you feel are the advantages and disadvantages of working with each group?
4. Would you feel comfortable referring a family member to a mental health clinician? What factors make you feel that way?
5. How do basic-level and advanced-practice psychiatric mental health nurses work together to provide the highest quality of care?
6. Would you consider joining a professional group or advocacy group that promotes mental health? Why or why not?

CHAPTER REVIEW

1. Resilience, the capacity to rebound from stressors via adaptive coping, is associated with positive mental health. Your friend has just been laid off from their job. Which of the following responses on your part would most likely contribute to their enhanced resilience?
   a. Using your connections to set up an interview with your employer
   b. Connecting him with a friend of the family who owns his own business
   c. Supporting him in arranging, preparing for, and completing multiple interviews
   d. Helping him to understand that the layoff resulted from troubles in the economy and is not his fault
2. Which of the following situations best supports the diathesis–stress model of mental illness development?
   a. The rate of suicide increases during times of national disaster and despair.
   b. A woman feels mildly anxious when asked to speak to a large group of people.
   c. A man with no prior mental health problems experiences sadness after his divorce.
   d. A man develops schizophrenia, but his identical twin remains free of mental illness.
3. Of the following statements about mental illness, identify all of the correct ones:
   a. About 20% of Canadians experience a mental disorder during their lifetime.
   b. Mental disorders and diagnoses occur very consistently across cultures.
   c. Most serious mental illnesses are psychological rather than biological in nature.
   d. The Mental Health Commission of Canada's report *Changing Directions, Changing Lives* outlines the mental health strategy for Canada.
4. Jane is a 32-year-old mother of four. She is active with her family and in her community despite having a diagnosis of severe anxiety. Refer to the mental health–mental illness continuum shown in Figure 1.2 and consider where you would place Jane.
   a. Optimal mental health with mental illness
   b. Optimal mental health without mental illness
   c. Poor mental health with mental illness
   d. Poor mental health without mental illness
5. Which of the following actions represent the primary focus of psychiatric nursing for a basic-level registered nurse? **Select all that apply**.
   a. Determining a patient's diagnosis according to the *DSM-5*
   b. Ordering diagnostic tests such as EEGs or MRI scans
   c. Identifying how a patient is coping with a symptom such as hallucinations
   d. Guiding a patient to learn and use a variety of stress-management techniques
   e. Helping a patient without personal transportation find a way to their treatment appointments
   f. Collecting petition signatures seeking the removal of stigmatizing images on television

 http://evolve.elsevier.com/Canada/Varcarolis/psychiatric/

REFERENCES

Alegría, M., NeMoyer, A., Falgàs Bagué, I., et al. (2018). Social determinants of mental health: Where we are and where we need to go. *Current Psychiatry Reports, 20*(11), 1–13. https://doi.org/10.1007/s11920-018-0969-9

American Psychiatric Association. (2013). *Diagnostic and statistical manual of mental disorders* (5th ed.).

Armstrong, P. (2018). Balancing the tension in long-term residential care. *Ageing International, 43*(1), 74–90. https://doi.org/10.1007/s12126-017-9284-8

Berrouiguet, S., Baca-García, E., Brandt, S., et al. (2016). Fundamentals for future mobile-health (mHealth): A systematic review of mobile phone and web-based text messaging in mental health. *Journal of Medical Internet Research, 18*(6), e135. https://doi.org/10.2196/jmir.5066

Black Lives Matter – Canada. (2020). *About us*. https://blacklivesmatter.ca/

Bray, N., & O'Donovan, M. (2018). The genetics of neuropsychiatric disorders. *Brain and Neuroscience Advances, 2*, 239821281879927. https://doi.org/10.1177/2398212818799271

Breen, G., Li, Q., Roth, B. L., et al. (2016). Translating genome-wide association findings into new therapeutics for psychiatry. *Nature Neuroscience, 19*(11), 1392–1396. https://doi.org/10.1038/nn.4411

Bull, P., Gadsby, J., & Williams, S. (2018). *Critical mental health nursing: observations from the inside.* Monmouth, UK: PCCS Books Ltd.

Burstow, B. (2015). *Psychiatry and the business of madness: An ethical and epistemological accounting.* New York: Palgrave Macmillan.

Butcher, H. K., Bulechek, G. M., Dochterman, J. M., et al. (2019). *Nursing Interventions Classification (NIC)* (7th ed.). St. Louis, MO: Mosby.

Canadian Federation of Mental Health Nurses. (2014). *Canadian standards for psychiatric-mental health nursing* (4th ed.). Toronto: Author.

Canadian Institute for Health Information. (2020). *International statistical classification of diseases and related health problems* (11th rev.). https://www.cihi.ca/en/submit-data-and-view-standards/codes-and-classifications/icd-11-international-statistical

Canadian Mental Health Association (CMHA). (2020). *About CMHA.* https://cmha.ca/about-cmha

Cénat, J. M. (2020). How to provide anti-racist mental health care. *The Lancet. Psychiatry, 7*(11), P929–P931. https://doi.org/10.1016/S2215-0366(20)30309-6

da Silva, A., Baldaçara, L., Cavalcante, D., et al. (2020). The impact of mental illness stigma on psychiatric emergencies. *Frontiers in Psychiatry, 11*, 573. https://doi.org/10.3389/fpsyt.2020.00573

Epp, J. (1988). *Mental health for Canadians: Striking a balance.* Ottawa: Minister of National Health and Welfare.

Gaebel, W., Rössler, W., & Sartorius, N. (2017). *The stigma of mental illness: End of the story?* Cham, Switzerland: Springer.

Hansson, E. Tuck, A. Lurie, S., et al. For the Task Group of the Services Systems Advisory Committee, Mental Health Commission of Canada. (2010). *Improving mental health services for immigrant, refugee, ethno-cultural and racialized groups: issues and options for service improvement.* https://www.mentalhealthcommission.ca/wp-content/uploads/drupal/Diversity_Issues_Options_Report_ENG_0_1.pdf

Harrist, A., & Gardner, B. (Eds.). (2019). *Biobehavioral markers in risk and resilience research.* Cham, Switzerland: Springer International Publishing. https://doi.org/10.1007/978-3-030-05952-1

Herdman, T. H., & Kamitsuru, S. (Eds.). (2018). *NANDA International nursing diagnoses: Definitions and classification, 2018–2020.* Oxford, UK: Wiley-Blackwell.

International Council of Nurses. (2017). *Nursing diagnosis and outcome statements.* https://www.icn.ch/sites/default/files/inline-files/icnp2017-dc.pdf

International Nursing Knowledge Association. (2020). *Glossary of terms.* https://nanda.org/nanda-i-resources/glossary-of-terms/

Jakubec, S. L., & Astle, B. J. (2021). *Research literacy for health and community practice* (2nd ed.). Toronto: Canadian Scholars' Press.

Leefmann, J., & Hildt, E. (2017). *The human sciences after the decade of the brain.* London, UK: Academic Press.

Mental Health Commission of Canada. (2009). *Toward recovery & well-being: A framework for a mental health strategy for Canada.* https://www.mentalhealthcommission.ca/wp-content/uploads/drupal/FNIM_Toward_Recovery_and_Well_Being_ENG_0_1.pdf

Mental Health Commission of Canada. (2012). *Changing directions, changing lives: The mental health strategy for Canada.* https://www.mentalhealthcommission.ca/wp-content/uploads/drupal/MHStrategy_Strategy_ENG.pdf

Mental Health Commission of Canada (2015). *Recovery guidelines.* Ottawa: Author. http://www.mentalhealthcommission.ca/sites/default/files/2016-07/MHCC_Recovery_Guidelines_2016_ENG.PDF

Mental Health Commission of Canada. (2017). *Advancing the mental health strategy for Canada: A framework for action 2017–2022.* http://www.mentalhealthcommission.ca/sites/default/files/2016-08/advancing_the_mental_health_strategy_for_canada_a_framework_for_action.pdf

Mental Health Commission of Canada. (2020a). *Recovery.* https://www.mentalhealthcommission.ca/English/recovery

Mental Health Commission of Canada. (2020b). *COVID-19 and mental health: Policy responses and emerging issues [environmental scan].* https://www.mentalhealthcommission.ca/sites/default/files/2020-06/COVID_19_policy_responses_emerging_issues_eng.pdf

Menzies, R. J., Reaume, G., & LeFrançois, B. A. (2013). *Mad matters: A critical reader in Canadian mad studies.* Toronto: Canadian Scholars' Press.

Moorhead, S., Swanson, E., Johnson, M., et al. (Eds.). (2018). *Nursing outcomes classification (NOC)* (6th ed.). St. Louis, MO: Mosby.

Morgan, C., Roberts, T., Donoghue, B. O., et al. (2020). Society and risk of psychosis. In A. Thompson, & M. Broome (Eds.), *Risk factors for psychosis: Paradigms, mechanisms, and prevention* (pp. 289–303). London: Academic Press.

Nolan, P. (1993). *A history of mental health nursing.* New York: Chapman and Hall.

Palay, J., Taillieu, T. L., Afifi, T. O., et al. (2019). Prevalence of Mental Disorders and Suicidality in Canadian Provinces. *Canadian Journal of Psychiatry, 64*(11), 761–769. https://doi.org/10.1177/0706743719878987

Porter, N. (1913). *Webster's revised unabridged dictionary.* Boston: Merriam.

Public Health Agency of Canada. (2015). *Report from the Canadian chronic disease surveillance system: Mental illness in Canada, 2015.* https://www.canada.ca/en/public-health/services/publications/diseases-conditions/report-canadian-chronic-disease-surveillance-system-mental-illness-canada-2015.html

Public Health Agency of Canada. (2017). *About mental illness.* https://www.canada.ca/en/public-health/services/about-mental-illness.html

Public Health Agency of Canada. (2019). *Promoting positive mental health.* https://www.canada.ca/en/public-health/services/promoting-positive-mental-health.html

Public Health Agency of Canada. (2020). *Social determinants of health and health inequalities.* https://www.canada.ca/en/public-health/services/health-promotion/population-health/what-determines-health.html

Renfrew, M., Morton, D., Morton, J., et al. (2020). A web- and mobile app–based mental health promotion intervention comparing email, short message service, and videoconferencing support for a healthy cohort: Randomized comparative study. *Journal of Medical Internet Research, 22*(1), e15592. https://doi.org/10.2196/15592

Rosen, A., Goldbloom, D., & McGeorge, P. (2010). Mental health commissions: Making the critical difference to the development and reform of mental health services. *Current Opinion in Psychiatry, 23*(6), 593.

Shim, R., & Compton, M. (2018). Addressing the social determinants of mental health: If not now, when? If not us, who?. *Psychiatric Services, 69*(8), 844–846. https://doi.org/10.1176/appi.ps.201800060

Stern, T. A., Freudenreich, O., Smith, F. A., et al. (2017). *Handbook of general hospital psychiatry* (7th ed.). Philadelphia: Elsevier.

Truth and Reconciliation Commission of Canada. (2015). *Truth and reconciliation commission of Canada calls to action.* https://ehprnh2mwo3.exactdn.com/wp-content/uploads/2021/01/Calls_to_Action_English2.pdf

Ungar, M. (2018). Systemic resilience: principles and processes for a science of change in contexts of adversity. *Ecology and Society, 23*(4), 34. https://doi.org/10.5751/ES-10385-230434

World Health Organization (WHO). (2018). *Mental health: Strengthening our response.* https://www.who.int/news-room/fact-sheets/detail/mental-health-strengthening-our-response

World Health Organization (2020). *International statistical classification of diseases and related health problems* (11th ed.). https://icd.who.int/en

Yellowlees, P., & Shore, J. (Eds.). (2018). *Telepsychiatry and health technologies : A guide for mental health professionals* (1st ed.). Washington: American Psychiatric Association Publishing

2

Historical Overview of Psychiatric Mental Health Nursing

Sandra Harrisson

 https://evolve.elsevier.com/Canada/Varcarolis/psychiatric/

OBJECTIVES

1. Identify the sociopolitical, economic, cultural, and religious factors that influenced the development of psychiatric mental health nursing.
2. Summarize the influence of psychiatric treatment trends on the role of the nurse.
3. Identify the factors that led to the separate designations of the registered nurse and registered psychiatric nurse.
4. Analyze the factors that have enhanced and delayed the professionalization of psychiatric mental health nursing.
5. Consider the future potentials and challenges for psychiatric mental health nursing in Canada.

KEY TERMS AND CONCEPTS

advanced-practice nursing
asylums
Canadian Federation of Mental Health Nurses
custodial care
deinstitutionalization
Dorothea Dix
moral treatment
Philippe Pinel
Registered Psychiatric Nurses of Canada
Weir Report
William Tuke

Exploring the history of nursing in Canada, and specifically of psychiatric mental health nursing, can enrich our understanding of the factors that have shaped the profession in the past and that will shape it in the future. Throughout history, the evolution of the role of nursing has been affected by sociopolitical, economic, cultural, medical, and religious trends in Canada and around the world. Although there has been much historical analysis of psychiatric mental health nursing in England, Holland, and the United States, Canadian nursing historians have only recently focused on the mental health field (see, for example, Boschma, 2012; Harrisson, 2017; Harrisson & Thifault, 2018; Hicks, 2011; Smith & Khanlou, 2013; Thifault & Kérouac, 2019). For many reasons, it is a convoluted history, unique to Canada and separate from that of generalist registered nursing. Understanding this history provides us with insights into the past challenges and accomplishments of psychiatric mental health nursing and prepares us for the continuing development of the role and further advanced-practice nursing (APN).

EARLY MENTAL ILLNESS CARE

Trends in approaches to the treatment of mental illness have significantly contributed to the emergence and evolution of the role of psychiatric nursing. These trends stem largely from societal values, politics, culture, and economics.

Madness has always been part of humanity. In the early years it was associated with disease of the soul, demons, sins, and mood unbalance. Responsibilities for these individuals fell on families and communities. In extreme cases of disturbance the mad person sees themself excluded from society and becomes errant. Without being necessarily dangerous, they may disrupt public order or sometimes shows signs of violence. To protect them and the population, it was decided to isolate them by locking them in religious communities, prisons, and eventually hospitals (Quétel, 2009).

Confinement in general hospitals was a European phenomenon in the fifteenth century. It accommodated the destitute, the old, the dying, and the mad. Treatments differed between quieter and more restless individuals (Quétel, 2009). Cases of extreme agitation necessitated surveillance personnel and isolation rooms. At that time, the deviants were transferred to new establishments called asylums. Patients in these settings were often chained or caged, and cruelty or neglect was not uncommon (Digby, 1983). This type of treatment reflected the societal view that people with mental illness were bestial or less human in nature and therefore required discipline and were immune to human discomforts such as hunger or cold (Digby, 1983).

Asylums, designed to be retreats from society, were built with the hope that, with early intervention and several months of rest, people with mental illness could be cured (Weir, 1932). In the late 1700s Philippe Pinel, a French physician, along with other humanitarians, began to advocate for more humane treatment of people with mental illness by literally removing the chains of the patients, talking to them, and providing a calmer, more soothing environment. Pinel and another reformer from England, William Tuke, described this use of social and psychological approaches to treatment as "moral treatment" (Digby, 1983). Critics such as French philosopher Michel Foucault argued that the asylum movement was little more than a shift from physical restraint to psychological and social control of people considered undesirable by societal norms (Foucault, 1971). Regardless, this revolutionary way of treating people with mental illness swept across Europe and influenced the design of early asylums in North America.

In Canada the country's size, location, and history have played a significant part in how people with mental illness are treated. Indigenous peoples in Canada had a variety of approaches to caring for people with mental illness. Most were holistic, treating mind, body, and soul, and included sweat lodges, animistic charms, potlatch, and Sundance (Kirkmayer et al., 2000). In the sixteenth century colonial settlers from France and, later, England brought with them their own approaches to mental illness care. As in their European homelands, much of the responsibility of caring for people with mental illness fell on the family and the asylums established in the communities (Cellard & Thifault, 2006). Some Canadian religious orders, such as the Grey Nuns, were early providers of care for people with mental illness (Hardill, 2006). Those who could not be cared for in the community, however, often ended up in jails, where they received minimal shelter at best and abuse at worst (Moran, 1998). By the 1800s, migration to Canada increased, as did its urbanization. This relocation of families to cities from isolated settlements changed support systems and families' ability to care for people with mental illness (Cellard & Thifault, 2006). In Europe the move to asylum care was well under way, and the Canadian colonies began to explore similar options.

Founded by Marguerite d'Youville in 1737 in Montreal, the Sisters of Charity, formally known as the Grey Nuns, is a Canadian religious institute that has been involved in the care of the poor, the development of health care services, and the nursing education. They created the school of nursing at the Notre-Dame Hospital (1898) in Montreal that constituted rapidly of a network all over the country. They took a leading role in the advancement of nurses' higher education with the establishment of the Institute of Marguerite d'Youville, affiliated with the University of Montreal, to offer the first French baccalaureate program (Paul, 1994). In 1893 the Quebec government entrusted the care and the custody of mentally ill persons of Saint-Michel-Archange asylum (Beauport) to the congregation. The increased demands for psychiatric care contributed to the development of these nursing speciality. The Grey Nuns were active in the psychiatric nursing education by creating their own school of nursing inside the institution in 1915 (Aubin, 2019). The deinstitutionalization movement and the disastrous reports issued by the different provinces in the 1960s raised the issues of overcrowding and poor quality of care inside psychiatric institutions and forced the religious communities to withdraw from the administration of the psychiatric hospital, including the Grey Nuns.

The poor life conditions of patients in custodial care caught the attention of many social reformers who, in the late nineteenth and early twentieth centuries, lobbied governments to create more humane environments of care for people with mental illness. Among them was Dorothea Dix, a retired schoolteacher from New England who became the superintendent of nurses during the American Civil War. Dix was educated in the asylum reform movements in England while she was there recuperating from tuberculosis. In 1841 during an encounter at a Boston jail, Dix was shocked to witness the degrading treatment of a woman with mental illness who was imprisoned there. Passionate about social reform, Dix began advocating for the improved treatment and public care of people with mental illness. She met with many politicians and even the Pope to push her agenda forward. Ultimately, she was influential in lobbying for the first public mental hospital in the United States and for reform in British and Canadian institutions. At that point, the asylums became peaceful and resourceful places focused on a therapeutic environment, until they became overcrowded.

Dorothea Dix, advocate, 1802–1887. (**Source:** Library of Congress Prints and Photographs Division. Washington, DC, 20540, USA.)

Early Canadian Asylums

The first asylum was created in Saint John, New Brunswick, in 1835 and became the Provincial Lunatic Asylum in 1848 (Wong, 2018). It housed patients with difficult conditions. Soon, more asylums were established in Upper and Lower Canada, the Maritime colonies, and Canada's West. Despite the creation of asylums, early historical records demonstrate that most families of people with a mental illness maintained the care of those individuals themselves (Cellard & Thifault, 2006), so the asylums predominantly housed patients who were poor and had no family support. Many asylums were built in countrylike settings on large parcels of land that could provide opportunity for occupational therapies such as farming. Toward the end of the nineteenth century, asylum care became more acceptable, and, with family support systems becoming diluted due to urbanization and relocation, the inpatient population grew exponentially (Cellard & Thifault, 2006). Although the moral treatment era had moved psychiatric treatment toward more humane treatment, the lack of success in treating mental illnesses combined with increased admissions to asylums led to overcrowding and less than humane conditions in many asylums. In most settings a large population of people received only minimal custodial care: assistance with performing the basic daily necessities of life, such as dressing, eating, using a toilet, walking, and so on.

EARLY PSYCHIATRIC TREATMENTS

By the end of the nineteenth century, the new field of psychiatry was being challenged to provide a medical cure for mental illness. Since there were few medications available other than heavily alcohol-based sedatives, doctors used many experimental treatments, for example, leeching (using bloodsucking worms), spinning (tying the patient to a chair and spinning it for hours), hydrotherapy (forced baths), and insulin shock treatment (injections of large doses of insulin to produce daily comas over several weeks). In the mid-twentieth century treatment choices expanded to include electroconvulsive therapy (see

Chapter 13) and lobotomies, through which nerve fibres in the frontal lobe were severed. As treatments became more invasive, the need for patient monitoring beyond custodial care led many medical superintendents to recruit nurses to work in their institutions.

THE INTRODUCTION OF NURSES TO ASYLUM CARE

In Canada prior to the late 1800s, there were no nurses working in psychiatric settings; instead, asylums used predominantly male attendants to provide custodial care for patients. Changes in treatment approaches and the increased medicalization of psychiatry prompted a need for more specially trained providers, especially for female patients (Connor, 1996). In 1888 Rockwood Asylum in Kingston, Ontario, became the first psychiatric institution in Canada to open a training program for nurses (Kerrigan, 2011). The 2-year program was overseen by the asylum's medical director and included one lecture a week combined with work experience training. The curriculum, taught by physicians, included courses in physiology, anatomy, nursing care of the sick, and nursing care of the insane (Legislature of the Province of Ontario, 1889). Consistent with societal beliefs of the time about women's innate caring capacity, the training was offered only to females. This exclusion of males from the program hindered the recognition of the importance of nursing knowledge and skills and lowered the status of male attendants at the time (Yonge et al., 2005). Both of these factors would greatly affect the future development of psychiatric mental health nursing in Canada.

Asylum-based training schools opened across Canada, and the training curriculum, similar to that of the hospital-based programs of generalist nurses, varied among institutions. Medical superintendents controlled the content and delivery of the programs, and hospital administrators highly valued the inexpensive labour provided by the female workforce, so much so that their cross-training in other medical settings was discouraged so as to maintain staffing supplies (Tipliski, 2004). The asylum-based programs were founded heavily on a medical model of training nurses to be obedient, orderly, and focused on

Nurses at Toronto Hospital for the Insane in 1910. (**Source:** RG 10-276-2-0-8. Ministry of Health. Queen Street Mental Health Centre miscellaneous historical materials. Queen Street Mental Health Centre miscellaneous photographs. Female infirmary at the Hospital for the Insane, Toronto, CA. 1910. Archives of Ontario, I0018987.)

the discipline of the inpatients (Cowles, 1916). Nursing duties at the beginning of the twentieth century often included extensive cleaning, serving meals, counting cutlery after meals, and assisting patients with hygiene activities, as well as administering treatments such as the long baths referred to as "hydrotherapy," sedation with alcohol, and postoperative care (Forchuk & Tweedell, 2001). Nurses also played a key role in the care of patients in the infirmary. The custodial environment of asylums did not promote a sense of professional knowledge for nurses and limited their ability to question the treatment approaches being offered at the time (Leishman, 2005).

SHIFTS IN CONTROL OVER NURSING

In the early part of the twentieth century nurses' lack of control over their own profession began to shift with changes to nursing education models and blossoming political advocacy by nursing groups across Canada, particularly with the formation of the Canadian National Association of Trained Nurses in 1908. This early group expanded, and by 1926, each province had an affiliate group, and the organization was renamed the Canadian Nurses Association (CNA). The CNA provided a united voice for nurses and increased advocacy for control over nursing by nurses (CNA, 2021a). At this time, nursing training programs still varied by institution, but many had long hours of hospital ward service taking precedence over instructional hours for students. The CNA's mandate included the professionalization of nursing, so it began to advocate for standardization of nursing education (Tipliski, 2004). This was a politically loaded issue for several reasons: physicians wanted control over nursing education, patriarchal society structures devalued nursing knowledge, nursing skills were seen as natural women's work, and hospitals relied on the economical service hours of nursing students (Anthony & Landeen, 2009).

In 1927 the Canadian Medical Association and the CNA performed a joint study on the state of nursing education in Canada. The result, known as the "Weir Report," was released in 1932 and concluded that drastic changes were needed in nursing education programs, including standardization of curriculum, work hours, and instructor training, and that care of

First graduating class of Rockwood Asylum Nursing School, Kingston, Ontario, 1890. (**Source:** Providence Care Archives, http://providencecarearchives.files.wordpress.com/2011/03/image2011-03-24-102507-1.jpg.)

people with mental illnesses needed to be integrated into all generalist programs (Fleming, 1932). The uptake of the recommendations varied across Canada and even within regions. Since psychiatric hospitals and asylums had a harder time recruiting nurses, the idea of giving up their workforce so that students could complete an affiliation in general hospital settings was considered very costly. The medical superintendent psychiatrists were protective of their asylum-based training programs, which they felt developed specialized skills compared to general nursing skills (Tipliski, 2004). They argued that a 3- to 6-month affiliation in psychiatry was too short to learn the skills required in their institutions.

At the time, provincial legislation in the form of nursing acts was coming into existence and further formalizing the title and licensure of the registered nurse. There were provincial differences in government-legislated power over licensure and nursing education as well as variable interest in psychiatric training by provincial nursing associations (Tipliski, 2004). This, combined with the political influence of some medical superintendents from provincial psychiatric hospitals, led registered nursing associations in Manitoba, Saskatchewan, Alberta, and British Columbia to be less inclusive of the psychiatric hospital–trained nurse than the associations in Eastern Canada were, which in turn led to the exclusion of registered nurse licensure for graduates of asylum programs. This division of perspectives eventually resulted in a split between Western and Eastern Canada in training programs and the creation in the western provinces of the specialty-focused psychiatric nursing training programs and the registered psychiatric nurse designation.

Eastern and Atlantic Canada

From the outset, the Registered Nurses' Association of Ontario (RNAO) accepted the asylum-based programs for licensing of prospective nurses who were affiliated with a general hospital (Tipliski, 2004). It also represented nurses working in asylum settings, providing them with advocacy and nursing leadership (Tipliski, 2004). With the support of nurse leaders like Nettie Fiddler and the publication of the Weir Report, more generalist hospital programs began adding a psychiatry rotation to the curriculum. Also influential in the addition of a psychiatry rotation was the RNAO addressing the nursing shortage in psychiatric settings and the care concerns of mentally ill patients at the organization's 1945 annual meeting (Tipliski, 2004). At this point, many psychiatric hospitals had large numbers of patients, inadequate staffing, and minimal enrollment of new students (Tipliski, 2004). The advocacy of nurse leaders, combined with the post–World War II mental hygiene movement, led to the addition of psychiatric nursing theory for all registered nurse education programs (Tipliski, 2004). Some asylum programs added training in general medical settings; however, by the 1950s, all of the psychiatric hospital training programs in Eastern Canada had closed. Nurses in psychiatric mental health were trained as generalist registered nurses with affiliations in psychiatry and the chance to specialize after graduation.

Western Canada

In the western provinces, where the population was much smaller and asylums were located in rural settings, recruiting an adequate labour force was a major concern. In the early 1900s British Columbia, Alberta, Saskatchewan, and Manitoba attempted different approaches to training nurses for psychiatric settings. Selkirk, Manitoba, opened the first asylum training school in Western Canada in 1920, followed closely by Brandon, Manitoba, in 1921 (Hicks, 2011). Manitoba implemented several combination programs between general hospitals and psychiatric hospitals, but similar attempts at other institutions in the western provinces failed due to lack of investment from administrators and nurse leadership groups and difficulty enticing nurses to remain in the psychiatric setting after their graduation (Hicks, 2011; Tipliski, 2004).

In the 1930s Saskatchewan's two provincial psychiatric hospitals began a training program for their attendants. Unlike in the rest of Canada, this training was offered to both male and female attendants and, upon completion, gave graduates the title "nursing attendant" (Tipliski, 2004). However, the specialized training did not bestow upon graduates any professional title or licensure, so several attendants lobbied for the creation of the designation "psychiatric nurse." The movement for the designation of the psychiatric nurse was supported by medical superintendents, unions, and politicians at the time, so despite opposition by provincial nursing leaders, the *Registered Psychiatric Nurses Act* was enacted in Saskatchewan in 1948 (Tipliski, 2004). This step toward professionalization of the role of the nurse in psychiatric hospitals was soon adopted by other western provinces. At the same time, the Saskatchewan Registered Nurses' Association's leader, Kathryn Ellis, was also trying to address the nursing shortage in mental

> ## RESEARCH HIGHLIGHT
>
> ### An Analysis of Canadian Psychiatric Mental Health Nursing: History and Possibilities
>
> **Problem**
> Given the need for increased accessibility to mental health care and treatment, there is a need to understand the circumstances of nurses with regard to occupational stress and barriers to advanced education in mental health nursing.
>
> **Purpose of Study**
> This study sought to compile a more complete analysis of what current Canadian mental health nursing looks like, considering important issues facing nurses regarding history, gender, education, and quality of work life.
>
> **Methods**
> An integrative review and historical analysis of existing literature was undertaken using a critical and gendered sociological lens.
>
> **Key Findings**
> Fourteen articles were selected, which provided a partial reflection of contemporary Canadian psychiatric mental health nursing. Findings included the identification of an association between gender and professional status, inconsistencies in psychiatric nursing education, and the limitations for Canadian nurse practitioners to advance the role of the psychiatric mental health nurse practitioner at this time.
>
> **Implications for Nursing Practice**
> The authors recommend facilitating advanced education in mental health so that people within primary care settings can benefit from the knowledge and expertise of nurses with additional mental health education. Additional educational opportunities for psychiatric nurses who wish to become advanced nurse practitioners and to prescribe psychiatric treatments or medications are encouraged. Partnerships are recommended for provincial and national nursing bodies to foster national standards and regulation for psychiatric mental health nursing education and bridging programs.
>
> **Source:** Smith, M., & Khanlou, N. (2013). An analysis of Canadian psychiatric mental health nursing through the junctures of history, gender, nursing education, and quality of work life in Ontario, Manitoba, Alberta, and Saskatchewan. *ISRN Nursing.* https://pubmed.ncbi.nlm.nih.gov/23710367/.
>
> **Other examples of mental health nursing research topics:** mental health promotion of individuals and families, forensic psychiatric nursing, substance use and addictions, marginalized people, stigmatization, trauma, harm reduction, motherhood and chronic mental disease, mental health community services, homelessness, psychiatric nursing role.

hospitals by convincing provincial hospitals to become more involved in training, but she was unable to negotiate satisfactory psychiatric or general hospital affiliations (Hicks, 2011; Tipliski, 2004).

Much of the professionalization movement was facilitated by the Canadian Council of Psychiatric Nurses (CCPN), an interprovincial organization of psychiatric nurses focused on increasing the standards and recognition of psychiatric nurse training (Hicks, 2011). The CCPN, along with the efforts of provincial psychiatrists, was successful in advocating for the registered psychiatric nurse specialty designation across the western provinces; subsequently, British Columbia passed its Psychiatric Nurses Act in 1951, Alberta followed in 1955, and Manitoba followed in 1960. To date, the separate designation has remained, although the CCPN evolved first into Registered Psychiatric Nurses of Canada (RPNC) and now is Registered Psychiatric Nurse Regulators of Canada (RPNRC). The organization has more than 5600 practising members (RPNRC, 2021), resulting in both registered nurses and registered psychiatric nurses working in psychiatric mental health settings in the four western provinces and Yukon.

DEINSTITUTIONALIZATION AND THE NURSING ROLE IN PSYCHIATRIC MENTAL HEALTH CARE

Psychiatric nursing continued to take place predominantly in hospital settings until the 1960s. The discovery of new neuroleptics, such as chlorpromazine, assured a permanent recovery, or at least symptoms' stabilization related to mental disorders. These new treatments allowed patients an early return home. The psychiatric deinstitutionalization movement, namely, the shift from caring for people with mental illness in institutions to caring for them in communities, began not only in Canada but all over the world. Psychiatric nurses had to redefine their role and their professional identity within the health care team as the treatment of patients underwent this transition (Harrisson, 2017, p. 37). (See Chapter 3 for further discussion of deinstitutionalization.) The "pioneer" community mental health nurses set up many programs and frameworks for the delivery of psychiatric mental health care in the community (Boschma, 2012) and in acute psychiatric wards of general hospitals (Harrisson, 2017). The wide range of community-based mental health services that eventually developed (e.g., crisis management, consultation-liaison, primary care psychiatry, day clinics) created new settings and skill requirements for psychiatric mental health nurses. The ability to assess and monitor patients and their environment changed nursing approaches toward mental health care. Assessment, autonomy, collaboration, crisis management, and resource finding became key skills for community-based nurses.

UNIVERSITY-BASED NURSING CURRICULUM

In 1919 the University of British Columbia (UBC) launched the first university-based program in nursing. The program was a "sandwich model," with 3 years of hospital-based nursing sandwiched between the first and final years of university studies (Anthony & Landeen, 2009). At the time, the idea of a university program for nursing was considered so risky that UBC refused to fund or administer the middle years of the program. A leader in nursing education at the time, E. Kathleen Russell at the University of Toronto, supported by the Rockefeller Foundation, set up one of the first university-based training programs in public health nursing, leadership, and education. This revolutionary post-diploma certification program for registered nurses was attended internationally. Later, in 1928 Russell coordinated the first solely university-based nursing program at the University of Toronto; in 1942 it began granting Bachelor of Science degrees in nursing (BScN)

(University of Toronto, 2011). These university programs initiated a critical change in nursing education: for the first time, education for nurses was separated from and prioritized over their service in the hospitals (Anthony & Landeen, 2009). Despite this revolution in nursing education, nursing programs remained under the control of medical faculties until 1962, when the University of Montreal set up the first independent nursing faculty (Anthony & Landeen, 2009).

Many other Canadian universities began to offer diploma programs in specialty areas such as public health. In the 1950s the University of Saskatchewan became the first to offer a 1-year post–registered nurse training diploma in advanced psychiatric nursing (University of Saskatchewan, 2011). The inception of university education for nurses led to the growth and formalization of nursing knowledge. The University of Western Ontario launched Canada's first graduate program in nursing in 1959, and the first PhD program in nursing began at the University of Alberta in 1991. The growth of graduate programs gave rise to increased research and theory in psychiatric nursing practice. The influence of nurse theorists such as American Hildegard Peplau, the first published nursing theorist since Florence Nightingale, contributed to the expansion of specialized nursing knowledge and related skills in the psychiatric mental health field. Much of Peplau's work focused on the role of the nurse in therapeutic relationships and anxiety management. The growth of academic study in nursing, in turn, influenced nursing in the practice setting: the Hamilton Psychiatric Hospital became the first health care institution in Canada to employ a clinical nurse specialist (CNS) and to require theory-based nursing practice (Forchuk & Tweedell, 2001).

Hildegard Peplau was born in 1909 in Reading, Pennsylvania. She graduated from Pottstown, Pennsylvania School of Nursing in 1931. She earned a Bachelor degree in Interpersonal Psychology in 1943 from Bennington College in Vermont. She served in the army as a nurse between 1943 and 1945. She was stationed in the School for Military Neuropsychiatry in the south of England and had the opportunity to work with William Menninger, psychiatric consultant of the US Army. After the war, she enrolled in the master program and completed her PhD (Smith, 2020).

She conceptualized the process of the nurse–patient interaction, advancing the idea that these interpersonal phenomena have a qualitative impact on patient outcome (Callaway, 2002; Peplau 1991). The development of a therapeutic relationship would allow a better understanding of the psychosocial behavioural problems of the patient rather than focusing on the mental illness diagnosis. "Her theory assists nurses to make sense of patients' experience and behaviour related to their health and illness, including mental illness. The development of her theoretical work coincided with the transition of care for mentally ill patients to the community and to short-term units in general hospitals." (Harrisson, 2017, p. 42). Peplau's theory is now taught in nursing programs as part of general knowledge for nurses, and not only as part of the psychiatric curriculum (Senn, 2013).

Currently, entry-to-practice mental health and addiction competencies for undergraduate nursing education in Canada have been established by the Canadian Association of Schools of Nursing and Canadian Federation of Mental Health Nurses (CASN & CFMHN, 2015). The CFMHN (2016) recommends that the curricula of all undergraduate nursing programs in Canada include entry-to-practice mental health and addiction competencies in both theoretical knowledge and clinical practice. The CFMHN recommends delivering mental health and addiction core competencies through a designated (stand-alone) theory course and a dedicated clinical experience. Regardless of pedagogical method, the obligatory outcome for undergraduate nurses is a strong knowledge base in mental health and addiction as outlined in the CFMHN practice standards (CFMHN, 2016). This body of core competency work and the nursing mandate to meet goals of key focus areas of the national mental health strategy (Mental Health Commission of Canada, 2021) are enhanced by growing nursing research. Nursing research in mental health continues to expand through the works of nurse researchers such as Bernie Pauly, Cheryl Forchuk, Dave Holmes, Kristin Cleverley, Cheryl L. Pollard, Nicole Letourneau, and Kimberley Ryan-Nicholls.

In Western Canada over the past 25 years, the shift to the role of the registered psychiatric nurse and the increased range of practice settings (i.e., away from inpatient facilities and into primary care and community-based clinics) have also brought about changes in educational programs. Registered psychiatric nursing programs have adjusted to ensure diversification of skills and knowledge base related to consumer-oriented primary health care and health promotion activities (Ryan-Nicholls, 2004). Registered psychiatric nurse training continued to be diploma based across the western provinces until 1995, when Brandon University began its baccalaureate program in psychiatric mental health nursing. Registered Psychiatric Nurses of Canada issued a position statement in 2012 advocating for baccalaureate degree entry to practice for registered psychiatric nurses due to the increasingly complex needs and roles of the registered psychiatric nurse (RPNC, 2012). The first graduate program in psychiatric nursing for registered psychiatric nurses began at Brandon University in January 2011.

NATIONAL ORGANIZATIONS FOR PSYCHIATRIC MENTAL HEALTH NURSING AND CANADIAN NURSES ASSOCIATION CERTIFICATION

The division of Eastern and Western Canada in psychiatric nursing training and designation resulted in separate organizational groups. Although having multiple organizations has led to some duplication and fragmentation of a voice for nurses in psychiatric settings, the groups have also worked collaboratively toward common goals. Since 1995, the CNA has offered registered nurses certification in psychiatric mental health nursing (CNA, 2021b). Under the umbrella of the CNA and with consumer input, the Canadian Federation of Mental Health Nurses, an organization of registered nurses across Canada who specialize in psychiatric mental health nursing, established the standards of practice for psychiatric mental health nursing, now in a fourth edition (see https://www.cna-aiic.ca/en/nursing/advanced-nursing-practice). The 2014 Standards for Psychiatric Mental Health Nursing build on the Canadian Nurses Association Code of Ethics (CNA, 2017). Despite the separations in licensure and professional bodies, in workplaces in Western Canada, registered nurses and registered psychiatric nurses work closely together in mental health settings and have many opportunities for collaboration and advocacy for the people they serve.

ADVANCED-PRACTICE NURSING IN PSYCHIATRIC MENTAL HEALTH CARE

Advanced-practice nursing includes the roles of nurse practitioner and CNS (CNA, 2019). Each province has its own regulations guiding the licensing and scope of practice for APN. The CNS's role has been well established in psychiatry since 1972, when Hamilton Psychiatric Hospital employed Pat Barry, a nurse with a graduate degree, to educate staff and increase theoretical-based nursing practice (Forchuk & Tweedell, 2001). CNSs can provide psychotherapy and have worked as consultants, educators, and clinicians in inpatient and outpatient psychiatry throughout Canada. Nurse practitioners, on the other hand, work as consultants or collaborative team members and can diagnose, prescribe and manage medications, and provide psychotherapy. While the role of psychiatric nurse practitioner has been well established in the United States, where specialized graduate programs and advanced certification exams are offered, the role has remained virtually non-existent in Canada, likely because the nurse practitioner role itself is relatively new to Canada compared to the United States, where it has been well established and regulated since the 1970s.

There has been a recent attempt in Canada to standardize the requirements for APN nationally through the use of exam certification. Currently, nurse practitioner certification falls under particular areas of specialization that are unique to certain provinces (Graduate Nursing EDU, 2021) and include adult, primary care, pediatric, and neonatal. All of these certifications are focused on physical health and mental health knowledge (CNA, 2021c). Further, differences in licensure for nurse practitioners exist among provinces due to hospital legislation and funding methodology for health care billing. Because of the strong need for psychiatric care throughout Canada and the lack of providers available, especially in rural areas, the role of the advanced-practice nurse in psychiatric mental health is expected to expand in the near future.

THE FUTURE OF PSYCHIATRIC MENTAL HEALTH NURSING

As its history has shown, the role of the nurse in psychiatric mental health care will continue to evolve and be influenced by societal trends. The change in the structure of health care delivery toward a primary health model and an integrative mental health care approach has led to new roles for nurses in psychiatric mental health, including shared-care roles in primary care and consultation-liaison psychiatry within the general hospital setting. The Association of Registered Nurses of Newfoundland and Labrador (2008) took some key steps in articulating the range of competencies and role development required for community mental health nursing in its 2008 policy paper *Advancing the Role of the Psychiatric–Mental Health Nurse in the Community*. These competencies and role development are in line with the CNA 2020 vision statement, which has called for an increased role for nurses working in integrative mental health care roles and primary care (Villeneuve & MacDonald, 2006). Career pathways for nurse practitioners who specifically work in mental health are lacking at this time in Canada. However, some provinces are rethinking this aspect in developing advanced nursing training at a graduate level. For example, Quebec has offered a diploma in mental health to nurse practitioners since 2019 (OIIQ, 2019). The changes in public perception of mental illness and efforts toward addressing stigma are placing a new emphasis on mental health promotion and illness prevention in schools and workplace settings (Mental Health Commission of Canada, 2021). Evidence-informed approaches to treatment, for example, concurrent treatment for people with mental illnesses and addictions, harm reduction, and dialectical behavioural therapy for people with borderline personality disorder, have led to the creation of related nursing roles, education, and research.

KEY POINTS TO REMEMBER

- Early asylum care for people with mental illness predominantly focused on containment and sometimes on punishment.
- Philippe Pinel and William Tuke were eighteenth-century reformers who introduced the moral treatment era of psychiatry, which

- attempted to focus on providing peaceful, nurturing environments for people with mental illness. Their theories influenced the rural, farmlike settings of early Canadian asylums.
- Nursing within asylums began in the late nineteenth century as a result of the increased medicalization of psychiatry.
- Psychiatric mental health nursing development in Canada was heavily influenced by societal values toward gender and toward mental illness, by politics, and by psychiatric care approaches.
- Early nursing roles in psychiatry were largely custodial until the introduction of new treatments such as electroconvulsive therapy, insulin shock therapy, and lobotomies.
- The division between western provinces and eastern provinces in the creation of the registered psychiatric nurse designation was largely related to differences in nursing leadership power, advocacy, and labour supply issues.
- The development of university-based programs in nursing in the 1920s was a key step in the professionalization of nursing and in the transition of nursing education from medical dominance to nursing-led knowledge development.
- Psychiatric mental health nursing led the way in reinforcing theory-based nursing practice with the use of clinical nurse specialists.
- Registered nurses work within psychiatric mental health settings across Canada.
- Registered psychiatric nurses work in psychiatric mental health settings in Manitoba, Saskatchewan, Alberta, British Columbia, and Yukon.
- The deinstitutionalization of patients in favour of community-based treatment led to the development of new nursing roles in psychiatric mental health care, including community mental health, crisis management, consultation-liaison, and primary care psychiatry.
- Advanced-practice nursing roles have had varied implementation in Canada. The clinical nurse specialist role has been well established, whereas the nurse practitioner role has had limited development.

CRITICAL THINKING

1. Consider the first students at Rockwood Asylum in 1888. What factors might have influenced their decision to enter into asylum nursing (a new program and role)?
2. How have educational programs for nurses evolved with the professionalization of nursing in Canada?
3. What are the potential implications of having two different designations and educational programs for nurses in psychiatric mental health nursing in four Canadian provinces?

CHAPTER REVIEW

1. Asylum care of people with mental illness in Canada began in which year?
   a. 1620
   b. 1932
   c. 1835
   d. 1798
2. The Weir Report was considered influential in which of the following areas?
   a. Asylum reform
   b. Nursing education curriculum reform
   c. Deinstitutionalization
   d. The establishment of the registered psychiatric nurse designation
3. Psychiatric mental health nursing in the community setting was influenced by which of the following factors?
   a. The Weir Report
   b. Deinstitutionalization
   c. The registered psychiatric nurse designation
   d. The increased medicalization of psychiatry

 https://evolve.elsevier.com/Canada/Varcarolis/psychiatric/

REFERENCES

Anthony, S. E., & Landeen, J. (2009). Evolution of Canadian nursing curricula: A critical retrospective analysis of power and caring. *International Journal of Nursing Education Scholarship, 69*, 1–14. https://doi.org/10.2202/1548-923X.1766

Association of Registered Nurses of Newfoundland and Labrador. (2008). *Advancing the role of the psychiatric–mental health nurse in the community (Policy paper)*. St. John's: Author.

Aubin, K. (2019). En quête de financement pour la création d'une clinique externe et d'un service social comme parachèvement de la désinstitutionnalisation à l'Hôpital Saint-Michel-Archange de Beauport, 1961–72. *CBMH/BCHM, 36*(2), 281–307.

Boschma, G. (2012). Community mental health nursing in Alberta, Canada: An oral history. *Nursing History Review, 20*(1), 103–135. https://doi.org/10.1891/1062-8061.20.103

Callaway, B. J. (2002). *Hildegard Peplau, psychiatric nurse of the century*. Springer Publishing Company.

Canadian Association of Schools of Nursing & Canadian Federation of Mental Health Nurses. (2015). *Entry-to-practice mental health and addiction competencies for undergraduate nursing education*. Ottawa, ON: Author. http://www.casn.ca/wp-content/uploads/2015/11/Mental-health-Competencies_EN_FINAL-3-Oct-26-2015.pdf

Canadian Federation of Mental Health Nurses. (2016). *CFMHN's 3rd position statement 2016: Mental health and addiction curriculum in undergraduate nursing education in Canada*. Toronto, ON: Author. https://www.cfmhn.ca/2019/05/14/cfmhn-2016-position-paper/

Canadian Nurses Association. (2017). *Code of ethics for registered nurses*. Ottawa: Author. https://www.cna-aiic.ca/en/nursing/regulated-nursing-in-canada/nursing-ethics

Canadian Nurses Association. (2019). *Advanced nursing practice: A national framework*. Ottawa: Author. https://www.cna-aiic.ca/en/nursing/advanced-nursing-practice

Canadian Nurses Association. (2021a). *Our history*. https://www.cna-aiic.ca/en/membership/who-we-are/our-history

Canadian Nurses Association. (2021b). *About certification*. https://www.cna-aiic.ca/en/certification/about-certification

Canadian Nurses Association. (2021c). *Nurse practitioners*. https://cna-aiic.ca/en/nursing-practice/the-practice-of-nursing/advanced-nursing-practice/nurse-practitioners

Cellard, A., & Thifault, M. C. (2006). The uses of asylums: Resistance, asylum propaganda and institutionalization strategies in turn of the century Quebec. In J. Moran (Ed.), *Mental illness and Canadian society: A historical perspective* (pp. 97–116). Montreal: McGill-Queen's University Press.

Connor, P. (1996). Neither courage nor perseverance enough": Attendants at the Asylum for the Insane, Kingston 1877–1905. *Ontario History, 88*(4), 251–272.

Cowles, E. (1916). Training schools for nurses and the first school in McLean Hospital. In H. Hurd (Ed.), *The institutional care of the* insane in the United States and Canada (pp. 289–300). New York: Arno Press.

Digby, A. (1983). Changes in the asylum: The case of York, 1777–1815. *Economic History Review, 36*, 218–239. https://doi.org/10.1111/j.1468-0289.1983.tb01230.x

Fleming, G. (1932). Survey on nursing education. *Canadian Medical Association Journal, 26*(4), 471–474.

Forchuk, C., & Tweedell, D. (2001). Celebrating our past. *Journal of Psychosocial and Mental Health Services, 39*(10), 16–24.

Foucault, M. (1971). *Madness and civilization: A history of insanity in the age of reason*. New York: Routledge.

Graduate Nursing EDU. (2021). *How to become an advanced practice nurse in Canada*. https://www.graduatenursingedu.org/canada/

Hardill, K. (2006). From the Grey Nuns to the streets: A critical history of outreach nursing in Canada. *Public Health Nursing, 24*(1), 91–97.

Harrisson, S. (2017). *Psychiatric nurses: An invisible role in the transition between the general hospital and the community*. In S. Dans Hähner-Rombach, & K. Nolte (Eds.), *Patients and social practice of psychiatric nursing in the 19th and 20th century*. Institute für Geschichte des Medezin Robert Bosh Stiftung. Stuttgart: Franz Steiner Verlag.

Harrisson, S., & Thifault, M.-C. (2018). L'infirmière psychiatrique: Témoin silencieux du processus de déshospitalisation. In H. Dans Guillemain, A. Klein, & M.-C. Thifault (Eds.), *La fin de l'asile? Histoire de la déshospitalisation psychiatrique dans l'espace francophone au XXe siècle*. Presses Universitaires de Rennes.

Hicks, B. (2011). Gender, politics, and regionalism: Factors in the evolution of registered psychiatric nursing in Manitoba, 1920–1960. *Nursing History Review, 19*, 103–126. https://doi.org/10.1891/1062-8061.19.103

Kerrigan, M. (2011). *Providence care family connection to Rockwood Nursing* [Blog post]. http://providencecarearchives.wordpress.com/2011/03/25/providence-care-family-connection-to-rockwood-nursing/

Kirkmayer, L. J., Brass, G. M., & Tait, C. L. (2000). The mental health of Aboriginal peoples: Transformations of identity and community. *The Canadian Journal of Psychiatry, 45*(7), 607–616.

Legislature of the Province of Ontario. (1889). *Sessional papers* (Vol. xxi, Part 1). Toronto: Queen's Printer.

Leishman, J. (2005). Back to the future: Making a case for including the history of mental health nursing in nurse education programmes. *The International Journal of Psychiatric Nursing Research, 10*(3), 1157–1164.

Mental Health Commission of Canada. (2021). *About us*. https://mentalhealthcommission.ca/about/

Moran, J. (1998). The ethics of farming-out: Ideology, the state, and the asylum in nineteenth-century Quebec. *Canadian Bulletin of Medical History, 15*, 297–316.

Ordre des Infirmières et Infirmiers du Québec (OIIQ). (2019). *Pratique clinique de l'infirmière praticienne spécialisée en santé mentale. Lignes directrices*. http://www.cmq.org/publications-pdf/p-1-2019-07-23-fr-lignes-dir-ips-sante-mentale.pdf

Paul, P. (1994). The contribution of the Grey Nuns to the development of nursing in Canada: Historiographical issues. *CBHM/BCHM, 11*, 207–217.

Peplau, H. (1991). *Interpersonal relations in nursing. A conceptual frame of reference for psychodynamic nursing*. New York: Springer Publishing Company.

Quétel, C. (2009). *Histoire de la folie, de l'antiquité à nos jours*. Tallander.

Registered Psychiatric Nurses of Canada. (2012). *Position statement on baccalaureate preparation as entry to practice in psychiatric nursing*. http://www.rpnc.ca/sites/default/files/resources/pdfs/BACCAL_Prep_PositionStatement_2012.pdf

Registered Psychiatric Nurse Regulators of Canada. (2021). *Registered psychiatric nursing in Canada*. http://www.rpnc.ca/registered-psychiatric-nursing-canada

Ryan-Nicholls, K. D. (2004). Impact of health reform on registered psychiatric nursing practice. *Journal of Psychiatric and Mental Health Nursing, 11*, 644–653. https://doi.org/10.1111/j.1365-2850.2004.00761.x

Senn, J. F. (2013). Peplau's theory of interpersonal relations: Application in emergency and rural nursing. *Nursing Science Quaterly, 26*(1), 31–35.

Smith, K. (2020). *Talking therapy. Knowledge and power in American psychiatric nursing*. Rutgers University Press.

Smith, M., & Khanlou, N. (2013). An analysis of Canadian psychiatric mental health nursing through the junctures of history, gender, nursing education, and quality of work life in Ontario, Manitoba, Alberta, and Saskatchewan. *ISRN Nursing*. https://pubmed.ncbi.nlm.nih.gov/23710367/

Thifault, M.-C., & Kérouac, L. (2019). Les infirmières psychiatriques témoins d'un mouvement d'humanisation au cours des premières et deuxièmes vagues de la désinstitutionnalisation au Québec (1960–1990). *Recherche en soins infirmiers, 139*(4), 99–108.

Tipliski, V. M. (2004). Parting at the crossroads: The emergence of education for psychiatric nursing in three Canadian provinces, 1909–1955. *Canadian Bulletin of Medical History, 21*(2), 253–279

University of Saskatchewan. (2011). *History of the College of Nursing*. http://www.usask.ca/nursing/college/history.php

University of Toronto. (2011). *Historic contributions*. http://bloomberg.nursing.utoronto.ca/about/history-of-the-faculty

Villeneuve, M., & MacDonald, J. (2006). *Toward 2020: Visions for nursing*. Ottawa: Canadian Nurses Association.

Weir, G. M. (1932). *Survey of nursing education in Canada*. Toronto: University of Toronto Press.

Wong, M. (2018). Centracare: A history of the New Brunswick Provincial Lunatic Asylum. *Dalhousie Medical Journal, 44*(2), 16–20.

Yonge, O., Boschma, G., & Mychajlunow, L. (2005). Gender and professional identity in psychiatric nursing practice in Alberta, Canada, 1930–1975. *Nursing Inquiry, 12*, 243–255. https://doi.org/10.1111/j.1440-1800.2005.00287

3

Overview of Psychiatric Mental Health Nursing Care Within Various Settings

Cheryl L. Pollard

 http://evolve.elsevier.com/Canada/Varcarolis/psychiatric/

OBJECTIVES

1. Identify key features of the Canadian health care system and funding structure.
2. Discuss the continuum of psychiatric treatment.
3. Describe primary, secondary, and tertiary treatment outcomes and interventions by setting.
4. Explain the evolution of the community mental health movement.
5. List the criteria for admission to inpatient care.
6. Explain the role and responsibilities of the nurse as care manager.
7. Discuss the process for preparing patients to return to the community for ongoing care.
8. Describe the role of the community psychiatric mental health nurse in disaster preparedness.
9. Discuss barriers to mental health treatment.
10. Examine influences on the future of community psychiatric mental health nursing.

KEY TERMS AND CONCEPTS

admission criteria
assertive community treatment
barriers to treatment
biopsychosocial model
case management
clinical pathway
continuum of psychiatric mental health treatment
decompensation
elopement
interdisciplinary
mental health-related disability
multidisciplinary
recovery

Mental illness is a significant problem faced by Canadians. Alterations in mental health have escalated during the COVID-19 pandemic. Findlay and Arim (2020) identify that "according to the recent Canadian Perspectives Survey Series (CPSS), 54% of Canadians aged 15 and older reported excellent or very good mental health during the COVID-19 period. This compares to the findings from the 2018 Canadian Community Health Survey (CCHS) when 68% of Canadians aged 15 and older said that their mental health was excellent or very good" (p. 1). Additionally, there are approximately 6.2 million Canadians, 15 years of age and older who live with disabilities (Morris et al., 2019). Of these Canadians, over 2 million have a mental health-related disability (Statistics Canada, 2020). **Mental health-related disability** is defined as limitations experienced in an individual's daily activities because of emotional, psychological, or mental conditions (Statistics Canada, 2020). Mental conditions include anxiety, depression, bipolar disorder, substance use, and anorexia. Mental health care services are accessed differently by men and women. Women generally tended to access counselling and support groups, while men were more likely to require access to addiction services (Statistics Canada, 2020). Most mental illnesses are treated today in the community. Community treatment services include mobile crisis intervention teams, psychologists, nurses, psychiatrics, social workers, addiction counsellors, other health professionals, and peer support groups. For those with more complex or urgent needs, mental health services are provided in general hospital psychiatric units or specialized provincial psychiatric organizations. Forensic psychiatric services are provided to individuals referred by the court system and are provided in both community and inpatient settings.

 HOW A NURSE HELPED ME

When Hope Fades

I'm Amanda, just 23 years old, but I reached a dark place where my life seemed intolerably painful and without hope. I felt weighted down by problems in my home community in Nunavut. At the same time, I felt the incredible pressure of my community, my family, and my own dream to complete a medical degree at McGill University Faculty of Medicine so that I could contribute to the healing of my people.

It was so strange and lonely at university. I felt isolated and without supports. I started to have trouble finding enough energy to keep up with the relentless pace of my studies. I couldn't concentrate, couldn't sleep, and couldn't be bothered eating, so I lost weight. I was anxious and afraid. In order to cope with my anxiety, I started to drink alone in my residence. I wanted to give up and felt I had no option other than suicide. I ate a whole bottle of Tylenol and drank it down with a bottle of gin.

When I was admitted to an acute care psychiatric facility, I felt so ashamed, so hopeless, and so angry. I just wanted to scream, but instead I was polite and withdrawn because that is expected from an Inuk. Luckily, a nurse, Andrea, reached out and helped me change my life. How? I think mostly by listening respectfully—that's important where I come from. When I whispered, "You can't understand my life," she said, "I know, but maybe I can help you understand your life better."

Andrea listened, but she also taught me about the symptoms of and treatment for depression. Andrea and I made a plan to keep me safe while I explored some options to make my life seem livable again. She was very clear that she had a responsibility to keep me safe while in hospital and explained the suicide precautions needed. I felt safe. Andrea helped me identify my health priorities (like getting back to healthy eating and sleeping), and she also helped me identify some community supports. I didn't know there was an Inuk medical resident at McGill. It was a huge relief to talk with him about university. Andrea also helped me talk with my family when they came all the way from home to visit me. Gradually, I began to see hope for life again. Andrea helped me by listening and respecting me. I will always be grateful for her care.

FUNDING PSYCHIATRIC MENTAL HEALTH CARE

The Canadian mental health care system has many areas of strength, for example, most citizens have access to mental health services; but it also has gaps, such as equitable access to specialized care at the primary, secondary, and tertiary levels. Canada has a predominately publicly financed and administered health care system whereby all eligible residents have reasonable access to medically necessary hospital and physician services. Federal government and provincial and territorial government roles and responsibilities for health care are set out, primarily, in the *Medicare Act* (1966) and the *Canada Health Act* (1984). Provincial and territorial governments are responsible for health care within their jurisdictions. The federal government is responsible for transferring health care funds to the provincial and territorial governments and for ensuring that insured health care services are publicly funded and administered by the provinces and territories according to five basic principles: public administration, comprehensiveness, universality, portability, and accessibility.

The federal government continues to maintain health care responsibility for select populations (specific First Nations and Inuit communities, armed forces, Royal Canadian Mounted Police, individuals in federal penitentiaries, and refugees) and select functions (such as health promotion, disease surveillance, and drug regulation). For instance, the federal government provides morale and welfare services programs across Canada for military members, veterans, and their families to help them cope with the psychological effects of stress and trauma associated with their military service. Operational Stress Injury Social Support (OSISS) is a national peer support network that can complement other mental health and family supports. (For more information on OSISS programs, visit https://www.cafconnection.ca/National/Programs-Services/Mental-Health/Operational-Stress-Injury-Social-Support.aspx).

Although the federal government is generally responsible for funding mental health services for Indigenous peoples, the Mental Health Strategy for Canada highlights the past and ongoing colonial systemic processes that have impacted the wellness of Indigenous individuals and communities, causing high rates of mental health problems, addictions, and suicides that are linked with complex issues such as family violence and involvement with the child welfare and criminal justice systems (Mental Health Commission of Canada, 2016). Indigenous peoples continue to experience the intergenerational impacts of Canada's colonial legacy: abuse, systemic racism, discrimination, displacement, the denial of culture and language, inequities in health, wellness, and socioeconomic factors, all of which have increased mental health challenges for individuals and for communities as a whole (Government of Canada, 2020). Despite funding being a federal responsibility, we all play a role in promoting a better understanding of the emotional and psychological distress and its relationship to childhood abuses.

Responsibility for health care services is further devolved from the provincial and territorial governments to regional organizations—for instance, regional health boards, regional health authorities, and hospitals—the type of which depend on the province or territory. Although differences that cause gaps in the continuum of mental health services exist among the various provinces or territories, mental health and addiction services generally include primary, secondary, and tertiary services that are provided in inpatient and outpatient psychiatric hospital settings and in community-based settings. These services may include mobile crisis response and intervention, emergency services, temporary and long-term housing, psychoeducational or support groups, and vocational or educational services. Services are generally delivered by a number of professionals, for example, registered nurses (RNs), registered psychiatric nurses (RPNs), licensed/registered practical nurses, psychiatrists, psychologists, counsellors, occupational therapists, recreation therapists, and social workers. Not all of these services, however, are publicly funded. Health expenditures vary across the provinces and territories, due in part to demographic differences, size and dispersion of the population, and cultural differences.

The Canadian Government spends 11.5% of the entire GDP on health care (Allin et al., 2020). Canadians pay directly or indirectly for all health care: 70% through taxation, 12% through private or employment insurance plans, 15% out of pocket, and another 3% through other means (Canadian Institute for Health Information, 2019). Of those with mental health–related disabilities, 52% have been disadvantaged as a result of their condition (Statistics Canada, 2020). Individuals with mental health problems often have financial challenges as a result of the signs and symptoms of their illness, which makes the private or employment health insurance plans difficult or impossible to access and out-of-pocket expenses, including medication costs, counselling, appropriate housing, re-entry to employment or education support, and dental care, which is burdensome.

THE CONTINUUM OF MENTAL HEALTH CARE

Health care services can generally be divided into three different levels: primary, secondary, and tertiary. Primary-level activities are delivered to healthy populations and include providing information and teaching coping skills to reduce stress, with the goal of avoiding mental illness (e.g., a nurse may teach parenting skills in a well-baby clinic). These services are generally provided in a community or outpatient setting. Secondary-level services involve the early detection and treatment of psychiatric symptoms, with the goal of minimizing impairment (e.g., a nurse may conduct screening for depression at a work site). These services are also generally provided in a community or outpatient setting. Tertiary-level services involve the treatment of psychiatric symptoms and address residual impairments in psychiatric patients in an effort to promote the highest level of community functioning. These are very specialized services that may be delivered in a clinic or a hospital (e.g., a nurse may provide long-term treatment in a clinic, or the person may be admitted to a specialized inpatient unit). In the past, tertiary care models focused on providing inpatient services.

Evolving Venues of Practice

Many psychiatric mental health nurses originally practised within tertiary care settings, but practice locations have evolved because of financial, technological, health care, regulatory, cultural, and population changes. Nurses are now providing primary mental health care at therapeutic day care centres, schools, PHPs, and shelters. In addition to these more traditional environments for care, psychiatric mental health nurses are entering forensic settings and drug and alcohol treatment centres. Box 3.1 presents examples of practice sites for the psychiatric mental health nurse.

BOX 3.1 Possible Community Mental Health Practice Sites

Primary Prevention
Adult and youth recreational centres
Churches, temples, synagogues, mosques
Day care centres
Ethnic cultural centres
Public health clinics
Schools

Secondary Prevention
Assisted-living facilities
Chemical dependency programs
Community outreach treatment programs
Correctional community facilities
Crisis centres
Early intervention psychosis programs
General inpatient units
Hospices and acquired immunodeficiency syndrome (AIDS) programs
Industry/work sites
Nursing homes
Partial hospitalization programs
Primary care networks
Shelters (homeless, women subjected to domestic violence, adolescents)
Youth residential treatment centres

Tertiary Prevention
Psychosocial rehabilitation programs
Specialized community mental health centres
Specialized inpatient units

⚡ SAFETY TIP
- Regardless of where mental health services are provided, nurses and other providers must be aware of their surroundings. Think about the environment.
- Are there other people nearby?
- Is there adequate lighting?
- Is there good ventilation?
- Is it hot, cold, raining, or windy?

Mobile mental health units have been developed in some service areas. In a growing number of communities, mental health programs are collaborating with other health or community services to provide integrated approaches to treatment. A prime example of this is the growth of concurrent disorder programming (programs that address the diagnosis of a mental illness and substance use disorder) at both mental health and chemical dependency clinics. Mobile crisis intervention teams is another example. These teams are typically collaborative partnerships between first responders (police) and health care agency staff (nurses, social workers, psychologists) who are specially trained to respond to individuals experiencing a mental health crisis.

The COVID-19 pandemic has presented serious accessibility and care continuity challenges for people with mental illness. Mental health service providers have had to pivot the modes of delivering critical services. In nearly all cases, the use of technology has been instrumental in offering a spectrum of services, integrating behavioural and physical healthcare and collaborative decision-making (Kopelovich et al., 2020). Telephone crisis counselling, telephone outreach, and the Internet are being used to support access to mental health services. Increased use of technologies has the potential to better leverage broader support systems, leverage natural supports, and can result in better integration of digital health interventions (Kopelovich et al., 2020). The Mental Health Commission of Canada (2020) identified that pivoting to virtual supports has been done to meet the needs of the general population. However, these offerings are not meeting the needs of some people who experience vulnerabilities; and the most significant impacts on mental health, substance use, and service systems will likely not be felt until the pandemic has ended.

Over the continuum of mental health and illness, patients may receive care from a range of psychiatric services. Figure 3.1 illustrates the continuum of psychiatric mental health treatment. A patient's movement along the continuum is fluid, from higher to lower levels of intensity of care, and changes are not necessarily made step by step. Upon discharge from acute hospital care or a 24-hour supervised crisis unit, many patients need intensive services to maintain their initial gains. Timely outpatient follow-up is critical to improving psychiatric outcomes and readmission rates for people who sought emergency psychiatric services (McCullumsmith et al., 2020). It is also notable that patients may pass through the continuum of treatment in the reverse direction; that is, if symptoms do not improve, a lower-intensity service may refer the patient to a higher level of care in an attempt to prevent decompensation (deterioration of mental health) and hospitalization.

PSYCHIATRIC MENTAL HEALTH CARE SETTINGS

The following sections describe various psychiatric settings, and each section offers examples of basic-level nursing interventions:
- Counselling—assessment interviews; crisis intervention; problem solving in individual, group, or family sessions

Fig. 3.1 The continuum of psychiatric mental health treatment.

- Promotion of self-care activities—fostering grooming, guidance in use of public transportation, instruction in budgeting (in home settings, the nurse may directly assist as necessary)
- Psychobiological interventions—medication administration, instruction in relaxation techniques, promotion of sound eating and sleep habits
- Health teaching and behaviour consultation—medication use, illness characteristics, coping skills, relapse prevention, behaviour change and lifestyle modification
- Case management—liaising with family, significant others, and other health care or community resource personnel of care regarding referrals, assistance with paperwork applications, connection to resources, and overall navigation of the health care system to coordinate an effective plan

Community Mental Health Centres

Since the 1950s, the trend of deinstitutionalization has occurred internationally (Lequin et al., 2020). In Canada, several factors contributed to this shift, including financial pressures on the provincially funded psychiatric hospitals, changing societal values, and new mental health treatment philosophies (LaJeunesse, 2002). Many hospitals were indeed grossly overcrowded, patients' rights were often disregarded, and seclusion and restraint were overused. Due to the largely custodial nature of inpatient treatment, patients were left with little incentive for growth or participation in their own care; this phenomenon became known as *institutionalization*. Grassroots efforts, increased advocacy, and legal initiatives on behalf of people with mental illness and their right to humane care resulted in the provincial health care systems looking for alternative treatment settings (LaJeunesse, 2002).

Policymakers came to believe that community care would be more humane and less expensive than hospital-based care, and the introduction of psychotropic drugs, beginning with chlorpromazine (Largactil), made community living a more realistic option for many people. Organizations like the Canadian Mental Health Association (CMHA) established housing and support services for people living with mental illness in the community. All Canadian provinces have implemented some type of deinstitutionalization of psychiatric services. The timing and degree of bed closures varied greatly across regions. For example, between 1965 and 1981, Canada saw a 70.6% decrease in psychiatry beds across the nation, but during that time, Saskatchewan had an 81.6% decrease and Prince Edward Island had only a 34.5% decrease (Sealy & Whitehead, 2004).

Government promises to expand funding for community services were not kept, mental health funding continued to decline, and patient needs outnumbered resources. Many patients with serious mental illness resisted treatment with available providers, so providers began to use up scarce resources for the less mentally disabled but more committed population. While deinstitutionalization, in principle, was largely considered to have been a step toward improved care for people with mental illness, the lack of funding and available community supports negated many of the benefits. In reality, many people with mental illness were discharged to inadequate supports, a situation that led to increased homelessness and criminalization (Paradis-Gagné, Jacob & Pariseau-Legault, 2020).

Through the 1990s, advocacy by the CMHA and others continued. Increasing awareness resulted in increasing pressure on government to redesign the mental health system in Canada and to ensure adequate community supports. The 2006 Senate report led by Michael Kirby and Wilbert Keon, *Out of the Shadows at Last*, was an optimistic step toward transforming the delivery system of mental health care. However, until 2012 Canada remained the only G7 country without a national mental health strategy. At that time, the Mental Health Commission of Canada (2012) issued *Changing Directions, Changing Lives: The Mental Health Strategy for Canada*, which was a call to action in an effort to unite people's efforts to improve mental health. Despite this call being made in the early 2010s, Canada continues to have lower rates of spending on mental health than most other G7 countries (Canadian Institute for Health Information, 2019).

Recovery is a critical aspect to improving the well-being and mental health of all Canadians. It is described as the ability of the individual to work, live, and participate in the community. It is a journey that provides patients with hope, empowerment, and confidence to take an active role in determining their own treatment paths. Ideally, recovery would be facilitated by interconnected community agencies that work in harmony to assist consumers of mental health care as they navigate an often-confusing system. Realistically, funding has always been an issue in treating people with mental illness, and current economic realities have not improved the situation. RNs and RPNs may be the answer to transforming an illness-driven and dependency-oriented system into one that emphasizes recovery and empowerment. Nurses are adept at understanding the system and coordinating care as well as taking a health-oriented approach.

Over the past 50 years, with advances in psychopharmacology and psychosocial treatments, psychiatric care in the community has become more sophisticated, with a continuum of care that provides more options for people with mental illness. The role of the psychiatric mental health nurse has grown to include service provision in a variety of community settings. Nurses may also provide care to individuals as they leave the criminal justice system and re-enter the community. The range of community services available varies but generally includes mobile crisis intervention teams, emergency services, and services for adults and children such as medication administration, treatment for concurrent disorders, individual therapy, group therapy, family therapy, psychoeducational services, and education to other professionals. A clinic may also be aligned with a psychosocial rehabilitation program that offers a structured day program, vocational services, and residential services. Some community mental health centres have an associated intensive case-management service to assist patients in finding housing or obtaining funding.

Community mental health centres often provide services using an interprofessional team model. The psychiatric mental health nurse will work with a number of patients. Patients are either self-referred or referred by inpatient units or primary care providers for long-term or short-term follow-up. Patients may attend the clinic for years or be discharged when they improve and reach desired goals. Each clinic varies in the design of service delivery; the nurse sees the majority of patients in the clinic but often will see patients in other settings such as primary care offices or their homes.

Walking into a person's home creates a different set of dynamics from that commonly seen in a clinical setting. Boundaries become important. The nurse may find it best to begin a visit informally by chatting about the patient's family events or by accepting refreshments offered. This interaction can be a strain for the nurse who has difficulty maintaining boundaries between the professional relationship and a personal one. However, there is great significance to the therapeutic use of self (i.e., the personality, insights, perceptions, and judgements of the nurse as part of the therapeutic process) in such circumstances to establish a level of comfort for the patient and family.

The vignette illustrates a typical day for a nurse in a community mental health centre.

Mobile Crisis Intervention Teams

When psychiatric mental health care moved to a community setting, the need to address some of the acute mental health care concerns of individuals living in the community increased. Initially, the necessary response was left to local police departments, which often felt unprepared to deal effectively with mental health concerns. Crisis intervention teams were set up in many communities across Canada to address this issue and are now considered an essential part of comprehensive community mental health services (Semple et al., 2020). Various service-delivery models for crisis intervention teams are being used. Common aspects of these models include the use of an interprofessional team, mobile units, and collaborative partnerships with police. Often the crisis intervention team is an interprofessional team made up of nurses, social workers, and psychologists. Psychiatrists often are used as consultants for the team. Crisis teams operate out of community clinics, emergency departments, or stand-alone offices.

Partnership with local police authorities has been found to be an extremely effective way to meet the needs of individuals in acute psychiatric crisis and has led to decreased criminalization and improved access to services for people with severe chronic mental illness (Semple et al., 2020). When required, the interprofessional team may act as consultants to the police. Some crisis intervention models in Canada even include specially trained police members on the interprofessional team. Crisis services offer 24/7 phone support and in-person mental health assessments in homes, public places, and emergency departments.

Nurses who work on crisis teams collaborate with other interprofessional members to assess patients in crisis; provide early intervention; provide crisis intervention counselling and support; offer short-term case management, including referrals to other resources; and advocate on behalf of families and patients.

The vignette describes a typical day of a nurse working on a crisis team.

> **VIGNETTE**
>
> Nita Desai is a nurse at a community mental health centre. She is on the adult team and carries a caseload of 80 patients diagnosed with chronic mental illness.
>
> **0830–0900:** Upon arriving at the clinic, Nita receives a voicemail message from Ms. DiTomasso, who is crying and says she is out of medication. Nita consults with the psychiatrist and calls Ms. DiTomasso to arrange for an emergency appointment later that day.
>
> **0900–0930:** Nita's first patient is Mr. Enright, a 35-year-old man diagnosed with schizophrenia, who has been in treatment at the clinic for 10 years. During their 30-minute counselling session, Nita assesses Mr. Enright for any exacerbation of psychotic symptoms (he has a history of grandiose delusions) and any changes in eating and sleep habits or social functioning in the psychosocial rehabilitation program that he attends 5 days a week. Today, he presents as stable. Nita gives Mr. Enright his haloperidol decanoate (Haldol Decanoate) injection and schedules a return appointment for a month from now, reminding him of his psychiatrist appointment the following week.
>
> **1000–1100:** Nita's second patient of the day is Susan, a 28-year-old mother with postpartum depression. Nita sees Susan weekly to assess her response to the antidepressant medication prescribed by her family physician and to work on anxiety coping strategies. She also spends time assessing Susan's attachment to her 6-month-old baby and provides education on any parenting questions that Susan may have. They discuss the idea of Susan attending a support group for postpartum depression as an adjunct to individual treatment. Susan is agreeable to the idea now that she is feeling less anxious and has more energy. Nita calls the group facilitator and arranges for Susan's intake for the following week.
>
> **1100–1200:** Nita writes progress and medication notes; responds to telephone calls from patients and other agencies, such as home care and public-health nursing agencies; and prepares for the team conference.
>
> **1200–1400:** All adult-team staff members attend the weekly intake meeting, at which new admissions are discussed and individual treatment plans are written with team input. Nita presents a patient intake, reading from the standardized interview form. She also gives nursing input about treatment for the other five newly admitted patients. The new patient she presented is assigned to her, and she plans to call him later in the afternoon to set up a first appointment.
>
> **1400–1500:** Nita co-leads a concurrent disorders therapy group with the addictions specialist, who is a social worker. The group is made up of seven patients who have concurrent diagnoses of substance use and a major psychiatric illness. The leaders take a psychoeducational approach, and today's planned topic is teaching about the physical effects of alcohol on the body. Nita focuses on risks associated with the interaction between alcohol and medications and answers the members' questions. Because this is an ongoing group, members take a more active role, and discussion may vary according to members' needs instead of following planned topics. After the session, the co-leaders discuss the group dynamics and write progress notes.
>
> **1530–1600:** Nita meets with Ms. DiTomasso, who arrives at the clinic tearful and agitated. Ms. DiTomasso says that she missed her appointment this month because her son died suddenly. Nita uses crisis intervention skills to assess Ms. DiTomasso's status (e.g., any risks for her safety related to her history of suicidal ideation). After helping Ms. DiTomasso clarify a plan to increase support from her family, Nita notes that insomnia is a new problem. She takes Ms. DiTomasso to the psychiatrist covering "emergency prescription time" and explains the change in the patient's status. The psychiatrist refills Ms. DiTomasso's usual antidepressant and adds a medication to aid sleep. Nita makes an appointment for the patient to return to see her in 1 week instead of the usual 1 month and also schedules her to meet with her assigned psychiatrist that same day.
>
> **1600–1630:** Nita completes all notes, makes necessary telephone calls to staff working with her patients in the psychosocial rehabilitation program, and phones her new patient to schedule an appointment.

Disaster Response Teams

Nurses who work in community mental health are often part of the intersectoral disaster response planning committee for the community in which they work. Following a disaster, the immediate goal is to ensure that those affected have shelter, food, and first aid as necessary. Then the community mental health nurse provides crisis management for victims and volunteers who are assisting in the relief efforts. After the crisis passes, the community psychiatric mental health nurse must find those individuals whose care was disrupted and help them to link back into the system. The nurse administers "psychological first aid" by assisting victims with meeting basic needs, listening to individuals who need to share their stories, directing individuals to agencies that can help, and providing compassion and appropriate hope. Mental health nurses take on a leadership role in disaster situations to enhance the biopsychosocial outcomes for people living in a disaster-affected community (Owen & Schimmels, 2020). Chapter 21 offers a more detailed discussion of crisis and disaster.

CHAPTER 3 Overview of Psychiatric Mental Health Nursing Care Within Various Settings

> **VIGNETTE**
>
> Ben Thien is a nurse working on the mobile crisis team in a large urban setting; the following describes a typical evening shift.
>
> **1500–1530:** Ben comes onto his shift and meets with the evening team to get a report from the day shift and plan for the evening shift. The team is told by day-shift staffers of any outstanding calls that have not been assessed and any updates regarding patients who are being case managed by the team currently. The team decides that Ben and Officer George will go out at 1700 hours to try to see a man whom a neighbour has called about today but who had not been at home when the day team went out earlier.
>
> **1530–1630:** Ben answers the phone and receives a call from a woman who is feeling very sad and hopeless. Ben conducts a mental status exam over the phone and assesses the woman for risk. The woman appears to be suffering from depression but is not currently suicidal, so Ben offers her support and some psychoeducation about depression and its treatment. He gives her a phone number for the mental health clinic in her area, and she agrees to follow up. Ben asks for permission to fax a copy of his assessment to her family physician to ensure continuity of care, and the patient agrees. Ben completes his documentation and then faxes the report to the family physician.
>
> **1630–1830:** Ben and his partner, Officer George, leave the office to follow up on the call from the day shift. They drive to the person's house in an unmarked police car. They both go to the door and ring the doorbell. A young man in his early 20s answers, and Ben explains who they are and that they would like to talk to him about how he has been feeling lately. The man agrees to speak to them. Officer George and Ben enter the house and assess it for any safety risks such as environmental issues, uncontrolled dogs, or other people present. Ben and George sit down at the kitchen table with the patient and begin the interview. The patient reports recent difficulties with his sleep and mood. He denies any history of mental illness or physical illness. He tells of his ability to control the weather and his fear that perhaps people in the government are out to get him. He denies any risk for harm or self-harm, and he agrees that this is a recent change for him but does not feel the need to seek medical treatment. He does not demonstrate any impulsive behaviour during the interview, but Ben notices that many of the kitchen appliances are wrapped in tin foil. The patient vaguely refers to this as "antiradar devices." At the completion of the interview, Ben concludes that although the patient seems to be showing signs of psychosis, he is not currently demonstrating risk and does not meet criteria under the mental health act for involuntary admission. Ben decides to try to engage the patient further and arranges a follow-up meeting for 2 days later. Prior to leaving, Ben ensures that the patient has adequate food supplies in his fridge and does some basic wellness teaching about sleep hygiene for the patient. Ben and George return to the office and document the visit.
>
> **1830–2030:** George receives a call from a fellow police officer requesting an assessment of a person in the community who was reported for disturbing the peace at a bus shelter. Ben and George leave to drive to the scene. On the way to the scene, Ben takes a crisis call over the cellphone from a young man looking for resources for panic attacks. Upon arrival at the scene, Ben and George meet briefly with the police officers on-site, who bring them up to date on the situation. According to witnesses, the woman has been pacing at the bus stop for the past 6 hours, occasionally stepping into traffic. George and Ben go into the bus shelter and begin talking to the woman, who is dressed in shorts despite the cold weather, is pacing back and forth muttering to herself, and refuses to go to the hospital, stating, "I've had enough of all you FBI agents." Ben conducts the mental status and risk assessment and then, conferring with George, decides that this woman does meet the criteria of the mental health act for an involuntary assessment because she appears to have a mental illness, is at risk for self-harm (walking into traffic, continued exposure to the cold weather) and further deterioration, and refuses to go to the hospital voluntarily. George and Ben explain that they need to take her to the hospital for an assessment. George puts her safely in the back of the police car, and Ben documents his assessment en route to the hospital. At the hospital, Ben informs the triage nurse of his assessment and arranges a secure room for the patient. Ben ensures that the patient is given food and fluids by the emergency staff and then discusses his assessment with the psychiatry resident on call. Ben and George then return to the office.
>
> **2030–2230:** Ben continues to answer the phone and provide support, referrals, and assessments to callers. He arranges a home visit for the following day for a woman who is concerned about her father-in-law and his recent changes in behaviour.
>
> **2230–2300:** Ben gets an update from the three other teams working the evening shift and then prepares his report for the night shift.

Partial Hospitalization Programs

Partial hospitalization programs (PHPs) offer intensive, short-term treatment similar to inpatient care, except that the patient is able to return home each day. Criteria for referral to a PHP include serious symptoms that otherwise could lead to hospitalization or step-down from acute inpatient treatment (Taube-Schiff et al., 2018). Referrals come from inpatient or outpatient providers. Patients receive 5 to 6 hours of treatment daily, usually 5 days a week, although some programs operate on weekends. The average length of stay is approximately 2 to 3 weeks, depending on the program, and the interprofessional team consists of a psychiatrist, RN or RPN, social worker, occupational therapist, and recreational therapist.

The following vignette illustrates a typical day for a psychiatric mental health nurse in a PHP.

> **VIGNETTE**
>
> Michael Sanders is a nurse in a partial hospitalization program (PHP) that is part of a general hospital's outpatient psychiatry department. Michael is the nurse member of the interprofessional team, and today his schedule is as follows:
>
> **0830–0900:** Michael arrives at the PHP and meets with the team to review the patients expected to arrive in the program today. He prepares to meet with the patients who are scheduled for medication review with the psychiatrist. He also prepares the teaching outline for his daily psychoeducational groups.
>
> **0900–1230:** Michael meets with a group of 10 patients and teaches them goal setting, medication management, and relapse prevention. Throughout the sessions, Michael assesses each patient's mental status and any concerns that have arisen.
>
> **1300–1400:** Michael conducts an intake interview with a newly admitted patient. Ms. Brown is a 50-year-old woman with a history of major depression who was hospitalized for 2 weeks after a drug overdose following an argument with her boyfriend. Michael completes the standardized interview form, paying extra attention to risk factors for suicide. When asked about substance use, Ms. Brown admits that she has been drinking heavily for the past 2 years, including the night she took the drug overdose. When the interview is completed, the patient is referred to the psychiatrist for a diagnostic evaluation.
>
> **1400–1500:** Michael meets with four patients scheduled to see the psychiatrist. He reviews the cases with the psychiatrist and ensures that the patients understand any changes in their medication regimens.
>
> **1500–1530:** Michael has a discharge meeting with Mr. Callaghan, a 48-year-old man with a diagnosis of schizophrenia. He was referred to the PHP by his clinic therapist to prevent hospitalization due to increasing paranoia and agitation. After 2 weeks in the PHP, he has restabilized and recognizes that he must adhere to his antipsychotic medication regimen. Michael finalizes Mr.

Callaghan's medication teaching and confirms his aftercare appointments with his previous therapist and psychiatrist.

1530–1600: To ensure Ms. Brown's safety, Michael meets with her again before she goes home, assessing her suicide risk potential. Michael also shares the preliminary individual treatment plan and begins a discussion of resources for alcohol treatment, including Alcoholics Anonymous.

1600–1700: Michael meets with the team for daily rounds. He presents Ms. Brown, and the team develops an individual treatment plan for her. In this treatment plan, the team notes discharge planning needs for referrals to a community mental health centre and an alcohol treatment program. As a critical member of the treatment team, Michael reviews the remaining cases and makes needed adjustments to their treatment plans. He completes his notes and discharge summary. He also makes case-management telephone calls to arrange for community referrals, communicate with families, and report to any mental health referral programs to review how often the patient has used the services.

Inpatient Psychiatric Mental Health Programs

Inpatient psychiatric care has undergone significant change over the past half-century. Consequences of deinstitutionalization have included a reduction in long-stay psychiatric beds (as these are concentrated in the provincial psychiatric hospitals), decreased lengths of hospital stay, increased use of crisis services, and an increase in the number of individuals with mental illness who are homeless or in the penitentiary system. Fewer psychiatric inpatient beds means that acuity within psychiatric facilities has been increasing, wait times for admission are increasing, and admission is commonly reserved for those people who are acutely suicidal, actively homicidal, or extremely disabled and in need of short-term acute care (Hensel et al., 2018).

Entry to Inpatient Care

Although some patients are admitted directly based on a psychiatrist or primary care provider referral, most people receiving inpatient acute psychiatric care are assessed in the emergency department (ED) first and then are admitted through the ED if they meet the established admission criteria. The average ED wait time for a patient in need of hospitalization is increasing; in some areas, the wait can be days. Nurses who work on psychiatric units should recognize that patients admitted from the ED may need additional patience and attention. They may have been deprived of medication, treatments, sleep, or proper food.

People with psychiatric symptoms are often isolated and ignored from the outset of their hospitalization. However, an increasing number of Canadian EDs are using nurses who have experience working with people with mental illness in the ED to assist with triage and care of patients with mental health problems.

In the ED, the patient is generally evaluated by an ED physician and a social worker, who will determine if the patient meets the criteria to justify admission. The admission criteria begin with the premise that the person is suffering from a mental illness and include evidence of one or more of the following:
- High risk of harming self
- High risk of harming others
- Inability to care for basic needs, which will likely cause substantial mental or physical deterioration or serious physical impairments

Patients who meet the admission criteria are then given the option of being admitted on a voluntary basis, which means that they agree with the need for treatment and hospitalization. The vast majority of patient admissions to psychiatric inpatient units are voluntary. If patients do not wish to be hospitalized but mental health care providers feel that admission is necessary, the patients can be admitted against their wishes, commonly known as an "involuntary admission." Involuntarily admitted patients, sometimes referred to as certified patients, still have rights: right to receive information on their rights in a timely manner, right to retain counsel, and right to an independent review of their committal (O'Reilly et al., 2010); Chapter 7 offers a more detailed discussion of this issue. If the admission is contested, a mental health review board (or panel or tribunal, depending on the province or territory) reviews the committal decision on behalf of the patient. Chapter 7 discusses legal requirements for admissions, commitment, and discharge procedures in more detail.

Preparation for Discharge to the Community

Discharge planning begins upon admission and is continually modified as required by the patient's condition until the time of discharge. The reduction of overt symptoms and the development of an adequate outpatient plan signal that discharge is imminent. As members of the health care team, nurses assist patients and their families with preparing for independent or assisted living in the community.

The treatment plans are influenced by the clinical pathway (when available), which is a guideline that outlines the clinical standards: the usual care provided for a patient undergoing a certain procedure or for a patient who has a certain illness. Since each patient is unique, each person's care will be customized to meet his or her needs while

> **VIGNETTE**
>
> Shane is a 22-year-old male who was brought to the emergency department by police after expressing thoughts of suicide. He reports having had difficulty sleeping and eating for the past several days and a weight loss of 5 pounds. He is restless and demanding. When approached, he becomes very irritable and threatening to the nurses and physicians, stating that he wants to leave and does not understand why he needs to be here. He states that he was tricked by his mother and brother, who are trying to have him admitted only so they can take his money. He is exhibiting poor judgement, insight, and impulse control. He has been nonadherent with his antipsychotic medication, risperidone, which he stopped taking 3 weeks ago because of adverse effects.
>
> Shane did not want to be admitted, and despite obvious mental health–related disability and several attempts by the nursing staff to encourage voluntary admission, he continued to refuse hospitalization. The decision was made to involuntarily admit him to the locked psychiatric inpatient unit. On arrival to the inpatient unit, Shane was informed of his rights and the fact that he was involuntarily committed to the unit.

RESEARCH HIGHLIGHT

Maternal Psychological Distress and Mental Health Service Use During the COVID-19 Pandemic

Problem

COVID-19 has impacted the lives of families. Previous research on epidemics/pandemics suggest that mothers may be at increased risk of experiencing mental health problems as compared to other members of the family

Purpose of Study

This study was conducted for three primary reasons: (1) describe prevalence rates of maternal depressive and anxiety symptoms from an online convenience sample during the COVID-19 pandemic, (2) identify risk and protective factors for elevated symptoms, and (3) describe current mental health service use and barriers.

> **Methods**
> In total, 641 mothers of children aged 0 to 8 years completed an online survey assessing mental health, sociodemographic, and COVID-19-related variables.
>
> **Key Findings**
> - Significant associations were identified between risk factors and maternal depression and anxiety in mothers of children 0 to 8 years.
>
> **Implications for Nursing Practice**
> The results of this study indicate that mothers have experienced a significant impact on their mental health related to their experience with COVID-19. Nurses in community clinics and emergency rooms need to ensure that a thorough mental status is completed to accurately assess the mental health care needs of the mother. Additionally, considering targeted early intervention strategies to prevent long-term impacts of COVID-19 on family well-being and child development is essential.
>
> **Source:** Cameron, E. E., Joyce, K. M., Delaquis, C. P., et al. (2020). Maternal psychological distress & mental health service use during the COVID-19 pandemic. *Journal of Affective Disorders, 276,* 765–774. https://doi.org/10.1016/j.jad.2020.07.081

keeping these guidelines in mind. The use of a clinical pathway is intended to improve patient care. The patient is expected to begin to progress toward a resolution of acute symptoms, assume personal responsibility, improve interpersonal functioning, and participate in discharge planning. Patients with prolonged mental illness benefit most from a seamless transition to community services. Such a transition is facilitated through collaboration with community mental health services and through the intensive case-management programs available there. Readiness for community re-entry should include preparation by members of the patient's support system for their role in enhancing the patient's mental health. Poverty, stigma, unemployment, and lack of appropriate housing are identified as major barriers to recovery of mental health. The nurse needs to consider these gaps when planning discharge for patients from acute care settings, as the gaps can delay discharge and increase the likelihood of readmission.

Assertive Community Treatment

Assertive community treatment (ACT) is an intensive type of case management developed in response to the community-living needs of people with serious, persistent psychiatric symptoms (Guan et al., 2021). Patients with severe symptoms are referred to ACT teams by inpatient or outpatient providers because of a pattern of repeated hospitalizations, along with an inability to participate in traditional treatment.

ACT teams work intensively with patients in their homes or in agencies, hospitals, or clinics, whatever settings patients find themselves in. Creative problem solving and interventions are hallmarks of the care provided by mobile teams. The ACT concept takes into account that people need support and resources after 1700 hours, and teams are on call 24 hours a day. ACT teams are interprofessional and typically composed of psychiatric mental health nurses, social workers, psychologists, advanced-practice RNs, and psychiatrists. One of these professionals (often the nurse) serves as the case manager and may have a caseload of up to 10 patients who require visits three to five times per week. Length of treatment may extend to years, until the patient is ready to accept transfer to a less intensive site for care.

The vignette illustrates a typical day for a psychiatric mental health nurse on an ACT team.

> **VIGNETTE**
> Tazmine meets with Shane and his mother on the day of discharge to review the aftercare arrangements. Tazmine reviews the goals that were established by the treatment team and Shane's own goal for hospitalization. She reviews the accomplishments Shane made during his hospitalization; reinforces the importance of medication adherence; reviews each prescription, highlighting how and when the medication must be taken; and tells Shane when and where his aftercare appointment is. Tazmine answers Shane's and his mother's questions.

Ensuring Safety

Safety is one of the most important aspects an overarching aspect of care in any setting. Protecting the patient is essential, but equally important is the safety of the staff and other patients. Nurses maintain safety primarily through collaborative teamwork, good patient assessment, respectful attention to patient concerns, and recognition and de-escalation of potentially dangerous situations.

Safety needs are identified and individualized interventions begin on admission. In a community, a thorough risk assessment is completed. In addition to this assessment in inpatient settings, staff should check all personal property and clothing to prevent any potentially harmful items from being taken onto the unit (e.g., medication, alcohol, sharp objects). Some people are at greater risk for suicide than others, and nurses must

> **VIGNETTE**
> Maria Restrepo is a nurse who works on an assertive community treatment (ACT) team at a large, inner-city university medical centre. She had 5 years of inpatient experience before joining the ACT team, and she works with two social workers, two psychiatrists, and a mental health worker.
>
> **0800–0930:** Maria starts the day at the clinic site with team rounds. Because she was on call over the weekend, she updates the team on three emergency department visits: two patients were able to return home after she met with them and the emergency department physician; one patient was admitted to the hospital because he made threats to his caregiver.
>
> **0930–1030:** Maria's first patient is Mr. Zaman, a 35-year-old man with a diagnosis of bipolar disorder and alcohol dependence. He lives with his mother and has a history of five hospitalizations with non-adherence to outpatient clinic treatment. Except during his manic episodes, he isolates himself at home or visits a friend in the neighbourhood, at whose house he drinks excessively. Today he is due for his biweekly haloperidol decanoate (Haldol Decanoate) injection (a long-acting anti-psychotic medication). Maria goes first to his house and learns that he is not at home. She speaks with his mother about his recent behaviour and an upcoming medical clinic appointment. Then she goes to the friend's house and finds Mr. Zaman playing cards and drinking a beer. He and his friend are courteous to her, and Mr. Zaman cooperates in receiving his injection. He listens as Maria repeats teaching about the risks of alcohol consumption. She encourages his attendance at an Alcoholics Anonymous meeting. He reports that he did go to one meeting yesterday. Maria praises him and encourages him and his friend to go again that night.
>
> **1100–1300:** The next patient is Ms. Abbott, a 53-year-old single woman with a diagnosis of schizoaffective disorder and hypertension. She lives alone in a building for older adults and has no contact with family. Ms. Abbott was referred by her clinic team because she experienced three hospitalizations for psychotic decompensation over a period of a year despite receiving monthly Haloperidol decanoate injections. The ACT team is now the payee for her disability cheque. Today, Maria is taking Ms. Abbott out to pay her bills and to see her primary care physician for a checkup. Ms. Abbott greets Maria warmly at the door, wearing excessive makeup and inappropriate summer clothing. With gentle encouragement, she agrees to wear warmer clothes. She is reluctant to show Maria her medication box and briefly gets irritable when Maria

points out that she has not taken her morning medications. As they stop by the apartment office to pay the rent, Maria talks with the manager briefly. This apartment manager is the team's only contact person and calls the team whenever any of the other residents report that Ms. Abbott is exhibiting unusual behaviour. Over the next hour and a half, Maria and Ms. Abbott drive to various stores and to Ms. Abbott's medical appointment.

1400–1630: The last patient visit of the day is with Mr. Hahn, a 60-year-old widowed man diagnosed with schizophrenia and cocaine dependence. Mr. Hahn was referred by the emergency department last year after repeated visits due to psychosis and intoxication. Initially he was homeless, but he now lives in a recovery house shelter and has been clean of illegal substances for 6 months. He receives a monthly decanoate injection and is socially isolated in the house. Now that he receives disability support payments, he is seeking an affordable apartment. Maria has made appointments at two apartment buildings. After greeting him, Maria notes that he is wearing the same clothes he had on 2 days earlier and his hair is uncombed. She suggests that he shower and change his clothes before they go out, and he agrees.

At the end of the day, Maria jots down information she will use to write her progress notes in patients' charts the next day when she returns to the clinic.

BOX 3.2 Patient Safety Goals in Mental Health Care Settings

- Improve the accuracy of patient identification:
  - Use at least two ways, such as the patient's name and date of birth, to identify patients.
- Improve the effectiveness of communication among caregivers:
  - Read back verbal orders.
  - Create a list of abbreviations and symbols that are not to be used.
  - Promptly report critical tests and critical results.
- Improve the safety of using medications:
  - Create a list of look-alike and sound-alike medications.
- Reduce the risk of health care–associated infections:
  - Follow hand-cleaning guidelines from the World Health Organization.
  - Record and report death or injury from infection.
- Accurately and completely reconcile medications across the continuum of care:
  - Compare current and newly ordered medications for compatibility.
  - Give a list of medications to the next provider and regular caregiver.
  - Provide a medication list to both the patient and the family.
- Encourage patients' active involvement in their own care:
  - Encourage patients and families to report safety concerns.
- Identify safety risks inherent in the patient population:
  - Identify individuals at risk for suicide.

Source: Adapted from Accreditation Canada. (2012). *Qmentum program standards*. Ottawa: Author.

---

be skillful in evaluating this risk through questions and observations. Understanding the types of precautions used in each setting is one of the most important tasks a new staff member or nursing student can learn.

Accreditation Canada (2020) publishes required patient safety practices for Canadian hospitals (also see Brickell et al., 2009, for developing work on patient safety guidelines specific to mental health care in Canada). Box 3.2 lists important safety goals for care in mental health settings.

Due to the increased acuity of patients receiving care on an inpatient unit, further precautions are taken. The nurse supervises the unit for overall safety. One of the most important interventions is tracking patients' whereabouts and activities. These checks are done periodically or continuously, depending on patients' risk for a health crisis or self-harm. Visitors are another potential safety hazard. Although visitors can contribute to patients' healing through socialization, acceptance, and familiarity, visits may be overwhelming or distressing. Also, visitors may unwittingly or purposefully provide patients with unsafe items such as sharp objects, glass, or drugs; bags and packages brought onto the unit should be inspected by unit staff. Sometimes unsafe items take the form of comfort foods from home or a favourite restaurant, and these should be monitored because they may be incompatible with prescribed diets or medications.

When the patient's illness is affecting insight and judgement, intimate relationships between patients are discouraged or expressly prohibited. There are risks for sexually transmitted infections, pregnancy, and emotional distress at a time when patients are vulnerable and may lack the capacity for consent.

Aggression and violence are also risks when a patient's illness affects perception, thinking, insight, judgement, and behaviour. This risk also increases if patients have reduced outlets for frustration. Aggression in the mental health workplace is an important concern (Geoffrion et al., 2020). Psychiatric staff should have specialized training to minimize hostility while maintaining an atmosphere that promotes healthy and appropriate expression of anger and other feelings. Many psychiatric units are locked since some patients are hospitalized involuntarily, and elopement (absence from the unit without leave) must be prevented in a way that avoids an atmosphere of imprisonment, which can increase the risk for agitation and aggression.

One of the most important safety aspects of a psychiatric service area is the design of patient care areas. These areas are usually less institutional looking than other hospital areas. Closets should be equipped with "break-bars" designed to hold a minimal amount of weight; windows, with shatterproof glass, are locked; beds are often platforms rather than mechanical hospital beds, which can be dangerous because of their crushing potential; and showers should have non–weight-bearing shower heads.

Differences in characteristics, treatment outcomes, and interventions between inpatient and community settings are outlined in Table 3.1. Note that all of these interventions fall within the practice domain of the basic-level RN or RPN.

PSYCHIATRIC MENTAL HEALTH NURSING: ROLES AND RESPONSIBILITIES

As noted in Chapter 1, psychiatric mental health nurses are educated at a variety of levels, including diploma, baccalaureate, master's, and doctoral. Perhaps the most significant distinction among the multiple levels of preparation is the extent to which the nurse acts autonomously and provides consultation to other providers, both inside and outside the particular workplace. The health professions acts of individual provinces and territories grant nurses authority to practice. Each Canadian nursing regulator also has additional codes that nurses must use to guide their practice. Table 3.2 describes the roles of psychiatric mental health nurses according to the level of education.

COMMUNITY PSYCHIATRIC MENTAL HEALTH NURSING

Psychiatric mental health nursing in the community setting requires strong problem-solving and clinical skills, cultural sensitivity, flexibility, solid knowledge of community resources, and comfort with functioning more autonomously than acute care nurses do. Patients need assistance with problems related to individual psychiatric symptoms,

TABLE 3.1 Characteristics, Treatment Outcomes, and Interventions by Setting

Inpatient Setting	Community Mental Health Setting
Characteristics	
Unit locked by staff	Home locked by patient
24-hour supervision	Intermittent supervision
Boundaries determined by staff	Boundaries negotiated with patient
Milieu with food, housekeeping, security services	Patient-controlled environment with self-care, safety risks
Treatment Outcomes	
Stabilization of symptoms and return to community	Stable or improved level of functioning in community
Interventions	
Develop short-term therapeutic relationship	Establish long-term therapeutic relationship
Develop comprehensive plan of care, with attention to sociocultural needs of patient	Develop comprehensive plan of care for patient and support system, with attention to sociocultural needs
Enforce boundaries by seclusion or restraint as needed	Negotiate boundaries with patient
Administer medication	Encourage adherence to medication regimen
Monitor nutrition and self-care, with assistance as needed	Teach and support adequate nutrition and self-care and provide referrals as needed
Provide health assessment and intervention as needed	Assist patient in self-assessment and self-management and provide referrals to meet health needs in community as needed
Offer structured socialization activities	Use creative strategies to refer patient to positive social activities
Plan for discharge to housing with family or significant other and plan for follow-up treatment	Communicate regularly with family or support system to assess and improve patient's level of functioning

family and support systems, and basic living needs, such as housing and financial support. Community treatment hinges on enhancing patients' strengths in the same environment in which they maintain their daily life, which makes individually tailored psychiatric care imperative. Treatment in the community permits patients and those involved in their support to learn new ways of coping with symptoms or situational difficulties. The result can be one of empowerment and self-management for patients and their support systems.

Biopsychosocial Assessment

Assessment of the needs and capacities of patients living in the community requires expansion of the general psychiatric mental health nursing assessment (see Chapter 6). To be able to plan and implement effective treatment, the community psychiatric mental health nurse must also develop a comprehensive understanding of the patient's ability to cope with the demands of living in the community. The **biopsychosocial model** is a system that can guide the nursing assessment and interventions in a holistic manner, viewing patients comprehensively, including their biology, social environment and skills, and psychological characteristics. Box 3.3 identifies the broad treatment team members involved in care, whether in the community or acute care. The biopsychosocial assessment depends on these interprofessional perspectives.

A well-communicated, strong biopsychosocial assessment is strongly related to the probability that the patient will experience successful outcomes in the community. Problems in any of the following areas require immediate attention because they can seriously influence mental health–related disability and impair the success of other treatment goals:

TABLE 3.2 Community Psychiatric Mental Health Nursing Roles Relevant to Educational Preparation

Role	Advanced Practice (MN, PhD)	Basic Practice (Diploma, BScN)
Practice	Nurse practitioner or clinical nurse specialist; manage patient care and prescribe or recommend interventions independently	Provide nursing care for patient and assist with medication management as prescribed, under direct supervision
Consultation	Act as consultant to staff about plan of care, to patient and family about options for care; collaborate with community agencies about service coordination and planning processes	Consult with staff about care planning and work with nurse practitioner or physician to promote health and mental health care; consult with patient and family about options for care; collaborate with community agencies about service coordination and planning processes; collaborate with staff from other agencies
Administration	Assume administrative or contract consultant role within mental health agencies or mental health authority	Take leadership role within mental health treatment team
Research and education	Take on role as educator or researcher within agency or mental health authority	Participate in research at agency or mental health authority; serve as preceptor to undergraduate nursing students

BOX 3.3 POTENTIAL MEMBERS OF PSYCHIATRIC MENTAL HEALTH TREATMENT TEAMS

Registered Psychiatric Nurses: Licensed professionals trained with an extensive focus on the knowledge and skills required for psychiatric mental health nursing (see the Registered Psychiatric Nurse Regulators of Canada website: http://www.rpnc.ca/pages/home.php).

Registered Nurses: Registered nurses working in psychiatric mental health care do not necessarily have specific certification, but many have some specialty experience. Registered nurses in Canada can complete a specialty certificate in psychiatric mental health nursing (see the Canadian Nurses Association certification program: http://www.nurseone.ca/Default.aspx?portlet=StaticHtmlViewerPortlet&plang=1&ptdi=153). Among the responsibilities of a registered nurse are diagnosing and treating responses to psychiatric disorders, coordinating care, counselling, giving medication and evaluating responses, and providing education.

Licensed Practical Nurses or Registered Practical Nurses: Provincial or territorial licensing or registration bodies regulate these professionals by determining entry-to-practice requirements and establishing and promoting standards for registration, practice, and professional conduct. These nurses are involved with the care of psychiatric patients by providing care within their scope of practice as determined by their provincial or territorial governing body.

Psychiatric Mental Health Advanced-Practice Nurses: Psychiatric mental health advanced-practice nurses work as nurse therapists, clinical nurse specialists, or education specialists by virtue of advanced training (e.g., master's or doctorate prepared) or recognized advanced level of experience. These nurses may be involved in conducting therapy, case management, consulting, education, or research.

Social Workers: Basic-level social workers help the patient prepare a support system that will promote mental health upon discharge from the hospital. They may help patients develop contacts with day treatment centres, employers, sources of financial aid, and landlords. Social workers can also undergo training in individual, family, and group therapies and function as primary care providers.

Counsellors: Counsellors prepared in disciplines such as psychology, rehabilitation counselling, nursing or psychiatric nursing, and addiction counselling may augment the treatment plan by co-leading groups, providing basic supportive counselling, or assisting in psychoeducational and recreational activities. Private counselling services in the community are not covered by Medicare.

Psychologists: In keeping with their doctoral degree preparation, psychologists conduct psychological testing, provide consultation for the team, and offer direct services such as specialized individual, family, or marital therapies. Psychologists' services in the community are not covered by Medicare.

Occupational, Recreational, Art, Music, and Dance Therapists: Based on their specialist preparation, these therapists assist patients in gaining skills that help them cope more effectively, gain or retain employment, use leisure time to the benefit of their mental health, and express themselves in healthy ways.

Psychiatrists: Depending on their specialty of preparation, psychiatrists may provide in-depth psychotherapy or medication therapy or head a team of mental health providers functioning as a community-based service. Psychiatrists may be employed by the hospital or may hold practice privileges in the facility. Because psychiatry is a medical specialty, treatment and care by psychiatrists—with the exception of psychoanalysis—is covered by Medicare. Because they have the legal power to prescribe and to write orders, psychiatrists often function as the leaders of the teams managing the care of patients individually assigned to them.

Medical Physicians: Medical physicians provide medical diagnoses and treatments on a consultation basis. Medical physicians will also provide referrals to psychiatrists, mental health nurses, psychologists, and social workers when needed. Occasionally, a physician trained as an addiction specialist may play a more direct role on a unit that offers treatment for addictive disease.

Health Care Aides: Health care aides function under the direction and supervision of nurses. They provide assistance to patients in meeting basic needs and also help the community to remain supportive, safe, and healthy.

Community Mental Health Workers: Community mental health workers are registered nurses or registered psychiatric nurses, social workers, or other trained professionals who offer case management and care in the community at various levels of intensity. Community mental health workers are sometimes involved in hospital-treatment-team and patient-discharge planning.

Pharmacists: In view of the intricacies of prescribing, coordinating, and administering combinations of psychotropic and other medications, the consulting pharmacist can offer a valuable safeguard. Physicians and nurses collaborate with the pharmacist regarding new medications, which are being introduced at a steady rate.

Spiritual Carers: Spiritual advisors can play an important role in addressing the spiritual, and sometimes cultural, aspects of patients' lives and support spirituality as a coping resource.

- Housing adequacy and stability: A patient who faces daily fears of homelessness will not be able to focus on the treatment.
- Income and source of income: A patient must have a basic income, whether from an entitlement, a relative, or other sources, to obtain necessary medication and meet daily needs for food and clothing.
- Family and support system: The presence of a family member, friend, or neighbour supports the patient's recovery and gives the nurse a contact person (with the patient's consent).
- Substance use history and current use: Often hidden or minimized during hospitalization, substance use can be a destructive force, undermining medication effectiveness and interfering with relationships, safety, community acceptance, and procurement of housing.
- Physical well-being: Factors that increase health risks and decrease lifespan for individuals with mental illnesses include decreased physical activity, smoking, adverse effects of medications, and absence of routine health exams.

Individual cultural characteristics are also very important to assess. For example, working with a patient who speaks a different language than the nurse does requires the nurse to consider the implications of language and cultural background. In such a case, the use of a translator or cultural consultant from the agency or from the family is essential (see Chapter 8).

Treatment Goals and Interventions

In the community setting, treatment goals and interventions are negotiated rather than imposed on the patient. To meet a broad range of patient needs, community psychiatric mental health nurses must approach interventions with flexibility and resourcefulness. Not unexpectedly, patient outcomes with regard to mental status and functional level have been found to be more positive and achieved with greater cost-effectiveness when the community psychiatric mental health nurse integrates case management into the professional role (Latimer et al., 2020). The complexity of navigating the mental health and social service funding systems is often overwhelming to patients. The 1980s brought increased emphasis on case management as a core nursing function in treating the patient with serious mental illness.

In the private domain as well, case management, or care management, found a niche. The intent was to charge case managers with designing individually tailored treatment services for patients and tracking outcomes of care. The new case management included assessing patient needs, developing a plan for service, linking the patient with necessary services, monitoring the effectiveness of services, and advocating for the patient as needed. Newer models, particularly team concepts, have since been developed and will be discussed later in this chapter.

Interprofessional Team Member

Interprofessional psychiatric nursing practice is one of the core mental health disciplines that work to the patient's benefit. In interprofessional team meetings, the individual and discipline-specific expertise of each member is recognized. Generally, the composition of the team reflects the availability of fiscal and professional resources in the area. The community psychiatric team may include psychiatrists, nurses, social workers, psychologists, addictions specialists, recreational therapists, occupational therapists, and mental health workers.

The nurse is able to integrate a strong nursing identity into the team perspective. At the basic- or advanced-practice level, the community psychiatric mental health nurse holds a critical position to link the biopsychosocial and spiritual components relevant to mental health care. The nurse also communicates a discipline-specific expertise in a manner that the patient, significant others, and other members of the health care team can understand. In particular, the management and administration of psychotropic medications have become significant tasks the community nurse is expected to perform.

Biopsychosocial Care Manager

The role of the community psychiatric mental health nurse includes coordinating mental health, physical health, spiritual health, social service, educational service, and vocational realms of care for the mental health patient. The reality of community practice in the new millennium is that few patients seeking treatment have uncomplicated symptoms of a single mental illness. The severity of illness has increased, and it is often accompanied by substance use, poverty, and stress. Repeated studies show that people with mental illnesses also have a higher risk for medical disorders than the general population (Gaulin et al., 2019).

The community psychiatric mental health nurse bridges the gap between the psychiatric and physical needs of the patient, meeting not only with the mental health treatment team but also with the patient's primary care team and serving as the liaison between the two.

Treatment Team

Psychiatric nursing practice is one of the core mental health disciplines that work with a patient to improve well-being. The health care team may include psychiatrists, nurses, social workers, psychologists, addictions specialists, recreational therapists, occupational therapists, and mental health workers. Generally, the composition of the team reflects the availability of fiscal and professional resources in the area.

In team meetings, the individual and discipline-specific expertise of each member is recognized (Box 3.3). The person with the mental illness is also an important member of the team. It is the nurse's responsibility to ensure that a space is created for this person's voice within the team. Input from the patient and family (if available and desirable) is critical in formulating treatment goals. To take part in decision making, though, a patient must be knowledgeable about the illness and treatment options. Research demonstrates that people with mental illness want more than watered-down and simplistic information. (Imagine a pamphlet titled *You and Your Mental Illness*.) To fully participate in the treatment plan, patients need current, evidence-informed information about their illness and treatment options (Hamlett et al., 2016). Incorporating the patient's feedback in developing the treatment plan goals increases the likelihood of the success of established care outcomes.

Members of each discipline are responsible for gathering data and participating in the planning of care. Patients may find meeting with so many people and answering similar questions from each of them extremely stressful or threatening; team members therefore must consider appropriate timing. The urgency of the need for data should be weighed against the patient's ability to tolerate assessment. Assessments, in particular, suicide assessments, made by the nurse often provide the basis for initial care. In many inpatient settings, the psychiatrist must evaluate the patient and provide orders within a limited time frame.

There are three regulated nursing professions in Canada: licensed practical nurse (LPN) or registered practical nurse (RPN), licensed registered nurse (RN), and licensed registered psychiatric nurse (RPN). The nurse has a leadership role in the team meetings. This nursing leadership reflects the holistic nature of nursing, as well as the fact that nursing is the discipline that is represented in the unit at all times. Nurses are in a unique position to advocate on behalf of the patient and to contribute valuable information such as continuous assessment findings, the patient's adjustment to the unit, and any health concerns, psychoeducational needs, and patient self-care deficits.

Multidisciplinary teams use their team members' individual levels of expertise to develop individual care plans. A care plan is developed by each discipline. For example, nursing develops a nursing care plan, and physiotherapy develops its own care plan. Although these plans of care may be housed in the same patient chart, they are discipline specific, and each discipline is responsible for obtaining its own goals. In contrast, an **interdisciplinary** team develops one care plan. All of the health care providers will work toward the same goals for the patient. For example, the goal may be for the patient to improve his or her self-concept; then nursing provides nursing interventions that lead to this outcome, and occupational therapy provides interventions that also lead to this outcome. With an interdisciplinary treatment plan, the overlap of professional scope of practice is recognized and shared goals are established. The team composes the plan of care, which is often based on the appropriate clinical pathway, revising the plan along the way if the patient's progress differs from that expected. A reduction in overt symptoms and the development of an adequate outpatient plan signal that discharge is near.

Within an interdisciplinary treatment team, the nurse may take on several roles. The role of the psychiatric mental health nurse includes coordinating mental health, physical health, spiritual health, social service, educational service, and vocational realms of care for the mental health patient. The reality of practice in the new millennium is that few patients seeking treatment have uncomplicated symptoms of a single mental illness. The severity of illness has increased, and it is often accompanied by substance use, poverty, and stress. Repeated studies show that people with mental illnesses also have a higher rate of mental–physical disorder comorbidity than the general population (Gaulin et al., 2019).

> **VIGNETTE**
>
> Joelle is assigned as Shane's primary nurse, with Tazmine as his evening-shift nurse. Joelle met with the treatment team to plan Shane's care during his hospitalization. The physician's diagnosis was major depression with psychotic features. The major problems the team identified, based on reports of the past 2 days and nursing assessments, were safety, paranoia, nonadherence to medication regimens, and hypertension. Joelle identified that the nursing diagnoses were risk for self-directed violence, disturbed thought processes, nonadherence, and deficient knowledge. Along with the treatment team, Joelle identified the therapy and psychoeducation groups that Shane should participate in and recommended that suicide-precaution monitoring be maintained, owing to Shane's inability to promise that he would not harm himself in the unit or that he would tell one of the staff members if his thoughts about suicide changed.

The psychiatric mental health nurse bridges the gap between the psychiatric and physical needs of the patient, meeting not only with the mental health treatment team but also with the patient's primary care team and serving as the liaison between the two. Case management includes the care coordination activities the nurse does with or for the patient and includes referrals, assistance with paperwork applications, connection to resources, and overall navigation of the health care system. The complexity of navigating the mental health and social service funding systems is often overwhelming to patients. The 1980s brought increased emphasis on case management as a core nursing function in treating the patient with serious mental illness. According to Latimer and colleagues (2020), integrating a nurse case manager to assist patients with primary care needs results in greater success with follow-up and attendance at appointments. Many case managers assess patient needs, design individually tailored treatment services for patients, link the patient with necessary services, monitor the effectiveness of services, and advocate for the patient as needed.

Nursing Care

Establishing a Therapeutic Relationship

Being admitted to a psychiatric mental health care service is anxiety provoking for anyone, but anxiety can be severe for patients admitted to an inpatient psychiatric unit. Especially for the first-time patient, admission often summons preconceptions about psychiatric hospitals and the negative stigma associated with them. Patients may experience shame, and families may be reluctant to be forthcoming with pertinent information. Psychiatric mental health nurses can be most effective when they are sensitive to both the patient and the family during the admission process. In this initial encounter with the patient, nurses must try to provide reassurance and hope.

Mental and Physical Health Assessment

Upon admission, the nurse will assess the patient with the goals of gathering information that will enable the treatment team to develop a suitable plan of care, ensuring that safety concerns are identified and addressed, identifying the learning needs of the patient so the nurse can prioritize the information needs, and initiating a therapeutic relationship between the nurse and the patient. Chapters 6 and 10 present a more detailed discussion of how to perform an admission assessment, as well as a mental status examination.

The nurse is in an excellent position to assess not only mental health but also physical health. Rates of metabolic syndrome, diabetes, and heart disease are all higher for individuals with mental health problems (Costa-Dookhan et al., 2020). Nurses can play a key role in assessing for these problems and initiating patient teaching, individual counselling and therapies, and supports for prevention and management.

Individuals with mental health problems may experience barriers to health care and healthy living practices necessary to maintain their health (Socias et al., 2016). Often, when patients with pre-existing or comorbid conditions seek treatment in the ED for a physical medical condition, health care providers will downplay or attribute the patient's physical complaints to the psychiatric condition. Patients also report reluctance to seek out health care providers, owing to the stigma they encounter when they reveal they are being treated for a comorbid psychiatric illness. This reluctance to seek treatment not only adversely affects the patient's quality of life but also contributes to a decreased life expectancy.

Milieu Management

A well-managed milieu offers patients a sense of security and comfort. Structured aspects of the milieu include activities, program and unit rules, reality orientation practices, and the environment. In addition to the structured components of the milieu, Peplau (1989) described other less tangible factors, such as the interactions that occur among patients and staff, patients and patients, and patients and visitors. This interactivity is quite different from the environment of medical inpatient units, where patients generally remain in their rooms, often with closed doors, and rarely interact with other patients or the milieu. On psychiatric units, patients are in constant contact with their peers and staff. These interactions help patients engage and can increase their sense of social competence and worth.

The therapeutic milieu can serve as a real-life training ground for learning about the self and practising communication and coping skills in preparation for a return to the community. Even events that seemingly distract from the program of therapies can be turned into valuable learning opportunities for the members of the milieu. Nurses can support the milieu and intervene when necessary. They usually develop an uncanny ability to assess the mood of the unit (e.g., calm, anxious, disengaged, or tense) and predict environmental risk. Nurses observe the dynamics of interactions, reinforce adaptive social skills, and redirect patients during negative interactions. Reports from shift to shift provide information on the emotional climate and level of tension in the unit.

Structured Group Activities

In most mental health programs, experienced psychiatric mental health nurses conduct specific, structured activities involving the therapeutic community, special groups, or families. Examples of these activities include morning goal-setting meetings and evening goal-review meetings. Community meetings may be held daily or at scheduled times during the week. At these meetings, new patients are greeted, and departing patients are given farewells; ideas for unit activities are discussed; community problems or successes are considered; and other business of the therapeutic community is conducted.

Nurses also offer psychoeducational groups for patients and families on topics such as stress management, coping skills, grieving, medication management, healthy-living practices, and communication skills. Group therapy is a specialized therapy led by a mental health practitioner with advanced training. This therapy addresses communication and sharing, helps patients explore life problems and decrease their isolation and anxiety, and engages patients in the recovery

> **VIGNETTE**
> During the evening shift, Tazmine observes that Shane is restless and pacing in the hallway. Tazmine recalls that when he was admitted, Shane was asked if he had been aggressive in the past. He stated that he had periods of being angry when he felt people were not listening to him or were telling him what to do. Tazmine also recalls that Shane said that he has never struck or hit anyone before and that he usually handles anger by taking a walk around the neighbourhood or going to his room.
> Tazmine asks Shane how things are going. He tells her he is upset because he told the doctor he wanted to be discharged, and the doctor said he was not ready yet. Tazmine affirms that this must be frustrating. She suggests that Shane practise some of the relaxation techniques he learned in the coping group today to manage his feelings of anger. Tazmine also asks Shane if he would like the medication that has been ordered to manage his feelings of agitation when necessary. Shane agrees to take 2 mg lorazepam (Lorazepam) orally and to relax in his room until he feels in better control of his anger. Tazmine goes to see Shane after 30 minutes. She provides positive feedback about his ability to successfully handle his aggressive feelings.

process. Chapter 33 presents a more detailed discussion of therapeutic groups led by nurses.

Documentation

Documentation of patient progress is the responsibility of the entire mental health care team. Although communication among team members and coordination of services are the primary goals when choosing a system for charting, practitioners in the inpatient setting must also consider professional standards, legal issues, and accreditation by regulatory agencies. Information must also be in a format that is retrievable for quality-assurance monitoring, utilization management, peer review, and research. Chapter 7 gives an overview of documentation options.

Medication Administration

The safe administration of medications and the monitoring of their effects is a responsibility for psychiatric mental health nurses, who are expected to have detailed knowledge of psychoactive medications and the interactions and psychological adverse effects of other medications. Nurse reports regarding the patient's adherence to the medication regimen, the presence or absence of adverse effects, and changes in the patient's behaviours exert great influence on the physician's medication decisions. For example, feedback about excessive sedation or increased agitation may lead to a decrease or increase in the dosage of an antipsychotic medication.

Nurses often have numerous decisions to make about medications that are prescribed to be administered p.r.n. (as needed). These decisions must be based on a combination of factors: the patient's wishes, the team's plan, attempts to use alternative methods of coping, and the nurse's judgements regarding timing and the patient's behaviour. Documentation for administering each p.r.n. medication must include the rationale for its use and its effects.

Medication adherence. One of the nurse's goals during hospitalization is to assist the patient with learning the importance of medication adherence during and after hospitalization. Taking medication regularly is a common challenge for psychiatric patients, often because of irritating adverse effects, lack of understanding about the medications, and lack of sufficient patient consultation in treatment decisions. Educating patients on how to recognize, report, and manage potential adverse effects can help empower patients and increase treatment success. This approach encourages the patient to seek out the nurse when it is time for medications to be administered and fosters responsibility and involvement in the treatment process.

Pain management. Just like others in the general population, psychiatric patients often suffer from medical problems that result in pain (e.g., neck, back, or spine problems; arthritis; migraine headaches). People with psychiatric conditions are often viewed as being unable to accurately assess their own sensations or are labelled "drug seeking," a situation that results in untreated or undertreated pain. Nurses can advocate for patients by stressing that relieving pain is a humanitarian consideration and that a patient in pain is less able to participate in formal activities in the unit and will have greater difficulty focusing on education. Psychological pain, which may manifest as anxiety, is equally distressing and can also decrease the ability of the individual to participate in activities of daily living and community life. Adequate assessment and treatment of pain within the psychiatric population may have a positive impact on the course of mental health disorders.

Crisis Management

Medical crises may occur in any setting; however, they are more common on inpatient units. Nurses anticipate, prevent, and manage emergencies and crises on the unit. These crises may be of a medical or behavioural nature.

Medical crises. Mental health units must be able to assess and stabilize the condition of a patient who experiences a medical crisis. Mental health or addictive disease units that manage detoxification (withdrawal from alcohol or other drugs) must anticipate several common medical crises associated with that process. Mental health units therefore store crash carts containing the emergency medications used to treat shock and cardiorespiratory arrest. Nurses must maintain their cardiopulmonary resuscitation skills and be able to use basic emergency equipment. To be effective and practise at a high level of competency, nurses are advised to attend in-service sessions and workshops designed to teach and maintain skills. Nurses must also be able to alert medical support systems quickly and mobilize transportation to the appropriate medical facility.

Behavioural crises. Behavioural crises can lead to patient violence toward self or others and are usually, but not always, observed to escalate through fairly predictable stages. Crisis prevention and management techniques are practised by staff in most mental health facilities (see the Registered Nurses' Association of Ontario's Best Practice Guideline for Crisis Intervention, https://rnao.ca/bpg/guidelines/crisis-intervention). Many psychiatric hospitals have special teams made up of nurses, psychiatric aides, and other professionals who respond to psychiatric emergencies. Each member of the team takes part in the team effort to defuse a crisis in its early stages. If preventive measures fail, each member of the team participates in a rapid, organized movement designed to immobilize, medicate, or seclude a patient. The nurse is most often this team's leader, not only organizing the plan but also timing the intervention and managing the concurrent use of p.r.n. medications. The nurse can initiate such an intervention in the absence of a physician but must secure a physician's order for restraint or seclusion within a specified time. The nurse also advocates for patients in crisis by ensuring that their legal rights are preserved, no matter how difficult it may be to manage their behaviour. Refer to Chapters 7 and 23 for further discussions about and protocols for the use of restraints and seclusion.

Crises are upsetting and threatening to uninvolved patients and staff as well. A designated staff member usually addresses the uninvolved patient concerns and feelings. This person removes other patients from the area of the crisis and helps them express their fears. Patients may be concerned for their own safety or the welfare of the patient involved in the crisis. They may fear that they, too, might experience such a loss of control. The noninvolved staff members, staff members of the code team, and the patient in crisis all benefit from debriefing after these difficult situations.

FUTURE ISSUES

Barriers to Treatment

Despite the current availability and variety of community psychiatric treatments in Canada, many patients in need of services still do not receive them because of various **barriers to treatment**, factors that impede access to psychiatric care, including stigma, geographical challenges, financial limitations, policy issues, and system shortcomings. Although the stigma of mental illness has lessened over the past 40 years, in part because mental illnesses are now recognized as biologically based and also because many well-known people have admitted to having received psychiatric treatment, many people still are afraid to disclose a psychiatric diagnosis. Instead, they seek medical care for vague somatic complaints from primary care providers, who too often fail to diagnose anxiety or depressive disorders.

In addition to stigma, as mentioned, geographical, financial, and systems factors can impede access to psychiatric care. Mental health services are scarce in some rural areas, and due to funding shortfalls, mental health treatment programs often have wait lists. The 2006 Senate report *Out of the Shadows at Last* (Kirby & Keon, 2006) identified national system and policy problems, including fragmented care for children and adults with serious mental illness, high unemployment and disability among those with serious mental illness, undertreatment of older adults, and lack of national priorities for mental health and suicide prevention. Provincial and other insurance plans do not reimburse for community mental health care at the same level that they cover other health care.

Meeting Changing Demands

It is increasingly recognized that people with mental illness are receiving care in all areas of the health care system. With high rates of mental–physical comorbidities, nurses in all areas need to have a strong foundation of mental health nursing assessment and basic treatment skills. Disaster nursing will also become an increasing area of focus within mental health. There is increasing recognition of the mental–physical needs of survivors of trauma and disaster. Certainly, many of these changing demands will occur within a context of a complex and adaptive health care system. As a result, nurses will need to become increasingly comfortable with ambiguity, have a willingness to be flexible, and become confident in their leadership skills.

KEY POINTS TO REMEMBER

- The basic-level community psychiatric mental health nurse practises in many sites.
- Inpatient psychiatric care is guaranteed for all Canadians, with costs and delivery responsibilities shared by regional, provincial or territorial, and federal governments.
- The continuum of psychiatric treatment includes numerous community treatment alternatives with varying degrees of intensity of care.
- Inpatient care has increasingly become more acute and short term.
- As part of the health care team, the psychiatric mental health nurse functions as a leader.
- Psychiatric mental health nurses require strong skills in management, communication, and collaboration.
- Discharge planning begins on the day of admission and requires input from the treatment team and the community mental health care provider.
- The nurse advocates for the patient and ensures that the patient's rights are protected.
- Monitoring the environment and mitigating risk factors are important components of good care for the patient and for the nurse.
- Basic-level psychiatric mental health nursing interventions include admission, provision of a safe environment, psychiatric and physical assessments, milieu management, documentation, medication administration, and preparation for discharge to the community.
- Documentation is an important form of communication to promote consistency in patient care and to justify the patient's stay in the hospital.
- Barriers to mental health care still exist, but the psychiatric mental health nurse may be able to diminish them.

CRITICAL THINKING

1. Imagine that you were asked for your opinion in regard to your patient's ability to make everyday decisions for himself. What sort of things would you consider as you weighed out safety versus autonomy and personal rights? How would you incorporate your knowledge of protective empowering?
2. If nurses function as equal members of the multidisciplinary mental health team, what differentiates the nurse from the other members of the team?
3. Identify gaps in community care that might affect patient discharge planning.
4. How might the community be affected when patients with serious mental illness live in group homes?

CHAPTER REVIEW

1. A friend recognizes that his depression has returned and tells you he is suicidal and concerned he will harm himself. He is afraid that if he seeks help, he will be involuntarily admitted to a psychiatric hospital, an idea that terrifies him. Which of the following responses best meets his immediate care needs?
   a. Provide emotional support and encourage him to contact his family.
   b. Express your concern for his safety, normalize psychiatric treatment as equal to treatment of any physical condition, and offer to accompany and support him through assessment at a nearby emergency department.
   c. Contact the police or a provincial/territorial magistrate to initiate involuntary assessment.
   d. Assist him with obtaining an outpatient counselling appointment at an area community mental health centre and call him frequently to ensure that he is safe until this appointment occurs.
2. You are about to interview a newly admitted patient on your inpatient mental health unit. This is his first experience with psychiatric treatment. Which of the following interventions would be appropriate for this patient? **Select all that apply.**
   a. Discuss outpatient care options for after discharge.
   b. Anticipate and address possible increased anxiety and shame.
   c. Ensure that the individual understands his rights as a patient on your unit.
   d. Assess the patient for physical health needs that may have been overlooked.
   e. Carefully check all clothing and possessions for potentially dangerous items.
3. Which of the following nursing actions are appropriate in maintaining a safe therapeutic inpatient milieu? Select all that apply.
   a. Interact frequently with both individuals and groups on the unit.
   b. Ensure that none of the unit fixtures can be used for suicide by hanging.
   c. Initiate and support group interactions via therapeutic groups and activities.
   d. Stock the unit with standard hospital beds and other sturdy hospital furnishings.
   e. Provide and encourage opportunities to practise social and other life skills.
   f. Collaborate with housekeeping to provide a safe, pleasant environment.
4. A patient becomes agitated and hostile, threatening to smash a chair into the nurses' station door. Which of the following responses would be most appropriate for the student nurse to make?
   a. Maintain a safe distance and attempt to de-escalate the patient verbally.
   b. When the response team arrives, assist in physically restraining the patient.

c. Assist in promptly moving other patients to a safe distance or separate location.
   d. Meet with the patient immediately after the crisis to help him process what happened.
5. A student is considering a career in mental health nursing. Which of the following statements accurately reflects the role and expectations of mental health nurses in acute care settings?
   a. The primary role of the nurse is to monitor the patients from the nurses' station.
   b. Psychiatric patients rarely need medical care, so nurses do not need medical nursing skills.
   c. The close relationships developed with patients can lead to later romantic relationships.
   d. Mental health nursing requires a high degree of interpersonal comfort and therapeutic skill.
6. You are a community mental health nurse meeting with a patient who has just been discharged from the hospital, where he had received psychiatric care for the first time. Which of the following activities would you expect to undertake in your role as the nurse on the treatment team caring for this patient?
   a. Take medications to the patient's home each day and administer them.
   b. Solve day-to-day problems for the patient to minimize his exposure to stress.
   c. Refer the patient to counsellors or other providers when he indicates a need to talk with someone.
   d. Take a ride on the local bus system with the patient to help him learn routes and schedules.
7. Mrs. Chan, a patient at the community mental health centre, tends to stop taking her medications at intervals, usually leading to decompensation. Which of the following interventions would most likely improve her adherence to her medications?
   a. Help Mrs. Chan understand her illness and allow her to share in decisions about her care.
   b. Advise Mrs. Chan that if she stops her medications, her doctor will hospitalize her.
   c. Arrange for Mrs. Chan to receive daily home care so that her use of medications is monitored.
   d. Discourage Mrs. Chan from focusing on adverse effects and other excuses for stopping her pills.

http://evolve.elsevier.com/Canada/Varcarolis/psychiatric/

REFERENCES

Accreditation Canada. (2020). *Required organizational practices: Handbook 2020*. Ottawa, ON: Author. https://store.accreditation.ca/products/required-organizational-practices-handbook-2017-version-2

Allin, S., Marchildon, G., & Peckman, A. (2020). *International health care system profiles*. International Health Systems. https://www.commonwealthfund.org/international-health-policy-center/countries/canada

Brickell, T. A., Nicholls, T. L., Procyshyn, R. M., McLean, C., Dempster, R. J., Lavoie, J. A. A., Sahlstrom, K. J., Tomita, T. M., & Wang, E. (2009). *Patient safety in mental health*. Edmonton: Canadian Patient Safety Institute and Ontario Hospital Association. https://www.patientsafetyinstitute.ca/en/toolsResources/Research/commissionedResearch/mentalHealthAndPatientSafety/Documents/Mental%20Health%20Paper.pdf

Canadian Institute for Health Information. (2019). *National health expenditure trends, 1975 to 2019*. https://www.cihi.ca/sites/default/files/document/nhex-trends-narrative-report-2019-en-web.pdf

Costa-Dookhan, K., Agarwal, S. M., Chintoh, A., Mackenzie, N., Casuccio-Treen, Q., Remington, G., Ward, K., & Hahn, M. (2020). Investigating metabolic dysfunction and metabolomic profile changes in antipsychotic naive patients. *Schizophrenia Bulletin, 46*, S68. https://doi.org/10.1093/schbul/sbaa031.155

Findlay, L., & Arim, R. (2020). *Canadians report lower self-perceived mental health during the COVID-19 pandemic*. Ottawa: Statistics Canada.

Gaulin, M., Simard, M., Candas, B., Lesage, A., & Sirois, C. (2019). Combined impacts of multimorbidity and mental disorders on frequent emergency department visits: A retrospective cohort study in Quebec, Canada. *CMAJ: Canadian Medical Association Journal, 191*(26), E724–E732. https://doi.org/10.1503/cmaj.181712

Geoffrion, S., Hills, D. J., Ross, H. M., Pich, J., Hill, A. T., Dalsbø, T. K., Riahi, S., Martínez-Jarreta, B., & Guay, S. (2020). Education and training for preventing and minimizing workplace aggression directed toward healthcare workers. *The Cochrane Database of Systematic Reviews, 9*, CD011860. https://doi.org/10.1002/14651858.CD011860.pub2

Government of Canada. (2020). *World mental health day 2020: Video*. Ottawa: Statistics Canada. https://www.sac-isc.gc.ca/eng/1602259188121/1602259217203

Guan, I., Kirwan, N., Beder, M., Levy, M., & Law, S. (2021). Adaptations and innovations to minimize service disruption for patients with severe mental Illness during COVID-19: Perspectives and reflections from an Assertive Community Psychiatry Program. *Community Mental Health Journal, 57*(1), 10–17. https://doi.org/10.1007/s10597-020-00710-8

Hamlett, N. M., Carr, E. R., & Hillbrand, M. (2016). Positive behavioral support planning in the inpatient treatment of severe disruptive behaviors: A description of service features. *Psychological Services, 13*(2), 178–182. https://doi.org/10.1037/ser0000070

Hensel, J. M., Taylor, V. H., Fung, K., Yang, R., & Vigod, S. N. (2018). Acute care use for ambulatory care-sensitive conditions in high-cost users of medical care with mental illness and addictions. *Canadian Journal of Psychiatry. Revue Canadienne de Psychiatrie, 63*(12), 816–825. https://doi.org/10.1177/0706743717752880

Kirby, M. L., & Keon, W. L. (2006). *Out of the shadows at last: Transforming mental health, mental illness and addiction services in Canada*. Ottawa: Standing Senate Committee on Social Affairs, Science and Technology. http://www.mentalhealthcommission.ca/sites/default/files/out_of_the_shadows_at_last_-_full_0_0.pdf

Kopelovich, S. L., Monroe-DeVita, M., Buck, B. E., Brenner, C., Moser, L., Jarskog, L. F., Harker, S., & Chwastiak, L. A. (2020). Community mental health care delivery during the COVID-19 pandemic: Practical strategies for improving care for people with serious mental illness. *Community Mental Health Journal, 57*, 405–415. https://doi.org/10.1007/s10597-020-00662-z

LaJeunesse, R. A. (2002). *Political asylums*. Edmonton: Muttart Foundation.

Latimer, E. A., Rabouin, D., Cao, Z., Ly, A., Powell, G., Aubry, T., Distasio, J., Hwang, S. W., Somers, J. M., Bayoumi, A. M., Mitton, C., Moodie, E. E. M., & Goering, P. N. (2020). Cost-effectiveness of housing first with assertive community treatment: Results from the Canadian At Home/Chez Soi trial. *Psychiatric Services, 71*(10), 1020–1030. https://doi.org/10.1176/appi.ps.202000029

Lequin, P., Golay, P., Herrera, F., Brisard, M. A., & Conus, P. (2021). Recovering the capacity to live outside of a psychiatric hospital: Impact of a specialized inpatient program. *The Psychiatric Quarterly, 92*(2), 751–759. https://doi.org/10.1007/s11126-020-09846-y

McCullumsmith, C., Tikhtman, R., & Benoit, S. C. (2020). Transition clinic: Reducing recidivism. In M. Fitz-Gerald, & J. Takeshita (Eds.), *Models of emergency psychiatric services that work. Integrating psychiatry and primary care* (pp. 85–93). Springer https://doi.org/10.1007/978-3-030-50808-1_8

Mental Health Commission of Canada. (2012). *Changing directions, changing lives: The mental health strategy for Canada*. Calgary: Author. https://www.mentalhealthcommission.ca/wp-content/uploads/drupal/MHStrategy_Strategy_ENG.pdf

Mental Health Commission of Canada. (2016). *Advancing the mental health strategy for Canada: A framework for action (2017–2022)*. Ottawa: Author.

Mental Health Commission of Canada. (2020). *COVID-19 and mental health: Policy responses and emerging issues [environmental scan]*. Ottawa: Author.

Morris, S., Fawcett, G., Timoney, L., & Hughes, J. (2019). *The dynamics of disability: Progressive, recurrent or fluctuating limitations*. Ottawa: Statistics Canada.

O'Reilly, R. L., Chaimowitz, G., Brunet, A., Looper, K., & Beck, P. (2010). Principles underlying mental health legislation [position paper]. *Canadian Journal of Psychiatry, 55*(10), 1–5. https://www.cpa-apc.org/wp-content/uploads/MH-Legislation-Principles-2010-49-web-EN.pdf

Owen, R. D., & Schimmels, J. (2020). Leadership after a crisis: The application of psychological first aid. *Journal of Nursing Administration, 50*(10), 505–507.

Paradis-Gagné, E., Jacob, J.-D., & Pariseau-Legault, P. (2020). What lies at the intersection of law and psychiatric nursing? Exploring the process of judiciarization in the context of mental health. *Witness: The Canadian Journal of Critical Nursing Discourse, 2*(2), 3–19. https://doi.org/10.25071/2291-5796.72

Peplau, H. E. (1989). Interpersonal constructs for nursing practice. In A. W. O'Toole, & S. R. Welt (Eds.), *Interpersonal theory in nursing practice: Selected works of Hildegard E. Peplau* (pp. 42–55). New York: Putnam.

Sealy, P., & Whitehead, P. C. (2004). Forty years of deinstitutionalization of psychiatric services in Canada: An empirical assessment. *Canadian Journal of Psychiatry, 49*(4), 249–257.

Semple, T., Tomlin, M., Bennell, C., & Jenkins, B. (2020). An evaluation of a community-based mobile crisis intervention team in a small Canadian police service. *Community Mental Health Journal, 57*, 567–578. https://doi.org/10.1007/s10597-020-00683-8

Socias, M. E., Shoveller, J., Bean, C., Nguyen, P., Montaner, J., & Shannon, K. (2016). Universal coverage without universal access: Institutional barriers to health care among women sex workers in Vancouver, Canada. *Public Library of Science One, 11*(5), 1–15. https://doi.org/10.1371/journal.pone.0155828

Statistics Canada. (2020). *Canadians with mental health-related disabilities*. Ottawa: Author.

Taube-Schiff, M., Mehak, A., Ferreira, N., Kalim, A., Ungar, T., & Mills, J. S. (2018). Treatment within an adult mental health day program: Examining psychosocial outcomes. *The Journal of Nervous and Mental Disease, 206*(7), 562–566. https://doi.org/10.1097/NMD.0000000000000847

4

Relevant Theories and Therapies for Nursing Practice

Cheryl L. Pollard
Originating US chapter by Margaret Jordan Halter

 http://evolve.elsevier.com/Canada/Varcarolis/psychiatric/

OBJECTIVES

1. Evaluate the premises behind the various therapeutic models discussed in this chapter.
2. Describe the evolution of therapies for psychiatric disorders.
3. Identify ways each theorist has contributed to the nurse's ability to assess a patient's behaviours.
4. Drawing on your experiences, provide the following:
   a. An example of how a patient's irrational beliefs influenced behaviour
   b. An example of counter-transference in your relationship with a patient
   c. An example of the use of behaviour modification with a patient
5. Identify Peplau's framework for the nurse–patient relationship.
6. Choose the therapeutic model that would be most useful for a particular patient or patient problem.

KEY TERMS AND CONCEPTS

automatic thoughts
behavioural therapy
biofeedback
classical conditioning
cognitive behavioural therapy
cognitive distortions
conditioning
conscious
counter-transference
defence mechanisms
dialectical behavioural therapy
ego
extinction
id
interpersonal psychotherapy
intrapsychic conflict
milieu therapy
negative reinforcement
operant conditioning
positive reinforcement
preconscious
psychodynamic therapy
punishment
reinforcement
superego
Tidal Model
transference
unconscious

Every professional discipline, from math, science, medicine, nursing, psychology, sociology, philosophy, to religious studies, bases its work and beliefs on theories. Grand theories are conceptual frameworks in which key concepts and principles are identified. Most of these theories can best be described as explanations, hypotheses, or hunches rather than as testable facts. For example, psychological theories provide us with plausible explanations for various behaviours. Philosophical theories provide us with ways to understand problems. And nursing theories provide us with ways to look at and link the person, health, environment, and nursing. Disciplines will use a variety of grand theories to help guide the development of more specific theories; middle-range theories to analyze a particular situation. The theories reviewed in this chapter are grand and mid-range theories developed by neurologists, psychiatrics, psychologists, sociologists, and nurses that are relevant to psychiatric mental health nursing.

Our patients challenge us to understand experiences that are complex and always unique. A broad base of knowledge about personality development, human needs, the determinants of mental health, contributing factors to mental illness, and the importance of relationships guide our nursing practice. This chapter provides you with a very brief overview of some of the most influential psychological and nursing theories relevant to mental health nursing. These theories include the work of Sigmund Freud on the psychodynamic perspective that emphasizes underlying unconscious psychological processes. Developmental theories are represented by Jean Piaget's research related to cognitive developmental theories that suggest that cognitive development is a process that occurs due to biological maturation and interaction with the environment. Lawrence Kolberg extended developmental theory by applying it to moral development. Also using a developmental approach, Erik Erikson focused on a psychosocial development perspective in which personality continues to evolve past the age of 5 and is influenced by culture and society. Interpersonal theories are represented most notably by Harry Stack Sullivan, Adolph Meyer, and Margaret Mahler. They based their work on the belief that our sense of security, self, and means of motivation are established through interactions with our significant others within our social context. Hildegard Peplau, a psychiatric nurse, built on these ideas as she developed an interpersonal relational model of nursing.

Most behavioural models build upon the works of Ivan Pavlov, B. F. Skinner, or J. B. Watson, which propose that behaviours are learned responses and can be modified through various means of reinforcement. Comparatively, cognitive theorists such as Albert Ellis or Aaron Beck believed that thoughts come before feelings and actions. Humanistic theories focus on the human potential and our ability to choose. One of the more famous humanistic theorists is Abraham Maslow. Although there is no specific person identified as the founder of the biological model/theory, this theoretical perspective guides many mental health practitioners today. The biological model views disease as a malfunction of the body and the goal of treatment is the correction of the malfunction. In addition to exploring the theories in more detail, this chapter also provides an overview of the treatment or therapy these theories inspired and the contributions they have made to our practice of psychiatric mental health nursing. The Canadian Standards for Psychiatric-Mental Health Nursing (Canadian Federation of Mental Health Nurses, 2014) (see Appendix) emphasizes that nurses should develop an evidence-informed practice built on evidence-based models and theories. This chapter will help provide a foundation for you to build your evidence-informed practice. It is important to note that although these theories provide a foundation for practice, they were developed at a different time in history and are written from a colonial perspective. See Chapter 8 for more information on the cultural implications for psychiatric mental health nursing.

PSYCHOANALYTIC THEORIES AND THERAPIES

Sigmund Freud's Psychoanalytic Theory

Sigmund Freud (1856–1939), an Austrian neurologist, revolutionized thinking about mental health disorders with his ground-breaking theory of personality structure, levels of awareness, anxiety, the role of defence mechanisms, and the stages of psychosexual development. Freud came to believe that the vast majority of mental health disorders were caused by unresolved issues that originated in childhood. He arrived at this conclusion through his experiences treating people with hysteria: individuals who were experiencing physical symptoms despite the absence of an apparent physiological cause.

As part of his treatment, Freud initially used hypnosis, but this therapy had mixed therapeutic results. He then changed his approach to talk therapy, known as the *cathartic method*. Today, we about catharsis as a way of "getting things off our chests." This talk therapy evolved to include "free association," which requires full and honest disclosure of thoughts and feelings as they come to mind. Freud (1961, 1969) concluded that talking about difficult emotional issues had the potential to heal the wounds causing mental illness. Viewing the success of these therapeutic approaches led Freud to construct his psychoanalytic theory.

Levels of Awareness

As Freud's psychoanalytic theory developed, he came to believe that there were three levels of psychological awareness. He offered a topographical theory of how the mind functions, using the image of an iceberg to describe three levels of awareness (Figure 4.1).

Conscious. Freud described the conscious part of the mind as the tip of the iceberg. It contains all of the material a person is aware of at any one time, including perceptions, memories, thoughts, fantasies, and feelings.

Preconscious. Just below the surface of awareness is the preconscious, which contains material that can be retrieved rather easily through conscious effort.

Unconscious. The unconscious includes all repressed memories, passions, and unacceptable urges lying deep below the surface. Freud believed that the memories and emotions associated with trauma are often "placed" in the unconscious because the individual finds it too painful to deal with them. The unconscious exerts a powerful yet unseen effect on the conscious thoughts and feelings of the individual. The individual is usually unable to retrieve unconscious material without the assistance of a trained therapist; however, with this assistance, unconscious material can be brought into conscious awareness.

Personality Structure

Freud (1960) delineated three major and distinct but interactive components of the personality: the id, the ego, and the superego.

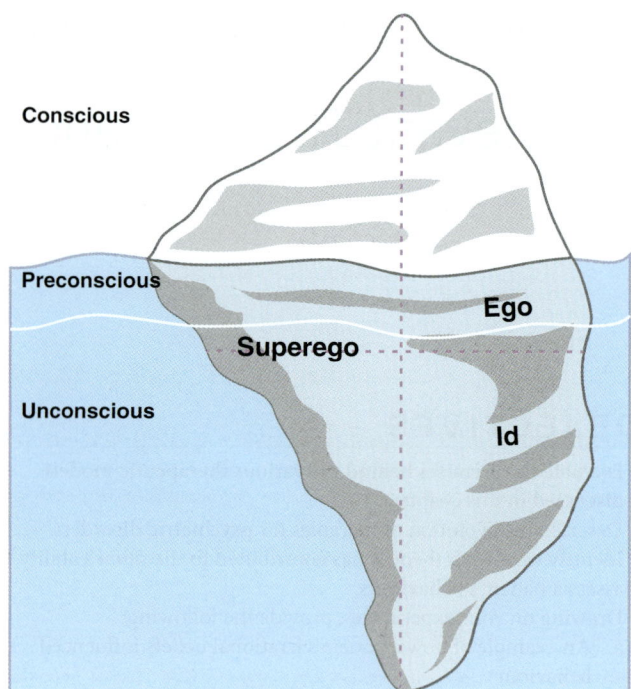

Fig. 4.1 The mind as an iceberg.

Id. At birth our personalities are all id. The id is the source of all drives, instincts, reflexes, needs, and wishes that motivate us. The id cannot tolerate frustration and seeks to discharge tension and return to a more comfortable state. The id lacks the ability to problem-solve; it is not logical and operates according to the pleasure principle. A hungry, screaming infant is the perfect example of id.

Ego. The ego develops because the needs, wishes, and demands of the id cannot be satisfactorily met through primary processes and reflex action. The ego emerges in the fourth or fifth month of life. It is the problem solver and reality tester. It is able to differentiate subjective experiences, memory images, and objective reality and attempts to negotiate a solution with the outside world. The ego follows the reality principle, which says to the id, "You have to delay gratification for right now," and then sets a course of action. For example, a hungry man feels tension arising from the id. His ego allows him not only to think about his hunger but also to plan where he can eat and to seek that destination. This process is known as *reality testing* because the individual is factoring in reality to implement a plan to decrease tension.

Superego. The superego, the last component of the personality to develop, represents the moral aspects of personality. The superego consists of the conscience (all the "should nots" internalized from parents) and the ego ideal (all the "shoulds" internalized from parents). The superego represents the ideal rather than the real; it seeks perfection, as opposed to seeking pleasure or engaging reason.

In a mature and well-adjusted individual the three components of the personality, namely, the id, the ego, and the superego, work together as a team under the administrative leadership of the ego. If the id is too powerful, the person will lack control over impulses; if the superego is too powerful, the person may be self-critical and suffer from feelings of inferiority.

Defence Mechanisms and Anxiety

Freud (1969) believed that anxiety is an inevitable part of living. The environment in which we live presents dangers, insecurities, threats, and satisfactions. It can produce pain and increase tension or produce pleasure and decrease tension. The ego develops defences, or

defence mechanisms, to ward off anxiety by preventing conscious awareness of threatening feelings.

Defence mechanisms share two common features: (1) they all deny, falsify, or distort reality to make it less threatening and (2) they (except suppression) operate on an unconscious level, and we are not aware of their operation. Although we cannot survive without defence mechanisms, it is possible for our defence mechanisms to distort reality to such a degree that we experience difficulty with healthy adjustment and personal growth. Chapter 12 offers further discussions of defence mechanisms.

Psychosexual Stages of Development

Psychoanalytic theorists believe that human development proceeds through five stages from infancy to adulthood. From this perspective, experiences that occur during the first 5 years of life determine an individual's lifetime adjustment patterns. In fact, many think that personality is formed by the time a child enters school and that subsequent growth consists of elaborating on this basic structure. The five psychosexual stages of development, proposed by Freud, are presented in Table 4.1.

Classical Psychoanalysis

Classical psychoanalysis, as developed by Sigmund Freud, is seldom used today. Freud's premise that all mental illness is caused by early **intrapsychic conflict**, a mental struggle, often unconscious, between the id, ego, and superego, is no longer widely thought to be valid, and such therapy requires a lengthy period of treatment, making it prohibitively expensive for most. However, there are two concepts from classic psychoanalysis that are used to guide contemporary mental health nursing practice: transference and counter-transference (Freud, 1969).

Transference develops when the patient experiences feelings toward the nurse or therapist that were originally held toward significant others in his or her life. When transference occurs, these feelings become available for exploration with the patient. Such exploration helps the patient to better understand certain feelings and behaviours. **Counter-transference** is the health care worker's unconscious personal response to the patient. For instance, if the patient reminds you of someone you do not like, you may unconsciously react as if the patient were that individual. Counter-transference underscores the importance of maintaining self-awareness and seeking supervisory guidance

TABLE 4.1 Freud's Psychosexual Stages of Development

Stage (Age)	Source of Satisfaction	Primary Conflict	Tasks	Desired Outcomes	Other Possible Personality Traits
Oral (0–1 year)	Mouth (sucking, biting, chewing)	Weaning	Mastery of gratification of oral needs; beginning of ego development (4–5 months)	Development of trust in the environment, with the realization that needs can be met	Fixation at the oral stage is associated with passivity, gullibility, and dependence; the use of sarcasm; and the development of orally focused habits (e.g., smoking, nail-biting)
Anal (1–3 years)	Anal region (expulsion and retention of feces)	Toilet training	Beginning of development of a sense of control over instinctual drives; ability to delay immediate gratification to gain a future goal	Control over impulses	Fixation at the anal stage is associated with anal retentiveness (stinginess, rigid thought patterns, obsessive-compulsive disorder) or anal-expulsive character (messiness, destructiveness, cruelty)
Phallic (oedipal) (3–6 years)	Genitals (masturbation)	Oedipus and Electra	Sexual identity with parent of same sex; beginning of superego development	Identification with parent of same sex	Lack of successful resolution may result in difficulties with sexual identity and difficulties with authority figures
Latency (6–12 years)	—	—	Growth of ego functions (social, intellectual, mechanical) and the ability to care about and relate to others outside the home (peers of the same sex)	The development of skills needed to cope with the environment	Fixations can result in difficulty identifying with others and in developing social skills, leading to a sense of inadequacy and inferiority
Genital (12 years and beyond)	Genitals (sexual intercourse)	—	Development of satisfying sexual and emotional relationships with members of the opposite sex; emancipation from parents—planning of life goals and development of a strong sense of personal identity	The ability to be creative and find pleasure in love and work	Inability to negotiate this stage could result in difficulties in becoming emotionally and financially independent, lack of strong personal identity and future goals, and inability to form satisfying intimate relationships

Source: Gleitman, H. (1981). *Psychology*. New York: W. W. Norton.

as therapeutic relationships progress. Chapter 9 talks more about counter-transference and the nurse–patient relationship.

Psychodynamic Therapy

Psychodynamic therapy uses many of the theoretical underpinnings of psychoanalytic models, such as unconscious conflicts, relational attachments, personality development, and the use of defence mechanisms. As a result, therapy is approached from a standpoint that unconscious dynamics exist within normal human consciousness and that it is possible in therapy to engage many aspects of the human psyche in ways that are useful, creative, and healing. Techniques used include active listening, reflection, support of ego strength, empathetic communication, and identification of past patterns. Psychodynamic therapy tends to last longer than other common therapeutic modalities and may extend 20 or more sessions.

Clinicians who use this approach when working with patients with psychosis, severe depression, borderline personality disorders, and severe character disorders require advanced training and work in collaboration with a practitioner who specializes in a biomedical approach. Supportive therapies, which are within the scope of practice of the basic-level psychiatric nurse, are useful for these patients. A variety of supportive therapies are described in chapters concerning specific disorders (see Chapters 12 to 20). Techniques common to the approaches discussed earlier and supportive therapies include identification of the presenting problem, identification of goals and values, open-ended questions, and psychoeducation.

Implications of Psychoanalytic Theory for Nursing Practice

Psychoanalytic theory has relevance to nursing practice at many junctures. It offers a comprehensive explanation of complex human processes and suggests that the formation of a patient's personality is influenced by many diverse sources rooted in past events. Freud's theory of the unconscious is particularly valuable as an explanation for understanding the complexity of human behaviour. By considering conscious and unconscious influences, a nurse can begin to think about meanings that might be behind certain behaviours. Psychoanalysts emphasize the importance of individual talk sessions characterized by attentive listening, with a focus on underlying themes as an important tool of healing in psychiatric care.

DEVELOPMENTAL THEORIES

Cognitive Development

Jean Piaget (1896–1980) was a Swiss psychologist and researcher. While working at a boys' school run by Alfred Binet, developer of the Binet Intelligence Test, Piaget helped to score these tests. He became fascinated by the fact that young children consistently gave wrong answers on intelligence tests, wrong answers that revealed a discernible pattern of cognitive processing that was different from that of older children and adults. He concluded that cognitive development was a dynamic progression from primitive awareness and simple reflexes to complex thought and responses. Our mental representations of the world, or schemata, depend on the cognitive stage we have reached.

- *Sensorimotor stage (birth–2 years).* Begins with basic reflexes and culminates with purposeful movement, spatial abilities, and hand–eye coordination. Physical interaction with the environment provides the child with a basic understanding of the world. By about 9 months, object permanence is achieved, and the child can conceptualize objects that are no longer visible. This explains the delight of the game of peek-a-boo as an emerging skill, as the child begins to anticipate the face hidden behind the hands.
- *Preoperational stage (2–7 years). Operations* is a term used to describe thinking about objects. Children are not yet able to think abstractly or generalize qualities in the absence of specific objects but rather think in a concrete fashion. Egocentric thinking is demonstrated through a tendency to expect others to view the world as they do. They are also unable to conserve mass, volume, or number. An example of this is thinking that a tall, thin glass holds more liquid than a short, wide glass.
- *Concrete operational stage (7–11 years).* Logical thought appears and abstract problem solving is possible. The child is able to see a situation from another's point of view and can take into account a variety of solutions to a problem. Conservation is possible. For example, two small cups of liquid are seen as being equal to a tall glass. The child is able to classify based on discrete characteristics, order objects in a pattern, and understand the concept of reversibility.
- *Formal operational stage (11 years–adulthood).* Conceptual reasoning commences at approximately the same time as does puberty. At this stage, the child's basic abilities to think abstractly and problem-solve mirror those of an adult.

Theory of Psychosocial Development

Erik Erikson (1902–1994), an American psychoanalyst, was a follower of Freud. However, Erikson (1963) believed that Freudian theory was restrictive and negative in its approach. He also stressed that factors other than the limited mother–child–father triangle influences an individual's development. According to Erikson, personality is not set in stone at age 5 but continues to develop throughout the lifespan and is influenced by culture and society.

Erikson described development as occurring in eight predetermined and consecutive life stages (psychosocial crises), each of which consists of two possible outcomes (e.g., industry versus inferiority). The successful or unsuccessful completion of each stage affects the individual's progression to the next (Table 4.2). For example, Erikson's crisis of industry versus inferiority occurs from the ages of 7 to 12. During this stage, the child's task is to gain a sense of personal abilities and competence and to expand relationships beyond the immediate family to include peers. The attainment of this task (industry) brings with it the virtue of confidence. The child who fails to navigate this stage successfully is unable to gain a mastery of age-appropriate tasks, cannot make a connection with peers, and will feel like a failure (inferiority).

Stages of Moral Development

Lawrence Kohlberg (1927–1987) was an American psychologist whose work reflected and expanded on Piaget's by applying his theory to moral development. While visiting Israel, Kohlberg became convinced that children living in a kibbutz had advanced moral development, and he believed that the atmosphere of trust, respect, and self-governance nurtured this development. In the United States he created schools or "just communities" that were grounded on these concepts. Based on interviews with youths, Kohlberg developed a theory of how people progressively develop a sense of morality (Kohlberg & Turiel, 1971).

His theory provides a framework for understanding the progression from black-and-white thinking about right and wrong to a complex, variable, and context-dependent decision-making process regarding the rightness or wrongness of action.

Preconventional Level

Stage 1: Obedience and punishment. The hallmarks of this stage are a focus on rules and on listening to authority. People at this stage believe that obedience is the method to avoid punishment.

TABLE 4.2 Erikson's Eight Stages of Development

Approximate Age	Developmental Task	Psychosocial Crisis	Successful Resolution of Crisis	Unsuccessful Resolution of Crisis
Infancy (0–1.5 years)	Forming attachment to mother, which lays foundation for later trust in others	Trust vs. mistrust	Sound basis for relating to other people; trust in people; faith and hope about environment and future, "I'm confident that my son will arrange for me to stay with his family until I'm able to live on my own again."	General difficulties relating to people effectively, suspicion, trust–fear conflict, fear of future, "I can't trust anyone; no one has ever been there when I needed them."
Early childhood (1.5–3 years)	Gaining some basic control of self and environment (e.g., toilet training, exploration)	Autonomy vs. shame and doubt	Sense of self-control and adequacy, willpower, "I'm sure that with the proper diet and exercise program, I can achieve my target weight."	Independence–fear conflict, severe feelings of self-doubt, "I could never lose the weight they want me to, so why even try?"
Late childhood (3–6 years)	Becoming purposeful and directive	Initiative vs. guilt	Ability to initiate one's own activities, sense of purpose, "I like to help Mom by setting the table for dinner."	Aggression–fear conflict, sense of inadequacy or guilt, "I know it's wrong, but I wanted the candy, so I took it."
School age (6–12 years)	Developing social, physical, and school skills	Industry vs. inferiority	Competence, ability to work, "I'm getting really good at swimming since I've been taking lessons."	Sense of inferiority, difficulty learning and working, "I can't read as well as the others in my class; I'm just dumb."
Adolescence (12–20 years)	Making transition from childhood to adulthood, developing sense of identity	Identity vs. role confusion	Sense of personal identity, fidelity, "I'm homosexual, and I'm okay with that."	Confusion about who one is, submersion of identity in relationships or group memberships, "I belong to the gang because without them, I'm nothing."
Early adulthood (20–35 years)	Establishing intimate bonds of love and friendship	Intimacy vs. isolation	Ability to love deeply and commit oneself, "My husband has been my best friend for 25 years."	Emotional isolation, egocentricity, "It's nearly impossible to find a man who is worth marrying."
Middle adulthood (35–65 years)	Fulfilling life goals that involve family, career, and society; developing concerns that embrace future generations	Generativity vs. self-absorption	Ability to give and to care for others, "I've arranged for a 6-month leave of absence to stay with my mother now that her illness is terminal."	Self-absorption, inability to grow as a person, "I've lived with this scar on my face for 3 years; it's worse than having cancer."
Later years (65 years–death)	Looking back over one's life and accepting its meaning	Integrity vs. despair	Sense of integrity and fulfillment, willingness to face death, wisdom, "I've led a happy, productive life, and I'm ready to die."	Dissatisfaction with life, denial of or despair over prospect of death, "I'm not ready to die; the doctors are wrong. You'll see they are wrong."

Sources: Altrocchi, J. (1980). *Abnormal psychology* (p. 196). New York: Harcourt Brace Jovanovich; and Erikson, E. H. (1963). *Childhood and society*. New York: W. W. Norton.

Stage 2: Individualism and exchange. Individuals become aware that not everyone thinks the way that they do and that different people see rules differently. If they or others decide to break the rules, they are risking punishment.

Conventional Level

Stage 3: Good interpersonal relationships. Children begin to view rightness or wrongness as related to motivations, personality, or the goodness or badness of the person. Generally speaking, people should get along and have similar values.

Stage 4: Maintaining the social order. A "rules are rules" mindset returns. However, the reasoning behind it is not simply to avoid punishment; it is because the person has begun to adopt a broader view of society. Listening to authority maintains the social order; bureaucracies and big government agencies often seem to operate with this tenet.

Postconventional Level

Stage 5: Social contract and individual rights. People in stage 5 still believe that the social order is important, but the social order must be *good*. For example, if the social order is corrupt, then rules should be changed, and it is a duty to protect the rights of others.

Stage 6: Universal ethical principles. Actions should create justice for everyone involved. We are obliged to break unjust laws.

Ethics of Care Theory

Carol Gilligan (born 1936) is an American psychologist, ethicist, and feminist who inspired the normative ethics of care theory. She worked with Kohlberg as he developed his theory of moral development and later criticized his work for being based on a sample of boys and men. In addition, she believed that he used a scoring method that favoured males' methods of reasoning, resulting in lower moral development scores for girls as compared with boys. Based on Gilligan's critique, Kohlberg later revised his scoring methods, which resulted in greater similarity between girls' and boys' scores.

Gilligan (1982) suggests that a morality of care should replace Kohlberg's "justice view" of morality, which maintains that we should do what is right no matter the personal cost or the cost to those we love. Gilligan's care view emphasizes the importance of forming relationships, banding together, and putting the needs of those for whom we care about above the needs of strangers. Gilligan asserts that a female approach to ethics has always been in existence but has been trivialized. Like Kohlberg, Gilligan asserts that moral development progresses through three major divisions: preconventional, conventional, and postconventional. These transitions are not dictated by cognitive ability but rather come about through personal development and changes in a sense of self.

Implications of Developmental Theories for Nursing Practice

Nurses continue to use developmental theories as an important part of patient assessment. For example, analysis of behaviour patterns using Erikson's framework can identify age-appropriate or arrested development of normal interpersonal skills. A developmental framework helps the nurse to know what types of interventions are most likely to be effective. For example, preschool and kindergarten-aged children in Piaget's preoperational stage of development respond best if they actively participate in imitative, imaginative, and dramatic play, and ask questions in order to learn how to do things. When this model is used with older patients, they may respond well to a life review strategy that focuses on the integrity of their life as a tapestry of experience. In the therapeutic encounter individual responsibility and the capacity for improving one's functioning are addressed. Treatment approaches and interventions can be tailored to the patient's developmental level.

INTERPERSONAL THEORIES AND THERAPIES

Theory of Object Relations

The theory of object relations was developed by interpersonal theorists who emphasize past relationships in influencing a person's sense of self as well as the nature and quality of relationships in the present. The term *object* refers to another person, particularly a significant person.

Margaret Mahler (1895–1985) was a Hungarian-born child psychologist who worked with emotionally disturbed children. She developed a framework for studying how an infant transitions from complete self-absorption, with an inability to separate from its mother, to a physically and psychologically differentiated toddler. Mahler and colleagues (1975) believed that psychological problems were largely the result of a disruption of this separation.

During the first 3 years of life, the significant other (e.g., the mother) provides a secure base of support that promotes enough confidence for the child to separate. This is achieved by a balance of holding (emotionally and physically) a child enough for the child to feel safe while encouraging independence and natural exploration.

Problems may arise in this process. If a toddler leaves their mother on the park bench and wanders off to the sandbox, the child should be encouraged with smiles and reassurance, "Go on honey. It's safe to go away a little." Then the mother needs to be reliably present when the toddler returns, thereby rewarding their efforts. Mahler notes that raising healthy children does not require that parents never make mistakes and that "good-enough parenting" will promote successful separation-individuation.

Interpersonal Theory

Harry Stack Sullivan (1892–1949), an American-born psychiatrist, initially approached patients using a Freudian framework, but he became frustrated by dealing with what he considered unseen and private mental processes within the individual. He turned his attention to interpersonal processes that could be observed in a social framework. Sullivan (1953) defined *personality* as behaviour that can be observed within interpersonal relationships.

According to Sullivan, the purpose of all behaviour is to get needs met through interpersonal interactions and to decrease or avoid anxiety. He defined *anxiety* as any painful feeling or emotion that arises from social insecurity or that prevents biological needs from being satisfied (Sullivan, 1953). Sullivan coined the term *security operations* to describe measures the individual uses to reduce anxiety and enhance security. For example, a person might imagine themself to be right, muster up anger to fuel this righteousness, and try to act to reduce anxiety. Collectively, the security operations an individual uses to defend against anxiety and ensure self-esteem make up the self-system.

There are many parallels between Sullivan's notion of security operations and Freud's concept of defence mechanisms. Both are unconscious processes, and both are ways we reduce anxiety. However, Freud's defence mechanism of repression is an intrapsychic activity, whereas Sullivan's security operations are interpersonal relationship activities that can be observed.

Interpersonal Psychotherapy

Interpersonal psychotherapy is an effective short-term therapy that originated with Adolph Meyer and Harry Stack Sullivan. The assumption is that psychiatric disorders are influenced by interpersonal interactions and the social context. The goal of interpersonal psychotherapy is to reduce or eliminate psychiatric symptoms (particularly depression and anxiety) by improving interpersonal functioning and underlying relational dynamics. Treatment is predicated on the notion that disturbances in important interpersonal relationships (or a deficit in one's capacity to form those relationships) can play a role in initiating or maintaining symptoms. In interpersonal psychotherapy the therapist identifies the nature of the problem to be resolved and then selects strategies consistent with that problem area.

Peplau's Theory of Interpersonal Relations

Hildegard Peplau (1909–1999) (Figure 4.2), influenced by the work of Sullivan and learning theory, developed the first systematic theoretical framework for psychiatric nursing in her ground-breaking book *Interpersonal Relations in Nursing*. Peplau was the first nurse to identify psychiatric mental health nursing both as an essential element of general nursing and as a specialty area that embraces specific governing principles. In shifting the focus from what nurses do *to* patients to what nurses do *with* patients Peplau (1989) engineered a major paradigm shift from a model focused on medical treatments to an interpersonal relational model of nursing practice. She viewed nursing as an educative instrument designed to help individuals and communities use their capacities to live more productively (Peplau, 1987). She believed that illness offered a unique opportunity for experiential learning, personal growth, and improved coping strategies and that psychiatric nurses play a unique role in facilitating this growth through the nurse–patient relationship (Peplau, 1982a, 1982b).

Peplau identified stages of the nurse–patient relationship (see Chapter 9) and also taught the technique of *process recording* to help her students hone their communication and relationship skills (see Table 10.4). The skills of the psychiatric nurse include observation, interpretation, and intervention. The nurse observes and listens to the patient, developing impressions about the meaning of the patient's situation. By employing this process, the nurse is able to view the patient as a unique individual. The nurse's inferences are then validated with the patient for accuracy. Peplau believed it was essential for nurses to observe the behaviour not only of the patient but also of themselves

Fig. 4.2 Hildegard Peplau. (Source: Courtesy Anne Peplau.)

and so proposed an approach in which nurses are both participants and observers in therapeutic conversations. This self-awareness on the part of the nurse is essential in keeping the focus on the patient, as well as in keeping the social and personal needs of the nurse out of the nurse–patient conversation.

Perhaps Peplau's most universal contribution to the everyday practice of psychiatric mental health nursing is her application of Sullivan's theory of anxiety to nursing practice. She described the effects of different levels of anxiety (mild, moderate, severe, and panic) on perception and learning. She promoted interventions to lower anxiety, with the aim of improving patients' abilities to think and function at more satisfactory levels. More on the application of Peplau's theory of anxiety and interventions is presented in Chapter 12. Table 4.3 lists selected nursing theorists and summarizes their major contributions and the impact of these contributions on psychiatric mental health nursing.

Building on the work of Peplau (1952), who emphasized the importance of understanding people's relationships with their illnesses and their health, the **Tidal Model** focuses on the interpersonal relationships as the context for recovery. Barker and Buchanan-Barker (2005) have defined the model as a philosophic approach leading to mental health. It relies heavily on metaphors that are used to empower people and uses each person's experience and wisdom to effect change. The Tidal Model emerged from the nursing practice. Through the use of this model, Barker and Buchanan-Barker (2005) suggest that mental well-being depends on individual experience or self, perceptions, thoughts, and actions. It is a recovery approach that can be used to inform person-centred collaborative care as listening to the person's "story" and experiences so that we can begin to understand and work out with the individual what might be done to help. The assumptions upon which this model is built are that people need to be encouraged to tell their story; in their own words, the account of their experiences must be listened to and respected, and it is through this sharing that assessments and collaborative care planning can occur. Each interaction is seen as an opportunity to repair, or damage still further, the person's vulnerable sense of self. When this model is used, assessment includes three primary questions: Why is this person experiencing this particular difficulty right now, how does the person see their problem, and what does the person think will work for or be counter-productive for them in the present circumstances? Nurses who use this model believe that the therapeutic relationship is crucial to the delivery of truly collaborative care and that mental pain is eased if a person feels listened to, understood, and reassured.

TABLE 4.3 Selected Nursing Theorists, Their Major Contributions, and Their Impact on Psychiatric Mental Health Nursing

Nursing Theorist	Focus of Theory	Contribution to Psychiatric Mental Health Nursing
Patricia Benner	"Caring" as foundation for nursing	Benner encourages nurses to provide caring and comforting interventions. She emphasizes the importance of the nurse–patient relationship and the importance of teaching and coaching the patient and bearing witness to suffering as the patient deals with illness.
Dorothea Orem	Goal of self-care as integral to the practice of nursing	Orem emphasizes the role of the nurse in promoting self-care activities of the patient; this has relevance to the seriously and persistently mentally ill patient.
Sister Callista Roy	Continual need for people to adapt physically, psychologically, and socially	Roy emphasizes the role of nursing in assisting patients to adapt so that they can cope more effectively with changes.
Betty Neuman	Impact of internal and external stressors on the equilibrium of the system	Neuman emphasizes the role of nursing in assisting patients to discover and use stress-reducing strategies.
Joyce Travelbee	Meaning in the nurse–patient relationship and the importance of communication	Travelbee emphasizes the role of nursing in affirming the suffering of the patient and in being able to alleviate that suffering through communication skills used appropriately throughout the stages of the nurse–patient relationship.

Sources: Benner, P., & Wrubel, J. (1989). *The primacy of caring: Stress and coping in health and illness.* Menlo Park: Addison-Wesley; Leddy, S., & Pepper, J. M. (1993). *Conceptual bases of professional nursing* (3rd ed., pp. 174–175). Philadelphia: Lippincott; Neuman, B., & Young, R. (1972). A model for teaching total-person approach to patient problems. *Nursing Research, 21*(3), 264–269; Orem, D. E. (1995). *Nursing: Concepts of practice* (5th ed.). New York: McGraw-Hill; Roy, C., & Andrews, H. A. (1991). *The Roy adaptation model: The definitive statement.* Norwalk: Appleton & Lange; and Travelbee, J. (1961). *Intervention in psychiatric nursing.* Philadelphia: F. A. Davis.

Implications of Interpersonal Theories for Nursing Practice

Sullivan's theory is the foundation for Hildegard Peplau's nursing theory of interpersonal relationships, which we examine later in this chapter. Believing that therapy should educate patients and assist them in gaining personal insight, Sullivan introduced the term *participant observer*, which underscores that professional helpers cannot be isolated from the therapeutic situation if they are to be effective. Sullivan would insist that the nurse interact with the patient as an authentic human being. Mutuality, respect for the patient, unconditional acceptance, and empathy, which are considered essential aspects of modern therapeutic relationships, were important aspects of Sullivan's theory of interpersonal therapy. Sullivan also demonstrated that a psychotherapeutic environment, characterized by an accepting atmosphere that provided numerous opportunities for practising interpersonal skills and developing relationships, is an invaluable treatment tool. Group psychotherapy, family therapy, and educational and skill training programs, as well as unstructured periods, can be incorporated into the design of a psychotherapeutic environment to facilitate healthy interactions. This method is used today in virtually all residential and day hospital settings.

BEHAVIOURAL THEORIES AND THERAPIES

Behaviourists have no concern with inner conflicts and argue that personality simply consists of learned behaviours. Consequently, if behaviour changes, so does the personality. Therefore contrary to what psychoanalyst theorists believe, a person's destiny was *not* carved in stone at a very early age.

The development of behavioural models began in the nineteenth century as a result of Ivan Pavlov's laboratory work with dogs. It continued into the twentieth century with John B. Watson's application of these models to shape behaviour and with B. F. Skinner's research on rat behaviour. These behavioural theorists developed systematic learning principles that could be applied to humans. Behavioural models emphasize the ways in which observable behavioural responses are learned and can be modified in a particular environment. Pavlov's, Watson's, and Skinner's models focus on the belief that behaviour can be influenced through a process referred to as *conditioning*. Conditioning involves pairing behaviour with a condition that reinforces or diminishes the behaviour's occurrence.

Classical Conditioning Theory

Ivan Pavlov (1849–1936) was a Russian physiologist. He won a Nobel Prize for his outstanding contributions to the physiology of digestion, which he studied through his well-known experiments with dogs. In incidental observation of the dogs Pavlov noticed that the dogs were able to anticipate when food would be forthcoming and would begin to salivate even before actually tasting the meat. Pavlov labelled this process *psychic secretion*. He hypothesized that the psychic component was a learned association between two events: the presence of the experimental apparatus and the serving of meat.

Pavlov formalized his observations of behaviours in dogs in a theory of classical conditioning. Pavlov (1928) found that when a neutral stimulus (a bell) was repeatedly paired with another stimulus (food that triggered salivation), eventually, the sound of the bell alone could elicit salivation in the dogs. An example of this response in humans is an individual who became very ill as a child after eating spoiled coleslaw at a picnic and later in life feels nauseated whenever he smells coleslaw. It is important to recognize that classical conditioned responses are involuntary, that is, not under conscious personal control, and are not spontaneous choices.

Behaviourism Theory

John B. Watson (1878–1958) was an American psychologist who rejected the unconscious motivation of psychoanalysis as being too subjective. He developed the school of thought referred to as behaviourism, which he believed was more objective or measurable. Watson contended that personality traits and responses, adaptive and maladaptive, were socially learned through classical conditioning (Watson, 1919). In a famous (but terrible) experiment Watson stood behind Little Albert, a 9-month-old who liked animals, and made a loud noise with a hammer every time the infant reached for a white rat. After this experiment, Little Albert became terrified at the sight of white fur or hair, even in the absence of a loud noise. Watson concluded that behaviour could be moulded by controlling the environment and that anyone could be trained to be anything, from a beggar to a merchant.

Operant Conditioning Theory

B. F. Skinner (1904–1990) represented the second wave of behavioural theorists. Skinner (1987) researched operant conditioning, in which voluntary behaviours are learned through consequences and behavioural responses are elicited through reinforcement, which causes a behaviour to occur more frequently. A consequence can be a positive reinforcement, such as receiving a reward (getting high marks after studying hard all semester), or a negative reinforcement, such as the removal of an objectionable or aversive stimulus (walking freely through a park once the vicious dog is picked up by animal services).

Other techniques can cause behaviours to occur less frequently. One technique is an unpleasant consequence, or punishment. Driving too fast may result in a speeding ticket, which, in mature and healthy individuals, decreases the chances that speeding will recur. The absence of reinforcement, or extinction, also decreases behaviour by withholding a reward that has become habitual. If a person tells a joke and no one laughs, for example, the person is less apt to tell jokes because his joke-telling behaviour is not being reinforced. Teachers employ this strategy in the classroom when they ignore acting-out behaviour that had previously been rewarded by more attention. Figure 4.3 illustrates the differences between classical conditioning (in which an involuntary reaction is caused by a stimulus) and operant conditioning (in which voluntary behaviour is learned through reinforcement).

Behavioural Therapy

Behavioural therapy is based on the assumption that changes in maladaptive behaviour can occur without insight into the underlying cause. This approach works best when it is directed at specific problems and the goals are well defined. Behavioural therapy is effective in treating people with phobias, alcoholism, schizophrenia, and many other conditions. Five types of behavioural therapy are discussed here: modelling, operant conditioning, systematic desensitization, aversion therapy, and biofeedback.

Fig. 4.3 Classical versus operant conditioning. (Source: Carson, V. B. (2000). *Mental health nursing: The nurse–patient journey* (2nd ed.). Philadelphia: Saunders.)

Modelling

In modelling, the therapist provides a role model for specific identified behaviours, and the patient learns through imitation. The therapist may do the modelling, provide another person to model the behaviours, or present a video for the purpose. Bandura et al. (1969) were able to help people lessen their phobias about nonpoisonous snakes by having them first view close-ups of filmed encounters between people and snakes that had successful outcomes and then view live encounters between people and snakes that also had successful outcomes. In a similar fashion some behavioural therapists use role-playing in the consulting room. For example, a student who does not know how to ask a professor for an extension on a term paper would watch the therapist portray a potentially effective way of making the request. The clinician would then help the student to practise the new skill in a similar role-playing situation.

Operant Conditioning

Operant conditioning is the basis for behaviour modification and uses positive reinforcement to increase desired behaviours. For example, when desired goals are achieved or behaviours are performed, patients might be rewarded with tokens. These tokens can be exchanged for food, small luxuries, or privileges. This reward system is known as a token economy.

Operant conditioning has been useful in improving the verbal behaviours of mute, autistic, and developmentally disabled children. In patients with severe and persistent mental illness behaviour modification has helped increase levels of self-care, social behaviour, group participation, and more.

We all use positive reinforcement in our everyday lives. A familiar case in point occurs when a mother takes her preschooler along to the grocery store, and the child starts acting out, demanding candy, nagging, crying, and yelling. Here are examples of three ways the child's behaviour can be reinforced:

Action	Result
1. The mother gives the child the candy.	The child continues to use this behaviour. This is positive reinforcement of negative behaviour.
2. The mother scolds the child.	Acting out may continue, because the child gets what he really wants—attention. This positively rewards negative behaviour.
3. The mother ignores the acting out but gives attention to the child when he is behaving appropriately.	The child gets a positive reward for appropriate behaviour.

Systematic Desensitization

Systematic desensitization is another form of behaviour modification therapy that involves the development of behavioural tasks customized to the patient's specific fears; these tasks are presented to the patient while using learned relaxation techniques. The process involves four steps:
1. The patient's fear is broken down into its components by exploring the particular stimulus cues to which the patient reacts. For example, certain situations may precipitate a phobic reaction, whereas others do not. Crowds at parties may be problematic, whereas similar numbers of people in other settings do not cause the same distress.
2. The patient is incrementally exposed to the fear. For example, a patient who has a fear of flying is introduced to short periods of visual presentations of flying, first with still pictures, then with videos, and finally in a busy airport. The situations are confronted while the patient is in a relaxed state. Gradually, over a period of time, exposure is increased until anxiety about or fear of the object or situation has ceased.
3. The patient is instructed on how to design a hierarchy of fears. For fear of flying, a patient might develop a set of statements representing the stages of a flight, order the statements from the most fearful to the least fearful, and use relaxation techniques to reach a state of relaxation as he or she progresses through the list.
4. The patient practises these techniques every day.

Aversion Therapy

Today, aversion therapy (which is akin to punishment) is used widely to treat behaviours such as alcoholism, sexual deviation, shoplifting, violent and aggressive behaviour, and self-mutilation. Aversion therapy is sometimes the treatment of choice when other less drastic measures have failed to produce the desired effects. The following are three paradigms for using aversive techniques:
1. Pairing of a maladaptive behaviour with a noxious stimulus (e.g., pairing the sight and smell of alcohol with electric shock) so that anxiety or fear becomes associated with the once-pleasurable stimulus
2. Punishment (e.g., punishment applied after the patient has had an alcoholic drink)
3. Avoidance training (e.g., patient avoids punishment by pushing a glass of alcohol away within a certain time limit)

Simple examples of extinguishing undesirable behaviour through aversion therapy include painting foul-tasting substances on the fingernails of nail biters or the thumbs of thumb suckers. Other examples of aversive stimuli are chemicals that induce nausea and vomiting, noxious odours, unpleasant verbal stimuli (e.g., descriptions of disturbing scenes), costs or fines in a token economy, and denial of positive reinforcement (e.g., isolation).

Before initiating any aversive protocol, the therapist, treatment team, or society *must* answer the following questions:
- Is this therapy in the best interest of the patient?
- Does its use violate the patient's rights?
- Is it in the best interest of society?

If aversion therapy is chosen as the most appropriate treatment, those administering it must provide ongoing supervision, support, and evaluation.

Biofeedback

Biofeedback is a form of behavioural therapy that uses sensitive instrumentation to acquire information about body functions such as muscle activity, brain waves, skin temperature, heart rate, and blood pressure. Biofeedback is successfully used today, especially for controlling the body's physiological response to stress and anxiety. This form of therapy is discussed in detail in Chapter 5.

Implications of Behavioural Theories for Nursing Practice

Behavioural models provide a concrete method for modifying or replacing behaviours. Behaviour management and modification programs based on these principles have proven to be successful in altering targeted behaviours. Programmed learning and token economies, in which tokens, or symbolic objects (e.g., check marks), can be exchanged for valued items, services, or privileges (e.g., food, passes out of the building, phone calls), represent extensions of thoughts on learning. Behavioural methods are particularly effective with children, adolescents, and individuals with many forms of chronic mental illness.

COGNITIVE THEORIES AND THERAPIES

While behaviourists focused on increasing, decreasing, or eliminating measurable behaviours, little attention was paid to the thoughts, or cognitions, that were involved in these behaviours. Rather than thinking of people as passive recipients of environmental conditioning, cognitive theorists proposed that there is a dynamic interplay between individuals and the environment. These theorists believe that thoughts come before feelings and actions and that thoughts about the world and our place in it are based on our own unique perspectives, which may or may not be based on reality. Two of the most influential theorists and their therapies are presented here.

Rational Emotive Behaviour Therapy

Rational emotive behaviour therapy (REBT) was developed by Albert Ellis (1913–2007) in 1955. The aim of REBT is to eradicate core irrational beliefs by helping people recognize thoughts that are not accurate, sensible, or useful. These thoughts tend to take the form of *should*s (e.g., "I should always be polite."), *ought*s (e.g., "I ought to consistently win my tennis games."), and *must*s (e.g., "I must be thin."). Ellis described negative thinking as a simple A-B-C process. *A* stands for the activating event, *B* stands for beliefs about the event, and *C* stands for the emotional consequence as a result of the event.

$$A \rightarrow B \rightarrow C$$
Activating Event Beliefs Emotional Consequence

Perception influences all thoughts, which in turn influence our behaviours. For example, imagine you have just received an invitation to a birthday party (activating event). You think, *I hate parties. Now I have to hang out with people who don't like me instead of watching my favourite television shows. They probably just invited me to get a gift* (beliefs). You will probably be miserable (emotional consequence) if you go. On the other hand, you may think, *I love parties!* (activating event). *This will be a great chance to meet new people, and it will be fun to shop for the perfect gift* (beliefs). You could have a delightful time (emotional consequence).

Although Ellis (Figure 4.4) admitted that the role of past experiences is instrumental in our current beliefs, the focus of REBT is on present attitudes, painful feelings, and dysfunctional behaviours. If our beliefs are negative and self-deprecating, we are more susceptible to depression and anxiety. Ellis noted that while we cannot change the past, we can change the way we are now. He was pragmatic in his approach to mental illness and colourful in his therapeutic advice: "It's too [darn] bad you panic, but you don't die from it! Get them over the panic about panic, you may find the panic disappears" (Ellis, 2000).

Cognitive Behavioural Therapy

Aaron T. Beck (Figure 4.4), another follower of Sigmund Freud, was originally trained in psychoanalysis but is regarded as a neo-Freudian. When he attempted to study depression from a psychoanalytic perspective, he became convinced that people with depression generally had stereotypical patterns of negative and self-critical thinking that seemed to distort their ability to think and process information. Cognitive behavioural therapy (CBT) is based on both cognitive psychology and behavioural theory. It is a commonly used, effective, and well-researched therapeutic tool.

Beck's method (Beck et al., 1979), the basis for CBT, is an active, directive, time-limited, structured approach used to treat a variety of psychiatric disorders (e.g., depression, anxiety, phobias, pain problems). It is based on the underlying theoretical principle that how people feel and behave is largely determined by the way they think about the world and their place in it (Beck, 1967). Their cognitions (verbal or pictorial events in their stream of consciousness) are based on attitudes or assumptions developed from previous experiences. These cognitions may be fairly accurate, or they may be distorted. According to Beck, we all have schemata or unique assumptions about ourselves, others, and the world around us. For example, a person who has the schema "The only person I can trust is myself" will have expectations that everyone else has questionable motives, will lie, and will eventually hurt them. Other negative schemata include incompetence, abandonment, evilness, and vulnerability. We are typically not aware of such cognitive biases but recognizing them as beliefs and attitudes based on distortions and misconceptions will help make apparent the dysfunctional schemata underlying our thinking.

Rapid, unthinking responses based on schemata are known as automatic thoughts. These responses are particularly intense and frequent in psychiatric disorders such as depression and anxiety. Often, automatic thoughts, or cognitive distortions, are irrational and lead to false assumptions and misinterpretations. For example, if a person interprets all experiences in terms of whether they are competent and adequate, thinking may be dominated by the cognitive distortion "Unless I do everything perfectly, I'm a failure." Consequently, the person reacts to situations in terms of adequacy, even when these situations are unrelated to whether they are personally competent. Table 4.4 describes common cognitive distortions.

The therapeutic techniques of the cognitive therapist are designed to identify, reality-test, and correct distorted conceptualizations and the dysfunctional beliefs underlying them. Patients are taught to challenge their own negative thinking and substitute it with positive, rational thoughts. They are taught to recognize when thinking is based on distortions and misconceptions. Homework assignments play an important role in CBT. A particularly effective technique is the use of a four-column format to record the precipitating event or situation, the resulting automatic thought, the proceeding feelings and behaviours, and, finally, a challenge to the negative thoughts based on rational evidence and thinking. The following is an example of the type of analysis done by a patient receiving CBT.

A 24-year-old nurse recently discharged from the hospital for severe depression presented this record (Beck et al., 1979):

Fig. 4.4 Aaron Beck *(left)* and Albert Ellis *(right).* (Source: Fenichel, 2002, APA Conference, http://www.fenichel.com/Beck-Ellis2002.shtml.)

TABLE 4.4 Common Cognitive Distortions

Distortion	Definition	Example
All-or-nothing thinking	Thinking in black and white, reducing complex outcomes into absolutes	Although Marcia earned the second highest score in the provincial figure-skating competition, she consistently referred to herself as "a loser."
Overgeneralization	Using a bad outcome (or a few bad outcomes) as evidence that nothing will ever go right again	Marty had a minor traffic accident. She refuses to drive and says, "I shouldn't be allowed on the road." When asked why, she answers, "I'm a horrible driver; I could have killed someone!"
Labelling	Generalizing a characteristic or event so that it becomes definitive and results in an overly harsh label for self or others	"Because I failed the advanced statistics exam, I am a failure. I should give up. I may as well quit my nursing program."
Mental filter	Focusing on a negative detail or bad event and allowing it to taint everything else	René's boss evaluated his work as exemplary and gave him a few suggestions for improvement. He obsessed about the suggestions and ignored the rest.
Disqualifying the positive	Maintaining a negative view by rejecting information that supports a positive view as being irrelevant, inaccurate, or accidental	"I've just been offered the job I've always wanted. No one else must have applied."
Emotional reasoning	Drawing a conclusion based on an emotional state	"I'm nervous about the exam. I must not be prepared. If I were, I wouldn't be afraid."
Jumping to conclusions	Making a negative interpretation despite the fact that there is little or no supporting evidence	"My fiancé, Ryan, didn't call me for 3 hours, which just proves he doesn't love me anymore."
a. Mind-reading	Inferring negative thoughts, responses, and motives of others	"The grocery store clerk was grouchy and barely made eye contact, so I must have done something wrong."
b. Fortune-telling error	Anticipating that things will turn out badly as an established fact	"I'll ask them out, but I know they won't have a good time."
Magnification or minimization	Exaggerating the importance of something (such as a personal failure or the success of others) or reducing the importance of something (such as a personal success or the failure of others)	"I'm alone on a Saturday night because no one likes me. When other people are alone, it's because they want to be."
a. Catastrophizing	Magnifying to the extreme so that the very worst is assumed to be a probable outcome.	"If I don't make a good impression on the boss at the company picnic, they will fire me."
Emotional reasoning	Drawing a conclusion based on an emotional state	"I'm nervous about the exam. I must not be prepared. If I were, I wouldn't be afraid."
Should and *must* statements	Assuming rigid self-directives that presume an unrealistic amount of control over external events	"My patient is worse today. I should give better care so that they will get better."
Personalization	Assuming responsibility for an external event or situation that was likely outside personal control.	"I'm sorry your party wasn't more fun. It's probably because I was there."

Source: Burns, D. D. (1989). *The feeling good handbook.* New York: William Morrow.

Event	Feeling	Cognitions	Other Possible Interpretations
While at a party, Jim asked me, "How are you feeling?" shortly after I was discharged from the hospital.	Anxious	Jim thinks I am a basket case. I must look really bad for him to be concerned.	He really cares about me. He noticed that I look better than before I went into the hospital and wants to know if I feel better too.

Box 4.1 presents an example of CBT, and Table 4.5 compares and contrasts psychodynamic, interpersonal, cognitive behavioural, and behavioural therapies.

Dialectical Behavioural Therapy

Dr. Marsha Linehan (1993) developed **dialectical behavioural therapy** (DBT), a specific type of cognitive behavioural psychotherapy. This model was developed for use with individuals with intractable behavioural disorders involving emotional dysregulation. DBT suggests that these individuals' arousal levels increase more quickly than that of others, obtain a higher level of emotional stimulation, and take significantly more time to return to baseline arousal levels after the emotional situation. More recently, DBT has been found to be an effective treatment modality for other mental health symptoms, such as depression, suicidal ideation, hopelessness, anger, substance dependence, and dissociation (Lenz et al., 2016). DBT focuses on teaching people methods to help them deal with swings in emotions, seeing the world in black and white, and seemingly jumping from one crisis to another. There are three primary characteristics of DBT. First, it is support oriented. Individuals are helped to identify their strengths. Second, it helps people to identify thoughts and beliefs that make life harder, such as "I am a failure," and to learn different ways of thinking. Third, this model requires constant attention to the therapeutic relationship. This model is used in individual and group settings. Individual sessions generally focus on decreasing and dealing with responses from previous trauma. Group sessions often focus on learning skills related to interpersonal effectiveness, distress tolerance, reality acceptance skills, emotional regulation, and mindfulness.

BOX 4.1 Example of Cognitive-Behavioural Therapy

The patient was an attractive woman in her early 20s. Her depression of 18 months' duration was precipitated by her boyfriend's leaving her. She had numerous automatic thoughts that she was ugly and undesirable. These automatic thoughts were handled in the following manner:

Therapist: Other than your subjective opinion, what evidence do you have that you are ugly?

Patient: Well, my sister always said I was ugly.

Therapist: Was she always right in these matters?

Patient: No. Actually, she had her own reasons for telling me this. But the real reason I know I'm ugly is that men don't ask me out. If I weren't ugly, I'd be dating now.

Therapist: That is a possible reason why you're not dating. But there's an alternative explanation. You told me that you work in an office by yourself all day and spend your nights alone at home. It doesn't seem like you're giving yourself opportunities to meet men.

Patient: I can see what you're saying, but still, if I weren't ugly, men would ask me out.

Therapist: I suggest we run an experiment: that is, for you to become more socially active, stop turning down invitations to parties and social events, and see what happens.

After the patient became more active and had more opportunities to meet men, she started to date. At this point, she no longer believed she was ugly.

Therapy then focused on her basic assumption that one's worth is determined by one's appearance. She readily agreed this didn't make sense. She also saw the falseness of the assumption that one must be beautiful to attract men or be loved. This discussion led to her basic assumption that she could not be happy without love (or attention from men). The latter part of treatment focused on helping her to change this belief.

Therapist: On what do you base this belief that you can't be happy without a man?

Patient: I was really depressed for a year and a half when I didn't have a man in my life.

Therapist: Is there another reason why you were depressed?

Patient: As we discussed, I was looking at everything in a distorted way. But I still don't know if I could be happy if no one was interested in me.

Therapist: I don't know either. Is there a way we could find out?

Patient: Well, as an experiment, I could not go out on dates for a while and see how I feel.

Therapist: I think that's a good idea. Although it has its flaws, the experimental method is still the best way currently available to discover the facts. You're fortunate in being able to run this type of experiment. Now, for the first time in your adult life, you aren't attached to a man. If you find you can be happy without a man, this will greatly strengthen you and also make your future relationships all the better.

In this case the patient was able to stick to a "cold turkey" regimen. After a brief period of dysphoria, she was delighted to find that her well-being was not dependent on another person.

There were similarities between these two interventions. In both the distorted conclusion or assumption was delineated, and the patient was asked for evidence to support it. An experiment to gather data was also suggested in both instances. However, to achieve the results, a contrasting version of the same experimental situation was required.

Source: Beck, A. T., Rush, A. J., Shaw, B. F., Emery, G. (1979). *Cognitive therapy of depression.* New York: Guilford Press.

TABLE 4.5 Comparison of Psychodynamic, Interpersonal, Cognitive Behavioural, and Behavioural Therapies

	Psychodynamic Therapy	Interpersonal Therapy	Cognitive Behavioural Therapy	Behavioural Therapy
Treatment focus	Unresolved past relationships and core conflicts	Current interpersonal relationships and social supports	Thoughts and cognitions	Learned maladaptive behaviour
Therapist role	Significant other transference object	Problem solver	Active, directive, challenging	Active, directive teacher
Primary disorders treated	Anxiety, depression, personality disorders	Depression	Depression, anxiety/panic, eating disorders	Post-traumatic stress disorder, obsessive-compulsive disorder, panic disorder
Length of therapy	20+ sessions	Short term (12–20 sessions)	Short term (5–20 sessions)	Varies; typically fewer than 10 sessions
Technique	Therapeutic alliance, free association, understanding transference, challenging defence mechanisms	Facilitate new patterns of communication and expectations for relationships	Evaluating thoughts and behaviours, modifying dysfunctional thoughts and behaviours	Relaxation, thought stopping, self-reassurance, seeking social support

Source: Dewan, M. J., Steenbarger, B. N., & Greenberg, R. P. (2008). Brief psychotherapies. In R. E. Hales, S. C. Yudofsky, & G. O. Gabbard (Eds.), *Textbook of psychiatry* (5th ed., pp. 1155–1170). American Psychiatric Publishing.

Implications of Cognitive Theories for Nursing Practice

Recognizing the interplay between events, negative thinking, and negative responses can be beneficial from both a patient care standpoint and a personal one. Workbooks are available to aid in the process of identifying cognitive distortions. Personal benefits from this cognitive approach could help the nurse to understand their own response to a variety of difficult situations. One example might be the anxiety that some students feel regarding the psychiatric nursing clinical rotation. Students may overgeneralize ("All psychiatric patients are dangerous.") or personalize ("My patient doesn't seem to be better; I'm probably not doing him any good.") the situation. The key to effectively using the CBT approach in clinical situations is to challenge the negative

> **BOX 4.2 Characteristics of Brief Therapies**
>
> At the start of treatment, the patient and therapist agree on what the focus will be and concentrate their work on that focus. Sessions are held weekly, and the total number of sessions to be held is determined at the outset of therapy. There is a rapid, back-and-forth pattern between patient and therapist, with both participating actively. The therapist intervenes constantly to keep the therapy on track, either by redirecting the patient's attention or by interpreting deviations from the focus to the patient.
>
> Brief therapies share the following common elements:
> - Assessment tends to be rapid and early.
> - Clear expectations are established for time-limited therapy with improvement demonstrated within a small number of sessions.
> - Goals are concrete and focus on improving the patient's worst symptoms, improving coping skills, and helping the patient to understand what is going on in their life.
> - Interpretations are directed toward present life circumstances and patient behaviour rather than toward the historical significance of feelings.
> - There is a general understanding that psychotherapy does not cure but that it can help troubled individuals learn to recognize that problems exist and can promote self-awareness as they deal with life's inevitable stressors.

thoughts that are not based on facts and then replace them with more realistic appraisals. Many cognitive therapy approaches use brief therapy modalities (Box 4.2).

HUMANISTIC THEORIES

In the 1950s humanistic theories arose as a protest against both the behavioural and the psychoanalytic schools, which were thought to be pessimistic, deterministic, and dehumanizing. Humanistic theories focus on human potential and free will to choose life patterns that are supportive of personal growth. Humanistic frameworks emphasize a person's capacity for self-actualization. This approach focuses on understanding the patient's perspective as they subjectively experience it. There are a number of humanistic theorists. We explore Abraham Maslow and his theory of self-actualization.

Abraham Maslow's Humanistic Psychology Theory

Abraham Maslow (1908–1970), considered the father of humanistic psychology, introduced the concept of a "self-actualized personality" associated with high productivity and enjoyment of life (Maslow, 1963, 1968). He criticized psychology for focusing too intently on humanity's frailties and not enough on its strengths. Maslow contended that the focus of psychology must go beyond experiences of hate, pain, misery, guilt, and conflict to include love, compassion, happiness, exhilaration, and well-being.

Hierarchy of Needs

Maslow conceptualized human motivation as a hierarchy of dynamic processes or needs that are critical for the development of all humans. Central to his theory is the assumption that humans are active rather than passive participants in life, striving for self-actualization. Maslow (1968) focused on human need fulfillment, which he categorized into six incremental stages, beginning with physiological survival needs and ending with self-transcendent needs (Figure 4.5). The hierarchy of needs is conceptualized as a pyramid, with the strongest, most fundamental needs placed on the lower levels. The more distinctly human needs occupy the top sections of the pyramid. When lower-level needs are met, higher needs are able to emerge.

- *Physiological needs.* The most basic needs are the physiological drives: food, oxygen, water, sleep, sex, and a constant body temperature. If all needs were deprived, this level would take priority over the rest.

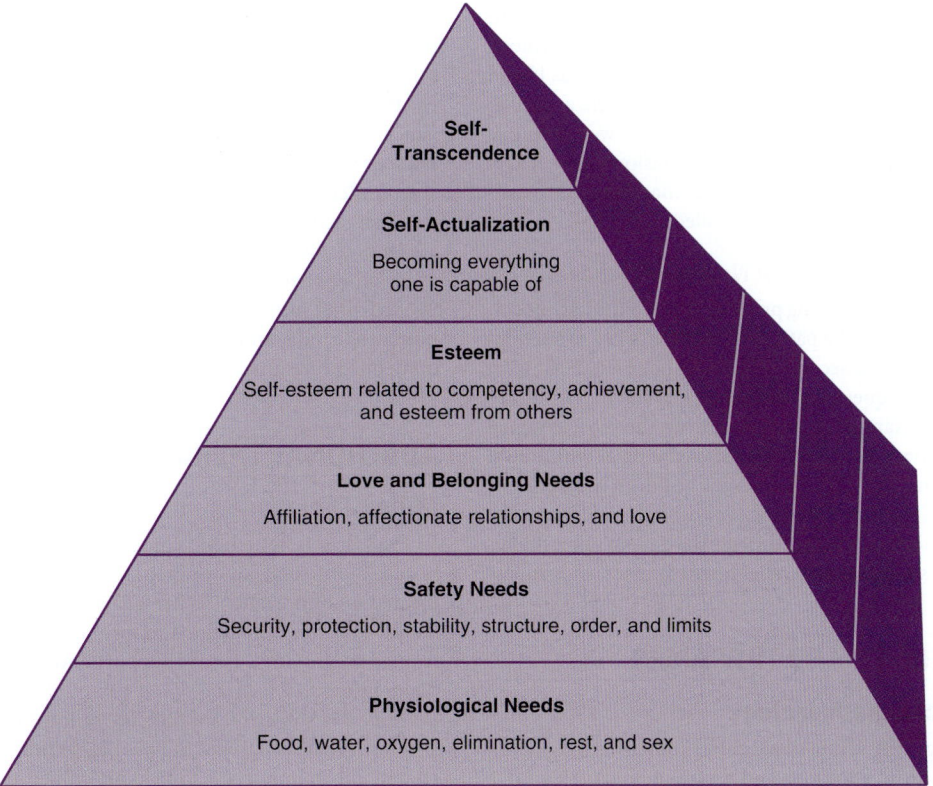

Fig. 4.5 Maslow's hierarchy of needs. (Source: Maslow, A. H. (1972). *The farther reaches of human nature.* New York: Viking.)

- *Safety needs.* Once physiological needs are met, safety needs emerge. They include security; protection; freedom from fear, anxiety, and chaos; and the need for law, order, and limits. Adults in a stable society usually feel safe, but they may feel threatened by debt, job insecurity, or lack of insurance. It is during times of crisis, such as war, disasters, assaults, and social breakdown, that safety needs really take precedence. Children, who are more vulnerable and dependent, respond far more readily and intensely to safety threats.
- *Belongingness and love needs.* People have a need for intimate relationships, love, affection, and belonging and will seek to overcome feelings of aloneness and alienation. Maslow stresses the importance of having a family and a home and of being part of an identifiable group.
- *Esteem needs.* People need to have a high self-regard and have it reflected to them from others. If self-esteem needs are met, we feel confident, valued, and valuable. When self-esteem is compromised, we feel inferior, worthless, and helpless.
- *Self-actualization.* We are preset to strive to be everything we are capable of becoming. Maslow said, "What a man *can* be, he *must* be." What we are capable of becoming is highly individual: an artist must paint, a writer must write, and a healer must heal. The drive to satisfy this need is felt as a sort of restlessness, a sense that something is missing. It is up to each person to choose a path that will bring about inner peace and fulfillment.

Although his early work included only five levels of needs, Maslow (1970) later took into account two additional factors: (1) cognitive needs (the desire to know and understand) and (2) aesthetic needs. He describes the acquisition of knowledge (our first priority) and the need to understand (our second priority) as being hard-wired and essential; he identified the aesthetic need for beauty and symmetry as universal. How else, after all, do we explain the impulse to straighten a crooked picture?

Maslow based his theory on the results of clinical investigations of people who represented self-actualized individuals, who moved in the direction of achieving and reaching their highest potentials. Among those, Maslow chose to investigate were historical figures such as Henry David Thoreau, Walt Whitman, and Ludwig von Beethoven, as well as others like Albert Einstein and Albert Schweitzer, who were living at the time they were studied. This investigation led Maslow (1963, 1970) to identify some basic personality characteristics that distinguish self-actualizing people from those who might be called "ordinary".

Implications of Motivation Theory for Nursing Practice

The value of Maslow's model in nursing practice is twofold. First, an emphasis on human potential and the patient's strengths is key to successful nurse–patient relationships. Second, the model helps establish what is most important in the sequencing of nursing actions in the nurse–patient relationship. For example, to collect any but the most essential information when a patient is struggling with acute drug withdrawal is inappropriate, as is managing public mental health in a disaster or pandemic such as the Covid-19 pandemic. Following Maslow's model as a way of prioritizing actions, the nurse meets the patient's physiological need for stable vital signs and pain relief before further assessment.

BIOLOGICAL THEORIES AND THERAPIES

The Advent of Psychopharmacology

In 1950 a French drug firm synthesized chlorpromazine (Largactil), a powerful antipsychotic medication, and psychiatry experienced a revolution. The advent of psychopharmacology presented a direct challenge to psychodynamic approaches to mental illness. The dramatic experience of observing patients freed from the bondage of psychosis and mania by powerful drugs such as chlorpromazine and lithium left witnesses convinced of the critical role of the brain in psychiatric illness.

Since the discovery of chlorpromazine, many other medications have proven effective in controlling psychosis, mania, depression, and anxiety. These medications greatly reduce the need for hospitalization and dramatically improve the lives of people with serious psychiatric difficulties. Today, we know that psychoactive medications exert differential effects on different neurotransmitters and help restore brain function, allowing patients with mental illness to continue living productive lives with greater satisfaction and far less emotional pain.

The Biological Model

A biological model of mental illness focuses on neurological, chemical, biological, and genetic issues and seeks to understand how the body and brain interact to create emotions, memories, and perceptual experiences. This perspective views abnormal behaviour as part of a disease process or a defect and seeks to stop or alter it. The biological model locates the illness or disease in the body, usually in the limbic system of the brain and the synapse receptor sites of the central nervous system, and targets the site of the illness using physical interventions such as medications, diet, or surgery.

The recognition that psychiatric illnesses are as physical in origin as diabetes and coronary heart disease serves to decrease the stigma surrounding them. Just as people with diabetes or heart disease cannot be held responsible for their illness, patients with schizophrenia or bipolar affective disorder are not to blame for theirs. It often happens that one of the most helpful things we can tell those whose lives are affected by psychiatric illness is that they are not responsible or to blame.

Implications of the Biological Model for Nursing Practice

Historically, psychiatric mental health nurses always have attended to the physical needs of psychiatric patients. Nurses administer medications; monitor sleep, activity, nutrition, hydration, elimination, and other functions; and prepare patients for somatic therapies, such as electroconvulsive therapy. They have continued to do so with the advancement of the biological model, which has not altered the basic nursing strategies: focusing on the qualities of a therapeutic relationship, understanding the patient's perspective, and communicating in a way that facilitates the patient's recovery.

One of the risks in adopting a biological model to the exclusion of all other theoretical perspectives is that such a theory ignores the myriad other influences, including social, environmental, cultural, economic, spiritual, and educational factors, that play a role in the development and treatment of mental illness.

ADDITIONAL THERAPIES

Milieu Therapy

In 1948 Bruno Bettelheim coined the term **milieu therapy** to describe his use of the total environment to treat disturbed children. Bettelheim created a comfortable, secure environment (or milieu) in which psychotic children were helped to form a new world. Staff members were trained to provide 24-hour support and understanding for each child on an individual basis.

Milieu is sometimes a difficult concept to grasp. It is an all-inclusive term that recognizes the people, setting, structure, and emotional climate all as important to healing. Milieu therapy uses naturally occurring events in the environment as rich learning opportunities for patients. There are certain basic characteristics of milieu therapy, regardless of whether the setting involves treatment of psychotic children, patients in a psychiatric hospital, drug abusers in a residential treatment centre, or psychiatric patients in a day hospital. Milieu therapy, or a therapeutic community, has as its focus a living, learning, or working environment. Such therapy may be based on any number of therapeutic modalities, from structured behavioural therapy to spontaneous, humanistic-oriented approaches.

Implications of Milieu Therapy for Nursing Practice

Milieu therapy is a basic intervention in nursing practice. Although most commonly associated with inpatient treatment (Nåvik et al., 2020), other examples of milieu therapy include providing a safe environment for the suicidal patient or for a patient with a cognitive disorder (e.g., Alzheimer's disease), referring people experiencing domestic abuse to safe houses, and advocating for children suspected of being abused in their home environments.

You will be introduced to other therapeutic approaches later in the book. Crisis intervention (see Chapter 21) is an approach you will find useful, not only in psychiatric mental health nursing but also in other nursing specialties. Group therapy (see Chapter 33) and family interventions (see Chapter 34), which are appropriate for the basic-level practitioner, will also be discussed.

Table 4.6 lists additional theorists whose contributions influence psychiatric mental health nursing.

TABLE 4.6 Additional Theorists Whose Contributions Influence Psychiatric Mental Health Nursing

Theorist	School of Thought	Major Contributions	Relevance to Psychiatric Mental Health Nursing
Carl Rogers	Humanism	Developed a person-centred model of psychotherapy; emphasized the concepts of: • Congruence—authenticity of the therapist in dealings with the patient • Unconditional acceptance and positive regard—climate in the therapeutic relationship that facilitates change • Empathic understanding—therapist's ability to apprehend the feelings and experiences of the patient as if these things were happening to the therapist	Encourages nurses to view each patient as unique; emphasizes attitudes of unconditional positive regard, empathic understanding, and genuineness that are essential to the nurse–patient relationship. *Example:* The nurse asks the patient, "What can I do to help you regain control over your anxiety?"
Jean Piaget	Cognitive development	Identified stages of cognitive development, including sensorimotor (0–2 years), preoperational (2–7 years), concrete operational (7–11 years), and formal operational (11 years–adulthood); these stages describe how cognitive development proceeds from reflex activity to application of logical solutions to all types of problems	Provides a broad base for cognitive interventions, especially with patients with negative self-views. *Example:* The nurse shows an 8-year-old all the equipment needed to start an intravenous when discussing the fact that they will need one prior to surgery.
Lawrence Kohlberg	Moral development	Posited a six-stage theory of moral development	Provides nurses with a framework for evaluating moral decisions. *Example:* In stage 5 the nurse views laws as social contracts that promote "the greatest good for the greatest number of people." The nurse would advocate access to universal health care.
Albert Ellis	Existentialism	Developed approach of rational emotive behavioural therapy that is active and cognitively oriented; confrontation used to force patients to assume responsibility for behaviour; patients are encouraged to accept themselves as they are and are taught to take risks and try out new behaviours	Encourages nurses to focus on here-and-now issues and to help the patient live fully in the present and look forward to the future. *Example:* The nurse encourages the patient to vacation with their family even though they will be in a wheelchair until their leg fracture heals.
Albert Bandura	Social learning theory	Responsible for concepts of modelling and self-efficacy, that is, a person's belief or expectation that they have the capacity to effect a desired outcome through their own efforts	Includes cognitive functioning with environmental factors, which provides nurses with a comprehensive view of how people learn. *Example:* The nurse helps the teenage patient identify three negative outcomes of tobacco use.

Continued

TABLE 4.6 Additional Theorists Whose Contributions Influence Psychiatric Mental Health Nursing—Cont'd

Theorist	School of Thought	Major Contributions	Relevance to Psychiatric Mental Health Nursing
Viktor Frankl	Existentialism	Developed "logotherapy," a future-oriented therapy offered to help people find their sense of self-respect, and focused on their need to find meaning and value in living as their most important life task	Focuses the nurse beyond mere behaviours to understanding the meaning of these behaviours to the patient's sense of life meaning. *Example:* The nurse listens attentively as the patient describes what life has been like since their daughter died.

Sources: Bandura, A. (1977). *Social learning theory.* Englewood Cliffs: Prentice-Hall; Bernard, M. E., & Wolfe, J. L. (Eds.). (1993). *The RET resource book for practitioners.* New York: Institute for Rational-Emotive Therapy; Ellis, A. (1989). *Inside rational emotive therapy.* San Diego: Academic Press; Frankl, V. (1969). *The will to meaning.* Cleveland: New American Library; Modgil, S., & Modgil, C. (1986). *Lawrence Kohlberg: Consensus and Controversy.* Philadelphia: Falmer Press; and Rogers, C. R. (1961). *On becoming a person.* Boston: Houghton Mifflin.

RESEARCH HIGHLIGHT

Mental Wellness Needs of Two Indigenous Communities: Bases for Culturally Competent Clinical Services

Problem

There is a lack of clear understanding of appropriate mental health services for Indigenous peoples. Mental health services are needed that respect Indigenous and non-Indigenous cultural values, traditions, beliefs, the impact of historical trauma, systemic racism and discrimination, and other practices that have arisen due to colonial oppression.

Purpose of Study

The primary purpose of the study was to explore the mental wellness needs of two Mi'kmaq communities within Prince Edward Island. The second goal was to provide mental wellness services in a manner that fit with the needs and expectations of the communities.

Methods

Using an Indigenous approach, relationships were built with both communities. Partnerships were established to cocreate the project and research methods. A relational paradigm was used that recognized the interconnected nature of individuals, experiences, and environment. A community-based participatory research method guided researcher activities. This collaborative approach recognizes that all persons involved are partners and contributors to the research process. A *two-eyed seeing* method was used that recognized that Indigenous and non-Indigenous knowledge is separate and distinct. When seeing from one eye, the strengths of Indigenous knowledge and ways of knowing are recognized, and from the other eye, the strengths of non-Indigenous knowledge and ways of knowing are seen. Photovoice was also used as a methodological approach to share stories and experiences through images, which allowed others to see the world through another's eyes. Research partners used the First Nation Mental Wellness Continuum Framework themes to guide photo-taking sessions around the themes of purpose, belonging, and meaning.

Key Findings

From the perspectives of these communities, wellness is a broader and more holistic concept than mental health and addiction. The decolonization of mental health practices with a focus on rebuilding respect and honour is an essential factor in providing mental wellness services. System-based recognition of the past and present impacts of forced assimilation on Indigenous culture is an important factor in delivering mental wellness services. Increased community cohesion, identity, and pride could also contribute to improving mental wellness. From an individual level, change efforts were identified that were related to increasing awareness of mental wellness.

Implications for Nursing Practice

When providing mental health care for Indigenous peoples, nurses and other health care providers must blend multiple cultural worldviews and healing approaches that value both Indigenous and non-Indigenous ways of knowing.

Source: Gould, B., MacQuarrie, C., O'Connell, M. E., & Bourassa, C. (2021). Mental wellness needs of two Indigenous communities: Bases for culturally competent clinical services. *Canadian Psychology/Psychologie Canadienne, 62*(3), 213–226. https://doi.org/10.1037/cap0000247

CHAPTER 4 Relevant Theories and Therapies for Nursing Practice

KEY POINTS TO REMEMBER

- Sigmund Freud advanced the first theory of personality development.
- Freud articulated levels of awareness (unconscious, preconscious, conscious) and demonstrated the influence of our unconscious behaviour on everyday life, as evidenced by the use of defence mechanisms.
- Freud identified three psychological processes of personality (id, ego, superego) and described how they operate and develop.
- Freud articulated one of the first modern developmental theories of personality, based on five psychosexual stages.
- Various psychoanalytic therapies have been used over the years. Currently, a short-term, time-limited version of psychotherapy is common.
- Erik Erikson expanded on Freud's developmental stages to include middle age through old age. Erikson called his stages *psychosocial stages* and emphasized the social aspect of personality development.
- Harry Stack Sullivan proposed the interpersonal theory of personality development, which focuses on interpersonal processes that can be observed in a social framework.
- Hildegard Peplau, a nursing theorist, developed an interpersonal theoretical framework that has become the foundation of psychiatric mental health nursing practice.
- Abraham Maslow, the founder of humanistic psychology, offered the theory of self-actualization and human motivation that is basic to all nursing education today.
- Cognitive behavioural therapy is the most commonly used, accepted, and empirically validated psychotherapeutic approach.
- A biological model of mental illness and treatment dominates care for psychiatric disorders.
- Milieu therapy is a philosophy of care in which all parts of the environment are considered to be therapeutic opportunities for growth and healing. The milieu includes the people (patients and staff), setting, structure, and emotional climate.

CRITICAL THINKING

1. Consider the theorists and theories discussed in this chapter. The following questions address how they may affect your nursing practice.
   a. How do Freud's concepts of the conscious, preconscious, and unconscious affect your understanding of patients' behaviours?
   b. Do you believe that Erikson's psychosocial stages represent a sound basis for identifying disruptions in stages of development in your patients? Support your position with a clinical example.
   c. What are the implications of Sullivan's focus on the importance of interpersonal relationships for your interactions with patients?
   d. Peplau believed that nurses must exercise self-awareness within the nurse–patient relationship. Describe situations in your student experience in which this self-awareness played a vital role in your relationships with patients.
   e. Identify someone you believe to be self-actualized. What characteristics does this person have that support your assessment?
   f. How do or will you make use of Maslow's hierarchy of needs in your nursing practice?
   g. What do you think about the behaviourist point of view that a change in behaviour results in a change in thinking? Can you give an example of this in your own life?
2. Which of the therapies described in this chapter do you think are or will be the most helpful to you in your nursing practice? Explain your choice.

CHAPTER REVIEW

1. The nurse is working with a patient who lacks the ability to problem-solve and seeks ways to self-satisfy without regard for others. Which system of the patient's personality is most pronounced?
   a. Id.
   b. Ego.
   c. Conscience (superego).
   d. Ego ideal (superego).
2. Which behaviour seen in a 30-year-old patient would alert the nurse to the fact that the patient is not in his appropriate developmental stage according to Erikson?
   a. States he is happily married.
   b. Frequently asks to call his brother "just to check in."
   c. Looks forward to visits from a coworker.
   d. Says, "I'm still trying to find myself."
3. A patient has difficulty sitting still and listening to others during group therapy. The therapist plans to use operant conditioning as a form of behavioural modification to assist the patient. Which action would the nurse expect to see in group therapy?
   a. The therapist will act as a role model for the patient by sitting still and listening.
   b. The patient will receive a token from the therapist for each session in which they sit still and listen.
   c. The patient will be required to sit in solitude for 30 minutes after each session in which they do not sit still or listen.
   d. The therapist will ask that the patient to sit still and listen for only 2 minutes at a time to begin with and will increase the time incrementally until the patient can sit and listen for 10 minutes at a time.
4. The nurse is planning care for a patient with anxiety who will be admitted to the unit shortly. Which nursing action is most important?
   a. Consider ways to assist the patient to feel valued during his stay on the unit.
   b. Choose a roommate for the patient so that a friendship can develop.
   c. Identify a room where the patient will have comfortable surroundings, and order a balanced meal plan.
   d. Plan methods of decreasing stimuli that could cause heightened anxiety in the patient.

http://evolve.elsevier.com/Canada/Varcarolis/psychiatric/

REFERENCES

Bandura, A., Blahard, E. B., & Ritter, B. (1969). Relative efficacy of desensitization and modeling approaches for inducing behavioural, affective, and attitudinal changes. *Journal of Personality and Social Psychology, 13,* 173–199. https://doi.org/10.1037/h0028276

Barker, P., & Buchanan-Barker, P. (2005). *The tidal model: A guide for mental health professionals.* New York: Brunner-Routledge.

Beck, A. T. (1967). *Depression: Clinical, experimental and theoretical aspects.* New York: Harper & Row.

Beck, A. T., Rush, A. J., Shaw, B. F., & Emery, G. (1979). *Cognitive therapy of depression.* New York: Guilford.

Canadian Federation of Mental Health Nurses. (2014). *Canadian standards for psychiatric-mental health nursing* (4th ed.). Toronto: Author.

Ellis, A. (2000). On therapy: A dialogue with Aaron T. Beck and Albert Ellis. *Symposium conducted at the American Psychological Association's 108th Convention.* Washington, DC.

Erikson, E. H. (1963). *Childhood and society.* New York: W. W. Norton.

Freud, S. (1960). *The ego and the id* (J. Strachey, Trans.). New York: W. W. Norton.

Freud, S. (1961). *The interpretation of dreams* (J. Strachey, Ed. & Trans.). New York: Scientific Editions.

Freud, S. (1969). *An outline of psychoanalysis* (J. Strachey, Trans.). New York: W. W. Norton.

Gilligan, C. (1982). *In a different voice.* Boston: Harvard University Press.

Kohlberg, L., & Turiel, E. (1971). Moral development and moral education. In G. S. Lesser (Ed.), *Psychology and educational practice* (pp. 410–465). Scott, Foresman, & Company.

Lenz, A. S., Del Conte, G., Hollenbaugh, K. M., & Callender, K. A. (2016). Emotional regulation and interpersonal effectiveness as mechanisms of change for treatment outcomes within a DBT program for adolescents. *Counseling Outcome Research, 7*(2), 73–85. https://doi.org/10.1177/2150137816642439

Linehan, M. M. (1993). *Cognitive behavioral treatment of borderline personality disorder.* New York: Guilford Press.

Mahler, M. S., Pine, F., & Bergman, A. (1975). *The psychological birth of the human infant.* New York: Basic Books.

Maslow, A. H. (1963). Self-actualizing people. In G. B. Levitas (Ed.), *The world of psychology Vol. 2.* New York: Braziller.

Maslow, A. H. (1968). *Toward a psychology of being.* Princeton: Van Nostrands.

Maslow, A. H. (1970). *Motivation and personality* (2nd ed.). New York: Harper & Row.

Nåvik, M., Hauge, S., & Sagen, U. (2020). Milieu therapy for hospitalized patients with late-life anxiety and depression: A qualitative study. *Nordic Journal of Psychiatry, 74*(7), 511–517. https://doi.org/10.1080/08039488.2020.1751879

Pavlov, I. (1928). In W. H. Grant (Ed.), *Lectures on conditioned reflexes.* New York: International Publishers.

Peplau, H. E. (1952). *Interpersonal relations in nursing: A conceptual frame of reference for psychodynamic nursing.* New York: Putnam.

Peplau, H. E. (1982a). Therapeutic concepts. In S. A. Smoyak, & S. Rouslin (Eds.), *A collection of classics in psychiatric nursing literature* (pp. 91–108). Slack.

Peplau, H. E. (1982b). Interpersonal techniques: The crux of psychiatric nursing. In S. A. Smoyak, & S. Rouslin (Eds.), *A collection of classics in psychiatric nursing literature* (pp. 276–281). Slack.

Peplau, H. E. (1987). Interpersonal constructs for nursing practice. *Nursing Education Today, 7*, 201–208. https://doi.org/10.1016/0260-6917(87)90002-5

Peplau, H. E. (1989). Future directions in psychiatric nursing from the perspective of history. *Journal of Psychosocial Nursing, 27*(2), 18–28.

Skinner, B. F. (1987). Whatever happened to psychology as the science of behavior?. *American Psychologist, 42*, 780–786. https://doi.org/10.1037/0003-066X.42.8.780

Sullivan, H. S. (1953). *The interpersonal theory of psychiatry.* New York: W. W. Norton.

Watson, J. B. (1919). *Psychology from the standpoint of a behaviourist.* Philadelphia: Lippincott.

Understanding Responses to Stress

Lisa-Marie Forcier
Originating US Chapter by Margaret Jordan Halter, Elizabeth M. Varcarolis

 http://evolve.elsevier.com/Canada/Varcarolis/psychiatric/

OBJECTIVES

1. Recognize the short- and long-term physiological consequences of stress.
2. Compare and contrast Cannon's fight-or-flight response, Selye's general adaptation syndrome, and the psychoneuroimmunological models of stress.
3. Describe how responses to stress are mediated through perception, personality, social support, culture, and spirituality.
4. Assess stress level using the Recent Life Changes Questionnaire.
5. Identify and describe holistic approaches to stress management.
6. Teach a classmate or patient a behavioural technique to help lower stress and anxiety.
7. Explain how cognitive techniques can help increase a person's tolerance for stressful events.

KEY TERMS AND CONCEPTS

Benson's relaxation technique
cognitive reframing
coping styles
distress
eustress
fight-or-flight response
general adaptation syndrome
guided imagery
journaling
meditation
mindfulness
physical stressors
progressive muscle relaxation
psychological stressors
psychoneuroimmunology
stressors

Before turning our attention to the clinical disorders presented in the chapters that follow, we explore the subject of stress as a foundation to understanding the context and experiences of distress. **Stress** is defined as an uncomfortable emotional experience accompanied by biochemical, physiological, and behavioural changes that occur during difficult or demanding circumstances or situations (Flores-Kanter et al., 2021; Nasso et al., 2020). Stress and our responses to it are central to psychiatric disorders and the provision of mental health care. The interplay among stress, the development of psychiatric disorders, and the exacerbation (worsening) of psychiatric symptoms has been widely researched. Early exposure to stressful events has been found to sensitize people to stress in later life. In other words, we know that people who are exposed to high levels of stress as children, especially during stress-sensitive developmental periods, have a greater incidence of all mental illnesses as adults (Paquola et al., 2017). While we all experience stress in our lives, which affects our mood, behaviour, and well-being (Flores-Kanter et al., 2021), it is important to recognize that severe stress is unhealthy and can weaken biological resistance to psychiatric pathology in any individual; however, stress is especially harmful to those who have a genetic predisposition to these disorders (Anisman, 2015). The inability to regulate daily stress is associated with the development of many psychological disorders such as major depression, substance use, and anxiety disorders (Flores-Kanter et al., 2021; Pulopulos et al., 2020).

While an understanding of the connection between stress and mental illness is essential in the psychiatric setting, it is also important when developing a plan of care for any patient, in any setting, with any diagnosis. Imagine having an appendectomy and being served with an eviction notice on the same day. How well could you cope with either situation, let alone both simultaneously? The nurse's role is to intervene to reduce stress by promoting a healing environment, facilitating successful coping, and developing future coping strategies. In this chapter we explore how we are equipped to respond to stress, what can go wrong with the stress response, and how to care for our patients and even ourselves during times of stress.

RESPONSES TO AND EFFECTS OF STRESS

Early Stress Response Theories

The earliest research into the stress response (Figure 5.1) began as a result of observations that stressors brought about physical disorders or made existing conditions worse. **Stressors** are psychological or physical stimuli that are incompatible with current functioning and require adaptation. Walter Cannon (1871–1945) methodically investigated the sympathetic nervous system as a pathway of the response to stress, known more commonly as fight (aggression) or flight (withdrawal). The well-known **fight-or-flight response** is the body's way of preparing for a situation perceived as a threat to survival. This response results in increased blood pressure, heart rate, and cardiac output.

While ground-breaking, Cannon's theory has been criticized for being simplistic since not all animals or people respond by fighting or fleeing. In the face of danger some animals (e.g., a deer) become still or freeze to avoid being noticed or to observe the environment in a state of heightened awareness. Also, Cannon's theory was developed primarily based on the responses of animals and men. Men and women, however, have different neural responses to stress. According to a study conducted by Goldfarb et al. (2019), throughout stressor

59

Fig. 5.1 The stress response. (Source: Brigham, D. D. (1994). *Imagery for getting well: Clinical applications of behavioural medicine.* New York: W. W. Norton.)

*Variable changes in β-endorphins, growth hormone, and prolactin (see text).
†Effects may be dependent on *amount* of cortisol and nature of the stressor.
‡Caused by protein catabolism in muscle, adipose tissue, skin, bones, lymphoid tissue.
ACTH, adrenocorticotropic hormone; *ADH*, antidiuretic hormone.

exposures, men showed higher responses in prefrontal regions, whereas women had higher responses in limbic/striatal areas. Such widespread differences are consistent with the influence of sex hormones (including estrogen and androgen) throughout the brain (Goldfarb et al., 2019, p. 8).

Hans Selye (1907–1982), another pioneer in stress research, introduced the concept of stress into both the scientific and popular literature. Selye (1974) expanded Cannon's 1956 theory of stress in his formulation of the *general adaptation syndrome* (GAS). The GAS occurs in three stages:

1. The *alarm* (or *acute stress*) stage is the initial, brief, and adaptive response (fight or flight) to the stressor. During the alarm stage, three principal *stress mediators* are involved:
   - The brain's cortex and hypothalamus signal the adrenal glands to release the catecholamine adrenaline. This release, in turn, increases sympathetic system activity (e.g., increased heart rate, respirations, and blood pressure) to enhance strength and speed. Pupils dilate for a broad view of the environment, and blood is shunted away from the digestive tract (resulting in dry mouth) and kidneys to more essential organs.
   - The hypothalamus also sends messages to the adrenal cortex. The adrenal cortex produces corticosteroids to help increase muscle endurance and stamina, whereas other nonessential functions (e.g., digestion) are decreased. Unfortunately, the corticosteroids also inhibit functions such as reproduction, growth, and immunity (Sadock & Sadock, 2017).
   - Endorphins that reduce sensitivity to pain and injury are released. The alarm stage is extremely intense, and no organism can sustain this level of reactivity and excitement for long. If the organism survives, the resistance stage follows.

2. The *resistance* stage could also be called the *adaptation stage*, because it is during this time that sustained and optimal resistance to the stressor occurs. Usually, stressors are successfully overcome; however, when they are not, the organism may experience the final stage: exhaustion.

3. The *exhaustion* stage occurs when attempts to resist the stressor prove futile. At this point, resources are depleted, and the stress may become chronic, producing a wide array of psychological and physiological responses and even death.

The body responds the same physiologically regardless of whether the stress is real or only perceived as a threat and whether the threat is physical, psychological, or social. In addition, the body cannot differentiate between the energy generated by positive and negative stimuli. Bienertova-Vasku et al. (2020) describe the reactions of distress and eustress:

- **Distress** is considered a negative stress where the individual can experience negative emotions. It is a draining energy that results in anxiety, depression, confusion, helplessness, hopelessness, and fatigue. Distress may be caused by such stressors as a death in the family, financial overload, or school or work demands.
- **Eustress** is considered a moderate, positive, beneficial energy that can stimulate the individual to feel happy or motivated. Eustress may be the result of a much-needed vacation, being called in for an interview, the birth of a baby, or buying a new car.

While Selye's GAS remains a popular theory, further research has offered and promoted a vast amount of knowledge in the stress field (McEwen et al., 2015).

Increased understanding of the exhaustion stage of the GAS has revealed that illness results from not only the depletion of reserves but also the stress mediators themselves. This finding is discussed in "Immune Stress Responses." Table 5.1 describes some reactions to acute and prolonged (chronic) stress.

TABLE 5.1 Some Reactions to Acute and Prolonged (Chronic) Stress

Acute Stress Can Cause	Prolonged (Chronic) Stress Can Cause
Uneasiness and concern	Anxiety and panic attacks
Sadness	Depression or melancholia
Loss of appetite	Anorexia or overeating
Suppression of the immune system	Lowered resistance to infections, leading to an increase in opportunistic viral and bacterial infections
Increased metabolism and use of body fats	Insulin-resistant diabetes
	Hypertension
Infertility	Amenorrhea or loss of sex drive
	Impotence, anovulation
Increased energy mobilization and use	Increased fatigue and irritability
	Decreased memory and learning
Increased cardiovascular tone	Increased risk for cardiac events (e.g., heart attack, angina, and sudden heart-related death)
	Increased risk for blood clots and stroke
Increased cardiopulmonary tone	Increased respiratory problems

Neurotransmitter Stress Responses

Serotonin is a brain catecholamine that plays an important role in mood, sleep, sexuality, appetite, and metabolism. It is one of the main neurotransmitters implicated in depression, and many medications used to treat depression do so by increasing the availability of serotonin (see Chapter 11). During times of stress, serotonin synthesis becomes more active. This stress-activated turnover of serotonin is at least partially mediated by the corticosteroids, and researchers believe this activation may dysregulate (impair) serotonin receptor sites and the brain's ability to use serotonin (Sadock & Sadock, 2017). The influence of stressful life events on the development of depression is well documented, but researchers still do not fully understand the relationship. This neurotransmitter stress response research sheds some new light on the process.

Immune Stress Responses

Cannon and Selye focused on the physical and mental responses of the nervous and endocrine systems to acute and chronic stress. Later work revealed that there is also an interaction between the nervous system and the immune system during the alarm phase of the GAS. In one classic study rats were given a mixture of saccharine and a drug that reduces the immune system (Ader & Cohen, 1975). Afterward, when given only the saccharine, the rats continued to have decreased immune responses, which indicated that stress itself negatively affects the body's ability to produce a protective structure. Researchers have discovered that the response to stressful stimuli is elaborated and triggered by the now-known *stress system*, which integrates a wide range of brain structures that, collectively, are able to detect situations and interpret them as either a real or potential threat: stressor (Godoy et al., 2018, p. 2).

Studies in *psychoneuroimmunology* (the study of the relationship between the mind, the nervous system, and the immune system) continue to provide evidence that stress, through the hypothalamic–pituitary–adrenal (HPA) and sympathetic–adrenal medullary axes, can induce changes in the immune system and are the two major components involved in the stress response (Godoy et al., 2018). Under stressful conditions, the HPA axis is activated, resulting in an increase in cortisol secretion that peaks between 20 and 40 minutes after initiation of the stressful event (Pulopulos et al., 2020). Along with this, individuals showing higher cortisol reactivity to stress are at greater risk for experiencing subsequent depressive symptoms (Pulopulos et al., 2020). This model helps explain what many researchers and clinicians have believed and witnessed for centuries: there are links between stress (biopsychosocial), the immune system, and disease, a clear mind–body connection that may alter health outcomes. Stress may result in malfunctions in the immune system that are implicated in autoimmune disorders, immunodeficiency, and hypersensitivities. Therefore when a stressful situation is anticipated, individuals make behavioral, cognitive, and physiological adjustments that facilitate the process of coping with the upcoming stressor (Pulopulos et al., 2018).

Stress influences the immune system in several complex ways. As discussed earlier, corticosteroids are released in response to stress and inhibit the immune system, which increases susceptibility to illness (Sadock & Sadock, 2017). Conversely, stress can enhance the immune system and prepare the body to respond to injury. Cytokines, which are proteins and glycoproteins used for communication between cells, are normally released by immune cells when a pathogen is detected; they serve to activate and recruit other immune cells. During times of stress, these cytokines are released, and immunity is profoundly activated. But the activation is limited since the cytokines stimulate the further release of corticosteroids, which inhibit the immune system.

The immune response and the resulting cytokine activity in the brain raise questions about their connection with psychological and cognitive states such as depression (Godoy et al., 2018). Some cancers are treated with a type of cytokine molecules known as interleukins. These chemotherapy drugs tend to cause or increase depression. Furthermore, elevated cytokines and immune activation are often seen during episodes of severe depression.

MEDIATORS OF THE STRESS RESPONSE

Stressors

A variety of situations, emotions, and circumstances (e.g., emotional arousal, fatigue, fear, loss, humiliation, loss of blood, extreme happiness, unexpected success) can produce stress and trigger the stress response. No individual factor can be singled out as the cause of the stress response; however, stressors can be divided into two categories: physical and psychological (Godoy et al., 2018). **Physical stressors** include changes to environmental conditions (e.g., environmental trauma or disaster, excessive cold or heat), as well as physical conditions (e.g., injury, illness, hunger, pain). **Psychological stressors** include cognitive- or emotion-based changes, such as divorce, loss of a job, unmanageable debt, the death of a loved one, retirement, and fear of violence, as well as changes we might consider positive, such as marriage, the arrival of a new baby, or unexpected success.

Perception

Researchers have looked at the degree to which various life events upset a specific individual and have found that the perception of a stressor determines the person's emotional and psychological reactions to it (Rahe et al., 2000). Epidemiological studies show that both experiencing an increased number of stressful life events and reporting high perceived stress over long periods of time are associated with worse mental and physical health and mortality (Crosswell & Lockwood, 2020; Epel et al., 2018). Responses to stress and anxiety are affected by factors such as age, gender, culture, life experience, and lifestyle, all of which may work to either lessen or increase the degree of emotional or physical influence and the sequel of stress. For example, a man in his 40s who has a new baby, has just purchased a home, and is laid off with 6 months' severance pay may feel the stress of the job loss more intensely than a man in his 60s who is financially secure and is asked to take an early retirement.

Personality

Afshar et al. (2015) show that personality traits are an important factor in identifying, responding, and approaching stress events. It has been found some personality traits can predict stress level. For example, maladaptive personality traits (e.g., neuroticism) are related to increased exposure to stressful life events and are likely to make individuals

---

RESEARCH HIGHLIGHT
Urban Tree Canopy and Stress Recovery

Background

Many *theories*, including Ulrich's stress reduction theory (1991), suggest, for evolutionary or psychological reasons, humans prefer greener environments because they help them survive and thrive. Further, many *empirical studies* report a significant association between greater tree coverage and healthier human functioning. Stress reduction is an important benefit of a greener environment. A recent study found "watching a 6-min 3-D video of residential streets with moderate eye-level tree cover density (29%) had a 3.1 times greater stress reduction effect assessed in psychological and hormonal measures than watching a similar video with a low tree cover density (2%)" (Jiang et al., 2016, p. 607). Another related study reported a "positive causal association between eye-level tree cover density and self-reported stress reduction" (Jiang et al., 2016, p. 607). These studies and several prior studies suggest that environments with higher tree cover density can produce greater stress reduction.

Problem

Although it is well established that viewing nature can help individuals to recover from illness or stressful experiences, the actual "dosage" or relationship of tree cover density and stress recovery is not known.

Purpose of Study

To determine the optimal urban tree canopy to aid in stress reduction.

Methods

An experiment was completed with 160 participants who engaged in a standard Trier Social Stress Test to induce stress. These participants were then randomly assigned to watch 1 of 10 three-dimensional videos of street scenes with varying degrees of tree cover density (2% to 62%). At three different points in the experiment, participants completed a Visual Analogue Scale.

Key Findings

Analysis revealed a positive, linear association between the density of urban street trees and self-reported stress recovery. In short, an increase in tree density yields greater self-reported stress reduction. Compared with watching a 6-minute video with 2% tree cover density, watching a 6-minute video with 62% tree cover density resulted in a 60% increase in stress recovery. This relationship held after controlling for gender, age, and baseline stress levels. Participants' written narratives revealed a similar but even stronger association.

Implications for Nursing Practice

These results can help nurses in encouraging nature immersion for patients recovering from stress-related disorders and in general mental health promotion. Nurses can also advocate for a greater investment in urban tree planting and community parks and landscape design based on these significant findings.

Source: Jiang, B., Li, D., Larsen, L., et al. (2016). A dose-response curve describing the relationship between urban tree cover density and self-reported stress recovery. *Environment and Behavior, 48*(4), 607–629. https://doi.org/10.1177/0013916514552321

susceptible to experience negative emotion and frustration, while adaptive personality traits (e.g., high extraversion and conscientiousness) are less affected by daily stresses. Personality traits can predict coping strategies and influence the coping strategies we choose (Afshar et al., 2015).

Social Support

Social support is a mediating factor with significant implications for nurses and other health care providers (Underwood, 2012). Strong social support from significant others can enhance mental and physical health and act as a significant buffer against distress. A shared identity, whether with a family, social network, or colleagues, helps people overcome stressors more adaptively (Newman & Roberts, 2013). Numerous studies have found a strong correlation between lower mortality rates and intact support systems (Koenig et al., 2012).

Self-Help Groups

The proliferation of self-help groups attests to the need for social supports, and the explosive growth of a great variety of support groups reflects their effectiveness for many people. Many of the support groups currently available are for people going through similar stressful life events, such as those experiencing grief and loss from death, suicide, divorce, or job loss and those seeking support through cancer survivorship, to note but a few.

Low- and High-Quality Support

It is important to differentiate between social support relationships of low quality and those of high quality. Low-quality support relationships (e.g., living in an abusive home situation or with a controlling and demeaning person) often negatively affect a person's coping effectiveness in a crisis. On the other hand, high-quality relationships have been linked to less loneliness, more supportive behaviour, and greater life satisfaction (Newman & Roberts, 2013). High-quality emotional support is a critical factor in enhancing a person's sense of control and in rebuilding feelings of self-esteem and competency after a stressful event. Supportive, high-quality relationships are relatively free from conflict and negative interactions and are close, confiding, and reciprocal (Newman & Roberts, 2013).

Diet

The relationship between diet and behavior is an area of significant interest and research. This includes the effects of diet on both mental and physical health, as well as related topics of the role of stress and obesity in these processes (Bremner et al., 2020). The relationship between diet and psychiatric disorders is often bidirectional. For example, changes in diet may influence psychiatric disorders through direct effects on mood, while the development of psychiatric disorders can lead to changes in eating habits (Bremner et al., 2020).

Dietary modification can prevent the development of cardiovascular disease, diabetes, and stress-related disorders, including major depression and post-traumatic stress disorder (Bremner et al., 2020).

Culture

Each culture not only emphasizes certain problems more than others but also interprets emotional problems differently from other cultures, even when similar concepts are used to describe a problem. For example, the idiom (or common expression) of distress, "thinking too much," was explored in a qualitative research synthesis. Exploring numerous studies, researchers found that the expression was used across multiple cultural groups to describe ruminating thoughts, worry, reliving trauma, and a host of other characteristics (Kaiser et al., 2015). Although Western European and North American cultures subscribe to a psychophysiological view of stress and somatic distress (e.g., feeling of sadness and anhedonia, negative thoughts about self [Huang et al., 2016]), it must be said that this view does not dominate in other cultures. The overwhelming majority of Asian, African, and Central American cultural groups experience and describe distress in somatic terms (e.g., appetite and sleep disturbance, agitation, shortness of breath [Huang et al., 2016]). Emerging evidence suggests that the somatic emphasis in most regions of the world may be due to differences in symptom reporting patterns, as opposed to the nature of the disorder in these regions (Huang et al., 2016). For more information about cultural implications for psychiatric mental health nursing, refer to Chapter 8.

Spirituality and Religious Beliefs

Spiritual and religious factors are strongly tied to a host of mental health characteristics, in both positive and negative ways (Rosmarin & Koenig, 2020).

Spirituality has many benefits for stress relief and overall mental health. It can serve as a coping mechanism, mediating negative impacts of traumatic stress on mental health; adding meaning, purpose and social support; and promoting general wellbeing (Reinert & Koenig, 2013).

Prayer can elicit the relaxation response (discussed later in this chapter), which is known to reduce stress physically and emotionally and to reduce stress on the immune system. Spiritual and religious organizations and pressures can, in some instances, bring judgment and social and cultural pressures, contributing to greater stress. Historical experiences of religious oppression and domination also contribute to stress, for example, for some South Asian and Indigenous people (Kent et al., 2021).

Figure 5.2 operationally defines the process of stress and the positive or negative results of attempts to relieve stress, including through spiritual practices. Box 5.1 identifies several stress busters that can be incorporated into our lives with little effort.

NURSING MANAGEMENT OF STRESS RESPONSES

Measuring Stress

Health indicators are a range of measures that can facilitate comparisons across time and place at national, provincial and territorial, and regional levels. Since 1999, Statistics Canada and the Canadian Institute for Health Information (CIHI) have collaborated on developing and providing a broad range of indicators for health regions across Canada. Life satisfaction is a personal subjective assessment of global well-being and it has become an important national health statistic in Canada. Responses have already been shown to have relevance for health care as a predictor both of future demands on the health care system and of subsequent morbidity and mortality (Helliwell et al., 2020). Using population-representative samples from the 2018 Canadian Community Health Survey and the June 2020 Canadian Perspectives Survey Series, from 2018 to June 2020, average life satisfaction in Canada declined from 8.09 to 6.71 on a 0-to-10 response scale, a decline of 1.38 points (Helliwell et al., 2020). This is the lowest level of life satisfaction observed in Canada over the 2003–2020 period for which comparable data are available (Helliwell et al., 2020).

In June 2020 40% of Canadians rated their life satisfaction as 8 or above on the scale, down from 72% in 2018; conversely, 40% of Canadians rated their life satisfaction as 6 or below, up from 12% (Helliwell et al., 2020). There was little difference in average life satisfaction reported by women and men (Helliwell et al., 2020). However, average life satisfaction changed far more across age groups, declining by 1.76 points among Canadians aged 15 to 29, by 1.32 points among those aged 30 to 59, and by 1.21 points among those aged 60 or older (Helliwell et al., 2020).

The Canadian Index of Wellbeing (CIW) also reports on key indicators that contribute to our understanding of the state of stress and resilience among Canadians. The 2016 CIW National Report titled *How Are*

Fig. 5.2 Stress and anxiety operationally defined.

BOX 5.1 Effective Stress Busters

Sleep
- Chronically stressed people are often fatigued, so go to sleep 30 to 60 minutes early each night for a few weeks.
- If you are still fatigued, try going to bed another 30 minutes earlier.
- Sleeping later in the morning is not helpful and can disrupt body rhythms.

Exercise (aerobic)
- Exercise:
  - Can dissipate chronic and acute stress
  - May decrease levels of anxiety, depression, and sensitivity to stress
  - Can decrease muscle tension and increase endorphin levels
- It is recommended that you exercise for at least 30 minutes three or more times a week.
- It is best to exercise at least 3 hours before bedtime.

Reduction or cessation of caffeine intake
- Lowering or stopping caffeine intake can lead to more energy and fewer muscle aches and help you feel more relaxed.
- Slowly wean off coffee, tea, colas, and chocolate drinks.

Music (classical or soft melodies of choice)
- Listening to music increases your sense of relaxation.
- Increased healing effects may result.
- Therapeutically, music can:
  - Decrease agitation and confusion in older adults
  - Increase quality of life in hospice settings

Pets
- Pets can bring joy and reduce stress.
- They can be an important social support.
- Pets can alleviate medical problems aggravated by stress.

Massage
- Massage can slow the heart rate and relax the body.
- Alertness may actually increase.

Canadians Really Doing? further highlights key stressors such as income inequality, time pressures, difficulties balancing commitments, poor sleep, less time with friends and at leisure, and poor self-reported health. Overall, Canadians reported conditions of increased stress and decreased life satisfaction in the reporting period (Canadian Index of Wellbeing, 2016). The report findings suggest the need for multiple levels of health promotion and stress-reduction interventions. The individual's level of stress illustrated in Figure 5.3 is expressed interpersonally, with family and friends, at work and community levels, and ultimately societally.

Take a few minutes to assess your stress level over the past 6 to 12 months using the *Recent Life Changes Questionnaire* (Table 5.2). Keep in mind that when you administer the questionnaire, you must take into account the following:
- Not all events are perceived to have the same degree of intensity or disruptiveness.
- Culture may dictate whether an event is stressful or how stressful it is.
- Different people may have different thresholds beyond which disruptions occur.
- The questionnaire equates change with stress.

Other stress scales that may be useful to nursing students have been developed. You might like to try the Perceived Stress Scale (Figure 5.4). Although there are no absolute scores, this scale measures how relatively uncontrollable, unpredictable, and overloaded you find your life. Try this scale in a clinical post-conference for comparison and discussion.

Adverse Childhood Experiences

According to a study by Karatekin (2018), adverse childhood experiences (ACEs) have been defined as moderately to severely stressful experiences during the first 18 years of life, including emotional, sexual and physical

Fig. 5.3 Canadians report high levels of stress and decreased life satisfaction. (Source: https://pixabay.com/en/adult-annoyed-blur-burnout-1850268/.)

abuse; neglect; parental psychopathology; parental incarceration; and parental separation or divorce. Over a third of adults in the general population report experiencing at least two ACEs. The cumulative impact of ACEs has been associated with many mental health problems, including anxiety and depression. Having at least one ACE has been estimated to account for two-thirds of suicide attempts in adults (Karatekin, 2018, p. 36).

Anniko et al. (2019) show that adolescent stress and stress-related mental health complaints are common and have been increasing over the past decades. In particular, females in adolescence report high levels of stress and stress-related symptoms such as anxiety, depressive symptoms, sleeping difficulties, and somatic complaints. According to the CIHI (2020), between 2008–2009 and 2018–2019, there was a 61% increase in visits to the emergency department and a 60% increase in hospitalizations for youth between the ages of 15 to 17 years old for mental health disorders (CIHI, 2020).

Studying the sources to which all adolescents attribute their stress, as well as cognitive mechanisms causing the development of increases in stress-related mental health problems, is an important effort as it will provide insight into possible targets for preventive intervention (Anniko et al., 2019, pp. 155–156).

Assessing Coping Styles

People cope with life stressors in a variety of ways, and a number of factors can act as effective mediators to decrease stress in our lives. Rahe (1995) identified four discrete personal attributes (**coping styles**) people can develop to help manage stress:

1. Health-sustaining habits (e.g., medical compliance, proper diet, relaxation, adequate rest and sleep, pacing one's energy)
2. Life satisfactions (e.g., occasional escapism, reading, movie watching, work, family, hobbies, humour, spiritual solace, arts, nature)
3. Social supports (e.g., talk with trusted friends, family, counsellors, or support groups)
4. Effective and healthy responses to stress (e.g., work off anger through physical activity, go for a walk, dig in the garden, do yoga)

Examining these four coping categories can help nurses identify areas to target for improving their patients' responses to stress. Table 5.3 presents positive and negative responses to stress.

Managing Stress Through Relaxation Techniques

Poor management of stress has been correlated with an increased incidence of a number of physical and emotional conditions, such as heart disease, poor diabetes control, chronic pain, and significant emotional distress (Thase et al., 2015). Psychoneuroimmunology provides the foundation for several integrative therapies, also referred to as mind–body therapies. There is now considerable evidence that many mind–body therapies rooted in ancient meditative traditions that incorporate controlled paced breathing (e.g., yoga, tai chi, qi gong) are therapeutic and can be used as effective adjuncts to conventional medical treatment for a number of common clinical conditions (Lavretsky & Feldman, 2021). Chapter 35 offers a more detailed discussion of holistic, mind–body, and integrative care.

Nurses should be aware of a variety of stress and anxiety reduction techniques they can teach their patients. The following are some of the known benefits of stress reduction:

- Alters the course of certain medical conditions, such as high blood pressure, arrhythmias, arthritis, cancer, and peptic ulcers
- Decreases the need for medications such as insulin, analgesics, and antihypertensives
- Diminishes or eliminates the urge for unhealthy and destructive behaviours, such as smoking, addiction to drugs, insomnia, and overeating
- Increases cognitive functions such as learning and concentration and improves study habits
- Breaks up static patterns of thinking and allows fresh and creative ways of perceiving life events
- Increases the sense of well-being through endorphin release
- Reduces anxiety, increases comfort, and helps decrease sleep disturbances

Because no single stress-management technique is right for everyone, employing a mixture of techniques brings the best results. All are useful in a variety of situations for specific individuals. Essentially, there are stress-reducing techniques for every personality type, situation, and level of stress. Give them a try. Practicing relaxation techniques will allow you not only to help your patients reduce their stress levels but also to manage your own physical responses to stressors. These techniques result in reduced heart and breathing rates, decreased blood pressure, improved oxygenation to major muscles, and reduced muscle tension. They also help manage subjective anxiety and improve appraisals of reality.

Relaxation Exercises

In 1938 Edmund Jacobson developed a rather simple procedure that elicits a relaxation response, which he coined **progressive muscle relaxation** (PMR) (Sadock & Sadock, 2017). This technique can be done without any external gauges or feedback and can be practiced almost anywhere. The premise behind PMR is that since anxiety results in tense muscles, one way to decrease anxiety is to nearly eliminate muscle contraction. This muscle relaxation is accomplished by tensing groups of muscles (beginning with the feet and ending with the face) as tightly as possible for 8 seconds and then suddenly releasing them. Considerable research supports the use of PMR as helpful for pain and a number of medical conditions, such as headaches and psychiatric disorders,

TABLE 5.2 Recent Life Changes Questionnaire

Life-Changing Event	Life Change Unit*	Life-Changing Event	Life Change Unit*
Health		Due to marriage	41
An injury or illness that:		For other reasons	45
Kept you in bed a week or more or sent you to the hospital	74	Change in arguments with spouse	50
Was less serious than above	44	In-law problems	38
Major dental work	26	*Change in the marital status of your parents:*	
Major change in eating habits	27	Divorce	59
Major change in sleeping habits	26	Remarriage	50
Major change in your usual type and/or amount of recreation	28	*Separation from spouse:*	
Work		Due to work	53
Change to a new type of work	51	Due to marital problems	76
Change in your work hours or conditions	35	Divorce	96
Change in your responsibilities at work:		Birth of grandchild	43
More responsibilities	29	Death of spouse	119
Fewer responsibilities	21	*Death of other family member:*	
Promotion	31	Child	123
Demotion	42	Brother or sister	102
Transfer	32	Parent	100
Troubles at work:		**Personal and Social**	
With your boss	29	Change in personal habits	26
With coworkers	35	Beginning or ending of school or college	38
With persons under your supervision	35	Change of school or college	35
Other work troubles	28	Change in political beliefs	24
Major business adjustment	60	Change in religious beliefs	29
Retirement	52	Change in social activities	27
Loss of job:		Vacation	24
Laid off from work	68	New close personal relationship	37
Fired from work	79	Engagement to marry	45
Correspondence course to help you in your work	18	Girlfriend or boyfriend problems	39
Home and Family		Sexual differences	44
Major change in living conditions	42	"Falling out" of a close personal relationship	47
Change in residence:		An accident	48
Move within the same town or city	25	Minor violation of the law	20
Move to a different town, city, or state	47	Being held in jail	75
Change in family get-togethers	25	Death of a close friend	70
Major change in health or behavior of family member	55	Major decision regarding your immediate future	51
Marriage	50	Major personal achievement	36
Pregnancy	67	**Financial**	
Miscarriage or abortion	65	*Major change in finances:*	
Gain of a new family member:		Increase in income	38
Birth of a child	66	Decrease in income	60
Adoption of a child	65	Investment and/or credit difficulties	56
A relative moving in with you	59	Loss or damage of personal property	43
Spouse beginning or ending work	46	Moderate purchase	20
Child leaving home:		Major purchase	37
To attend college	41	Foreclosure on a mortgage or loan	58

*One-year totals ≥500 life change units are considered indications of high recent life stress.

Source: Miller, M. A., & Rahe, R. H. (1997). Life changes scaling for the 1990s. *Journal of Psychosomatic Research, 43*(3), 279–292. doi:10.1016/S0022-3999(97)00118-9.

Instructions: The questions in this scale ask you about your feelings and thoughts during the last month. In each case please indicate with a check how often you felt or thought a certain way.

1. In the last month how often have you been upset because of something that happened unexpectedly?
   ___0 never   ___1 almost never   ___2 sometimes   ___3 fairly often   ___4 very often
2. In the last month how often have you felt that you were unable to control the important things in your life?
   ___0 never   ___1 almost never   ___2 sometimes   ___3 fairly often   ___4 very often
3. In the last month how often have you felt nervous and "stressed"?
   ___0 never   ___1 almost never   ___2 sometimes   ___3 fairly often   ___4 very often
4. In the last month how often have you felt confident about your ability to handle your personal problems?
   ___0 never   ___1 almost never   ___2 sometimes   ___3 fairly often   ___4 very often
5. In the last month how often have you felt that things were going your way?
   ___0 never   ___1 almost never   ___2 sometimes   ___3 fairly often   ___4 very often
6. In the last month how often have you found that you could not cope with all the things that you had to do?
   ___0 never   ___1 almost never   ___2 sometimes   ___3 fairly often   ___4 very often
7. In the last month how often have you been able to control irritations in your life?
   ___0 never   ___1 almost never   ___2 sometimes   ___3 fairly often   ___4 very often
8. In the last month how often have you felt that you were on top of things?
   ___0 never   ___1 almost never   ___2 sometimes   ___3 fairly often   ___4 very often
9. In the last month how often have you been angered because of things that were outside of your control?
   ___0 never   ___1 almost never   ___2 sometimes   ___3 fairly often   ___4 very often
10. In the last month how often have you felt difficulties were piling up so high that you could not overcome them?
    ___0 never   ___1 almost never   ___2 sometimes   ___3 fairly often   ___4 very often

Perceived stress scale scoring
Items 4, 5, 7, and 8 are the positively stated items. PSS-10 scores are obtained by reversing the scores on the positive items—e.g., 0 = 4, 1 = 3, 2 = 2, etc.—and then adding all 10 items.

Fig. 5.4 Perceived stress scale—10 item (PSS-10). (Source: Cohen, S., Kamarck, T., & Mermelstein, R. (1983). A global measure of perceived stress. *Journal of Health and Social Behavior, 24*(4), Appendix A.)

TABLE 5.3 Positive and Negative Responses to Stress

Positive Stress Responses	Negative Stress Responses
Problem solving—figuring out how to navigate the situation	Avoidance—choosing not to deal with the situation, letting negative feelings and situations fester and continue to become chronic
Using social support—calling in others who are caring and may be helpful	Self-blame—faulting oneself, which keeps the focus on minimizing one's self-esteem and prevents positive action toward resolution or working through the feelings related to the event
Reframing—redefining the situation to see both positive and negative sides, as well as the way to use the situation to one's advantage	Wishful thinking—believing that things will resolve themselves and that "everything will be fine" (a form of denial)

Source: Lazarus, R. S. (2012). Evolution of a model of stress, coping, and discrete emotions. In V. H. Rice (Ed.), *Handbook of stress, coping, and health: Implications for nursing research, theory, and practice* (2nd ed., pp. 199–225). Sage.

especially those with anxiety components (Unger et al., 2017). Many good PMR scripts are available online.

Herbert Benson (1975) expanded on Jacobson's work by incorporating a state of mind that is conducive to relaxation. His technique, influenced by Eastern practices, is achieved by adopting a calm and passive attitude and focusing on a pleasant mental image in a calm and peaceful environment. **Benson's relaxation technique** allows the patient to switch from the sympathetic mode of the autonomic nervous system (fight-or-flight response) to the parasympathetic mode (a state of relaxation). Follow the steps in Box 5.2 to practice the relaxation response. Benson's relaxation technique has been combined successfully with meditation and visual imagery to treat symptoms of numerous disorders, such as diabetes, high blood pressure, migraine headaches, cancer, and peptic ulcers.

Meditation

Meditation follows the basic guidelines described for the relaxation response. It is a discipline for training the mind to develop greater calm and then using that calm to bring penetrative insight into one's experience. Meditation can be used to help people reach their deep inner resources for healing, to calm the mind, and to operate more efficiently in the world. It can help people develop strategies to cope with stress, make sensible adaptive choices under pressure, and feel more engaged in life (Donnelly, 2013; Galante et al., 2014).

Meditation elicits a relaxation response by creating a hypometabolic state of quieting the sympathetic nervous system. Some people

> **BOX 5.2 Benson's Relaxation Technique**
>
> - Choose any word or brief phrase that reflects your belief system, such as *love, unity in faith and love, joy, shalom, one God, peace*.
> - Sit in a comfortable position.
> - Close your eyes.
> - Deeply relax all your muscles, beginning at your feet and progressing up to your face. Keep them relaxed.
> - Breathe through your nose. Become aware of your breathing. As you breathe out, say your word or phrase silently to yourself. For example, breathe IN … OUT (phrase), IN … OUT (phrase), and so forth. Breathe easily and naturally.
> - Continue for 10 to 20 minutes. You may open your eyes and check the time, but do not use an alarm. When you finish, sit quietly for several minutes, at first with your eyes closed and then with your eyes open. Do not stand up for a few minutes.
> - Do not worry about whether you are successful in achieving a deep level of relaxation. Maintain a passive attitude, and permit relaxation to occur at its own pace. When distracting thoughts occur, try to ignore them by not dwelling on them, and return to repeating your word or phrase. With practice, the response should come with little effort. Practise the technique once or twice daily, but not within 2 hours after any meal, because the digestive process seems to interfere with the elicitation of the relaxation response.
>
> **Source:** Benson, H. (1975). *The relaxation response.* New York: William Morrow & Company.

> **BOX 5.3 Script for Guided Imagery**
>
> - Imagine releasing all the tension in your body … letting it go.
> - Now, with every breath you take, feel your body drifting down deeper and deeper into relaxation … floating down … deeper and deeper.
> - Imagine a peaceful scene. You are sitting beside a clear, blue mountain stream. You are barefoot, and you feel the sun-warmed rock under your feet. You hear the sound of the stream tumbling over the rocks. The sound is hypnotic, and you relax more and more. You see the tall pine trees on the opposite shore bending in the gentle breeze. Breathe the clean, scented air, with each breath moving you deeper and deeper into relaxation. The sun warms your face.
> - You are very comfortable. There is nothing to disturb you. You experience a feeling of well-being.
> - You can return to this peaceful scene by taking time to relax. The positive feelings can grow stronger and stronger each time you choose to relax.
> - You can return to your activities now, feeling relaxed and refreshed.

> **BOX 5.4 Deep-Breathing Exercise**
>
> - Find a comfortable position.
> - Relax your shoulders and chest; let your body relax.
> - Shift to relaxed, abdominal breathing. Take a deep breath through your mouth, expanding the abdomen. Hold it for 3 seconds and then exhale slowly through the nose; exhale completely, telling yourself to relax.
> - With every breath, turn attention to the muscular sensations that accompany the expansion of the belly.
> - As you concentrate on your breathing, you will start to feel focused.
> - Repeat this exercise for 2–5 minutes.

meditate using a visual object or a sound to help them focus. Others may find it useful to concentrate on their breathing while meditating. There are many meditation techniques, some with a mindfulness or awareness base and some with a spiritual base, such as Siddha meditation or prayer. Meditation is easy to practice anywhere. Some students find that meditating on the morning of a test helps them to focus and lessens anxiety. Keep in mind that meditation, like most other skills, must be practiced to produce the relaxation response.

Guided Imagery

Guided imagery is a process whereby a person is led to envision images that are both calming and health enhancing. It can be used in conjunction with Benson's relaxation technique. The content of the imagery exercises is shaped by the person helping with the imagery process. A person who has dysfunctional images can be helped to generate more effective and functional coping images to replace the depression- or anxiety-producing ones (Bigham et al., 2014). Often, audio recordings are made specifically for patients and their particular situations. However, many generic guided-imagery CDs, podcasts, and MP3s are available to patients and health care workers. An example of a script for guided imagery can be found in Box 5.3.

Breathing Exercises

Respiratory retraining, usually in the form of learning abdominal (diaphragmatic) breathing, has numerous merits in the modification of stress and anxiety reactions (Perciavalle et al., 2017). Self-regulation of breathing through patterns or cycles of breathing as a yoga exercise to modulate the stress response has been studied (Jerath et al., 2015). Another breathing exercise that has proved helpful for many patients with anxiety disorders has two parts: the first part focuses on abdominal breathing, while the second part helps patients to interrupt trains of thought, thereby quieting mental noise (Box 5.4). With increasing skill, breathing becomes a tool for dampening the cognitive processes likely to induce stress and anxiety reactions.

Physical Exercise

Physical exercise can lead to protection from the harmful effects of stress on both physical and mental states. In addition to its good effects for depression and anxiety, there is evidence to suggest that regular exercise and being physically fit can reduce stress levels generally. There are mixed results regarding the level of intensity (high or moderate exercise intensity) required to avoid stress, but aerobic exercise seems to have a better effect than strength training (Pedersen & Saltin, 2015). Yoga, an ancient form of exercise, has been found to be helpful for depression when used in conjunction with medication (Sharma, 2014). Forest bathing, also called "Shinrin-yoku" in Japanese, is a traditional practice characterized by walking in a forest environment, watching it, and breathing its air (Antonelli et al., 2019). In Japan forest bathing is considered an "art" and a type of meditation, with its origins deeply rooted in local traditions (Antonelli et al., 2019). Antonelli et al. (2019) illustrate how previous reviews of the scientific literature have indicated that forest bathing in particular can be useful for the immune system function; for cardiovascular and respiratory diseases; and for depression, anxiety, attention-deficit/hyperactivity disorder, and stress (Hansen et al., 2017; Lee et al., 2017; Oh et al., 2017). Other popular forms of exercise that show promise for stress reduction are walking, tai chi, dancing, drumming, cycling, aerobics, and water exercise. There are many considerations regarding motivation, energy, and other barriers, despite the benefits, particularly when patients are acutely unwell or struggling with serious and persistent anxiety, depression, or psychosis (Cooney et al., 2013). Although there are considerable benefits, motivating factors and barriers must also be addressed as nurses encourage physical exercise in the treatment and prevention of stress (Firth et al., 2016).

Biofeedback

Through the use of sensitive instrumentation, biofeedback provides immediate and exact information about muscle activity, brain waves, skin temperature, heart rate, blood pressure, and other bodily functions. Indicators of the particular internal physiological process are detected and amplified by a sensitive recording device. An individual can achieve greater voluntary control over phenomena once considered to be exclusively involuntary if they know instantaneously, through an auditory or visual signal, whether a somatic activity is increasing or decreasing.

Using biofeedback requires special training, and the technique is thought to be most effective for people with low to moderate hypnotic ability. For people with higher hypnotic ability, meditation, PMR, and other cognitive behavioural therapy techniques produce the most rapid reduction in clinical symptoms.

With increasing recognition of the role of stress in a variety of medical illnesses, including diseases affected by immune dysfunction, biofeedback has emerged as an effective strategy for stress management. The need to use the complex instrumentation required to detect minute levels of muscle tension or certain patterns of electroencephalographic activity is uncertain, but it has been confirmed that teaching people to relax deeply and apply these skills in response to real-life stressors can be helpful in lowering stress levels.

Cognitive Reframing

Cognitive reframing is a technique used to revise perceptions of a negative, distorted, or self-defeating belief with a goal of changing behaviours or improving well-being (Robson & Troutman-Jordan, 2014). The practice has been found to be positively correlated with greater positive affect and higher self-esteem. The goal of cognitive reframing is for an individual to change their perceptions of stress by reassessing a situation and replacing irrational beliefs ("I can't pass this course.") with more positive self-statements ("If I choose to study for this course, I will increase my chances of success."). We can learn from most situations by asking ourselves:

- What positive things came out of this situation or experience?
- What did I learn in this situation?
- What would I have done differently?

The desired result is to reframe a disturbing event or experience as less disturbing and to give the patient a sense of control over the situation. When the perception of the disturbing event is changed, there is less stimulation to the sympathetic nervous system, which in turn reduces the secretion of cortisol and catecholamines that destroy the balance of the immune system (Robson & Troutman-Jordan, 2014).

Cognitive distortions occur when our mind convinces us of something that is not really true. These incorrect thoughts help to reinforce negative thinking or emotions. These thoughts sound rational and accurate but really only reinforce the bad feeling we have about ourselves (Beck, 1976). They often include overgeneralizations ("He always …" or "I'll never …") and "should" statements ("I should have done better" or "She shouldn't have said that").

Table 5.4 shows some examples of cognitive reframing of anxiety-producing thoughts. Often cognitive reframing is used along with PMR and guided imagery to reduce stress.

Mindfulness

Mindfulness, a centuries-old form of meditation, has been dated back to Buddhist treatises. Mindfulness is a heightened state of awareness and attention derived from focusing on present moment experiences in a nonjudgmental and accepting way (Grover et al., 2017). Mindfulness is related to meditation, but the terms are not synonymous. Moreover, mindfulness consists of formal meditation exercises (e.g., paying attention to the body or walking slowly with a sense of awareness of one's surroundings) as well as informal exercises (e.g., paying full attention to what one is doing or experiencing at a certain moment) (Janssen et al., 2018, p. 1). Research shows that mindfulness reduces stress for chronically ill people (Grover et al., 2017). Mental activity often occurs unchecked; thoughts can become negative, untrue, and unrealistic and result in anxiety, depression, and lack of focus. Happiness or lack of happiness is not caused by outside forces but by our own perceptions and interpretations of reality.

Practitioners suggest that, to become mindful, we observe and monitor the content of our consciousness and recognize that thoughts are just thoughts. Mindfulness interventions vary in delivery mode (e.g., face-to-face, online) and target clinical populations (e.g., various mental disorders [eating disorders, personality disorders, anxiety]) and non-clinical populations (e.g., workplace functioning) (Janssen et al., 2018).

The various aspects of mindfulness include attention to the present moment, acting with awareness and intentionality, a lack of reactivity and negative judgment toward one's own inner experiences, and the ability to describe one's own thoughts, emotional states, and physical sensations (O'Loughlin et al., 2019, p. 122).

This moment-to-moment awareness also extends to the outer world. Being mindful includes being in the moment by paying attention to what is going on around you: what you are seeing, feeling, and hearing. Imagine how much you miss during an ordinary walk to class if you spend it staring straight ahead as your mind wanders from one concern to the next. You miss the pattern of sunlight filtered through the leaves, the warmth of the sunshine on your skin, and the sounds of birds calling out to one another. By focusing on the here and now rather than on the past and future, you are meditating and practicing mindfulness.

Journaling

Journaling or *expressive writing* is an extremely useful therapeutic means used to reduce depression, anxiety, and distress, as well as improve overall well-being (Kim-Godwin, 2021). Similarly, gratitude writing focuses on the positive aspects of life and has been found to effectively manage depression and stress as well as improve happiness and mental health

TABLE 5.4 Cognitive Reframing of Irrational Thoughts

Irrational Thought	Positive Statements
"I have so many problems, I'll never find a partner who will accept me for who I am."	"If a potential partner doesn't seem to understand all of my issues and problems right away, that is fine, I can slowly help them to learn more."
	"If someone I seek as a partner rejects me in some way, that will seem unfortunate, but it is not the end of the world."
	"If a person I care for can't accept me, including my flaws, I can devote more time and energy to others who will."
	"If no one I care for fully accepts or appreciates me for me, I can still find enjoyment in friendships, family, hobbies, work, and other things."
"Considering all I do for my partner, they should do more to appreciate me."	"I would like to be recognized when I go out of my way to support others. I don't support others simply for recognition; I get a good feeling by doing things for those I care about. I am free to make choices about where I spend my time and give of myself. If people take advantage of my generosity, I can redirect my acts of service to others."

outcomes (Kim-Godwin, 2021; O'Leary & Dockray, 2015; Wong et al., 2018). Keeping an informal diary of daily events and activities can reveal surprising information about sources of daily stress. Simply noting which activities put a strain on energy and time, which trigger anger or anxiety, and which precipitate a negative physical experience (e.g., headache, backache, fatigue) can be an important first step in stress reduction.

Humour

The use of humour as a cognitive approach is a good example of how a stressful situation can be "turned upside down." The intensity attached to a stressful thought or situation can be dissipated when it is made to appear absurd or comical. Essentially, the bee loses its sting.

KEY POINTS TO REMEMBER

- Stress is a universal experience and an important concept when caring for any patient in any setting.
- The body responds similarly whether stressors are real or perceived and whether the stressor is negative or positive.
- Physiologically, the body reacts to anxiety and fear by arousal of the sympathetic nervous system. Specific symptoms include rapid heart rate, increased blood pressure, diaphoresis, peripheral vasoconstriction, restlessness, repetitive questioning, feelings of frustration, and difficulty concentrating.
- Cannon introduced the fight-or-flight model of stress, and Selye, a Canadian endocrinologist, introduced the widely known general adaptation syndrome (GAS).
- The psychoneuroimmunology model describes the immune system's response to stress and its effect on neural pathways in the brain.
- Prolonged stress can lead to chronic psychological and physiological responses when not mitigated at an early stage (Table 5.1).
- There are basically two categories of stressors: physical (e.g., heat, hunger, cold, noise, trauma) and psychological (e.g., death of a loved one, loss of job, schoolwork, humiliation).
- Age, gender, culture, life experience, and lifestyle are all important in identifying the degree of stress a person is experiencing.
- Lowering the effects of chronic stress can alter the course of many physical conditions; decrease the need for some medications; diminish or eliminate the urge for unhealthy and destructive behaviours such as smoking, insomnia, and drug addiction; and increase a person's cognitive functioning.
- Perhaps the most important factor for a nurse to assess is a person's support system. Studies have shown that high-quality social and intimate supports can go a long way toward minimizing the long-term effects of stress.
- Cultural differences exist in the extent to which people perceive an event as stressful and in the behaviours they consider appropriate to deal with a stressful event.
- Spiritual practices have been found to lead to an enhanced immune system and a sense of well-being.
- A variety of relaxation techniques are available to reduce the stress response and elicit the relaxation response, which results in improved physical and psychological functioning.

CRITICAL THINKING

1. Assess your level of stress using the Recent Life Changes Questionnaire found in Table 5.2, and evaluate your potential for illness in the coming year. Identify stress-reduction techniques you think would be useful to learn.
2. Teach a classmate the deep-breathing exercise identified in this chapter (Box 5.4).
3. Assess a classmate's coping styles, and have that same classmate assess yours. Discuss the relevance of your findings.
4. Using Figure 5.1, explain to a classmate the short-term effects of stress on the sympathetic–adrenal medulla system, and identify three long-term effects if the stress is not relieved. How would you use this information to provide patient teaching? If your classmate were the patient, how would their response indicate that effective learning had taken place?
5. Using Figure 5.1, have a classmate explain to you the short-term effects of stress on the hypothalamus–pituitary–adrenal cortex and the eventual long-term effects if the stress becomes chronic. Summarize to your classmate your understanding of what was presented. Using your knowledge of the short-term effects of stress on the hypothalamus–pituitary–adrenal cortex and the long-term effects of stress, develop and present to your clinical group a patient education model related to stress.
6. In clinical post-conference discuss a patient you have cared for who had one of the stress-related effects identified in Figure 5.1. See if you can identify some stressors in the patient's life and possible ways to lower chronic stress levels.
7. Assess the number of positive emotions, especially happiness, that you have experienced over the past week. Note the activities you were engaged in at the time. How might you increase the number of positive emotions in order to reduce your potential for illness in the coming year?

CHAPTER REVIEW

1. The nurse is caring for a patient who is experiencing a crisis. Which symptoms would indicate that the patient is in the stage of alarm?
    a. Constricted pupils.
    b. Dry mouth.
    c. Decrease in heart rate.
    d. Sudden drop in blood pressure.
2. If it is determined that a patient will benefit from guided imagery, what teaching should the nurse provide?
    a. Focus on a visual object or sound.
    b. Become acutely aware of your breathing pattern.
    c. Envision an image of a place that is peaceful.
    d. Develop deep abdominal breathing.
3. A patient is going to undergo biofeedback. Which patient statement requires further teaching by the nurse?
    a. "This will measure my muscle activity, heart rate, and blood pressure."
    b. "It will help me recognize how my body responds to stress."
    c. "I will feel a small shock of electricity if I tell a lie."
    d. "The instruments will know if my skin temperature changes."
4. A patient has told the nurse that she knows she is going to lose her job, which scares her because she needs to work to pay her bills. Which nursing response reflects the positive stress response of problem solving?
    a. "What are your plans to find a new job?"
    b. "Can you call your parents to support you during this time?"
    c. "Is it possible that this job loss is an opportunity to find a better-paying job?"
    d. "I'm sure everything will turn out just fine."
5. The nurse is caring for four patients. Which patient would be at highest risk for psychosocial compromise? The patient who has experienced:
    a. The death of a friend.
    b. A divorce.
    c. A recent job layoff.
    d. The death of a spouse.

http://evolve.elsevier.com/Canada/Varcarolis/psychiatric/

REFERENCES

Ader, R., & Cohen, N. (1975). Behaviourally conditioned immunosuppression. *Psychosomatic Medicine, 37*(4), 333–340.

Afshar, H., Roohafza, H. R., Keshteli, A. H., Mazaheri, M., Feizi, A., & Adibi, P. (2015). The association of personality traits and coping styles according to stress level. *Journal of Research in Medical Sciences: The Official Journal of Isfahan University of Medical Sciences, 20*(4), 353–358.

Anisman, H. (2015). *Stress and your health: From vulnerability to resilience.* Malden: Wiley Blackwell.

Anniko, M. K., Boersma, K., & Tillfors, M. (2019). Sources of stress and worry in the development of stress-related mental health problems: A longitudinal investigation from early-to mid-adolescence. *Anxiety, Stress and Coping, 32*(2), 155–167.

Antonelli, M., Barbieri, G., & Donelli, D. (2019). Effects of forest bathing (shinrin-yoku) on levels of cortisol as a stress biomarker: A systematic review and meta-analysis. *International Journal of Biometeorology, 63*(8), 1117–1134. http://centennial.idm.oclc.org/10.1007/s00484-019-01717-x

Beck, A. T. (1976). *Cognitive therapies and emotional disorders.* New York: New American Library.

Benson, H. (1975). *The relaxation response* (2nd ed.). New York: William Morrow & Company.

Bienertova-Vasku, J., Lenart, P., & Scheringer, M. (2020). Eustress and distress: Neither good nor bad, but rather the same. *BioEssays.* https://doi.org/10.1002/bies.201900238

Bigham, E., McDannel, L., Luciano, I., & Salgado-Lopez, G. (2014). Effect of a brief guided imagery on stress. *Biofeedback, 42*(1), 28.

Bremner, J. D., Moazzami, K., Wittbrodt, M. T., Nye, J. A., Lima, B. B., Gillespie, C. F., Rapaport, M. H., Pearce, B. D., Shah, A. J., & Vaccarino, V. (2020). Diet, stress and mental health. *Nutrients, 12*(8), 2428. https://pubmed.ncbi.nlm.nih.gov/32823562/

Canadian Index of Wellbeing. (2016). *How are Canadians really doing? The 2016 CIW National Report.* Canadian Index of Wellbeing and University of Waterloo. https://uwaterloo.ca/canadian-index-wellbeing/sites/ca.canadian-index-wellbeing/files/uploads/files/c011676-nationalreport-ciw_final-s_0.pdf

Canadian Institute for Health Information (CIHI). (2020). *Child and youth mental health in Canada—Infographic.* https://www.cihi.ca/en/child-and-youth-mental-health-in-canada-infographic

Cooney, G. M., Dwan, K., Greig, C. A., Lawlor, D. A., Rimer, J., Waugh, F. R., McMurdo, M., & Mead, G. E. (2013). Exercise for depression. *The Cochrane Database of Systematic Reviews, 9*, CD004366.

Crosswell, A. D., & Lockwood, K. G. (2020). Best practices for stress measurement: How to measure psychological stress in health research. *Health Psychology Open, 7*(2), 2055102920933072. https://doi.org/10.1177/2055102920933072

Donnelly, G. F. (2013). Health benefits of emptying the mind: Rediscovering meditation. *Holistic Nursing Practice, 27*(2), 57–58. https://doi.org/10.1097/HNP.0b013e3182837d64

Epel, E. S., Crosswell, A. D., Mayer, S. E., Prather, A. A., Slavich, G. M., Puterman, E., & Mendes, W. B. (2018). More than a feeling: A unified view of stress measurement for population science. *Frontiers of Neuroendocrinology, 49*, 146–169.

Firth, J., Rosenbaum, S., Stubbs, B., Gorczynski, P., Yung, A. R., & Vancampfort, D. (2016). Motivating factors and barriers towards exercise in severe mental illness: A systematic review and meta-analysis. *Psychological Medicine, 46*(14), 2869–2881. https://doi.org/10.1017/S0033291716001732

Flores-Kanter, P. E., Moretti, L., & Medrano, L. A. (2021). A narrative review of emotion regulation process in stress and recovery phases. *Heliyon, 7*(6), e07218. https://www.sciencedirect.com/science/article/pii/S2405844021013219

Galante, J., Galante, I., Bekkers, M., & John, G. (2014). Effect of kindness-based meditation on health and well-being: A systematic review and meta-analysis. *Journal of Consulting and Clinical Psychology, 82*(6), 1101–1114. https://doi.org/10.1037/a0037249

Godoy, L. D., Rossignoli, M. T., Delfino-Pereira, P., Garcia-Cairasco, N., & Umeoka, E. H. L. (2018). A comprehensive overview on stress neurobiology: Basic concepts and clinical implications. *Frontiers in Behavioral Neuroscience, 12*, 127. https://doi.org/10.3389/fnbeh.2018.00127

Goldfarb, E. V., Seo, D., & Sinha, R. (2019). Sex differences in neuronal stress responses and correlation with subjective stress and stress regulation. *Neurobiology of Stress.* https://doi.org/10.1016/j.ynstr.2019.100177

Grover, S. L., Teo, S. T. T., Pick, D., & Roche, M. (2017). Mindfulness as a personal resource to reduce work stress in the job demands-resources model. *Stress and Health, 33*(4), 426–436

Hansen, M. M., Jones, R., & Tocchini, K. (2017). Shinrin-yoku (forest bathing) and nature therapy: A state-of-the-art review. *International Journal of Environmental Research and Public Health, 14*(8), 851. https://doi.org/10.3390/ijerph14080851

Helliwell, J. F., Schellenberg, G., & Fonberg, J. (2020). *Life satisfaction in Canada before and during the COVID-19 pandemic.* Statistics Canada. https://www150.statcan.gc.ca/n1/pub/11f0019m/11f0019m2020020-eng.htm

Huang, V., Beshai, S., & Yu, M. (2016). The effects of the gender-culture interaction on self-reports of depressive symptoms: Cross-cultural study among Egyptians and Canadians. *PeerJ, 4*, e2783. https://www.ncbi.nlm.nih.gov/pmc/articles/PMC5147018/

Janssen, M., Heerkens, Y., Kuijer, W., van der Heijden, B., & Engels, J. (2018). Effects of mindfulness-based stress reduction on employees' mental health: A systematic review. *Public Library of Science, 13*(1), e0191332. https://doi.org/10.1371/journal.pone.0191332

Jerath, R., Crawford, M. W., Barnes, V. A., & Harden, K. (2015). Self-regulation of breathing as a primary treatment for anxiety. *Applied Psychophysiology and Biofeedback, 40*(2), 107–115. https://doi.org/10.1007/s10484-015-9279-8

Kaiser, B. N., Haroz, E. E., Kohrt, B. A., Bolton, P. A., Bass, J. K., & Hinton, D. E. (2015). Thinking too much": A systematic review of a common idiom of distress. *Social Science & Medicine, 147*, 170–183. https://doi.org/10.1016/j.socscimed.2015.10.044

Karatekin, C. (2018). Adverse childhood experiences (ACEs), stress and mental health in college students. *Stress and Health, 34*(1), 36–45.

Kent, B. V., Davidson, J. C., Zhang, Y., Pargament, K. I., VanderWeele, T. J., Koenig, H. G., Underwood, L. G., Krause, N., Kanaya, A. M., Tworoger, S. S., Schachter, A. B., Cole, S. A., O'Leary, M., Cozier, Y. C., Daviglus, M. L., Giachello, A. L., Zacher, T., Palmer, J. R., & Shields, A. E. (2021). Religion and spirituality among American Indian, South Asian, Black, Hispanic/Latina, and White women in the study on stress, spirituality, and health. *Journal for the Scientific Study of Religion, 60*(1), 198–215. https://doi.org/10.1111/jssr.12695

Kim-Godwin, Y. (2021). Beliefs and experience of journaling in mothers of adult children with substance use problems. *Journal of Addictions Nursing.* Advance online publication. https://doi.org/10.1097/JAN.0000000000000410

Koenig, H. G., King, D. E., & Carson, V. B. (2012). *Handbook of religion and health* (2nd ed.). New York: Oxford University Press.

Lavretsky, H., & Feldman, J. L. (2021). Precision medicine for breath-focused mind-body therapies for stress and anxiety: Are we ready yet?. *Global Advances in Health and Medicine, 10.* https://doi.org/10.1177/2164956120986129

Lee, I., Choi, H., Bang, K. S., Kim, S., Song, M., & Lee, B. (2017). Effects of forest therapy on depressive symptoms among adults: A systematic review. *International Journal of Environmental Research & Public Health, 14*(3), 321. https://doi.org/10.3390/ijerph14030321

McEwen, B. S., Gray, J. D., & Nasca, C. (2015). 60 years of neuroendocrinology: Redefining neuroendocrinology: Stress, sex and cognitive emotional regulation. *Journal of Endocrinology, 226,* T67–T83. https://doi.org/10.1530/joe-15-0121

Nasso, S., Vanderhasselt, M. A., Schettino, A., & De Raedt, R. (2020). The role of cognitive reappraisal and expectations in dealing with social feedback. *Emotion.* Advance online publication. https://doi.org/10.1037/emo0000825

Newman, M. L., & Roberts, N. A. (2013). *Health and social relationships: The good, the bad, and the complicated* (1st ed.). Washington, DC: American Psychological Association.

Oh, B., Lee, K. J., Zaslawski, C., Yeung, A., Rosenthal, D., Larkey, L., & Back, M. (2017). Health and well-being benefits of spending time in forests: Systematic review. *Environmental Health Prevention Medicine, 22*(1), 71. https://doi.org/10.1186/s12199-017-0677-9

O'Leary, K., & Dockray, S. (2015). The effects of two novel gratitude and mindfulness interventions on well-being. *The Journal of Alternative and Complementary Medicine, 21,* 243–245.

O'Loughlin, R. E., Fryer, J. W., & Zuckerman, M. (2019). Mindfulness and stress appraisals mediate the effect of neuroticism on physical health. *Personality and Individual Differences, 142,* 122–131.

Paquola, C., Bennett, M. R., Hatton, S. N., Hermens, D. F., & Lagopoulos, J. (2017). Utility of the cumulative stress and mismatch hypotheses in understanding the neurobiological impacts of childhood abuse and recent stress in youth with emerging mental disorder. *Human Brain Mapping, 38*(5), 2709–2721. https://doi.org/10.1002/hbm.23554

Pedersen, B. K., & Saltin, B. (2015). Exercise as medicine—Evidence for prescribing exercise as therapy in 26 different chronic diseases. *Scandinavian Journal of Medicine & Science in Sports, 25*(S3), 1–72. https://doi.org/10.1111/sms.12581

Perciavalle, V., Blandini, M., Fecarotta, P., Fecarotta, P., Buscemi, A., Corrado, D. D., Bertolo, L., Fichera, F., & Coco, M. (2017). The role of deep breathing on stress. *Neurological Sciences, 38*(3), 451–458. https://doi.org/10.1007/s10072-016-2790-8

Pulopulos, M. M., Baeken, C., & De Raedt, R. (2020). Cortisol response to stress: The role of expectancy and anticipatory stress regulation. *Hormones and Behaviour, 117,* 104587. https://doi.org/10.1016/j.yhbeh.2019.104587

Pulopulos, M. M., Hidalgo, V., Puig-Perez, S., & Salvador, A. (2018). Psychophysiological response to social stressors: Relevance of sex and age. *Psicothema, 30*(2), 171–176. https://pubmed.ncbi.nlm.nih.gov/29694317/

Rahe, R. H. (1995). Stress and psychiatry. In H. I. Kaplan, & B. J. Sadock (Eds.), *Comprehensive textbook of psychiatry/VI* (Vol. 2 6th ed., pp. 1545–1559). Williams & Wilkins.

Rahe, R. H., Veach, T. L., Tolles, R. L., & Murakami, K. (2000). The stress and coping inventory: An educational and research instrument. *Stress Medicine, 16*(4), 199–208. https://doi.org/10.1002/1099-1700(200007)16:4<199::AID-SMI848>3.0.CO;2-D

Rahe, R. H., Veach, T. L., Tolles, R. L., & Murakami, K. (2000). The stress and coping inventory: An educational and research instrument. *Stress Medicine, 16*(4), 199–208. https://doi.org/10.1002/1099-1700(200007)16:4<199::AID-SMI848>3.0.CO;2-D

Reinert, K. G., & Koenig, H. G. (2013). Re-examining definitions of spirituality in nursing research. *Journal of Advanced Nursing, 69*(12), 2622–2634. https://doi.org/10.1111/jan.12152

Robson, J. P., & Troutman-Jordan, M. (2014). A concept analysis of cognitive reframing. *Journal of Theory Construction & Testing, 18*(2), 55.

Rosmarin, D., & Koenig, H. (2020). *Handbook of spirituality, religion and mental health* (2nd ed.). London: Academic Press (Elsevier).

Sadock, V. A., & Sadock, B. J. (2017). *Kaplan and Sadock's concise textbook of clinical psychiatry* (4th ed.). Philadelphia: Wolters Kluwer Health/Lippincott Williams & Wilkins.

Selye, H. (1974). *Stress without distress.* Philadelphia: Lippincott.

Sharma, M. (2014). Yoga as an alternative and complementary approach for stress management: A systematic review. *Journal of Evidence-Based Complementary & Alternative Medicine, 19*(1), 59–67. https://doi.org/10.1177/2156587213503344

Thase, M. E., Wright, J. H., Friedman, E. S., & Russ, E. (2015). Cognitive and behavioural therapies. In A. Tasman, J. Kay, J. A. Lieberman, M. B. First, & M. B. Riba (Eds.), *Psychiatry* (4th ed., pp. 1836–1858). Wiley.

Underwood, P. (2012). Social support: The promise and reality. In V. H. Rice (Ed.), *Handbook of stress, coping, and health: Implications for nursing research, theory, and practice* (2nd ed., pp. 355–380). Sage.

Unger, C. A., Busse, D., & Yim, I. S. (2017). The effect of guided relaxation on cortisol and affect: Stress reactivity as a moderator. *Journal of Health Psychology, 22*(1), 29–38. https://doi.org/10.1177/1359105315595118

Wong, Y. J., Owen, J., Gabana, N. T., Brown, J. W., McInnis, S., Toth, P., & Gilman, L. (2018). Does gratitude writing improve the mental health of psychotherapy clients? Evidence from a randomized controlled trial. *Psychotherapy Research, 28,* 192–202.

UNIT 2

Foundations in Practice

6. The Nursing Process and Standards of Care for Psychiatric Mental Health Nursing

7. Ethical Responsibilities and Legal Obligations for Psychiatric Mental Health Nursing Practice

8. Cultural Implications for Psychiatric Mental Health Nursing: A Critical Cultural Perspective

6

The Nursing Process and Standards of Care for Psychiatric Mental Health Nursing

Lisa-Marie Forcier, Eric MacMullin
Originating US chapter by Margaret Jordan Halter, Elizabeth M. Varcarolis

 http://evolve.elsevier.com/Canada/Varcarolis/psychiatric/

OBJECTIVES

1. Compare the approaches you would consider when performing an assessment with a child, an adolescent, and an older adult.
2. Differentiate between the use of an interpreter and the use of a translator when performing an assessment with a non–English-speaking patient.
3. Understand the nursing process steps used in psychiatric mental health nursing.
4. Conduct a mental status examination (MSE).
5. Perform a psychosocial assessment, including brief cultural and spiritual components.
6. Explain three principles a nurse follows in planning actions to meet agreed-upon outcome criteria.
7. Construct a plan of care for a patient with a mental or emotional health problem.
8. Identify two advanced-practice psychiatric mental health nursing interventions.
9. Demonstrate basic nursing interventions and evaluation of care.
10. Compare and contrast *Nursing Interventions Classification* (NIC), *Nursing Outcomes Classification* (NOC), and evidence-informed practice.

KEY TERMS AND CONCEPTS

evidence-informed decision making
health teaching
mental status examination
outcome criteria
psychosocial assessment
self-care activities
standards of nursing practice

The nursing process is a six-step problem-solving approach that is the cornerstone of clinical decision making in nursing. The nursing process is intended to facilitate and identify appropriate, safe, culturally competent, developmentally relevant, and quality care for individuals, families, groups, or communities. To develop competency within nursing, the nurse must know that the nursing process is not a linear but a continuous process of assessing, planning, implementing, and evaluating. Within the standards of practice for psychiatric mental health nursing it is important that the nurse knows not only the nursing process but is able to practice nursing judgements and behaviours based on this framework (Figure 6.1). Particularly, in psychiatric mental health nursing it is critical for the nurse to know that central to the nursing process is the therapeutic nurse–patient relationship and therapeutic communication.

The use of the nursing process in psychiatric mental health nursing is aligned with **standards of nursing practice**, as outlined in the *Code of Ethics and Standards of Psychiatric Nursing Practice* (Registered Psychiatric Nurses of Canada, 2019) and *Canadian Standards for Psychiatric-Mental Health Nursing* (Canadian Federation of Mental Health Nurses, 2014). Regardless of practice area, standards of practice "guide the professional knowledge, skills and judgment needed to practice nursing safely" (College of Registered Nurses of Nova Scotia, 2017, p. 4). Both the code of ethics and the standards of practice are provided in the Appendix of this book.

Nursing care planning is a collaborative process undertaken with people (individual patients, families, groups, or communities), working toward mutually-agreed-upon definitions of problems, desired outcomes, and interventions. Utilizing therapeutic communication engagement and collaboration in a patient-centred, therapeutic relationship is fundamental to the practice of Psychiatric Mental Health Nursing and the Standards of Care (refer to Chapter 9 for more on relational practice and therapeutic relationships). Each step in the nursing process includes collaboration with the patient:

- *Data gathering/assessment* is a transparent process (the patient is aware of when, how, what, and why data are gathered about them, typically through interview or observation approaches).
- *Nursing diagnosis* is a process that includes the patient's definition of problems and patient education on the nursing perception of problems.
- *Outcome identification* is mutually negotiated and respects the patient's goals.
- *Planning* includes interventions to achieve goals and health teaching on best practice interventions.
- *Implementation* includes patient actions.
- *Evaluation* includes patient evaluation of progress toward goals.

Taken together, the process incorporates the arts of mental health nursing and recovery practice and the science of evidence-informed decision making ((Varcarolis & Fosbre, 2021). See also Addiction and Mental Health Collaborative Project Steering Committee (2015) for a report on collaboration as inherent in evidence-informed practices aligned with recovery principles. The steps, activities, and considerations of the psychiatric mental health nursing process are explored in detail as follows.

CHAPTER 6 The Nursing Process and Standards of Care for Psychiatric Mental Health Nursing

NURSING ASSESSMENT

The assessment interview requires culturally effective communication skills and encompasses a large database (e.g., significant support system; family; cultural and community system; spiritual and philosophical values, strengths, and health beliefs and practices).

1. ASSESSMENT
- Construct database:
  - Mental status examination (MSE)
  - Psychosocial assessment
  - Physical examination
  - History taking
  - Interviews
  - Standardized rating scales
- Verify the data

2. DIAGNOSIS
- Identify problem and etiology
- Construct nursing diagnoses and problem list
- Prioritize nursing diagnoses

3. OUTCOMES IDENTIFICATION
- Identify attainable and culturally expected outcomes
- Document expected outcomes as measurable goals
- Include time estimate for expected outcomes

4. PLANNING
- Identify safe, pertinent, evidence-informed actions
- Strive to use interventions that are culturally relevant and compatible with health beliefs and practices
- Document plan using recognized terminology

5. IMPLEMENTATION
- Basic-level and advanced-practice interventions:
  - Coordination of care
  - Health teaching and health promotion
  - Milieu therapy
  - Pharmacological, biological, and integrative therapies
- Advanced-practice interventions:
  - Prescriptive authority and treatment
  - Psychotherapy
  - Consultation

6. EVALUATION
- Document results of evaluation
- If outcomes have not been achieved at desired level:
  - Additional data gathering
  - Reassessment
  - Revision of plan

Fig. 6.1 The nursing process in psychiatric mental health nursing.

ASSESSMENT

A view of the individual as a complex blend of many parts is consistent with nurses' holistic approach to care. Nurses who care for people with physical illnesses ideally maintain a holistic view that involves an awareness of psychological, social, cultural, and spiritual issues. Likewise, nurses who work in the psychiatric mental health field need to assess or have access to reports on past and present medical history, a recent physical examination, and any physical complaints, as well as document any observable physical conditions or behaviours (e.g., unsteady gait, abnormal breathing patterns, wincing as if in pain, doubling over to relieve discomfort). The assessment process begins with the initial patient encounter and continues throughout the duration of caring for the patient. To develop a basis for the plan of care and plan for discharge, every patient should have a thorough, formal nursing assessment upon entering treatment. Subsequent to the formal assessment, data are collected continually and systematically as the patient's condition changes and, it is to be hoped, improves. For example, a patient may have come into treatment feeling actively suicidal, and the initial focus of care was on protection from injury; through regular assessment, it may be determined that although suicidal ideation has diminished, negative self-evaluation is still certainly a problem.

Assessments are conducted interprofessionally by a variety of practitioners, including nurses, psychiatrists, psychologists, social workers, recreation therapists, dietitians, and others. Building your confidence to conduct your assessment and to share your interpretations with the

HOW A NURSE HELPED ME
They Told Us He Has Schizophrenia

My brother lived next door to my parents for years. After Dad died, Mom said it was nice to have my brother so close so he could help her with the yard work. Although I knew that my brother had some "strange ideas" and had always preferred to be by himself, he seemed to be doing okay. It was really only after Mom died that I fully understood how much she had been helping him.

My brother had been afraid of the police and the spies that, he was convinced, were tracking him. He had piled up old papers and magazines in front of his windows so no one could look in. Although he had been prescribed medication to help reduce these fears, he was not taking it. Soon, my brother also stopped eating because of his belief that his food was being poisoned. He was admitted to hospital. After several weeks, he was discharged and came to live with me and my family. He was not happy about this arrangement, and, frankly, neither was I. We soon moved him into an apartment a few blocks from my home. As part of the hospital discharge plan, my brother and I saw a nurse at our local community mental health office. She met with us and helped us understand what schizophrenia is and how it would affect our lives. The question she asked that was most helpful was, "What action by your brother would let you know you didn't need to worry so much about him?" I told her his coming over for Sunday supper. My brother was surprised by my response. He thought that I was going to say his taking his medication. The nurse also helped my brother understand the purpose of the medication and how it would help reduce some of his worries, helped him get to his appointments, and helped him plan his meals. But most importantly, the nurse helped me reconnect with my brother as sister and brother rather than as caregiver and a person who needed care.

broad interprofessional team is essential to patient outcomes (Registered Nurses' Association of Ontario [RNAO], 2013). Virtually all inpatient and outpatient health centres have standardized nursing assessment forms to aid in organization and consistency among reviewers. These forms may be paper or electronic versions, according to the resources and preferences of the institution. The time required for the nursing interview, a standard aspect of the formal nursing assessment, varies, depending on the assessment form and the patient's response pattern (e.g., speaks at great length or rambles, is prone to tangential thought, has memory disturbances, or gives markedly slow responses).

Refer to Chapter 10 for sound guidelines on setting up and conducting a clinical interview.

Emergency situations may require immediate intervention based on a minimal amount of data and the emergency sharing of personal health information. However, health care workers are required to adhere to legislation regulating the collection of, use of, and access to patient information. Protection of personal health information is a provincial and territorial legislative responsibility, as mandated by the federal *Personal Information Protection and Electronic Documents Act* (Government of Canada, 2021); therefore each province and territory has specific health information legislation (Table 6.1).

The nurse's primary source for data collection is the patient; however, there may be times when it is necessary to supplement or rely completely on another for the assessment information. These secondary sources can be invaluable when caring for a patient experiencing psychosis, muteness, agitation, or catatonia. Such secondary sources may include members of the family, friends, neighbours, police, health care workers, and medical records. It may be appropriate to conduct a nursing family assessment with the patient and their significant others in order to understand more fully the resources, supports, and problems in the patient's life (Shajani & Snell, 2019).

The best atmosphere in which to conduct an assessment is one of minimal anxiety. Therefore if an individual becomes upset, defensive, or embarrassed about any topic, the topic should be abandoned. The nurse can acknowledge that the subject makes the patient uncomfortable and suggest within the medical record that the topic be discussed when the patient feels more comfortable. It is important that the nurse does not probe, pry, or push for information that is difficult for the patient to discuss. However, it should be recognized that increased anxiety about any subject is data in itself and should be noted in the assessment even without obtaining any further information.

Age Considerations
Assessment of Children

When assessing children, it is important to gather data from a variety of sources. Although the child is the best source for determining emotions, the caregivers (parents or guardians) often can best describe the behaviour, performance, and attitude of the child. Caregivers also are helpful in interpreting the child's words and responses. However, an interview separate from caregivers is advisable when an older child is

TABLE 6.1 Provincial and Territorial Health Information Acts

Province or Territory	Website Link
Alberta	https://www.alberta.ca/health-information-act.aspx
British Columbia	http://www.bclaws.ca/EPLibraries/bclaws_new/document/ID/freeside/00_03063_01
Manitoba	http://www.gov.mb.ca/health/phia/
New Brunswick	http://www2.gnb.ca/content/gnb/en/services/services_renderer.201227.Access_to_Personal_Health_Information.html
Newfoundland and Labrador	https://www.health.gov.nl.ca/health/PHIA/
Northwest Territories	http://www.priv.gc.ca/resource/prov/index_e.asp#006
Nova Scotia	http://novascotia.ca/dhw/phia/
Nunavut	http://www.priv.gc.ca/resource/prov/index_e.asp#008
Ontario	http://www.e-laws.gov.on.ca/html/statutes/english/elaws_statutes_04p03_e.htm
Prince Edward Island	http://www.healthpei.ca/index.php3?number=1020297&lang=E
Quebec	http://www.publicationsduquebec.gouv.qc.ca/fre/products/61184
Saskatchewan	https://publications.saskatchewan.ca/#/products/4523
Yukon	http://www.hss.gov.yk.ca/healthprivacy.php

reluctant to share information, especially in cases of suspected abuse (Arnold & Boggs, 2020).

Developmental levels should be considered in the evaluation of children. One of the hallmarks of psychiatric disorders in children is the tendency to regress (return to a previous level of development). Although it is developmentally appropriate for toddlers to suck their thumbs, such a gesture in an older child is unusual.

Age-appropriate communication strategies are perhaps the most important factor in establishing successful communication (Arnold & Boggs, 2020). Assessment of children should be accomplished by a combination of interview and observation. Watching children at play provides important clues to their functioning. From a psychodynamic view, supported play (play encouraged to a level with which the child is comfortable) is a safe way for the child to act out thoughts and emotions and to release pent-up emotions, for example, having a child act out their story (or family's story) with the use of anatomically correct dolls. Asking the child to tell a story, draw a picture, or engage in specific therapeutic games can be useful assessment tools in determining critical concerns and painful issues a child may have difficulty expressing. Usually, a clinician with special training in child and adolescent psychiatry works with young children. Chapter 27 presents a more extensive overview of assessing children.

Assessment of Adolescents

Adolescents are especially concerned with confidentiality and may fear that anything they say to the nurse will be repeated to their parents. Lack of confidentiality can become a barrier to care with this population. Adolescents need to know that their records are private, and they must receive an explanation as to how information will be shared among the treatment team. The adolescent may be hesitant to answer questions related to such topics as substance use and sexual activity. Therefore these must be asked in a nonjudgemental manner. If the answers to these questions do not indicate that the adolescent is at risk for harm, the answers may be handled confidentially (Arnold & Boggs, 2020). However, threats of suicide, homicide, sexual abuse, or behaviours that put the patient or others at risk for harm must be shared with other professionals, as well as with the parents and any other agencies that may be appropriate (e.g., a children's aid society). Because identifying risk factors is one of the key objectives when assessing adolescents, it is helpful to use a brief, structured interview technique such as the HEADSSS interview (Box 6.1). Chapter 27 offers more on the assessment of adolescents.

Assessment of Older Adults

As we get older, our five senses (taste, touch, sight, hearing, and smell) and brain function begin to diminish, but the extent to which this affects each person varies. Your patient may be a spry and alert 80-year-old or a frail and confused 60-year-old. Therefore it is important not to stigmatize older adults or expect them to be physically or mentally deficient. For example, the tendency may be to jump to the conclusion that someone who is hard of hearing is cognitively impaired, an assumption that should be avoided. However, it is true that many older adults need special attention. The nurse needs to be aware of any physical limitations, for example, any sensory condition (difficulty seeing or hearing), motor condition (difficulty walking or maintaining balance), or medical condition (back pain, cardiac, or pulmonary deficits), that could cause increased anxiety, stress, or physical discomfort for the patient during the assessment of mental and emotional needs. It is wise to identify any physical deficits at the onset of the assessment and make accommodations for them. If the patient is hard of hearing, speak a little more slowly in clear, louder tones (but not too loud) and seat the patient close to you without invading their personal space. Often, a voice that is lower in pitch is easier for older adults to hear, and a higher-pitched voice may convey anxiety to some.

Language Barriers

It is becoming more and more apparent that psychiatric mental health nurses can best serve their patients if they have a thorough understanding of the complex cultural and social factors that influence health and illness. Awareness of individual cultural beliefs and health care practices can help nurses minimize stigma and assumptions that can lead to ineffective care and interfere with the ability to evaluate care. There are many opportunities for misunderstandings when assessing a patient from a different cultural or social background from your own, particularly if the clinical interview is conducted in a language that is not the patient's primary language. To understand the patient's history and health care needs, health care providers often require translation and, at times, lay interpreters are used to communicate when there are language barriers. Such interpreters are often other staff or family members or friends who stand in to interpret back and forth from the patient to the mental health care team and vice versa. There are risks of these interpreters inserting their own understanding of what is being said, leading to potential misinterpretation and misunderstanding. There are further concerns related to confidentiality and ethics in this mode of interpretation (Elkington & Talbot, 2016). In this way it is always preferred to use the services of trained translators, who are skilled in direct translation whenever possible.

Although there is no federal legislation mandating the use of trained translators for patients whose English or French proficiency is limited, Canadian health care organizations and providers recognize that language barriers compromise health and patient care and consider access to translators as a health care priority. Unfortunately, professional translators are not always readily available in many health care facilities.

Psychiatric Mental Health Nursing Assessment

The purposes of the psychiatric mental health nursing assessment are to:
- Establish rapport
- Obtain an understanding of the current problem and/or chief complaint
- Review physical status and obtain baseline vital signs
- Assess for risk factors affecting the safety of the patient or others
- Perform a mental status examination (MSE)
- Assess psychosocial status
- Identify mutual goals for treatment
- Formulate a plan of care

Gathering Data

Review of systems. The mind–body connection is significant in the understanding and treatment of psychiatric disorders. Many

---

> **BOX 6.1 The HEADSSS Psychosocial Interview Technique**
>
> **H**—Home environment (e.g., relationships with parents and siblings)
> **E**—Education and employment (e.g., school performance)
> **A**—Activities (e.g., sports participation, after-school activities, peer relations)
> **D**—Drug, alcohol, or tobacco use
> **S**—Sexuality (e.g., whether the patient is sexually active, practices safer sex, uses contraception)
> **S**—Suicide risk or symptoms of depression or other mental health disorder
> **S**—Signs of violence, abuse, or aggression

patients who are admitted for treatment of psychiatric conditions also are given a thorough physical examination by a primary care provider. Likewise, most nursing assessments include a baseline set of vital signs, a historical and current review of body systems, and a documentation of allergic responses.

Martin (2016) points out that several medical conditions and physical illnesses may mimic psychiatric illnesses (Box 6.2). Therefore physical causes of symptoms must be ruled out. Conversely, psychiatric disorders can result in physical or somatic symptoms such as stomach aches, headaches, lethargy, insomnia, intense fatigue, and even pain. When depression is secondary to a known physical medical condition, it often goes unrecognized and thus untreated.

Therefore all patients who come into the health care system need to have both a medical and a mental health evaluation to ensure correct diagnoses and appropriate care.

Individuals with certain physical conditions may be more prone to psychiatric disorders such as depression. It is believed, for example, that the disease process of multiple sclerosis or other autoimmune diseases may actually bring about depression. Other physical diseases typically associated with depression are coronary artery disease, diabetes, and stroke. Individuals need to be evaluated for any medical origins of their depression or anxiety.

When evidence suggests the presence of mental confusion or organic mental disease, an MSE, discussed below, should be performed.

BOX 6.2 Some Medical Conditions That May Mimic Psychiatric Illness

Depression

Neurological disorders:
- Cerebrovascular accident (stroke)
- Alzheimer's disease
- Brain tumour
- Huntington's disease
- Epilepsy (seizure disorder)
- Multiple sclerosis
- Parkinson's disease

Infections:
- Mononucleosis
- Encephalitis
- Hepatitis
- Tertiary syphilis
- Human immunodeficiency virus (HIV)

Endocrine disorders:
- Hypothyroidism (similar clinical features to depression)
- Hyperthyroidism (similar clinical features to anxiety, depression, and bipolar disorders)
- Cushing's syndrome
- Addison's disease
- Parathyroid disease

Gastrointestinal disorders:
- Liver cirrhosis
- Pancreatitis

Cardiovascular disorders:
- Hypoxia
- Heart failure

Respiratory disorders:
- Sleep apnea

Nutritional disorders:
- Thiamine deficiency
- Protein deficiency
- B_{12} deficiency
- B_6 deficiency
- Folate deficiency

Collagen vascular diseases:
- Lupus erythematosus
- Rheumatoid arthritis

Cancer

Anxiety

Neurological disorders:
- Alzheimer's disease
- Brain tumour
- Stroke
- Huntington's disease

Infections:
- Encephalitis
- Meningitis
- Neurosyphilis
- Septicemia

Endocrine disorders:
- Hypothyroidism and hyperthyroidism
- Hypoparathyroidism
- Hypoglycemia
- Pheochromocytoma
- Carcinoid

Metabolic disorders:
- Low calcium
- Low potassium
- Acute intermittent porphyria
- Liver failure

Cardiovascular disorders:
- Angina
- Heart failure
- Pulmonary embolus

Respiratory disorders:
- Pneumothorax
- Acute asthma
- Emphysema

Drug effects:
- Stimulants
- Sedatives (withdrawal)

Lead, mercury poisoning

Psychosis

Medical conditions:
- Temporal lobe epilepsy
- Migraine headaches
- Temporal arteritis
- Occipital tumours
- Narcolepsy
- Encephalitis
- Hypothyroidism
- Addison's disease
- HIV

Drug effects:
- Marijuana
- Heroin/methadone
- Alcohol withdrawal
- Stimulants
- Cocaine
- Corticosteroids

Laboratory data. While hypothyroidism and depression share some similar clinical features (Talaei et al., 2017), the most common clinical features associated with hyperthyroidism are anxiety and depression. However, in a study conducted by Hu (2013, para. 5) hyperthyroidism may also increase the risk of developing bipolar disorders. Therefore it is important to complete laboratory testing as part of data gathering. A simple blood test (thyroid-stimulating hormone [TSH]) can usually differentiate thyroid problems and potential psychiatric concerns. Abnormal liver enzyme levels can explain irritability, depression, and lethargy. People who have chronic renal disease often suffer from the same symptoms when their blood urea nitrogen and electrolyte levels are abnormal. A toxicology screen for the presence of either prescription or illegal drugs also may provide useful information. Further information on the psychological needs of patients with medical conditions is found in Chapter 30.

Mental status examination. Fundamental to the psychiatric mental health nursing assessment is a **mental status examination**. In fact, an MSE is part of the assessment in all areas of health care. The MSE in psychiatry is analogous to the physical examination in general medicine, and the purpose is to evaluate an individual's current cognitive, affective (emotional), and behavioural functioning. For acutely ill patients, it is not unusual for the mental health clinician to administer MSEs every day. It is the key assessment tool used by all members of the mental health team for ongoing assessment of the patient and to establish treatment effectiveness, as well as certain aspects of recovery (Mental Health Commission of Canada, 2016). It is also the key assessment tool used to communicate assessment data across the interprofessional team (RNAO, 2017). Box 6.3 provides an example of the basic structure of and some descriptors for an MSE.

BOX 6.3 Mental Status Examination

A. Appearance (observed)
A person's appearance provides useful clues to their quality of self-care, lifestyle, and daily living skills. Assessment is observed in the following domains:
1. Grooming and dress
2. Level of hygiene
3. Pupil dilation or constriction
4. Facial expression
5. Height, weight, nutritional status
6. Presence of body piercing or tattoos, scars, etc.
7. Relationship between appearance and age

B. Behaviour (observed)
Along with noting what a person is actually doing during the examination, attention should be given to *nonverbal communication*, which reveals much about a person's emotional state and attitude.
1. Excessive or reduced body movements
2. Peculiar body movements (e.g., scanning of the environment, odd or repetitive gestures, mannerisms, balance and gait)
3. Abnormal movements (e.g., tardive dyskinesia, tremors)
4. Level of eye contact (keep cultural differences in mind; see Chapter 8)
5. Rapport (openness to the interview; e.g., if the patient is resistive versus open)

C. Speech (observed)
Speech can be a particularly revealing feature of a person's mental state and should be described behaviourally as well as having its content considered (see also "E. Thought"). Unusual speech is sometimes associated with mood and anxiety problems, schizophrenia, and organic pathology.
1. Rate (e.g., slow, rapid, pressured, normal)
2. Volume (e.g., loud, soft, normal)
3. Tonality (e.g., monotone, tremulous, varied)
4. Articulation (e.g., slurring, stuttering, mumbling)
5. Organization (e.g., disorganized, tongue-tied speech)
6. Quantity (e.g., poverty of speech, minimal, plentiful, voluminous)

D. Mood (observed and inquired)
The relationship of emotional affect and mood can be considered as being similar to that of the weather (affect) and the season (mood). Affect refers to immediate expressions of emotion (observed), whereas mood refers to emotional experience over a more prolonged period of time (inquired).
1. Affect (observed):
   - Range (e.g., restricted, blunted, flat, expansive)
   - Appropriateness (e.g., appropriate to conversation or setting, inappropriate, incongruous)
   - Stability (e.g., stable, labile)
2. Mood (inquired): sad, euphoric, duration, degree, stability
   - Tone (e.g., sad, euphoric, depressed, elevated, lowered)
   - Degree (e.g., extreme, moderate, mild, minor)
   - Irritability (e.g., explosive, irritable, calm)
   - Stability or duration (e.g., rapid, delayed)

E. Thought (observed and inquired)
Thinking is generally evaluated according to a person's thought *content* or *nature* and thought *form* or *process*.
1. Thought content (e.g., delusions such as grandeur, jealousy, thought control/withdrawal/insertion; obsessions or preoccupations)
2. Thought process (e.g., disorganized, coherent, flight of ideas, neologisms, thought blocking, circumstantiality)

F. Perception (observed and inquired)
Assessment of perceptual disturbance is critical for detecting serious mental health problems like psychosis, severe anxiety, organic brain disorders, and mood disorders. It is also important in trauma or substance use. Perceptual disturbances are typically notable and may be disturbing or frightening. Consider the nature, timing, and triggers or precursors.
1. Hallucinations
   - Sensory involvement (e.g., auditory, visual, tactile, gustatory)
   - Content of auditory hallucination (e.g., conspiratory, command hallucinations telling a person to do something such as harm oneself or others)
   - Level of discernment of reality (e.g., questions the reality of the hallucination, hallucination is undistinguished from reality)
   - Level of associated distress (e.g., amused, distracted, fearful, extreme fear)
2. Illusions (similar to hallucinations but involving misperception of a real stimulus; e.g., perception of insects coming from pattern in wallpaper)
3. Dissociations (e.g., derealization, or feeling that the world or one's surroundings are not real; depersonalization, or feeling detached from oneself)

G. Cognition (inquired)
Cognitive assessment is in reference to a person's current capacity to process information. It is important because it is often sensitive (though in young people usually secondary) to mental health problems. Note that insight and judgement are particularly important in evaluating safety.
1. Orientation to reality (expressed as orientation to time, place, and person; e.g., awareness of the time/day/date, where they are, ability to provide personal details)
2. Level of consciousness (e.g., alert, drowsy, confused, clouded, stuporous, unconscious, comatose)
3. Memory functioning (e.g., immediate or short-term memory, memory for recent and remote information or events)

> **BOX 6.3 Mental Status Examination—cont'd**
>
> 4. Fund of knowledge or intelligence (e.g., general knowledge as compared to the average person in a given society)
> 5. Language (e.g., naming objects, following instructions)
> 6. Abstraction (e.g., ability to describe similarity between two things—i.e., an apple and an orange; ability to explain the meaning of simple proverbs—i.e., "measure twice, cut once")
> 7. Attention and concentration: performance on serial sevens (counting down from 100 by increments of 7), serial threes (counting down from 20 by increments of 3), digit span tests (recalling in order a series of digits)
> 8. Visual or spatial processing (e.g., copying a diagram, drawing a bicycle, drawing a clock with the hands at 9 o'clock)
> 9. Insight (e.g., patient's acknowledgement and understanding of problems; potential pathological events—e.g., hallucinations, suicidal thoughts, and potential treatment. Evaluated by exploring questions such as "What do you believe is contributing to the problems you are experiencing or that others are identifying?" "What might be the outcomes of the problems you are experiencing?")
> 10. Judgement (e.g., patient's general problem-solving ability. Evaluated by exploring recent decision making or by posing a practical dilemma such as "What would you do if you saw smoke coming out of a house?")
>
> **H. Ideas of Harming Self or Others (inquired)**
> Every mental status examination requires an assessment of thought content regarding self-harm and suicidal and homicidal ideation. The same must be documented. Further, if police are notified or children's aid is notified, this must be documented as well. Ideation, intent, and plan are all examined and explore the following (described in further detail in Chapter 22):
> 1. Target of ideation (e.g., the person—self or other, i.e., wife, boss, etc.)
> 2. Frequency of ideation (e.g., fleeting, constant, preoccupying)
> 3. Intent (an evaluation of whether the ideation is a reflection of wishing or thinking about death or harm versus an intent to kill oneself or another; e.g., general thoughts, presence of a plan)
> 4. Plan
>   a. Level of specificity (e.g., vague, general, detailed, specific, secretive)
>   b. Lethality of means (e.g., violent, lethal method)
>   c. Means to carry out the plan (e.g., possesses a gun and ammunition, possesses a vehicle, has stockpiled medication)
>   d. Opportunity to carry out the plan

The MSE, by and large, aids in collecting and organizing objective data of the here-and-now experience of the patient. The nurse both observes and asks directly about the patient's physical behaviour, nonverbal communication, appearance, speech patterns, mood and affect, thought content, perceptions, cognitive ability, and insight and judgement.

The MSE is much more than simply a means of gathering information; however, it is also a vehicle for relationship building and communication (see Chapters 9 and 10). Often a first or routine contact with a patient, the MSE sets the stage for your supportive care of a patient who may be agitated, depressed, suspicious, frightened, or angry. Choosing the time, place, and your approach to the MSE are all crucial to successful implementation (RNAO, 2017).

Psychosocial assessment. A psychosocial assessment (also called a mental health assessment) provides additional information from which to develop a plan of care. It may involve a more comprehensive assessment than the MSE and may involve collateral information from family or others (Coombs et al., 2013). A comprehensive mental health assessment includes the following information about the patient:
- Central or chief complaint (in the patient's own words)
- History of violent, suicidal, or self-mutilating behaviours
- Alcohol or substance use
- Family psychiatric history
- Personal psychiatric treatment, including medications and complementary therapies
- Stressors and coping methods
- Quality of activities of daily living
- Personal background (including any trauma the patient may want to disclose)
- Social background, including support system
- Strengths, areas patient wants to develop, and goals for treatment
- Ethnic and cultural beliefs and practices (it is important that healthcare providers engage in cultural safety during assessments)
- Screening of gender-related needs
- Spiritual beliefs or religious practices

The patient's psychosocial history is most often the subjective part of the assessment. The focus of the history is the patient's perceptions and recollections of current lifestyle and life in general (family, friends, education, work experience, coping styles, and spiritual and cultural beliefs).

Foundational to the mental health assessment are trauma-informed care practices and approaches. It is critical for nurses to understand that patients arrive with complex trauma histories (including multigenerational trauma) and experiences. By utilizing trauma-informed approaches, healthcare providers offer patients choice, control, and safety. These are critical for the development of the therapeutic nurse–patient relationship.

According to the Government of Canada (2018) trauma and violence-informed approaches are policies and practices that recognize the connections between violence, trauma, negative health outcomes, and behaviours. These approaches increase safety, control, and resilience for people who are seeking services in relation to experiences of violence and/or have a history of experiencing violence. The following are key policy and practice principles:
1. Understand trauma and violence, and their impacts on peoples' lives and behaviours
2. Create emotionally and physically safe environments
3. Foster opportunities for choice, collaboration, and connection
4. Provide a strengths-based and capacity-building approach to support patient coping and resilience (Government of Canada, 2018, p. 1)

Further, a psychosocial assessment elicits information about the person's social functioning and the systems in which a person operates. To conduct a mental health assessment, the nurse should have fundamental knowledge of growth and development, basic cultural and religious practices, pathophysiology, psychopathology, and pharmacology. Box 6.4 provides a basic psychosocial assessment tool.

Spiritual or religious assessment. Gomi and colleagues (2014) stress the importance of a spiritual or religious assessment to a holistic mental health assessment and for patient recovery. The idea that spirituality or religious involvement is recognized as an important influence on a person's health and behaviour has long been recognized. Spirituality and religious beliefs have the potential to exert a positive influence on patients' views of themselves and on how they interact with and respond to others (Chaze et al., 2015; Starnino, 2016).

Spirituality and religion are, however, quite different in their influences. *Spirituality* may offer a way for patients to cope with symptoms and difficulties by serving as stress relieving, instilling a sense of hope,

BOX 6.4 Psychosocial Assessment

A. Previous hospitalizations
B. Educational background
C. Occupational background
  1. Employed? Where? What length of time?
  2. Special skills
D. Social patterns
  1. Describe family
  2. Describe friends
  3. With whom does the patient live?
  4. To whom does the patient go in times of crisis?
  5. Describe a typical day
E. Sexual patterns
  1. Sexually active? Practices safer sex? Practices birth control?
  2. Sexual orientation?
  3. Sexual difficulties?
F. Interests and abilities
  1. What does the patient do in their spare time?
  2. What sport, hobby, or leisure activity is the patient good at?
  3. What gives the patient pleasure?
G. Substance use
  1. What medications does the patient take? How often? How much?
  2. What herbal or over-the-counter medications does the patient take (e.g., caffeine, anti-inflammatory or cough medicines, an herbal sleep aid or weight loss supplement)? How often? How much?
  3. What psychotropic medications does the patient take? How often? How much?
  4. How many drinks of alcohol does the patient have per day? Per week?
  5. What recreational drugs does the patient use (e.g., club drugs, marijuana, stimulants, heroin, steroids)? How often? How much?
  6. Does the patient overuse prescription medications (benzodiazepines, pain medications)?
  7. Does the patient identify the use of drugs as a problem?
H. Coping abilities
  1. What does the patient do when they get upset?
  2. To whom can the patient talk?
  3. What usually helps to relieve stress?
  4. What did the patient try this time?
I. Spiritual assessment
  1. What importance does religion or spirituality have in the patient's life?
  2. Do the patient's religious or spiritual beliefs relate to the way the patient takes care of themself or the illness? How does the patient's spiritual life contribute to recovery (meaning, purpose, joy, belonging, and so on)?
  3. Does the patient's faith help the patient in stressful situations?
  4. Whom does the patient see when they are medically ill? Mentally upset?
  5. Are there special health care practices within the patient's spiritual or cultural community that address their particular mental problem?

---

or offering a perspective of oneself outside of being a patient (Milner et al., 2020). Spirituality in children has been described in terms of experiences of wonder and joy in life, the nurturing of moral sensitivities, early experiences of wisdom and compassion, and expressions of the sacred qualities in life (Michaelson et al., 2019). Four relational domains of spirituality include connections to self; others; nature; and some kind of transcendent, or larger meaning to life (Michaelson et al., 2019). Spirituality can increase healthy behaviours, social support, and a sense of meaning, which are linked to decreased overall mental and physical illness (Starnino, 2016).

Religion is a multidimensional construct, with public and private aspects. Religious service attendance is commonly distinguished from private dimensions of religiosity, namely the strength of beliefs and the frequency of prayer (Dilmaghani, 2018). Private dimensions of religion and spirituality are suggested to provide meaning, optimism, and comfort, all of which are predictors of a better mental health (Dilmaghani, 2018). A religious community can provide support during difficult times, and prayer can be a source of hope, comfort, and support in healing.

Addressing patients' spiritual needs is an indispensable element in nursing care, necessary from the patient's point of view, and is prominent for health maintenance (Minton et al., 2018). As an element of holistic care, spiritual care is deeper than psychosocial care (Minton et al., 2018, p. 174).

The following questions may be included in a spiritual or religious assessment:
- Who or what supplies you with strength and hope?
- Do you have a religious affiliation?
- Do you practice any spiritual activities (yoga, tai chi, meditation, prayer)?
- Do you participate in any religious activities?
- What role does religion or spiritual practice play in your life?
- Does your faith help you in stressful situations?
- Has your illness affected your religious or spiritual practices?
- Would you like to have someone from your faith (church, synagogue, or temple) or from our facility visit you?

Cultural and social assessment. Canada is rich in cultural diversity. According to Statistics Canada (2020), since the very first censuses, Statistics Canada has collected data on the origins of the population. In 1871, the year of the first Canadian census following Confederation, approximately 20 origins were enumerated in the Canadian population. At that time, 60.5% of the population reported origins from the British Isles, 31.1% reported French origins, and less than 1% reported Indigenous origins. In 2016 over 250 origins were reported and 41.1% of the Canadian population recorded more than one origin. In 2016 close to 20 million people reported European origins. In the entire Canadian population three Asian origins were among the 20 most reported origins: Chinese (close to 1.8 million people), East Indian (approximately 1.4 million), and Filipino (837 130). In 2016 just over 1 million people reported African origins; 749 155 reported Caribbean origins; and 674 640 reported Latin, Central, or South American origins (Statistics Canada 2020).

Canada's official policy of multiculturalism means that cultural diversity is respected and the privilege of one culture over another is challenged. With rapid changes in the ethnic diversities and multicultural and linguistic groups in the population, health care providers must develop awareness and knowledge about different attitudes and beliefs that can influence their psychological thought processes (Fogel et al., 2020). The multicultural context requires a particular focus on Indigenous models of health and well-being and on addressing the mental health needs of immigrants and refugees (Paniagua & Yamada, 2013), as well as a particular focus on spirituality and religion (Chaze et al., 2015). Chapter 8 offers a detailed discussion of the cultural implications for psychiatric mental health nursing and further information needed to conduct a cultural and social assessment in the Canadian context with a focus on Indigenous peoples and refugee and immigrant mental health. Four principles should be considered to develop understanding and the treatment of culture, according to Fogel et al. (2020):

- understanding the importance of avoiding stereotypes about individuals and groups
- learning how to ask the right questions and improving the nurses' skills for active listening and eliciting culturally relevant information
- improving cultural competence in a way that is coextensive with the nurses' emerging clinical skills in other areas
- improving the nurses' insight and acceptance of cultural competence as integral to the assessment and clinical care of every patient (p. 3).

Not addressing cultural concerns when assessing patients may lead to unnecessary or even incorrect treatment modalities (Fogel et al., 2020).

According to the Canadian Nurses Association (2020), nurses and all other health care providers are just as susceptible to unconscious racial bias or inappropriate beliefs that can affect interactions with patients, communities, and even fellow coworkers. Systemic anti-Black racism within the health care system has also affected access to services, with some people reluctant to seek care due to racist and discriminatory experiences and therefore potential under-screening. In particular, patients can lose trust in the system when access to mental health services is limited or linked to interactions with police. Trust can also be undermined when clinical tools fail to address unique risk protective factors of Black communities (Canadian Nurses Association, 2020).

Some questions that psychiatric mental health nurses can ask to help with a cultural and social assessment are:

- What is your primary language? Would you like a translator?
- How would you describe your cultural background and experiences that have been part of your history?
- Who are you close to?
- Who do you seek in times of crisis?
- How do people support one another at times of illness in your cultural, religious, or spiritual community?
- Who do you live with? How are activities at home organized in your cultural background?
- Who do you seek when you are medically ill? Mentally upset or concerned?
- What do you do to get better when you have physical problems?
- What are the attitudes toward emotional or social problems in your culture?
- How is your current mental health viewed by your culture?
- Do you have a special diet? Any dietary restrictions?
- Are there special healthcare (or religious or spiritual) practices within your culture that address your particular mental or emotional health problem?
- Are there any special cultural beliefs about your experience that might help me understand and provide care for you?
- Are there cultural practices we can incorporate into your care?

After the cultural and social assessment, it is useful to summarize pertinent data with the patient. This summary provides patients with reassurance that they have been heard and gives them the opportunity to clarify any misinformation. The patient should be told what will happen next. For example, if the initial assessment takes place in the hospital, you should tell the patient who else they will be seeing. If you believe a referral is necessary, discuss this recommendation with the patient.

Validating the Assessment

To gain an even clearer understanding of your patient, it is helpful to look to outside sources. Emergency department records can be a valuable resource in understanding an individual's presenting behaviour and problems. Police reports may be available in cases in which hostility and legal altercations occurred. Old medical records, most now electronically accessible, are of great help in validating information you already have or in adding new information to your database. If the patient was admitted to a psychiatric unit in the past, information about the patient's previous level of functioning and behaviour gives you a baseline for making clinical judgements. Check with your provincial or territorial personal health information act to find out when signed consent of the patient or an appropriate relative is necessary to obtain access to records. All personal health information legislation requires nurses to obtain verbal consent from patients before discussing confidential information and treatment with their families; however, nurses have the skills and a responsibility to facilitate the involvement of families where appropriate.

Using Rating Scales

A number of standardized rating scales are useful for psychiatric evaluation and monitoring. Rating scales are often administered by a clinician, but many are self-administered. Table 6.2 lists some that are in common use. Many of the clinical chapters in this book include a rating scale.

NURSING DIAGNOSIS

A nursing diagnosis is a clinical judgement about a patient's response, needs, actual and potential psychiatric disorders, mental health problems, and potential comorbid physical illnesses. A well-chosen and well-stated nursing diagnosis is the basis for selecting therapeutic outcomes and interventions (Herdman et al., 2021).

A nursing diagnosis has three structural components:
1. Problem (unmet need)
2. Etiology (probable cause)
3. Supporting data (signs and symptoms)

The *problem*, or unmet need, describes the state of the patient at present. Problems that are within the nurse's domain to treat are termed *nursing diagnoses*. The nursing diagnostic title states what should change. Example: *Hopelessness*.

Etiology, or probable cause, is linked to the diagnostic title with the words *related to*. Stating the etiology or probable cause tells what needs to be addressed to effect the change and identifies causes the nurse can treat through nursing interventions. Example: *Hopelessness related to multiple losses*.

Supporting data, or signs and symptoms, state what the patient's condition is like at present. It may be linked to the diagnosis and etiology with the words *as evidenced by*. Supporting data (defining characteristics) that validate the diagnosis may include:

- The patient's statement (e.g., "It's no use; *nothing will change*.")
- Lack of involvement with family and friends
- Lack of motivation to care for self or environment

The complete nursing diagnosis might be *Hopelessness related to multiple losses, as evidenced by lack of motivation to care for self*.

OUTCOMES IDENTIFICATION

Outcome criteria are the hoped-for outcomes that reflect the maximal level of patient health that can realistically be achieved through nursing interventions. Whereas nursing diagnoses identify problems, outcomes reflect desired changes. The expected outcomes provide direction for continuity of care (American Nurses Association [ANA] et al., 2014). Outcomes should take into account the patient's culture, values, ethical beliefs, and personal goals. Specifically, outcomes are stated in attainable and measurable terms and include a time estimate for attainment (ANA et al., 2014). Moorhead and colleagues (2018) have compiled a standardized list of nursing outcomes in the *Nursing Outcomes Classification (NOC)* (see Chapter 1). *NOC* includes a total of 385 standardized outcomes that provide a mechanism for

TABLE 6.2 Standardized Rating Scales[a]

Use	Scale
Depression	Beck Inventory
	Brief Patient Health Questionnaire (Brief PHQ)
	Geriatric Depression Scale (GDS)
	Hamilton Depression Scale
	Zung Self-Report Inventory
	Patient Health Questionnaire–9 (PHQ-9)
Anxiety	Brief Patient Health Questionnaire (Brief PHQ)
	Generalized Anxiety Disorder–7 (GAD-7)
	Modified Spielberger State Anxiety Scale
	Hamilton Anxiety Scale
Substance use disorders	CAGE[b] (see Ewing, 1984; O'Brien, 2008)
	Addiction Severity Index (ASI)
	Recovery Attitude and Treatment Evaluator (RAATE)
	Brief Drug Abuse Screen Test (B-DAST)
	Clinical Institute Withdrawal Assessment for Alcohol—Revised (CIWA-AR) and Clinical Opiate Withdrawal Scale (COWS)
Obsessive-compulsive behaviour	Yale-Brown Obsessive-Compulsive Scale (Y-BOCS)
Mania	Mania Rating Scale
Schizophrenia	Scale for Assessment of Negative Symptoms (SANS)
	Brief Psychiatric Rating Scale (BPRS)
Abnormal movements	Abnormal Involuntary Movement Scale (AIMS)
	Simpson Neurological Rating Scale
General psychiatric assessment	Brief Psychiatric Rating Scale (BPRS)
	Global Assessment of Functioning Scale (GAF)
Cognitive function	Mini-Mental State Examination (MMSE)
	St. Louis University Mental Status Examination (SLUMS)
	Cognitive Capacity Screening Examination (CCSE)
	Alzheimer's Disease Rating Scale (ADRS)
	Memory and Behavior Problem Checklist
	Functional Assessment Screening Tool (FAST)
	Global Deterioration Scale (GDS)
	Montreal Cognitive Assessment (MoCA)
Family assessment	McMaster Family Assessment Device
Eating disorders	Eating Disorders Inventory (EDI)
	Body Attitude Test
	Diagnostic Survey for Eating Disorders
Suicidality	SAD PERSONS scale
	Suicide Assessment Five-Step Evaluation and Triage (SAFE-T)

[a]These rating scales highlight important areas in psychiatric assessment. Because many of the answers are subjective, experienced clinicians use these tools as a guide when planning care and also draw on their knowledge of their patients and their patients' perception of their own experience.
[b]This acronym helps the clinician remember to ask questions about **c**utting down, **a**nnoyance by criticism related to substance use, feelings of **g**uilt related to substance use, and if the substance is needed to "get going" in the morning—the **e**ye opener.

communicating the effect of nursing interventions on the well-being of patients, families, and communities. Each outcome has an associated group of indicators used to determine patient status in relation to the outcome. Whether nursing outcomes are derived from *NOC*, a psychiatric mental health nursing care plan text, evidence-based practice, or other sources, it is important that criteria are individualized and documented as obtainable goals.

It is helpful to use long- and short-term outcomes, often stated as goals, when assessing the effectiveness of nursing interventions. The use of long- and short-term outcomes or goals is particularly helpful for teaching and learning purposes. It is also valuable in providing guidelines for appropriate interventions. The use of goals guides nurses in building incremental steps toward meeting the desired outcome. All outcomes (goals) are written in positive terms. Table 6.3 shows how specific outcome criteria might be stated for a suicidal individual with a nursing diagnosis of *Risk for suicide related to depression*.

PLANNING

The nurse considers the following specific principles when planning care:
- *Safe*—Interventions must be safe for the patient, as well as for other patients, staff, and family.
- *Compatible and appropriate*—Interventions must be compatible with other therapies and with the patient's personal goals and cultural values, as well as with institutional rules.
- *Realistic and individualized*—Interventions should be (1) within the patient's capabilities, given the patient's age, physical strength, condition, and willingness to change; (2) based on the number of staff available; (3) reflective of the actual available community resources; and (4) within the student's or nurse's capabilities.
- *Evidence-informed*—Interventions should be based on scientific evidence and principles when available.

In an evidence-informed practice model the practitioner bases treatment decisions on a blend of information gleaned from empirical evidence, patient values, and practitioner expertise and skills (Jakubec & Astle, 2021). While empirical evidence is an important aspect of nursing practice, the Canadian Nurses Association promotes the use of the term **evidence-informed decision making** in nursing practice because it includes other elements that affect clinical decision making, such as professional clinical judgement, patient preference, and collaboration with other key health stakeholders (Canadian Nurses Association, 2018). Certainly, there are elements within the nursing process for psychiatric mental health care whereby empirical evidence is simply not available, for example, in the area of spiritual and religious assessment and support (Michaelson et al., 2019; Milner et al., 2020). Yet this does not mean that we cannot intervene appropriately and safely in the best interest of the patient. Box 6.5 lists several online resources for evidence-informed decision making and nursing practice.

> ⚡ **SAFETY TIP: Planning for recovery shapes patient safety.**
>
> Interventions planned must be acceptable and appropriate to the individual patient, and some care and interventions focus on harm reduction. Psychiatric mental health nurses must keep the principles of recovery, anchored by harm reduction, participation, and choice (Baklien & Bongaardt, 2014; Mental Health Commission of Canada, 2016), front of mind when planning care. It is often this approach of "walking alongside" (Ness et al., 2014) that facilitates improved outcomes of interventions, including outcomes of healthy risk taking and choices of patients (Higgins et al., 2016).

TABLE 6.3 Examples of Long- and Short-Term Goals for a Suicidal Patient

Long-Term Goals or Outcomes	Short-Term Goals or Outcomes
1. Patient will remain free from injury throughout the hospital stay.	a. Patient will state that they understand the rationale and procedure of the unit's protocol for suicide precautions shortly after admission. b. Patient will sign a "no-suicide" contract for the next 24 hours, renewable at the end of every 24-hour period (if approved for use by the mental health facility). c. Patient will seek out staff when feeling overwhelmed or self-destructive during hospitalization.
2. By discharge, patient will state that they no longer wish to die and that they have at least two people to contact if suicidal thoughts arise.	a. Patient will meet with social worker to find supportive resources in the community before discharge and work on trigger issues (e.g., housing, job). b. By discharge, patient will state the purpose of medication, time and dose, adverse effects, and who to call with questions or concerns. c. Patient will have the written name and telephone numbers of at least two people to turn to if feeling overwhelmed or self-destructive. d. Patient will have a follow-up appointment to meet with a mental health professional by discharge.

BOX 6.5 Useful Evidence-Informed Decision Making and Nursing Practice Websites and Links

- Canadian Best Practices Portal: https://cbpp-pcpe.phac-aspc.gc.ca/
- Canadian Nurses Association: Evidence-Informed Decision-Making: https://www.cna-aiic.ca/en/policy-advocacy/policy-support-tools/position-statements
- Practice of Psychological Treatments: http://www.cpa.ca/docs/File/Practice/Report_of_the_EBP_Task_Force_FINAL_Board_Approved_2012.pdf
- National Collaborating Centre for Methods and Tools: https://www.nccmt.ca/
- Academic Center for Evidence-Based Practice (ACE): https://brilliantnursingpapers.com/wp-content/uploads/2018/08/The-ACE-Star-Model.pdf
- The Cochrane Collaboration: https://www.cochrane.org
- The Joanna Briggs Institute: https://jbi.global

The *Nursing Interventions Classification (NIC)* (Butcher et al., 2019) is a research-based, standardized listing of 565 interventions reflective of current clinical practice that the nurse can use to plan care (see Chapter 1). Nurses in all settings can use *NIC* to support quality patient care and incorporate evidence-informed nursing actions. Although many safe and appropriate interventions may not be included in *NIC*, it is a useful guide for standardized care. Individualizing interventions to meet a patient's special needs, with patient input, should always be part of planning care.

When choosing nursing interventions from *NIC*, psychiatric nursing care plan texts, or other sources, the nurse uses not just those that fit the nursing diagnosis (e.g., risk for suicide) but also interventions that match the defining data. Although the outcome criteria might be similar or the same (e.g., suicide self-restraint), the safe and appropriate interventions may be totally different because of the defining data. For example, consider the nursing diagnosis *Risk for suicide related to feelings of despair, as evidenced by two recent suicide attempts and repeated statements that "I want to die."* The planning of appropriate nursing interventions might include:

- Initiate suicide precautions (e.g., ongoing observations and monitoring of the patient, provision of a protective environment) for the person who is at serious risk for suicide.
- Search the newly hospitalized patient and personal belongings for weapons or potential weapons during the inpatient admission procedure, as appropriate.
- Use protective interventions (e.g., area restriction seclusion, physical restraints) if the patient lacks the restraint to refrain from harming self, as needed.
- Assign the hospitalized patient to a room located near the nursing station for ease of observation, as appropriate.

However, if the defining data are different, the appropriate interventions will be as well, for example: *Risk for suicide related to loss of spouse, as evidenced by lack of self-care and statements evidencing loneliness.* The nurse might choose the following interventions for this patient's plan of care:

- Determine the presence and degree of suicide risk.
- Facilitate support of the patient by family and friends.
- Consider strategies to decrease isolation and the opportunity to act on harmful thoughts.
- Assist the patient in identifying a network of supportive personnel and resources within the community (e.g., support groups, grief counselling, clergy, care providers).
- Provide information about available community resources and outreach programs.

Chapter 22 addresses assessment of and interventions for suicidal patients in more depth.

IMPLEMENTATION

The therapeutic interpersonal relationship is recognized as the first standard of practice by both the Registered Psychiatric Nurses of Canada (2019) and the Canadian Federation of Mental Health Nurses (2014), emphasizing the critical importance of this fundamental competency. The basic implementation skills are accomplished through the nurse–patient relationship and therapeutic interventions. The nurse implements the plan using evidence-informed practice whenever possible, uses community resources, and collaborates with nursing colleagues. Recent graduates and practitioners new to the psychiatric setting practice at the "entry to practice" level with the guidance and support of more experienced health care providers. The Registered Psychiatric Nurse Regulators of Canada (2014) outline that the level of education, experience, and context of employment all shape the characteristics of entry to practice expectations. Entry-level psychiatric mental health nurses enter practice working in a variety of practice settings, with diverse populations. They are responsible for practicing within the context of their legislated scope of practice, the law, regulatory standards, employer policies, and their individual competence.

Basic-Level Interventions

Coordination of Care

The psychiatric mental health nurse coordinates the implementation of the plan and provides documentation.

Health Teaching and Health Promotion

Psychiatric mental health nurses use a variety of health teaching methods, which they adapt to the patient's needs (e.g., age, culture, ability to learn, readiness), integrating current knowledge and research and seeking opportunities for feedback and effectiveness of care. Health teaching includes identifying the health education needs of the patient and teaching basic principles of physical and mental health, such as giving information about coping, interpersonal relationships, social skills, mental health disorders, the treatments for such illnesses and their effects on daily living, relapse prevention, problem-solving skills, stress management, crisis intervention, and self-care activities. The last of these, self-care activities, assist the patient in assuming personal responsibility for activities of daily living and focuses on improving the patient's mental and physical well-being.

Milieu Therapy

Milieu therapy requires managing the environment in which treatment takes place so that patients feel comfortable, safe, and respected (see Chapter 3). Milieu management includes orienting patients to their rights and responsibilities, selecting specific activities that meet patients' physical and mental health needs, and ensuring that patients are maintained in the least restrictive environment that safety permits. It also includes informing patients about the need for limits and the conditions necessary to set limits in a culturally competent manner (see Chapter 8).

Pharmacological, Biological, and Integrative Therapies

Nurses need to know the intended action, therapeutic dosage, adverse reactions, and safe blood levels of medications being administered and must monitor them when appropriate (e.g., blood levels for lithium). The nurse is expected to discuss and provide medication teaching tools to the patient and family regarding drug action, adverse effects, dietary restrictions, and drug interactions and to provide time for questions. The nurse's assessment of the patient's response to psychobiological interventions is communicated to other members of the multidisciplinary mental health team. Interventions are also aimed at alleviating untoward effects of medication. For more information on psychotropic drugs, refer to Chapter 11.

Advanced-Practice Interventions

Some registered nurses, registered practical nurses, and registered psychiatric nurses are educationally and clinically prepared to conduct advanced interventions such as offering psychotherapy to individuals, couples, groups, and families and providing consultation to other disciplines using evidence-informed psychotherapeutic frameworks and nurse–patient therapeutic relationships. These assessment and intervention skills require advanced training and supervision (Rhoads & Murphy, 2014; Wheeler, 2020). Refer to Chapter 4 for an overview of various psychotherapies, Chapter 33 for a discussion of therapeutic groups, Chapter 34 for a discussion of family interventions, and Chapter 35 for a discussion of integrative therapies.

EVALUATION

Unfortunately, the evaluation of patient outcomes is often the most neglected part of the nursing process. Evaluation of the individual's response to treatment should be systematic, ongoing, and criteria based. Supporting data are included to clarify the evaluation. Patient input is essential during the evaluation and establishment of next steps for the patient's recovery plan (Mental Health Commission of Canada, 2015). Simply asking the following is valuable in the evaluation of patient outcomes: "*How do you see things now?*" "*Have you observed any particular changes?*" "*Is there anything that you'd like to discuss about your recovery and plans?*" Ongoing assessment of data allows for revisions of nursing diagnoses, changes to more realistic outcomes, or identification of more appropriate interventions when outcomes are not met.

DOCUMENTATION

Documentation could be considered the seventh step in the nursing process. Keep in mind that medical records are legal documents and may be used in a court of law. (Chapter 7 provides further information on the various purposes and guidelines for the use of medical records.) Besides the evaluation of stated outcomes, the medical record should include changes in patient condition, informed consents (for medications and treatments), reaction to medication, documentation of symptoms (verbatim when appropriate), concerns of the patient, safety concerns (thoughts of harm to self or others), incidents of mandatory reporting (children's aid society, police), and any untoward incidents in the healthcare setting. Documentation of patient progress is the responsibility of the entire mental health team (Doenges et al., 2019).

Information also must be in a format that is retrievable for quality-assurance monitoring, utilization management, peer review, accreditation by regulatory agencies, and research. Electronic medical records are increasingly used in both inpatient and outpatient settings. Whatever format is used, documentation must be focused, organized, and pertinent and must conform to certain legal and other generally accepted principles (Box 6.6). The College and Association of Registered Nurses of Alberta (2013), the Nurses Association of New Brunswick (2020), and the College of Nurses of Ontario (2019) are among the provincial professional associations that have published nursing documentation guidelines.

BOX 6.6 Legal Considerations for Documentation of Care

Do

- Chart in a timely manner all pertinent and factual information.
- Be familiar with the nursing documentation policy in your facility, and make your charting conform to this standard. The policy generally states the method; frequency; and pertinent assessments, interventions, and outcomes to be recorded. If your employer's policies and procedures do not encourage or allow for quality documentation, bring the need for change to the administration's attention. See documentation standards for provincial regulatory bodies.
- Chart legibly in ink.
- Chart facts fully, descriptively, and accurately.
- Chart what you see, hear, and smell.
- Chart pertinent observations: psychosocial observations, physical symptoms pertinent to the medical diagnosis, and behaviours pertinent to the nursing diagnosis.
- Chart follow-up care provided when a problem has been identified in earlier documentation. For example, if a patient has fallen and injured a leg, describe how the wound is healing.

BOX 6.6 Legal Considerations for Documentation of Care—cont'd

- Chart fully the facts surrounding unusual occurrences and incidents.
- Chart all nursing interventions, treatments, and outcomes (including teaching efforts and patient responses) and safety and patient-protection interventions.
- Chart the patient's expressed subjective feelings.
- Chart each time you notify a physician, and record the reason for notification, the information that was communicated, the accurate time, the physician's instructions or orders, and the follow-up activity.
- Chart when nursing supervisors are consulted or informed about the patient, and record the reason for notification, information communicated, time, and any instructions or follow-up.
- Chart when fulfilling duty to report (children's aid society, police).
- Chart when family are notified of occurrences.
- Chart physicians' visits and treatments.
- Chart discharge medications and instructions given for use, as well as all discharge teaching performed, and note which family members were included in the process.
- Ensure all documentation includes your full name, signature, and designation.

Do not

- Do not chart opinions that are not supported by facts.
- Do not defame patients by calling them names or making derogatory statements about them (e.g., "an unlikeable patient who is demanding unnecessary attention").
- Do not chart before an event occurs.
- Do not chart generalizations, suppositions, or pat phrases (e.g., "patient in good spirits," "patient appears to be sleeping," "it seems patient is not eating").
- Do not obliterate, erase, alter, or destroy a record. If an error is made, draw one line through the error, write "mistaken entry," record the date, and initial the clarification. Follow your employer's and regulatory body's guidelines closely.
- Do not leave blank spaces for chronological notes. If you must chart out of sequence, chart "late entry." Identify the time and date of the entry and the time and date of the occurrence.
- If an incident report is filed, do not note in the chart that one was filed. This form is generally a privileged communication between the hospital and the hospital's attorney. Describing it in the chart may destroy the privileged nature of the communication.

According to the Canadian Nurses Protective Society (2020, para. 2), the primary purpose of documenting in the patient's chart (electronic or paper) is to record relevant information so that the patient receives the best and most personalized care.

Documentation is necessary for:

- Communication between healthcare providers
- Promoting continuity of care
- Meeting legislative and professional requirements
- Showing accountability for the professional practice, and outlining the nurse's commitment to providing safe, effective, and ethical care
- Quality improvement
- Research
- Acting as legal proof of health care provided

Source: Canadian Nurses Protective Society. (2020). Quality documentation: Your best defence. https://cnps.ca/article/quality-documentation/#:~:text=Quality%20Documentation%3A%20Your%20Best%20Defence%20The%20Canadian%20Nurses,to%20documentation%2C%20whether%20in%20paper%20or%20electronic%20form

KEY POINTS TO REMEMBER

- The nursing process is a six-step problem-solving approach to patient care.
- The primary source of assessment is the patient. Secondary sources of information include family members, neighbours, friends, police, and other members of the health care team.
- A professional translator often is needed to prevent serious misunderstandings during assessment, treatment, and evaluation with non–English- or non–French-speaking patients.
- The assessment interview includes gathering objective data (mental or emotional status) and subjective data (psychosocial assessment).
- Medical examination, history, and systems review round out a complete assessment.
- Trauma-informed care approaches are central to developing the therapeutic nurse–patient relationship and offer the patient choice, control, and safety.
- Assessment tools and standardized rating scales may be used to evaluate and monitor a patient's progress.
- Determination of the nursing diagnosis defines the practice of nursing, improves communication between staff members, and assists in accountability of care.
- A nursing diagnosis consists of (1) an unmet need or problem, (2) an etiology or probable cause, and (3) supporting data.
- Outcomes are variable, measurable, and stated in terms that reflect a patient's actual state. Planning involves determining desired outcomes.
- Behavioural goals support outcomes. Goals are short, specific, and measurable; indicate the desired patient behaviours; and include a set time for achievement.
- Planning nursing actions (using *NIC*, psychiatric nursing care plan texts, evidence-informed practice, or other sources) to achieve outcomes include the use of specific principles. The plan should be (1) safe, (2) compatible with and appropriate for implementation with other therapies, (3) realistic and individualized, and (4) evidence informed whenever possible.
- Psychiatric mental health nursing practice includes four basic-level interventions: (1) coordination of care; (2) health teaching and health promotion; (3) milieu therapy; and (4) pharmacological, biological, and integrative therapies.
- Advanced-practice interventions (e.g., psychotherapy, consulting work) are carried out by a nurse with advanced education or experience.
- The evaluation of care is a continual process of determining to what extent the outcome criteria have been achieved. The plan of care may be revised based on the evaluation.
- Documentation of patient progress through evaluation of the outcome criteria is crucial. The medical record is a legal document and should accurately reflect the patient's condition, medications, treatment, tests, responses, reporting to agencies (children's aid, police) and any untoward incidents.

CRITICAL THINKING

1. Martin Redbird, a 47-year-old Cree man, arrives by ambulance from a supermarket, where he had fallen. On his arrival to the emergency department (ED), his breath smells "fruity." He appears confused and anxious, saying that "they put a curse on me, they want me to die … they are yelling, they are yelling … no, no, I'm not bad. Oh God, don't let them get me!" Martin is from a reserve

community 700 km north of the city in which he is being treated. When his nephew (closest next of kin) is contacted by the ED by phone, he tells the staff that Martin has diabetes and a diagnosis of paranoid schizophrenia and that this happens when he doesn't take his medications or eat properly. In a group or in collaboration with a classmate respond to the following:

a. A number of nursing diagnoses are possible in this scenario. Given the above information, formulate at least two nursing diagnoses (problems); include *related to* and *as evidenced by* statements.
b. For each of your nursing diagnoses, write one long-term outcome (the problem, what should change, etc.). Include a time frame, desired change, and three criteria that will help you evaluate whether the outcome has been met, not met, or partially met.
c. What specific needs might you take into account when planning nursing care for Mr. Redbird?
d. Formulate an initial nurse's note for Mr. Redbird.

CHAPTER REVIEW

1. The nurse is assessing a 6-year-old patient. When assessing a child's perception of a difficult issue, which methods of assessment are appropriate? **Select all that apply.**
   a. Engage the child in a specific therapeutic game.
   b. Ask the child to draw a picture.
   c. Provide the child with an anatomically correct doll to act out a story.
   d. Allow the child to tell a story.
2. Which are the purposes of a thorough mental health nursing assessment? **Select all that apply.**
   a. Establish a rapport between the nurse and patient.
   b. Assess for risk factors affecting the safety of the patient or others.
   c. Allow the nurse the chance to provide counselling to the patient.
   d. Identify the nurse's goals for treatment.
   e. Formulate a plan of care.
3. The nurse is performing a spiritual assessment on a patient. Which patient statement would indicate to the nurse that there is an experiential concern in the patient's spiritual life?
   a. "I really believe that my spouse loves me."
   b. "My sister will never forgive me for what I did."
   c. "I try to find time every day to pray, even though it's not easy."
   d. "I am happy with my life choices, even if my mother is not."
4. The nurse is caring for a patient who states that he has "given up on life." His wife left him, he was fired from his job, and he is four payments behind on his mortgage, meaning he will soon lose his house. Which nursing diagnosis is appropriate?
   a. Anxiety related to multiple losses.
   b. Defensive coping related to multiple losses.
   c. Ineffective denial related to multiple losses.
   d. Hopelessness related to multiple losses.
5. The nurse is documenting. Which statement is appropriate to include in the patient's chart?
   a. "Patient states, 'I am going to end my life.'"
   b. "Patient is in good spirits today."
   c. "Patient has been nasty to the nursing staff this afternoon."
   d. "Patient is demanding and uncooperative."

http://evolve.elsevier.com/Canada/Varcarolis/psychiatric/

REFERENCES

Addiction and Mental Health Collaborative Project Steering Committee. (2015). *Collaboration for addiction and mental health care: Best advice*. Canadian Centre on Substance Abuse. http://www.ccsa.ca/Resource%20Library/CCSA-Collaboration-Addiction-Mental-Health-Best-Advice-Report-2015-en.pdf

American Nurses Association (ANA), American Psychiatric Nurses Association, & International Society of Psychiatric-Mental Health Nurses. (2014). *Psychiatric–mental health nursing: Scope and standards of practice* (2nd ed.). Washington, DC: Nursebooks.org.

Arnold, E. C., & Boggs, K. U. (2020). *Interpersonal relationships: Professional communication skills for nurses* (8th ed.). St. Louis: Saunders.

Baklien, B., & Bongaardt, R. (2014). The quest for choice and the need for relational care in mental health work. *Medicine, Health Care, and Philosophy, 17*(4), 625–632. https://doi.org/10.1007/s11019-014-9563-z

Butcher, H. K., Bulechek, G. M., McCloskely Docherman, J. M., & Wagner, C. M. (2019). *Nursing Interventions Classification (NIC)* (7th ed.). St. Louis: Elsevier.

Canadian Federation of Mental Health Nurses. (2014). *Canadian standards for psychiatric-mental health nursing* (4th ed.). Toronto: Author. https://www.cfmhn.ca/2019/05/07/cfmhn-2014-standards/

Canadian Nurses Association. (2018). *Position statement: Evidence-informed decision-making and nursing practice*. Ottawa: Author. https://www.cna-aiic.ca/en/policy-advocacy/policy-support-tools/position-statements

Canadian Nurses Association. (2020). *CNA's key messages on anti-Black racism in nursing and health*. https://www.cna-aiic.ca/-/media/cna/page-content/pdf-en/anti-racism-key-messages_e.pdf?la=en&hash=413A57BA251745BD496E88FF8AAE81DEC761A7AF

Canadian Nurses Protective Society. (2020). *Quality documentation: Your best defence*. https://cnps.ca/article/quality-documentation/#:~:text=Quality%20Documentation%3A%20Your%20Best%20Defence%20The%20Canadian%20Nurses,to%20documentation%2C%20whether%20in%20paper%20or%20electronic%20form

Chaze, F., Thomson, M. S., George, U., & Guruge, S. (2015). Role of cultural beliefs, religion, and spirituality in mental health and/or service utilization among immigrants in Canada: A scoping review. *Canadian Journal of Community Mental Health, 34*(3), 1–15. https://doi.org/10.7870/cjcmh-2015-015

College and Association of Registered Nurses of Alberta. (2013). *Documentation standards for regulated members*. https://nurses.ab.ca/docs/default-source/document-library/standards/practice-standards-for-regulated-members.pdf?sfvrsn=d4893bb4_16

College of Nurses of Ontario. (2019). *Documentation, revised 2008*. https://www.cno.org/globalassets/docs/prac/41001_documentation.pdf

College of Registered Nurses of Nova Scotia. (2017). *Standards of practice for registered nurses 2017*. Halifax: Author. http://crnns.ca/wp-content/uploads/2015/02/RNStandards.pdf

Coombs, T., Curtis, J., & Crookes, P. (2013). What is the process of a comprehensive mental health nursing assessment? Results from a qualitative study: Process of mental health nursing assessment. *International Nursing Review, 60*(1), 96–102. https://doi.org/10.1111/j.1466-7657.2012.01036.x

Dilmaghani, M. (2018). Importance of religion or spirituality and mental health in Canada. *Journal of Religion and Health, 57*(1), 120–135.

Doenges, M. E., Moorhouse, M. F., & Murr, A. C. (2019). *Nursing diagnosis manual: Planning, individualizing, and documenting patient care* (6th ed.). Philadelphia: F. A. Davis.

Elkington, E. J., & Talbot, K. M. (2016). The role of interpreters in mental health care. *South African Journal of Psychology, 46*(3), 364–375. https://doi.org/10.1177/0081246315619833

Ewing, J. A. (1984). Detecting alcoholism: The CAGE questionnaire. *Journal of the American Medical Association, 252*(14), 1905–1907. https://doi.org/10.1001/jama.252.14.1905

Fogel, A., Nazir, S., Hirapara, K., & Ray, S. (2020). *Cultural assessment and treatment of psychiatric patients*: NCBI Bookshelf. StatPearls [Internet]. https://www.statpearls.com/articlelibrary/viewarticle/20169/

Gomi, S., Starnino, V. R., & Canda, E. R. (2014). Spiritual assessment in mental health recovery. *Community Mental Health Journal, 50*(4), 447–453. https://doi.org/10.1007/s10597-013-9653-z

Government of Canada. (2018). *Trauma and violence-informed approaches to policy and practice*. https://www.canada.ca/en/public-health/services/publications/health-risks-safety/trauma-violence-informed-approaches-policy-practice.html

Government of Canada. (2021). *Personal Information Protection and Electronic Documents Act*. http://laws-lois.justice.gc.ca/eng/acts/P-8.6/

Herdman, T. H., Kamitsuru, S., & Lopez, C. (2021). *NANDA international nursing diagnoses: Definitions and classification, 2021–2023*. Oxford: Wiley-Blackwell.

Higgins, A., Doyle, L., Downes, C., Morrissey, J., Costello, P., Brennan, M., & Nash, M. (2016). There is more to risk and safety planning than dramatic risks: Mental health nurses' risk assessment and safety-management practice. *International Journal of Mental Health Nursing, 25*(2), 159–170. https://doi.org/10.1111/inm.12180

Hu, L. Y., Shen, C. C., Hu, Y. W., Chen, M. H., Tsai, C. F., Chiang, H. L., Yeh, C. M., Wang, W. S., Chen, P. M., Hu, T. M., Chen, T. J., Su, T. P., & Liu, C. J. (2013). Hyperthyroidism and risk for bipolar disorders: A nationwide population-based study. *PLOS One, 8*(8), e73057. https://doi.org/10.1371/journal.pone.0073057

Jakubec, S. L., & Astle, B. J. (2021). *Research literacy for health and community practice*. (2nd ed.). Toronto: Canadian Scholars' Press.

Martin, C. T. (2016). The value of physical examination in mental health nursing. *Nurse Education in Practice, 17*, 91–96. https://doi.org/10.1016/j.nepr.2015.11.001

Mental Health Commission of Canada. (2016). *Recovery guidelines*. Ottawa: Author. http://www.mentalhealthcommission.ca/sites/default/files/2016-07/MHCC_Recovery_Guidelines_2016_ENG.PDF

Michaelson, V., King, N., Inchley, J., Currie, D., Brooks, F., & Pickett, W. (2019). Domains of spirituality and their associations with positive mental health: A study of adolescents in Canada, England and Scotland. *Preventive Medicine, 125*, 12–18.

Milner, K., Crawford, P., Edgley, A., Hare-Duke, L., & Slade, M. (2020). The experiences of spirituality among adults with mental health difficulties: A qualitative systematic review. *Epidemiology and Psychiatric Science, 29*, e34.

Minton, M. E., Isaacson, M. J., Varilek, B., Stadick, J. L., & O'Connell-Persaud, S. (2018). A willingness to go there: Nurses and spiritual care. *Journal of Clinical Nursing, 27*(1–2), 173–181.

Moorhead, S., Johnson, M., Maas, M. L., & Swanson, E. (2018). *Nursing Outcomes Classification (NOC)* (6th ed.). St. Louis: Mosby.

Ness, O., Borg, M., Semb, R., & Karlsson, B. (2014). "Walking alongside:" Collaborative practices in mental health and substance use care. *International Journal of Mental Health Systems, 8*(1), 55. https://doi.org/10.1186/1752-4458-8-55

Nurses Association of New Brunswick. (2020). *Standards for documentation*. http://www.nanb.nb.ca/media/resource/NANB-Standards-Documentation-May20-E.pdf

O'Brien, C. P. (2008). The CAGE Questionnaire for detection of alcoholism. *Journal of the American Medical Association, 300*(17), 2054–2056. https://doi.org/10.1001/jama.2008.570

Paniagua, F. A., & Yamada, A. M. (2013). *Handbook of multicultural mental health: Assessment and treatment of diverse populations* (2nd ed.). Amsterdam: Elsevier.

Registered Nurses' Association of Ontario. (2013). *Developing and sustaining interprofessional health care: Optimizing patients/clients, organizational, and system outcomes*. Toronto: Author.

Registered Nurses' Association of Ontario. (2017). *Nursing best practice guidelines: Components of mental status assessment*. https://pda.rnao.ca/content/components-mental-status-assessment

Registered Psychiatric Nurse Regulators of Canada. (2014). *Registered psychiatric nurse entry-level competencies*. http://www.rpnc.ca/sites/default/files/resources/pdfs/RPNRC-ENGLISH%20Compdoc%20%28Nov6-14%29.pdf

Registered Psychiatric Nurses of Canada. (2019). *Standards of psychiatric nursing practice*. https://crpnm.mb.ca/wp-content/uploads/2019/10/Standards-of-Psychiatric-Nursing-Practice-FINAL-October-2019.pdf

Rhoads, J., & Murphy, P. J. M. (2014). *Clinical consult to psychiatric nursing for advanced practice*. New York: Springer.

Shajani, Z., & Snell, D. (2019). *Wright & Leahey's nurses and families: A guide to family assessment and intervention* (7th ed.). F. A. Davis.

Starnino, V. R. (2016). Conceptualizing spirituality and religion for mental health practice: Perspectives of consumers with serious mental illness. *Families in Society, 97*(4), 295–304. https://doi.org/10.1606/1044-3894.2016.97.36

Statistics Canada. (2020). *2021 Census Fact Sheets*. https://www12.statcan.gc.ca/census-recensement/2021/ref/98-20-0001/982000012020002-eng.cfm

Talaei, A., Rafee, N., & Chahrei, A. (2017). TSH cut off based on depression in hypothyroid patients. *BMC Psychiatry, 17*(327). https://doi.org/10.1186/s12888-017-1478-9

Varcarolis, E. M., & Fosbre, C. D. (2021). *Essentials of psychiatric mental health nursing: A communication approach to evidence-based care*. (4th ed.). Philadelphia: Elsevier.

Wheeler, K. (2020). *Psychotherapy for the advanced practice psychiatric nurse: A how-to guide for evidence-based practice* (3rd ed.). New York: Springer.

7

Ethical Responsibilities and Legal Obligations for Psychiatric Mental Health Nursing Practice

Cheryl L. Pollard

 http://evolve.elsevier.com/Canada/Varcarolis/psychiatric/

OBJECTIVES

1. Identify the differences between ethical responsibilities and legal obligations within the practice of psychiatric mental health nursing.
2. Describe key elements of the common approaches that inform health care ethics.
3. Identify the ethical nursing responsibilities related to psychiatric mental health research.
4. Identify relevant legislation enacted to protect, promote, and improve the lives of Canadians with mental illness.
5. Describe the rights of the patient in a psychiatric setting.
6. Discuss the meaning of standard care in a psychiatric setting.

KEY TERMS AND CONCEPTS

abandonment
advance directives
assault
autonomy
battery
beneficence
bioethics
competency
confidentiality
consequentialist theory
conscientious objection
deontology
duty to protect

duty to warn
engagement
ethics
false imprisonment
guardianship
implied consent
informed consent
intentional torts
justice
malpractice
moral agent
moral distress
moral residue

moral resilience
moral uncertainty
negligence
nonmaleficence
relational ethics
respect for autonomy
right to privacy
right to refuse treatment
tort law
unintentional torts
utilitarianism
virtue ethics
virtues

Every nurse will face dilemmas in which values, responsibilities, and obligations seem to conflict, in which there is no clear path to "doing good" or determining what is "most fitting." The purpose of this chapter is to help nurses think about the ethical responsibilities and the legal obligations of their practice. It is important to recognize that in professional nursing, ethical responsibilities and legal obligations are distinct areas, but they often have overlapping influences on clinical practice. Nursing ethics is unique in that it is an expression of the values and beliefs that guide nursing practice. Nurses must think about ethical issues on an individual level, professional level, and systems level as they respond to clinical questions.

In contrast, legislation, the foundation of legal obligations, is a means used within society to meet objectives and consolidate values. For example, provincial health protection acts define the scope of practice for health care providers. Mental health legislation is designed to protect and provide safeguards and supervision to improve the lives and mental well-being of citizens. This legislation generally acknowledges the fundamental value of mental health and aims to ensure that the rights of individuals are protected. The type and form of legislative text varies from country to country and, within Canada, between jurisdictions. Jurisdictions may organize their laws related to the protection of rights for people with mental illness within a single statute or within a variety of different legislative measures. In Canada the laws are dispersed within a variety of legislative measures, which include the *Canada Health Act*, the *Employment Equity Act*, and provincial or territorial legislation regarding social welfare and benefits, disability, guardianship, employment, housing, and involuntary admission and treatment of individuals with mental illness. Although the legislation that affects the social determinants of health for people with mental illness is important, the focus of the discussion of legal implications in this chapter relates to the involuntary admission and involuntary treatment of people with mental illness.

ETHICAL CONCEPTS

"Like other kinds of growth, moral development is more likely to occur in the right environment—one that provides models, mentors, heroes and antiheroes; support, guidance and correction; relevant experiences and time for healing, and reflection, and building" (Andre, 2000, p. 61).

Ethics are an expression of the values and beliefs that guide practice. Manitoba Provincial Health Ethics Network (2016) has developed a decision-making guide for patient care ethics (Figure 7.1).

Fig. 7.1 Making ethical decisions. (**Source:** Manitoba Provincial Health Ethics Network. (2016). *Patient care ethics: Decision-making guide: Framework for clinical or patient-care issues.* Winnipeg: Author.)

Three types of moral theories have traditionally been used as a foundation for the development of nursing ethics: deontological theory, consequentialist theory, and virtue theory. More recently, the developing theory of relational ethics, an ethical theory with the core elements of mutual respect, engagement, embodied knowledge, interdependent environment, and uncertainty (Bergum & Dossetor, 2004), has also affected the application of ethics within nursing.

Deontology is a system of ethics with the central concepts of reason and duty: there is an obligation to act in accordance with particular rules and principles. The Canadian Nurses Association (CNA, 2017) code of ethics (Box 7.1), and the standards of psychiatric nursing practice developed jointly by the British Columbia College of Nursing Professionals, College of Registered Psychiatric Nurses of Alberta, Registered Psychiatric Nurses Association of Saskatchewan, and the College of Registered Psychiatric Nurses of Manitoba (2019) (Box 7.2) are written from this perspective. Immanuel Kant (1724–1804), a prominent deontologist, believed that people were free to make choices and that those choices should be based not on emotion but on reason alone. Within the paradigm of deontology, Beauchamp and Childress (2019) outlined several fundamental principles that are irreducible and must be balanced in clinical situations (referred to as **bioethics**). The basic principles are:

1. **Respect for autonomy**—respecting the rights of others to make their own decisions (e.g., acknowledging the patient's right to refuse medication).

> **BOX 7.1 Canadian Nurses' Values and Ethical Responsibilities**
>
> The ethical responsibilities of Canadian registered nurses are articulated through seven primary values
> 1. Providing safe, compassionate, competent, and ethical care
> 2. Promoting health and well-being
> 3. Promoting and respecting informed decision making
> 4. Honouring dignity
> 5. Maintaining privacy and confidentiality
> 6. Promoting justice
> 7. Being accountable
>
> **Source:** Canadian Nurses Association. (2017). *Code of ethics for registered nurses.* Ottawa: Author. Copyright © 2021, Canadian Nurses Association. Reprinted with permission. Further reproduction prohibited.

2. **Nonmaleficence**—the duty to minimize harm and do no wrong to the patient (e.g., by maintaining expertise in nursing skill through nursing education).
3. **Beneficence**—the duty to act to benefit or promote the good of others (e.g., spending extra time to help calm an extremely anxious patient).

BOX 7.2 Standards of Psychiatric Nursing Practice

Psychiatric nursing is regulated as a distinct profession in Canada by the provinces of Alberta, British Columbia, Manitoba, and Saskatchewan, as well as the territory of Yukon. Registered psychiatric nurses provide services relating to mental, physical, and developmental health and engage in various roles providing health care services to individuals, families, groups, and communities. The practice of psychiatric nursing occurs within the domains of direct practice, education, administration, and research. The standards provide a guide to the knowledge, skills, values, judgement, and attitudes that psychiatric nurses need to practise safely. There are four standards of psychiatric nursing practice:

1. The registered psychiatric nurse establishes collaborative professional, interpersonal, and therapeutic relationships with patients.
2. The registered psychiatric nurse continually acquires and integrates evidence-informed knowledge and builds on psychiatric nursing education and lifelong learning.
3. The registered psychiatric nurse is accountable and responsible for safe, competent, and ethical psychiatric nursing practice that meets the standards of the profession and legislated requirements.
4. The registered psychiatric nurse enhances the safety, quality, and effectiveness of psychiatric nursing practice through leadership and collaboration.
5. The registered psychiatric nurse understands, upholds, and incorporates the profession's Code of Ethics into their professional practice.

Source: British Columbia College of Nursing Professionals, College of Registered Psychiatric Nurses of Alberta, Registered Psychiatric Nurses Association of Saskatchewan, & the College of Registered Psychiatric Nurses of Manitoba. (2019). *Standards of psychiatric nursing practice.* Winnipeg: Author.

---

4. Justice—the duty to distribute resources or care equally, regardless of personal attributes (e.g., an intensive care nurse devotes equal attention to someone who has attempted suicide as to someone who has suffered a brain aneurysm).

Other pluralistic deontologists have identified two other principles to consider when making ethical decisions in clinical settings. These additional principles are:

5. Principle of impossibility—the principle that a right or obligation that cannot be met within the current situation is no longer an obligation (e.g., a person does not have a right to receive magnetic resonance imaging [MRI] if MRI is not available, or a person does not have a right to be cured of schizophrenia when there are currently no permanent cures).
6. Principle of fidelity or best action—maintaining loyalty and commitment to the patient to perform your duty in the best manner possible (e.g., if a patient requires a dressing change, it is your duty to use the greatest skill and care possible).

The consequentialist theory is based on the belief that every person in society has the right to be happy and that we have an obligation to make sure happiness results from our actions. Within this theory, happiness is the maximization of pleasure and the minimization of pain. Accordingly, this theory's central concept relates to bringing about the greatest good and the least harm for the greatest number of people (called utilitarianism). John Stuart Mill (1806–1873) referred to this idea as the *principle of utility*. This type of approach is used when decisions are based on the outcomes of a cost–benefit analysis.

Critics of consequentialism argue that consequentialist theories fail to take into account how people are affected by actions. Elizabeth Anscombe (1919–2001) argued that consequentialism does not provide guidance on what ought to be done and that it is through the use of virtues that decisions can be made. Virtues provide guidance on what one ought to do. Religiously based ethics, and more recently, moral psychology, moral virtue, and facts of human nature, have been used by virtue ethicists to identify virtues relevant to ethical decision making.

Unlike deontology or utilitarianism theorists, who use duties and obligations to guide decision making, virtue theorists do not. The ancient philosopher Aristotle believed that virtuous people would make decisions that would maximize their own and others' well-being. Similarly, the central premise of virtue ethics is that good people will make good decisions. Virtues are attitudes, dispositions, or character traits (e.g., honesty, courage, compassion, generosity, fidelity, integrity, fairness, self-control) that enable us to be and to act in ways that develop ethical potential and ensure ethical outcomes. The most prevalent and most valued virtues in health care are compassion and care. Just as the ability to run a marathon develops through much training and practice, so too does our capacity to be fair, to be courageous, and to be compassionate. Virtues, fostered through learning, practice, and self-discipline, enable us to use these attitudes and traits to guide decisions.

Relational ethics, an action-based ethics, requires nurses to appreciate the context in which an ethical issue arises. Context, though, is not a mathematical equation to be figured out, nor is it a black-and-white phenomenon to be described. Context is a dynamic and fluid interaction of the participants, and it is this interaction that inspires (requires) responsibility (Olthuis, 1997). This responsibility, in turn, evokes ethical action. From the perspective of relational ethics, the fulcrum for action (how to be and how to act) is the relationship (Austin et al., 2003). When using a relational ethics approach, the core question to be answered in an ethical situation is "What action or decision is most fitting?" Understanding the relationship and the actions to be taken requires knowledge of traditions, universal principles, rationality, our subjectivity, and our interconnectedness (Rodney et al., 2012). As researchers explored relational ethics, they found five core elements that are cornerstones for ethical action (Austin et al., 2003):

1. Mutual respect—an intersubjective experience arising from a non-oppositional perception of difference. There is a recognition that individuals are affected by how others view and react to them as well as by their attitudes toward themselves and others.
2. Engagement—the connection between the self and another. It is through this connection that nurses can develop a meaningful understanding of another person's experience, perspective, and vulnerability.
3. Embodied knowledge—our understanding of the other, incorporated with a scientific body of knowledge. Nursing knowledge and compassion are given equal weight; therefore emotions and feelings are viewed to be as important as physical signs and symptoms.
4. Interdependent environment—the recognition that we are not separate entities but that we exist as part of a larger community, society, and system. We are not merely affected by our environment; each action we take affects the environment, too.
5. Uncertainty or vulnerability—a recognition that ethical dilemmas exist and, furthermore, that ethical deliberation and contemplation are difficult and at times unpleasant.

From a relational ethics perspective, the consequences of uncertainty or vulnerability are ethical dilemmas. An ethical dilemma results when a choice must be made between two mutually exclusive courses of action, each of which has favourable and unfavourable consequences. How we respond to these dilemmas is based partly on our own morals (beliefs of right and wrong) and values. The nurse is a moral agent who has the power and capacity to direct their motives and actions to some ethical end: essentially, doing what is good and right (CNA, 2017). Suppose you are caring for a pregnant woman with schizophrenia who wants to carry the baby to term but whose family insists she get an abortion. To promote fetal safety, her antipsychotic medication will need to be reduced, putting her at risk for exacerbation of the illness. Furthermore, there is a question as to whether she can safely care for the child. If you rely on the ethical principle of autonomy (the right to make decisions for oneself), you may conclude that she has the right to decide. Would other ethical principles be in conflict with autonomy in this case? At times, your personal values may be in conflict with the value system of the institution. This situation further complicates the decision-making process and necessitates careful consideration of the patient's desires. For example, you may experience a conflict of values in a setting where older adult patients are routinely tranquilized to a degree you are not comfortable with. Whenever one's value system is challenged, increased stress results.

Consequently, psychiatric mental health nurses may develop moral (or ethical) distress, moral uncertainty, moral residue, or a combination of these stressors. Rodney (2017) identifies that feelings of **moral distress** develop from situations where nurses know or believe they know the right thing to do but, for various reasons (including fear or circumstances beyond their control), do not or cannot take the right action or prevent a particular harm. This is in comparison to **moral uncertainty**, which occurs when a nurse feels indecision or [has] a lack of clarity or is unable to even know what the moral problem is or which moral principles apply (Dorman & Bouchal, 2020). When involved in repeated situations that cause moral distress, there is a crescendo effect leading to **moral residue**. Moral residue builds with each morally distressing situation and can lead to moral numbing, conscious objection to an increasing number of circumstances, and/or burnout (Arnold, 2020). Lachman (2016) has identified various means of coping with moral distress and moral residue: moral resilience. **Moral resilience** is the ability and willingness to speak and take the most fitting action in the presence of moral and ethical dilemmas (Lachman, 2016, p. 122). See Box 7.3 for strategies to develop moral resilience.

There may be particular times in nurses' careers when they are unable to align their own understanding of ethical principles, duties, or required virtues with those of their patients. In these situations professional organizations and health care organizations may have policies that will help guide the nurse to balance professional obligations and personal values. **Conscientious objection** is the action a health care practitioner takes when their belief that the procedure requested by a patient or the employer is morally wrong (Neal & Fovargue, 2019). Most professional codes of conduct and organizational policies attempt to forge a means of compromising between individual conscience and professional responsibilities. However, if the health care provider is responsible for the patient's care, the provider must ensure that the patient's needs are met until another provider takes over responsibility for care provision (CNA, 2017).

⚡ SAFETY TIP
Delivering health care services to patients is never straightforward and there are not always answers or results that leave us feeling proud of the work we do. When situations arise where the right action cannot be taken, utilize your support systems. These can include talking with your instructor or a more experienced nurse or health professional. It is important that you remember that you are not alone. Nursing is a team sport.

The last area of ethical consideration to be discussed in this chapter is research ethics. The code of ethics of the CNA (2017) outlines ethical standards of practice, among them, for research. Actions and ethical responsibilities of the nurse can include ensuring that patients are informed of their rights with regard to research; however, the CNA code of ethics also contains rules and regulations to ensure that nursing research is conducted legally and ethically. These rules and regulations apply to all areas of nursing and parallel the *Tri-Council Policy Statement: Ethical Conduct for Research Involving Humans* (Canadian Institutes of Health Research, Natural Sciences and Engineering Research Council of Canada, & Social Sciences and Humanities Research Council of Canada, 2018) core principles of respect for persons, concern for welfare, and justice. Research within a mental health setting raises unique ethical considerations. People with a mental illness are potentially very vulnerable. "Vulnerability is often caused by limited decision-making capacity, or limited access to social goods, such as rights, opportunities and power" (Canadian Institutes of Health Research, Natural Sciences and Engineering Research Council of Canada, & Social Sciences and Humanities Research Council of Canada, 2018, p. 8). There is a strong research tradition in Canada. As nurses continue to transform their practices using evidence-informed knowledge, they must be aware of the consequences of not adhering to ethical standards. An example is included in the following Research Highlight.

BOX 7.3 Developing Moral Resilience
1. Identify your beliefs and values.
2. Compare these to your professional code of ethics.
3. Compare these to your organizational values.
4. Identify if there are any differences.
   a. Identify potential responsibilities that may result in a conscientious objection.
   b. Articulate morally distressing concerns.
   c. Act as an advocate for resolution of these concerns.
5. Engage in ethical consultations.
6. Make a decision that balances your beliefs with professional responsibilities.
7. Identify emotional reactions after the decision has been made and an action has been taken.
8. Explore these reactions.
9. Explore the complexity of the situation.
10. Connect with others.

Source: Adapted from Lachman, V. D. (2016). Ethics, law, and policy. Moral resilience: Managing and preventing moral distress and moral residue. *Medsurg Nursing, 25*(2), 121–124. http://www.medsurgnursing.net/cgi-bin/WebObjects/MSNJournal.woa

🔬 RESEARCH HIGHLIGHT
Exploring Relationships Among Moral Distress, Moral Courage, and Moral Resilience in Undergraduate Nursing Students

Problem
Nurses are faced with complex ethical situations within complex and fluid health care systems. An increasing number of studies report that moral distress is common among health care providers who face constraints that result in conflicting professional values or are perceived to compromise patient care. Moral distress also occurs in students when they perceive differences between the principles they learned in an academic setting and those they observe during their clinical experiences. Eliminating moral distress is not possible. However, moral courage and moral resilience are means of mitigating the negative effects of moral distress.

Purpose of Study
This study addressed four primary questions: (1) Do nursing students with greater moral resilience and moral courage report significantly less moral distress? (2) Do students with higher moral resilience have less moral distress?

(3) Do students with higher moral courage have less moral distress? and (4) Does moral courage predict moral distress more than moral resiliency?

Methods
A descriptive correlational design was used to investigate the interrelationships of moral distress, moral courage, and moral resilience among undergraduate nursing students. Moral courage, moral resilience, and moral distress were assessed using the Moral Courage Scale for Physicians (MCSP) (Martinez et al., 2016), the Connor-Davidson Resilience Scale (CD-RISC) (Connor & Davidson, 2003), and the Moral Distress Thermometer (MDT) (Wocial & Weaver, 2013).

Key Findings
Nursing students with greater moral resilience and moral courage did not experience less moral distress than those with less moral resilience and moral courage. However, those with higher moral courage generally also had higher moral resilience scores. Interestingly, researchers have identified that there is a statistically significant positive correlation between age and developing moral distress.

Implications for Nursing Practice
Moral distress is present in both clinical and academic settings. A knowledge gap exists related to understanding how moral distress is manifested and what educational experiences and factors can affect students most strongly. Nursing education programs should not underestimate the importance of developing competencies related to moral courage and resilience as a means of coping with situations that may create moral distress. Nursing programs may also want to reflect on who they are recruiting to be the next generation of nurses.

Source: Gibson, E., Duke, G., & Alfred, D. (2020). Exploring the relationships among moral distress, moral courage, and moral resilience in undergraduate nursing students. *Journal of Nursing Education, 59*(7), 392–395. https://doi.org/10.3928/01484834-20200617-07

Additional citations:
Connor, K. M., & Davidson, J. R. T. (2003). Development of a new resilience scale: The Connor-Davidson Resilience Scale (CD-RISC). *Depression and Anxiety, 18*(2), 76–82. https://doi.org/10.1002/da.10113

Martinez, W., Bell, S. K., Etchegaray, J. M., & Lehmann, L. S. (2016). Measuring moral courage for interns and residents: Scale development and initial psychometrics. *Academic Medicine, 91*(10), 1431–1438. https://doi.org/10.1097/ACM.0000000000001288

Wocial, L. D., & Weaver, M. T. (2013). Development and psychometric testing of a new tool for detecting moral distress: The moral distress thermometer. *Journal of Advanced Nursing, 69*(1), 167–174. https://doi.org/10.1111/j.1365-2648.2012.06036.x

MENTAL HEALTH LEGISLATION

Nurses must consider both the ethical and the legal dimensions of practice, which are distinct. Ideally, the system of law would be completely compatible with the CNA's code of ethics; however, there may be times when nurses will need to collaborate with others to change a law or policy that is incompatible with ethical practice. When this occurs, the relevant codes of ethics can guide and support nurses' actions as they advocate for changes to law, policy, or practice. These "code[s] can be powerful political instrument[s] for nurses when they are concerned about being able to practice ethically" (CNA, 2017, p. 4).

Canada is a society that respects and cares for its people. As a result, legislation that protects vulnerable citizens has been developed. People with mental health disorders are, or can be, particularly vulnerable to abuse and violation of rights because of the embedded structural stigma and systemic discrimination. As a result, all provinces and territories have laws that protect the rights of people with mental illness and of others whose lives may be directly affected by another's mental illness.

Historically, in Canada mental health legislation was developed to protect members of the public from so-called mentally deranged and dangerous patients. Legislation ensured that these "dangerous" individuals were isolated from the public rather than ensuring that their rights as people and Canadian citizens were protected. Early legislation, when interpreted using today's societal values, allowed for violations of human rights. For example, there was legislation that permitted long-term custodial care for people who were deemed to be "a danger" and were unable to care for themselves. This type of legislation heightened the burden of stigma and discrimination faced by people with mental illness. The Supreme Court of Canada has also recognized the disadvantages endured by people with mental illness. In *Battlefords and District Co-operative Ltd. v. Gibbs* (1996), the court recognized that it was discriminatory to differentiate between physical and mental disability. The court further recognized that individuals with mental illness are subjected to treatment that people with other illnesses are not and determined this treatment to be discriminatory *Battlefords and District Co-operative Ltd. v. Gibbs* (1996). The United Nations Universal Declaration of Human Rights, written in 1948, and other international agreements provide the foundation for current mental health legislation. The fundamental basis for current mental health legislation is respecting human rights, and the key rights and principles reflected related to equality and nondiscrimination, the right to privacy and individual autonomy, freedom from inhuman and degrading treatment, the principle of least restrictive environment, and the rights to information and participation. Many Canadian jurisdictions have used the core principles to guide the revision of old and the development of new mental health legislation (Box 7.4.).

Legislation consolidates fundamental principles, values, goals, and objectives of mental health policies and programs. It provides a legal framework to ensure that critical issues affecting the lives of people with mental health disorders, in facilities and in the community, are addressed. In Canada there are 13 different mental health acts, all of which allow for the involuntary confinement of people with mental illness to protect them from themselves and others from them. Each of the provinces and territories has developed its mental health act from a perspective that prioritizes either the respect of persons (autonomy) or the concern for welfare (beneficence). As a result, the acts differ in many ways. However, the primary areas of difference are related to

---

BOX 7.4 Mental Health Care Law: Ten Basic Principles

These principles were developed from a comparative analysis of national mental health laws in 45 countries worldwide conducted by the World Health Organization. The selection of principles drew from the Principles for the Protection of Persons with Mental Illness and the Improvement of Mental Health Care adopted by the UN General Assembly Resolution 46/119 of December 17, 1991.

1. Promotion of mental health and prevention of mental health disorders
2. Access to basic mental health care
3. Mental health assessments in accordance with internationally accepted principles
4. Provision of the least restrictive type of mental health care
5. Self-determination
6. Right to be assisted in the exercise of self-determination
7. Availability of review procedure
8. Automatic periodical review mechanism
9. Qualified decision-maker
10. Respect of the rule of law

Source: World Health Organization. (1996). *Mental health care law: Ten basic principles.* Geneva: Author.

when the rights of an individual become secondary to the safety of self and others and who has the authority to authorize treatment. You are encouraged to review your province's or territory's act to better understand the legal climate in which you will practise (Table 7.1). As you review the act relevant to your province, you will notice that there is different paperwork, or forms, required to enact various parts of the acts.

As people started to receive their psychiatric care while living in the community, provincial and territorial acts have changed to reflect a shift in emphasis from institutional care of people with mental illness to community-based care delivery models. Along with this shift in setting has come the more widespread use of psychotropic drugs in the treatment of mental illness, which has enabled many people to integrate more readily into the larger community, and an increasing awareness of the need to provide mentally ill patients with care that respects their human rights. However, the increased use of psychotropic drugs has resulted in more discussions, and debate, about the ethical use of medication.

ESTABLISHING BEST PRACTICE

Each province and territory provides a regulatory framework for the governance of health professions and gives professional bodies their mandates and powers. In many provinces this legislation is referred to as the Health Professions Act (HPA); however, a number of provinces continue to use legislation that is specific to each registering body, such as registered nurses, registered psychiatric nurses, or registered practical nurses. HPAs, or similar legislation, also authorize professional bodies to create and enforce bylaws, standards of practice, and professional ethics. This type of regulation also sets out reserved titles and scopes of practice for professional registrants, including restricted activities for general and certified registered or licensed nursing practice as well as for nurse practitioner practice. You are encouraged to review your province's or territory's legislation to better understand the legal climate in which you will practise (Table 7.2).

TABLE 7.1 Provincial and Territorial Mental Health Acts

Province or Territory	Website Link
Alberta	http://www.qp.alberta.ca/574.cfm?page=M13.cfm&leg_type=Acts&isbncln=0779748727
British Columbia	http://www.bclaws.ca/EPLibraries/bclaws_new/document/ID/freeside/00_96288_01
Manitoba	http://web2.gov.mb.ca/laws/statutes/ccsm/m110e.php
New Brunswick	http://laws.gnb.ca/en/ShowTdm/cs/M-10//
Newfoundland and Labrador	http://www.assembly.nl.ca/legislation/sr/statutes/m09-1.htm
Northwest Territories	https://www.justice.gov.nt.ca/en/files/legislation/mental-health/mental-health.a.pdf
Nova Scotia	http://novascotia.ca/dhw/mental-health/involuntary-psychiatric-treatment-act.asp
Nunavut	https://assembly.nu.ca/sites/default/files/Bill-36-Mental-Health-Act-Reprint-EN-FR.pdf
	(The Government of Nunavut accepted this new bill in 2021 after consolidation and consultation over several years.)
Ontario	http://www.e-laws.gov.on.ca/html/statutes/english/elaws_statutes_90m07_e.htm
Prince Edward Island	http://www.gov.pe.ca/law/statutes/pdf/m-06_1.pdf
Quebec	http://legisquebec.gouv.qc.ca/fr/ShowDoc/cs/P-38.001
Saskatchewan	http://www.qp.gov.sk.ca/documents/English/Statutes/Statutes/M13-1.pdf
Yukon	https://laws.yukon.ca/cms/images/LEGISLATION/PRINCIPAL/2002/2002-0150/2002-0150.pdf

TABLE 7.2 Provincial and Territorial Health Professions Acts

Province or Territory	Website Link
Alberta	http://www.qp.alberta.ca/documents/acts/h07.pdf
British Columbia	http://www.bclaws.ca/EPLibraries/bclaws_new/document/ID/freeside/00_96183_01
Manitoba	http://www.gov.mb.ca/health/rhpa/index.html
New Brunswick	https://www.canlii.org/en/nb/laws/stat/rsnb-2014-c-112/latest/rsnb-2014-c-112.html
Newfoundland and Labrador	http://www.assembly.nl.ca/legislation/sr/annualstatutes/2010/h01-02.c10.htm
Northwest Territories	http://www.assembly.gov.nt.ca/sites/default/files/15-02-25bill36_amended.pdf
Nova Scotia	http://www.novascotia.ca/just/regulations/index.htm
Nunavut	https://www.gov.nu.ca/health/information/legislation-and-policy-0
Ontario	https://www.ontario.ca/laws/statute/91r18?search=health+professions
Prince Edward Island	https://www.princeedwardisland.ca/en/legislation/regulated-health-professions-act
Quebec	https://professions-quebec.org/en/quebec-interprofessional-council/about-us/members/
Saskatchewan	https://www.srna.org/about-us/how-we-govern/act-bylaws/
Yukon	http://www.gov.yk.ca/legislation/acts/hepr_c.pdf

Standards of Practice

The standards of practice, determined by professional associations and regulatory bodies, differ from the minimal qualifications set forth by provincial or territorial licensure for entry into the profession of nursing because the primary purposes of each are different. Regulatory bodies establish acceptable qualifications for entry to practice. These provide consumer protection by ensuring that all practising nurses have successfully completed an approved nursing program and passed the national licensing examination. Whereas the professional association's primary focus is to elevate the practise of its members by setting standards of excellence.

Standards of Care

Nurses are held to a basic standard of care that is based on what other nurses who possess the same degree of skill or knowledge would do in the same or similar circumstances. Psychiatric patients, whether in a large, small, rural, or urban facility, have a right to the standard of care recognized by professional bodies governing nursing. Nurses must participate in continuing education courses to stay current with existing standards of care.

Policies and Procedures

Hospital policies and procedures define institutional criteria for care, which may be introduced in legal proceedings to prove that a nurse met or failed to meet them. The weakness of individual institutions setting such criteria is that a particular hospital's policy may be substandard. Substandard institutional policies, however, do not absolve the individual nurse of responsibility to practise on the basis of professional standards of nursing care.

Traditional Practice Knowledge

Like hospital policies and procedures, traditional practice knowledge can be used as evidence of a standard of care. But using traditional practice knowledge to establish a standard of care may result in the same defect as using hospital policies and procedures: traditional practice knowledge may not adhere to the laws, recommendations of the accrediting body, or other recognized standards of care. Traditional practice knowledge must be carefully and regularly evaluated to ensure that substandard routines have not developed.

GUIDELINES FOR ENSURING ADHERENCE TO STANDARDS OF CARE

Students or practising nurses may encounter situations in which they suspect negligence on the part of a peer. In most provinces and territories nurses have a legal duty to report such risks for harm. It is also important for nurses to document the evidence clearly and accurately before making serious accusations against a peer. If you question any regulated health provider's orders or actions, it is wise to communicate these concerns directly to the person involved. If the risky behaviour continues, you have an obligation to communicate your concerns to a supervisor, who should then intervene to ensure that the patient's rights and well-being are protected.

If you suspect a peer of being chemically impaired or of practising irresponsibly, you have an obligation to protect not only the rights of the peer but also the rights of all patients who could be harmed by this person. If the danger persists after you have reported suspected behaviour of concern to a supervisor, you have a duty to report the concern to someone at the next level of authority. It is important to follow the channels of communication in an organization, but it is also important to protect the safety of the patients. To that end, if supervisors' actions or inactions do not rectify the dangerous situation, you have a continuing duty to report the behaviour of concern to the appropriate authority, such as the provincial or territorial nursing college or association.

The CNA and the Canadian Federation of Mental Health Nurses have useful information related to standards of practice on their websites.

The issues become more complex when a professional colleague's conduct (including that of a student nurse) is criminally unlawful. Specific examples include the diversion of drugs from the hospital and sexual misconduct with patients. Increasing media attention and the recognition of substance use as an occupational hazard for health professionals have led to the establishment of substance use programs for health care workers in many provinces or territories. These programs provide appropriate treatment for impaired health care providers to protect the public from harm and to rehabilitate the provider.

The problem of reporting impaired colleagues becomes a difficult one, particularly when no direct harm has occurred to any patients. Concern for professional reputations, damaged careers, and personal privacy has generated a code of silence among health care providers regarding substance use. Chapter 18 deals more fully with issues related to the chemically impaired nurse.

PATIENTS' RIGHTS UNDER THE LAW

Authorization of Treatment

Two models of decision making are supported by legislation. The first, the state (civil government) model, is used to build a system wherein the psychiatrists make the decisions (paternalism). The premise of this model is that the education and experience of a psychiatrist enable them to make better treatment decisions than would the patient's family members. Thus treatment can be started immediately and without delay. The second is the private model. Within this model, the patient or their family member is viewed as the most appropriate authority for making treatment decisions. In Canada in physical medicine the private model is used exclusively, based on a civil liberties perspective (Browne, 2010). However, legislation regarding authorization of treatment of mental illnesses has been developed using either a state model or a private model, depending on the jurisdiction. Both models have consequences for the provision of mental health nursing care. Therefore nurses need to reflect on the impact that the current legislation in use in their province or territory has on autonomy, beneficence, non-maleficence, engagement, mutual respect, reciprocity, and an interdependent environment.

> **VIGNETTE**
> Elizabeth is a 50-year-old woman with a long history of admissions to psychiatric hospitals. During previous hospitalizations, she was diagnosed with paranoid schizophrenia. She has refused visits from her case worker and stopped taking medication, and her young-adult children have become increasingly concerned about her behaviour. When they visit her, she is unkempt and smells bad, her apartment is filthy and filled with cats, and there is no food in the refrigerator except for ketchup and an old container of yogurt; as well, she is not paying her bills. Elizabeth accuses her children of spying on her and of being in collusion with the government to get at her secrets of mind control and oil-rationing plans. Elizabeth is making vague threats to the local officials, claiming that the people who have caused the problems need to be "taken care of." Her daughter contacts her psychiatrist with this information, and a decision is made to begin emergency involuntary admission proceedings.

Autonomy

Consent

The principle of *informed consent* is based on a person's right to self-determination and the ethical principle of autonomy. An essential aspect of informed consent is that it must occur without coercion. Proper orders for specific therapies and treatments are required and must be documented in the patient's medical record. Consent for surgery, electroconvulsive treatment, or the use of experimental medications or procedures must be obtained. Patients have the right to refuse participation in experimental treatments or research and the right to voice grievances and recommend changes in policies or services offered by the facility without fear of punishment or reprisal.

For consent to be effective, it must be informed. Generally, the informed consent of the patient must be obtained by the physician or other health care provider before a treatment or procedure is performed. Methods of obtaining informed consent vary based on patient age or their ability to understand the consequences of their decision. For example, when working with children, informed consent will be sought from the guardian or parent. Assent, an expression of willingness, would be sought from the child. Without coercion, patients must be informed of:

- The nature of their problem or condition
- The nature and purpose of a proposed treatment
- The risks and benefits of that treatment
- The alternative treatment options
- The probability of success of the proposed treatment
- The risks of not consenting to treatment

It is important that psychiatric mental health nurses know that the presence of psychotic thinking does not mean that the patient is mentally incompetent or incapable of understanding; they are still able to provide or deny consent.

Competency is the capacity to understand the consequences of one's decisions. Patients must be considered legally competent until they have been declared incompetent through a legal proceeding. If found incompetent, the patient may be appointed a legal guardian or representative, who is legally responsible for giving or refusing consent for the patient while always considering the patient's wishes. Guardians are typically selected from among family members. The order of selection is usually (1) spouse, (2) adult children or grandchildren, (3) parents, (4) adult siblings, and (5) adult nieces and nephews. If a family member is either unavailable or unwilling to serve as guardian, the court may also appoint a court-trained and court-approved social worker, representing the province or territory, or a member of the community.

Many procedures nurses perform have an element of *implied consent* attached. For example, if you approach the patient with a medication in hand, and the patient indicates a willingness to receive the medication, implied consent has occurred. The fact that you may not have a legal duty to be the person to inform the patient of the associated risks and benefits of a particular medical procedure, however, does not excuse you from clarifying the procedure to the patient and ensuring their expressed or implied consent. When providing care, via implied consent, the nurse must be confident that the person understands, to the best of their abilities, the procedure, risks, and benefits.

The Right to Refuse Treatment

Admission to the hospital, whether voluntary or involuntary, is not synonymous with the commencement of treatment. "In some jurisdictions, treatment can begin as soon as admission is deemed appropriate, that is, after the confirmation by the second physician. In others, it cannot begin until all the appeals have been exhausted" (Browne, 2010, pp. 292–293). At the core of the *right to refuse treatment* is a person's ability to understand and appreciate their condition. The importance of this right was highlighted in 2003 in the case of *Starson v. Swayze*, discussed in Box 7.5.

Community treatment orders (CTOs) are legal mechanisms by which individuals can be mandated against their will to undergo psychiatric treatment in an outpatient setting" (Jager & Perron, 2020). There are several ethical implications related to the enactment of a CTO. The principles of respect for autonomy/paternalism, beneficence/nonmaleficence, and justice must be considered when working with an individual affected by a CTO. From a relational ethics perspective, this

---

BOX 7.5 Facts: *Starson v. Swayze* (2003)

Scott Starson (born Schutzman, 1956) was diagnosed with bipolar disorder with psychosis and was hospitalized many times from young adulthood onward. He had no formal education in physics but his interest in it led to copublication of articles in the field. In the late 1990s he was arrested for uttering death threats, as he had done many times before. In 1998 he was found not criminally responsible for uttering more death threats and was once again arrested and taken to the Centre for Addiction and Mental Health in Toronto. There his treatment plan included neuroleptic medication, which he refused. Because Starson's physicians felt strongly that he needed this medication, the issue was taken to the Ontario Consent and Capacity Board and then to the courts above it. In January 1999 the Ontario Consent and Capacity Board found Starson incapable to refuse medication. Starson appealed the decision and, later that same year, won his case in the Superior Court of Ontario, which deemed him capable. The physicians appealed that ruling, taking the case first to the Ontario Court of Appeal (2001) and ultimately to the Supreme Court of Canada (SCC) (p. 53).

All of these decisions turned on how the board, and then the courts, interpreted Ontario's *Health Care Consent Act*, s. 4(1). Under that law, an individual is capable to refuse (in this case) treatment if they can understand information relevant to making a decision about treatment, and if they can appreciate that the information applies to the patient themself and does not exist in the abstract or apply to a third party.

Decision of the Supreme Court of Canada

The SCC majority (six judges) interpreted the mental capacity test as being fairly low, or easy to pass. They found that Starson was capable to refuse treatment. They found that Starson's "enthusiasm" for (in Starson's words) his own "not normal" mental functioning was a sign that he was aware of the nature of the psychiatric diagnosis given to him and that he simply disagreed with the medical treatment plan (pp. 67–68). By contrast, the SCC dissent (three judges) found that Starson's very enthusiasm for his condition was a sign that, despite obvious intelligence, he could neither understand nor appreciate the severity of his deteriorating condition and the need for treatment. The dissent found that the mental capacity test was not a general intelligence test but very specifically related to information tailored to the individual. Even a highly intelligent person can fail it (pp. 69–70).

Effects on Mr. Starson

With the SCC decision, Scott Starson continued to refuse treatment, and his condition declined markedly. He believed that his nonexistent son would be tortured if he ate or drank. He nearly died and was found without capacity in 2005. His mother became his substitute decision maker and allowed him to be treated with neuroleptic medication. His condition improved and he spent 2 years living in a community-based supportive housing setting while under a community treatment order. In April 2008 he appealed his incapacity finding. Treatment was suspended, his condition deteriorated, and he was again hospitalized involuntarily. Starson appealed his incapacity finding to the Ontario Superior Court. The court upheld the finding of incapacity (pp. 77–78).

Source: Dull, M. W. (2009). Starson v. Swayze, 2003–2008: Appreciating the judicial consequences. *Health Law Journal, 17*, 51–79.

type of "forced treatment" or coercive relationship affects the power dynamics between the nurse and the person with mental illness. Therefore special consideration needs to be given to the aspects of engagement, mutual respect, the environment, and uncertainty.

Beneficence and Nonmaleficence

Involuntary Admission Criteria

All provinces and territories have written legislation that enables the legally sanctioned violation of human rights for a person with mental illness. This violation occurs when an individual is involuntarily admitted to a mental health facility. Every mental health act in Canada specifies the data, assessment findings, or symptoms that must be present for an involuntary admission. For example, in Alberta a person must be (1) suffering from a mental health disorder, (2) is likely to cause harm to themself or others or to suffer substantial mental or physical deterioration or serious physical impairment, and (3) has the potential to benefit from treatment of the mental health disorder (Province of Alberta, 2021). However, in all provinces and territories coupled with the criteria for the original involuntary commitment are safeguards for inappropriately detaining a person in hospital by mandating the completion of an independent examination by a second physician before the person can be kept in hospital. Many jurisdictions stipulate that this physician must be a psychiatrist.

Provision of the Least Restrictive Type of Mental Health Care

As previously mentioned, the use of the least restrictive means of restraint for the shortest duration is always the general rule. Using verbal interventions such as asking the patient for cooperation is the first approach, and medications are considered if verbal interventions fail. Chemical interventions (i.e., medications) are usually considered less restrictive than physical or mechanical interventions (e.g., restraints, seclusion), but they can have a greater impact on the patient's ability to relate to the environment because medication alters our ability to think and produces other effects. However, when used judiciously, psychopharmacology is extremely effective and helpful as an alternative to physical methods of restraint.

The history of using mechanical restraints and seclusion is marked by abuse, overuse, and even a tendency to use restraint as punishment, especially prior to the 1950s, when there were no effective chemical treatments. Most mental health acts in Canada now legislate that clinicians attempting to bring under control people with a mental illness who are a danger to themselves or others are to use a minimal amount of force or treatment in order to protect the patient and others. Nurses must know under which circumstances the use of seclusion and restraints is contraindicated (Box 7.6).

When in restraints, the patient must be protected from all sources of harm. The behaviour leading to restraint or seclusion and the time the patient is placed in and released from restraint must be documented. The patient in restraint must be assessed at regular and frequent intervals (e.g., every 5 to 15 minutes) for physical needs (e.g., food, hydration, toileting), safety, and comfort, and these observations must also be documented. The patient must be removed from restraints when safer and quieter behaviour is observed.

> **BOX 7.6 Contraindications to Seclusion and Restraint**
> - Psychological inability to tolerate the experience of confinement or isolation
> - Physical condition that may be exacerbated by restraint application
> - Desire for punishment of patient or convenience of staff

Agencies have continued to revise their policies and procedures regarding restraint and seclusion, further limiting these practices after recent changes in laws.

Advance Directives

Since the 1960s, the public's desire to participate in decision making about health care has increased. Most provinces and territories have passed legislation that establishes the right of a person to provide directions (advance directives) for clinicians to follow in the event of a serious illness. Such a directive indicates preferences for the types of medical care or extent of treatment desired. The directive comes into effect should physical or mental incapacitation prevent the patient from making health care decisions. Health care institutions are required to (1) provide to each patient at the time of admission written information regarding their right to execute advance health care directives and (2) inquire if the patient has made such directives. The patient's admission records should state whether such directives exist.

Patients concerned that they may be subject to involuntary admission can prepare an advance directive document that will express their treatment choices. The advance directive for mental health decision making should be followed by health care providers when the patient is not competent to make informed decisions. This document can clarify the patient's choice of a surrogate decision maker and instructions about hospital choices, medications, treatment options, provider preferences, and emergency interventions.

Nursing responsibilities with advance directives. The nurse is often responsible for explaining the legal policies of the institution to both the patient and the family and can help them understand advance directives. The nurse serves as an advocate and knowledgeable resource for the patient and family and encourages the patient to verbalize thoughts and feelings during this sensitive time of decision making.

Nurses must be knowledgeable about both the provincial or territorial regulations on advance directives and the potential obstacles in completing the directives for the province or territory in which they practise. Maintaining an open and continuing dialogue among patient, family, nurse, and physician is of principal importance. The nurse supports any surrogates appointed to act on the patient's behalf and seeks consultation for ethical issues the nurse feels unprepared to handle.

Nurses must prepare themselves to deal with the legal, ethical, and moral issues involved when counselling about advance directives. The law does not specify who should talk with patients about treatment decisions, but in many facilities nurses are asked to discuss such issues with the patient. If the advance directive of a patient is not being followed, the nurse should intervene on the patient's behalf. If the problem cannot be resolved with the physician, the nurse must follow the facility's protocol providing for notification of the appropriate supervisor.

Although nurses may discuss options with their patients, they may not assist patients in writing advance directives because doing so is considered a conflict of interest. The existence of an advance directive serves as a guide to health care providers in advocating for the patient's rightful wishes in this process.

Guardianship

A guardianship is an involuntary trust relationship in which one party, the *guardian*, acts on behalf of an individual, the *ward*. The law regards the ward as incapable of managing their own person or affairs. Through investigation and an evaluation process, probate court determines if guardianship is warranted. A physician's expert opinion indicating incompetence is required to initiate the proceeding. Many people with mental illness, intellectual disability, traumatic brain injuries, and organic brain disorders such as dementia have guardians. It is important that health care providers identify patients who have guardians and communicate with the guardians when health care decisions are being made.

Rights Regarding Confidentiality

Confidentiality (the right to privacy of information) of care and treatment is also an important right for all patients, particularly psychiatric patients. Any discussion or consultation involving a patient should be conducted discreetly and only with individuals who have a need and a right to know this privileged information.

The CNA (2017) asserts that it is a duty of the nurse to protect confidential patient information (Box 7.1). The fundamental principle underlying the code on confidentiality is a person's right to privacy, that is, the assurance that only those with a right to know will have access to privileged information. Failure to provide this protection may harm the nurse–patient relationship as well as the patient's well-being. However, the CNA's code of ethics clarifies that this duty is not absolute. In some situations disclosure may be mandated to protect the patient, other persons, or public health. The following four situations warrant the violation of this right to privacy by the nurse:

1. There is the potential for suspected harm to another.
2. There is suspected harm to a child.
3. There is the potential for harm to the patient's self (suicide risk).
4. There is the presence of a reportable communicable disease.

Duty to Warn and Protect Third Parties

Although the following event occurred in the United States, it also had an impact in Canada. The California Supreme Court, in its 1974 landmark decision *Tarasoff v. Regents of the University of California*, ruled that a psychotherapist has a duty to warn a patient's potential victim of potential harm. A university student who was in counselling at the University of California was despondent over being rejected by Tatiana Tarasoff, whom he had once kissed. The psychologist notified police verbally and in writing that the young man might pose a danger to Tarasoff. The police questioned the student, found him to be rational, and secured his promise to stay away from Tarasoff. The student murdered Tarasoff 2 months later.

The *Tarasoff* case acknowledged that generally there is no common-law duty to aid third persons, except when special relationships exist, and the court found the patient–therapist relationship sufficient to create a duty of the therapist to aid Ms. Tarasoff, the victim. It asserted that the duty to protect the intended victim from danger arises when the therapist determines, or, pursuant to professional standards, should have determined, that the patient presents a serious danger to another.

This case created much controversy and confusion in the psychiatric and medical communities over (1) breach of patient confidentiality and its impact on the therapeutic relationship in psychiatric care and (2) the ability of the therapist to predict when a patient is truly dangerous. Nevertheless, many jurisdictions have adopted or modified the California rule despite objections from the psychiatric community.

The California Supreme Court held a second hearing in 1976 in the case of *Tarasoff v. Regents of the University of California* (now known as *Tarasoff II*). It delivered a second ruling that broadened the earlier duty to warn: when a therapist determines that a patient presents a serious danger of violence to another, the therapist has the duty to protect that other person; in providing protection, it may be necessary for the therapist to call and warn the intended victim, the victim's family, or the police or to take whatever steps are reasonably necessary under the circumstances.

Most areas have similar laws regarding the duty to protect third parties from potential life threats. The duty to protect usually includes:

- Assessing and predicting the patient's danger of violence toward another
- Identifying the specific persons being threatened
- Taking appropriate action to protect the identified potential victims

As this trend toward the therapist's duty to warn third persons of potential harm continues to gain wider acceptance, it is important for nurses to understand its implications for nursing practice. Although none of these cases has dealt with nurses, it is fair to assume that in jurisdictions that have adopted the *Tarasoff* doctrine, the duty to warn third persons will be applied to advanced-practice psychiatric mental health nurses who engage in individual therapy in private practice. If a staff nurse, who is a member of a team of psychiatrists, psychologists, psychiatric social workers, and other nurses, does not report to other members of the team a patient's threats of harm against specified victims or classes of victims, this failure is considered substandard nursing care.

Failure to communicate and record relevant information from police, relatives, or the patient's old records may also be deemed negligent. Breach of patient–nurse confidentiality should not pose ethical or legal dilemmas for nurses in these situations, because a team approach to the delivery of psychiatric care presumes communication of pertinent information to other staff members to develop a treatment plan in the patient's best interest.

The nurse's assessment of the patient's potential for violence must be documented and acted on if it suggests legitimate concern about a patient discussing or exhibiting potentially violent behaviour. The psychiatric mental health nurse must communicate their observations to the medical staff when discharge decisions are being considered.

Collaboration of Treatment Team

Health care providers have a responsibility to communicate assessment findings and treatment plans to other members of the treatment team. For example, a health care provider who believes that a patient is going to try to kill themself has a duty to try to mitigate the risk for that person. Strategies to mitigate this risk would include informing other treatment team members. The nurse working on an inpatient unit who has assessed a patient as acutely suicidal would, in consultation with the other team members, develop a plan of care to mitigate the potential for that person to commit suicide.

Documentation of care. The purposes of the medical record are to provide accurate and complete information about the care and treatment of patients and to give health care personnel a means of communicating with each other, supporting continuity of care. A record's usefulness is determined by its accuracy and thoroughness in portraying the patient's behavioural status at the time it was written. For example, if a psychiatric patient describes to a nurse a plan to harm themself or another person and that nurse fails to document the information, including the need to protect the patient or the identified victim, the information will be lost when the nurse leaves work. If the patient's plan is carried out, the harm caused could be linked directly to the nurse's failure to communicate this important information. Even though documentation takes time away from the patient, the importance of communicating and preserving the nurse's memory through the medical record cannot be overemphasized.

Patients have the right to see their medical records, but records belong to the institution. Patients must follow appropriate protocol to view their records.

Guidelines for electronic documentation. Electronic documentation, now common, has created new challenges for protecting the confidentiality of records of psychiatric patients. While ensuring the appropriate sharing of information, institutions must, at the same time, protect against intrusions into patient-record systems. Sensitive information regarding treatment for mental illness can adversely affect patients who are employed, seeking employment, insurance, or credit (Ricciardelli et al., 2020).

Concerns for the privacy of patients' records have been addressed by provincial, territorial, and federal laws that provide guidelines for agencies that use electronic documentation. These guidelines include the recommendation that staff members be assigned individual passwords for entering patients' records to allow for the identification of persons who have accessed confidential information. Only health care providers who have a legitimate need for information about the patient are authorized to access a patient's electronic medical record. There are penalties, including termination of employment, for staff members who access a record without authorization. For this reason, it is important to keep your password private. You are responsible for all entries into records using your password. Various systems allow for specific time frames within which the nurse must make corrections if a documentation error is made.

Any documentation method that improves communication between health care providers should be encouraged. Courts assume that nurses and physicians read each other's notes on patient progress. Many courts take the attitude that if care is not documented, it did not occur. Your documentation also serves as a valuable memory refresher if the patient sues years after the care has been rendered. In providing complete and timely information on the care and treatment of patients the medical record enhances communication among health care providers. Internal institutional audits of records can improve the quality of care rendered. Chapter 6 describes common documentation forms, provides examples, and gives the pros and cons of each.

Organizational use of medical records. The medical record has many uses aside from providing information on the course of the patient's care and treatment by health care providers. A retrospective medical record review can offer an organization valuable information on the quality of care given and on ways to improve that care. An organization may conduct reviews for risk-management purposes to determine areas of potential liability and to evaluate methods of reducing the organization's exposure to liability. For example, risk managers may review documentation of the use of restraints and seclusion for psychiatric patients, or a medical record may be used to evaluate care for quality assurance or peer review. Utilization review analysts use the medical record to determine appropriate use of hospital and staff resources consistent with reimbursement schedules. Insurance companies and other reimbursement agencies rely on the medical record in determining what payments they will make on the patient's behalf.

Medical records as evidence. From a legal perspective, the medical record is a recording of data and opinions made in the normal course of the patient's hospital care. It is deemed to be good evidence because it is presumed to be true, honest, and untainted by memory lapses. Accordingly, the medical record finds its way into a variety of legal cases for a variety of reasons. Some examples of its use include determining (1) the extent of the patient's damages and pain and suffering in personal injury cases, such as when a psychiatric patient attempts suicide while under the protective care of a hospital; (2) the nature and extent of injuries in child abuse or elder abuse cases; (3) the nature and extent of physical or mental disability in disability cases; and (4) the nature and extent of injury and rehabilitative potential in workers' compensation cases.

Medical records may also be used in police investigations, competency hearings, and involuntary-admission procedures. In provinces and territories that mandate mental health legal services or a patients' rights advocacy program audits of medical records may be performed to determine the facility's adherence to provincial or territorial law or violation of patients' rights. Finally, medical records may be used in professional and hospital negligence cases.

During the initial, or discovery, phase of litigation, the medical record is a pivotal source of information for lawyers in determining whether a cause of action exists in a professional negligence or hospital negligence case. Evidence of the nursing care rendered will be found in what the nurse documented.

BOX 7.7 How Does a Nurse Report Child Abuse?

Institutions usually have policies for reporting abuse. Often the responsibility goes to social workers who have expertise in these matters and know how to navigate the system. However, if you are caring for a child covered in old and new bruises or who has a broken bone or decaying teeth, and you suspect abuse, it is your legal and ethical responsibility to make a report to your province's or territory's child welfare agency. You should also let the child's parents or guardians know that you are filing the report. Whether the physician or your peers agree with you or not, if you report suspected child abuse in good faith, you will be protected from criminal or civil liability. More importantly, you may save a child from further suffering.

Reporting Suspected Child Abuse

All provinces and territories have enacted child abuse reporting legislation. Although these statutes differ among provinces and territories, they generally include a definition of *child abuse*, a list of persons required or encouraged to report abuse, and the governmental agency designated to receive and investigate these reports. Most statutes include the consequences of failure to report. Many provinces and territories specifically require nurses to report cases of suspected abuse. Refer to Box 7.7 for some guidelines on how to report abuse.

As incidents of abuse in society surface, some jurisdictions may require health care providers to report other kinds of abuse. A growing number of provinces and territories are enacting "protection for persons in care" legislation, which requires registered nurses and others to report cases of abuse of people who are receiving care or support services. Under most provincial or territorial law, a person who is required to report suspected abuse, neglect, or exploitation of a person in care and willfully does not do so is guilty of a misdemeanour crime. Most provincial or territorial legislation provides protection to anyone who makes a report in good faith, ensuring immunity from civil liability in connection with the report. Because provincial and territorial laws vary, students are encouraged to become familiar with the requirements of their province or territory.

Confidentiality and Communicable Diseases

All provinces and territories have enacted legislation that requires health care providers to report suspected or confirmed cases of selected communicable diseases. Examples of these are Creutzfeldt-Jakob disease, human immunodeficiency virus (HIV), syphilis, tuberculosis, and West Nile virus infections. In addition, some provinces and territories have enacted mandatory or permissive legislation that directs health care providers to warn a spouse if a partner tests positive for HIV. Nurses must understand the laws in their jurisdiction of practice regarding privileged communications and warnings of infectious disease exposure.

Confidentiality After Death

A person's reputation can be damaged even after death. Therefore it is important after a person's death not to divulge information that you would not have been able to share legally before the person's death.

CIVIL OBLIGATIONS AND RESPONSIBILITIES

Legal issues common in psychiatric mental health nursing relate to the failure to protect the safety of patients (Table 7.3). Miscommunications and medication errors are common in all facets of nursing, including

TABLE 7.3 Common Liability Issues

Issue	Examples
Patient safety	Failure to take notice of or take action on suicide risks
	Failure to use restraints properly or to monitor the restrained patient
	Miscommunication
	Medication errors
	Violation of boundaries (e.g., sexual misconduct)
	Misdiagnosis
Intentional torts	Voluntary acts intended to bring a physical or mental consequence
	Purposeful acts
	Recklessness
	Not obtaining patient consent
Negligence or malpractice	Carelessness
	Foreseeability of harm
Assault and battery	Reasonable belief that a person means to cause one harm (assault) through harmful or offensive touching (battery)
	Threat to use force, along with opportunity and ability to carry out threat
	Giving treatment without patient's consent
False imprisonment	Intent to confine to a specific area
	Indefensible use of seclusion or restraints
	Detention of voluntarily admitted patient, with no agency or legal policies to support detaining
Defamation of character:	Sharing private information with people who are not directly involved with care
• Slander (spoken)	Posting information on social media sites that identifies specific individuals or organizations and that has the potential to damage their reputation
• Libel (written)	Confidential documents shared with people who are not directly involved with care
Invasion of privacy	Taking a picture of your patient without permission
Supervisory liability (vicarious liability)	Inappropriate delegation of duties
	Lack of supervision of those supervising

psychiatric care. Another common area of liability in psychiatry is abuse of the therapist–patient relationship. Issues of sexual misconduct during the therapeutic relationship have become a source of concern in the psychiatric community. Diagnosing a patient, and avoiding misdiagnosing, also requires ethical, moral, and legal responsibility of the treatment team.

Tort Law

Tort law is a law developed from obligations to another. Although these laws are not based on nurses' professional codes of ethics, they have many similarities. Both describe the nurse's obligations and responsibilities to the patient. The difference is that tort laws have a much broader applicability. They apply to all Canadians.

Intentional Torts

Nurses in psychiatric settings may encounter provocative, threatening, or violent behaviour that may require the use of restraint or seclusion. However, such interventions must be carefully determined and used only in the most extreme situations. As discussed earlier in this chapter, restraint and seclusion historically were used with little regard to patients' rights, and overuse and abuses were common. Stories of patients restrained and left to lie in their own excrement or locked in seclusion for days for being annoying have resulted in strict laws. Accordingly, the nurse in the psychiatric setting should understand **intentional torts**, which are willful or intentional acts that violate another person's rights or property. Some examples of intentional torts are **assault** (reasonable belief that a person means to cause one harm), **battery** (offensive or harmful touching), and **false imprisonment** (detention of a patient with no agency or legal policies to support detention) (Table 7.3).

Other types of intentional torts may hurt a person's sense of self or financial status. These include invasion of privacy and defamation of character. Invasion of privacy in health care has to do with breaking a person's confidences or taking photographs without explicit permission. Defamation of character includes slander (verbal), such as talking about patients on the elevator with others around, and libel (printed), such as sharing written information about the patient with people outside the professional setting.

Unintentional Torts

Unintentional torts are unintended acts that produce injury or harm to another person. **Negligence** (carelessness) is a general tort for which anyone may be found responsible. For example, if you do not shovel the snow from your driveway, and a visitor falls and breaks a hip, you may be found liable for negligence. Health care providers who fail to act in accordance with professional standards, or who fail to foresee consequences that other professionals with similar skills and education would foresee, can be found responsible as a result of professional negligence, or **malpractice**. Malpractice is an act or omission to act that breaches the duty of due care and results in or is responsible for a person's injuries. The five elements required to prove negligence are

(1) duty, (2) breach of duty, (3) cause in fact, (4) proximate cause, and (5) damages. Foreseeability, or likelihood of harm, is also evaluated.

Duty. When nurses represent themselves as being capable of caring for psychiatric patients and accept employment, a duty of care has been assumed. As a psychiatric mental health nurse, you have the duty to understand the theory and medications used in the care of psychiatric patients, whether they are being treated in a community clinic, general practitioner's office, medical unit, or psychiatric treatment unit. The staff nurse who is responsible for care delivery must be knowledgeable enough to assume a reasonable or safe duty of care for the patients.

The nurse's duty of care includes a duty to intervene when the safety or well-being of the patient or another person is obviously at risk. When caring for individuals within a healthcare facility, if the nurse believes the patient is being harmed, regardless of age, the nurse must take steps to protect this individual. For example, a nurse who knowingly follows an incorrect or possibly harmful order is responsible for any harm that results to the patient. If you have information that leads you to believe that the physician's orders need to be clarified or changed, it is your duty to intervene and protect the patient. It is important that you communicate the concern to the physician who has ordered the treatment. If the treating physician does not appear willing to consider your concerns, you should carry out your duty to intervene through other appropriate channels. The following vignette illustrates two possible outcomes of a nurse's intervention in a medication issue.

> ### VIGNETTE
> Monia is a new nurse on the crisis management unit. She completed the hospital and unit orientations 2 weeks ago and has begun to care for patients independently. As she prepares to give her 1700 hours medications, Monia notices that Greg Thorn, a 55-year-old man admitted after a suicide attempt, has been given a new order for the antidepressant sertraline (Zoloft). Monia remembers that Mr. Thorn had been taking phenelzine (Nardil) before his admission and seems to recall something unsafe about mixing these two medications. She looks up the antidepressants in her drug guide and realizes that Nardil is a monoamine oxidase inhibitor and that adding this second antidepressant within 2 weeks of discontinuing the Nardil could result in severe adverse effects and possibly a lethal response.
>
> After clarifying with Mr. Thorn that he had been on Nardil and discussing the issue with another nurse, Monia realizes that she needs to put the medication on hold and contact Mr. Thorn's psychiatrist, Dr. Cruz. Monia phones him and begins by saying, "I see that Mr. Thorn has been ordered Zoloft. I am looking at his nursing admission assessment, and it says that he had been taking Nardil up until a few days ago. However, I don't see it listed on the medical assessment that was done by the resident."
>
> **First Possible Outcome**
> Dr. Cruz responds, "Thank you for calling that to my attention. When I make my rounds in the morning, I'll decide what to do with his medications. For now, please put a hold on the Zoloft." Monia clarifies what Dr. Cruz has said, writes the order, and documents what happened in the nurses' notes.
>
> **Second Possible Outcome**
> Dr. Cruz responds, "Are you telling me how to do my job? If it wasn't on the medical assessment, then he wasn't taking it. A nurse must have made a mistake—again. I wrote an order for Zoloft, so give him the Zoloft." He hangs up. Monia documents the exchange, determines that the safest and most appropriate response is to hold the medication for now, and contacts her nursing supervisor. The supervisor supports her decision and follows up with the chief of psychiatry.

The duty to intervene on the patient's behalf poses legal and ethical dilemmas for nurses in the workplace. Institutions with a chain-of-command policy or other reporting mechanisms offer some assurance that the proper authorities in the administration are notified of nursing concerns. Most patient-care issues regarding physicians' orders or treatments can be settled fairly early in the process through the nurse discussing any concerns with the physician. However, if further intervention by the nurse is required to protect the patient, generally, the nurse would notify their immediate nursing supervisor, who would discuss the problem with the physician and subsequently, if necessary, the chief of staff of a particular service until a resolution is reached. If there is no time to resolve the issue through the normal process because of a life-threatening situation, the nurse has no choice but to act to protect the patient's life. It is important to follow employer policies and procedures for reporting differences of opinion. If you fail to intervene and the patient is injured, you may be partly liable for the injuries that result because of your failure to use safe nursing practice and good professional judgement.

Breach of duty. Breach of duty is any conduct that exposes a patient to an unreasonable risk of harm, through either commission or omission of acts by the nurse. If you are not capable of providing the standard of care that other nurses would be expected to supply under similar circumstances, you have breached the duty of care. Or if you do not have the required education and experience to provide certain interventions, you have breached the duty by neglecting or omitting the provision of necessary care.

The legal concept of *abandonment* is another concern of nurses. When a nurse is given an assignment to care for a patient, they must provide the care or ensure that the patient is safely reassigned to another nurse, or abandonment occurs. Abandonment also takes place in the absence of accurate, timely, and thorough reporting and in the absence of follow-through of care on which the patient relies.

The same principles apply to the psychiatric mental health nurse working in a community setting. For example, if a suicidal patient refuses to go to the hospital for treatment, you must take the necessary steps to ensure the patient's safety. These actions may include enlisting the assistance of the law in involuntarily admitting the patient on a temporary basis.

Cause in fact, proximate cause, damages, and foreseeability. Cause in fact may be evaluated by asking, "Would this injury have occurred without the nurse's actions?" If the answer is no, the nurse is guilty of causing the injury.

Proximate cause, or legal cause, may be evaluated by determining whether any intervening actions or persons, other than the nurse, were, in fact, the cause of harm to the patient. If it is determined that the harm resulted from intervening persons or actions, the nurse is not guilty of proximate cause.

Damages include actual damages (e.g., loss of earnings, medical expenses, property damage), as well as pain and suffering. They also include incidental or consequential damages. For example, giving a patient the wrong medication may incur actual damage of a complicated hospital stay, but it also may result in permanent disability, which could require such needs as special education and special accommodations in the home. Furthermore, incidental damages may deprive others of the benefits of life with the injured person, such as losing a normal relationship with a husband or father.

Foreseeability of harm evaluates the likelihood of the outcome under the circumstances. If the average, reasonable person could foresee that injury could result from the action or inaction, the injury was foreseeable.

The Canadian Nurses Protective Society (CNPS) (https://cnps.ca/) is a not-for-profit society that offers legal advice and assistance related to nursing practice in Canada. This includes information about professional obligations, responsibilities, and liability. In addition to providing legal advice, the CNPS also publishes material to help nurses understand our professional legal obligations and manage risks within our nursing practice.

KEY POINTS TO REMEMBER

- Deontology, consequentialist theory, virtue ethics, and relational ethics have provided the foundation for nursing ethics and nursing standards of practice.
- Psychiatric mental health nurses frequently encounter ethical dilemmas.
- The provinces and territories have enacted laws (mental health acts) for public health and safety and for the care of those unable to care for themselves. Within these acts are provisions for involuntary admissions to a psychiatric hospital or unit.
- The principle of respect of persons provides the foundation for a person's right to self-determination.
- Provincial, territorial, and federal legislation provides the framework for the development of mental health policies and programs.
- The nurse's privilege to practise carries with it the responsibility to practise safely, competently, and according to provincial, territorial, and federal laws.
- Best practices are determined by standards of practice, standards of care, policies and procedures, and the use of traditional practice knowledge.
- Knowledge of the law, nursing codes of ethics, and the standards of practice for psychiatric mental health nursing are essential for providing safe, effective psychiatric mental health nursing care and will serve as a framework for decision making.

CRITICAL THINKING

1. Noskye and Beth are nurses who have worked together on the psychiatric unit for 2 years. Beth confided to Noskye that her marital situation has become particularly difficult over the past 6 months. He expressed concern and shared his observation that she seems to be distracted and not as happy lately. Privately, Noskye concludes that this explains why Beth has become so irritable and distracted. As Noskye prepares the medication for the evening shift, he notices that two of his patients' medications are missing; both are bedtime lorazepam (Ativan). When he phones the pharmacy to request the missing medications, the pharmacist responds, "You people need to watch your carts more carefully because this has become a pattern." Shortly after, another patient complains to Noskye that he did not receive his 1700 hours alprazolam (Xanax). On the medication administration record, Beth has recorded that she has given the drugs. Noskye suspects that Beth may be diverting the drugs.
    a. What action, if any, should Noskye take? Should he confront Beth with his suspicions?
    b. If Beth admits that she has been diverting the drugs, should Noskye's next step be to report Beth to their supervisor or to the board of nursing?
    c. When Noskye talks to the nursing supervisor, should he identify Beth or should he state his suspicions in general terms?
    d. How does the nature of the drugs affect your responses? That is, if the drugs were to treat a "physical" condition such as hypertension, would you be more concerned?
    e. What does the nurse practice act in your province or territory mandate regarding reporting the illegal use of drugs by a nurse?

2. A 40-year-old man is admitted to the emergency department for a severe nosebleed and has both of his nostrils packed. Because of a history of alcoholism and the possibility of developing delirium tremens (withdrawal), the patient is transferred to the psychiatric unit. His physician has ordered a private room, restraints, continuous monitoring, and 15-minute checks of vital signs and other indicators. At the first 15-minute check, the nurse discovers that the patient has no pulse or respiration. He had apparently inhaled the nasal packing and suffocated.
    a. Does it sound as though the nurse was responsible for the patient's death?
    b. Was the order for the restraint appropriate for this type of patient?
    c. What factors did you consider in making your determination in (b)?

3. Assume that there are no mandatory-reporting laws for impaired or incompetent colleagues in the following clinical situation. A 15-year-old boy is admitted to a psychiatric facility voluntarily at the request of his parents because of violent, explosive behaviour. This behaviour began after his father's recent remarriage that followed his parents' divorce. In group therapy he has become incredibly angry in response to a discussion about weekend passes for Mother's Day. "Everyone has abandoned me. No one cares!" he screamed. Several weeks later, on the day before his discharge, he convinces his nurse to keep his plan to kill his mother confidential. Consider the CNA code of ethics on patient confidentiality, the principles of psychiatric nursing, and the duty to warn third parties in answering the following questions:
    a. Did the nurse use appropriate judgement in promising confidentiality?
    b. Does the nurse have a legal duty to warn the patient's mother of her son's threat?
    c. Is the duty owed to the patient's father and stepmother?
    d. Would a change in the admission status from voluntary to involuntary (based on an assessment determining that he is a danger to himself or others, has a mental health disorder, and is unwilling to voluntarily remain in hospital) protect the patient's mother without violating the patient's confidentiality?
    e. What nursing action, if any, should the nurse take after this disclosure by the patient?

4. Patients admitted to an inpatient psychiatric unit are being recruited for research on a new drug that is hoped to have an impact on the negative symptoms of schizophrenia. The attending psychiatrists are all involved in the research. One of the patients asks a nurse about the experimental medication.
    a. Does the nurse have a responsibility to explain the research to the patient?
    b. Why are the patients involved in this research considered vulnerable?
    c. How can the nurse advocate for vulnerable patients?
    d. What are the documentation responsibilities of the nurses when they observe a medication adverse effect in one of the patients involved in the research?

CHAPTER REVIEW

1. A patient with depression presents with her family in the emergency department. The family feels she should be admitted because "she might hurt herself." An assessment indicates moderate depression with no risk factors for suicide other than the depressed mood itself, and the patient denies any intent or thoughts of self-harm. The family agrees that the patient has not done or said anything

to suggest that she might be a danger to herself. Which of the following responses is consistent with the concept of "least restrictive alternative" doctrine?
   a. Admit the patient as a temporary inpatient admission.
   b. Persuade the patient to agree to a voluntary inpatient admission.
   c. Admit the patient involuntarily to an inpatient mental health treatment unit.
   d. Arrange for an emergency outpatient counselling appointment the next day.
2. An advanced-practice nurse wishes to initiate treatment with an antipsychotic medication that, although very likely to benefit the patient, in a small percentage of patients may cause a dangerous adverse effect. The nurse explains the purpose, expected benefits, and possible risks of the medication. The patient readily signs a form accepting the medication, stating, "These pills will poison the demons inside of me." Although he has been informed of the risk for adverse effects, he is unable to state what these are and simply reports, "I won't have side effects because I am iron and cannot be killed." Which of the following responses would be most appropriate under these circumstances?
   a. Begin administration of the medications based on his signed permission because he has legally consented to treatment.
   b. Petition the court to appoint a guardian for the patient because he is unable to comprehend the proposed treatment.
   c. Administer the medications even though consent is unclear because the patient is clearly psychotic and in need of the medications.
   d. Withhold the medication until the patient is able to identify the benefits and risks of both consenting and refusing consent to the medications.
3. A patient incidentally shares with you that he has difficulty controlling his anger when around children because their play irritates him, leading to resentment and fantasies about attacking them. He has a history of impulsiveness and assault, escalates easily on the unit, and has a poor tolerance for frustration. This weekend he has an overnight pass, which he will use to see his sister and her family. As you meet with the patient and his sister just prior to his getting the pass, the sister mentions that she has missed her brother because he usually helps her watch the children, and she has to work this weekend and needs him to babysit. The patient becomes visibly apprehensive upon hearing this. Which of the following responses would best reflect appropriate nursing practice relative to the conflict this situation presents between safety and the patient's right to confidentiality?
   a. Cancel the pass without explanation to the sister, and reschedule it for a time when babysitting would not be required of the patient.
   b. Suggest that the sister make other arrangements for child care, but withhold the information the patient shared regarding his concerns about harming children.
   c. Speak with the patient about the safety risk involved in babysitting, seeking his permission to share this information and advising against the pass if he declines to share the information.
   d. Meet with the patient's sister, sharing with her the patient's disclosure about his anger toward children and the resultant risk that his babysitting would present.
4. Mrs. Fujiwara was admitted for treatment of depression with suicidal ideation triggered by marital discord. She has spoken with staff about her fears that the marriage will end, has indicated that she does not know how she could cope if her marriage ended, and has a history of suicide attempts when the marriage seemed threatened in the past. Her spouse visits one night and informs Mrs. Fujiwara that he has decided to file for divorce. Staff members, though aware of the visit and the husband's intentions regarding divorce, take no action, feeling that the 15-minute suicide checks Mrs. Fujiwara is already on are sufficient. Thirty minutes after the visit ends, staff make rounds and discover that Mrs. Fujiwara has hanged herself in her bathroom using hospital pyjamas she had tied together into a rope. Which of the following statements best describes this situation? **Select all that apply.**
   a. The nurses have created liability for themselves and their employer by failing in their duty to protect Mrs. Fujiwara.
   b. The nurses have breached their duty to reassess Mrs. Fujiwara for increased suicide risk after her husband's visit.
   c. Given Mrs. Fujiwara's history, the nurses should have expected an increased risk for suicide after the husband's announcement.
   d. The nurses correctly reasoned that suicides cannot always be prevented and did their best to keep Mrs. Fujiwara safe via the 15-minute checks.
   e. The nurses are subject to a tort of professional negligence for failing to increase the suicide precautions in response to Mrs. Fujiwara's increased risk.
   f. Had the nurses restricted Mrs. Fujiwara's movements or increased their checks on her, they would have been liable for false imprisonment and invasion of privacy, respectively.

 http://evolve.elsevier.com/Canada/Varcarolis/psychiatric/

REFERENCES

Andre, J. (2000). Humility reconsidered. In S. B. Rubin, & L. Zoloth (Eds.), *Margin of error: The ethics of mistakes in the practice of medicine* (pp. 59–72). Hagerstown: University Publishing Group.

Arnold, T. C. (2020). Moral distress in emergency and critical care nurses: A metaethnography. *Nursing Ethics, 27*(8), 1681–1693. https://doi.org/10.1177/0969733020935952

Austin, W., Bergum, V., & Dossetor, J. (2003). Relational ethics. In V. Tshudin (Ed.), *Approaches to ethics* (pp. 45–52). Woburn: Butterworth-Heinemann.

Battlefords and District Co-operative Ltd. v. Gibbs. (1996). 1996 CanLII 187 (Supreme Court of Canada), 3 SCR 566. https://canlii.ca/t/1fr6c

Beauchamp, T. L., & Childress, J. F. (2019). *Principles of biomedical ethics* (8th ed.). New York: Oxford University Press.

Bergum, V., & Dossetor, J. (2004). *Relational ethics: The full meaning of respect.* Hagerstown: University Publishing Group.

British Columbia College of Nursing Professionals, College of Registered Psychiatric Nurses of Alberta, Registered Psychiatric Nurses Association of Saskatchewan, & the College of Registered Psychiatric Nurses of Manitoba. (2019). *Standards of psychiatric nursing practice.* Winnipeg: Authors.

Browne, A. (2010). Mental health acts in Canada. *Cambridge Quarterly of Healthcare Ethics, 19,* 290–298. https://doi.org/10.1017/S096318011000006X

Canadian Institutes of Health Research, Natural Sciences and Engineering Research Council of Canada, & Social Sciences and Humanities Research Council of Canada. (2018). *Tri-council policy statement: Ethical conduct for research involving humans.* Ottawa: Author.

Canadian Nurses Association (CNA). (2017). *Code of ethics for registered nurses.* Ottawa: Author.

Dorman, J. D., & Raffin Bouchal, S (2020). Moral distress and moral uncertainty in medical assistance in dying: A simultaneous evolutionary concept analysis. *Nursing Forum, 55*(3), 320–330. https://doi.org/10.1111/nuf.12431

Jager, F., & Perron, A. (2020). The social utility of community treatment orders: Applying Girard's mimetic theory to community-based mandated mental health care. *Nursing Philosophy, 21*(2), 1–9. https://doi.org/10.1111/nup.12280

Lachman, V. D. (2016). Ethics, law, and policy. Moral resilience: Managing and preventing moral distress and moral residue. *Medsurg Nursing, 25*(2), 121–124. http://www.medsurgnursing.net/cgi-bin/WebObjects/MSNJournal.woa

Manitoba Provincial Health Ethics Network. (2016). *Patient care ethics: Decision-making guide: Framework for clinical or patient-care issues*. Winnipeg: Author.

Neal, M., & Fovargue, S. (2019). Is conscientious objection incompatible with healthcare professionalism? *New Bioethics, 25*(3), 221–235. https://doi.org/10.1080/20502877.2019.1651935

Olthuis, J. H. (1997). Face-to-face: Ethical asymmetry or the symmetry of mutuality? In J. H. Olthuis (Ed.), *Knowing otherwise: Philosophy at the threshold of spirituality* (pp. 131–158). New York: Fordham University Press.

Province of Alberta. (2021). *Mental Health Act. Revised Statues of Alberta 2000*. Chapter M-13. https://www.qp.alberta.ca/documents/Acts/M13.pdf

Ricciardelli, R., Carleton, R. N., Mooney, T., & Cramm, H. (2020). "Playing the system": Structural factors potentiating mental health stigma, challenging awareness, and creating barriers to care for Canadian public safety personnel. *Health: An Interdisciplinary Journal for the Social Study of Health, Illness & Medicine, 24*(3), 259–278. https://doi.org/10.1177/1363459318800167

Rodney, P. A. (2017). What we know about moral distress [Supplemental material]. *American Journal of Nursing, 117*(2), S7–S10. https://doi.org/10.1097/01.NAJ.0000512204.85973.04

Rodney, P., Burgess, M., McPherson, G., & Brown, H. (2012). Our theoretical landscape: A brief history of health care ethics. In J. Storch, R. Starzomski, & P. Rodney (Eds.), *Toward a moral horizon: Nursing ethics for leadership and practice* (2nd ed., pp. 77–97). Toronto: Pearson Education Canada.

Tarasoff v. Regents of the University of California. (1974). 529 P.2d 553, 118 Cal Rptr 129.

Tarasoff v. Regents of the University of California. (1976). 551 P.2d 334, 131 Cal Rptr 14.

8

Cultural Implications for Psychiatric Mental Health Nursing: A Critical Cultural Perspective

Victoria Smye, Abe Oudshoorn

 http://evolve.elsevier.com/Canada/Varcarolis/psychiatric/

OBJECTIVES

1. Define key concepts central to understanding critical cultural considerations in psychiatric mental health nursing.
2. Distinguish between cultural sensitivity, cultural competence, and cultural safety and consider the implications for psychiatric mental health nursing.
3. Define the key dimensions of equity-oriented health care: cultural safety and trauma- and violence-informed care.
4. Consider the intersection of culture and stigma (self and social) and their influence on mental health/well-being.
5. Describe the influence of culture on mental health/illness experiences of immigrants, refugees, and Indigenous peoples.

KEY TERMS AND CONCEPTS

collectivist (collectivism)
colonization
cultural competence
cultural diversity
cultural humility
cultural safety
cultural sensitivity
culture
diaspora
dominant culture
equity-oriented health care

ethnicity
ethnocentrism
health inequity
health equity
immigrant
Indigenous peoples
individualism
medicine wheel
multi-culturalism
race
racialization

racism
recovery-oriented
refugee
social determinants of health
stereotyping
stigma
trauma-informed practice
structural violence
violence-informed practice
Western tradition
world view

UNDERSTANDING THE LANDSCAPE OF CULTURE IN MENTAL HEALTH

Canadian psychiatric mental health nursing practice takes place within rich Indigenous and multi-cultural contexts. In these contexts and in keeping with nursing's social mandate equity-oriented practice is a goal anchored by approaches to relational inquiry (Doane & Varcoe, 2020) and culturally safe practice (Browne et al., 2018; Ford-Gilboe et al., 2018; Levine et al., 2020). In this chapter we introduce the concepts of culture, cultural influences on the conceptualization of mental health and well-being and illness, and ultimately, culturally safe, and trauma- and violence-informed care of patients, families, and communities who may be experiencing mental illness or mental health problems.

Culture, Race, Ethnicity, and the Social Determinants of Health

We understand culture as relational; it is dynamic and ever-changing, dependent on our history, past experiences, social, professional, and gendered locations, and our perceptions of how we are viewed by others in society. All people are influenced by culture. Culture also can be a site of push and pull as groups struggling for power attempt to restrict meanings, categories, and practices. Culture and intersecting categories, such as ethnicity, race, gender, sexuality, religion, etc., have multiple and shifting meanings that influence social power and position. **Dominant culture** refers to those deeply rooted understandings that tend to be taken up as "truths" about individuals, society, and social relationships. Notably, this does not mean there is a single dominant culture that all people belong to or that these ideas are fixed, rather, these ideas permeate our everyday lives in multiple and often hard to see ways.

Traditional theorizing in the domain of *difference* and *culture* in nursing was led in large part by nursing scholar Madeleine Leininger (e.g., 1985; 1988) who developed the Culture Care Diversity and Universality theory and what she coined as, "transcultural nursing." Leininger drew nurses' attention to the notion of culture as an important interest in nursing in order to understand the "other" thus the concepts of cultural diversity, cultural sensitivity, and cultural competence emerged within nursing. **Cultural diversity** refers to existence of a number of cultures that exist simultaneously in one space. **Cultural sensitivity** reflects the idea that people have culturally based understandings, practices, and customs and that health care providers need

105

to be aware of those understandings. Being culturally sensitive can be useful if taken up in a way that does not stereotype people because they are different from that of the dominant culture (Browne & Varcoe, 2019). **Cultural competence** has been taken up widely in Canada, for example, by the Canadian Nurses Association (CNA) as "the application of knowledge, skills, attitudes or personal attributes required by nurses to maximize respectful relationships with diverse populations of clients and coworkers" (CNA, 2010, p. 1). CNA asserts the position that cultural competence should be an entry-to-practice level competency and the belief that cultural competence promotes cultural safety. CNA (2010; 2018) also recognizes that culture is intertwined with socioeconomic and political issues and that social justice is central to nursing. The CNA's position on cultural competence is that both cultural competence and cultural safety are integral parts of providing "high quality, safe, and equitable nursing care" (CNA, 2018, pp. 1–2).

Unfortunately, culture has often been simplified into a formula for practice (Browne & Varcoe, 2019). Although cultural sensitivity and cultural competency models have helped nurses to recognize difference, there has been a tendency to stop at identifying difference and common practices of certain people that has resulted in stereotyping, and to create a them versus us—or an "othering" mindset—understood as "culturalist" (Browne & Varcoe). A *stereotype* is an overgeneralized, fixed, conscious or unconscious, conceptualization of a group of people that does not allow for individual differences within the group; by **stereotyping** we infer that a person has a whole range of characteristics and health practices that we assume all members of that group possess. Regardless of the good intention behind this conceptualization of culture, it also runs the risk of conflating culture with notions of ethnicity and race and other forms of difference. **Ethnocentrism** often works in tandem with stereotyping; it is the belief (sometimes unconscious) that a person's own culture and worldview are superior to those of others from different cultural, ethnic, or racial backgrounds; carrying this kind of perspective can have a negative effect on the nurse–patient relationship.

In addition to these concerns, current cultural competency theories and conceptual models tend to focus on the individual patient and do little to address the social/structural determinants of health and there is little evidence that their existence has made a difference in terms of addressing health inequities (Drevdahl, 2018).

Because of these concerns, Leininger's work has been enhanced by an array of nursing and other scholars who further conceptualized and critiqued notions of culture, cultural sensitivity, and cultural competence (e.g., Drevdahl, 2018) and have added **cultural safety** (e.g., Berg et al., 2019; Browne & Varcoe, 2019; Downey, 2020; Gerlach, Browne, & Greenwood, 2017; Greenwood, 2019; Greenwood et al., 2017; Urbanoski et al., 2020) and **cultural humility** (e.g., First Nations Health Authority, 2018; Yeager & Bauer-Wu, 2013).

As Hartrick Doane and Varcoe (2020) illustrate in their recent book on relational inquiry, attending to cultural differences remains central to nurses' ability to provide high-quality care to increasingly diverse patient groups; as they note, differences cannot be overlooked or trivialized. However, they also underline the importance of not conflating all "difference" with cultural difference and an understanding that there are individual differences *within* groups.

Assumptions about what culture is or how to attend to issues of culture have implications for nursing, patients, and health care more generally (Browne & Varcoe, 2019). When we see culture as a relational experience, the nurse is not located outside of the culture of the other, the nurse shapes and participates in culture, "culture is happening as patients and nurses relate" (Doane & Varcoe, 2005, p. 88). As an example, when meeting with an Indigenous patient, the psychiatric mental health nurse enters into the relationship within multiple and shifting cultures; the relationship occurs within webs of power (and meaning) (e.g., the culture of the nurse and the patient, the culture of health care, and colonial Canadian culture).

A critical cultural perspective shifts our attention beyond the individual to how power operates through structures (e.g., policies and legislation), systems (e.g., education, health, justice, social and child welfare), and direct services (e.g., mental health services, housing). It also shifts our focus from the culture of the "other" to the culture of "health care" as the site for needed transformational change. For example, in our studies it has not been uncommon to hear health care providers attach negative characteristics to Indigenous people as the cause of their health care issues instead of looking to the system and its inflexibility or lack of attention to how it might respond in a good way to what is being seen. In this chapter Aboriginal or **Indigenous peoples** refer to First Nations, Inuit, and/or Métis peoples. Indigenous peoples in Canada also refer to themselves by their specific tribal affiliation (such as Mi'kmaq, Cree, Innu, Ojibwa) and/or as First Nations, Native, Indian, Inuit, or Métis (Allan & Smylie, 2015, p. ii). Aboriginal is only used in this chapter when using a citation where this terminology is utilized.

To add to the complexities associated with the notion of culture, the concepts of ethnicity and race often are conflated with culture. **Ethnicity**, also a complex concept, refers to the sharing of common traits and customs across groups who have a common heritage, history, and worldview. Ethnic identity also may shift dependent on immigration and other experiences. **Race** refers to a *socially constructed* category of "difference" without biological meaning. However, although the concept of distinct "races" has generally been rejected, the notion of **racism** remains important. Racism can be defined as a set of attitudes and behaviours in which social groups are identified, separated, treated as inferior or superior, and given differential access to power and other valued resources; racism often intersects with other forms of discrimination such as sexism, ageism, homophobia, and classism; a means of creating "them/other" versus "us" categorizations and distancing. **Racialization** is a process of differentiation underpinned by the assumption that "race" is the primary, natural, and neutral means of categorization. From this perspective, behavioral characteristics are also linked with race (Ahmad, 1993, p. 18, as cited in Tang & Browne, 2008, p. 113). Power is exerted through everyday actions and attitudes and from institutionalized policies and practice that disadvantage individuals and groups on the basis of presumed biological, physical, or genetic differences. Racialization also is closely linked to culturalism that was defined earlier (Browne & Varcoe, 2019, p. 31).

Equity-Oriented Health Care (EOHC): Cultural Safety and Trauma- and Violence-Informed Care

Foundational theories derived from Western ideology have guided mental health service delivery and the formation of the Canadian mental health system. However, a disconnect often exists between those accessing services and the services themselves because of differences in worldview/perspectives (i.e., services may not fit everyone). **Health equity** can be understood as a social justice goal focused on pursuing the highest possible standard of health and health care for all people, with particular attention paid to those at greatest risk of poor health, and taking into account broader socio-political and economic influences on health and access to care. **Health inequity** can be understood as socially constructed, unjust, and avoidable differences in health and well-being between and within groups of people (Braveman, 2014; Krieger, 2014). Simplistic perspectives on culture have limited our work as nurses to reduce inequities such as those caused by racialization. Health equity interventions can be implemented at multiple levels, including within health services (Wyatt et al., 2016), and have been shown, through prior and ongoing research in primary health care (i.e., EQUIP Health Care, www.equiphealthcare.ca), to be associated with positive health outcomes, including better quality of life, less chronic pain, and fewer depressive and post-traumatic stress symptoms over time. Equity-oriented health care, is comprised of three *intersecting* key dimensions: cultural safety, trauma- and violence-informed care (TVIC), and harm reduction (Browne et al., 2018; Ford-Gilboe et al., 2018). Harm Reduction is discussed in Chapter 18.

Understanding culture and mental health care in the context of Indigenous peoples helps us see the promise of equity-oriented care practices for enhancing the work that nurses do in multi-cultural contexts. Downey (2020) draws attention to the impact colonialism and racism have on the health and well-being of First Nations, Métis, and Inuit peoples and the need to address the unique social, political, and historical determinants of Indigenous mental health (e.g., **structural violence**) in a culturally safe way (p. 99). Recently disclosed racism and discrimination in Canada surrounding the tragic death of an Indigenous woman in a Quebec hospital, Ms. Joyce Echaquan (https://www.cbc.ca/news/canada/montreal/joyce-echaquan-coroner-inquest-may-19-1.6032387) and the over-a-decade-long investigation into the tragic death of Mr. Brian Sinclair, an Indigenous man with a urinary tract infection who waited for 34 hours without being seen in a Manitoba emergency department, have brought renewed attention to the harms of Indigenous-specific racism, which unfortunately is an everyday reality in Canadian society (Azpiri, 2020; Brian Sinclair Working Group, 2017; Lowrie & Malone, 2020). Jordan's Principle is named in honour of Jordan River Anderson, a young First Nations boy from Norway House Cree Nation in northern Manitoba, who spent his entire life in hospital while caught in a jurisdictional dispute between the governments of Canada and Manitoba, which both refused to pay for the in-home medical care necessary for Jordan to live in his home and community. Jordan's Principle is a response to structural violence. Jordan's Principle is not a policy or program, rather it is a legal requirement resulting from the Orders of the Canadian Human Rights Tribunal (CHRT). "Jordan's Principle is a child-first principle that aims to eliminate service inequities and delays for First Nations children. Jordan's Principle states that any public service ordinarily available to all other children must be made available to First Nations children without delay or denial" (Assembly of First Nations, 2018a, 2018b). These principles alongside the context of unequal power, racism, and discrimination are the context in which the CNA (2021) established a Nursing Declaration Against Anti-Indigenous Racism in Nursing and Health Care.

Structural violence refers to the existence of unequal power, restricted access to resources, and systematic oppression resulting in the denial of basic needs. Racism is structural when acts are embedded within political and economic organizations/systems (e.g., education, health, child welfare, and justice) and they are *violent* because they shape individual experience, deny basic human rights, and cause injury to people (Farmer et al., 2007; Gerlach et al., 2017).

As noted earlier, transcultural nursing as a theoretical approach to cultural skills education was an approach developed from largely Eurocentric perspectives. Cultural safety, on the other hand, was proposed by a Māori nurse in New Zealand (NZ) in response to the glaring health inequities between Māori (the Indigenous people of NZ) and non-Māori persons (Ramsden 1993; 2000). As an explicitly anti-racist stance (Smye & Browne, 2002), cultural safety was intended to draw attention to how power operates in a health care context and create health system transformation (Greenwood, 2019). These shifts are important in light of the continued Indigenous experience of colonization, structural violence, and racism.

Broadly, **colonization** is the invasion, dispossession, forced **assimilation**, and subjugation of peoples by the dominant force/power for the political and economic benefit of the colonizing country; processes that remain active today.

Awareness of cultural safety means that psychiatric mental health nurses are aware of their position in the context of colonization and racialization; they recognize that they are in a powerful role as a health care provider and that power in this relationship needs to be negotiated with the patient (Kurtz et al., 2014). Culturally safe practice moves beyond cultural sensitivity to explicitly address inequitable power relations, racism, discrimination, and the ongoing impacts of historical and current inequities in health care encounters (Greenwood, 2019; Varcoe & Browne, 2015). In this way cultural safety (Box 8.1) and trauma- and violence-informed care (Box 8.2) are pivotal considerations in psychiatric mental health nursing practice.

Closely aligned with cultural safety, **cultural humility** is an awareness of your own limitations as a provider regarding what you can actually know about the culture of another person. Culture is a lived, dynamic experience so we can only know what someone chooses to share with us. This means we need to be curious in our relationships with others; we need to be willing to seek out information in a respectful and nonjudgmental manner.

Trauma- and violence-informed practice reflects a recognition of the impacts of previous traumatic events on current health and mental

---

BOX 8.1 Cultural Safety and Relational Practice in Psychiatric Mental Health Nursing

Cultural safety asks you to be more attentive to the judgements and assumptions that may be driving your thoughts, actions, and practices. It also asks you to attend to how power operates in the relational space. When we see "culture" as relational, we begin our relationships with our patients by asking questions like:

- Who am I? Where do I come from? What is my background (social, cultural, family)? How do I identify in terms of those categorizations such as ethnicity, etc.? What are the assumptions I carry about others based on my social, professional, and other experiences?
- Where is my attention focussed? What am I missing?
- Put yourself in your patient's shoes and imagine what it might be like for them to be in this physical and social space. Is this a place where they will feel they belong? Where they experience safety? How are they welcomed here? What are the assumptions lived out in this space?

Remember, cultural safety is not what is deemed as culturally safe by the health care provider, it is what is deemed as culturally safe by the person receiving care.

BOX 8.2 Trauma- and Violence-Informed Care and Psychiatric Mental Health Nursing

There are four, inter-related principles of Trauma- and Violence-Informed Care:
- Understand trauma and violence and its impacts on peoples' lives and behaviours
- Create emotionally and physically safe environments for all patients and providers
- Foster opportunities for choice, collaboration, and connection
- Use a strengths-based and capacity-building approach to support patients
To see what this means for your individual interactions with patients and for your organization, link to the following:
https://gtvincubator.uwo.ca/wp-content/uploads/sites/22/2019/07/EQUIP_GTV_TVIC_Principles.pdf, and https://equiphealthcare.ca/resources/tvic-workshop/.

health situations. This approach concentrates on relationship building; engagement and choice; awareness; and skills building across individual, interpersonal, and system levels of mental health service. A key aspect of trauma-informed practice is understanding how trauma can be experienced differently by immigrants and refugees, people with developmental disabilities, women, men, children, and youth, Indigenous peoples, and other populations (BC Provincial Mental Health and Substance Use Planning Council, 2013).

Given the extent of violence and trauma in society and its strong association with negative health effects, psychiatric mental health nurses need to assume a universal approach to trauma and violence (i.e., they must assume that anyone, anytime could have been or currently is being exposed to violence). Nursing practice also needs to reflect the understanding that mental health issues can overlap with problematic substance use and trauma and violence and that these challenges need to be seen within the context of social and structural determinants of health to ensure the provision of integrated care (British Columbia Centre of Excellence for Women's Health, 2016; Salmon et al., 2006; as cited in Oudshoorn & Smye, 2019) and a harm reduction approach (Smye et al., 2011).

In summary, equity-oriented health care is fundamentally about creating safe and respectful care environments and processes, while tailoring care to fit with the needs, priorities, histories, and contexts of diverse people and populations served: it points to the need for respectful engagement that includes attention to structures (policies), systems, and services to enable this work.

Culture and Our Worldviews

The values that make up the foundation of how nurses see the world are often quite hidden. Psychiatric mental health nursing practice in Canada has historically been informed by borrowed theories from disciplines, such as psychology, that are grounded in the values and belief systems of the dominant culture. The attitudes and assumptions nurses hold are deeply entrenched in dominant culture; they are not simply an individual perspective, rather they reflect those conversations and assumptions embedded in broader society and reinforced through media, institutional policies, everyday practice (Browne, 2009, p. 185), and texts, and other sources.

Therefore nursing knowledge and practice cannot be abstracted from broader cultural norms (Hilario et al., 2017). For example, nursing knowledge of psychology, human growth and development, and mental health and illness is based on traditions from Greek, Roman, and Judeo-Christian thought and the philosophy of body–mind dualism. Mind and body dualism represents the stance that mind and body are two distinct substances, each with a different essential nature. This perspective is dominant in health care, for example in medicine (Meeta, 2011) and nursing (Keller, 2020). From this perspective, mind and body generally are treated by different practitioners. However, there are many peoples in our world with a different worldview. For example, although there are many different Indigenous peoples and perspectives, common to the Indigenous worldview is natural law and the widespread Indigenous belief that the physical, emotional, mental, and spiritual aspects of the individual are inseparable and interconnected (Bellamy & Hardy, 2015) and when in balance, the individual is whole and healthy (McCormick, 1996). The **medicine wheel** is an ancient symbol and way of knowing these dimensions that represents a wholistic world view of health, well-being, and illness based on deep personal connections to the natural world and the collective (Figure 8.1). In keeping with this wholistic perspective the First Nations Mental Wellness Continuum Framework (the Framework) document (Box 8.3) puts forward the definition of mental wellness as "a balance of the mental, physical, spiritual, and emotional" (Health Canada, 2015, p. 4); in many of the discussions held in support of the development of the Framework, the four directions provided guidance for exploring the meaning of mental wellness within First Nations communities (p. 4).

A Western worldview (often referred to as the dominant culture worldview) is underpinned by a focus on the individual called **individualism**. However, many ethnocultural populations across the globe embrace a **collectivist (collectivism)** stance; that is, a worldview that is underpinned by the perspective that the interests of the group have priority over the interests of the individual (i.e., the self is connected to a group and this connection is essential to how the self can function) (Ong-Flaherty, 2015). As Ong-Flaherty notes, from this perspective, actions reflect not just one individual but everyone connected to that individual. The worldview of "self" in the contexts of collectivism and individualism affect mental health practices. For example, clinical decision-making from a collectivist stance *may* involve family and/or community members, whereas, from an individualist perspective, whereby autonomy and independence are highly valued, this *may* not be the case.

The worldview of a group or population provides a framework for how its members explain and define their responses to life events, their position in the universe, and their understanding of health (Andrews & Boyle, 2016). Worldviews shape perceptions about time, health and well-being and illness, rights and obligations in society, and acceptable ways of behaving in relation to others and to nature. Consider how your assumptions about personality development, emotional expression, ego boundaries, and interpersonal relationships were formed and how they affect your clinical judgements. Psychiatric mental health nurses come from diverse cultural backgrounds themselves and are likely to engage with people who have worldviews that differ from their own or from the dominant philosophical traditions of Western cultures. Being open to the rich diversity of worldviews and their impact on mental health, well-being, and illness is fundamental to culturally safe nursing care. Failing to consider or attempt to understand the worldview of patients and their families will lead to an inability to establish a relational connection, trust, and the therapeutic alliance, the cornerstone of psychiatric mental health nursing. As nurses begin to acknowledge that many of the concepts and interventions enshrined in psychiatric mental health nursing are based on beliefs different from those of many patients and families, they are more likely to progress towards culturally safe practice.

Finally, it is important to understand that worldviews are fluid, dynamic, and not mutually exclusive. Our experiences and social, political, and historical processes shape/shift our cultural identities. In addition, worldviews are not necessarily discrete categories. One example of this fluidity is an Indigenous view put forward by Mi'kmaq Elder Albert Marshall entitled, Two-Eyed Seeing, which is a guiding principle found in Mi'kmaq Knowledge known as "Etuaptmumk," whereby two knowledges are brought together; it is the gift of multiple perspectives treasured by many Indigenous peoples. Two-Eyed Seeing refers to learning to see from one eye with the strengths of Indigenous knowledges and ways of knowing, and from the other eye with the strengths of Western knowledges and ways of knowing and learning to use both these eyes together, for the benefit of all (Ermine et al., 2004; Hogue & Bartlett, 2014). The advantage of Two-Eyed Seeing is that you are always fine-tuning your mind into different places at once, you are always looking for another perspective (Institute for Integrative Science and Health, 2004) (Box 8.4 is an example of an Indigenous Mental Wellness Pathway Program underpinned by a Two-Eyed Seeing Approach entitled, *Biigajiiskaan*).

CHAPTER 8 Cultural Implications for Psychiatric Mental Health Nursing: A Critical Cultural Perspective

Fig. 8.1 An Indigenous Wellness Framework based on the Medicine Wheel by Elder Jim Dumont. (https://thunderbirdpf.org/wp-content/uploads/2015/07/4_Indigenous_Wellness_Framework.pdf.)

Critical Thinking: Who Do You Position as Different?

Imagine you are now beginning your practicum in a psychiatric mental health setting. Consider each of the following scenarios. Attend to and note your thoughts, feelings, and inner responses (the embodied experience) as you read each one. (Note: Where there is a gendered pronoun, individuals identified as male or female on their intake.)

- Willow is an Asian graduate student in her mid-twenties who has recently been diagnosed with schizophrenia. She has experienced three psychotic episodes in the past 2 years. Willow plans to go on to complete her PhD as soon as she is able to do so. She has been struggling with her medications; she finds the medications she is currently taking make it difficult for her to concentrate and does not consistently take them. Most recently, she has become increasingly depressed.
- Leslie is a 24-year-old Black person who lives with a mood disorder. Leslie identifies as a member of the LGBTQ2 community. They are single and live in an apartment in a large urban centre. Leslie works as an office manager close by. Leslie has come into the clinic complaining of serious and persistent anxiety and depression which has flared in the past couple of weeks.
- John, who identifies as Saulteaux-Ojibwe/Cree, is a 52-year-old married man with two grown children. John grew up in an urban setting dislocated from his Indigenous heritage. Over the past 2 decades he has been exploring his Indigenous roots and has been requesting connection with an Indigenous elder during his

> **BOX 8.3 The First Nations Mental Wellness Continuum Framework (FNMWC)**
>
> The FNMWC Framework is a national framework that addresses mental wellness among First Nations in Canada. It identifies ways to enhance service coordination among various systems and supports culturally safe delivery of services. The *FNMWC* Framework was developed through collaboration between the Assembly of First Nations, Health Canada's First Nations and Inuit Health Branch, the National Native Addictions Partnership Foundation, the Native Mental Health Association, and other community mental health leaders.
>
> https://thunderbirdpf.org/first-nations-mental-wellness-continuum-framework/.

> **BOX 8.4 Biigajiiskaan: An Indigenous Pathway to Mental Wellness**
>
> Biigajiiskaan is an Indigenous-led, innovative partnership program, underpinned by a two-eyed seeing approach, between Atlohsa Family Healing Services, an Indigenous community organization, and St. Joseph's Health Care (Parkwood Mental Health, an acute care hospital) in London, Ontario. Grounded in culture as care and healing, the Biigajiiskaan program is creating Indigenous-informed pathways that combine Elder-guided psychiatry and traditional healing practices and knowledges with current hospital-based mental health care practices through the Okwari: Kowa Healing Space at Parkwood Mental Health Institute, a Mobile Outreach Team, and the development of an Urban Healing Lodge.

hospitalization. He also uses some Indigenous remedies, for example, to manage a serious skin condition he has had since he was in his teens (psoriasis).
- Saleema is a 72-year-old South Asian Muslim woman, who immigrated from Pakistan 20 years ago. She lives with her 95-year-old mother for whom she is the caretaker because her mother's physical ability has recently declined (i.e., she has become quite frail). Saleema's youngest sister also lives with them, however, Saleema assumes most of the caregiving responsibilities; her sister Fatima continues to be employed as a registered nurse full-time. Saleema has been struggling with serious and persistent depression for several years.
- William is a 32-year-old male who has been struggling with an addiction to heroin for the past decade. He has been in and out of several rehabilitation programs since that time. He also struggles with a mood disorder. He is disconnected from family and has been living rough on the streets for the past 2 years.

Culture of Health Care, Mental Illness, Social and Structural Inequity, and Stigma

Cultures are dynamic and ever-changing and shaped by social, political, and historical realities. For example, our recent world-wide pandemic (COVID-19) has shaped how we think about space and place and being in relationship. Not everyone has a safe place to isolate or to live (e.g., long-term care facilities, where many older adults have contracted the virus, and the homeless). In addition, social isolation is a well-understood determinant of (mental) health.

As noted earlier, culturally safe practice entails an understanding of culture as a relational experience; thus every psychiatric mental health nurse–patient encounter is a cultural encounter (i.e., a bringing together of multiple cultural experiences), shaped by multiple intersecting factors. Culture is an influencing factor related to beliefs and attitudes regarding mental health and illness. For example, a scoping review of the mental health issues and service needs of older immigrants revealed that the key social determinants of mental health are *culture*, health services, and gender and that older immigrants use fewer mental health services than their Canadian-born counterparts due to *cultural beliefs and values*, lack of culturally and linguistically appropriate services, financial difficulties, and ageism (Guruge et al., 2015). For some older immigrants, societal and internalized stigma associated with mental illness and accessing mental health services acts as a significant barrier to reaching out and receiving mental health care (Guruge et al., 2015).

Stigma associated with mental illness is an ongoing concern in Western societies (e.g., Link & Phelan, 2006, 2014; Mental Health Commission of Canada [MHCC], 2012; Phelan et al., 2014; Stuart & Arboleda-Flórez, 2012) and internationally (e.g., World Health Organization, 2019). This contributes to the burden and marginalization of mental illness (e.g., Heflinger & Hinshaw, 2010). In addition, it also has acted as a major barrier to access to mental health treatment and recovery and poorer quality physical care for persons with mental illness (e.g., Henderson et al., 2014; Knaak et al., 2015). For example, using data from the Canadian Community Health Survey (Goldie, 2013; Heart and Stroke Foundation, 2014), a nurse, Dr. Katie Goldie, explored the associations between cardiovascular risk and disease, mental health disorders, and the use of psychiatric medication. The study found that: (1) people who have had a mental health disorder at any point in their life were twice as likely to have had heart disease or have experienced a stroke; (2) those who have not developed heart disease or had a stroke are more likely to be at a high long-term risk of developing cardiovascular disease when compared to the general population; and, (3) people who used psychiatric medications were twice as likely to have heart disease and three times as likely to have had a stroke compared to those not taking these medications. This heightened risk is associated with a number of factors including: higher tobacco use; psychiatric medications and their association with obesity, high cholesterol and diabetes; communication difficulties associated with illness; a lack of integration and communication between primary and mental health services; and the fact that *mental illness stigma* also can affect the care health professionals provide.

Reducing stigma and discrimination is at the heart of Canada's mental health strategy, *Changing Directions, Changing Lives* (MHCC, 2012). Research provides insights into how stigma manifests in mental health care institutions as taken-for-granted, discriminatory practices that place people at risk of harm when interfacing with the mental health care system (e.g., Henderson et al., 2014; Knaak et al., 2015; Knaak, Mantler, & Szeto, 2017). In response, growing anti-stigma activities aim to reduce societal stigma and health care provider stigma (Knaak & Patten, 2014) with increased research occurring in these areas (Knaak, 2018; Knaak et al., 2017). For example, an evaluation of the Mental Health Commission of Canada's online anti-stigma program *Destigmatizing Practices and Mental Illness* (https://www.mdcme.ca/courseinfo.asp?id=167) showed it can reduce health care provider stigma against mental illness, specifically among nurses and nursing students (Knaak, 2018). Research findings related to the stigma of mental illness held by health care providers in health care settings, including in nurses working in mental health settings (e.g., Ross & Goldner, 2009), highlights the importance of addressing stigma and discrimination in mental health care settings as both a fight for mental health, and for social justice and equity in mental health (Stuart, 2016; Stuart & Arboleda-Flórez, 2012). In addition, a key element of anti-stigma practice is engaging in **recovery-oriented** approaches to mental illness, that is, those approaches underpinned by a belief that recovery is increasingly possible, including significant improvements in symptoms and quality of life when the right services, treatments, and supports are provided (Mental Health Commission of Canada, 2015). However, while recovery-oriented care is a best practice approach generating considerable interest in Canada, its adoption has been challenging (Park et al., 2014). Stereotypes attributed to people with a mental illness (e.g., that they can never be well enough to make decisions, or are dangerous), and pessimism about the possibility of recovery remain common among health care providers (Caldwell & Jorm, 2001), contributing to stigma and creating barriers to recovery (Knaak & Patten, 2014; Mental Health Commission of Canada, 2009, 2015; Stuart, 2016).

Diagnostic assessment of a mental illness is based on the interpretation of clinical behaviours and is guided by criteria from the *Diagnostic and Statistical Manual of Mental Disorders (DSM)*, which historically has undervalued sociocultural interpretations of mental health and mental illness. Due to globalization, migration, and the international use of the *DSM-IV*, the new *DSM-5* has broadened the sociocultural considerations within assessment and diagnoses (Alarcon et al., 2009). This effort addresses in part the critiques of insensitivity to the context of people's lives and a lack of cultural awareness within previous editions (O'Mahony & Donnelly, 2007).

THE CULTURAL LANDSCAPE OF CANADA

Indigenous Peoples, Multi-culturalism, and Equity

All Canadians, with the exception of Indigenous peoples, entered this nation from other countries (British Columbia Public Service Agency, 2021). In 2016 there were more than 1 673 785 "Aboriginal" people in Canada, accounting for 4.9% of the total population. This is an increase from 3.8% in 2006 and 2.8% in 1996 (Statistics Canada, 2017a) representing a 42.5% increase since 2006, more than more than four times the growth rate of the non-Aboriginal population over the same period; attributed to natural growth, increased life expectancy, and relatively high fertility rates, and more people newly identifying as Aboriginal on the census, a continuation of a trend over time.

A large body of literature has documented the impact of ongoing colonialism and racism and the negative impact on the health and well-being of Indigenous peoples. However, not only have Indigenous peoples resisted these forces, they have engaged in powerful struggles for self-determination and revitalization of traditional Indigenous languages, culture, medicine, healing, and knowledge systems (Greenwood et al., 2017, p. 181). As Greenwood et al. note, this resilience and resurgence has been a powerful force directly challenging the Government of Canada to recognize and redress the harms associated with colonialism in a number of government-led agreements/commissions and reports including the Royal Commission on Aboriginal Peoples (RCAP, 1996), the United Nations Declaration on the Rights of Indigenous Peoples (UNDRIP) (United Nations, 2007), and, more recently, the Truth and Reconciliation Commission of Canada (TRC, 2015). Both RCAP and the TRC resulted in a series of recommendations to assist with moving towards reconciliation and healing associated with the significant harms incurred on Indigenous peoples in Canada; several of those recommendations relate to health and a focus on the health care system.

Multi-culturalism is a concept or philosophy with the aim of emphasizing promotion and recognition of diversity, participation of all individuals in Canadian society, respect for inclusivity, equal treatment, and appreciation of diverse cultures (Hilario et al., 2017; Lee, 2013). Unfortunately, multi-culturalism as often presented in Canadian society tends towards culturalist and essentialist perspectives on culture, and rarely goes beyond ideas of "tolerance" (Anderson & Kirkham, 1998). This means there is a gap in analysis of how dominant culture impacts how this policy is lived out. Multi-culturalism should not be just about saying X people eat Y food, rather, it should be about ensuring a society where all people can be safe and free to achieve their optimum physical and mental health together. As noted earlier, when we employ a critical cultural perspective and see culture as dynamic and relational, it takes us to a very different place in nursing. It shifts our attention beyond the individual or interpersonal level to an analysis of structural and ideological influences on intersecting health inequities, to the root causes of those inequities, racism, ableism, sexism, poverty, homelessness, etc. This is not an indictment of multi-culturalism per se, however, it is a reminder of our need as psychiatric mental health nurses to ensure that we do not get caught in the trap of reinforcing systems of inequity by putting our focus in the wrong place. Instead of focussing on the culture of the "other," we need to focus our attention on the ways that the culture of health care can limit safe access and treatment.

Immigrants are those persons born outside of Canada who have been granted the right to live in Canada permanently (Statistics Canada, 2017a) and **refugees** are people, who because of persecution for reasons of race, religion, nationality, membership in a particular social group or political opinion, decide to leave due to fear and/or an inability to seek safety in their country of origin (United Nations High Commissioner for Refugees, 1951; as cited in McKenzie et al., 2016).

Between 2011 and 2016, Canada had 1 212 075 new immigrants who had permanently settled in Canada (Statistics Canada, 2017b). Newcomers, immigrants, and refugees resettled in Canada make up to 20% of the national population. Recent immigrants represented 3.5% of Canada's total population in 2016. The majority (60.3%) of these new immigrants were admitted under the economic category, 26.8% were admitted under the family class to join family already in the country, and 11.6% were admitted to Canada as refugees. In 2016 there was an increase in refugees to Canada because of the influx of refugees from Syria during that year.

In psychiatric mental health nursing the lives of many people who live with mental illness have been impacted by their illness in multiple ways; mental illness in and of itself has created marginalizing experiences, such as loss of employment and income and challenges to continuing with education and safe and comfortable housing, language barriers and a lack of easily accessible, safe interpreters within health care settings, to name only a few. Tensions and inequities also sometimes arise because of perceived differences across populations and groups, for example, for those people who do not speak either French or English (Canada's official languages) or are most likely to be racialized because of their colour. Many immigrants and refugees end up working at the lower ends of the labor market, with lower pay and higher levels of casualization than the general population. As such, they experience much higher levels of income inequality within these countries, inequalities that in turn impact negatively on mental health and wellbeing.

MENTAL HEALTH CONCERNS OF INDIGENOUS PEOPLES

High proportions of the First Nations, Inuit, and Métis peoples have been marginalized by systemic racism, discrimination, and intergenerational and historical traumas resulting from residential schooling and other colonial policies and practices (Allan & Smylie, 2015; Gone, 2013; Linklater & Mehl-Madrona, 2014). Residential schools have been the most often cited cause of the mental health and substance use issues for Indigenous peoples (but certainly not the only cause) (Nelson

& Wilson, 2017; Wilk, et al., 2017). Not surprisingly, residential school experiences have been linked to post-traumatic disorder (most common) and substance use, major depression, dysthymia, and anxiety disorders (Elias, et al., 2012; Hackett et al., 2016; Nelson & Wilson, 2017; Wilk, et al., 2017). Adverse childhood experiences have been well-documented as strongly linked to problematic substance use, chronic pain, and a wide range of other health effects in adulthood, including early mortality (Anda, et al., 2006; Felliti & Anda, 2010).

However, despite these realities, it is also important to note that many First Nations, Inuit, and Métis are living well; as noted in the First Nations Mental Wellness Continuum report, "First Nations have maintained their cultural knowledge in their ways of living (with the land and with each other) and in their language. These foundations have ensured First Nations people have strength, laughter, and resilience" (Health Canada, 2015, p. 1). In fact, cultural continuity has been put forward as a determinant of Indigenous peoples' health (Auger, 2017). In addition, statistics related to Indigenous health need to be understood as variable; the impact of colonialism, racism, etc. has not been the same for all Indigenous peoples/communities, rather health/well-being has been shown to be associated with variation in access to education, housing, food security, employment and health care, and protective features such as connectedness to culture, to name several (Allan & Smylie, 2015; Auger, 2017; Chandler and Lalonde, 2008; Downey, 2020; MacDonald, et al., 2013; Napoleon, 2009).

Historical Trauma

For more than 500 years since first contact between the Indigenous peoples of Canada and dominant immigrant settler nations, Indigenous communities were displaced and disconnected from their traditional ways (Linklater & Mehl-Madrona, 2014). Consequent government policies and legislation signalled forced cultural genocide and attempts at assimilation of Indigenous peoples who had lived peacefully on the land for thousands of years prior to first contact with colonization and foreign settlers. The *Indian Act* of 1876 (race-based legislation) laid the foundation that would drastically change traditional Indigenous lives in Canada. Rather than remaining self-sufficient, "the Indian" became subjects of Canada considered inferior to their non-Indigenous counterparts and monitored by a system of constant surveillance (Government of Canada, 2016a, 2016b). The legacy of historical social and political injustices characterized by cultural oppression (including language disruption), displacement from traditional lands, incarceration of children in government-run Indian Residential Schools (IRSs), and removal of children by child welfare authorities (Bourque-Bearskin & Jakubec, 2022) was created. The ongoing regulation of the lives of First Nations peoples and restrictions created by the Indian Act related to self-government, land claims, and economic development continue to shape the well-being and social status of individuals and families (Browne & Varcoe, 2019, p. 35). The legacy of colonialism has resulted in intergenerational loss of traditional family values, leading to a breakdown of the family and community structures and to consequent social and economic challenges (Gone, 2013). Colonialism is responsible for much of the trauma experienced by Indigenous people and its effects continue to this day (Center for Suicide Prevention, 2017; Linklater & Mehl-Madrona, 2014).

Trauma places people at higher risk for additional mental health issues such as depression and substance use issues, and as Nelson and Wilson (2017) argue Indigenous people in Canada carry a "disproportionate burden of mental and physical illness" as a consequence of historical trauma (p. 93). People who have experienced historical trauma are also at greater risk for depression and mental illness, suicide, sexual and physical abuse, including domestic violence, feelings of hopelessness, and substance use (Center for Suicide Prevention, 2017).

Suicide

Although there were no suicides reported in 60% of Indigenous First Nations communities between 2011 and 2016, suicide rates remain significantly higher for Indigenous, Métis, and Inuit peoples than for non-Indigenous Canadians; the suicide rates and disparities were highest in youth and young adults (15–24 years of age) among Indigenous males and Inuit males and females. These rates are particularly alarming given that nearly 40% of Indigenous peoples in Canada are under 25 years of age (Statistics Canada, 2015). Notably, in a study by Chandler and Lalonde in 1998, rates of suicide were found to vary dramatically across communities and were related to markers of cultural continuity (i.e., what they deemed as "protective" factors such as land claim negotiations, self-government, education services, police and fire services, health services, and cultural facilities).

Interpersonal and Structural Violence

As noted earlier in this Chapter, the "violence" noted in trauma- and violence-informed care (TVIC) remind us of the powerful intersection between interpersonal and structural violence and the long-standing effects of cumulative and ongoing trauma: violence is never over and it is not something you simply "get over". The impact of the enactment of colonization and ongoing racism is largely felt.

In Canada 52.2% of children in foster care are Indigenous, but account for only 7.7% of the child population according to Census 2016. This means 14 970 out of 28 665 foster children in private homes under the age of 15 are Indigenous. Racism and structural violence are embedded in our systems of care, including child welfare (Department of Justice, 2019); understandably fear and mistrust are associated with child welfare authorities, a mistrust that began with the forced removal of Indigenous children from their homes into residential schools and the removal of large numbers of children of Indigenous ancestry from their families who were placed for adoption in the 1960s (referred to as the 60s Scoop) (Duff et al., 2014).

While Indigenous children continue to be over-represented in the child welfare system, women experience disproportionately higher levels of violence in terms of both incidence and severity and are disproportionately represented in the number of missing and murdered women across Canada (Oppal, 2012). In addition, Indigenous people are overrepresented in virtually all aspects of the justice system. There is widespread bias against Indigenous people within Canada, (i.e., "[t]here is evidence that this widespread racism has translated into systemic discrimination in the criminal justice system") (*R. v. Gladue*, 1999).

Indigenous women face severe marginalization associated with a multiplicity of inequities (Allan & Smylie, 2015, p. ii), including poverty, under-housing or homelessness, unemployment, violence, and incarceration (Smye et al., 2020). The epidemic of violence against Indigenous women profoundly threatens the health of women and subsequently their families (Allan & Smylie, p. 16).

Thus high rates of family violence, sexual abuse, incarceration, and emotional distress underscore the significance of historical trauma and ongoing structural violence on the current mental health and societal problems facing many Indigenous peoples. Notably, interpersonal violence is widespread in our society. It has nothing to do with culture. It is about the misuse of power and power inequities/imbalance; one of the manifestations is gender-based violence. The multiple traumas and revictimization that many Indigenous people endure are linked to complex trauma responses, which require strong, culturally appropriate intervention programs.

Lastly, relationship and community violence experienced among Indigenous communities have not always been met with a thorough response by policing and legal systems (Carbone-Lopez, 2013; McCall & Lauridsen-Hoegh, 2014; Oppal, 2012). In 2016 a long-awaited inquiry into the root causes of the disproportionate rates of violent crime against Indigenous women and girls was initiated (Narine, 2016) and the final report was released in 2019 (National Inquiry into Missing and Murdered Indigenous Women and Girls, 2019). For further discussion, see Chapter 25.

Substance Use

Higher rates of illicit drug and other substance use have been reported in Indigenous peoples compared with non-Indigenous people. In addition, although a smaller proportion of Indigenous peoples actually consume alcohol than in the general population, the rate of "problem drinking" is higher in the Indigenous population (Statistics Canada, 2015). From a critical cultural perspective, we understand these challenges not to be inherent in the Indigenous culture but rather to be results of historic and ongoing colonialism, discrimination, and racism. Culturally based interventions and community-owned services have demonstrated promise for achieving gains in population health and reducing disparities among Indigenous communities. However, the need for tailored services does not negate the need for broader structural and systemic change to address socioeconomic disparities and to remove the social and political barriers that continue to have a negative impact on the health of Indigenous communities in Canada (Urbanoski, 2017).

As an integral part of the healing process, the National Native Alcohol and Drug Abuse Program provides Indigenous-specific programs and inpatient, outpatient, and residential treatment for addictions. It provides direction and identifies opportunities to ensure that individuals, families, and communities have access to appropriate, culturally relevant services. There are approximately 53 Indigenous addiction treatment centres across the country that are not only used by Indigenous people but also open to other funding agencies. Barriers to access and cumbersome referral processes that require many pages of information and consents often hinder recovery. Like other specialist services, wait lists as long as 6 months and limited local detoxification resources continue to challenge many health authorities.

MENTAL HEALTH CONCERNS OF IMMIGRANTS AND REFUGEES

In a recent report prepared for the MHCC and based on the findings of three literature reviews and a secondary analysis of existing data, McKenzie et al. (2016) examined the mental health of immigrant, refugee, ethnocultural, and racialized populations. Not surprisingly, they found that the rates of mental health problems and illnesses vary considerably among different immigrant and refugee populations and within particular groups; variances that they assert likely reflect differences in exposure to and effects of social risk factors on subpopulations and groups within these populations (p. 9). For example, it was found that context matters: the same group may have different rates dependent on different circumstances (e.g., asylum seekers who are detained in immigration holding centres upon arrival in Canada report significantly higher rates of post-traumatic stress disorder [PTSD] [31.97%], depression [77.87%], and anxiety [63.11%], compared with asylum seekers who have never been detained [PTSD: 18.18%; depression: 51.52%; anxiety: 46.97%]) (Cleveland & Rousseau, 2013, as cited in McKenzie et al., 2016). In addition, intergroup and intragroup differences are common within immigrant and refugee groups in Canada. For example, while immigrants generally report lower rates of mental health problems in Canada, one study found that South Asian immigrants report statistically significantly higher rates of diagnosed anxiety (3.44%) than the South Asian population born in Canada (1.09%) (Islam et al., 2014, as cited in McKenzie

> **BOX 8.5 Migrant Workers and Health: A Largely Forgotten Population**
>
> **See RNAO "Doris Blog":** Migrant agricultural workers are important members of our communities; they deserve respect and protection during the COVID-19 crisis.
> https://doris-blog.rnao.ca/taxonomy/term/57
>
> **See RNAO Article:** Harvesting for Good Health. Registered nurses who care for migrant farm workers are helping to mitigate barriers and manage health concerns for those temporarily living far from home.
> Dr. Constanzo, M. (2014). Harvesting for good health. *Registered Nurse Journal* (July/Aug), 12–16. https://rnao.ca/sites/rnao-ca/files/Harvesting_good_health.pdf

et al., 2016). The time people have spent in Canada also makes a difference. For example, recent immigrants to Canada are less likely to report depression than longer-term immigrants whose reported rates are more similar to the Canadian-born population (Muldoon et al., 2013, as cited in McKenzie et al., 2016). Evidence also suggests that immigrants from racialized groups and refugees are at risk for deteriorating health soon after arrival (e.g., Gushulak et al., 2011, as cited in McKenzie et al., 2016). Immigrant resettlement experiences are varied with some populations experiencing more challenges than others.

In many instances the rates of mental health problems are lower in immigrant groups than in the general population. There are, however, elevated rates of PTSD and common mental health disorders (anxiety and depression) among refugees; and increased risk of substance use and suicide in some second and third-generation immigrant groups (e.g., Bourque, van der Ven, & Malia, 2011, as cited in McKenzie et al., 2016). Among people living with mental health problems or illnesses from immigrant populations, health service use is low, although in general, service use by immigrant populations is increasing. As McKenzie et al. (2016) note, low use of health services in general may mask higher use of costly, more intensive services, such as inpatient care (patient care provided in a hospital or other facility) and emergency services (Box 8.5).

Social determinants of health are clearly linked to health and achievement of health equity for all. However, in the examination of the literature noted above McKenzie et al. (2016) report particular risk factors to be considered as they relate to health outcomes:
- Safety from or exposure to victimization or violence;
- Parents' mental health or substance use problems;
- Food (security or insecurity); and
- Caregiver burden or health of a family member (p. 11).

As the authors note, although these risk factors are not unique to the populations under study, these groups are more likely to be exposed to them. In addition, these factors may have increased impact because they interact with each other and other determinants of health to create more or less stress.

> **RESEARCH HIGHLIGHT**
>
> ***Belonging and Mental Wellbeing Among a Rural Indian–Canadian Diaspora: Navigating Tensions in "Finding a Space of Our Own"***
>
> **Problem**
> Belonging is linked to a variety of positive health outcomes. Yet this relationship is not well understood, particularly among rural immigrant diasporas. **Diaspora** refers to any group dispersed outside of their original geographic homeland.

> **Purpose of the Study**
> In this article the researchers explore the experiences of community belonging and wellbeing among a rural Indian–Canadian diaspora in the Interior of British Columbia, Canada, The central research questions were: "What are the experiences of belonging in this community? How does a sense of belonging (or lack of) shape mental health and wellbeing among local residents?"
>
> **Methods**
> A qualitative research design informed by a socioecological lens was employed. The researchers used a blended narrative and situational analysis research approach as well as participatory action research design.
>
> **Key Findings**
> Local residents navigated several tensions shaping belonging and mental well-being within an overarching reality of "finding a space of their own."
> - Tight-knitedness amid isolation; people longed for a sense of closeness/ and varying levels of connectedness. Creating closeness was challenged by language barriers, intergenerational conflict, economic hardships, and having access to local knowledge.
> - Culture was an important source of belonging and mental well-being for all participants and all wanted to create a space for this to happen in Canada. For many, there was a strong connection between their Sikh spirituality and Punjabi culture. For some, visiting the homeland (the Punjab) was an important feature of cultural renewal. The need for connection outside the Punjabi community varied. For some, connection to their home in Canada and the land was more important than connecting with the wider community.
> - Key barriers to connection were the agricultural seasonal cycle and worklife, language and communication, and socio-cultural differences and contexts.
> - Small town standards/resources were limited; there was a lack of culturally specific or relevant services
>
> **Implications for Nursing Practice**
> - Creative service provision, collaborative decision making, and diversity-informed program planning are key elements in the provision of services.
> - Geographic location (rurality) is a determinant of health.
> - There are within-group differences that need to be understood by engaging in respectful, relational processes in practice.
> - Consider both spiritual and cultural aspects of identity to promote mental well-being.
> - Providers need to have a broader understanding of cultural safety and appropriateness.
>
> **Source:** Caxaj, C. S., & Gill, N. K. (2017). Belonging and mental wellbeing among a rural Indian-Canadian diaspora: Navigating tensions in "Finding a Space of Our Own." *Qualitative Health Research, 27*(8), 1119–1132. https://doi.org/10.1177/1049732316648129

BARRIERS AND PATHWAYS TO MENTAL HEALTH CARE IN A MULTI-CULTURAL CONTEXT

A multi-cultural context, means there are potential barriers to mental health care that need to be addressed including stigma and discrimination, communication barriers, patient self-stigma about using mental health services or receiving a psychiatric diagnostic label, a lack of culturally safe and appropriate services (McCall & Lauridsen-Hoegh, 2014), misdiagnosis due to unrecognized cultural differences, and ethnic variations in pharmacodynamics, all of which influence the mental health status of Indigenous, immigrant, and refugee peoples and their use of health care services.

The reality of recovery from mental illness is further complicated within many cultural contexts. Among cultural groups that emphasize the interdependence and harmony of the family, mental illness may be perceived as a failure of the family. Influenced by these values and perceptions, the pressures on both the person experiencing a mental illness and their family are increased since the illness is thought to reflect on the character of all family members. Stigma and shame can result in avoidance of the formal health care system; therefore people from cultures where this shame predominates may enter the mental health care system only at an advanced stage of illness, when the family has exhausted its ability to cope with the problem (Na et al., 2016). Although great strides have been made through numerous campaigns and expanded global awareness, misunderstanding and stigmatization continue to be experienced on a number of personal, cultural, and institutional levels (Gaebel et al., 2017), warranting nursing care and community interventions related specifically to stigma.

Guidelines for Clinical Practice: Communication

Relational inquiry centers on building trust, engaging through listening, conveying respect for difference, and paying attention to the contextual features of people's lives (Browne & Varcoe, 2019).

Building trust can take time; any kind of inquiry needs to be conducted in a non-judgmental, respectful manner. Inquiry that is person-centered will be tailored to the patient and their needs. For example, the sharing of personal information may create fear based on recent or past experiences; there may be fear of reprisal (rejection) or judgement or for some, a fear related to a possible disruption in their immigration status. For others, inquiry of this kind may create mistrust, for example, for some Indigenous people, mental health professionals may be seen as part of the problem, both from a historical perspective as well as in their roles within the State (e.g., in the child welfare and justice systems) (Gopalkrishnan, 2018). To minimize this risk, during an assessment you might say something like, "What do you believe is happening right now?"; "What have you found most helpful?" To find a connection, it might be helpful to demonstrate an interest in a person's life by asking related questions such as in the case of an Indigenous patient, you might ask "What nation or community are you from?" or with a newcomer to Canada, "In what country were you born?"; "Tell me a little bit about the country where you were born."

As noted numerous times in this chapter, *conveying respect for difference* is an essential element of the relational process. This can be as simple as asking questions focussed on the patient and those things that are meaningful to them. For example, "Have you found any treatments or medications that have helped you in the past?"; "Are you using any medicines at this time that you find helpful." Some people use complementary and alternative healing health care practices so you may want to ask questions about traditional medicines or healing methods that they may have found helpful, and if so, if they have access to them or are using them at this time.

Lastly, *paying attention to the social and economic context of peoples' lives* is a key element of relational inquiry; you want to inquire how the patient is managing in their day-to-day life. This attention to life circumstances can be a powerful point of connection and a source of important information. Genuine interest in the patient and their circumstances can mitigate against being perceived as intrusive. For example, you could say something like: "Tell me about how you are managing your health/illness?"; "Is there anything particularly challenging or difficult at this time related to your health/illness?"; "What kinds of supports do you have in or outside of the home to assist you?"; "What kinds of supports would be useful?"; "Is there anything you need that you have had difficulty accessing?"; "Are you working at this time?"; "What kind of work do you enjoy?"; "Are you able to access the things you need at this time?"

When difference in language poses a significant challenge to communication, it is important to seek professional interpreters whenever possible (instead of family members or friends) to ensure patient safety and freedom of speech. Cross-language facilitation also can be supported by avoiding the use of complex words and jargon; the provision of an explanation regarding why you need to ask questions; checking that you have understood the words the person is using and whether you have been understood (particularly important when providing directions regarding medication use); using diagrams, models, film/video, and images to explain concepts, instructions, and terms; being cautious about using traditional languages or words unless you have excellent understanding; and if this is an Indigenous patient who speaks their Indigenous language, you may want to seek assistance from an Indigenous elder or community member that the patient trusts.

Misdiagnosis

Reasons for misdiagnosis of mental illness within culturally diverse populations include the use of culturally inappropriate psychometric instruments and diagnostic tools and the lack of consideration of and attention to cultural variations in the expression and conceptualization of mental health/illness, including the different meanings people attach to the symptoms of mental illness. As Gopalkrishnan (2018) notes, there is an extensive body of research literature that emphasizes the fact that health and illness are perceived differently across cultures with real consequences for whether people seek treatment; the ways in which they cope with symptoms; the support they will receive from family and community; where and how they seek help (mental health specialist, primary care provider, clergy, traditional healer); and the health outcomes (Office of the Surgeon General (US), Center for Mental Health Services (US), & National Institute of Mental Health (US), 2001, p. 19; as cited in Gopalkrishnan).

Many available diagnostic tools have been validated using study participants of European origin and underpinned by Western conceptualizations of health. These tools tend to focus on individual pathology (an individualist and deficit-focused stance) rather than on community or familial processes (a collectivist stance), and strengths-based approaches and cognitive rather than physical symptoms. For example, in response to the lack of culturally safe diagnostic tools and interventions, the Native Wellness Assessment Tool, an Indigenous knowledge-based instrument, was developed through the Thunderbird Partnership that demonstrates the effectiveness of First Nations culture as a health intervention in addressing substance use and mental health issues; it also is a strengths-based approach to mental (health) wellness.

Examples of diversity in conceptualizations are helpful, but we also warn against assuming anyone from any particular culture holds these particular beliefs. For some people, mental illness takes the form of emotional expression and for others, physical symptoms, such as headaches, backaches, or stomach discomfort; this is referred to as somatization. For example, *Hwa-Byung* and neurasthenia have many similarities to depression (Park et al., 2001), but because the somatic complaints are prominent, and patients deny feelings of sadness or depression, the symptoms may not fit the *DSM-5* diagnostic criteria for depression. *Ataque de nervios* and ghost sickness are characterized by abnormal behaviours culturally understood as illness and are culturally acceptable ways to express overwhelming stress.

Perceptions of etiology of disease can be very different across cultures; illness causality is seen by some at the individual level and by others in the natural or social world. Some people may ascribe the onset of disease to possession by spirits, the "evil eye," black magic or the breaking of taboos, which falls under the purview of traditional healers, elders, or other significant people in the community. Religion and spirituality often play a key role in these perceptions by juxtaposing hardship with a higher order good and the solutions are accordingly sought within these systems of thought and belief. Examples of these would be the healing temples in India or other religious pilgrimage sites across the world that are visited every day by thousands of people experiencing mental health issues (Gopalkrishnan, 2018).

Susto, or "soul loss," is believed by some to occur after a traumatic incident (Lim, 2006). From a Western perspective, the patient may be experiencing depression, anxiety, or PTSD, but the patient believes that they are experiencing the illness of soul loss. Similarly, some Indigenous people will strongly believe that their symptoms are caused by "bad medicine" deliberately sent to harm them. Authors have examined the socio-cultural-political views of anorexia and bulimia over time, revealing layers of cultural meaning that underlie body ideals (whether thin or fit), media messages, as well as health and wellbeing influences (Eli & Warin, 2018).

Culture affects the way we express our thoughts, behaviors, and emotions. Thus it makes sense that there may be differences in the expression of mental health illness and the meanings given to them. If culture is not considered in diagnosis and treatment, practitioners also are more likely to see culturally normal behaviour as "abnormal" instead of merely different from their own. For example, what some may view as delusional or hallucinatory behaviour may be part of a vision quest from an Indigenous perspective.

Better understanding of idioms of distress can assist in understanding and in communication from cultural (rather than pathologizing) perspectives (Kaiser et al., 2015). Cultural concepts of distress or illnesses may seem foreign to Canadian-trained nurses, as these illnesses are poorly conceptualized in the Western biomedical perspective. However, these illnesses are well understood by the cultural group, which can name the problem, its etiology, its course, and its treatment. Accounts of illness are often told in a cultural narrative, a person's story that is well articulated and involves all significant psychosocial relationships and egocentric elements. When treated in corresponding culturally prescribed ways, the remedies are frequently effective.

Nurses often work in environments that are dominated by biomedical perspectives, which may dismiss other potential perspectives and subtly (or not so subtly) create barriers to cultural safety. Negotiations between the patient, family, and health care provider are critical and must consider the culture, history, and environment of the patient.

KEY POINTS TO REMEMBER

- Culture is dynamic and ever-changing. It is a relational concept.
- Culture is cocreated through the nurse–patient interaction.
- Nurses and patients are shaped by their own personal and professional cultures.
- Psychiatric mental health nursing is based on personality and developmental theories largely grounded in Western cultural ideals and values.
- In a shifting multi-cultural Canadian context nurses are caring for more people from diverse cultural populations.
- Nurses must guard against stereotyping, racialization, and ethnocentrism by beginning with a reflection on their own assumptions and biases.
- Nurses are challenged to deliver culturally safe and trauma- and violence-informed care, inclusive of appropriate assessments and interventions.
- Trauma- and violence-informed care reflects an understanding that anyone could have a trauma history (universality) and that trauma/violence has a cumulative and ongoing impact on health and wellbeing. Trauma/violence is not something you simply "get over."
- Colonization, including the residential school system and national assimilation policies, has resulted in historical trauma of Indigenous peoples in Canada, significantly contributing to the social and mental health issues experienced by Indigenous populations.
- Regardless of the severity of impact, many Indigenous peoples in Canada are enjoying well-being.

- Immigrants and refugees may experience stress related to resettlement. Refugees sometimes develop post-traumatic stress disorder as a consequence of trauma/violence experiences.
- Barriers to quality mental health care include mental illness stigma and discrimination, communication barriers, ethnic variations in psychotropic drug metabolism, and misdiagnoses caused by culturally inappropriate diagnostic tools and miscommunication related to a lack of attention to differences between people.

CRITICAL THINKING

1. Describe the cultural and other factors that have influenced the development of Western psychiatric mental health nursing practice.
2. Some of you have grown up in contexts that mirrored the Western individualist worldview that historically undergirds most of the concepts, processes, and perspectives in nursing and the health professions more broadly. Others may come from cultural backgrounds that uphold a collectivist worldview. Create ways of knowing, being, and doing inherent in each of these perspectives. Generate as many specific points as you can. Remember that these are not necessarily discrete categories of difference.
3. Discuss the impact of colonization and assimilation policies such as the residential school system on the current mental health and social problems of Indigenous peoples in Canada.
4. Discuss the impact of immigration and refugee experiences on mental health/well-being.
5. Analyze the effects that cultural safety (or unsafety) can have on psychiatric mental health nurses, their patients, and their patients' families.
6. Identify what nurses can do to overcome communication barriers and the risk of misdiagnosis?
7. Consider what types of programs might reinforce street youth's resilience and survival skills.

CHAPTER REVIEW

1. Mr. Yeung, a recent immigrant from China, has been admitted to the observation unit for investigation of unspecified physical malaise. His family tells the nurse that Mr. Yeung began to exhibit certain behaviours when his import business declined and his creditors demanded money. He has subsequently made vague physical complaints for the past 6 weeks. Which patient behaviour would alert the nurse to the potential for somatization?
    a. Patients who somatize often discuss physical ailments but do not make mention of feelings.
    b. Showing the medication he uses to the nurse is not an expression of somatization.
    c. Somatization is psychological distress manifested as physical problems. Instead of perceiving the distress as emotional or affective, the patient perceives psychological distress in the body.
    d. Discussing the diagnosis of bipolar disorder is not an expression of somatization.
2. Mr. Oliva has been admitted to the psychiatric ward for depression and substance use, mainly of alcohol and recreational drugs. As you are explaining his diagnoses and the potential treatment plan to him, his wife and he state that the problem is "ghost sickness," which came about when his mother died. What is the most therapeutic nursing response?
    a. "I have no idea what 'ghost sickness' is."
    b. "Please explain what you mean by 'ghost sickness.'"
    c. "There is not a disorder known as 'ghost sickness.'"
    d. "Why do you believe in evil spirits?"
3. You are a nurse in an outpatient well-baby clinic. You are planning care for a young Cree mother and her infant. The young mother has been identified as at risk for post-partum depression. Which intervention is most appropriate?
    a. Engage relationally with the young mother; get to know who she is and what is important to her.
    b. Contact an elder from Indigenous Services.
    c. Discuss the medicine wheel concept of healing with the patient.
    d. Contact a "singer" to provide a healing ritual within 3 days of admission.
4. You are a nurse on a busy medical unit with a multi-cultural clientele. In your orientation to the unit, you learn that individualism is a concept closely aligned with North American values. When caring for patients with diverse cultural backgrounds, which general nursing action would be most appropriate?
    a. This response assumes that constant eye contact is important.
    b. This response makes assumptions about the required personal space of others.
    c. Beliefs about control over self and predestination need to be further explored before this response is used.
    d. While the predominant status quo belief in Canada places value on individualism, a significant number of ethnic groups in our multicultural society value a group focus. Thus, family may be actively involved in patient care, decision making, and information sharing. The nurse can assess how much the family wants and expects to be involved and what level of family involvement is comfortable for the patient.
5. You are a flight nurse who is bringing a young Inuit man from Nunavut for psychiatric assessment in a Winnipeg hospital. You assess the patient as acutely suicidal. Which goal is appropriate?
    a. Patient will visit with a cultural leader from the Inuit community.
    b. Patient will experience rebalance of yin–yang by discharge.
    c. Patient will identify sources that increase "cold wind" within 24 hours of admission.
    d. Patient will be put on suicidal observation and ongoing assessment.

 http://evolve.elsevier.com/Canada/Varcarolis/psychiatric/

REFERENCES

Ahmad, W. I. U. (1993). Making Black people sick: "Race", ideology and health research. In W. I. U. Ahmad (Ed.), *"Race" and health in contemporary Britain* (pp. 11–33). Open University Press.

Alarcon, R. D., Becker, A. E., Lewis-Fernandez, R., Like, R. C., Desai, P., Foulks, E., Gonzales, J., Hansen, H., Kopelowicz, A., Lu, F. G., Oquendo, M. A., & Primm, A., & Cultural Psychiatry Committee of the Group for the Advancement of Psychiatry. (2009). Issues for DSM-V: The role of culture in psychiatric diagnosis. *The Journal of Nervous and Mental Disease, 197*(8), 559–560. https://doi.org/10.1097/NMD.0b013e3181b0cbff

Allan, B., & Smylie, J. (2015). *First Peoples, second class treatment: The role of racism in the health and well-being of Indigenous peoples in Canada*. Toronto: The Wellesley Institute.

Anda, R. F., Felliti, V. J., Bremner, J. D., Walker, J. D., Whitfield, C., Perry, B. D., Dube, S. R., & Giles, W. H. (2006). The enduring effects of abuse and related adverse experiences in childhood: A convergence of evidence from neurobiology and epidemiology. *European Archives of Psychiatry & Clinical Neuroscience, 256*(3), 174–186.

Anderson, J., & Kirkham, R. S (1998). Constructing nation: The gendering and racializing of the Canadian health care system. In S. Grace, J. Anderson, V. Strong-Boag, & A. Eisenberg (Eds.), *Painting the maple: Essays on race, gender, and the construction of Canada* (pp. 242–261). Vancouver: University of British Columbia Press.

Andrews, M. M., & Boyle, J. S. (2016). *Transcultural concepts in nursing care* (7th ed.). Philadelphia: Wolters Kluwer.

Assembly of First Nations. (2018a). *Jordon's Principle*. Author. Retrieved from https://www.afn.ca/policy-sectors/social-secretariat/jordans-principle/

Assembly of First Nations. (2018b). *Jordan's Principle Summit Report. Sharing, learning and growing: Imagining the future of Jordan's Principle*. September 12–13. Author. Retrieved from https://www.afn.ca/uploads/Social_Development/Jordan%27s%20Principle%20Summit%20Report_en.pdf

Auger, M. D. (2017). Cultural continuity as a determinant of Indigenous peoples' health: A metasynthesis of qualitative research in Canada and the United States. *The International Indigenous Policy Journal, 7*(4). https://doi.org/10.18584/iipj.2016.7.4.3

BC Provincial Mental Health and Substance Use Planning Council. (2013). *Trauma-informed practice guide*. Author. Retrieved from http://bccewh.bc.ca/wp-content/uploads/2012/05/2013_TIP-Guide.pdf

Bellamy, S., & Hardy, C. (2015). *Understanding depression in Aboriginal communities and families*. National Collaborating Centre for Aboriginal Health.

Berg, K., McLane, P., Eshkakogan, N., Mantha, J., Lee, T., Crowshoe, C., & Phillips, A. (2019). Perspectives on Indigenous cultural competency and safety in Canadian hospital emergency departments: A scoping review. *International Emergency Nursing, 43*, 133–140. https://doi.org/10.1016/j.ienj.2019.01.004

Bourque, F., van der Ven, E., & Malla, A. (2011). A meta-analysis of the risk for psychotic disorders among first- and second-generation immigrants. *Psychological Medicine, 41*(5), 897–910.

Bourque-Bearskin, L., & Jakubec, S. L (2022). Indigenous health: Working with First Nations people, Inuit and Metis. In S. A. Pike-MacDonald & S. L. Jakubec (Eds.), *Stanhope and Lancaster's community health nursing in Canada* (4th ed.) (pp. 324–350). Toronto: Elsevier.

Braveman, P. (2014). What are health disparities and health equity? We need to be clear. *Public Health Report, 129*(2), 5–8.

British Columbia Centre of Excellence for Women's Health. (2016). *Trauma-informed online tool: Coalescing on Women and Substance Use—Linking Research, Practice and Policy*. Retrieved from https://yourexperiencesmatter.com/wp-content/uploads/2016/01/R_181.pdf

British Columbia Public Service Agency. (2021). *Indigenous relations behavioural competencies*. Retrieved from https://www2.gov.bc.ca/gov/content/careers-myhr/job-seekers/about-competencies/indigenous-relations

Browne, A. J. (2009). Discourses influencing nurses' perceptions of First Nations patients. *Canadian Journal of Nursing Research, 41*(1), 166–191.

Browne, A. J., & Varcoe, C (2019). Cultural and social considerations in health assessment. In A. J. Browne, J. MacDonald-Jenkins, & M. Luctkar-Flude (Eds.), *Physical examination and health assessment by C. Jarvis* (3rd Canadian ed.) (pp. 28–45). Elsevier.

Browne, A. J., Varcoe, C., Ford-Gilboe, M., Wathen, C. N., Smye, V., Jackson, B. E., Wallace, B., Pauly, B. B., Herbert, C. P., Lavoie, J. G., Wong, S. T., & Garneau, A. B. (2018). Disruption as opportunity: Impacts of an organizational health equity intervention in primary care clinics. *International Journal for Equity in Health, 17*(1), 154. https://doi.org/10.1186/s12939-018-0820-2

Caldwell, T. M., & Jorm, A. F. (2001). Mental health nurses' beliefs about likely outcomes for people with schizophrenia or depression: A comparison with the public and other healthcare professionals. *International Journal of Mental Health Nursing, 10*(1), 42–54.

Canadian Nurses Association. (2010). *Social justice… A means to an end, an end in itself* (2nd ed.). Retrieved from https://central.bac-lac.gc.ca/.item?id=social_justice_e&op=pdf&app=Library

Canadian Nurses Association. (2018). *Position statement: Promoting cultural competence in nursing*. Retrieved from https://hl-prod-ca-oc-download.s3-ca-central-1.amazonaws.com/CNA/2f975e7e-4a40-45ca-863c-5ebf0a138d5e/UploadedImages/documents/Position_Statement_Promoting_Cultural_Competence_in_Nursing.pdf

Canadian Nurses Association. (2021). *Nursing declaration against anti-indigenous racism in nursing and health care*. Retrieved from https://hl-prod-ca-oc-download.s3-ca-central-1.amazonaws.com/CNA/2f975e7e-4a40-45ca-863c-5ebf0a138d5e/UploadedImages/documents/Nursing_Declaration_Anti-Indigenous_Racism_November_8_2021_ENG_Copy.pdf

Carbone-Lopez, K. (2013). Across racial/ethnic boundaries: Investigating intimate violence within a national sample. *Journal of Interpersonal Violence, 28*(1), 3–24. https://doi.org/10.1177/0886260512448850

Centre for Suicide Prevention. (2017). *A suicide prevention toolkit: Indigenous people, trauma and suicide prevention*. Retrieved from https://www.suicideinfo.ca/wp-content/uploads/2017/04/Indigenous-people-trauma-and-suicide.pdf

Chandler, M. J., & Lalonde, C. (1998). Cultural continuity as a Hedge against suicide in Canada's First Nations. *Transcultural Psychiatry, 35*(2), 191–219. https://doi.org/10.1177/136346159803500202

Chandler, M., & Lalonde, C. (2008). Cultural continuity as a protective factor against suicide in First Nations youth. *Horizons, 10*(I), 68–72.

Cleveland, J., & Rousseau, C. (2013). Psychiatric symptoms associated with brief detention of adult asylum seekers in Canada. *Canadian Journal of Psychiatry, 58*(7), 409–416.

Department of Justice. (2019). Understanding the Overrepresentation of Indigenous People in the Criminal Justice System. *Government of Canada*. Retrieved from https://www.justice.gc.ca/socjs-esjp/en/ind-aut/uo-cs

Doane, G. H., & Varcoe, C. (2005). Towards compassionate action: Pragmatism and the inseparability of theory/practice. *Advances in Nursing Science, 28*(1), 81–90. https://doi.org/10.1097/00012272-200501000-00009

Doane, G. H., & Varcoe, C. (2020). *How to nurse: Relational inquiry in action* (2nd ed.). Philadelphia: Wolters Kluwer.

Downey, B. (2020). Completing the circle: Towards the achievement of IND-equity—A culturally relevant health equity model by/for Indigenous populations. *Witness: The Canadian Journal of Critical Nursing Discourse, 2*(1), 97–110. https://doi.org/10.25071/2291-5796.59

Drevdahl, D. J. (2018). Culture shifts: From cultural to structural theorizing in nursing. *Nurse Researcher, 67*(2), 146–160. https://doi.org/10.1097/NNR.0000000000000262

Duff, P., Bingham, B., Simo, A., Jury, D., Reading, C., & Shannon, K. (2014). The "stolen generations" of mothers and daughters: Child apprehension and enhanced HIV vulnerabilities for sex workers of Aboriginal ancestry. *PLoS ONE, 9*(6), e99664. https://doi.org/10.1371/journal.pone.0099664

Eli, K., & Warin, M. (2018). Anthropological perspectives on eating disorders: Deciphering cultural logics. *Transcultural Psychiatry, 55*(4), 443–453. https://doi.org/10.1177/1363461518784385

Elias, B., Mignone, J., Hall, M., Hong, S. P., Hart, L., & Sareen, J. (2012). Trauma and suicide behaviour histories among a

Canadian Indigenous population: An empirical exploration of the potential role of Canada's residential school system. *Social Science & Medicine, 74*(10), 1560–1569. https://doi.org/10.1016/j.socscimed.2012.01.026

Ermine, W., Sinclair, R., & Jeffrey, B. (2004). *The ethics of research involving Indigenous peoples.* Report of the Indigenous Peoples' Health Research Centre to the Interagency Advisory Panel on Research Ethics. Retrieved from https://drc.usask.ca/projects/legal_aid/file/resource385-2c4c0417.pdf

Farmer, P. E., Nizeye, B., Stulac, S., & Keshavjee, S. (2007). Structural violence and clinical medicine. *PLoS Medicine, 3*(10), 1686–1691. https://doi.org/10.1371/journal.pmed.0030449

Felitti, V., & Anda, R. F. (2010). *The relationship of adverse childhood experiences to adult medical disease, psychiatric disorders, and sexual behavior: Implications for healthcare.* https://doi.org/10.1017/CBO9780511777042.010

First Nations Health Authority. (2018). *It starts with me: FNHA's commitments to cultural safety and cultural humility.* Retrieved from http://www.fnha.ca/documents/fnha-policy-statement-cultural-safety-and-humility.pdf

Ford-Gilboe, M., Wathen, N., Varcoe, C., Herbert, C., Jackson, B., Lavoie, J. G., Pauly, B. B., Perrin, N. A., Smye, V., Wallace, B., & Wong, S. T. (2018). How equity-oriented health care affects health: Key mechanisms and implications for primary health care practice and policy. *The Milbank Quarterly, 96*(4), 635–671. https://doi.org/10.1111/1468-0009.12349

Gaebel, W., Rössler, W., & Sartorius, N. (2017). *The stigma of mental illness: End of the story?.* Cham: Springer.

Gerlach, A. J., Browne, A. J., & Greenwood, M. (2017). Engaging Indigenous families in a community-based Indigenous early childhood programme in British Columbia, Canada: A cultural safety perspective. *Health & Social Care in the Community, 25*(6), 1763–1773. https://doi.org/10.1111/hsc.12450

Gerlach, A. J., Browne, A. J., Sinha, V., & Elliott, D. (2017). Navigating structural violence with Indigenous families: The contested terrain of early childhood intervention and the child welfare system in Canada. *The International Indigenous Policy Journal, 8*(3). Retrieved from https://ojs.lib.uwo.ca/index.php/iipj/article/view/7526

Goldie, C. L. (2013). *Cardiovascular risk and disease among people with mental health disorders in Canada.* University of British Columbia [Unpublished dissertation]. Retrieved from http://Users/vickismye/Downloads/ubc_2014_spring_goldie_catherine-1.pdf

Gone, J. P. (2013). Redressing First Nations historical trauma: Theorizing mechanisms for indigenous culture as mental health treatment. *Transcultural Psychiatry, 50*(5), 683–706. https://doi.org/10.1177/1363461513487669

Gopalkrishnan, N. (2018). Cultural diversity and mental health: Considerations for policy and practice. *Frontiers in Public Health, 6*, 179. https://doi.org/10.3389/fpubh.2018.00179

Government of Canada. (2016a). *Indian Act.* Ottawa: Minster of Justice. Retrieved from http://laws-lois.justice.gc.ca/PDF/I-5.pdf

Government of Canada. (2016b). *Indigenous peoples and human rights.* Retrieved from https://www.canada.ca/en/canadian-heritage/services/rights-indigenous-peoples.html

Greenwood, M. (2019). Modelling change and cultural safety: A case study in Northern British Columbia health system transformation. *Healthcare Management Forum, 32*(1), 11–14. https://doi.org/10.1177/0840470418807948

Greenwood, M., Lindsay, N., King, J., & Loewen, D. (2017). Ethical spaces and places: Indigenous cultural safety in British Columbia health care. *Alter Native: An International Journal of Indigenous Peoples, 13*(3), 179–189. https://doi.org/10.1177/1177180117714411

Guruge, S., Thomson, M. S., & Seifi, S. G. (2015). Mental health and service issues faced by older immigrants in Canada: A scoping review. *Canadian Journal on Aging, 34*(4), 431–444. https://doi.org/10.1017/S0714980815000379

Gushulak, B. D., Pottie, K., Roberts, J. H., Torres, S., & DesMeules, M. (2011). On behalf of the Canadian Collaboration for Immigrant and Refugee Health. Migration and health in Canada: Health in the global village. *Canadian Medical Association Journal, 183*(12), E952–E958.

Hackett, C., Feeny, D., & Tompa, E. (2016). Canada's residential school system: Measuring the intergenerational impact of familial attendance on health and mental health outcomes. *Journal of Epidemiology and Community Health, 70*(11), 1096–1105. https://dx.doi.org/10.1136/jech-2016-207380

Health Canada. (2015). *First Nations mental wellness continuum framework—Full report.* Ottawa: Author. Retrieved from https://thunderbirdpf.org/wp-content/uploads/2015/01/24-14-1273-FN-Mental-Wellness-Framework-EN05_low.pdf

Heflinger, C. A., & Hinshaw, S. P. (2010). Stigma in child and adolescent mental health services research: Understanding professional and institutional stigmatization of youth with mental health problems and their families. *Administration and Policy in Mental Health and Mental Health Services Research, 37*(1–2), 61–70.

Henderson, C., Noblett, J., Parke, H., Clement, S., Caffrey, A., Gale-Grant, O., Schulze, B., Druss, B., & Thornicroft, G. (2014). Mental health-related stigma in health care and mental health-care settings. *The Lancet Psychiatry, 1*(6), 467–482.

Hilario, C., Browne, A. J., & McFadden, A. (2017). The influence of democratic racism in nursing inquiry. *Nursing Inquiry, 25*(1), e12213. https://doi.org/10.1111/nin.12213

Hogue, M., & Bartlett, C. (2014). Two-eyed seeing: Creating a new liminal space in education. *Canada Education, 56*(3), 30–31.

Islam, F., Khanlou, N., & Tamim, H. (2014). South Asian populations in Canada: Migration and mental health. *BMC Psychiatry, 14*, 154.

Kaiser, B. N., Haroz, E. E., Kohrt, B. A., Bolton, P. A., Bass, J. K., & Hintone, D. E. (2015). "Thinking too much": A systematic review of a common idiom of distress. *Social Science & Medicine, 147*, 170–183. https://doi.org/10.1016/j.socscimed.2015.10.044

Keller, K. (2020). The body as machine and the lived body in nursing. *Collegian, 27*, 238–244.

Knaak, S. (2018). *Destigmatizing practices and mental illness: An evaluation report.* Ottawa: Mental Health Commission of Canada.

Knaak, S., Mantler, E., & Szeto, A. (2017). Mental illness-related stigma in healthcare: Barriers to access and care and evidence-based solutions. *Healthcare Management Forum, 30*(2), 111–116. https://doi.org/10.1177/0840470416679413

Knaak, S., & Patten, S. (2014). *Building and delivering successful anti-stigma programs for healthcare providers: Results of a qualitative study.* Ottawa: Mental Health Commission of Canada. Retrieved from https://www.mentalhealthcommission.ca/wp-content/uploads/drupal/qualitative_model_report_feb_2015_0.pdf

Knaak, S., Szeto, A., Kassam, A., Hamer, A., Modgill, G., & Patten, S. (2017). Understanding stigma: A pooled analysis of a national program aimed at healthcare providers to reduce stigma towards patients with a mental illness. *Journal of Mental Health and Addiction Nursing, 1*(1). https://doi.org/10.22374/jmhan.v1i1.19

Knaak, S., Ungar, T., & Patten, S. (2015). Mental illness stigma as a quality of care problem. *The Lancet Psychiatry, 2*, 863–864.

Krieger, N. (2014). Discrimination and health inequities. *International Journal of Health Services, 44*(4), 643–710. https://doi.org/10.2190/HS.44.4.b

Kurtz, D. L. M., Turner, D., Nyberg, J., & Moar, D. (2014). Social justice and health equity: Urban aboriginal women's action for health forum. *The International Journal of Health, Wellness, and Society, 3*(4), 13–26.

Lee, E. (2013). *A critique of Canadian multiculturalism as a state policy and its effects on Canadian subjects*: University of Toronto [Unpublished master's thesis].

Leininger, M. (1985). Transcultural care diversity and universality: A theory of nursing. *Nursing and Health Care, 6*(4), 209–212.

Leininger, M. (1988). Leininger's theory of nursing: Cultural care diversity and universality. *Nursing Science Quarterly, 1*(4), 152–160.

Levine, S., Varcoe, C., & Browne, A. J. (2020). "We went as a team closer to the truth": Impacts of interprofessional education on trauma- and violence- informed care for staff in primary care settings. *Journal of Interprofessional Care 35*(1), 46–54. https://doi.org/10.1080/13561820.2019.1708871

Lim, R. F. (2006). *Clinical manual of cultural psychiatry*. Arlington: American Psychiatric Publishing.

Link, B. G., & Phelan, J. C. (2006). Stigma and its public health implications. *The Lancet, 367*(9509), 528–529.

Link, B. G., & Phelan, J. (2014). Stigma power. *Social Science & Medicine, 103*, 24–32.

Linklater, R., & Mehl-Madrona, L. (2014). *Decolonizing trauma work: Indigenous stories and strategies*. Winnipeg: Fernwood Publishing.

McCall, J., & Lauridsen-Hoegh, P. (2014). Trauma and cultural safety: Providing quality care to HIV-infected women of Aboriginal descent. *The Journal of the Association of Nurses in AIDS Care, 25*(1S), S70–S78. https://dx.doi.org/10.1016/j.jana.2013.05.005

McCormick, R. (1996). Culturally appropriate means and ends of counselling as described by the First Nations people in British Columbia. *International Journal for the Advancement of Counselling, 18*, 163–172.

McKenzie, K., Agic, B., Tuck, A., & Antwi, M. (2016). *The case for diversity: Building the case to improve mental health services for immigrant, refugee, ethno-cultural and racialized populations*. Ottawa: MHCC Report to the Mental Health Commission of Canada (MHCC).

MacDonald, J. P., Ford, J. D., Willox, A. C., & Ross, N. A. (2013). A review of protective factors and causal mechanisms that enhance the mental health of Indigenous circumpolar youth. *International Journal of Circumpolar Health, 72*(1), 21775. https://doi.org/10.3402/ijch.v72i0.21775

Meeta, N. (2011). Mind-body dualism: A critique from a health perspective. *Mens Sana Monographs, 9*(1), 202–209. https://doi.org/10.4103/0973-1229.77436

Mental Health Commission of Canada. (2009). *Toward recovery and wellbeing: A framework for a mental health strategy in Canada*. Retrieved from https://www.mentalhealthcommission.ca/wp-content/uploads/drupal/FNIM_Toward_Recovery_and_Well_Being_ENG_0_1.pdf

Mental Health Commission of Canada (MHCC). (2012). *Changing directions, changing lives: The mental health strategy for Canada*. Calgary: Author. Retrieved from https://www.mentalhealthcommission.ca/wp-content/uploads/drupal/MHStrategy_Strategy_ENG.pdf

Mental Health Commisssion of Canada (MHCC). (2015). *Guidelines for recovery-oriented practice*. Ottawa: Author. Retrieved from https://www.mentalhealthcommission.ca/sites/default/files/2016-07/MHCC_Recovery_Guidelines_2016_ENG.PDF

Muldoon, K. A., Duff, P. K., Fielden, S., & Anema, A. (2013). Food insufficiency is associated with psychiatric morbidity in a nationally representative study of mental illness among food insecure Canadians. *Social Psychiatry and Psychiatric Epidemiology, 48*, 795–803.

Na, S., Ryder, A. G., & Kirmayer, L. J. (2016). Toward a culturally responsive model of mental health literacy: Facilitating help-seeking among east Asian immigrants to North America. *American Journal of Community Psychology, 58*(1–2), 211–225. https://doi.org/10.1002/ajcp.12085

Napoleon, A. (2009). Language and culture as protective factors for at-risk communities. *Journal of Aboriginal Health*. (November, 2009), 6–25. Retrieved from http://www.ecdip.org/docs/pdf/McIvor_Napoleon%202009.pdf

Narine, S. (2016). Missing and murdered Indigenous women and girls: Commission has authority to conduct MMIWG inquiry as "they see fit." *Windspeaker*. Retrieved from https://windspeaker.com/news/windspeaker-news/commission-has-authority-to-conduct-mmiwg-inquiry-as-they-see-fit

National Inquiry into Missing and Murdered Indigenous Women and Girls. (2019). *Reclaiming power and place. The final report of the national inquiry into missing and murdered indigenous women and girls. The National Inquiry*. Retrieved from https://www.mmiwg-ffada.ca/final-report/

Nelson, S. E., & Wilson, K. (2017). The mental health of Indigenous peoples in Canada: A critical review of research. *Social Science and Medicine, 176*, 93–112. https://doi.org/10.1016/j.socscimed.2017.01.021

Office of the Surgeon General (US), Center for Mental Health Services (US), & National Institute of Mental Health (US). (2001). Mental health: Culture, race, and ethnicity: A supplement to mental health: A report of the Surgeon General. *Substance Abuse and Mental Health Services Administration (US)*. Retrieved from https://pubmed.ncbi.nlm.nih.gov/20669516/

O'Mahony, J. M., & Donnelly, T. T. (2007). Health care providers' perspective of the gender influences on immigrant women's mental health care experiences. *Issues in Mental Health Nursing, 28*(10), 1171–1188. https://doi.org/10.1080/01612840701581289

Ong-Flaherty, C. (2015). Critical cultural awareness and diversity in nursing: *A minority perspective. Nurse Leader, 13*(15), 58–62. https://doi.org/10.1016/j.mnl.2015.03.012

Oppal, W. (2012). *Forsaken: The report of the Missing Women Commission of Inquiry: Executive summary*. Victoria: Government of British Columbia. Retrieved from https://www2.gov.bc.ca/assets/gov/law-crime-and-justice/about-bc-justice-system/inquiries/forsaken-vol_3.pdf

Oudshoorn, A., & Smye, V. L. (2019). Substance use: A critical perspective. In L. L. Stamler, L. Yiu, A. Dosani, J. Etowa, & C. van Daalen-Smith (Eds.), *Community health nursing: A Canadian perspective* (5th ed., Chapter 30, pp. 537–556). Toronto: Pearson.

Park, Y.-J., Kim, H. S., Kang, H.-C., & Kim, J. W. (2001). A survey of Hwa-Byung in middle-age Korean women. *Journal of Transcultural Nursing, 12*, 115–122. https://doi.org/10.1177/104365960101200205

Park, M. M., Zafran, H., Stewart, J., Salsberg, J., Ells, C., Rouleau, S., Esterin, O., & Valente, T. W. (2014). Transforming mental health services: A participatory mixed methods study to promote and evaluate the implementation of recovery-oriented services. *Implementation Science, 9*(1), 119. https://doi.org/10.1186/s13012-014-0119-7

Phelan, J. C., Lucas, J. W., Ridgeway, C. L., & Taylor, C. J. (2014). Stigma, status, and population health. *Social Science & Medicine, 103*, 15–23.

Ramsden, I. (1993). Kawa Whakaruruhau: Cultural safety in nursing education in Aotearoa, New Zealand. *Nursing Praxis in New Zealand, 8*(3), 4–10.

Ramsden, I. (2000). Cultural safety/Kawa whakaruruhau ten years on: A personal overview. *Nursing Praxis in New Zealand, 15*(1), 4–12.

Ross, C. A., & Goldner, E. M. (2009). Stigma, negative attitudes and discrimination towards mental illness within the nursing profession: A review of the literature. *Journal of Psychiatric and Mental Health Nursing, 16*(6), 558–567.

Royal Commission on Aboriginal Peoples. (1996). *Report of the Royal Commission on Aboriginal peoples*. Ottawa: Author. Retrieved from https://www.bac-lac.gc.ca/eng/discover/aboriginal-heritage/royal-commission-aboriginal-peoples/Pages/final-report.aspx

Salmon, A., Poole, N., Morrow, M., Greaves, L., Ingram, R., & Pederson, A. (2006). *Improving conditions: Integrating sex and gender into federal mental health and addictions policy*. Vancouver: The British Columbia Centre of Excellence for Women's Health.

Smye, V., & Browne, A. J. (2002). Cultural safety' and the analysis of health policy affecting Aboriginal people. *Nurse Researcher: The International Journal of Research Methodology in Nursing and Health Care, 9*(3), 42–56. https://doi.org/10.7748/nr2002.04.9.3.42.c6188

Smye, V. L., Browne, A. J., Varcoe, C., & Josewski, V. (2011). Harm reduction, methadone maintenance treatment and the root causes of health and social inequities: An intersectional lens in the Canadian context. *Harm Reduction Journal, 8*, 17. https://doi.org/10.1186/1477-7517-8-17

Smye, V., Varcoe, C., Browne, A., Dion Stout, M., Josewski, V., Ford-Gilboe, M., & Keith, B (2020). Violence at the intersections of women's lives: Indigenous women's experiences of leaving and/or staying with an abusive partner. *Violence Against Women*, 1–22. https://doi.org/10.1177/1077801220947183

Statistics Canada. (2015). *Aboriginal peoples fact sheet for Canada*. Retrieved from https://www150.statcan.gc.ca/n1/pub/89-656-x/89-656-x2015001-eng.htm

Statistics Canada. (2017a). *Statistics on Indigenous peoples*. Retrieved from https://www.statcan.gc.ca/eng/subjects-start/indigenous_peoples

Statistics Canada. (2017b). *Immigration and ethnocultural diversity: Key results from the 2016 Census*. Retrieved from https://www150.statcan.gc.ca/n1/daily-quotidien/171025/dq171025b-eng.htm?indid=14428-1&indgeo=0

Stuart, H., & Arboleda-Flórez, J. (2012). A public health perspective on the stigmatization of mental illness. *Public Health Reviews, 34*(2). https://doi.org/10.1007/BF03391680

Stuart, H. (2016). Reducing the stigma of mental illness. *Global mental health* (Cambridge, England), 3, e17. https://doi.org/10.1017/gmh.2016.11

Tang, S., & Browne, A. J. (2008). "Race" matters: Racialization and egalitarian discourses involving Aboriginal people in the Canadian health care context. *Ethnicity & Health, 2*, 109–127. https://doi.org/10.1080/13557850701830307

Truth and Reconciliation Commission of Canada (TRC). (2015). *Honouring the truth, reconciling for the future: Summary of the final report of the Truth and Reconciliation Commission of Canada*: Author. Retrieved from www.trc.ca

United Nations. (2007). *The United Nations declaration on the rights of Indigenous peoples*. Retrieved from http://www.un.org/esa/socdev/unpfii/documents/DRIPS_en.pdf

United Nations High Commissioner for Refugees. (1951). *Convention relating to the status of refugees*. Retrieved from https://www.ohchr.org/EN/ProfessionalInterest/Pages/StatusOfRefugees.aspx

Urbanoski, K. A. (2017). Need for equity in treatment of substance use among Indigenous people in Canada. *Canadian Medical Associate Journal, 189*(44), E1350–E1351. https://doi.org/10.1503/cmaj.171002

Urbanoski, K., Pauly, B., Inglis, D., Cameron, F., Haddad, T., Phillips, J., Phillips, P., Rosen, C., Schlotter, G., & Hartney, E. (2020). Defining culturally safe primary care for people who use substances: A participatory concept mapping study. *BMC Health Services Research, 20*, 1060. https://doi.org/10.1186/s12913-020-05915-x

Varcoe, C., & Browne, A. J. (2015). Culture and cultural safety: Beyond cultural inventories. In D. Gregory, T. Stephens, C. Raymond-Seniuk, & L. Patrick (Eds.), *Fundamentals: Perspectives on the art and science of Canadian nursing* (pp. 216–231). Philadelphia: Lippincott.

Wilk, P., Maltby, A., & Cook, M. (2017). Residential schools and the effects on Indigenous health and well-being in Canada—A scoping review. *Public Health Reviews, 8*, 38. https://doi.org/10.1186/s40985-017-0055-6

World Health Organization. (2019). *Mental health*. Retrieved from https://www.who.int/health-topics/mental-health#tab=tab_3

Wyatt, R., Laderman, M., Botwinick, L., & Mate, K. (2016). *Achieving health equity: A guide for health care organizations*: IHI. [White paper]. Retrieved from http://www.ihi.org/resources/Pages/IHIWhitePapers/Achieving-Health-Equity.aspx

Yeager, K. A., & Bauer-Wu, S. (2013). Cultural humility: Essential foundation for clinical researchers. *Applied Nursing Research, 26*(4), 251–256. https://doi.org/10.1016/j.apnr.2013.06.008

RESOURCES/NEWS RELEASES

Azpiri, J. (2020). Allegations of B.C. health staff guessing alcohol levels prompt calls to address systemic racism. *Global News*. Retrieved from https://globalnews.ca/news/7089480/bc-health-racist-allegations/

Brian Sinclair Working Group. (2017). *Out of sight*. Manitoba: Author. Retrieved from https://www.dropbox.com/s/wxf3v5uh2pun0pf/Out%20of%20Sight%20Final.pdf?dl=0

Gladue. R. v. (1999). 1999 CanLII 679 (Supreme Court of Canada), 1 SCR 688. Retrieved November 03, 2021 from https://canlii.ca/t/1fqp2

Institute for Integrative Science and Health. (2004). *Two-eyed seeing*: Cape Breton University. Retrieved from http://www.integrativescience.ca/Principles/TwoEyedSeeing/

Lowrie, M., & Malone, K. G. (2020). Joyce Echaquan's death highlights systemic racism in health care, experts say. *CTV News*. Retrieved from https://www.ctvnews.ca/health/joyce-echaquan-s-death-highlights-systemic-racism-in-health-care-experts-say-1.5132146

UNIT 3

Biopsychosocial Interventions

9. Therapeutic Relationships

10. Communication and the Clinical Interview

11. Psychotropic Drugs

9

Therapeutic Relationships

Cheryl L. Pollard
Originating US chapter by Margaret Jordan Halter, Elizabeth M. Varcarolis

 http://evolve.elsevier.com/Canada/Varcarolis/psychiatric/

OBJECTIVES

1. Compare and contrast the three phases of the nurse–patient relationship and the dimensions of the helping relationship.
2. Compare and contrast a social relationship and a therapeutic relationship in terms of purpose, focus, communications style, and goals.
3. Identify at least four patient behaviours a psychiatric nurse may encounter in the clinical setting.
4. Explore qualities that foster a therapeutic nurse–patient relationship and qualities that contribute to a non-therapeutic psychiatric nursing interactive process.
5. Define and discuss the importance of empathy, genuineness, and positive regard in a nurse–patient relationship.
6. Identify two attitudes and four actions that may reflect the nurse's positive regard for a patient.
7. Analyze what is meant by boundaries and the influence of transference and counter-transference on boundary blurring.
8. Understand the use of non-verbal behaviour or body language in the context of the psychiatric nurse–patient relationship of attending behaviours.
9. Discuss the influences of disparate values and cultural beliefs on the therapeutic relationship.

KEY TERMS AND CONCEPTS

clinical supervision
contract
empathy
genuineness
orientation phase
pre-orientation phase
rapport
social relationship
termination phase
therapeutic encounter
therapeutic relationship
therapeutic use of self
values
working phase

Psychiatric mental health nurses practise in a variety of contexts, providing care to individuals, groups, families, and communities. Psychiatric nursing care is both an art and a science. Knowledge of anatomy, physiology, microbiology, and chemistry is the basis for providing safe and effective physiological nursing care. Knowledge of pharmacology, that is, a medication's mechanism of action, indications for use, and adverse effects, based on evidence-informed studies and trials, is central to safe and competent psychiatric nursing practice. However, it is the nurse–patient relationship and the development of the interpersonal skills needed to enhance and maintain such a therapeutic relationship that comprise the art of psychiatric nursing. Moral duties and professional responsibilities are generated from this relationship (Steuber & Pollard, 2018).

♥ HOW A NURSE HELPED ME

Dan's Story: "Our Friend Is Really a Well-Put-Together Guy!"

Our friend Dan was staying at our rural cottage for a long weekend. He had been increasingly stressed in his management job at an engineering firm in the city, where he was responsible for making big decisions that affected a number of employees. We knew Dan had not been sleeping or eating well and was finding his work increasingly difficult, so we offered our place as a sort of retreat while we were away.

When we returned on the Sunday afternoon, it was clear that Dan was in a very bad mental state. He recognized us, but he had not bathed or showered and could not really respond sensibly to any questions—it was almost as though he was speaking another language! My wife and I immediately drove Dan to our regional hospital's emergency department, where a psychiatric mental health nurse met with him. Dan could barely speak at this stage, so my wife and I were included in the interview. We had brought his belongings in with us and discovered he had been taking a strong herbal sleep aid that, in the end, was found to have contributed to the extreme changes—I guess it was a sort of drug reaction.

We were terribly frightened by the whole thing. We had never seen Dan like this before! Throughout the interview, the nurse paused often, spoke in a relaxed way, breathed, and made sure we took breaks to eat at mealtimes. She asked Dan questions directly, even though he was not really taking it all in. When he was unable to answer, the nurse would invite my wife and me to think about our own possible responses. It was the most calming way of helping us all.

At the start of the interview, the nurse told us that "sometimes any number of things can create difficulties in the mood, behaviour, and thinking of people who are normally well put together." I remember my wife and I both spoke at the same time: "You are exactly right. Dan is normally the most well-put-together guy. This is something very out of the ordinary—please help sort it out!" This simple respect for Dan's dignity and acknowledgement of how seriously we took the situation allowed us to establish a good relationship with the nurse, helped get to the root of the problem, and started Dan's treatment in a way that made this complicated mess seem manageable. We felt Dan was in a good position to recover from the acute drug reaction and also his poor sleep and other stress-related troubles. Despite it being a very bad time for Dan—and us, as his friends—we will never forget how the nurse showed us all so much respect and dignity. What could have been an even more stressful as well as embarrassing experience for Dan ended up being okay.

CONCEPTS OF THE NURSE–PATIENT RELATIONSHIP

The nurse–patient relationship is the basis of all psychiatric mental health nursing care, regardless of the specific goals of patient care (Peplau, 1952). To establish a relational practice, the nurse must be self-aware. In addition to understanding the patient's needs, nurses must be aware of their own needs. Relationships are established when boundaries intersect. Therapeutic relationships are grounded in empathy, trust, and respect.

It is argued that many psychiatric disorders, for example, schizophrenia, bipolar disorder, and major depression, have strong biochemical and genetic elements of origin. However, many accompanying emotional problems, such as altered self-concept and self-image, low self-esteem, and difficulties with adherence to a treatment regimen, can be significantly improved through a therapeutic relationship (Knox, 2019). All too often, patients entering psychiatric treatment have exhausted their familial and social resources and find themselves isolated and in need of emotional and spiritual support.

Therapeutic Use of Self

The psychiatric nurse–patient relationship is a creative process unique to each nurse and patient. The notion of the **therapeutic use of self** is rooted within one's individual, genuine ways of being with another person based on one's personal values and beliefs of humanity and enhanced by the application of micro-communication skills (such as warmth, respect, and empathy) to guide the process of developing, maintaining, and terminating a therapeutic relationship. Travelbee (1971) defined therapeutic use of self as "the ability to use one's personality consciously and in full awareness in an attempt to establish relatedness and to structure nursing interventions" (p. 19). It is important to note that the efficacy of this therapeutic use of self has been scientifically substantiated as an evidence-informed intervention (Fisher, 2020).

> **RESEARCH HIGHLIGHT**
>
> **Narrative Descriptions of Miyo-Mahcihoyān (Physical, Emotional, Mental, and Spiritual Well-Being) From a Contemporary Néhiyawak (Plains Cree) Perspective**
>
> **Problem**
> It is unclear why the health and mental status of Indigenous people continue to lag behind those of non-Indigenous people in Canada. The answer is embedded in the Indigenous/non-Indigenous historical relationship, specifically colonization.
>
> **Purpose of Study**
> The primary goal of this research project was to explore factors that improve the mental health and well-being of the néhiyawak from Thunderchild First Nation and what they perceived as necessary to attain optimal mental health and well-being. Second, the first author, an Indigenous woman, wanted to conduct research that was strength based and would give voice to contemporary Indigenous (Plains Cree) people from her community of Thunderchild First Nation, Saskatchewan.
>
> **Methods**
> Narrative inquiry was used to guide the research process, and thematic narrative analysis was used to analyze the data.
>
> **Key Findings**
> The researchers revealed four overarching themes that highlighted what positively affected mental health and well-being. These were (1) relationships, (2) spiritual beliefs and cultural practices, (3) tānisī si wāpahtaman pimātisiwin (world view), and (4) ēkwa ō hi kikwaya piko ka-ispayiki kī spin ka-nohtē-miyo-mahcihoyān (these are the things that need to happen if I want to be healthy).
>
> **Implications for Nursing Practice**
> For Indigenous peoples, honouring Indigenous values and perspectives, which include interconnectedness, reciprocity, language, and ceremony, is the cornerstone of a collaborative therapeutic relationship. The insight gathered from an Indigenous perspective is essential for planning effective health care delivery strategies.
>
> **Source:** Graham, H., & Martin, S. (2016). Narrative descriptions of miyo-mahcihoyān (physical, emotional, mental, and spiritual well-being) from a contemporary néhiyawak (Plains Cree) perspective. *International Journal of Mental Health Systems, 10*(58), 1–12. https://doi.org/10.1186/s13033-016-0086-2

Relationships

A relationship is an interpersonal process that involves two or more people. Throughout life, we meet people in a variety of settings and share a variety of experiences. With some individuals, we develop long-term relationships; with others, the relationship lasts only a short time. Naturally, the kinds of relationships we enter vary from person to person and from situation to situation. Generally, relationships can be defined as intimate, social, or therapeutic. Intimate relationships occur between people who have an emotional commitment to each other. Within intimate relationships, mutual needs are met and intimate desires and fantasies are shared. For our purposes in this chapter, we limit our exploration to the aspects of social and therapeutic relationships.

The psychiatric nurse's needs must be met outside the relationship. When psychiatric nurses begin to want the patient to "like them," "do as they suggest," "be nice to them," or "give them recognition," the needs of the patient cannot be adequately met, and the interaction transitions from being therapeutic to being detrimental (non-therapeutic) to the patient.

Social Relationships

A **social relationship** can be defined as a relationship that is initiated primarily for the purpose of friendship, socialization, enjoyment, or accomplishment of a task. Mutual needs are met during social interaction (e.g., participants share ideas, feelings, and experiences). Communication skills may include giving advice, such as relationship advice, and, sometimes, meeting basic dependency needs, such as offering a listening ear or material support during a stressful time. Social relationships may occur in any type of setting. Generally, there is a relatively equal distribution of power, but this is determined by a variety of social, political, spiritual, and financial factors. For these types of relationships to endure, both individuals have the responsibility to maintain the relationship. Empathy and trust are often present in social relationships; however, the degree of empathy and trust experienced may change as the relationship evolves.

Therapeutic Relationships

Communication skills and knowledge of the stages and phenomena in a therapeutic relationship are critical tools in the formation and maintenance of the therapeutic relationship. A **therapeutic relationship** is defined as a helping relationship based on trust, respect, empathy, compassion, and authenticity. While assisting others in meeting their needs, within this type of relationship, the nurse is goal directed and sensitive to self and others. Additionally, the nurse is keenly aware of power differences between themself and the patient. Many believe that the best treatment for most psychological stressors is a combination of medication and therapeutic approach that has a therapeutic relationship as its foundation. Cognitive behavioural therapy, in particular, has met with great success in the treatment of depression, phobias, obsessive-compulsive disorders, and others.

Establishing a therapeutic relationship with a patient takes time. Competency in relationship building is developed from understanding communication theory and applying it within the context of nursing. With experience and mentoring from experts, nurses will develop expertise along the communication continuum from novice to expert (Benner, 2000). Within the context of a therapeutic relationship, the following occur:

- The needs of the patient are identified and explored.
- Clear boundaries are established.
- Alternative problem-solving approaches are taken.
- New coping skills may be developed.
- Insight is developed, and behavioural change is encouraged.

Upon meeting with the patient, the nurse will begin to explore the patient's ideas, experiences, feelings, and personal issues. The nurse and the patient co-identify areas that need exploration, periodically evaluate the degree of change in the patient's understanding of the stressors, and pinpoint strategies to manage them differently. Although the psychiatric nurse may assume a variety of roles (e.g., teacher, counsellor, socializing agent, liaison), the relationship is consistently focused on the patient's issues, problems, and needs.

Sometimes the type of relationship that occurs may be informal and short lived, such as when the psychiatric nurse and patient meet for only a few sessions. However, even though it is brief, the relationship may be substantial, useful, and important for the patient. This limited relationship is often referred to as a **therapeutic encounter**. When the nurse shows genuine concern for another's circumstances (empathy and compassion), even a short encounter can have a powerful effect. At other times, the encounters may be longer and more formal, such as in inpatient settings, mental health units, crisis centres, and mental health facilities. This longer time span allows the therapeutic nurse–patient relationship to be more fully developed.

Relationship Boundaries

All nurses and nursing students need to approach identifying our boundaries as a reflective exercise focused on self-awareness. All will struggle with the boundaries between social and therapeutic relationships because there is a fine line between the two. In fact, students often feel more comfortable "being a friend" because it is a more familiar role, especially with people close to their own age. However, before a social relationship takes root, the psychiatric nurse or student needs to make it clear (to themself and to the patient) that the relationship is a therapeutic one. This does not mean that the nurse is not friendly toward the patient, and it does not mean that talking about everyday topics (television, weather, children's pictures) is forbidden. It does mean, however, that the nurse must follow the prior stated guidelines regarding a therapeutic relationship: essentially, the focus is on the patient, and the relationship is not designed to meet the psychiatric nurse's needs. The patient's problems and concerns are explored, potential solutions are discussed by both patient and psychiatric nurse, and solutions are implemented by the patient, as in the following example. The Friend responses represent a social relationship.

Patient: "Oh, gosh, I just hate to be alone. It's getting me down, and sometimes it hurts so much."

Nurse: "Loneliness can be painful. Tell me what is going on now that you are feeling so alone."

Friend: "When I feel like that I go skating."

Patient: "Well, my mom died 2 years ago, and last month, my—oh, I am so scared." (Takes a deep breath, looks down, and looks as though she might cry)

Nurse: (Sits in silence while the patient recovers) "Go on … tell me more."

Friend: "Come skating with me. Guaranteed you'll feel better. I have an extra pair of skates that will fit you."

Patient: "My boyfriend left for Afghanistan with his regiment 6 months ago. I haven't heard from him, and they say he's missing. He was my best friend, and we were going to get married, and if he dies, I don't want to live."

Nurse: "Have you thought of wanting to end your life?"

Friend: "Oh my gosh! You didn't tell me that before. No wonder you're depressed. You need to get out of here for a while."

Patient: "Well, if he dies, … I can't live without him."

Nurse: "Have you ever felt like this before?"

Friend: "Come on. You will get through it. I'll be here for you."

Patient: "Yes, when my mom died. I was depressed for about a year until I met my boyfriend."

Nurse: "It sounds as though you are worried, scared, and uncertain whether your boyfriend is alive because you have not heard from him. Perhaps you and I can talk some more and come up with some ways for you to feel less anxious, scared, and overwhelmed. Let's take some time to talk more about this together."

Friend: "You met him when you started to go out again. Didn't you meet him skating?"

For further information on the differences between social and therapeutic relationships, you can visit the College of Nurses of Ontario's website: http://www.cno.org/en/learn-about-standards-guidelines/educational-tools/ask-practice/social-versus-professional-relationships/. The Canadian Nurses Association also has developed a practice standard related to the therapeutic nurse–patient relationship that can be accessed on their website: https://www.cno.org/globalassets/docs/prac/41033_therapeutic.pdf.

Establishing Boundaries

Health care providers will discuss and negotiate boundaries very early in the therapeutic relationship as they use a patient-centred model to guide their practice. From a bioethical perspective, boundaries are necessary primarily to protect the patient from harm: non-maleficence. Establishing and maintaining boundaries is an essential competency for psychiatric mental health nurses. Within therapeutic relationships, boundaries are commonly established to protect the space between the professional's power and the patient's vulnerability.

Sharing of the patient's ideas, thoughts, feelings, and behaviours, thus providing the opportunity to develop insight and explore barriers to achieving patient goals, is a very powerful experience. To ensure that the nurse or patient is not harmed within a therapeutic relationship, clear boundaries must be established. Boundaries are commonly established using strategies from the following four areas.

- Treatment planning and delivery: anticipated length of treatment or service delivery, limits of confidentiality, members of treatment team, limits on interactions, how frequently you meet, etc.
- Space: personal space, physical space, emotional space, agreement between nurse and patient as to roles and responsibilities of all involved in the therapeutic relationship (nurse, patient, and family), and so forth.
- Comportment: act on the belief that dress and language reflect the nurse's respect for whom they provide care. Other examples include professional dress, language, how you react to others, limited self-disclosure, social media use, means of identification, and professional image.
- Location of service delivery: inpatient unit, community clinic, home visits, treatment room, conference room, and other such places.

Health professionals need to constantly assess the effectiveness of their boundaries. When there is a shift in the dynamics of the relationship associated with power and vulnerability, the boundaries become blurred and the resulting shift in the psychiatric nurse–patient relationship may lead to non-therapeutic dynamics. Two common circumstances in which nursing boundaries are blurred occur (1) when the relationship becomes social and (2) when the nurse's needs (for attention, affection, money, sex, emotional or spiritual support) are met at the expense of the patient. Breaches in therapeutic boundaries, whether intentional or not, result in patient harm.

Blurring of Boundaries

The most egregious boundary violations are those related to physical or sexual abuse. These types of violations result in malpractice actions and may result in the loss of professional licensure on the part of the nurse. Other boundary issues are not as obvious. Table 9.1 illustrates some examples of patient and psychiatric nurse behaviours that reflect blurred boundaries.

Transference. Patients experience positive or negative thoughts, feelings, and reactions that are realistic and appropriate and not a result of transference onto the health care provider. Most therapeutic relationships are not negatively impacted because of transference. For example, if a nurse makes promises to the patient that are not kept (e.g., not showing up for a scheduled meeting), the patient may feel resentment for and mistrust of the nurse. Transference, originally identified by Sigmund Freud when he used psychoanalysis to treat patients, occurs when the patient unconsciously and inappropriately displaces (transfers) onto the nurse the patient's feelings and behaviours related to significant figures in the patient's past (see Chapter 4). The patient may even say, "You remind me of my (mother, sister, father, brother, or so on)."

Patient: "Oh, you are so high and mighty. Did anyone ever tell you that you are a cold, unfeeling machine, just like others I know?"

Nurse: "Tell me about one person who is cold and unfeeling toward you." (In this example the patient is experiencing the nurse in the same way he experienced a significant other or others during his formative years. In this case the patient's mother was very aloof, leaving him with feelings of isolation, worthlessness, and anger.)

Although transference occurs to some degree in all relationships, it is intensified in relationships of authority. One theory is that transference occurs in therapeutic relationships because parental figures were the original figures of authority. Physicians, nurses, and social workers are all potential objects of transference. This transference may be positive or negative. The following is an example of how to address "positive" transference. If a patient is motivated to work with you, completes all assignments between sessions, and shares feelings openly and easily, the nurse should engage in self-reflection. The self-reflection would include asking yourself, "Is the speed of progress and improvement related to some transference issues?" "How do these patient behaviours compare to others?" "If there is a difference, what might contribute to this difference?" "How is this difference affecting me?" "Is the care I'm providing different?"

Negative forms of transference include the desire for affection or respect and the gratification of dependency needs. Other transferred feelings are hostility, jealousy, competitiveness, and love. The nurse and patient will explore these feelings within the context of the therapeutic relationship. It is not uncommon for nurses to experience a counter-transference reaction when the nurse has not accurately assessed the signs and symptoms of transference or when there is a lack of self-awareness.

Counter-transference. Counter-transference occurs when the nurse unconsciously displaces feelings and behaviours related to significant figures and relationships in the nurse's past onto the patient. When exhibiting counter-transference, the nurse's ability to utilize their emotional intelligence is inhibited. For example, it is normal to feel angry when attacked persistently, annoyed when frustrated unreasonably, or flattered when idealized. However, when personally attacked and the nurse feels rage, this could be a result of counter-transference. Another example is the nurse who is flattered by a patient and feels desirable and physically attractive. Counter-transference, even though unconscious, precipitates stigma, discrimination, and alienation. For example:

TABLE 9.1 Patient and Nurse Behaviours That Reflect Blurred Boundaries

When the Psychiatric Nurse Is Overly Involved	When the Psychiatric Nurse Is Not Involved
More frequent requests for assistance by the patient, which causes increased dependency on the psychiatric nurse	Patient's increased verbal or physical expression of isolation (depression)
Inability of the patient to perform tasks that they are known to have been capable of prior to the psychiatric nurse's help, which causes regression	Lack of mutually agreed-upon goals
Unwillingness on the part of the patient to maintain performance or progress in the psychiatric nurse's absence	Lack of progress toward goals
Expressions of anger by other staff who do not agree with the psychiatric nurse's interventions or perceptions of the patient	Psychiatric nurse's avoidance of spending time with the patient
Psychiatric nurse's keeping of secrets about the psychiatric nurse–patient relationship	Failure of the psychiatric nurse to follow through on agreed-upon interventions

Source: Pilette, P. C., Berck, C. B., & Achber, L. C. (1995). Therapeutic management of helping boundaries. *Journal of Psychosocial Nursing and Mental Health Services, 33*(1), 40–47. Reprinted with permission from SLACK Incorporated.

Patient: "Yeah, well I decided not to go to that dumb group. 'Hi, I'm so-and-so, and I'm an alcoholic.' Who cares?" (Sits slumped in a chair chewing gum, non-chalantly looking around)

Nurse: (In a very impassioned tone) "You always sabotage your chances. You need AA to get in control of your life. Last week you were going to go, and now you've disappointed everyone." (Here the nurse is reminded of his mother, who was an alcoholic. He had tried everything to get his mother into treatment and took it as a personal failure and deep disappointment that his mother never sought recovery. After the psychiatric nurse sorts out his thoughts and feelings and realizes that the frustration and feelings of disappointment and failure belonged with his mother and not the patient, he starts the next session with the following approach.)

Nurse: "Look, I was thinking about last week, and I realize the decision to go to AA or find other help is solely up to you. It's true that I would like you to live a fuller and more satisfying life, but it's your decision. I'm wondering, however, what happened to change your mind about going to AA."

A nurse feeling either a strongly positive or a strongly negative reaction to a patient most often signals counter-transference and needs further investigation. One common sign of counter-transference is over-identification with the patient. In this situation the nurse may have difficulty recognizing or objectively seeing patient problems that are similar to the nurse's own problems. The patient is at risk for harm if counter-transference is not closely examined and actions taken to minimize the risk. For example, a nurse who is struggling with an alcoholic family member may feel uninterested in, cold toward, or disgusted by an alcoholic patient. This nurse would consult with other members of the team or a more experienced clinician about the dynamics of the relationship. Other indicators of counter-transference are the nurse's becoming involved in an argument with the patient or their family or the nurse applying employer rules without regard for individual patient experiences and resources. Table 9.2 lists some common counter-transference reactions.

Identifying and working through various transference and counter-transference issues is central to working therapeutically with the patient. In order for the nurse to achieve professional growth and meet the patient's needs, transference and counter-transference issues must be effectively managed. Transference and counter-transference, as well as numerous other issues, are best dealt with through the use of mentorship, sometimes referred to as clinical supervision, by either the peer group or the therapeutic team. Besides helping with boundary issues, clinical supervision supplies practical and emotional support, education, and guidance regarding ethical issues. Regular mentorship and clinical supervision sessions provide the psychiatric nurse with the opportunity to increase self-awareness and improve clinical skills to better meet patient needs and growth, as well as allow for the continued growth of the patient.

Self-Check on Boundaries

It is useful for all of us to take time out to be reflective and aware of our thoughts and actions with patients, as well as with colleagues, friends, and family. Figure 9.1 is a helpful boundary self-test you can use throughout your career, no matter what area of nursing you choose.

VALUES, BELIEFS, AND SELF-AWARENESS

Values are abstract standards that represent an ideal, either positive or negative. It is crucial that we have an understanding of our own values and attitudes so that we may become aware of the beliefs or attitudes we hold that may interfere with establishing positive therapeutic relationships with patient groups.

When working with patients, it is important for nurses to understand that their values and beliefs are not necessarily "right" and certainly are not right for everyone. It is helpful to realize that our values and beliefs (1) reflect our own culture or sub-culture, (2) are derived from a range of choices, and (3) are those we have chosen for ourselves from a variety of influences and role models. These chosen values (religious, cultural, societal) guide us in making decisions and taking actions that we hope will make our lives meaningful, rewarding, and fulfilling.

Interviewing others whose values, beliefs, cultures, or lifestyles are radically different from our own can be a challenge. Several topics that cause controversy in society in general, including religion, gender roles, abortion, war, politics, money, drugs, alcohol, sex, and corporal punishment, also can cause conflict between nurses and patients.

Although we emphasize that the patient and nurse should identify outcomes together, what happens when the psychiatric nurse's values, beliefs, and interpretive system are very different from those of a patient? How can nurses develop working relationships and help patients solve problems when patients' values, goals, and interpretive systems are so different from their own? Self-awareness requires that we understand what we value and the beliefs that guide our own behaviour. It is critical that as nurses, we not only understand and accept our own values and beliefs but also are sensitive to and accepting of the unique and different values and beliefs of others. Supervision by an experienced colleague can prove invaluable in helping us to develop this sensitivity. Chapter 7 explores this further as it relates to conscientious objection.

PEPLAU'S MODEL OF THE NURSE–PATIENT RELATIONSHIP

Hildegard Peplau introduced the concept of the nurse–patient relationship in 1952 in her ground-breaking book *Interpersonal Relations in Nursing*. This model of the nurse–patient relationship is well accepted in the United States and Canada (Registered Nurses' Association of Ontario, 2002) and has become an important tool for all nursing practice. A professional nurse–patient relationship includes a mutually engaged relationship. This is a nurse who has skills and expertise and a patient who wants to alleviate suffering, find solutions to problems, explore different avenues to an improved quality of life, find an advocate, or do any combination of these.

Peplau (1952) proposed that the nurse–patient relationship "facilitates forward movement" for both the nurse and the patient (p. 12). The ability of the nurse to engage in interpersonal interactions in a goal-directed manner to assist patients with their emotional, spiritual, or physical health needs is the foundation of the therapeutic nurse–patient relationship. The following are necessary behaviours of all health care workers, including nurses:

- Accountability—Psychiatric nurses assume responsibility for their conduct and the consequences of their actions.
- Focus on patient needs—The interest of the patient, rather than that of the nurse, other health care workers, or the institution, is given first consideration. The psychiatric nurse's role is that of patient advocate.
- Clinical competence—The criteria on which the nurse bases their conduct are principles of knowledge and the most appropriate actions for specific situations. This knowledge and action involve awareness and incorporation of the latest knowledge available from research (evidence-informed practice).
- Delaying judgement—Ideally, nurses refrain from judging patients and avoid inflicting their own values and beliefs on others.
- Reflection—Reflection is ideally done with the guidance of an experienced clinician or team and is essential to developing self-awareness and clinical competence in establishing therapeutic relationships.

TABLE 9.2 Common Counter-Transference Reactions

As a nurse, you will sometimes experience counter-transference feelings. Once you are aware of them, use them for self-analysis to understand those feelings that may inhibit productive nurse–patient communication.

Reaction To Patient	Behaviours Characteristic of the Reaction	Self-Analysis	Solution
Boredom (indifference)	Showing inattention Frequently asking the patient to repeat statements Making inappropriate responses	Is the content of what the patient presents uninteresting? Or is it the style of communication? Does the patient exhibit an offensive style of communication? Have you anything else on your mind that may be distracting you from the patient's needs? Is the patient discussing an issue that makes you anxious?	Redirect the patient if they provide more information than you need or go "off track" Clarify information with the patient Confront ineffective modes of communication
Rescue	Reaching for unattainable goals Resisting peer feedback and supervisory recommendations Giving advice	What behaviour stimulates your perceived need to rescue the patient? Has anyone evoked such feelings in you in the past? What are your fears or fantasies about failing to meet the patient's needs? Why do you want to rescue this patient?	Avoid secret alliances Develop realistic goals Do not alter the meeting schedule Let the patient guide the interaction Facilitate patient problem solving
Overinvolvement	Coming to work early, leaving late Ignoring peer suggestions, resisting assistance Buying the patient clothes or other gifts Accepting the patient's gifts Behaving judgementally at family interventions Keeping secrets Calling the patient when off duty	What particular patient characteristics are attractive? Does the patient remind you of someone? Who? Does your current behaviour differ from your treatment of similar patients in the past? What are you getting out of this situation? What needs of yours are being met?	Establish firm treatment boundaries, goals, and nursing expectations Avoid self-disclosure Avoid calling the patient when off duty
Overidentification	Having a special agenda, keeping secrets Increasing self-disclosure Feeling omnipotent Experiencing physical attraction	With which of the patient's physical, emotional, cognitive, or situational characteristics do you identify? Recall similar circumstances in your own life. How did you deal with the issues now being created by the patient?	Allow the patient to direct issues Encourage a problem-solving approach from the patient's perspective Avoid self-disclosure
Misuse of honesty	Withholding information Lying	Why are you protecting the patient? What are your fears about the patient learning the truth?	Be clear in your responses and aware of your hesitation; do not hedge If you can provide information, tell the patient and give your rationale Avoid keeping secrets Reinforce the interdisciplinary nature of treatment
Anger	Withdrawing Speaking loudly Using profanity Asking to be taken off the case	What patient behaviours are offensive to you? What dynamic from your past may this patient be re-creating?	Determine the origin of the anger (nurse, patient, or both) Explore the roots of patient anger Avoid contact with the patient if you do not understand the roots of the anger
Helplessness or hopelessness	Feeling sadness	Which patient behaviours evoke these feelings in you? Has anyone evoked similar feelings in the past? Who? What past expectations were placed on you (verbally and non-verbally) by this patient?	Maintain therapeutic involvement Explore and focus on the patient's experience rather than on your own

Source: Aromando, L. (1995). *Mental health and psychiatric nursing* (2nd ed.). Springhouse: Springhouse.

NURSING BOUNDARY INDEX SELF-CHECK

Please rate yourself according to the frequency with which the following statements reflect your behavior, thoughts, or feelings within the past 2 years while providing patient care.*

	Never	Rarely	Sometimes	Often
1. Have you ever received any feedback about your behavior being overly intrusive with patients and their families?	____	____	____	____
2. Do you ever have difficulty setting limits with patients?	____	____	____	____
3. Do you ever arrive early or stay late to be with your patient for a longer period?	____	____	____	____
4. Do you ever find yourself relating to patients or peers as you might to a family member?	____	____	____	____
5. Have you ever acted on sexual feelings you have for a patient?	____	____	____	____
6. Do you feel that you are the only one who understands the patient?	____	____	____	____
7. Have you ever received feedback that you get "too involved" with patients or families?	____	____	____	____
8. Do you derive conscious satisfaction from patients' praise, appreciation, or affection?	____	____	____	____
9. Do you ever feel that other staff members are too critical of "your" patient?	____	____	____	____
10. Do you ever feel that other staff members are jealous of your relationship with your patient?	____	____	____	____
11. Have you ever tried to "match-make" a patient with one of your friends?	____	____	____	____
12. Do you find it difficult to handle patients' unreasonable requests for assistance, verbal abuse, or sexual language?	____	____	____	____

*Any item that is responded to with "Sometimes" or "Often" should alert the nurse to a possible area of vulnerability. If the item is responded to with "Rarely," the nurse should determine whether it is an isolated event or a possible pattern of behavior.

Fig. 9.1 Nursing Boundary Index Self-Check. (**Source:** Pilette, P., Berck, C., & Achber, L. (1995). Therapeutic management of helping boundaries. *Journal of Psychosocial Nursing and Mental Health Services, 33*(1), 45. Reprinted with permission from SLACK Incorporated.)

Peplau (1952, 1997) described the nurse–patient relationship as evolving through distinct interlocking and overlapping phases, generally recognized as:
1. Orientation phase
2. Working phase
3. Termination phase

An additional **pre-orientation phase**, during which the nurse prepares for the orientation phase, for instance, by familiarizing themself with the patient's background or engaging in self-reflection and other learning, has also since been identified. Most likely, you will not have time to develop all phases of the nurse–patient relationship in a brief student practice experience. However, it is important to be aware of these phases in order to recognize and consciously engage in them in your nursing practice and in the patient's experience with the treatment team. It is also important to remember that any contact that is caring, respectful, and demonstrative of concern for the situation of another person can have an enormous positive impact, as illustrated by Dan's story earlier in this chapter (see How a Nurse Helped Me box earlier).

Pre-orientation Phase

Even before the first meeting, the psychiatric nurse may have many thoughts and feelings related to the first clinical session. Novice health care providers typically experience concerns and anxiety on their first practice days. These universal concerns include being afraid of people with psychiatric problems, saying "the wrong thing," and not knowing what to do in response to certain patient behaviours. Table 9.3 identifies common patient behaviours (e.g., crying, asking the nurse to keep a secret, threatening to commit suicide, giving a gift, wanting physical contact with the nurse) and gives examples of possible reactions by the nurse and suggested responses.

Talking with an instructor and participating in supervised peer group discussion will promote confidence and produce feedback and suggestions to prepare students for clinical practice. To prepare you for your first clinical day, your instructor will set the ground rules for safety. For example, do not go into a patient's room alone, know if there are any patients not to engage, stay in an open area where other people are around, and know the signs and symptoms of escalating anxiety. You should always trust your own instincts. If you feel uncomfortable for any reason, excuse yourself for a moment and discuss your feelings with your instructor or a staff member. In addition to getting reassurance and support, students can often provide valuable information about the patient's condition by sharing their perceptions.

Most experienced psychiatric mental health nursing faculty and staff are able to skillfully assess the unit atmosphere and behaviours that may indicate escalating tension. They are trained in crisis intervention, and formal security is often available on-site to give the staff support.

TABLE 9.3 Common Patient Behaviours, Possible Nurse Reactions, and Suggested Nurse Responses

Possible Reactions	Useful Responses
If the Patient Threatens Suicide ...	
The nurse may feel overwhelmed or responsible for "talking the patient out of it."	The nurse assesses whether the patient has a plan and the lethality of the plan.
The nurse may pick up some of the patient's feelings of hopelessness.	The nurse tells the patient that this situation is serious, that the nurse does not want harm to come to the patient, and that this information needs to be shared with other staff: "This is very serious, Mr. Lamb. I don't want any harm to come to you. I'll have to share this with the other staff."
	The nurse can then discuss with the patient the feelings and circumstances that led to this decision. (Refer to Chapter 22 for strategies for suicide intervention.)
If the Patient Asks the Nurse to Keep a Secret ...	
The nurse may feel conflict because they want the patient to share important information but are unsure about making such a promise.	The nurse cannot make such a promise. The information may be important to the health or safety of the patient or others: "I cannot make that promise. It might be important for me to share the information with other staff."
	The patient then decides whether to share the information
If the Patient Asks the Nurse a Personal Question ...	
The nurse may think that it is rude not to answer the patient's question.	The nurse may or may not answer the patient's query. If the nurse decides to answer a natural question, they answer in a word or two, then return the focus to the patient:
A new psychiatric nurse might feel relieved to put off having to start the interview.	*Patient:* Are you married?
The nurse may feel put on the spot and want to leave the situation.	*Nurse:* Yes. Do you have a spouse? *Patient:* Do you have any children?
New nurses are often manipulated by a patient into changing roles, thereby keeping the focus off the patient and preventing the building of a relationship.	*Nurse:* This time is for you. Tell me about yourself. *Patient:* You can just tell me if you have any children. *Nurse:* This is your time to focus on your concerns. Tell me something about your family.
If the Patient Makes Sexual Advances ...	
The nurse feels uncomfortable but may feel conflicted about "rejecting" the patient or making them feel "unattractive" or "not good enough."	The nurse needs to set clear limits on expected behaviour: "I'm not comfortable having you touch (kiss) me. This time is for you to focus on your problems and concerns."
	Frequently restating the nurse's role throughout the relationship can help maintain boundaries. If the patient does not stop the behaviour, the nurse might say: "If you can't stop this behaviour, I'll have to leave. I'll be back at [time] to spend time with you then."
	Leaving gives the patient time to gain control. The nurse returns at the stated time.
If the Patient Cries ...	
The nurse may feel uncomfortable and experience increased anxiety or feel somehow responsible for making the person cry.	The nurse should stay with the patient and reinforce that it is all right to cry. Often, it is at that time that feelings are closest to the surface and can be best identified:
	"You seem ready to cry."
	"You are still upset about your brother's death."
	"Tell me what you are thinking right now."
	The psychiatric nurse offers tissues when appropriate.
If the Patient Leaves Before the Session Is Over ...	
The nurse may feel rejected, thinking it was something that they did. The nurse may experience increased anxiety or feel abandoned by the patient.	Some patients are not able to relate for long periods without experiencing an increase in anxiety.
	Some patients may be testing the nurse: "I'll wait for you here for 15 minutes, until our time is up."
	During this time, the nurse does not engage in conversation with any other patient or even with the staff.
	When the time is up, the nurse approaches the patient, says the time is up, and restates the day and time of their next meeting.
If the Patient Does Not Want to Talk ...	
The nurse new to this situation may feel rejected or ineffectual.	At first, the nurse might say something to this effect: "It's all right. I would like to spend time with you. We don't have to talk."
	The nurse might spend short, frequent periods (e.g., 5 minutes) with the patient throughout the day: "Our 5 minutes is up. I'll be back at 10 o'clock and stay with you 5 more minutes."
	This response gives the patient the opportunity to understand that the nurse means what they say and consistently returns on time. It also gives the patient time between visits to assess how they feel, to formulate thoughts about the nurse, and perhaps to feel less threatened.

Continued

TABLE 9.3 Common Patient Behaviours, Possible Nurse Reactions, and Suggested Nurse Responses—cont'd

Possible Reactions	Useful Responses
If the Patient Gives the Nurse a Present …	
The nurse may feel uncomfortable when offered a gift. The meaning needs to be examined. Is the gift (1) a way of getting better care, (2) a way to maintain self-esteem, (3) a way of making the nurse feel guilty, (4) a sincere expression of thanks, or (5) a cultural expectation?	Possible guidelines: If the gift is expensive, the only policy is to graciously refuse. If it is inexpensive, then (1) if it is given at the end of hospitalization when a relationship has developed, graciously accept; (2) if it is given at the beginning of the relationship, graciously refuse and explore the meaning behind the present: "Thank you, but it is our job to care for our patients. Are you concerned that some aspect of your care will be overlooked?" If the gift is money, it is always graciously refused.
If Another Patient Interrupts During Time With Your Current Patient …	
The nurse may feel a conflict: they do not want to appear rude. Sometimes the nurse tries to engage both patients in conversation.	The time the nurse had contracted with a selected patient is that patient's time. By keeping their part of the contract, the nurse demonstrates commitment and conviction that the sessions are important: "I am with Mr. Rob for the next 20 minutes. At 10 o'clock, after our time is up, I can talk to you for 5 minutes."

TABLE 9.4 Guidelines for Maintaining Safety When a Patient's Anger Escalates

Nursing Intervention	Rationale
Pay attention to angry and aggressive behaviour. Respond as early as possible.	Minimization of angry behaviours and ineffective limit setting are the most frequent factors contributing to the escalation of violence.
Assess for and provide for personal safety. Pay attention to the environment: • Leave door open or use hallway. Interact with the patient in a quiet place that is visible to staff. • Have a quick exit available. The more angry the patient, the more space they will need to feel comfortable. Never turn your back on an angry patient. Leave immediately if there are signs that behaviour is escalating out of control or if you are uncomfortable. State, "I am leaving now. I will be back in 10 minutes," and seek out your clinical instructor or another staff member right away.	Exercising basic caution is essential to protecting yourself. Although the risk for violence may be minimal, it is easier to prevent a problem than to get out of a bad situation. These precautions are similar to using universal precautions (gloves, masks, gowns, etc.) on medical floors.
Appear calm and in control.	The perception that someone is in control can be comforting and calming to an individual whose anxiety is beginning to escalate.
Speak softly in a non-provocative, non-judgemental manner.	When tone of voice is low and calm and the words are spoken slowly, anxiety levels in others may decrease.
Demonstrate genuineness and concern.	Even the most psychotic individual with schizophrenia may respond to non-provocative interpersonal contact and expressions of concern and caring.
If patient is willing, both the psychiatric nurse and the patient should sit at a 45-degree angle. Do not tower over or stare at the patient.	Sitting at a 45-degree angle puts you both on the same level but allows for frequent breaks in eye contact. Towering over or staring at someone can be interpreted as threatening or controlling by paranoid individuals.
When the patient begins to talk, listen. Use clarification techniques.	Active listening allows the patient to feel heard and understood, helps build rapport, and can productively channel energy.

There are actions a psychiatric nurse can take if a patient's anger begins to escalate, many of which are presented in Table 9.4. Chapter 23 offers a more detailed discussion of maintaining personal safety, recognizing potential agitation, and intervening with angry or aggressive patients. Refer to Chapter 10 for a detailed discussion of communication strategies used in clinical practice.

Orientation Phase

The orientation phase can last for a few meetings or extend over a longer period. It marks the first time the nurse and the patient meet and is the phase during which the nurse conducts the initial interview (see Chapter 10). When strangers meet, they interact according to their own backgrounds, standards, values, and experiences. The fact that each person has a unique frame of reference underlies the need for self-awareness on the part of the nurse. The initial interview includes the following aspects:

- An atmosphere is established in which rapport can grow.
- The nurse's role is clarified, and the responsibilities (parameters) of both the patient and the nurse are defined.
- The contract containing the time, place, date, and duration of the meetings is discussed.
- Confidentiality is discussed and assumed.

- The terms of termination are introduced (these are also discussed throughout the orientation phase and beyond).
- The nurse becomes aware of transference and counter-transference issues.
- Patient problems are articulated, and mutually agreed-upon goals are established.

Establishing Rapport

A major emphasis during the first few encounters with the patient is on providing an atmosphere in which trust and understanding, or rapport, can grow. As in any relationship, **rapport** can be nurtured by demonstrating genuineness and empathy, developing positive regard, showing consistency, and offering assistance in problem solving and providing support.

Parameters of the Relationship

The patient needs to know about the psychiatric mental health nurse (who the nurse is and the nurse's background) and the purpose of the meetings. For example, a student might provide the following information:

    Student: "Hello, Mrs. Almodovar. I am Jim Thompson from the university. I am in my psychiatric rotation and will be coming here for the next six Thursdays. I would like to spend time with you each Thursday while you are here. I'm here to be a support person for you as you work on your treatment goals."

Formal or Informal Contract

A contract emphasizes the patient's participation and responsibility because it shows that the psychiatric nurse does something *with* the patient rather than *for* the patient. The **contract**, either stated or written, contains the place, time, date, and duration of the meetings. During the orientation phase, the patient may begin to express thoughts and feelings, identify problems, and discuss realistic goals. Mutual agreement about those goals is also part of the contract. Students also make this contract with patients they interact with.

    Student: "Mrs. Almodovar, we will meet at 10 o'clock each Thursday in the consultation room at the clinic for 45 minutes. We can use that time for further discussion of your feelings of loneliness and anger and explore some strategies you could use to make the situation better for yourself."

Confidentiality

The patient has a right to know (1) that specific information may be shared with others on the treatment team and (2) who else will be given the information (e.g., a clinical supervisor, the physician, the staff, or, if the nurse is in training, other students in conference). The patient also needs to know that the information will not be shared with relatives, friends, or others outside the treatment team, except in extreme situations. Extreme situations include (1) child or elder abuse, (2) threats of self-harm or of harm to others, and (3) intention not to follow through with the treatment plan.

If information must be shared with others, it is usually the physician who will share it, according to legal guidelines (see Chapter 7). The psychiatric nurse must be aware of the patient's right to confidentiality and must not violate that right. Safeguarding the privacy and confidentiality of patients is not only an ethical obligation but a legal responsibility as well (Wong et al., 2015). For example, a student may say:

    Student: "Mrs. Almodovar, I will be sharing some of what we discuss with my nursing instructor, and at times I may discuss certain concerns with my peers in conference or with the staff. However, I will not be sharing this information with your husband or any other members of your family or anyone outside the hospital without your permission."

Planning for Terms of Termination

Termination is the last phase in Peplau's model, but planning for termination actually begins in the orientation phase. It also may be mentioned, when appropriate, during the working phase if the nature of the relationship is time limited (e.g., six or nine sessions). The date of the termination should be clear from the beginning. In some situations the nurse–patient contract may be renegotiated once the termination date has been reached. In other situations when the therapeutic psychiatric nurse–patient relationship is an open-ended one, the termination date is not known.

    Student: "Mrs. Almodovar, as I mentioned earlier, our last meeting will be on October 25. We will have three more meetings after today."

Working Phase

The development of a strong working relationship can provide support and safety for the patient, who may experience increased levels of anxiety and demonstrate dysfunctional behaviours while trying out new and more adaptive coping behaviours. In Moore and Hartman (1988, pp. 92–117) identified specific tasks of the **working phase** of the nurse–patient relationship that remain relevant in current practice:

- Maintain the relationship.
- Gather further data.
- Promote the patient's problem-solving skills, self-esteem, and use of language.
- Facilitate behavioural change.
- Overcome resistance behaviours.
- Evaluate problems and goals, and redefine them as necessary.
- Promote practice and expression of alternative adaptive behaviours.

During the working phase, the psychiatric nurse and patient together identify and explore areas that are causing problems in the patient's life. Often the patient's present ways of handling situations stem from earlier means of coping devised to survive in a chaotic and dysfunctional family environment. Although certain coping methods may have worked for the patient at an earlier age, they now interfere with the patient's interpersonal relationships and prevent the attainment of current goals. The patient's dysfunctional behaviours and basic assumptions about the world are often defensive, and the patient is usually unable to change the dysfunctional behaviour at will. Therefore most of the problem behaviours or thoughts continue because of unconscious motivations and needs that are beyond the patient's awareness.

The psychiatric nurse can work with the patient to identify unconscious motivations and assumptions that keep the patient from finding satisfaction and reaching their potential. Describing, and often re-experiencing, old conflicts generally awakens high levels of anxiety. Patients may use various defences against anxiety and displace their feelings onto the nurse. Therefore during the working phase, intense emotions such as anxiety, anger, self-hate, hopelessness, and helplessness may surface. Defence mechanisms, such as acting out anger inappropriately, withdrawing, intellectualizing, manipulating, and denying are to be expected.

During the working phase, the patient may unconsciously transfer strong feelings about or for significant others from the past into the present and onto the nurse (transference). The emotional responses and behaviours of the patient may also awaken strong counter-transference feelings in the psychiatric nurse. The nurse's awareness of these personal feelings and of reactions to the patient are vital for effective interaction with the patient.

Termination Phase

The **termination phase** is the final, integral phase of the nurse–patient relationship. Termination is discussed during the first interview and

again during the working stage at appropriate times. Termination occurs when the patient is discharged. The tasks of termination are to:
- Summarize the goals and objectives achieved in the relationship.
- Discuss ways for the patient to incorporate into daily life any new coping strategies learned.
- Review situations that occurred during the nurse–patient relationship.
- Exchange memories, which can help validate the experience for both the nurse and the patient and facilitate closure of the relationship.

Termination can stimulate strong feelings in both the nurse and the patient. Termination of the relationship signifies a loss for both, although the intensity and meaning of termination may be different for each. If a patient has unresolved feelings of abandonment, loneliness, being unwanted, or rejection, these feelings may be re-awakened during the termination process. This process can be an opportunity for the patient to express these feelings, perhaps for the first time.

Important reasons for the nurse to engage consciously in the termination phase of the therapeutic relationship include the following:
- Feelings are aroused in both the patient and the nurse about the experience they have had; when these feelings are recognized and shared, patients learn that it is acceptable to feel sadness and loss when someone they care about leaves.
- Termination can be a learning experience; patients can learn that they are important to at least one person, and psychiatric nurses learn continually from each clinical experience and patient encounter.
- By sharing the termination experience with the patient, the psychiatric nurse demonstrates genuineness and caring for the patient.
- This encounter may be the first successful termination experience for the patient.

If a psychiatric nurse has been working with a patient for a while, it is important for the nurse to bring into awareness any feelings or reactions the patient may be experiencing related to separations. If a patient denies that the termination is having an effect (assuming that the nurse–patient relationship was strong), the nurse may say something like, "Goodbyes are difficult for people. Often they remind us of other goodbyes. Tell me about another separation in your past." If the patient appears to be displacing anger, either by withdrawing or by being overtly angry at the nurse, the nurse may use generalized statements such as "People may experience anger when saying goodbye. Sometimes they are angry with the person who is leaving. Tell me how you feel about my leaving."

New practitioners and students in a psychiatric nursing setting need to give serious thought to their final clinical experience with a patient and work with their supervisor or instructor to facilitate communication during this time. A common response of beginning practitioners and of students is feeling guilty about terminating the relationship. These feelings may, in rare cases, be manifested by the student's giving the patient their telephone number, making plans to get together for coffee after the patient is discharged, continuing to see the patient afterward, or exchanging emails or other communications. Often such actions are in response to the student's need to feel less guilty for using the patient to meet learning needs, to maintain a feeling of being important to the patient, or to sustain the illusion that the student is the only one who understands the patient, among other student-centred rationales. Maintaining contact with a patient after discharge, however, is not acceptable and is in opposition to the goals of a therapeutic relationship.

Indeed, part of the termination process may be to explore, after discussion with the patient's case manager, the patient's plans for the future: where the patient can go for help, which agencies to contact, and which people may best help the patient find appropriate and helpful resources.

WHAT HINDERS AND WHAT HELPS THE NURSE–PATIENT RELATIONSHIP

Not all nurse–patient relationships follow the classic phases outlined by Peplau. Some start in the orientation phase and move to a mutually frustrating phase and finally to mutual withdrawal (Figure 9.2).

Forchuk and colleagues (2000) conducted a qualitative study of the nurse–patient relationship. They examined the phases of both therapeutic and non-therapeutic relationships. From this study, they identified certain behaviours that were beneficial to the progression of the nurse–patient relationship, as well as those that hampered its development. The study emphasized that consistent, regular, and private interactions with patients are essential to the development of a therapeutic relationship. Nurses in this study stressed the importance of consistency, pacing, and listening. Specifically, the study found evidence that the following factors enhanced the nurse–patient relationship, allowing it to progress in a mutually satisfying manner:

- Consistency—ensuring that a nurse is always assigned to the same patient and that the patient has a regular routine for activities. Interactions are facilitated when they are frequent and regular in duration, format, and location. The importance of consistency extends to the nurse's being honest and consistent (congruent) in what is said to the patient.
- Pacing—letting the patient set the pace and letting the pace be adjusted to fit the patient's moods. A slow approach helps reduce pressure; at times, it is necessary to step back and realize that developing a strong relationship may take a long time.
- Listening—letting the patient talk when needed. The nurse becomes a sounding board for the patient's concerns and issues. Listening is perhaps the most important skill for nurses to master. Truly listening to another person (i.e., attending to what is behind the words) is a learned skill.
- Initial impressions, especially positive initial attitudes and preconceptions, are significant considerations in how the relationship will progress. Pre-conceived negative impressions and feelings toward the patient (e.g., the nurse's feeling that the patient is "interesting" or a "challenge") usually bode poorly for the positive growth of the relationship. In contrast, an inherent positive regard for the patient as a person is usually a favourable sign for the developing therapeutic relationship.
- Promoting patient comfort and balancing control usually reflect caring behaviours. *Control* refers to keeping a balance in the relationship: not too strict and not too lenient.

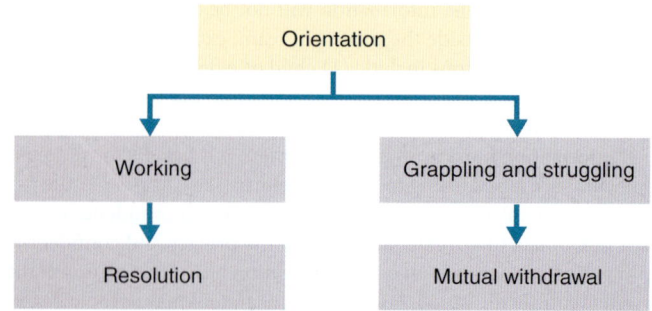

FIG. 9.2 Phases of therapeutic and non-therapeutic relationships. (**Source:** Forchuk, C., Westwell, J., Martin, M., Bamber-Azzapardi, W., Kosterewa-Tolman, D., & Hux, M. (2000). The developing nurse–client relationship: Nurses' perspectives. *Journal of the American Psychiatric Nurses Association, 6*(1), 3–10. https://doi.org/10.1177/107839030000600102.) Copyright © 2000 by SAGE Publications. Reprinted by Permission of SAGE Publications.

- Patient factors that seem to enhance the relationship include trust on the part of the patient and the patient's active participation in the nurse–patient relationship.

In addition to patient factors, nurse factors are also key to establishing an effective therapeutic relationship. Nurses can enhance the therapeutic relationship by ensuring they are present during the interaction. Being present means focusing on the patient, listening to what they are saying, and suspending judgement.

> **⚡ SAFETY TIP**
>
> As nurses engage and are present with patients, it requires that they are able to focus on the patient. Nurses who have been able to find methods to promote their own mental well-being are more effective engaging with patients. When nurses are more actively engaged with patients they are more easily able to pick up cues that the patient's emotions or behaviours may be escalating or that the patient is "shutting down." General strategies used to promote personal mental well-being include: physical activity, allowing time for meditation, starting the interaction with ceremony, finding ways to ground yourself prior to entering the patient room, or inviting the patient into your office or meeting space.

In relationships that did not progress to therapeutic levels there seemed to be two major factors that hampered the development of positive relationships: inconsistency and unavailability (e.g., lack of contact, infrequent meetings, meetings in the hallway) on the part of the nurse, patient, or both. When nurse and patient are reluctant to spend time together, and meeting times become sporadic or superficial, the term *mutual avoidance* is used. This is clearly a lose-lose situation.

The nurse's personal feelings and lack of self-awareness are major elements that contribute to the lack of progression toward a positive, relationship. Negative pre-conceived ideas and feelings (e.g., discomfort, dislike, fear, avoidance) about the patient seem to be a constant in relationships that end in frustration and mutual withdrawal. Sometimes these feelings are known, and sometimes the nurse is only vaguely aware of them.

FACTORS THAT ENCOURAGE AND PROMOTE PATIENTS' GROWTH

Rogers and Truax (1967) identified three personal characteristics of the nurse that help promote change and growth in patients, factors still valued today as vital components for establishing a therapeutic relationship: genuineness, empathy, and positive regard. These are some of the intangibles that are at the heart of the art of nursing.

Genuineness

Genuineness, or self-awareness of one's feelings as they arise within the relationship and the ability to communicate them when appropriate, is a key ingredient in building trust. When a person is genuine, one gets the sense that what the person displays is congruent with their internal processes. Genuineness is conveyed by listening to and communicating with patients without distorting their messages and being clear and concrete in communications. Being genuine in a therapeutic relationship implies the ability to use therapeutic communication tools in an appropriately spontaneous manner, rather than rigidly or in a parrotlike fashion.

Empathy

Empathy is a complex multi-dimensional concept in which the helping person attempts to understand the world from the patient's perspective. Essentially, it means "temporarily living in the other's life, moving about in it delicately without making judgments" (Rogers, 1980, p. 142). You sense others' emotions, and you imagine what they are thinking and feeling. It is not how the nurse feels.

In the past empathy was thought of as the nurse accurately perceiving the patient's situation, perspective, and feelings; however, as relational ways of caring are being developed further, the concept of empathy is shifting to include the idea of care and responsiveness that supports people's health and healing (Doane & Varcoe, 2010). The ability to empathize is developed through practising relational competencies related to understanding the meaning and complexity of experience. There is a relationship intersubjectivity that is developed between the patient and the nurse. It is that relationship that becomes the foundation of being, knowing, and doing.

Empathy Versus Sympathy

There is much confusion regarding empathy versus sympathy. A simple way to distinguish them is to recognize that in empathy we *imagine* the feelings of others; in sympathy we *feel* the feelings of others. When a nurse is feeling sympathy for another, objectivity is lost, and the ability to assist the patient in solving a personal problem ceases. Furthermore, sympathy is associated with feelings of pity and commiseration. Feelings of sympathy can be a symptom of counter-transference.

The following examples are given to clarify the distinction between empathy and sympathy. A friend tells you that her mother was just diagnosed with inoperable cancer. Your friend then begins to cry and pounds the table with her fist.

Sympathetic response: "I feel so sorry for you. I know exactly how you feel. My mother was hospitalized last year, and it was awful. I was so depressed. I still get upset just thinking about it." (You go on to tell your friend about the incident.)

Sometimes when psychiatric nurses try to be sympathetic, they are apt to project their own feelings onto the patient's, which can limit the patient's range of responses. A more useful response might be:

Empathic response: "It sounds as though you are feeling upset and angry having learned about your mother's inoperable cancer diagnosis. Tell me what thoughts and feelings you are having." (You continue to stay with your friend and listen to her thoughts and feelings.)

Empathy is not a technique but rather an attitude that conveys respect, acceptance, and validation of the patient's strengths.

Positive Regard

Positive regard implies respect. It is the ability to view another person as being worthy of being cared about and as someone who has strengths and achievement potential. Positive regard is usually communicated indirectly by attitudes and actions rather than directly by words.

Attitudes

One attitude through which a nurse might convey positive regard, or respect, is willingness to work with the patient. That is, the nurse takes the patient and the relationship seriously. The experience is viewed not as a job, part of a course, or time spent talking but as an opportunity to work with patients to help them develop personal resources and actualize more of their potential in living.

Actions

Some actions that manifest an attitude of respect are attending, suspending value judgements, calling the individual by their first or last name, and helping patients develop their own resources.

Attending. Attending behaviour is the foundation of interviewing. *Attending* is a special kind of listening that refers to an intensity of presence, or of being with the patient. At times, simply being with another person during a painful time can make a difference. Posture, eye contact, and body language are non-verbal behaviours that reflect a person's degree of attending and are highly influenced by culture. Refer to Chapter 10 for a more detailed discussion of the cultural implications of the clinical interview.

Suspending value judgements. Although we will always have personal opinions, nurses are more effective when they guard against using their own value systems to judge patients' thoughts, feelings, or behaviours. For example, if a patient is taking drugs or is involved in risky sexual behaviour, the nurse may recognize that these behaviours are hindering the patient from living a more satisfying life, posing a potential health threat, or preventing the patient from developing satisfying relationships. However, labelling these activities as bad or good is not useful. Rather, the nurse should focus on exploring the behaviour and work toward identifying the thoughts and feelings that influence this behaviour. Judgement on the part of the nurse will most likely interfere with further exploration.

The first steps in eliminating judgemental thinking and behaviours are to (1) recognize their presence, (2) identify how or where you learned these responses to the patient's behaviour, and (3) construct alternative ways to view the patient's thinking and behaviour. Denying judgemental thinking will only compound the problem.

Patient: "I guess you could consider me an addictive personality. I love to gamble when I have money and spend most of my time in the casino. It seems as though I'm hooking up with a different woman every time I'm there, and it always ends in sex. This has been going on for at least 3 years."

A judgemental response would be:

Nurse A: "So your compulsive gambling and promiscuous sexual behaviours really haven't brought you much happiness, have they? You're running away from your problems and could end up with sexually transmitted infections and no money."

A more helpful response would be:

Nurse B: "So your sexual and gambling activities are part of the picture also. You make it sound as though these activities are not making you happy."

In this example nurse B focuses on the patient's behaviours and the possible meaning they might have to the patient. This nurse does not introduce personal value statements or prejudices regarding promiscuous behaviour as nurse A does. Empathy and positive regard are essential qualities in a successful nurse–patient relationship.

Helping patients develop resources. The nurse becomes aware of patients' strengths and encourages patients to work at their optimal level of functioning. This support can be seen as one form of collaboration with the patient. The psychiatric nurse does not act for patients unless absolutely necessary, and even then only as a step toward helping them to act on their own. It is important that patients remain as independent as possible to develop new resources for problem solving. The following are examples of helping the patient to develop independence:

Patient: "This medication makes my mouth so dry. Could you get me something to drink?"

Nurse: "There is juice in the refrigerator. I'll wait here for you until you get back" *or* "I'll walk with you while you get some juice from the refrigerator."

Patient: "Could you ask the doctor to let me have a pass for the weekend?"

Nurse: "Your doctor will be on the unit this afternoon. I'll let her know that you want to speak with her."

Consistently encouraging patients to use their own resources helps minimize the patients' feelings of helplessness and dependency and validates their potential for change.

KEY POINTS TO REMEMBER

- The nurse–patient relationship is well defined, and the roles of the nurse and the patient must be clearly stated.
- It is important that the nurse be aware of the differences between a therapeutic relationship and a social or intimate relationship. In a therapeutic psychiatric nurse–patient relationship the focus is on the patient's needs, thoughts, feelings, and goals. The psychiatric nurse is expected to meet personal needs outside this relationship.
- Although the boundaries and roles of the nurse–patient relationship generally are clearly defined, they can become blurred; this blurring can be insidious and may occur on an unconscious level. Usually, transference and counter-transference phenomena are operating when boundaries are blurred.
- It is important to have a grasp of common counter-transferential feelings and behaviours and of the psychiatric nursing actions to counteract these phenomena.
- Supervision aids in promoting both the professional growth of the psychiatric nurse and the psychiatric nurse–patient relationship, allowing the patient's goals to be worked on and met.
- The phases of the psychiatric nurse–patient relationship include pre-orientation, orientation, working, and termination.
- Genuineness, empathy, and positive regard are personal strengths of effective helpers who are able to foster growth and change in others.

CRITICAL THINKING

1. On your first clinical day, you are assigned to work with an older person, Mrs. Schneider, who is depressed. Your first impression is, "Oh my, she looks like my nasty aunt Helen. She even sits like her." You approach her with a vague feeling of uneasiness and say hello. Mrs. Schneider responds, "Who are you, and how can you help me?" You answer by providing your name and telling her that you are a nursing student and will be working with her today. She tells you that "a student" could never understand what she is going through. She then says, "If you really want to help me, you would get me a good job after I leave here."
   a. Identify transference and counter-transference issues in this situation. What is your most important course of action?
   b. How could you best respond to Mrs. Schneider's question about who you are? What other information will you give her during this first clinical encounter? Be specific.
   c. What are some useful responses you could give Mrs. Schneider regarding her legitimate questions about ways you could be of help to her?
   d. Analyze Mrs. Schneider's request that you find her a job. Keeping in mind the aim of Peplau's interactive nurse–patient process, describe some useful ways you could respond to this request.
   e. Consider how your response and ongoing discussions with Mrs. Schneider can convey key characteristics of a therapeutic relationship: respect, positive regard, genuineness, and empathy.
2. You are interviewing Tom Stone, a 17-year-old who was admitted to a psychiatric unit after a suicide attempt. How would you best respond to each of the following patient requests and behaviours?
   a. "I would feel so much better if you would sit closer to me and hold my hand."
   b. "I will tell you if I still feel like killing myself, but you have to promise not to tell anyone else. If you do, I just can't trust you, ever."
   c. "I don't want to talk to you. I have absolutely nothing to say."

d. "I will be going home tomorrow, and you have been so helpful and good to me. I want you to have my watch to remember me by."
e. Tom breaks down and starts sobbing.

CHAPTER REVIEW

1. Which of the following actions best represents the basis or foundation of all other psychiatric nursing care?
   a. The nurse assesses the patient at regular intervals.
   b. The nurse administers psychotropic medications.
   c. The nurse spends time sitting with a withdrawn patient.
   d. The nurse participates in team meetings with other professionals.
2. A male patient frequently inquires about the female student nurse's boyfriend, social activities, and school experiences. Which of the following initial responses by the student best addresses the issue raised by this behaviour?
   a. The student requests assignment to a patient of the same gender as the student.
   b. The student points out to the patient that he is making social inquiries and explores this behaviour.
   c. The student tells the patient that she cannot talk about her personal life and returns the focus to his issues.
   d. The student explains that if the patient persists in focusing on her, she cannot work with him.
3. Mary, a patient in the psychiatric unit, had a very rejecting and abusive father and a difficult childhood but, from age 10 on, was raised by a very warm and supportive grandmother who recently passed away. Mary frequently comments on how hard her nurse, Jessa, works and on how other staff do not seem to care as much about their patients as Jessa does. Jessa finds herself agreeing with Mary and appreciating her insightfulness, recalling to herself that except for her former head nurse, other staff do not seem to appreciate how hard she works and seem to take her for granted. Jessa enjoys the time she spends with Mary and seeks out opportunities to interact with her. What phenomenon is occurring here, and which response by Jessa would most benefit her and the patient?
   a. Mary is experiencing transference; Jessa should help Mary to understand that she is emphasizing in Jessa those qualities that were missing in her father.
   b. Jessa is idealizing Mary, seeing in her strengths and abilities that Mary does not really possess; Jessa should temporarily distance herself somewhat from Mary.
   c. Mary is overidentifying with Jessa, seeing similarities that do not in reality exist; Jessa should label and explore this phenomenon in her interactions with Mary.
   d. Jessa is experiencing counter-transference in response to Mary's meeting Jessa's needs for greater appreciation; Jessa should seek clinical supervision to explore these dynamics.
4. Which of the following statements would be appropriate during the orientation phase of the nurse–patient relationship? **Select all that apply.**
   a. "My name is Sarah, and I am a student nurse here to learn about mental health."
   b. "I will be here each Thursday from 8 a.m. until noon if you would like to talk."
   c. "Tell me about what you think would best help you to cope with the loss of your wife."
   d. "Let's talk today about how our plan for improving your sleep has been working."
   e. "We will meet weekly for 1 hour, during which we will discuss how to meet your goals."
   f. "Being home alone while your wife was hospitalized must have been very difficult for you."
5. A student nurse exhibits the following behaviours or actions while interacting with her patient. Which of these is appropriate as part of a therapeutic relationship?
   a. Sitting attentively in silence with a withdrawn patient until the patient chooses to speak.
   b. Offering the patient advice on how they could cope more effectively with stress.
   c. Controlling the pace of the relationship by selecting topics for each interaction.
   d. Limiting the discussion of termination issues so as not to sadden the patient unduly.

https://evolve.elsevier.com/Canada/Varcarolis/psychiatric/

REFERENCES

Benner, P. (2000). *From novice to expert: Excellence and power in clinical nursing practice* (commemorative ed). Upper Saddle River: Prentice-Hall.

Doane, G. H., & Varcoe, C. (2010). Boundaries and the culture of theorizing in nursing. *Nursing Science Quarterly, 23*(2), 130–137. https://doi.org/10.1177/0894318410362544

Fisher, M. J. (2020). Navigating professional boundaries: The use of the therapeutic self in rehabilitation nursing. *Journal of the Australasian Rehabilitation Nurses' Association, 23*(1), 2–3. https://doi.org/10.33235/jarna.23.1.2-3

Forchuk, C., Westwell, J., Martin, M-L., Bamber-Azzapardi, W., Kosterewa-Tolman, D., & Hux, M. (2000). The developing nurse–client relationship: Nurses' perspectives. *Journal of the American Psychiatric Nurses Association, 6*(1), 3–10. https://doi.org/10.1177/107839030000600102

Knox, J. (2019). The harmful effects of psychotherapy: When the therapeutic alliance fails. *British Journal of Psychotherapy, 35*(2), 245–262. https://doi.org/10.1111/bjp.12445

Moore, J. C., & Hartman, C. R. (1988). Developing a therapeutic relationship. In C. K. Beck, R. P. Rawlins, & S. R. Williams (Eds.), *Mental health–psychiatric nursing* (pp. 92–117). St. Louis: Mosby.

Peplau, H. E. (1952). *Interpersonal relations in nursing: A conceptual frame of reference for psychodynamic nursing* (pp. 92–117). New York: Putnam.

Peplau, H. E. (1997). Peplau's theory of interpersonal relations. *Nursing Science Quarterly, 10*, 162–167.

Registered Nurses' Association of Ontario. (2002). *Nursing best practice guidelines: Establishing therapeutic relationships*. Toronto: Author. https://rnao.ca/bpg/guidelines/establishing-therapeutic-relationships

Rogers, C. R. (1980). *A way of being*. Boston: Houghton Mifflin.

Rogers, C. R., & Truax, C. B (1967). The therapeutic conditions antecedent to change: A theoretical view. In C. R. Rogers (Ed.), *The therapeutic relationship and its impact* (pp. 97–108). Madison: University of Wisconsin Press.

Steuber, P., & Pollard, C. (2018). Building a therapeutic relationship: How much is too much self-disclosure?. *International Journal of Caring Sciences, 11*(2), 651–657.

Travelbee, J. (1971). *Interpersonal aspects of nursing* (2nd ed.). Philadelphia: F. A. Davis Co.

Wong, S. T., Lavoie, J. G., Browne, A. J., MacLeod, M. L. P., & Chongo, M. (2015). Patient confidentiality within the context of group medical visits: Is there cause for concern?. *Health Expectations, 18*(5), 727–739. https://doi.org/10.1111/hex.12156

10

Communication and the Clinical Interview

Erin Ziegler
Originating US chapter by Margaret Jordan Halter, Elizabeth M. Varcarolis

 https://evolve.elsevier.com/Canada/Varcarolis/psychiatric/

OBJECTIVES

1. Identify three personal and two environmental factors that can impede communication.
2. Discuss the differences between verbal and non-verbal communication and identify five examples of non-verbal communication.
3. Identify two attending behaviours the psychiatric nurse might focus on to increase communication skills.
4. Compare and contrast the range of verbal and non-verbal communication of different cultural groups in the areas of communication style, eye contact, and touch.
5. Relate problems that can arise when nurses are insensitive to cultural aspects of patients' communication styles.
6. Demonstrate the use of four techniques that can enhance communication, highlighting what makes them effective.
7. Demonstrate the use of four techniques that can obstruct communication, highlighting what makes them ineffective.
8. Identify and give rationales for suggested setting, seating, and methods for beginning the psychiatric nurse–patient interaction.
9. Explain the importance of clinical supervision.

KEY TERMS AND CONCEPTS

active listening
closed-ended questions
cultural filters
debriefing
double messages
double-bind messages
feedback
non-therapeutic communication techniques
non-verbal behaviours
nonv-erbal communication
open-ended questions
therapeutic communication skills and strategies
verbal communication

Humans have a built-in need to relate to others, and our advanced ability to communicate contributes to the substance and meaning in our lives. Our need to express ourselves to others is powerful; it is the foundation on which we form happy and productive relationships in our adult lives. At the same time, stress and negative feelings within a relationship are often the result of ineffective communication. All of our actions, words, and facial expressions convey meaning to others. It has been said that we cannot not communicate. Even silence can convey acceptance, anger, or thoughtfulness.

In the provision of psychiatric nursing care communication takes on a new emphasis. Just as social relationships are different from therapeutic relationships (see Chapter 9), *basic communication* is different from professional, patient-centred, goal-directed, and scientifically based *therapeutic communication*.

The ability to form therapeutic relationships is fundamental and essential to effective psychiatric nursing care, and therapeutic communication is central to the formation of a therapeutic relationship. Determining levels of pain in the post-operative patient; listening as parents express feelings of fear concerning their child's diagnosis; or understanding, without words, the needs of the intubated patient in the intensive care unit are essential skills in providing quality nursing care.

Psychiatric patients experience more positive outcomes when engaged in therapeutic relationships with nurses (Hartley et al., 2020). Ideally, therapeutic communication is a professional skill you learn and practise early in your nursing curriculum. But in psychiatric mental health nursing, communication skills take on a different and new emphasis. Psychiatric disorders cause not only physical responses (fatigue, loss of appetite, insomnia) but also emotional responses (sadness, anger, hopelessness, euphoria) that affect a patient's ability to relate to others.

It is often during a psychiatric nursing practice experience that students discover the utility of therapeutic communication and begin to rely on techniques they once considered artificial. For example, restating may seem like a funny thing to do. Using it in a practice session between students ("I felt sad when my dog ran away." "You felt sad when your dog ran away?") can derail communication and end the seriousness with laughter. Yet in the clinical setting, restating can become a powerful and profound communication strategy in building a therapeutic alliance:

Patient: "At the moment they told me my daughter would never be able to walk like her twin sister, I felt as though I couldn't go on."

Nurse: (After a short silence) "You felt uncertain that you could go on when you learned your daughter would never be able to walk like her twin sister."

The technique, and the empathy it conveys, is appreciated in such a situation. Developing therapeutic communication skills takes time, and with continued practice, you will develop your own style and rhythm. Eventually, these communication skills and strategies will become a part of the way you instinctively communicate with others in the clinical setting and in your personal life as you integrate them into your way of being with others.

Beginning psychiatric practitioners are often concerned that they may say the wrong thing, especially when learning to apply therapeutic techniques. Will you say the wrong thing? Yes, you probably will, but that is how we all learn to find more useful and effective ways of helping individuals to reach their goals. The challenge is to recover from your mistakes and use them for learning and growth (Sommers-Flanagan & Sommers-Flanagan, 2016).

One of the most common concerns students have is that they will say the one thing that will "push the patient over the edge" or maybe even be the cause for the patient to give up on living. This is highly unlikely. Consider that behaviours associated with psychiatric disorders, such as irritability, agitation, negativity, disinterest in communication, and being hypertalkative, often frustrate and alienate friends and family. It is likely that the interactions the patient has had to date have not always been pleasant and supportive. Patients often see a well-meaning person who conveys genuine acceptance, respect, empathy, and concern for their well-being as a gift. Even if mistakes in communication are made or the "wrong thing" is said, there is little chance that the comments will do actual harm. With reflection and supervision, mistakes in communication can be corrected and repaired. When a nurse explains their errors in communication and repairs the miscommunication, this show of humility and genuineness may even strengthen the therapeutic relationship.

THE COMMUNICATION PROCESS

Communication is an interactive process between two or more people who send and receive messages to one another. The following is a simplified model of communication (Berlo, 1960):

1. One person has a need to communicate with another (*stimulus*) for information, comfort, or advice.
2. The person sending the message (*sender*) initiates interpersonal contact.
3. The *message* is the information sent or expressed to another. The clearest messages are those that are well organized and expressed in a manner familiar to the receiver.
4. The message can be sent through a variety of media, including auditory (hearing), visual (seeing), tactile (touch), smell, or any combination of these.
5. The person receiving the message (*receiver*) then interprets the message and responds to the sender by providing **feedback** (communication of impressions of and reactions to the sender's actions or verbalizations). Validating the accuracy of the sender's message is extremely important. The nature of the feedback often indicates whether the meaning of the message sent has been correctly interpreted by the receiver. An accuracy check may be obtained by simply asking the sender, "Is this what you mean?" or "I notice you turn away when we talk about your going back to college. Is there a conflict there?"

Figure 10.1 shows this simple model of communication, along with some of the many factors that affect it.

Effective communication in therapeutic relationships depends on nurses knowing what they are trying to convey (the purpose of the message), communicating to the patient what is really meant, and comprehending the meaning of what the patient intentionally or unintentionally conveys (Arnold & Boggs, 2019). Peplau (2004) identified two main principles that can guide the communication process during the nurse–patient interview (discussed in detail later in this chapter): (1) clarity, which ensures that the meaning of the message is accurately understood by both parties in an ongoing mutual effort, and (2) continuity, which promotes the connections among relevant ideas and encourages a shared understanding of the activities, emotions, and context of those ideas. Maintaining this clarity and continuity requires particular concentration and attention when patients are acutely mentally ill and possibly experiencing symptoms impairing their communication.

RESEARCH HIGHLIGHT
Supplementing Goal Setting for Families Using Motivational Interviewing

Problem
Communication with and for families around healthy eating and behaviours can be challenging, and it is unclear what kind of interviewing will be most effective to support change in food choices and habits of family meals.

Purpose of Study
The purpose of the study was to describe how motivational interviewing (a style of communication that prepares people for change through questions and interviewing to enhance intrinsic motivation, building confidence for change) can be used to support parents to facilitate health behaviour change, particularly around healthy eating, family meals, and obesity prevention.

Methods
A motivational interviewing (MI) intervention (focused on healthy homes and meals) was part of a randomized controlled trial that included 81 families (children 8 to 12 years old and their parents) in the intervention group. The intervention included 10 monthly 2-hour group sessions and 5 bi-monthly motivational or goal-setting phone calls. Data were collected for intervention families only at each of the goal-setting calls, and a behaviour change assessment was administered at the tenth and final group session.

Key Findings
Descriptive statistics were used to analyze the MI call data and behaviour assessment. Overall group attendance was high (68% attending ≥7 sessions). Motivational or goal-setting phone calls were well accepted by parents, with an 87% average completion rate. More than 85% of the time, families reported meeting their chosen goal between calls. Families completing the behavioural assessment reported the most change in having family meals more often and improving home food healthfulness.

Implications for Nursing Practice
A combination of delivery methods using MI may be useful when implementing behaviour change programs for families to promote goal setting.

Source: Draxten, M., Flattum, C., & Fulkerson, J. (2016). An example of how to supplement goal setting to promote behavior change for families using motivational interviewing. *Health Communication, 31*(10), 1276–1283. https://doi.org/10.1080/10410236.2015.1062975

FACTORS THAT AFFECT COMMUNICATION

Personal Factors

Personal factors that can impede accurate transmission or interpretation of messages include emotional factors (e.g., mood, responses to stress, personal bias), social factors (e.g., previous experience, cultural differences, language differences), and cognitive factors (e.g., problem-solving ability, knowledge level, language use).

Environmental Factors

Environmental factors that may affect communication include physical factors (e.g., background noise, lack of privacy, uncomfortable accommodations) and societal determinants (e.g., sociopolitical, historical, and economic factors; the presence of others; expectations of others).

Relationship Factors

Relationship factors refer to the status of individuals in terms of social standing, power, roles, responsibilities, age, and so on. Communication

Fig. 10.1 Operational Definition of *Communication*. (**Source:** Data from Ellis, R., & McClintock, A. (1990). *If you take my meaning*. London: Arnold.)

is influenced by all of these factors. Consider how you would describe your day in the clinical setting to your instructor, compared to how you would describe it to your friend. The fact that your instructor has more education than you and is in an evaluative role would likely influence how much you share and your choice of words.

Now think about the relationship between you and your patient. Your patient may be older or younger than you are, more or less educated, richer or poorer, successful at work or unemployed. These factors play into the dynamics of the communication, whether at a conscious or an unconscious level, and recognizing their influence is important. It may be difficult for you to work with a woman your mother's age or one your own age, or you may feel impatient with a patient who is unemployed and abuses alcohol.

It is sometimes difficult for students to grasp or remember that patients, regardless of these relationship factors, are in a position of vulnerability. Wearing a hospital identification band or stepping through the door of a community mental health clinic formally indicates a need for care, and as a caregiver, you are viewed to be in a role of authority. Part of the art of therapeutic communication is finding a balance between your role as a professional and your role as a human being who has been socialized into complex patterns of interactions based, at least in part, on status.

Students sometimes fall back into time-tested and comfortable roles. As such, one of the most common responses of nursing students to nurse–patient relationships is treating the patient as a friend. Imagine a male nursing student walking into the unit, seeing his assigned patient, and saying, "Hey, how's it going today?" while giving the patient a high-five. Or consider the female nursing student assigned to a 60-year-old woman who used to work as a registered nurse. This relationship has the potential to become unbalanced and non-therapeutic if the patient shifts the focus away from his or her own concerns and onto the student nurse's interests and concerns (see Chapter 9).

VERBAL AND NON-VERBAL COMMUNICATION

Verbal Communication

Verbal communication consists of all the words a person speaks. We live in a society of symbols, and our main social symbols are words. Talking is our most common activity. It is our public link to one another, the primary instrument of instruction, a need, an art, and one of the most personal aspects of our private lives. When we speak, we:
- Communicate our beliefs and values
- Communicate perceptions and meanings
- Convey interest and understanding or insult and judgement
- Convey messages clearly or convey conflicting or implied messages
- Convey clear, honest feelings or disguised, distorted feelings

Words are culturally perceived; therefore clarifying the intent of certain words is very important. Even if the nurse and patient have a similar cultural background, the mental image that each has for a given word may not be the same. Although they believe they are talking about the same thing, the nurse and patient may be talking about two quite different things. While they produce mental images, words are also symbols for emotions.

Non-verbal Communication

Non-verbal communication (often called *cues*) are those messages expressed through directly observable behaviours such as physical appearance, facial expressions, body posture, amount of eye contact, eye cast (e.g., emotion expressed in the eyes), hand gestures, sighs, fidgeting, and yawning. A person's tone of voice, emphasis on certain words, and pacing of speech are also examples of non-verbal behaviours. Sometimes these behaviours operate outside of the awareness of the person exhibiting the behaviours, or unconsciously. It is often said that "it's not what you say but how you say it." In other words, it is the non-verbal behaviours that may be communicating the "real" message (Table 10.1). Non-verbal behaviours must be observed and interpreted considering a person's culture, class, gender, age, sexual orientation, and spiritual beliefs. Cultural influences on communication are addressed later in this chapter.

Interaction of Verbal and Non-verbal Communication

Shawn Shea (2017), a nationally renowned psychiatrist and communication workshop leader, suggests that communication is roughly 10% verbal and 90% non-verbal. Our interpretation of feelings and attitudes may account for the high percentage of communication attributed to non-verbal behaviours. While it would be difficult to watch a foreign film and understand 90% of its meaning based solely on body language and vocal tones, non-verbal behaviours and cues do influence communication to a surprising degree in nurse–patient interactions. Communication thus involves two radically different but highly interdependent kinds of symbols: verbal and non-verbal.

Spoken words can be straightforward or may distort, conceal, deny, or disguise true feelings. Whereas spoken words represent our public selves, non-verbal behaviours (e.g., how a person listens and uses silence and sense of touch) can convey important information about the private self that is not available from conversation alone, especially in consideration of cultural norms.

Some elements of non-verbal communication, such as facial expressions, seem to be biologically based and are similar across cultures. The facial expression of anger, sadness, happiness, fear, surprise, and disgust are considered universal; however, differences in other facial expressions may differ across cultures (Lorié et al., 2017).

Messages are not always simple; they can appear to be one thing when, in fact, they are another (Shea, 2017). Often people have greater conscious awareness of their verbal messages than of their non-verbal behaviours. The verbal message is sometimes referred to as the *content* of the message (what is said), and the non-verbal behaviour is called the *process* of the message (non-verbal cues a person gives to substantiate or contradict the verbal message, or how it is said). When the content is congruent with the process, the communication is more clearly understood and is considered healthy. For example, a student saying, "It's important that I get good grades in this class" is content. The student buying the required books, taking good notes, and working with a study buddy is process. The content and process in this example are congruent and straightforward, and there is a "healthy" message. If, however, the verbal message is not reinforced or is, in fact, contradicted by the non-verbal behaviour, the message is confusing. For example, the student not buying the books, skipping several classes, and not studying is also process, but in this case the student is sending two different messages.

TABLE 10.1	Non-verbal Behaviours	
Behaviour	**Possible Non-verbal Cues**	**Example**
Body behaviours	Posture, body movements, gestures, gait	The patient is slumped in a chair, puts their face in their hands, and occasionally taps their right foot.
Facial expressions	Frowns, smiles, grimaces, raised eyebrows, pursed lips, licking of lips, tongue movements	The patient grimaces when speaking to the nurse; when alone, they smile and giggle to themself.
Eye cast	Angry, suspicious, and accusatory looks	The patient's eyes harden with suspicion.
Voice-related behaviours	Tone, pitch, level, intensity, inflection, stuttering, pauses, silences, fluency	The patient talks in a loud singsong voice.
Observable autonomic physiological responses	Increase in respirations, diaphoresis, pupil dilation, blushing, paleness	When the patient mentions discharge, they become pale, their respirations increase, and their face becomes diaphoretic.
Personal appearance	Grooming, dress, hygiene	The patient is dressed in a wrinkled shirt, their pants are stained, their socks are dirty, and they are unshaven.
Physical characteristics	Height, weight, physique, complexion	The patient is grossly overweight, and their muscles appear flabby.

Messages are sent to create meaning but also can be used defensively to hide what is actually going on, create confusion, and attack relatedness (Shea, 2017). Conflicting messages are known as **double messages** or *mixed messages*. One way a nurse can respond to verbal and non-verbal incongruity is to reflect and validate the patient's feelings. For example, the nurse could say to the student, "you say you are upset you did not pass this semester, but I notice you look more relaxed and less conflicted than you have all term. What do you see as some of the pros and cons of not passing the course this semester?"

Bateson and colleagues (1956) coined the term **double-bind messages**. A double-bind message is a contradictory mix of content and process that communicates both nurturing and hurtful expressions. The following vignette gives an example of a double-bind message.

> **VIGNETTE**
> A 21-year-old female who lives at home with her chronically ill mother wants to go out for an evening with her friends. She is told by her frail but not helpless mother: "Oh, go ahead, have fun. I'll just sit here by myself, and I can always call 911 if I don't feel well, but you go ahead and have fun." The mother says this while looking sad, eyes downcast, slumped in her chair, and letting her cane drop to the floor.

The recipient of this double-bind message is caught inside contradictory statements, so she cannot decide what is right. If she goes, the implication is that she is being selfish by leaving her sick mother alone. But if she stays, the mother could say, "I told you to go have fun." If she does go, the chances are she will not have much fun because of concern for her mother. The daughter is trapped in a no-win situation of which she may not be fully aware.

With experience, nurses become increasingly aware of patients' verbal and non-verbal communication and compare the two to gain important clues about the real message. What individuals do may either express and reinforce or contradict what they say. So, as in the saying "Actions speak louder than words," actions often reveal the true meaning of a person's intent, whether the intent is conscious or unconscious.

COMMUNICATION SKILLS FOR NURSES

Therapeutic Communication Strategies

The nurse must establish and maintain a therapeutic relationship in which the patient will feel safe and hopeful that positive change is possible. A study by Unhjem et al. (2018) found that the nurse–patient relationship within the mental health setting was strengthened when the nurse self-disclosed some personal information. Done in a positive way, self-disclosure can build rapport and make the patient more comfortable, creating a more open, honest, reciprocal, and equal relationship.

Once a therapeutic relationship is established, specific needs and problems can be identified, and the nurse can work with the patient on increasing self-awareness, developing insight and problem-solving skills, learning new coping behaviours, and experiencing more appropriate and satisfying ways of relating to others. To do this, the nurse must have a sound knowledge of communication theory and skills. Therefore nurses must become more aware of their own interpersonal methods, eliminating obstructive, non-therapeutic communication techniques and strategies, and developing additional responses that maximize the nurse–patient interactions and increase the use of **therapeutic communication skills and strategies** (e.g., skills such as warmth, respect, and empathy and strategies such as using silence, recognizing strengths, and making observations). Helpful tools for nurses when communicating with their patients are silence, active listening, and clarifying techniques.

Silence

Silence can sometimes intimidate both interviewers and patients (Sommers-Flanagan & Sommers-Flanagan, 2016). In Canada there is an emphasis on action and a high level of verbal activity. Students and practising nurses alike may find that when the flow of words stops, they become uncomfortable. They may rush to fill the void with "questions or chatter," thus cutting off potentially important thoughts and feelings the patient might be taking time to think about before articulating. Silence is not the absence of communication but a specific channel for transmitting and receiving messages; therefore the practitioner needs to understand that silence is a significant means of influencing and being influenced by others.

Talking is a highly individualized practice. Some people find phone calls a nuisance, whereas others believe they cannot live without speaking on the phone and having their phone always available. In the initial interview patients may be reluctant to speak because of the newness of the situation; the fact that the nurse is a stranger; or feelings of distrust, self-consciousness, embarrassment, or shyness. The nurse must recognize and respect individual differences in styles and tempos of responding. People who are quiet, those who have a language barrier or speech disorder, older persons, and those who lack confidence in their ability to express themselves may communicate a need for support and encouragement through their silence.

Although there is no universal rule concerning how much silence is too much, silence has been said to be worthwhile only as long as it is serving some function and not frightening the patient. Knowing when to speak during the interview depends largely on one's perception about what is being conveyed through the silence. Icy silence may be an expression of anger and hostility; being ignored or given "the silent treatment" is recognized as an insult and is a particularly hurtful form of communication.

Silence may provide meaningful moments of reflection for both participants, giving an opportunity to contemplate thoughtfully what has been said and felt, weigh alternatives, formulate new ideas, and gain a new perspective on the matter under discussion. If the nurse waits to speak and allows the patient to break the silence, the patient may share thoughts and feelings that would otherwise have been withheld. Nurses who feel compelled to fill every void with words often do so because of their own anxiety, self-consciousness, and embarrassment. This action, however, prioritizes the nurse's need for comfort over the needs of the patient.

It is crucial to recognize that for some individuals living with a psychiatric disorder, such as major depression or schizophrenia, medications may cause an overall slowing of thought processes. This slowing may be so severe that it may seem like an eternity before the patient responds. Patience and gentle prompting (e.g., "You were saying that you would like to get a pass this weekend to visit your niece") can help patients gather their thoughts.

Silence is not always therapeutic. Prolonged and frequent silences by the psychiatric nurse may hinder an interview that requires verbal articulation. Although a less talkative nurse may be comfortable with silence, this mode of communication may make the patient feel like a fountain of information to be drained dry. Moreover, without feedback, patients have no way of knowing whether what they said was understood. In addition, children and adolescents tend to feel uncomfortable with silence.

Active Listening

People want more than just a physical presence in human communication. Most people want the other person to be there for them psychologically, socially, emotionally, and spiritually. **Active listening** in the nurse–patient relationship includes the following aspects:
- Observing the patient's non-verbal behaviours
- Understanding and reflecting on the patient's verbal message

- Understanding the patient in the context of the social setting of the patient's life
- Detecting "false notes" (e.g., inconsistencies or things the patient says that need more clarification)
- Providing constructive feedback about the patient that they might not be aware

Effective interviewers learn to become active listeners not only when the patient is talking but also when the patient becomes silent. During active listening, psychiatric nurses carefully note verbal and non-verbal patient responses and monitor their own non-verbal responses. Using silence effectively and learning to listen actively, both to the patient and to your own thoughts and reactions, are key ingredients in effective communication. Both skills take time to develop but can be learned; you will become more proficient with guidance and practice.

Some important principles of active listening include (Mohl & Carr, 2015):

- The answer is always inside the patient.
- Objective truth is never as simple as it seems.
- Everything you hear is modified by the patient's filters.
- Everything you hear is modified by your own filters.
- It is okay to feel confused and uncertain.
- Listen to yourself, too.

Active listening helps strengthen the patient's ability to solve problems. By giving the patient undivided attention, the nurse communicates that the patient is not alone. This kind of intervention enhances self-esteem and encourages the patient to direct energy towards finding ways to deal with problems. Serving as a sounding board, the nurse listens as the patient tests thoughts by voicing them aloud. This form of interpersonal interaction often enables the patient to clarify thinking, link ideas, and tentatively decide what should be done and how best to do it.

Listening with empathy. Wheeler (2020) identifies empathy as the most important element in therapeutic communication. Research indicates that the connectedness that results from empathy improves brain function by increasing brain plasticity. Wheeler describes the empathic process as the nurse entering and feeling the patient's world, the patient perceiving their own understanding of the world, and the patient experiencing acceptance and confirmation of themself.

It is not enough for the nurse to feel empathy; an important part of this process is the communication of empathy to the patient. Egan and Reese (2018) suggested that the communication of empathy is achieved by connecting to the emotions, experiences, and thoughts of our patients and, to this end, proposed two forms of empathic statements, demonstrated through these examples:

1. "You feel _____ (name the emotion) because _____ (describe the *experiences*, thoughts, and behaviours)."
2. "Your _____ (name the emotion) is an outcome of _____ (describe the *context* of the experiences)."

If we plug in a scenario to the first statement, emphasizing the experience, it could sound something like this: "You feel like a failure because you have let your father down by joining the Canadian Armed Forces rather than becoming a lawyer." Now, try composing an empathic statement for the same scenario that encompasses the emotion considering a particular context.

It is not always easy to be empathic and communicate a connection to the experiences, emotions, thoughts, behaviours, and contexts of our patients. Patients may describe experiences of brutal physical or sexual abuse, feelings of torment watching a loved one die, hate and anger towards another person, or acts of violence or hurtful inconsideration they have committed. When people are self-pitying, critical, angry, sarcastic, or demeaning, the nurse's ability to connect to these experiences and communicate empathy may also be challenged. Chapter 9 offers a more detailed discussion of empathy.

Clarifying Techniques

Understanding depends on clear communication, which is aided by the nurse's verifying their own interpretation of the patient's messages. The nurse can request feedback on the accuracy of the message received from verbal and non-verbal cues. The use of clarifying techniques helps both participants identify major differences in their frame of reference, giving them the opportunity to correct misperceptions before they cause any serious misunderstandings. The patient who is asked to elaborate on or clarify vague or ambiguous messages needs to know that the purpose is to promote mutual understanding.

Paraphrasing. To clarify, the nurse might use *paraphrasing*, or explaining in different (often fewer) words the basic content of a patient's message (Sommers-Flanagan & Sommers-Flanagan, 2016). Using simple, precise, and culturally relevant terms, the nurse may readily confirm interpretation of the patient's previous message before the interview proceeds. By prefacing statements with a phrase such as "I'm not sure I understand" or "In other words, you seem to be saying …," the nurse helps the patient form a clearer perception of what may be a bewildering mass of details. After paraphrasing, the nurse must validate the accuracy of the restatement and its helpfulness to the discussion. The patient may confirm or deny the perceptions through non-verbal cues or by direct response to a question from the nurse, such as "Was I correct in saying … ?" As a result, the patient is made aware that the interviewer is actively involved in the search for understanding.

Restating. In *restating* the nurse mirrors the patient's overt and covert messages, so the technique may be used to echo feeling as well as content or context. Restating differs from paraphrasing in that it involves repeating the same key words the patient has just spoken. If a patient remarks, "My life is empty … it has no meaning," additional information may be gained by restating, "Your life has no meaning?" The purpose of this technique is to explore more thoroughly subjects that may be significant.

Too frequent and indiscriminate use of restating, however, may be interpreted by patients as inattention or disinterest. It is easy to overuse this tool so that its application becomes mechanical. As well, parroting or mimicking what another has said may be perceived as poking fun at the person; therefore the use of this non-direct approach can become a definite barrier to communication. To avoid overuse of restating, the nurse can combine restatements with direct questions that encourage descriptions: "What is lacking in your life?" "What are you missing in your life?" "Describe a day in your life that felt empty to you."

Reflecting. Reflection is a means of assisting people to better understand their own thoughts and feelings. Reflecting may take the form of a question or a simple statement that conveys the nurse's observations of the patient when sensitive issues are being discussed. The nurse might then describe briefly to the patient the apparent meaning of the emotional tone of the patient's verbal and non-verbal behaviour. For example, to reflect a patient's feelings about their life, a good beginning might be, "You sound as if you have had many disappointments."

Sharing observations with a patient shows that you accept them and that the patient has your full attention. When you reflect, you make the patient aware of their inner feelings and encourage the patient to own them. For example, you may say to a patient, "You look sad." Perceiving your concern may allow the patient to spontaneously share feelings. The use of a question in response to the patient's question is another reflective technique (Arnold & Boggs, 2019). For example:

Patient: "Nurse, do you think I really need to be hospitalized?"
Nurse: "What do you think, Jane?"
Patient: "I don't know—that's why I'm asking you."
Nurse: "I'll be willing to share my impression with you at the end of this first session. However, you've probably thought about hospitalization and have some feelings about it. I wonder what they are."

Exploring. A technique that enables the nurse to examine important ideas, experiences, or relationships more fully is *exploring*. For example, if a patient tells you he does not get along well with his wife, you will want to further explore this area. Possible openers include:

"*Tell me more* about your relationship with your wife."

"*Describe* your relationship with your wife."

"*Give me an example* of how you and your wife don't get along."

Asking for an example can greatly clarify a vague or generic statement made by a patient.

Patient: "No one likes me."

Nurse: "Give me an example of one person who doesn't like you."

or

Patient: "Everything I do is wrong."

Nurse: "Give me an example of one thing you do that you think is wrong."

Table 10.2 lists more examples of therapeutic communication techniques.

Asking Questions and Eliciting Patient Responses

Open-ended questions. Many of the questions cited as examples above and in Table 10.2 are open ended. Open-ended questions and comments encourage lengthy responses and facilitate the expression of thoughts, feelings, and information about experiences, perceptions, or responses to a situation. For example:

- "What do you perceive as your biggest problem right now?"
- "Give me an example of some of the stresses you are under right now."
- "Tell me more about your relationship with your wife."

Since open-ended questions are not intrusive and do not put the patient on the defensive, they help the clinician elicit information, especially at the beginning of an interview or when a patient is guarded or resistant to answering questions. They are particularly useful when establishing rapport with a person.

Closed-ended questions. Nurses are usually urged to ask open-ended questions to elicit more than a "yes" or "no" response. However, closed-ended questions, when used sparingly, can give you specific and needed information. Closed-ended questions (those requiring only a "yes" or "no" response) are most useful during an initial assessment or intake interview, to obtain concrete responses to specific assessment data such as a suicide risk assessment, or to determine outcomes of interventions (e.g., "Are the medications helping you?" "When did you start hearing voices?" "Did you seek therapy after your first suicide attempt?"). Care needs to be exercised with this technique. Frequent use of closed-ended questions with a patient leaves the patient feeling interrogated and can close down an interview rapidly, especially in the case of patients who are guarded or resist engaging in interactions.

Non-therapeutic Communication Techniques

Although people may use "non-therapeutic," or ineffective, communication techniques in their daily lives, these techniques can cause problems for nurses because they tend to impede or shut down the nurse–patient interaction. Table 10.3 describes non-therapeutic communication techniques and suggests more helpful responses.

Excessive Questioning

Excessive questioning, that is, asking multiple questions (particularly closed-ended questions) consecutively or very rapidly, casts the nurse in the role of an interrogator who demands information without respect for the patient's willingness or readiness to respond. This approach conveys a lack of respect for and sensitivity to the patient's needs. Excessive questioning controls the range and nature of the responses, can easily result in a therapeutic stall, or may completely shut down an interview. It is a controlling tactic and may reflect the interviewer's lack of security in letting the patient tell their own story. It is better to ask more open-ended questions and follow the patient's lead. For example:

Excessive questioning: "Why did you leave your wife? Did you feel angry at her? What did she do to you? Are you going back to her?"

A more therapeutic approach: "Tell me about the situation between you and your wife."

Giving Approval or Disapproval

"I'm proud of the way you controlled your temper at lunch." "That's a great quilt you made." What could be bad about giving someone a pat on the back once in a while? Nothing, if it is done without conveying a positive or negative judgement. We often give our friends and family approval when they do something well. However, in a nurse–patient relationship, giving praise and approval becomes much more complex.

A patient may be feeling overwhelmed, experiencing low self-esteem, feeling unsure of where their life is going, or desperately seeking recognition, approval, and attention. Yet when people are feeling vulnerable, a value comment may be misinterpreted. For example, the nurse may say, "You did a great job in group telling John just what you thought about how rudely he treated you." This message implies that the nurse was pleased by the manner in which the patient talked to John. The patient then sees such a response as "doing the right thing" and as a way to please the nurse. To continue to please the nurse (and get approval), the patient may continue the behaviour. The behaviour may indeed be useful for the patient, but when done to please another person, it is not coming from the individual's own volition or conviction. Also, when the person the patient needs to please is not around, the motivation for the new behaviour may not be either. Thus the new response really is not a change in behaviour as much as a ploy to win approval and acceptance from another.

Giving approval also cuts off further communication. A more therapeutic approach may be to say, "I noticed that you spoke up to John in group yesterday about his rude behaviour. How did it feel to be more assertive?" This response opens the way for finding out if the patient was scared, was comfortable, wants to work more on assertiveness, and so on. It also suggests that this behaviour was a self-choice made by the patient. While the patient is recognized for the change in behaviour, the topic is also opened for further discussion.

Giving disapproval (e.g., "You really should not cheat, even if you think everyone else is doing it") implies that the nurse has the right to judge the patient's thoughts or feelings. Again, an observation should be made instead (e.g., "Can you give me two examples of how cheating could negatively affect your goal of graduating?").

Giving Advice

Although we ask for and give advice all the time in daily life, giving advice to a patient is rarely helpful. Often when we ask for advice, our real motive is to discover whether we are thinking along the same lines as someone else or if they would agree with us. When a nurse gives advice or offers solutions to a patient, the nurse is interfering with the patient's ability to make personal decisions. The patient may eventually begin to think the nurse does not view them as capable of making effective decisions. People often feel inadequate when they are given no choices over decisions in their lives. Not only can giving advice to patients undermine the patient's sense of competence and adequacy, it can also foster dependency ("I'll have to ask the nurse what to do about …").

However, people do need information and time to reflect in order to make informed decisions. Often you can help a patient define a problem and identify what information might be needed to come

TABLE 10.2　Therapeutic Communication Techniques

Therapeutic Technique	Description	Example
Using silence	Gives the person time to collect thoughts or think through a point	Encouraging a person to talk by waiting for the answers
Accepting	Indicates that the person has been understood; an accepting statement does not necessarily indicate agreement but it is non-judgemental (The nurse should not imply understanding when they do not understand.)	"Yes." "Uh-huh." "I follow what you say."
Giving recognition	Indicates awareness of change and personal efforts; does not imply good or bad, right or wrong	"Good morning, Mr. James." "You've combed your hair today." "I see you've eaten your whole lunch."
Offering self	Offers presence, interest, and a desire to understand; is not offered to get the person to talk or behave in a specific way	"I would like to spend time with you." "I'll stay here and sit with you awhile."
Offering general leads	Allows the other person to take direction in the discussion; indicates interest in what comes next	"Go on." "And then?" "Tell me about it."
Giving broad openings	Clarifies that the lead is to be taken by the patient; however, the nurse discourages pleasantries and small talk	"Where would you like to begin?" "What are you thinking about?" "What would you like to discuss?"
Placing the events in time or sequence	Puts events and actions in better perspective; notes cause-and-effect relationships and identifies patterns of interpersonal difficulties	"What happened before?" "When did this happen?"
Making observations	Calls attention to the person's behaviour (e.g., trembling, nail biting, restless mannerisms); encourages patient to notice the behaviour and describe thoughts and feelings for mutual understanding; helpful with mute and withdrawn people	"You appear tense." "I notice you're biting your lips." "You appear nervous whenever John enters the room."
Encouraging description of perception	Increases the nurse's understanding of the patient's perceptions; talking about feelings and difficulties can lessen the need to act them out inappropriately	"Tell me, what do these voices seem to be saying?" "What is happening now?" "Tell me when you feel anxious."
Encouraging comparison	Brings out recurring themes in experiences or interpersonal relationships; helps the person clarify similarities and differences	"Has this ever happened before?" "Is this how you felt when … ?" "Was it something like … ?"
Restating	Repeats the main idea expressed; gives the patient an idea of what has been communicated; if the message has been misunderstood, the patient can clarify it	*Patient:* "I can't sleep. I stay awake all night." *Nurse:* "You have difficulty sleeping?" or *Patient:* "I don't know … he always has some excuse for not coming over or keeping our appointments." *Nurse:* "You think he no longer wants to see you?"
Reflecting	Directs questions, feelings, and ideas back to the patient; encourages the patient to accept their own ideas and feelings; acknowledges the patient's right to have opinions and make decisions and encourages the patient to think of self as a capable person	*Patient:* "What should I do about my husband's affair?" *Nurse:* "What do you think you should do?" or *Patient:* "My brother spends all of my money and then has the nerve to ask for more." *Nurse:* "You feel angry when this happens?"
Focusing	Concentrates attention on a single point; especially useful when the patient jumps from topic to topic; if a person is experiencing a severe level of anxiety, the nurse should not persist until the anxiety lessens	"This point you are making about leaving school seems worth looking at more closely." "You've mentioned many things. Let's go back to your thinking of 'ending it all.'"
Exploring	Examines certain ideas, experiences, or relationships more fully; if the patient chooses not to elaborate by answering no, the nurse does not probe or pry but instead respects the patient's wishes	"Tell me more about that." "Would you describe it more fully?" "Could you talk about how you learnt your mom was dying of cancer?"

Continued

TABLE 10.2	Therapeutic Communication Techniques—cont'd	
Therapeutic Technique	Description	Example
Giving information	Makes available facts the person needs; supplies knowledge from which decisions can be made or conclusions can be drawn—for example, the patient needs to know the role of the nurse; the purpose of the nurse–patient relationship; and the time, place, and duration of the meetings	"My purpose for being here is …" "This medication is for …" "The test will determine … "
Seeking clarification	Helps patients clarify their own thoughts and maximizes mutual understanding between nurse and patient	"I am not sure I follow you." "What would you say is the main point of what you just said?" "Give an example of a time you thought everyone hated you."
Presenting reality	Indicates what is real; the nurse does not argue or try to convince the patient but just describes personal perceptions or facts in the situation	"That was Dr. Todd, not a man from the Mafia." "That was the sound of a car backfiring." "Your mother is not here; I am a nurse."
Voicing doubt	Undermines the patient's beliefs by not reinforcing the exaggerated or false perceptions	"Isn't that unusual?" "Really?" "That's hard to believe."
Seeking consensual validation	Clarifies that both the nurse and the patient share mutual understanding of communications; helps the patient see more clearly what they are thinking	"Tell me whether my understanding agrees with yours."
Verbalizing the implied	Puts into concrete terms what the patient implies, making the patient's communication more explicit	Patient: "I can't talk to you or anyone else. It's a waste of time." Nurse: "Do you perceive that no one understands?"
Encouraging evaluation	Aids the patient in considering people and events from the perspective of the patient's own set of values	"How do you feel about … ?" "What did it mean to you when he said he couldn't stay?"
Attempting to translate into feelings	Responds to the feelings expressed, not just the content; often termed *decoding*	Patient: "I am dead inside." Nurse: "Are you saying that you feel lifeless? Does life seem meaningless to you?"
Suggesting collaboration	Emphasizes working with the patient, not doing things for the patient; encourages the view that change is possible through collaboration	"Perhaps you and I can discover what produces your anxiety." "Perhaps by working together, we can come up with some ideas that might improve your communications with your spouse."
Summarizing	Brings together important points of discussion to enhance understanding; also allows the opportunity to clarify communications so that both nurse and patient leave the interview with the same ideas in mind	"Have I got this straight?" "You said that …" "During the past hour, you and I have discussed …"
Encouraging formulation of a plan of action	Allows the patient to identify alternative actions for interpersonal situations the patient finds disturbing (e.g., when anger or anxiety is provoked)	"What could you do to let anger out harmlessly?" "The next time this comes up, what might you do to handle it?" "What are some other ways you can approach your boss?"

Source: Adapted from Hays, J. S., & Larson, K. (1963). *Interacting with patients*. New York: Macmillan.

to an informed decision. A useful approach would be to ask, "What do you see as some possible actions you can take?" It is much more respectful and ultimately constructive to encourage problem solving by the patient than simply to provide solutions. Sometimes, though, you might suggest several alternatives a patient could consider (e.g., "What are your thoughts on telling your friend about the incident?"). When you open up the conversation in this way, the patient is free to express their thoughts and feelings about such a disclosure, giving the nurse an opportunity to explore other potential alternatives and to support the patient in their decision.

Asking "Why" Questions

"Why did you come late?" "Why didn't you go to the funeral?" "Why didn't you study for the exam?" Very often, "why" questions imply criticism. We may ask our friends or family such questions, and in the context of a solid relationship, the "why" may be understood more as "What happened?" With people we do not know, especially those who may be anxious or overwhelmed, a "why" question from a person in authority (e.g., nurse, psychiatrist, teacher) can be perceived as intrusive and judgemental, serving only to make the person feel the need to justify behaviour and respond defensively.

TABLE 10.3 Non-therapeutic Communication Techniques

Non-therapeutic Technique	Description	Example	More Helpful Response
Giving premature advice	Assumes the nurse knows best and the patient can't think for self; inhibits problem solving and fosters dependency	"Get out of this situation immediately."	*Encouraging problem solving:* "What are the pros and cons of your situation?" "What were some of the actions you thought you might take?" "What are some of the ways you have thought of to meet your goals?"
Minimizing feelings	Indicates that the nurse is unable to understand or empathize with the patient; the patient's feelings or experiences are being belittled, which can cause the patient to feel small or insignificant and devalued	*Patient:* "I wish I were dead." *Nurse:* "Everyone gets down in the dumps." "I know what you mean." "You should feel happy you're getting better." "Things get worse before they get better."	*Empathizing and exploring:* "You must be feeling very upset. Are you thinking of hurting yourself?"
Falsely reassuring	Under-rates a person's feelings and belittles a person's concerns; may cause the patient to stop sharing feelings if they expect to be ridiculed or not taken seriously	"I wouldn't worry about that." "Everything will be all right." "You will do just fine—you'll see."	*Clarifying the patient's message:* "What specifically are you worried about?" "What do you think could go wrong?" "What are you concerned might happen?"
Making value judgements	Prevents problem solving; can make the patient feel guilty, angry, misunderstood, not supported, or anxious to leave	"Why do you still smoke when your wife has lung cancer?"	*Making observations:* "I notice you are still smoking even though your wife has lung cancer. Is this a problem?"
Asking "why" questions	Implies criticism; often has the effect of making the patient feel a need to justify behaviour and leaves the patient feeling defensive	"Why did you stop taking your medication?"	*Asking open-ended questions; giving a broad opening:* "Tell me some of the events that led up to your not taking your medications."
Asking excessive questions	Results in the patient not knowing which question to answer and possibly being confused about what is being asked	*Nurse:* "How's your appetite? Are you losing weight? Are you eating enough?" *Patient:* "No."	*Clarifying:* "Tell me about your eating habits since you've been depressed."
Giving approval, agreeing	Implies the patient is doing the right thing—and that not doing it is wrong; may lead the patient to focus on pleasing the nurse or clinician; denies the patient the opportunity to change their mind or decision	"I'm proud of you for applying for that job." "I agree with your decision."	*Making observations:* "I noticed that you applied for that job. What factors might contribute to your choice one way or the other?" *Asking open-ended questions; giving a broad opening:* "What led to that decision?"
Disapproving; disagreeing	Can make a person defensive	"You really should have shown up for the medication group." "I disagree with that."	*Exploring:* "What was going on with you when you decided not to come to your medication group?" "That's one point of view. How did you arrive at that conclusion?"
Changing the subject	May invalidate the patient's feelings and needs; can leave the patient feeling alienated and isolated and increase feelings of hopelessness	*Patient:* "I'd like to die." *Nurse:* "Did you go to Alcoholics Anonymous like we discussed?"	*Validating and exploring:* *Patient:* "I'd like to die." *Nurse:* "This sounds serious. Have you thought of harming yourself?"

Source: Adapted from Hays, J. S., & Larson, K. (1963). *Interacting with patients.* New York: Macmillan.

It is much more useful to ask *what* is happening than *why* it is happening. Questions that focus on who, what, where, and when often elicit important information that can facilitate problem solving and further the communication process. See Table 10.3 for additional ineffective communication techniques, as well as statements that would better facilitate interaction and patient comfort.

Cultural Considerations

Canada is becoming increasingly culturally diverse, and health care providers need to be familiar with the verbal and non-verbal communication characteristics of a multicultural national population. The nurse's awareness of cultural meanings of certain verbal and non-verbal communications in initial face-to-face encounters with a patient can lead to the formation of a positive therapeutic relationship (Ehrmin, 2019).

Unrecognized differences in cultural identities can result in assessment and interventions that are not optimally respectful of the patient and can be inadvertently biased or prejudiced. Health care workers need to have not only knowledge of various patients' cultures but also awareness of their own cultural identities. Especially important are nurses' attitudes and beliefs about those from cultures other than their own, because these will affect their relationships with patients (Ehrmin, 2019). Four areas that may prove problematic for the nurse trying to interpret specific verbal and non-verbal messages of the patient are:
1. Communication style
2. Use of eye contact
3. Perception of touch
4. Cultural filters

Further information about working with people of various cultures is presented in Chapter 8.

Communication Style

People may communicate in an intense and highly emotional manner. Some may consider it normal to use dramatic body language when describing emotional problems, and others may perceive such behaviour as being out of control or reflective of some degree of pathology. For example, within the Hispanic community, intensely emotional styles of communication often are culturally appropriate and expected (Ehrmin, 2019). Similarly, French and Italian Canadians typically use animated facial expressions and expressive hand gestures during communication, which can be misinterpreted by others.

In other cultures a calm façade may mask severe distress. For example, in many South Asian cultures, expression of positive or negative emotions is a private affair, and open expression of them is considered to be in bad taste and possibly a weakness. A quiet smile by a South Asian Canadian may express joy, an apology, stoicism, or even anger. German and British Canadians also tend to value highly the concept of self-control and may show little facial emotion in the presence of great distress or emotional turmoil.

Eye Contact

The presence or absence of eye contact should not be used to assess attentiveness, judge truthfulness, or make assumptions about the degree of engagement one has with a patient. Cultural norms often dictate a person's comfort or lack of comfort with direct eye contact. Some cultures consider direct eye contact disrespectful and improper. For example, Indigenous individuals have traditionally been taught to avoid eye contact with authority figures, including nurses, physicians, and other health care providers; avoidance of direct eye contact is seen as a sign of respect to those in authority, but it could be misinterpreted as a lack of interest or even as a lack of respect.

In Japanese culture making direct eye contact is also considered a lack of respect and a personal affront; the preference is for shifting or downcast eyes or a focus on the speaker's neck. For many Chinese people, gazing around and looking to one side when listening to another is considered polite. In some Middle Eastern cultures a woman making direct eye contact with a man may imply a sexual interest or even promiscuity. On the other hand, most Canadians of European descent maintain eye contact during conversation and may interpret avoidance of eye contact by another person as a lack of interest, a show of dishonesty, or avoiding the sharing of important information.

Touch

The therapeutic use of touch is a basic aspect of the nurse–patient relationship and is generally considered a gesture of warmth and friendship; however, the degree to which a patient is comfortable with the use of touch is often culturally determined. People from some cultures, Indigenous people, for example, are accustomed to frequent physical contact. Holding an Indigenous patient's hand in response to a distressing situation or giving the patient a reassuring pat on the shoulder may be experienced as supportive and thus facilitate openness (Ehrmin, 2019). People from Italian or French backgrounds may also be accustomed to frequent touching during conversation, and in the Russian culture touch is an important part of non-verbal communication used freely with intimate and close friends (Giger & Haddad, 2020).

However, in other cultures personal touch within the context of an interview may be perceived as an invasion of privacy or as patronizing, intrusive, aggressive, or sexually inviting. Among German, Swedish, and British Canadians, touch practices are infrequent, although a handshake may be common at the beginning and end of an interaction. Chinese Canadians may not like to be touched by strangers. Within the Muslim culture, touch between members of the opposite gender is discouraged and should be avoided unless required for a clinical examination (Attum et al., 2021).

Even among people from similar cultures, the use of touch has different interpretations and rules regarding gender and class. Nurses and nursing students are urged to find out if their facility has a "no touch" policy, particularly with adolescents and children who have experienced inappropriate touch and may not know how to interpret therapeutic touch from the health care provider.

Cultural Filters

It is important to recognize that it is impossible to listen to people in an unbiased way. In the process of socialization we develop **cultural filters** through which we listen to ourselves, others, and the world around us (Egan & Reese, 2018). Cultural filters are a form of cultural bias or cultural prejudice that determine what we pay attention to and what we ignore. Egan and Reese (2018) stated that we need these cultural filters to provide structure for our lives and help us interpret and interact with the world. However, these cultural filters also unavoidably introduce various forms of bias into our communication, because they are bound to influence our personal, professional, familial, and sociological values and interpretations.

We all need a frame of reference to help us function in our world, but at the same time, we must understand that other people use other frames of reference to help them function in their worlds. Acknowledging that everyone views the world differently and understanding that these various views affect each person's beliefs and behaviours can go a long way toward minimizing our personal distortions in listening. Building acceptance and understanding of cultural diversity is a skill that can be learned. Chapter 8 has a more in-depth discussion of cultural considerations in nursing.

Assertive Communication

Openness and patient-centred communication has been introduced and likely practised to date. Another aspect of communication for psychiatric mental health nursing that must be emphasized is *assertive communication*. Assertive communication means clearly expressing what you need, with respectful language and behaviour (Balzer-Riley, 2021). Psychiatric mental health nurses must face anger and depression, psychosis and dementia, intense elation and despair, and behaviour that may be bizarre or at time self-destructive. In this work nurses hear and witness some of the worst experiences of people's lives, and assertive communication is important to maintain clarity of purpose to meet goals of empathy while also addressing immediate needs for information, care, and safety.

At times assertive communication will mean challenging patients who may be inhibiting their own success or in denial of the problems they are facing. Assertive communication may be necessary to deescalate the agitation a patient is experiencing and to avoid aggression. At other times, assertive communication will establish an avenue for thought-provoking or alternative viewpoints for families or colleagues in a team meeting.

Working as advocates, and as part of interprofessional teams, where not everyone shares the same priorities, goals, or views, psychiatric mental health nurses must routinely practise assertive communication. Psychiatric mental health nurses must be assertive to maintain clarity; ask the right questions; and respect themselves and the dignity of their patients, families, and colleagues. Finally, psychiatric mental health nurses must draw on assertive communication to communicate their own needs and to establish balance in their lives (Balzer-Riley, 2021).

Assertiveness for these purposes can be accomplished with a calm mind, careful thought, and attention to maintaining therapeutic and professional relationships with the utmost respect for all concerned. Asking questions in a humble inquiry (e.g., asking "Have you thought about ..." or "What might happen if we took the _____ approach?") can be an effective part of assertive communication (Schein, 2014).

Evaluation of Communication Skills

After you have had some introductory clinical experience, you may find the facilitative skills checklist in Figure 10.2 useful for evaluating your progress in developing interviewing and assessment skills.

Note that some of the items might not be relevant for some of your patients (e.g., numbers 11 to 13 may not be possible when a patient is experiencing psychosis [disordered thought, delusions, or hallucinations]). Self-evaluation of clinical skills is a way to focus on therapeutic improvement. Role-playing can help prepare you for clinical experience and provide practice in using effective and professional communication skills.

THE CLINICAL INTERVIEW

Ideally, the content and direction of the clinical interview are decided and led by the patient. The nurse uses communication skills and active listening to better understand the patient's situation. During the clinical interview, the nurse can conduct key assessments including the mental status examination and psychosocial assessment (see Chapter 6).

Preparing for the Interview
Pace
Helping a person with an emotional or medical problem is rarely a straightforward task, and the goal of assisting a patient in regaining psychological or physiological stability can be difficult to achieve. Extremely important to any kind of counselling is permitting the patient to set the pace of the interview, no matter how slow or halting the progress may be (Arnold & Boggs, 2019).

Setting
Effective communication can take place almost anywhere. However, the quality of the interaction, whether in a clinic, a clinical unit, an office, or the patient's home, depends on the degree to which the nurse and patient feel safe; establishing a setting that enhances feelings of security is important to the therapeutic relationship. A health care setting, a conference room, or a quiet part of the unit that has relative privacy but is within view of others is ideal, but when the interview

---

Facilitation Skills Checklist

The following list identifies several different facilitation skills. Think about a clinical experience in which you were trying to facilitate a conversation or discussion. Place a check mark by each of the skills you believe you did well. Circle the ones you would like to improve.

Communication
_____ Invites quiet participants to contribute.
_____ Asks open questions to stimulate discussion.
_____ Paraphrases ideas and suggestions.
_____ Maintains open, balanced and clear communication.

Keeping on Track
_____ Allows time to address process issues.
_____ Keeps group on track to achieve objectives in given time frame.
_____ Establishes and reminds group members of norms for meeting behaviour.

Goals and Roles
_____ Clarifies goals and objectives of interaction or discussion.
_____ Checks and ensures common understanding of goals.
_____ Provides time to discuss, clarify, or modify or negotiate goals.
_____ Ensures roles are assigned and understood.

Conflict Management
_____ Steers conflict away from personalities and towards task-related issues.
_____ Summarizes opposing or differing positions.
_____ Determines when members are suppressing their ideas to avoid conflict.
_____ Determines whether conflict is constructive and task related.

Fig. 10.2 Facilitative Skills Checklist.

takes place in the patient's home, the nurse has a valuable opportunity to assess the patient in the context of everyday life.

Seating

In all settings chairs should be arranged so that conversation can take place in a normal tone of voice and eye contact can be comfortably maintained or avoided. A non-threatening physical environment for both nurse and patient involves:

- Assuming the same height, either both sitting or both standing
- Avoiding a face-to-face stance when possible; a 90- to 120-degree angle or side-by-side position may be less intense, and the patient and nurse can look away from each other without discomfort
- Providing safety and psychological comfort in terms of exiting the room; the patient should not be positioned between the nurse and the door, nor should the nurse be positioned in such a way that the patient feels trapped in the room
- Avoiding a desk barrier between the nurse and the patient

Introductions

In the orientation phase nurses introduce themselves to their patients, describe the purpose of the meeting, and explain for how long and at what times they will be meeting with the patient. This introduction process sets an important tone and is crucial to later interventions and outcomes (Shajani & Snell 2019). The issue of confidentiality is brought up during the initial interview. Remember that all health care providers must respect the private, personal, and confidential nature of the patient's communication, except in the specific situations outlined earlier (e.g., harm to self or others, child abuse, elder abuse). What is discussed with fellow staff and your clinical group in conference should not be discussed outside with others, no matter who they are (e.g., patient's relatives, news media, friends). The patient needs to know that whatever is discussed will stay confidential unless permission is given for it to be disclosed. Refer to Chapter 9 to review the nurse's responsibilities in the orientation phase.

Ask the patient how they would like to be addressed. This question conveys respect and gives the patient direct control over an important ego issue. Some patients like to be called by their last names; others prefer being on a first-name basis with the nurse (Arnold & Boggs, 2019).

Initiating the Interview

Once introductions have been made, you can turn the interview over to the patient by using one of a number of open-ended questions or statements:

- "Where should we start?"
- "Tell me a little about what has been going on with you."
- "What are some of the stresses you have been coping with recently?"
- "Tell me a little about what has been happening in the past couple of weeks."
- "Perhaps you can begin by letting me know what some of your concerns have been recently."
- "Tell me about your difficulties."

Communication can be facilitated by appropriately offering leads (e.g., "Go on"), making statements of acceptance (e.g., "Uh-huh"), or otherwise conveying interest.

Tactics to Avoid

Certain behaviours are counterproductive and should be avoided. For example:

Do Not …	Try To …
Argue with, minimize, or challenge the patient	Keep the focus on facts and the patient's perceptions
Give false reassurance	Make observations of the patient's behaviour (e.g., "Change is always possible.")
Interpret situations for the patient or speculate on interpersonal dynamics	Listen attentively, use silence, and try to clarify the patient's problems
Question or probe patients about sensitive topics they do not wish to discuss	Pay attention to non-verbal communication; strive to keep the patient's anxiety to a minimum
Try to sell the patient on accepting treatment	Encourage the patient to look at pros and cons
Join in attacks that patients launch on their mates, parents, friends, or associates	Focus on facts and the patient's perceptions; be aware of non-verbal communication
Participate in criticism of another nurse or any other staff member	Focus on facts and the patient's perceptions; check out serious accusations with the nurse or staff member; have the patient meet with the nurse or staff member in question in the presence of a senior staff member and clarify perceptions

Helpful Guidelines

Meier and Davis (2019) offer some guidelines for conducting the initial interview:

- Speak briefly.
- When you do not know what to say, say nothing.
- When in doubt, focus on feelings.
- Avoid giving advice.
- Avoid relying on questions.
- Pay attention to non-verbal cues.
- Keep the focus on the patient.

Attending Behaviours: The Foundation of Interviewing

Engaging in attending behaviours and actively listening are two key principles of counselling on which almost everyone can agree (Sommers-Flanagan & Sommers-Flanagan, 2016). Positive attending behaviours serve to open up communication and encourage free expression, whereas negative attending behaviours are more likely to inhibit expression. All behaviours must be evaluated in terms of cultural patterns and past experiences of both the interviewer and the interviewee. There are no universals; however, there are guidelines that students can follow.

Eye Contact

As previously discussed, cultural and individual variations influence a patient's comfort with eye contact. For some patients and interviewers, sustained eye contact is normal and comfortable. For others, it may be more comfortable and natural to make brief eye contact but look away or down much of the time. In most situations it is appropriate for nurses to maintain more eye contact when the patient speaks and less constant eye contact when the nurse speaks (Sommers-Flanagan & Sommers-Flanagan, 2016).

Body Language

Body language involves two elements: kinesics and proxemics. *Kinesics* is associated with physical characteristics, such as body movements and postures. Facial expressions; eye contact or lack thereof; and the way someone holds the head, legs, and shoulders convey a multitude of messages. A person who slumps in a chair, rolls their eyes, and sits with arms crossed in front of the chest can be perceived as resistant and unreceptive to what another wants to communicate. On the other hand, a person who leans in slightly towards the speaker, maintains a relaxed and attentive posture, makes appropriate eye contact, makes hand gestures that are unobtrusive and smooth while minimizing the number of other movements, and whose facial expressions match their feelings or the patient's feelings can be perceived as open to and respectful of the communication.

Proxemics refers to the study of personal space and the significance of the physical distance between individuals. Proxemics considers that these distances may be different for different cultural groups. Intimate distance in Canada is 0 to 45 centimetres and is reserved for those we trust most and with whom we feel most safe. Personal distance (45 to 120 centimetres) is for personal communications, such as those with friends or colleagues. Social distance (120 to 360 centimetres, or approximately 3.5 metres) applies to strangers or acquaintances, often in public places or formal social gatherings. Public distance (3.5 metres) relates to public space (e.g., public speaking). In public space one may hail another, and the parties may move about while communicating.

Vocal Quality

Vocal quality, or paralinguistics, encompasses voice loudness, pitch, rate, and fluency and can improve rapport, demonstrate empathy and interest, and add emphasis to words or concepts (Sommers-Flanagan & Sommers-Flanagan, 2016). Speaking in soft and gentle tones is apt to encourage a person to share thoughts and feelings, whereas speaking in a rapid, high-pitched tone may convey anxiety and create it in the patient. Consider, for example, how tonal quality can affect communication in a simple sentence like "I will see you tonight."

1. "*I* will see you tonight." (I will be the one who sees you tonight.)
2. "I *will* see you tonight." (No matter what happens, or whether you like it or not, I will see you tonight.)
3. "I will see *you* tonight." (Even though others are present, it is you I want to see.)
4. "I will see you *tonight*." (It is definite; tonight is the night we will meet.)

Verbal Tracking

Verbal tracking is just that: tracking what the patient is saying. Individuals cannot know if you are hearing or understanding what they are saying unless you provide them with cues. Verbal tracking offers neutral feedback in the form of simply restating or summarizing what the patient has already said without personal or professional opinions, judgements, or comments (Sommers-Flanagan & Sommers-Flanagan, 2016). For example:

Patient: "I don't know what the fuss is about. I smoke marijuana to relax, and everyone makes a fuss."
Nurse: "Do you see the use of marijuana as a problem for you?"
Patient: "No, I don't. It doesn't affect my work ... well, most of the time, anyway. I mean, of course, if I have to think things out and make important decisions, then obviously it can get in the way. But most of the time, I'm cool."
Nurse: "So when important decisions have to be made, then it interferes; otherwise, you don't see it affecting your functioning."
Patient: "Yeah, well, most of the time, I'm cool."

Meier and Davis (2019) stated that verbal tracking involves checking one's understanding with the patient by restating—as much as possible, in one's own words—in order to confirm the patient's speech content (as well as to clarify the meaning of speech volume and tone, as discussed earlier). It can be difficult to know which leads to follow if the patient introduces many topics at once. When this happens, the nurse can summarize what they have heard; reflect the emotions, experiences, thoughts, and contexts as much as possible; and help the patient focus on and explore a specific topic or goal. "With everything going on in your life recently, you must really feel overwhelmed. You're $2000 in debt and don't have a job, you've gained 15 kg in 6 months, and your wife is frustrated with your drinking. Let's talk more about what is going on with your wife and her concerns about alcohol."

Clinical Supervision

Communication and interviewing techniques are acquired skills. You will learn to improve these abilities through practice and clinical supervision. With clinical supervision, the focus is on the nurse's behaviour in the nurse–patient relationship; the nurse and supervisor have opportunities to examine and analyze the nurse's feelings and reactions to the patient and the way they affect the relationship. Clinical supervision for students in psychiatric mental health practice can occur in a one-to-one conversation or as part of a group discussion in post-conference. The rationale for and importance of clinical supervision is stressed in Chapter 9.

An increasingly popular method of providing clinical supervision is debriefing. According to the National League for Nursing (2015), debriefing is such an excellent learning method that it should be incorporated into all clinical experiences. **Debriefing** refers to a critical conversation and reflection regarding an experience that results in growth and learning. Debriefing supports essential learning along a continuum of "knowing what" to "knowing how" and "knowing why" (Varcarolis, 2017).

The opportunity to examine interactions, obtain insights, and devise alternative strategies for dealing with various clinical issues enhances clinical growth and minimizes frustration and burnout. Clinical supervision and debriefing are necessary professional activities that foster professional growth and curiosity and help minimize the development of non-therapeutic nurse–patient relationships.

Process Recordings

The best way to improve communication and interviewing skills is to review your clinical interactions exactly as they occur. This process offers the opportunity to identify themes and patterns in both your own and your patients' communications. As students, clinical review helps you learn to deal with the variety of situations that arise in the clinical interview.

Process recordings are written records of a segment of the nurse–patient session that reflect as closely as possible the verbal and nonverbal behaviours of both patient and nurse. Process recordings have some disadvantages because they rely on memory and are subject to distortions. However, they can be a useful tool for identifying communication patterns. Sometimes an observing clinician takes notes during the interview, but this practice also has disadvantages in that it may be distracting for both interviewer and patient. Some patients (especially those with a paranoid disorder) may resent or misunderstand the observer's intent.

It is usually best to write notes verbatim (word for word) in a private area immediately after the interaction has taken place. You can carefully record your words and the patient's words, identify whether your responses are therapeutic, and recall your thinking and emotions at the time.

Videotaped simulations with professional actors or in role-play may also provide students with an opportunity to analyze their communication skills using a process recording.

Table 10.4 gives an example of a process recording.

TABLE 10.4 Example of a Process Recording

Nurse	Patient	Communication Technique	Nurse's Thoughts and Feelings
"Good morning, Mr. Long."		**Therapeutic.** Giving recognition. Acknowledging a patient by name can enhance self-esteem and communicates that the nurse views the patient as an individual.	I was feeling nervous. He had attempted suicide, and I didn't know if I could help him. Initially I was feeling somewhat overwhelmed.
	"Who are you, and where the devil am I?" (Gazes around with a confused look on his face—quickly sits on the edge of the bed)		
"I am Ms. Rossi. I am your nurse, and you are at St. Paul's Hospital. I would like to spend some time with you today."		**Therapeutic.** Giving information. Informing the patient of facts needed to make decisions or come to realistic conclusions. **Therapeutic.** Offering self. Making oneself available to the patient.	
	"What am I doing here? How did I get here?" (Spoken in a loud, demanding voice)		I felt a bit intimidated when he raised his voice.
"You were brought in by your wife last night after swallowing a bottle of aspirin. You had to have your stomach pumped."		**Therapeutic.** Giving information. Giving needed facts so that the patient can orient himself and better evaluate his situation.	
	"Oh … yeah." (Silence for 2 minutes; shoulders slumped, Mr. Long stares at the floor and drops his head and eyes)		I was uncomfortable with the silence, but since I didn't have anything useful to say, I stayed with him in silence for the 2 minutes.
"You seem upset, Mr. Long. What are you thinking about?"		**Therapeutic.** Making observations. **Therapeutic.** Giving broad openings in an attempt to get at his feelings.	I began to feel sorry for him; he looked so sad and helpless.
	"Yeah, I just remembered. … I wanted to kill myself." (Said in a low tone almost to himself)		
"Oh, Mr. Long, you have so much to live for. You have such a loving family."		**Non-therapeutic.** Defending **Non-therapeutic.** Introducing an unrelated topic.	I felt overwhelmed. I didn't know what to say—his talking about killing himself made me nervous. I could have said, "You must be very upset" (verbalizing the implied) or "Tell me more about this" (exploring).
	"What do you know about my life? You want to know about my family? My wife is leaving me, that's what." (Faces the nurse with an angry expression on his face and speaks in loud tones)		Again, I felt intimidated by his anger, but now I linked it with his wife's leaving him, so I didn't take it as personally as I did the first time.
"I didn't know. You must be terribly upset by her leaving."		**Therapeutic.** Reflective. Observing the angry tone and content of the patient's message and reflecting the patient's feelings.	I really felt for him, and now I thought that encouraging him to talk more about this could be useful for him.

KEY POINTS TO REMEMBER

- Knowledge of communication and interviewing techniques is the foundation for the development of any nurse–patient relationship. Goal-directed professional communication is referred to as *therapeutic communication*.
- Communication is a complex process. Berlo's (1960) communication model has five parts: stimulus, sender, message, medium, and receiver.
- Feedback is a vital component of the communication process for validating the accuracy of the sender's message.
- Several factors can minimize, enhance, or otherwise influence the communication process: culture, language, knowledge level, noise, lack of privacy, presence of others, and expectations.
- There are verbal and non-verbal elements in communication; the non-verbal elements often play the larger role in conveying a person's message. Verbal communication consists of all words a person speaks. Non-verbal communication consists of the behaviours displayed by an individual, outside the actual content of speech.
- Communication has two levels: the content level (verbal speech) and the process level (non-verbal behaviour). When content is congruent with process, the communication is said to be healthy. When the verbal message is not reinforced by the communicator's actions, the message is ambiguous and incongruent; this is called a double (or mixed) message, leaving the responder in a double-bind situation.
- Cultural background (as well as individual differences) has a great deal to do with what non-verbal behaviour means to different individuals. The degree of eye contact and the use of touch are two non-verbal behaviours that can be misunderstood by individuals of different cultures.
- There are several therapeutic communication techniques nurses can use to enhance their nursing practices (see Table 10.2).
- There are also several non-therapeutic communication techniques that nurses can learn to avoid and to enhance their effectiveness in therapeutic relationships (see Table 10.3).
- Most nurses are most effective when they use non-threatening and open-ended communication techniques.
- Effective communication is a skill that develops over time and is integral to the establishment and maintenance of a therapeutic relationship.
- The clinical interview is a key component of psychiatric mental health nursing, and the nurse must establish a safe setting and plan for appropriate seating, introductions, and initiation of the interview.
- Attending behaviours (e.g., eye contact, body language, vocal qualities, verbal tracking) are key elements in effective communication.
- A meaningful therapeutic relationship is facilitated when values and cultural influences are considered. It is the nurse's responsibility to seek to understand the patient's perceptions.

CRITICAL THINKING

1. Keep a written log of a conversation you have with a patient. In your log identify the therapeutic and non-therapeutic techniques you noticed yourself using. Then rewrite the non-therapeutic communications using statements that would better facilitate discussion of thoughts and feelings. Share your log and discuss the changes you are working on with one classmate.
2. Role-play with a classmate at least five non-verbal communications, and have your partner identify the message they received.
3. With the other students in your class watching, plan and role-play a nurse–patient conversation that lasts about 3 minutes. Use both therapeutic and non-therapeutic techniques. When you are finished, have your other classmates try to identify the techniques you used. Discuss ways in which a reliance on colleagues or other subtle institutional concerns might factor into the communication.
4. Demonstrate how the nurse would use touch and eye contact when working with patients from three different cultural groups.

CHAPTER REVIEW

1. You have been working closely with a patient for the past month. Today, he tells you he is looking forward to meeting with his new psychiatrist but frowns and avoids eye contact while reporting this to you. Which of the following responses would most likely be therapeutic?
   a. "A new psychiatrist is a chance to start fresh. I'm sure it will go well for you."
   b. "You say you look forward to the meeting, but you appear anxious or unhappy."
   c. "I notice that you frowned and avoided eye contact just now—don't you feel well?"
   d. "I get the impression you don't really want to see your psychiatrist—can you tell me why?"
2. Which behaviour is consistent with therapeutic communication?
   a. Offering your opinion when asked in order to convey support.
   b. Summarizing the essence of the patient's comments in your own words.
   c. Interrupting periods of silence before they become awkward for the patient.
   d. Telling the patient they did well when you approve of their statements or actions.
3. Which statement about non-verbal behaviour is accurate?
   a. A calm expression means that the patient is experiencing low levels of anxiety.
   b. Patients respond more consistently to therapeutic touch than to verbal interventions.
   c. The meaning of non-verbal behaviours varies with cultural and individual differences.
   d. Eye contact is a reliable measure of the patient's degree of attentiveness and engagement.
4. A nurse stops in to interview a patient on a medical unit and finds the patient lying supine in her bed with the head elevated at 10 degrees. Which initial response would most enhance the chances of achieving a therapeutic interaction?
   a. Apologize for the differential in height and proceed while standing to avoid delay.
   b. If permitted, raise the head of the bed and, with the patient's permission, sit on the bed.
   c. If permitted, raise the head of the bed to approximate the nurse's height while standing.
   d. Sit in whatever chair is available in the room to convey informality and increase comfort.
5. A patient with schizophrenia approaches staff arriving for the day shift and anxiously reports, "Last night, demons came to my room and tried to rape me." Which response would be most therapeutic?
   a. "There are no such things as demons; what you saw were hallucinations."
   b. "It is not possible for anyone to enter your room at night; you are safe here."
   c. "You seem very upset; please tell me more about what you experienced last night."
   d. "That must have been very frightening, but we'll check on you at night, and you'll be safe."

https://evolve.elsevier.com/Canada/Varcarolis/psychiatric/

REFERENCES

Arnold, E. C., & Boggs, K. U. (2019). *Interpersonal relationships: Professional communication skills for nurses* (8th ed.). St. Louis: Elsevier.

Attum, B., Hafiz, S., Malik, A., & Shamoon, A. (2021). Cultural competence in the care of Muslim patients and their families. https://www.ncbi.nlm.nih.gov/books/NBK499933/

Balzer-Riley, J. W. (2021). *Communication in nursing* (9th ed.). St. Louis: Elsevier.

Bateson, G., Jackson, D. D., Haley, J., & Weakland, J. (1956). Toward a theory of schizophrenia. *Behavioural Sciences, 1*, 251–264.

Berlo, D. K. (1960). *The process of communication*. San Francisco: Reinhart Press.

Egan, G., & Reese, R. (2018). *The skilled helper: A problem-management approach and opportunity-development approach to helping* (11th ed.). Belmont: Brooks/Cole, Cengage Learning.

Ehrmin, J. T. (2019). Transcultural perspectives in mental health nursing. In M. M. Andrews, J. S. Boyle, & J. Collins (Eds.), *Transcultural concepts in nursing care* (8th ed.) (pp. 299–332). Philadelphia: Lippincott Williams & Wilkins.

Giger, J. N., & Haddad, L. (2020). *Transcultural nursing: Assessment and intervention* (8th ed.). Philadelphia: Elsevier.

Hartley, S., Raphael, J., Lovell, K., & Berry, K. (2020). Effective nurse–patient relationships in mental health care: A systematic review of interventions to improve therapeutic alliance. *International Journal of Nursing Studies, 102*(103490), 1–9. https://doi.org/10.1016/j.ijnurstu.2019.103490

Lorié, Á., Reinero, D. A., Phillips, M., Zhang, L., & Riess, H. (2017). Culture and non-verbal expressions of empathy in clinical settings: A systematic review. *Patient Education and Counseling, 100*(3), 411–424. https://dx.doi.org/10.1016/j.pec.2016.09.018

Meier, S. T., & Davis, S. R. (2019). *The elements of counseling* (8th ed.). Long Grove: Waveland Press Inc.

Mohl, P. C., & Carr, R. B. (2015). Listening to the patient. In A. Tasman, J. Kay, J. A. Lieberman, M. B. First, & M. B. Riba (Eds.), *Psychiatry* (4th ed.) (pp. 1–19). Chichester: Wiley. https://doi.org/10.1002/9781118753378.ch1

National League for Nursing. (2015). *Debriefing across the curriculum*. http://www.nln.org/docs/default-source/about/nln-vision-series-(position-statements)/nln-vision-debriefing-across-the-curriculum.pdf?sfvrsn=0

Peplau, H. E. (2004). *Interpersonal relations in nursing: A conceptual frame of reference for psychodynamic nursing*. New York: Springer.

Schein, E. H. (2014). *Humble inquiry: The gentle art of asking instead of telling*. San Francisco: Berrett-Koehler.

Shajani, Z., & Snell, D. (2019). *Wright and Leahey's nurses and families: A guide to family assessment and intervention* (7th ed.). Philadelphia: F. A. Davis Company.

Shea, S. C. (2017). *Psychiatric interviewing: The art of understanding* (3rd ed.). Philadelphia: Elsevier.

Sommers-Flanagan, J., & Sommers-Flanagan, R. (2016). *Clinical interviewing* (6th ed.). Hoboken: Wiley.

Unhjem, J. V., Vatne, S., & Hem, M. H. (2018). Transforming nurse–patient relationships—A qualitative study of nurse self-disclosure in mental health care. *Journal of Clinical Nursing, 27*(5–6), e798–e807. https://doi.org/10.1111/jocn.14191

Varcarolis, E. M. (2017). *Essentials of psychiatric mental health nursing: A communication approach to evidence-based care*. Philadelphia: Elsevier.

Wheeler, K. (2020). *Psychotherapy for the advanced practice psychiatric nurse: A how-to guide for evidence-based practice* (2nd ed.). New York: Springer.

11

Psychotropic Drugs

Martin Davies, Paul M. Kerr

 https://evolve.elsevier.com/Canada/Varcarolis/psychiatric/

OBJECTIVES

1. Identify the functions of the brain and discuss how these functions can be altered by psychotropic drugs.
2. Describe how a neurotransmitter functions as a chemical messenger.
3. Identify the functions of the three major areas of the brain.
4. Explain how specific brain functions are altered in mental health disorders such as depression, anxiety, bipolar disorder, and schizophrenia.
5. Describe how imaging techniques are used to study brain structure and function in individuals with mental health disorders.
6. Describe the result of blockage of muscarinic receptors and α_1-adrenergic receptors by drugs used to treat psychosis.
7. Identify the main neurotransmitters affected by the following psychotropic drugs and their subgroups:
   a. Anti-anxiety drugs
   b. Sedative–hypnotic drugs
   c. Anti-depressant drugs
   d. Mood stabilizers
   e. Anti-psychotic drugs
   f. Anti-cholinesterase drugs
8. Discuss dietary and drug restrictions for a patient taking a monoamine oxidase inhibitor.
9. Identify specific cautions for a patient taking natural health products and psychotropic drugs.
10. Explore the relevance of pharmacogenetics (i.e., variations in effects and therapeutic actions of medications among different ethnic groups) in the use of psychotropic drugs.

KEY TERMS AND CONCEPTS

agonist
antagonist
anti-anxiety (anxiolytic) drugs
anti-cholinesterase drugs
biopsychiatry
circadian rhythms
first-generation antipsychotic drugs
hypnotic
limbic system
lithium carbonate
metabolites
monoamine oxidase inhibitors
mood stabilizer
neurons
neurotransmitters
pharmacodynamics
pharmacogenetics
pharmacokinetics
receptors
reticular activating system
reuptake
second-generation antipsychotic drugs
selective serotonin reuptake inhibitors
serotonin–norepinephrine reuptake inhibitor
synapse
therapeutic index
tricyclic anti-depressants

One in every five Canadians will have a mental health problem at some point in their lives.

Biopsychiatry, sometimes referred to as the *biological approach*, is a theoretical approach to understanding mental health disorders as biological malfunctions of the nervous system. Implied in this approach is the idea that brain function is related to, and can be affected by, several factors; these include genetics, neurodevelopmental factors, drugs, infection, and psychosocial experience, either alone or in combination with one another. Clinicians using this approach believe that abnormal changes in a patient's behaviour and mental and emotional experiences are caused by disturbances in normal brain function. For example, when the brain is not working as it should, the way it produces and responds to neurotransmitters, the "chemical messengers" of the nervous system, changes. These changes can, in turn, result in symptoms of depression, anxiety, post-traumatic stress disorder (PTSD), or any other combination of behavioural, emotional, or mental health disorders.

The primary goal of drug therapy is to restore "balance" to a malfunctioning brain. In recent years, there has been an explosion of information about the efficacy of psychotropic drugs (medication to treat mental illness); however, a full understanding of how these drugs improve symptoms continues to elude investigators. Early theories, such as the dopamine theory of schizophrenia and the monoamine theory of depression, are currently seen as overly simplistic because a large number of other neurotransmitters, hormones, and coregulators are now thought to play important and complex roles. Indeed, evidence suggests that some clinically useful drugs may be working by additional pathways at the genetic level that lead to long-term changes in brain structure and function. Current research, therefore, is focused on refining our understanding of how drugs can be used to alter the brain's responses to neurotransmitters, hormones, and coregulators, either by making more of the chemical available in the brain or by making the brain more sensitive to the chemical that is already there. In addition, as our understanding of these drugs grows, research is focusing more and more on how they bring about long-term changes in neuronal survival and connectivity via effects at the genetic level.

Included in this chapter is an overview of the major drugs used to treat mental health disorders and an explanation of how they work. Additional and detailed information regarding adverse and toxic effects, dosage, nursing implications, and teaching tools are presented in the appropriate clinical chapters (see Chapters 12–20).

Despite new knowledge about complex brain functions, there is still much to be clarified in understanding the ways in which the brain carries out its normal functions, is altered during disease, and is improved by pharmacological intervention. After reading this chapter, you should have a neurobiological framework into which you can place existing, as well as future, information about mental illness and its treatment.

 HOW A NURSE HELPED ME
When the Adverse Effects Are Too Much to Take

> A patient with a mental health disorder faces numerous challenges during the search for the correct medication and treatment regimen. At 19, my brother was hearing voices and felt that others were talking about him or trying to watch him through windows. A number of factors were thought to contribute to his strange behaviours, among them, his being stressed over a recent breakup with a girlfriend and using marijuana. However, he was diagnosed with paranoid schizophrenia. It was an extremely stressful time for my family, who had difficulty understanding and coping with his seemingly irrational and illogical behaviours.
>
> He was admitted to hospital and started on first-generation antipsychotics. After a psychiatric nurse met my parents, she assessed that they needed assistance in understanding my brother's illness. Specifically, she explained that my brother's behaviours were symptoms of his illness and also how the medications would help ease his symptoms. She also outlined the common adverse effects that he might experience as a consequence of taking the medication. As well, she listened to my parents' worries about the future.
>
> My brother was started on fluphenazine decanoate, a medication administered by injection, and his symptoms improved. The drug was administered for 2 years, but then he stopped taking it because of the adverse effects he was experiencing. We learned that restlessness, dry mouth, fatigue, tremors, and dizziness are not uncommon for people who are being treated with this kind of medication. It has been 40 years now since my brother's diagnosis, and he has not been on any medications for treatment since. Unfortunately, without any medication, he has been homeless for many years.
>
> If my brother resumes psychopharmacological treatment in the future, the nurse will need to identify what factors will affect his decision to continue to take the prescribed medication. The nurse will need to listen to my brother's preferences about when he takes the medication, and his level of tolerance for various adverse effects will need to be considered when making decisions about possible interventions. The treatment team will also have to examine ways to predict how my brother will respond to the medication so as to optimize initial treatment selections. It will be important to select the medication that will have the best effect on his schizophrenia and the one with the fewest adverse effects, because they may get only one more chance.

STRUCTURE AND FUNCTION OF THE BRAIN

Functions and Activities of the Brain

Regulating behaviour and carrying out mental processes are two of the many important responsibilities of the brain. Some of the major functions and activities of the brain are summarized in Box 11.1. Because these brain functions are carried out by similar mechanisms (interactions between neurons) and often in similar locations, mental health disturbances are often associated with alterations in other brain

> **BOX 11.1 Functions of the Brain**
> - Monitor changes in the external world
> - Monitor the composition of body fluids
> - Regulate the contractions of skeletal muscles
> - Regulate the internal organs
> - Initiate and regulate the basic drives: hunger, thirst, sex, aggressive self-protection
> - Mediate conscious sensation
> - Store and retrieve memories
> - Regulate mood (affect) and emotions
> - Think and perform intellectual functions
> - Regulate the sleep cycle
> - Produce and interpret language
> - Process visual and auditory data

functions, and the drugs used to treat mental disturbances can interfere with other activities of the brain.

Maintenance of Homeostasis

The brain serves as the coordinator and director of the body's response to both internal and external changes. Appropriate responses require a constant monitoring of the environment, interpretation and integration of the incoming information, and control over the appropriate organs of response. The goal of these responses is to maintain homeostasis and thus to maintain life.

Information about the external world is relayed from various sense organs to the brain by the peripheral nerves. This information, at first received as stimuli such as light, sound, or touch, must ultimately be interpreted into a picture, a train whistle, or a hand on the back. Interestingly, a component of major psychiatric disturbance (e.g., schizophrenia) is an alteration of sensory experience. Thus the patient may experience a sensation that does not originate in the external world. For example, people with schizophrenia may hear voices talking to them (auditory hallucination).

To respond to external changes, the brain has control over the skeletal muscles. This control involves the ability not only to initiate contraction (e.g., to contract the biceps and flex the arm) but also to fine-tune and coordinate contraction so a person can, for example, guide the fingers to the correct keys on a piano. Unfortunately, both psychiatric disease and the treatment of psychiatric disease with psychotropic drugs are associated with movement disturbances. It is important to remember that the skeletal muscles controlled by the brain include the diaphragm, essential for breathing, and the muscles of the throat, tongue, and mouth, essential for speech. Therefore drugs that affect brain function can, for example, stimulate or depress respiration or lead to slurred speech.

The brain not only makes sense of the external world but also keeps a close watch on internal functions. Information about blood pressure, body temperature, blood gases, and the chemical composition of body fluids are continuously received by the brain, allowing it to send the responses required to maintain homeostasis. Adjustments to changes within the body require that the brain exert control over the various internal organs. For example, if blood pressure drops, the brain must direct the heart to pump more blood and the smooth muscle cells of arterioles to constrict. This increase in cardiac output and vasoconstriction allows the body to return blood pressure to its normal level.

Regulation of the Autonomic Nervous System and Endocrine System

The autonomic nervous system and the endocrine system serve as the communication links between the brain and the internal organs of the body (Figure 11.1). If the brain needs to stimulate the heart, it must

Fig. 11.1 The autonomic nervous system has two divisions: the sympathetic and the parasympathetic. The sympathetic division is dominant in stressful situations such as those that incite fear or anger, known as the *fight-or-flight response*.

activate the sympathetic nerves to the sinoatrial node and the ventricular myocardium. If the brain needs to bring about vasoconstriction, it must activate sympathetic nerves that innervate the smooth muscle cells of arterioles.

The linkage between the brain and the internal organs that allows for the maintenance of homeostasis may also serve to translate mental health disturbances, such as anxiety, into alterations of internal function. For example, anxiety in some people can cause inappropriate activation of parasympathetic nerves to the digestive tract, leading to hypermotility and diarrhea. Likewise, anxiety can activate the sympathetic nerves innervating cardiac muscle, leading to a pounding, fast heart rate, and arterioles, leading to vasoconstriction and hypertension.

The brain also exerts influence over the internal organs by regulating hormonal secretions of the pituitary gland, which in turn regulates other glands. The hypothalamus is involved in several functions of the brain. It secretes hormones that act on the pituitary gland to stimulate or inhibit the synthesis and release of pituitary hormones. Once in the general circulation, these hormones influence various internal activities. For example, when gonadotropin-releasing hormone is secreted by the hypothalamus at puberty, this hormone stimulates the release of two gonadotropins, follicle-stimulating hormone and luteinizing hormone, by the pituitary gland, which consequently activate the ovaries or testes.

The relationship between the brain, the pituitary gland, and the adrenal glands is particularly important in determining normal and abnormal mental function. Specifically, the hypothalamus secretes corticotropin-releasing hormone (CRH), which stimulates the pituitary gland to release corticotropin, which in turn stimulates the cortex of each adrenal gland to secrete the hormone cortisol. This system is activated as part of the normal response to a variety of mental and physical stresses. Among many other actions, all three hormones, CRH, corticotropin, and cortisol, influence the functions of the nerve cells of the brain. There is considerable evidence that in both anxiety and depression this system is overactive and does not respond properly to negative feedback.

Control of Biological Drives and Behaviour

Apart from the many higher cognitive tasks in which the brain engages, it is also responsible for the basic drives such as sex and hunger that play a strong role in moulding behaviour. Disturbances in these drives, which may be manifested as eating disorders or loss of sexual interest, can be an indication of an underlying mental health disorder such as depression. By understanding why these disturbances occur, we may start to unravel the underlying pathology of these illnesses and establish a rational framework from which to approach treatment.

Cycle of sleep and wakefulness. The entire cycle of sleep and wakefulness, as well as the intensity of alertness while the person is awake, is regulated and coordinated by various regions of the brain. Although the true homeostatic function of sleep is not well understood, sleep is known to be essential for both physiological and psychological well-being. Assessment of sleep patterns is part of what is required to determine a diagnosis of a mental health disorder.

Unfortunately, many of the drugs used to treat mental health problems interfere with the normal regulation of sleep and alertness. Drugs with a sedative–hypnotic effect can blunt the degree to which a person feels alert and focused and can cause drowsiness. Because of the sedative–hypnotic effect, caution is necessary for using these drugs while engaging in activities that require a great deal of attention, such as driving a car or operating machinery. One way of minimizing the danger is to take such drugs at night just before bedtime.

Circadian rhythms. The cycle of sleep and wakefulness is only one aspect of circadian rhythms, the fluctuation of various physiological and behavioural parameters over a 24-hour cycle. Other variations include changes in body temperature, secretion of hormones such as corticotropin and cortisol, and secretion of neurotransmitters, chemicals that transmit signals from one neuron to another across a synapse, such as norepinephrine and serotonin. Both norepinephrine and serotonin are thought to be involved in mood, and daily fluctuations of mood may be related in part to circadian variations in these neurotransmitters. There is evidence that the circadian rhythm of neurotransmitter secretion is altered in mental health disorders, particularly in those that involve mood.

Conscious Mental Activity

All aspects of conscious mental experience and sense of self originate from the neurophysiological activity of the brain. Conscious mental activity can be a basic, meandering, stream-of-consciousness flow among thoughts of future responsibilities, memories, fantasy, and so on. Conscious mental activity can also be much more complex when it is applied to problem solving and the interpretation of the external world. Both the random stream of consciousness and the complex problem solving and interpretation of the environment can become distorted in mental health disorders. For instance, a person with schizophrenia may have chaotic and incoherent speech and thought patterns (e.g., a jumble of unrelated words known as *word salad*, unconnected phrases and topics known as *looseness of association*) and delusional interpretations of personal interactions (e.g., beliefs about people or events that are not supported by data or reality).

Memory

Memory, the ability to retain and recall past experience, is a crucial component of mental activity. From both an anatomical and a physiological perspective, there is thought to be a major difference in the processing of short- and long-term memory. This can be seen dramatically in some forms of cognitive mental health disorders such as dementia, in which a person has no recall of the events of the previous 10 minutes but may have vivid recall of events that occurred decades earlier.

Social Skills

An important and often neglected aspect of brain functioning involves the social skills that make interpersonal relationships possible. In almost all types of mental health disorders, from mild anxiety to severe schizophrenia, difficulties in interpersonal relationships are an important characteristic, and improvements in these relationships are important gauges of progress. The connection between brain activity and social behaviour is an area of intense research and is believed to be influenced by a combination of genetic makeup and individual experience.

Cellular Composition of the Brain

The brain is composed of approximately 100 billion neurons, nerve cells that conduct electrical impulses, as well as other types of cells that surround the neurons. Most functions of the brain, from regulation of blood pressure to the conscious sense of self, are thought to result from the actions of individual neurons and the interconnections between them. Although neurons come in a great variety of shapes and sizes, all carry out the same three types of physiological actions: (1) they respond to stimuli; (2) they conduct electrical impulses; and (3) they release chemicals called *neurotransmitters*.

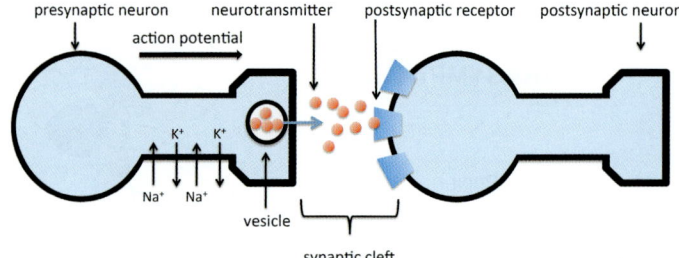

Fig. 11.2 Activities of neurons. Conduction of an action potential along a neuron involves the inward movement of sodium ions (Na+) followed by the outward movement of potassium ions (K+). When the action potential reaches the end of the neuron, neurotransmitter is released from vesicles (storage compartments). The neurotransmitter crosses the synapse and binds to a receptor on the postsynaptic cell. The interaction of neurotransmitter and receptor either stimulates or inhibits the postsynaptic cell.

An essential feature of neurons is their ability to conduct an electrical impulse (action potential) from one end of the cell to the other. The action potential consists of a change in membrane permeability that first allows the inward flow of sodium ions and then the outward flow of potassium ions. The inward flow of sodium ions changes the polarity of the membrane potential from negative to positive with respect to the outside. Movement of potassium ions out of the cell re-establishes the negative membrane potential readying the cell to generate the next action potential. Because these electrical charges are self-propagating, a change at one end of the cell is conducted along the membrane until it reaches the other end (Figure 11.2). The functional significance of this propagation is that the electrical impulse serves as a means of communication between one part of the body and another.

Once action potentials reach the end of a neuron, the neurotransmitter is released. Neurotransmitters are released from storage compartments called vesicles in the axon terminal of the *presynaptic neuron* (the term for the neuron from which the neurotransmitter is released). This neurotransmitter then diffuses across a space, or synapse, to an adjacent *postsynaptic neuron* (the neuron receiving the neurotransmitter), where it binds to receptors (protein molecules embedded in a cell membrane). A postsynaptic neuron may have a variety of receptors that allow for multiple neurotransmitters to affect its function. This communication between neurons by way of neurotransmitter–receptor interaction allows the activity of one neuron to influence the activity of other neurons. Depending on the chemical structure of the neurotransmitter and the specific type of receptor to which it binds, the postsynaptic cell will be rendered either more or less likely to initiate an action potential. The interaction between neurotransmitter and receptor is a major target of drugs used to treat mental health disorders. Important neurotransmitters and the types of receptors to which they bind are identified in Table 11.1. Also identified are the mental health disorders associated with an increase or decrease in these neurotransmitters.

The signal from the presynaptic to postsynaptic neuron is terminated by a reduction in the amount of neurotransmitter in the synapse. There are two basic mechanisms by which this is achieved: (1) Some neurotransmitters, such as acetylcholine are degraded by specific enzymes in the synapse. Acetylcholinesterase is the enzyme that destroys acetylcholine. (2) Other neurotransmitters, such as norepinephrine, are taken back into the presynaptic neuron from which they were originally released, a process called cellular reuptake. The neurotransmitters are then either reused or degraded by intracellular enzymes. In the case of the monoamine neurotransmitters (e.g., norepinephrine, dopamine, serotonin) the degrading enzyme is called *monoamine oxidase* (MAO). The processes of neurotransmitter removal are described further in Box 11.2.

TABLE 11.1 Transmitters and Receptors

Transmitters	Receptors	Effects/Comments	Association With Mental Health Disorders
Monoamines			
Dopamine (DA)	D_1, D_2, D_3, D_4, D_5	Involved in fine muscle movement Involved in integration of emotions and thoughts Involved in decision making Stimulates hypothalamus to release hormones (sex, thyroid, adrenal)	*Decreases:* Parkinson's disease Depression *Increases:* Schizophrenia Mania
Norepinephrine (NE) (noradrenaline)	α_1, α_2, β_1, β_2	Causes changes in mood Causes changes in attention and arousal Stimulates sympathetic branch of autonomic nervous system for fight or flight in response to stress	*Decreases:* Depression *Increases:* Mania Anxiety states Schizophrenia
Serotonin (5-hydroxytryptophan [5-HT])	$5\text{-}HT_1$, $5\text{-}HT_2$, $5\text{-}HT_3$, $5\text{-}HT_4$	Plays a role in sleep regulation, hunger, mood states, and pain perception Alters hormonal activity Plays a role in aggression and sexual behaviour	*Decreases:* Depression *Increases:* Anxiety states
Histamine	H_1, H_2	Involved in alertness Involved in inflammatory response Stimulates gastric secretion	*Decreases:* Sedation Weight gain
Amino Acids			
Gamma-aminobutyric acid (GABA)	$GABA_A$, $GABA_B$	Plays a role in inhibition; reduces aggression, excitation, and anxiety May play a role in pain perception Has anticonvulsant and muscle-relaxing properties May impair cognition and psychomotor functioning	*Decreases:* Anxiety disorders Schizophrenia Mania Huntington's disease *Increases:* Reduction of anxiety
Glutamate	N-methyl-d-aspartate (NMDA), α-amino-3-hydroxy-5-methyl-4-isoxazolepropionic acid (AMPA)	Is excitatory AMPA plays a role in learning and memory	*Decreases (NMDA):* Psychosis *Increases (NMDA):* Prolonged increased state can be neurotoxic Neurodegeneration in Alzheimer's disease *Increases (AMPA):* Improvement of cognitive performance in behavioural tasks
Cholinergics			
Acetylcholine (ACh)	Nicotinic, muscarinic (M_1, M_2, M_3)	Plays a role in learning, memory Regulates mood, mania, sexual aggression Affects sexual and aggressive behaviour Stimulates parasympathetic nervous system	*Decreases:* Alzheimer's disease Huntington's disease Parkinson's disease *Increases:* Depression
Peptides (Neuromodulators)			
Substance P (SP)	Neurokinin 1 receptor (NK1)	Has antidepressant and anti-anxiety effects in depression Promotes and reinforces memory Enhances sensitivity of pain receptors	Involved in regulation of mood and anxiety Plays a role in pain management
Somatostatin (SST, somatotropin release–inhibiting factor [SRIF])	SST_1, SST_2, SST_3, SST_4, SST_5	Alters cognition, memory, and mood	*Decreases:* Alzheimer's disease Decreased levels of SRIF in spinal fluid of some depressed patients *Increases:* Huntington's disease
Neurotensin (NT)	$NTSR_1$, $NTSR_2$	Has endogenous antipsychotic-like properties	Decreased levels in spinal fluid of schizophrenic patients

> ### BOX 11.2 Reduction of Neurotransmitters in the Synapse
>
> A full explanation of the various ways in which psychotropic drugs alter neuronal activity requires a brief review of the manner in which neurotransmitter levels are reduced in the synapse to avoid continuous and prolonged action on the postsynaptic cell.
> Following release of neurotransmitter from vesicles in the presynaptic neuron, the neurotransmitter is dealt with in one of two ways.
>
> 1. Degradation of the neurotransmitter in the synapse. An example of this method of destruction is the action of the enzyme acetylcholinesterase (AChE) on the neurotransmitter acetylcholine. AChE is located on the pre- and postsynaptic membrane and breaks down acetylcholine.
>
>
>
> 2. Neurotransmitter is taken back into the presynaptic neuron. Following release of neurotransmitter into the synapse, it re-enters the presynaptic neuron via a transporter in the cell membrane. This process, referred to as *reuptake*, is a target for many drugs. Once inside the presynaptic neuron, the neurotransmitter is either recycled into vesicles or inactivated by an enzyme within the cell. The monoamine neurotransmitters norepinephrine, dopamine, and serotonin are all inactivated in this manner by the enzyme monoamine oxidase (MAO).
>
>

As a means of fine control of communication between neurons, the amount of neurotransmitter released from presynaptic nerve terminals can be regulated by presynaptic neurotransmitter receptors. Autoreceptors are presynaptic receptors that bind to the very neurotransmitter that the nerve ending is releasing, and their activation typically inhibits further neurotransmitter release. On the other hand, some presynaptic receptors respond to different neurotransmitters released from adjacent neurons, and their activation can inhibit or stimulate further neurotransmitter release.

Researchers have found that in many cases, neurons release more than one chemical at the same time. Neurotransmitters such as norepinephrine or acetylcholine, which have immediate effects on postsynaptic neurons, are often accompanied by larger molecules, neuropeptides, that may initiate long-term changes in the postsynaptic neurons. These changes may involve basic cell functions, such as genetic expression, and lead to modifications of cell shape and responsiveness to stimuli. Ultimately, this means that the action of one neuron on another affects not only the immediate response of that neuron but also its sensitivity to future influence. The long-term implications of this for neural development, normal and abnormal mental health, and the treatment of mental health disorders are being investigated.

The communication between neurons at a synapse is not unidirectional. *Neurotrophic factors*, proteins and even simple gases, such as carbon monoxide and nitric oxide, are released by postsynaptic cells and influence the growth, shape, and activity of presynaptic cells. These factors are thought to be particularly important during the development of the fetal brain, guiding the growing brain to form the proper neuronal connections. However, it is now apparent that the brain retains anatomical plasticity throughout life and that internal and external influences can alter synaptic networks of the brain. The role of altered genetic expression or environmental trauma in the action of these factors and the negative and positive consequences of these changes on mental function and psychiatric disease are areas of much research.

The development and responsiveness of neurons are dependent not only on chemicals released by other neurons but also on chemicals, particularly the steroid hormones, carried to the brain in the blood. Estrogen, testosterone, and cortisol can bind to receptors in neurons, where they can cause short- and long-term changes in neuronal activity. A clear example of this is seen in the psychosis that can sometimes result from the hypersecretion of cortisol in Cushing's disease or from the use of prednisone in high doses to treat chronic inflammatory disease.

Organization of the Brain
Brainstem
The brainstem is responsible for such vital functions as the regulation of internal organs, blood gases, and blood pressure. It also serves as a crucial psychosomatic link between higher brain activities, such as thought and emotion, and the functioning of the internal organs. The brainstem also functions as an initial processing centre for sensory information that is then sent on to the cerebral cortex. Through projections of the **reticular activating system** (RAS), the brainstem regulates the entire cycle of sleep and wakefulness and the ability of the cerebrum to carry out conscious mental activity.

Other ascending pathways, referred to as *mesolimbic* and *mesocortical pathways*, seem to play a strong role in modulating the emotional value of sensory material. These pathways project to those areas of the cerebrum, the hypothalamus, amygdala, and hippocampus, collectively known as the **limbic system**, that play a crucial role in emotional status and psychological function. The hypothalamus, a small area in the ventral superior portion of the brainstem, plays a vital role in such basic drives as hunger, thirst, and sex. The pathways use norepinephrine, serotonin, and dopamine as their neurotransmitters. Much attention has been paid to the role of these pathways in normal and abnormal mental activity. For example, it is thought that the release of dopamine from the *ventral tegmental pathway* plays a role in psychological reward and substance dependence. The neurotransmitters released by the neurons in the mesolimbic and mesocortical pathways are major targets of the drugs used to treat mental health disorders.

Cerebellum

Located posteriorly to the brainstem, the cerebellum (Figure 11.3) is primarily involved in the regulation of skeletal muscle coordination and contraction and the maintenance of equilibrium. It plays a crucial role in coordinating contractions so that movement is accomplished in a smooth and directed manner.

Cerebrum

The human brainstem and cerebellum are similar in both structure and function to these same structures in other mammals. The development of a much larger and more elaborate cerebrum is what distinguishes human beings from the rest of the animal kingdom.

The cerebrum, situated on top of and surrounding the brainstem, is responsible for mental activities and a conscious sense of being, including our conscious perception of the external world and our own body, emotional status, memory, and control of skeletal muscles that allows willful direction of movement. It is also responsible for language and the ability to communicate.

The cerebrum (the cerebral cortex and basal ganglia) consists of both the surface and deep areas of undulating grey matter and the connecting tracts of white matter that link these areas with each other and the rest of the nervous system. The cerebral cortex, which forms the outer layer of the brain, is responsible for conscious sensation and the initiation of movement. Specific areas of the cortex are responsible for specific sensations: the parietal cortex for touch, the temporal cortex for sound, the occipital cortex for vision, and so on. The initiation of skeletal muscle contraction is controlled by a specific area of the frontal cortex. All areas of the cortex are interconnected to enable an appropriate picture of the world to be formed and, if necessary, linked to a proper response (Figure 11.4).

Specialized areas of the cerebral cortex are responsible for language in both its sensory and its motor aspects. Sensory language functions include the ability to read, understand spoken language, and know the names of objects perceived by the senses. Motor functions involve the physical ability to use muscles properly for speech and writing. In both neurological and psychological dysfunction the use of language may

Fig. 11.3 The functions of the brainstem and cerebellum.

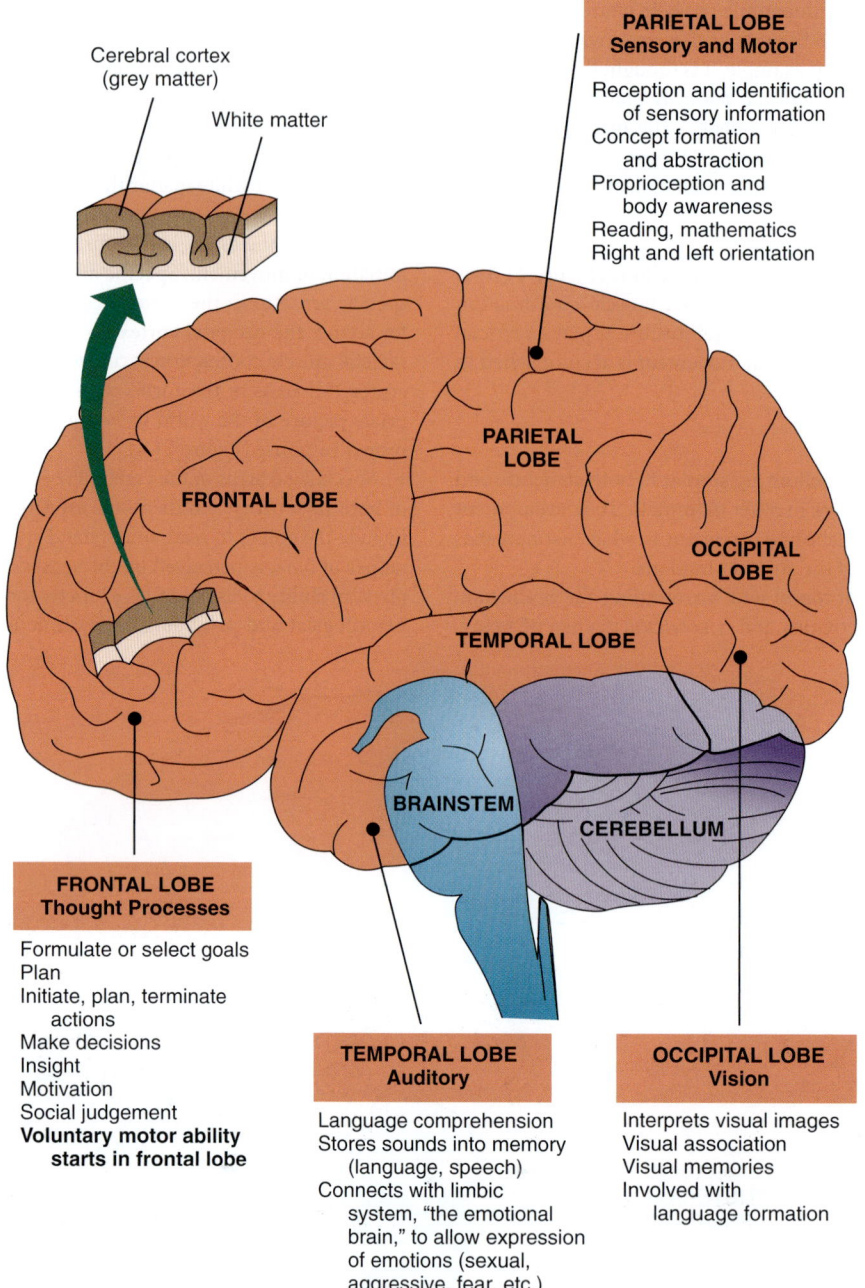

Fig. 11.4 The functions of the cerebral lobes: frontal, parietal, temporal, and occipital.

become compromised or distorted. A change in linguistic ability may be a factor in determining a diagnosis.

The basal ganglia are located deep within the grey matter of the cerebrum; they are involved in the regulation of movement. Other structures, the amygdala and hippocampus, are involved in emotions, learning, memory, and basic drives. Significantly, there is an overlap of these various areas both anatomically and in the types of neurotransmitters employed. One consequence of this overlap is that drugs used to treat emotional disturbances may cause movement disorders, and drugs used to treat movement disorders may cause emotional changes.

Visualizing the Brain

Various non-invasive imaging techniques can be used to visualize brain structure, function, and biological activity. Some common brain imaging techniques and preliminary findings as they relate to psychiatry are identified in Table 11.2. There are basically two types of information that can be obtained using neuroimaging techniques: structural and functional. By obtaining structural information from people with a specific disease and comparing it to those free of the disease, investigators can determine whether differences in the structure or volume of specific brain regions may be tied to the disease (Lui et al., 2016). Techniques such as computed tomography (CT) and magnetic resonance imaging (MRI) are often used in these types of studies. Functional information can reveal whether people suffering from psychiatric illness display changes in communication between different brain regions, alterations in blood flow and glucose metabolism, or differences in the function of specific neurotransmitter systems. For these types of studies, positron emission tomography (PET) and single-photon emission computed tomography (SPECT) are commonly used, as is a variant of MRI called functional magnetic resonance imaging (fMRI).

TABLE 11.2 Common Brain Imaging Techniques

Technique	Description	Detection	Psychiatric Relevance and Preliminary Findings
Structural: Show Gross Anatomical Details of Brain Structures			
Computed tomography (CT)	A series of X-ray images of the brain is taken, and computer analysis produces "slices," providing a precise 3D-like reconstruction of each segment	Lesions Abrasions Areas of infarct Aneurysm	*Schizophrenia:* Cortical atrophy Third ventricle enlargement *Cognitive disorders:* Abnormalities
Magnetic resonance imaging (MRI)	A magnetic field is applied to the brain; nuclei of hydrogen atoms absorb and emit radio waves that are analyzed by computer, providing 3D visualization of the brain's structure in sectional images	Brain edema Ischemia Infection Neoplasm Trauma	*Schizophrenia:* Enlarged ventricles Reduction in temporal lobe and prefrontal lobe
Functional magnetic resonance imaging (fMRI)	Functional imaging approach avoids exposure to ionizing radiation	(See MRI)	(See MRI)
Functional: Show Some Activity of the Brain			
Positron emission tomography (PET)	Radioactive substance (tracer) injected, travels to the brain, and shows up as bright spots on the scan; data collected by detectors are relayed to a computer, which produces images of the activity and 3D visualization of CNS	Oxygen use Glucose metabolism Blood flow Neurotransmitter–receptor interaction	*Schizophrenia:* Increased D_2, D_3 receptors in caudate nucleus Abnormalities in limbic system *Mood disorders:* Abnormalities in temporal lobes *Adult ADHD:* Decreased use of glucose
Single-photon emission computed tomography (SPECT)	Similar to PET but uses radionuclides that emit gamma radiation (photons); measures various aspects of brain functioning and provides images of multiple layers of the CNS (as does PET)	Circulation of cerebrospinal fluid Similar functions to PET	(See PET)

ADHD, Attention-deficit/hyperactivity disorder; CNS, central nervous system; 3D, three-dimensional; D2/3 receptors mediate specific dopamine neurotransmission impacting locomotion, attention, sleep, memory, learning (D2) and cognition, impulse control, attention, sleep (D3).

PET scans are particularly useful in identifying physiological and biochemical changes as they occur in living tissue. Usually there is not the potential for dependence that a radioactive "tag" is used to trace compounds such as glucose. Because neurons rely on glucose as their primary energy source, the tagged glucose can be followed to see which parts of the brain are most active. For example, in patients with untreated schizophrenia, PET scans may show a decreased use of glucose in the frontal lobes. Figure 11.5 shows lower brain activity in the frontal lobe of an identical twin diagnosed with schizophrenia than in that of the asymptomatic twin. The area affected in the frontal cortex of the twin with schizophrenia is an area associated with reasoning skills, which are greatly impaired in people with schizophrenia. Scans such as these suggest a location in the frontal cortex as the site of functional impairment in people with schizophrenia.

In one study of people with obsessive-compulsive disorder (OCD) PET scans revealed abnormally high activity in certain parts of the frontal cortex. This is illustrated in Figure 11.6, which shows increased use of glucose in these regions in an individual with OCD when compared with a control. This indicates that these parts of the brain are working harder than is usual.

Similarly, changes in activity in discrete brain regions have been shown in people diagnosed with depression. Figure 11.7 illustrates findings from a PET study with depressed people showing decreased glucose use (and therefore lower activity) in the prefrontal cortex and other areas of the brain. Finally, Figure 11.8 shows PET scans of the brain of a patient with Alzheimer's disease at ages 56 and 58. In this study investigators used a radioactive chemical to detect β-amyloid, the protein that is a hallmark of the disease. The scans indicate increased amounts of β-amyloid in various brain regions as the patient ages, and this was associated with diminished cognitive performance as assessed by a Mini-Mental State Examination (MMSE). In a separate experiment this study also showed that there was a strong correlation between a decrease in MMSE scores and a decrease in cerebral glucose metabolism as assessed by PET.

Modern imaging techniques have also become important tools in assessing molecular changes in mental health disorders and in marking the receptor sites of drug action. It is important to be able to understand which brain areas are associated with psychopathology and which biological functions are altered in psychiatric disease states in order to develop new therapies, as well as to improve the use of those currently available. While these imaging techniques have greatly increased our understanding of psychiatric diseases, they still cannot be used in isolation to diagnose these diseases. However, it is hoped that as these techniques mature and become more sophisticated, they can be used in the early diagnosis of various conditions and to monitor changes that occur in response to pharmacotherapy in order to personalize drug treatment. In conjunction with other validated diagnostic tools this could lead to a powerful new approach to disease management (Fu & Costafreda, 2013).

Fig. 11.5 Positron emission tomography (PET) scans of blood flow in identical twins, one of whom has schizophrenia, illustrate that individuals with this illness have reduced brain activity in the frontal lobes when asked to perform a reasoning task that requires activation of this area. Patients with schizophrenia perform poorly on the task. This suggests a site of functional impairment in schizophrenia. (From Karen Berman, MD, Courtesy National Institute of Mental Health, Clinical Brain Disorders Branch.)

Fig. 11.6 Positron emission tomography (PET) scans show increased brain metabolism (brighter colours), particularly in the frontal cortex, in a patient with obsessive-compulsive disorder (OCD), compared with a control. This suggests altered brain function in OCD. (From Lewis Baxter, MD, University of California, Los Angeles.)

Fig. 11.7 Positron emission tomography (PET) scans of a patient with depression *(right)* and a person without depression *(left)* reveal reduced brain activity (darker colours) in depression, especially in the prefrontal cortex. A form of radioactively tagged glucose was used as a tracer to visualize levels of brain activity. (From Mark George, MD, Courtesy National Institute of Mental Health, Biological Psychiatry Branch.)

Fig. 11.8 Positron emission tomography (PET) scan of a patient with Alzheimer's disease demonstrates the retention of ^{11}C-PIB, a marker for amyloid protein. Scans of the same patient at ages 56 and 58 show a consistently high amyloid load in various brain regions. Note that as the disease progresses, a drop in her cognitive abilities is reflected in a lower score in the mini-mental standard evaluation (MMSE). (From Kadir, A., Marutle, A., Gonzalez, D., et al. [2011]. Positron emission tomography imaging and clinical progression in relation to molecular pathology in the first Pittsburgh Compound B positron emission tomography patient with Alzheimer's disease. *Brain, 134*, 301–317. By permission of Oxford University Press.)

Disturbances of Mental Function

The origin of most mental health dysfunction is unknown. Among known biological causes are drugs (e.g., lysergic acid diethylamide [LSD]), long-term use of prednisone, unusually high levels of hormones (e.g., thyroxine, cortisol), infection (e.g., encephalitis, acquired immunodeficiency syndrome [AIDS]), and physical trauma. However, even when the cause is known, the mechanistic link between the causative factors, biological and psychosocial, and the mental health dysfunction is far from understood.

Evidence suggests that many people with psychiatric disorders are genetically predisposed to them. The incidence of both thought and mood disorders is higher in relatives of people with these diseases than in the general population. Evidence has also shown a strong concordance among identical twins, even when they are raised apart. *Concordance* refers to how often one twin will be affected by the same illness as the other. Psychosocial stress, either in the family of origin or in contacts with society at large, increases the likelihood of mental health problems, including biological changes, as does physical disease. Genetics and environment interact in complex ways so that some people are better able to cope with stress than others (Amstadter et al., 2014; Palix Foundation, 2022).

Researchers ultimately want to be able to understand mental health dysfunction in terms of altered activity of neurons in specific areas of the brain. The hope is that such an understanding will lead to better treatments and possible prevention of mental health disorders. Current interest is focused on certain neurotransmitters and their receptors, particularly those in the limbic system: norepinephrine, dopamine, serotonin, gamma-aminobutyric acid (GABA), and glutamate.

As shown in Figure 11.9, dysfunction of these neurotransmitter systems may be due to a deficiency in neurotransmitter release by the presynaptic cell or an inability of postsynaptic receptors to respond to neurotransmitters. Changes in neurotransmitter release and receptor response can be both a cause and a consequence of disease states, and it has proven to be difficult to determine which happens first. Thought disorders such as schizophrenia are associated physiologically with excess transmission of the neurotransmitter dopamine, among other changes. As illustrated in Figure 11.10, this change in dopamine transmission may be due to either an excess release of neurotransmitter or an increase in receptor responsiveness.

Fig. 11.9 (A) Normal neurotransmission can be affected by both how much neurotransmitter is released and the number of receptors to which it binds. Deficiency in neurotransmission may be due to a decrease in neurotransmitter release, as shown in (B), or to a reduction in the number of postsynaptic receptors, as shown in (C).

Fig. 11.10 Causes of increased signalling between neurons. Normal dopamine transmission (A) balances release to reception of the neurochemical. Increased neurotransmission may be due to excess release of neurotransmitter, as shown in (B), or to increased numbers of receptors, as shown in (C).

The neurotransmitter GABA plays a central role in modulating neuronal excitability. Abnormalities in GABA-related neurotransmission have been linked to anxiety. Not surprisingly, many **anti-anxiety (anxiolytic) drugs** act by increasing the effectiveness of this neurotransmitter, primarily by increasing receptor responsiveness.

It is important to keep in mind that the various areas of the brain are interconnected structurally and functionally by a vast network of neurons. This network serves to integrate the many and varied activities of the brain. A limited number of neurotransmitters are used in the brain, and thus a particular neurotransmitter is often used by different neurons and neuronal circuits to carry out quite different activities. For example, dopamine is used by neuronal circuitry involved not only in mood and reward but also in the regulation of movement. Because one neurotransmitter can mediate multiple brain functions, alterations in its activity due to a mental disturbance or to the drugs used to treat the disturbance can produce multiple effects that at first glance may seem unrelated to one another. In other words alterations in one particular aspect of brain function, whether arising from disease or from medication, are often accompanied by changes in basic drives, sleep patterns, body movement, and autonomic functions.

USE OF PSYCHOTROPIC DRUGS

The concepts of **pharmacodynamics** and **pharmacokinetics** are central to the understanding of the therapeutic actions and properties of drugs. Pharmacodynamics refers to the biochemical and physiological effects of drugs on the body, which include the mechanisms of drug action and its effect. When discussing the pharmacodynamics of a drug, the terms **agonist** and **antagonist** may be used to describe the actions of the drug at its target. A drug that is an agonist is one that binds to and activates its target and produces a response. On the other hand, a drug that is an antagonist binds to, but does not activate, its target. Rather, antagonists typically prevent other molecules such as neurotransmitters from binding to and activating the target protein. Antagonists produce no measurable effect by themselves. Pharmacokinetics refers to the actions of the body on the drug and involves four key aspects: (1) absorption (how much of the drug enters the circulation following administration); (2) distribution of an administered drug to body tissues; (3) metabolism of the drug (chemical change of the drug by the body); and (4) excretion of the drug or its **metabolites** (the products of metabolism). The major organ responsible for drug metabolism is the liver, and the major route of excretion is via urine produced by the kidneys. Ultimately, pharmacokinetics determines the change in blood level of a drug with time and is used to guide the dosage schedule. It is also used to determine the appropriate characteristics and doses of drugs that can safely be used in patients with liver and kidney disease.

The processes of pharmacokinetics and pharmacodynamics play an extensive role in how genetic factors give rise to variations in drug response among individuals and among ethnic groups. Pharmacogenetics is an approach to treatment that takes into consideration individual genetic differences when determining which and how much medication to prescribe (see Considering Culture box).

CONSIDERING CULTURE
Pharmacogenetics

Pharmacogenetic researchers are attempting to explain how genetic variations lead to clinical differences in drug responses for different individuals and ethnic groups (Zhang & Nebert, 2017). For example, different metabolizer phenotypes have significant differences in drug metabolism rates due to variations in the genes that code for their cytochrome P450 (CYP450) liver enzymes (Bertilsson, 2007). Of the more than 50 different CYP450 enzymes identified in humans, seven metabolize greater than 90% of the clinically most important drugs. For example, CYP2D6 (cytochrome P450 2D6, an enzyme encoded by the *CYP2D6* gene) alone is involved in the metabolism of 25 to 30% of all prescribed drugs, including those used to treat depression and schizophrenia (Lewis, 2004). Because of this, variations in any of the genes that code for these seven enzymes can have significant effects on drug metabolism, which, in turn, affects circulating levels of the drug. There are variations in the CYP2D6 enzyme within any given population that result in some people being poor metabolizers of some drugs while others are so-called ultra-metabolizers because they metabolize certain drugs more rapidly than expected (Gaedigk, 2013). Poor metabolizers may experience adverse effects due to higher than expected circulating levels of the drug, whereas ultra-metabolizers may receive fewer therapeutic benefits than expected due to lower circulating levels of the drug (Teh & Bertilsson, 2012). The differences in genes that influence drug response are the key to the idea of personalized medicine, the goal of which is to tailor drug treatments (specific drugs, and doses) to the particular genetic makeup of individuals in order for them to receive the maximum benefit from any therapeutic treatment plan. Although the costs of obtaining genetic information of individuals continue to fall and the techniques used to obtain the information become more powerful, we are probably still far away from achieving a genetics-based approach to therapy (Zhang & Nebert, 2017).

In addition to adverse effects related to genetic factors, many other factors influence adherence to a medical regimen. For example, cultural and ethnic beliefs surrounding mental health disorders, attitudes toward the mental health system, and the cultural practices of an ethnic group all greatly affect a patient's degree of engagement with and adherence to the medical regimen. Cultural factors are discussed more fully in Chapter 8.

Sources: Bertilsson, L. (2007). Metabolism of antidepressant and neuroleptic drugs by cytochrome P450s: Clinical and interethnic aspects. *Clinical Pharmacology and Therapeutics, 82*(5), 606–609. https://doi.org/10.1038/sj.clpt.6100358; Gaedigk, A. (2013). Complexities of CYP2D6 gene analysis and interpretation. *International Review of Psychiatry, 25*(5), 534–553. https://doi.org/10.3109/09540261.2013.825581; Lewis, D. F. (2004). 57 varieties: The human cytochromes P450. *Pharmacogenomics, 5*(3), 305–318. https://doi.org/10.1517/phgs.5.3.305.29827; Teh, L. K., & Bertilsson, L. (2012). Pharmacogenomics of CYP2D6: Molecular genetics, interethnic differences and clinical importance. *Drug Metabolism and Pharmacokinetics, 27*(1), 55–67; and Zhang, G., & Nebert, D. W. (2017). Personalized medicine: Genetic risk prediction of drug response. *Pharmacology and Therapeutics, 175*, 75–90. https://doi.org/10.1016/j.

An ideal psychiatric drug would relieve the mental health disturbance of the patient without inducing additional cerebral (mental) or somatic (physical) effects. Unfortunately, in psychopharmacology, as in most areas of pharmacology, no drugs are both fully effective and free of unwanted effects. Nevertheless, researchers are working toward developing medications that target the symptoms while producing no or few adverse effects.

The development of new drugs or treatment protocols with existing drugs that minimize adverse effects are important goals, as experiencing adverse effects is frequently listed as a reason why many patients stop taking their psychotropic medications. Non-adherence to medications (i.e., primarily medication non-persistence and the lack of consistency in adhering to the prescribed regimen) is a significant barrier to the successful treatment of mental health disorders. For example, a systematic review of adherence to antipsychotic medications in schizophrenia reveals adherence rates ranging from 47% to 95% (Sendt et al., 2015). Similarly, adherence to medications for the treatment of depression is often poor, resulting in an increased risk of relapse and hospitalization (Ho et al., 2016). Non-adherence is typically due to a combination of the patient experiencing adverse effects and a lack of efficacy (Leucht et al., 2013).

Because all functions of the brain involve activity of neurons, neurotransmitters, and receptors, these are the targets of pharmacological intervention. Most psychotropic drugs act by either increasing or decreasing the activity of certain neurotransmitter–receptor systems. It is generally agreed that the dysfunctional neurotransmitter–receptor systems differ depending on a person's mental health condition. These differences offer more specific targets for drug action. In fact, much of what is known about the relationship between specific neurotransmitters and specific disturbances has been derived from knowledge of the pharmacology of the drugs used to treat these conditions. For example, most drugs that are effective in reducing the delusions and hallucinations of schizophrenia block D_2 dopamine receptors. Therefore we can infer that delusions and hallucinations result from overactivity of dopamine pathways in the brain. In turn, this type of understanding subsequently leads to the development of drugs that are more selective for these targets.

Drugs Used to Treat Anxiety and Insomnia

GABA is the major inhibitory (calming) neurotransmitter in the central nervous system (CNS). There are three major types of GABA receptors: $GABA_A$, $GABA_B$, and $GABA_C$ receptors. The family of $GABA_A$ receptors contains several different subtypes (versions) of receptor, each with its own particular drug recognition properties. Specific members of the $GABA_A$ receptor family are the targets of benzodiazepines, barbiturates, and alcohol. Drugs that enhance the actions of GABA at $GABA_A$ receptors exert a sedative–hypnotic action on brain function. The most commonly used anti-anxiety drugs are the benzodiazepines and, more recently, the selective serotonin reuptake inhibitors (SSRIs) and serotonin–norepinephrine reuptake inhibitors (SNRIs), which were originally introduced for the treatment of depression.

Benzodiazepines

Benzodiazepines enhance the actions of GABA by binding to a specific location on the $GABA_A$ receptor complex. They only have an effect if GABA is also bound to its binding sites on the receptor complex. This interaction decreases the probability that the neuron on which the receptors are found will depolarize and thus leads to an overall decrease in neuronal excitability. As shown in Figure 11.11, benzodiazepines, such as diazepam (Valium), clonazepam (Rivotril), and alprazolam (Xanax), bind to $GABA_A$ receptors. The receptors are common in the limbic system, the brain's emotional centre, and enhanced GABA activity is important for decreasing anxiety.

Fig. 11.11 Action of benzodiazepines. Drugs in this group bind to a site that is part of the $GABA_A$ receptor complex to which gamma-aminobutyric acid (GABA) itself binds. Clinically useful benzodiazepines enhance the inhibitory effects of GABA. Benzodiazepines do not produce an inhibitory effect in the absence of GABA. Both must simultaneously bind to the receptor for any clinical effect to occur.

At higher doses, all benzodiazepines can cause sedation. There are six benzodiazepines used in Canada for treatment of insomnia, lorazepam (Ativan), nitrazepam (Mogadon), oxazepam (Serax), temazepam (Restoril), triazolam (Halcion), and flurazepam (Dalmane), with a predominantly **hypnotic** (sleep-inducing) effect. Used at lower doses, lorazepam (Ativan) and alprazolam (Xanax) can reduce anxiety without being as *soporific* (sleep producing).

The fact that the benzodiazepines promote the ability of GABA to decrease neuronal excitability probably accounts for their efficacy in the treatment of seizures and for their ability to reduce the neuronal overexcitement that is characteristic of alcohol withdrawal. While being efficacious at treating seizures and convulsions, benzodiazepines cannot be used prophylactically due to their tendency to quickly induce tolerance in those that use them. When used in the absence of other CNS depressant drugs, even at high dosages, these drugs rarely inhibit the brain to the degree that respiratory depression, coma, and death result, and so they are considered relatively safe drugs. However, when combined with other CNS depressants, such as alcohol, opioids, or **tricyclic anti-depressants** (TCAs), the inhibitory actions of the benzodiazepines can lead to life-threatening respiratory and CNS depression.

Any drug that inhibits electrical activity in the brain can interfere with motor ability, attention, and judgement. A patient taking benzodiazepines must be cautioned about engaging in activities that could be dangerous if reflexes and attention are impaired, including specialized activities such as working in construction and more common activities such as driving a car. In older persons the use of benzodiazepines may contribute to falls and broken bones. Ataxia is a common adverse effect secondary to the abundance of GABA receptors in the cerebellum.

Short-Acting Sedative–Hypnotic Sleep Drugs

Zopiclone (Imovane) is a member of a newer class of benzodiazepine-like hypnotics. It and the other benzodiazepine-like drugs, zaleplon and zolpidem, have been grouped together into a class colloquially called the *Z-drugs*. Structurally, zopiclone is not a true benzodiazepine; however, zopiclone displays similar actions as the true benzodiazepines at $GABA_A$ receptors. Thus its use also results in a decrease in neuronal excitability. As a result, zopiclone has sedative effects as well as hypnotic, anxiolytic, anti-convulsant, and muscle-relaxant effects. The onset of action is faster than that of most benzodiazepines. It is important to inform patients taking non-benzodiazepine hypnotic drugs about the quick onset and advise them to take the drug only when they are ready to go to sleep.

Zopiclone reaches peak plasma concentration within 2 hours and has a short half-life (the amount of time it takes the body to eliminate half of the drug). Zopiclone also has the unique adverse effect of an unpleasant bitter taste upon awakening. Severe drowsiness or impaired coordination are signs of drug intolerance or excessive doses. Because of the potential for misuse, zopiclone should not be taken for more than 7 to 10 consecutive days and should be used with caution in those who misuse alcohol and other substances.

Buspirone

Buspirone (Bustab) is an anxiolytic drug that is useful for bringing about the short-term relief of excessive anxiety without producing strong sedative–hypnotic effects. Because this drug does not leave the patient sleepy or sluggish, it is often much better tolerated than the benzodiazepines. It is not a CNS depressant, and so the danger of it interacting with other CNS depressants such as alcohol is minimal. Also, there is not the potential for dependence that exists with benzodiazepines.

Although, at present, the mechanism of action of buspirone is not clearly understood, one possibility is illustrated in Figure 11.12. Buspirone is a partial agonist (a drug that is unable to fully activate a receptor) at 5-hydroxytryptamine ($5\text{-}HT_{1A}$) receptors. These receptors are known to modulate the release of a number of neurotransmitters, including serotonin and dopamine. Buspirone may also enhance dopamine release from nerve endings via its action as an antagonist at presynaptic dopamine D_2 autoreceptors.

Refer to Chapter 12 for a discussion of adverse reactions, dosages, nursing implications, and patient and family teaching related to the drugs used to treat anxiety and related disorders.

Treating Anxiety Disorders With Anti-depressant Drugs

The symptoms, neurotransmitters, and circuits associated with anxiety disorders overlap extensively with those of depressive disorders (see Chapter 13), and many drugs used to treat depression have proven to be effective treatments for anxiety disorders (Curtis et al., 2017). **SSRIs**, medications that preferentially act to increase serotonin levels in the synapse, are often used to treat OCD, social anxiety disorder (SAD), generalized anxiety disorder (GAD), panic disorder (PD), and PTSD. The **SNRI** venlafaxine (Effexor XR) is used to treat GAD, SAD, and PD. Duloxetine (Cymbalta), another SNRI, is approved for GAD.

Fig. 11.12 Proposed mechanism of action of buspirone. *Top,* In a normal state excessive serotonin release is prevented when serotonin binds to the presynaptic $5\text{-}HT_{1A}$ autoreceptors. The inhibitory effect of these autoreceptors on release is indicated by the red arrow. *Bottom,* Feedback inhibition by serotonin is blocked when buspirone binds and occupies $5\text{-}HT_{1A}$ receptors, leading to a loss of inhibition on serotonin release from the presynaptic cell as indicated by the dashed red line. This leads to an increase in serotonin levels in the synaptic cleft.

Drug Treatment for Depression

Understanding of the neurophysiological basis of depression is far from complete. However, some theories have been proposed to explain why this disease occurs. The monoamine theory of depression suggests that depression occurs as a result of a deficit in the monoamine neurotransmitters serotonin (sometimes called 5-hydroxytryptamine and abbreviated as 5-HT) and norepinephrine. This theory arose from the findings that drugs used to treat various disease states that had the adverse effect of altering monoamine levels also affected mood. Further investigation revealed that by deliberately decreasing monoamine neurotransmitter levels, mood could be depressed, with the opposite effect occurring when monoamine levels were deliberately elevated. Thus arose the idea that depressed mood is tied to deficits in monoamine neurotransmitter signalling. These findings ultimately led to the development of various types of drugs whose mode of action was to elevate serotonin or norepinephrine in the brain through a number of different mechanisms. Since their introduction into clinical practice, there has been much debate on the effectiveness of anti-depressant drugs. However, a major review of drug trials involving adults with depression suggests that all drugs studied were more effective than placebo (Cipriani et al., 2018). While these drugs have successfully treated many people with depression, it should be noted that a significant proportion of those suffering from depression is resistant to current pharmacological interventions. Figure 11.13 identifies the effects these drugs produce via interactions with a variety of drug targets that are responsible for both therapeutic and non-therapeutic effects. Figure 11.14 illustrates the processes of normal release, reuptake, and degradation of the monoamine neurotransmitters. A grasp of this underlying physiology

Fig. 11.14 The cycle of release, reuptake, and degradation of the monoamine neurotransmitters. Neurotransmitter release occurs when vesicles containing neurotransmitter fuse with the membrane of the nerve ending. The neurotransmitter is released into the synaptic cleft where it can bind to postsynaptic receptors. To terminate this process, the monoamine is removed from the synaptic cleft by a reuptake protein. The neurotransmitter can then be degraded by monoamine oxidase (MAO).

is essential for understanding the mechanisms by which the antidepressant drugs are thought to act.

Tricyclic Anti-depressants

Tricyclic and heterocyclic anti-depressants were widely used prior to the development of SSRIs. TCAs are no longer considered first-line treatment for depression since they have more adverse effects, take longer to reach an optimal dose, and have a greater potential for lethality when taken in overdose situations. They have more recently found a place in the treatment of neuropathic pain. The TCAs are thought to act primarily by blocking the reuptake of serotonin and norepinephrine. TCAs that contain a secondary amine in their structure (e.g., nortriptyline [Aventyl, Norventyl]) primarily block the reuptake of

Fig. 11.13 Potential receptor interactions of drugs used to treat depression. Note that the therapeutic targets of these drugs (e.g., 5-HT$_2$ receptors and 5-HT transporters) may be involved in both wanted and unwanted effects of these drugs. This diagram reflects all possible interactions and resulting side effects; most drugs will manifest only a limited number of these.

Fig. 11.15 Drugs that block the reuptake process increase neurotransmitter levels in the synaptic cleft. *Top,* In the undrugged state neurotransmitter is removed from the synaptic cleft by reuptake proteins into the presynaptic terminal, where it can then be degraded by monoamine oxidase (MAO). *Bottom,* In the presence of an uptake inhibitor this process is interrupted and the neurotransmitter can no longer be removed, thus leading to greater availability in the synaptic cleft.

norepinephrine, whereas those that possess a tertiary amine in their structure (e.g., amitriptyline [Elavil, Levate], imipramine [Impril]) can block the reuptake of both norepinephrine and serotonin. As shown in Figure 11.15, this block of reuptake processes results in the accumulation of neurotransmitter in the synapse.

Many of the tricyclic drugs produce adverse effects by acting as antagonists at muscarinic acetylcholine receptors. Acetylcholine, as mentioned, is the neurotransmitter released by postganglionic neurons of the parasympathetic nervous system. Through its binding to muscarinic acetylcholine receptors on internal organs, it serves to help regulate many important physiological functions. Antagonism of muscarinic receptors by tricyclic drugs, as well as a wide variety of other psychotropic drugs, can lead to a constellation of untoward effects, which are predictable based on knowledge of which physiological systems are regulated by the parasympathetic nervous system. These adverse effects usually involve blurred vision, dry mouth, constipation, and urinary hesitancy. Because of the central role of acetylcholine in memory and cognition, these drugs can also result in deficits in these processes. These adverse effects can be troubling to patients and may limit their adherence to the regimen.

Depending on the individual drug, these drugs can also act as antagonists at histamine (H_1) receptors in the brain. Antagonism of these receptors by any drug causes sedation and drowsiness, an unwelcome adverse effect in daily use (see Figure 11.13). People taking the TCAs often have adherence issues because of these issues. TCA overdose can be fatal, secondary to cardiac conduction disturbances from excessive sodium channel and calcium channel blockade.

Selective Serotonin Reuptake Inhibitors

The SSRIs were introduced in hopes of providing a useful tool in the treatment of depression that would display fewer adverse effects than the TCAs. As the name implies, SSRIs such as fluoxetine (Prozac), paroxetine (Paxil), citalopram (Celexa), escitalopram (Cipralex), and fluvoxamine (Luvox) preferentially block the reuptake of serotonin from the synaptic cleft. Sertraline (Zoloft) inhibits the neuronal reuptake of serotonin but to a lesser degree also inhibits norepinephrine and dopamine neuronal reuptake. SSRIs bind more poorly to acetylcholine muscarinic and H_1 receptors than the TCAs and so tend to have fewer adverse effects in comparison. They seem to show comparable efficacy in treating depression without the anti-cholinergic and sedating adverse effects that limit patient adherence to other drug regimens. However, SSRIs have other adverse effects: inappropriate stimulation of various serotonin receptors due to increased serotonin levels may lead to insomnia, low libido and failure of orgasm, and nausea or vomiting (Rang et al., 2016) (Figure 11.13). While much less likely to cause cardiotoxicity in comparison to TCAs in overdose situations, SSRIs in high doses can cause ventricular arrhythmias that can lead to death.

Serotonin–Norepinephrine Reuptake Inhibitors

SNRIs are medications that increase both serotonin and norepinephrine levels in the brain. Venlafaxine (Effexor XR) and desvenlafaxine (Pristiq) are effective inhibitors of neuronal serotonin and norepinephrine reuptake and weak inhibitors of dopamine reuptake. Thus these neurotransmitters will accumulate in the synapse. Venlafaxine has the dual mechanism of working as an SSRI at lower doses (75 mg/day), affecting the reuptake of serotonin, and as an SNRI at higher doses (150–225 mg/day), affecting the reuptake of both serotonin and norepinephrine.

Duloxetine (Cymbalta) affects norepinephrine and serotonin reuptake equally. Thus it has a greater noradrenergic effect than does venlafaxine at lower doses. This SNRI is indicated for acute and maintenance treatment of major depressive disorder, for acute treatment of GAD, for managing fibromyalgia, and for managing neuropathic pain associated with diabetic peripheral neuropathy. In fact, many SNRIs, as with the TCAs, have therapeutic effects on neuropathic pain. The common underlying mechanism of *neuropathic pain* is nerve injury or dysfunction. The mechanism by which TCAs and SNRIs reduce neuropathic pain is through activation of the descending norepinephrine and serotonin pathways to the spinal cord, thereby limiting pain signals ascending to the brain.

Serotonin Modulator and Stimulator

Vortioxetine (Trintellix) is a serotonin modulator and stimulator. It affects many different serotonin receptors by inhibiting serotonin reuptake like the SSRIs, activating 5-HT_{1A} receptors like buspirone, acting as a partial agonist at 5-HT_{1B} receptor, and blocking 5-HT_3, 5-HT_{1D}, and 5-HT_7 receptors. Geriatric patients may experience an improvement of cognitive deficits independent of its anti-depressant properties. Common adverse effects include constipation, nausea, and vomiting. More serious side effects are hyponatremia and, rarely, induction of hypomania or mania.

Serotonin and Norepinephrine Disinhibitors

The class of drugs described as serotonin and norepinephrine disinhibitors (SNDIs) is represented by only one drug, mirtazapine (Remeron). This unique drug increases norepinephrine, dopamine, and serotonin transmission by acting as an antagonist at central presynaptic $α_2$-adrenergic receptors. The normal function of these receptors is to inhibit neurotransmitter release when norepinephrine binds to them. Thus any drug that prevents noradrenaline from binding to these receptors will potentiate neurotransmitter release. This is why this drug is called a disinhibitor. Mirtazapine tends to have a more rapid onset of effect than do single neurotransmitter anti-depressant drugs, and this may be because it can simultaneously affect several neurotransmitter systems. Mirtazapine is a potent antagonist of 5-HT_{2C} receptors, which may account for its anti-anxiety and anti-depressant effects, as these receptors, when activated by serotonin, typically inhibit norepinephrine and dopamine release. In addition, this drug acts as an antagonist at 5-HT_{2A} and 5-HT_3 receptors, activation of which are thought to mediate sexual dysfunction and nausea. Thus these effects are less likely to occur, and this is an advantage compared to other drugs used in depression. Mirtazapine is also a potent H_1-receptor antagonist, which accounts for drowsiness and increased appetite resulting in weight gain being the most common adverse effects. Patients may also experience orthostatic hypotension and the occasional occurrence of anti-cholinergic adverse effects. When discontinuing use of any anti-depressant drug, but particularly SSRIs or SNRIs, patients should be weaned gradually over several weeks rather than abruptly due to the risk of discontinuation symptoms such as dizziness, agitation, anxiety, sleeping difficulties, nausea, excessive sweating, and fatigue. These symptoms do not indicate that an addiction has developed. Most people taking anti-depressant drugs never develop a "craving" or feel the need to increase the dose. What these symptoms do indicate is that the brain has adapted to drug-induced changes in neurotransmitter levels. These symptoms typically resolve within 4 to 6 weeks after discontinuation of the drug. However, if the symptoms persist beyond this time frame, there is the potential that depression is still present and that the drugs are still needed.

Monoamine Oxidase Inhibitors

Monoamine oxidase inhibitors (MAOIs) are a group of drugs used to treat depression that prevent the destruction of monoamines by inhibiting the action of MAO. MAOIs illustrate the principle that drugs can have a desired and beneficial effect in the brain, while at the same time having possibly dangerous effects elsewhere in the body. To understand the action of these drugs, keep in mind the following definitions:

- *Monoamines* are a type of organic compound and include the neurotransmitters norepinephrine, epinephrine, dopamine, and serotonin, as well as many different food substances and drugs.
- *MAO* is an enzyme that degrades monoamines and is located in the nerve endings that release dopamine, serotonin, and noradrenaline.
- *MAOIs* inhibit the action of MAO and thereby prevent the degradation of monoamines.

The monoamine neurotransmitters, as well as any monoamine food substance or drug, are destroyed by the enzyme MAO, which is located in neurons and in the liver. Anti-depressant drugs such as phenelzine (Nardil), tranylcypromine (Parnate), and selegiline (Eldapryl) are MAOIs that act by inhibiting the enzyme and interfering with the degradation of the monoamine neurotransmitters. This action, in turn, increases the presynaptic availability of the neurotransmitters, which leads to the neurotransmitter leaking out of the nerve endings and into the synaptic cleft. This is the mechanism by which synaptic levels of neurotransmitters are increased and by which the anti-depressant effects of these drugs are thought to occur (Figure 11.16).

The use of MAO-inhibiting drugs is complicated by the fact that MAO is also present in the liver and is responsible for destroying monoamines that enter the body via food or drugs. Of particular importance

Fig. 11.16 Monoamine oxidase inhibitors (MAOIs) prevent the breakdown of monoamines and increase the availability of neurotransmitter in the presynaptic nerve terminal. This increased availability leads to an increase in neurotransmitter concentrations in the synaptic cleft.

is the monoamine tyramine, which is present in many food substances, such as aged cheeses, pickled or smoked fish, chocolate, many types of beans, and beer and wine. Tyramine, which is normally metabolized by liver and gut MAO and so never reaches a concentration in the blood high enough to cause any issues, poses a threat of hypertensive crisis when MAO is inhibited. The displacement of norepinephrine from neuronal storage vesicles by elevated tyramine levels and the resulting increase in norepinephrine availability are thought to cause an increase in blood pressure (pressor response). In severe cases, a hypertensive crisis can occur.

A substantial number of drugs are chemically monoamines. The dosages of these drugs are determined by the rate at which they are metabolized by MAO in the liver. In a patient taking MAOIs, the blood level of monoamine drugs can reach high levels and cause serious toxicity. Therefore MAOIs are contraindicated with concurrent use of any other anti-depressant or sympathomimetic drugs (those that affect the sympathetic nervous system). Concurrent use with some over-the-counter products with sympathomimetic properties (e.g., oral decongestants) should also be avoided.

Because of the serious dangers that result from inhibition of hepatic MAO, patients taking MAOIs *must* be given a list of foods high in tyramine and drugs that must be avoided. Chapter 13 contains a list of these foods, along with nursing measures and instructions for patient teaching.

Other Drugs Used to Treat Depression

Bupropion is effective both as a treatment for depression and as a smoking cessation aid. It seems to act as a dopamine–norepinephrine reuptake inhibitor and also as an antagonist at nicotinic acetylcholine receptors. Since bupropion has no serotonergic action, it does not cause sexual dysfunction. Adverse effects include insomnia, tremor, anorexia, and weight loss. Bupropion is contraindicated in patients with a seizure disorder, in patients with a current or prior diagnosis of bulimia or anorexia nervosa, and in patients undergoing abrupt discontinuation of alcohol or sedatives (including benzodiazepines), owing to the increased seizure risk.

Trazodone (Trazodone) is a serotonin antagonist and reuptake inhibitor (SARI) and is not a first choice for treatment of depression. Its anti-depressant effects are seen only at high therapeutic doses. An adverse effect of trazadone is sedation, which arises from its ability to act as a potent H_1-receptor antagonist. However, this can prove to be useful in those patients who suffer from insomnia. Another common adverse effect is orthostatic hypotension due to α_1-adrenergic receptor antagonism. Its potent blockade of these receptors can lead to rare cases of priapism (painful, prolonged penile erection).

Ketamine is a potential new drug treatment for depression and has been called one of the most important discoveries in mood research over the last half century (Wei et al., 2020). Unlike traditional anti-depressant drugs, ketamine induces a rapid, long-lasting reversal of symptoms and appears to treat suicidal ideation (Duman, 2018). Additionally, these effects occur in patients resistant to traditional depression medications.

Ketamine is a dissociative anesthetic that is used in selective medical procedures. Its widespread use as an anesthetic is limited because it can induce hallucinations and delirium during emergence from anesthesia in some patients. This property is sought after in those that use ketamine illicitly and ketamine has become a popular "club drug."

Ketamine is known to block a type of glutamate receptor (the *N*-methyl-d-aspartate [NMDA] receptor). While this appears to be an important mechanism in its anti-depressant effects, it is clearly not the whole story as other drugs that block these receptors do not show the same effects on depression. Experimental evidence suggests that a number of additional targets, including the brain-derived neurotrophic factor (BDNF) system, likely play a role (Hashimoto, 2020; Zanos & Gould, 2018).

While there is a great deal of optimism surrounding this drug, it should be noted that some of the effects sought after by those who use ketamine as a club drug have been experienced by those using it as a therapeutic drug. These side effects include hallucination, dissociation, and cognitive deficits. There is also some concern regarding the potential for addiction and abuse as this can occur when ketamine is used illicitly. Lastly, there are no studies regarding the long-term safety of the drug when used as an anti-depressant drug.

Is the Monoamine Theory of Depression Still Valid?

The monoamine theory of depression served as a useful lens through which to view the underlying pathology leading to depression. Indeed, it resulted in many clinically useful drugs whose main mechanism of action was to elevate monoamine neurotransmitter release in brain tissue being brought to market. However, physicians noted an interesting phenomenon in patients prescribed these drugs. There was a delay of several weeks before the patients experienced a relief in symptoms. Drugs such as the SSRIs will block serotonin reuptake almost immediately after entering the brain, so why the delay in clinical response? This question led scientists to explore the idea that mechanisms occurring after the initial drug effect or separate from the proposed mechanism of the drug were bringing about their clinical efficacy. A re-investigation of these drugs revealed that their therapeutic benefit may be a result of their ability to increase levels of BDNF, a peptide that is essential for the survival and growth of neurons (Castren & Kojima, 2017). The concentration of this peptide is low in people with depression and increases in those who receive anti-depressant drug therapy. The time scale of this effect fits better with the alleviation of depressive symptoms due to anti-depressant drug treatment. In addition, BDNF supports the growth of new neurons in the hippocampus. A number of lines of evidence suggest that depressed people have lower levels of hippocampal neurogenesis compared to non-depressed people (Wilner et al., 2013). In addition, animal models have revealed that anti-depressant drugs can promote neurogenesis and lessen behaviours associated with depression (Castren & Kojima, 2017).

Another explanation for the delay in symptom relief is that clinical efficacy is not due to the initial increase in monoamine levels that most of these drugs provide, but rather due to this effect bringing about a loss of neurotransmitter receptor responsiveness over time, a process called receptor desensitization (Rang et al., 2016). For example, 5-HT_{1A} receptors can act as presynaptic autoreceptors to inhibit serotonin release. Therefore once desensitized by high levels of serotonin, there will be less inhibitory action on further serotonin release, and the overall levels of this neurotransmitter will increase. Again, the timeline of this type of effect correlates better with the onset of clinical relief brought about by these drugs.

Pathways other than those using monoamines as neurotransmitters are likely involved in the pathophysiology of depression. The ability of ketamine to rapidly reverse some of the clinical manifestations of depression strongly suggests that dysfunction of pathways involving the neurotransmitter glutamate and its receptors is also likely a component of this disorder.

Suicide Risk and Anti-depressant Drugs

There is concern that anti-depressant drug use results in an increased risk of suicide. Since first reported, many studies have investigated this relationship. The results of these studies have often been contradictory or inconclusive and have been difficult to reconcile with one another. This is partly because these events are rare and also because of inconsistency in how these events are reported. However, the evidence thus far suggests that suicide risk in adults is likely not increased, and the data are most consistent in showing an increased risk in children and adolescents (Brent, 2016; Sharma et al., 2016), although even this relationship has been questioned (Dubicka et al., 2016; Garland et al., 2016). Health Canada requires a warning on drug labels for users of all ages but specifically for SSRIs and SNRIs. In addition, a warning about being aware of potentially dangerous changes in behaviour must be included in drug information sheets and labels.

Drug Treatment for Bipolar Disorders
Lithium Carbonate

Although the efficacy of **lithium carbonate** (Carbolith, Lithane, Lithmax) as a "**mood stabilizer**" in patients with bipolar disorders has been established for many years (Lithium is still a first-line option in the treatment of patients with bipolar disorder, Yatham et al., 2018), its mechanism of action is still far from understood. While it was originally believed to exert its clinical effects via a non-specific disruption of neurotransmission, recent evidence suggests that it may be enhancing neuroprotective pathways and decreasing neuronal injury and death (Forlenza et al., 2014). One target that may play a key role in mediating the effects of lithium is glycogen synthase kinase 3ß (GSK3ß). This enzyme can affect a number of neuroprotective pathways, and its inhibition by lithium appears to trigger those that bring about a clinical response. In addition, lithium appears to increase levels of BDNF, which is thought to be neuroprotective. Another target affected by lithium is inositol monophosphatase 1, an enzyme involved in the phosphatidylinositol second messenger pathway. Lithium has been shown to inhibit inositol monophosphatase activity, resulting in a disruption of the entire signalling pathway. This is thought to lead to less intracellular signalling from receptor activation and to lessen the risk of neuronal cell death by improving mitochondrial health. Lastly, there is evidence that lithium decreases excitatory neurotransmission by decreasing glutamate release and acting as an antagonist at certain glutamate receptors. Excessive glutamate release can lead to neuronal injury and death, and so these effects are thought to prevent neuronal harm that may arise from excessive glutamatergic activity (Malhi & Outhred, 2016).

While it is not known exactly how lithium works, many of its adverse effects are thought to arise from the fact that it mimics the role of sodium in neurons and thus alters the electrical properties of neuronal membranes. By altering electrical conductivity, lithium represents a potential threat to all body functions regulated by electrical currents. Foremost among these functions is cardiac contraction; lithium can induce, although not commonly, sinus bradycardia. Overdose causes extreme alteration of cerebral conductivity, which can lead to convulsions. Changes in nerve and muscle conduction can commonly lead to tremor at therapeutic doses or to more extreme motor dysfunction with overdose.

Lithium commonly induces polyuria (the output of large volumes of urine) as a consequence of decreasing the effectiveness of vasopressin on renal function. Long-term use of lithium can result in thyroid gland enlargement (goiter) and, possibly, hypothyroidism in some patients. In addition, hyponatremia can increase the risk of lithium toxicity because increased kidney reabsorption of sodium leads to increased reabsorption of lithium as well.

Primarily because of its effects on electrical conductivity, lithium has a low **therapeutic index**. The therapeutic index is a measure of overall drug safety with respect to the risk for overdose or toxicity. It can be expressed as the ratio between the median lethal dose and the median effective dose. A low therapeutic index means that the dose of the drug that can cause death is not that much greater than the dose required for therapeutic effectiveness. This risk mandates that the blood level of lithium be monitored on a regular basis to ensure that the drug is not accumulating and rising to dangerous levels. See Table 11.3 for a list of some of the adverse and toxic effects of lithium. Chapter 14 contains a more in-depth discussion of lithium carbonate treatment and

TABLE 11.3 Adverse and Toxic Effects of Lithium

System	Adverse and Toxic Effects
Nervous and muscular	Tremor, ataxia, confusion, convulsions
Digestive	Nausea, vomiting, diarrhea
Cardiac	Arrhythmias
Fluid and electrolyte	Polyuria, polydipsia, edema
Endocrine	Goiter and hypothyroidism

specific dose-related adverse and toxic effects, nursing implications, and the patient teaching plan.

Other Drugs Used to Treat Bipolar Disorders

While lithium has played a central role in the pharmacological management of bipolar depression for many years, drugs that were once used primarily to treat seizure disorders have also emerged as useful therapeutic drugs (Corrado & Walsh, 2016). These drugs work through several different mechanisms but all share the common property of decreasing neuronal excitability. The major modes of action for these drugs include (1) inhibition of sodium channel activity, (2) inhibition of calcium channel activity, (3) enhancement of GABAergic neurotransmission pathways, and (4) inhibition of glutamatergic neurotransmission pathways. Although some drugs work almost exclusively via a single one of these mechanisms, a number of the drugs in this group work through a combination of these effects. Three drugs used in the treatment of seizure disorders, valproate (Depakene), carbamazepine (Tegretol), and lamotrigine (Lamictal, Lamotrigine), have displayed efficacy in the treatment of bipolar disorder and, in the context of this disease, are considered to be mood stabilizers. It is thought that their ability to re-establish a balance between excitatory and inhibitory neuronal pathways has a stabilizing effect on mood. More recent evidence suggests that, much like lithium, these drugs that are efficacious in treating bipolar disorders are also able to inhibit GSK3ß activity.

Carbamazepine

The primary mechanism of action of carbamazepine is to inhibit neuronal sodium channels during depolarization events, hence reducing neuronal excitability. Interestingly, this blocking action is greater in neurons that fire frequently and repetitively, and so the drug is effective at reducing inappropriate excitability. Because of this mechanistic characteristic, carbamazepine does not have as strong of an effect on neurons that are behaving normally and is therefore less likely to affect normal neuronal function. Common adverse effects include anticholinergic effects (e.g., dry mouth, constipation, urinary retention, blurred vision), orthostatic hypotension, sedation, and ataxia. Rash may occur in 10% of patients (Sadock et al., 2015). Recommended baseline laboratory work includes liver function tests, complete blood count (CBC), electrocardiogram, and electrolyte levels. Blood levels are monitored to avoid toxicity, but there are no established therapeutic blood levels for carbamazepine in the treatment of bipolar disorder.

Valproate

As with carbamazepine, valproate also displays efficacy in treating bipolar disorders. Valproate works through a number of the mechanisms listed earlier. It blocks both sodium and calcium channels and may elevate GABA levels by inhibiting the enzyme that normally degrades this neurotransmitter. Common adverse effects include tremor, weight gain, and sedation. More rarely occurring but serious adverse effects include thrombocytopenia, pancreatitis, and hepatic failure. In addition, this drug has been demonstrated to be a potent teratogen. Because of its potential to cause hepatotoxicity, baseline levels are established for liver function indicators and a CBC is obtained before an individual is started on this medication. These measurements are then repeated periodically. In addition, the level of the drug in the blood is monitored to ensure that it stays within the recommended therapeutic range.

Lamotrigine

Lamotrigine (Lamictal) is perhaps the most effective drug for maintenance therapy of bipolar disorder, but it is not as effective in acute mania (Preston et al., 2013). Lamotrigine is best known for its ability to treat the depressive phase of bipolar disorder, with less risk of causing a switch into mania when compared to anti-depressant drugs (Prabhavalkar et al., 2015). It inhibits neuronal sodium and calcium channels and modulates the release of the excitatory neurotransmitters glutamate and aspartate. Patients should promptly report any rashes, which could be a sign of life-threatening Stevens–Johnson syndrome. This risk can be minimized by slow titration to therapeutic doses.

Other Anti-seizure Drugs

Because these drugs work by inhibiting neuronal excitability, they have found a home in the treatment of other disorders. Along with their use with bipolar disorders (as discussed above), some of these drugs show efficacy in treating neuropathic pain, anxiety, and migraines.

Other anti-seizure drugs used as mood stabilizers are gabapentin (Neurontin), topiramate (Topamax), and oxcarbazepine (Trileptal). None of them have Health Canada approval as mood stabilizers, and studies have not provided strong support for their use as primary treatments for bipolar disorders. However, they are used for their calming effects during mania. Chapter 14 offers a more detailed discussion of these medications.

Drugs Used to Treat Psychosis

First-Generation (Conventional) Antipsychotic Drugs

First-generation antipsychotic drugs, introduced into clinical practice in the 1950s and also referred to as conventional or typical antipsychotic drugs, are antagonists or weak partial agonists at the D_2 type of dopamine receptors. By binding to these receptors and therefore preventing dopamine from doing so, these drugs reduce dopaminergic neurotransmission. It has been postulated that an overactivity of the dopamine system in certain areas of the mesolimbic system may be responsible for at least some of the symptoms of schizophrenia; thus antagonism of certain dopamine receptors should reduce these symptoms, particularly the "positive" symptoms of schizophrenia, such as delusions (e.g., paranoid and grandiose ideas) and hallucinations (e.g., hearing or seeing things not present in reality). While these drugs are relatively selective for certain types of dopamine receptors, as with many therapeutic drugs, they can interact with other receptors such as those for acetylcholine, α_1-adrenergic receptors to which norepinephrine binds, and H_1 receptors. It is not clear if any of these interactions leads to a clinical benefit, but many of the adverse effects associated with the use of first-generation antipsychotic drugs come from these interactions. See Chapter 15 for a more detailed discussion of schizophrenia and its symptoms.

The proposed mechanism of action of the first generation of antipsychotic drugs, which includes the phenothiazines (e.g., chlorpromazine), thioxanthenes (e.g., thiothixene), butyrophenones (e.g., haloperidol), and pharmacologically related drugs, is illustrated in Figure 11.17. As summarized in Figure 11.18, many of the untoward adverse effects of these drugs can be understood as a logical extension of their receptor antagonism profile, which varies from drug to drug. Because dopamine

Fig. 11.17 The first generation of drugs to show efficacy in treating psychosis work, at least in part, by acting as antagonists at dopamine D_2 receptors. These drugs bind to the receptors but do not activate them. Rather, they prevent dopamine from binding to and activating these receptors.

in the basal ganglia plays a major role in the regulation of movement, it is not surprising that inhibition of dopamine signalling through its receptors can lead to acute drug-induced motor abnormalities (extrapyramidal side effects [EPS]) such as parkinsonism, akinesia, akathisia, dyskinesia, and delayed EPS (tardive dyskinesia). The extent of the EPS varies between drugs. While chlorpromazine and haloperidol are equally effective in treating the symptoms of psychosis, haloperidol is associated with a greater risk of developing acute EPS. Risks of tardive dyskinesia are the same for all first-generation drugs. Normally there is a balance between dopamine and acetylcholine signalling in the striatum. Dopamine antagonists upset this balance and allow acetylcholine signalling to predominate, thus leading to EPS. With this in mind, muscarinic acetylcholine receptor antagonists, such as benztropine, are often prescribed to prevent or treat these antipsychotic drug–induced extrapyramidal symptoms. Nurses and physicians often monitor patients for evidence of involuntary movements after administration of the first-generation antipsychotic drugs. One commonly used scale is the Abnormal Involuntary Movement Scale (AIMS). See Chapter 15 for an example of AIMS and a discussion of the clinical use of antipsychotic drugs, adverse effects, specific nursing interventions, and patient teaching strategies.

An important physiological function of dopamine is to act as the hypothalamic factor that inhibits the release of prolactin from the anterior pituitary gland. A blockade of dopaminergic neurotransmission can lead to increased pituitary secretion of prolactin. In women this drug-induced hyperprolactinemia can result in amenorrhea (absence of the menses) or galactorrhea (breast milk flow); in men, it can lead to gynecomastia (development of the male mammary glands).

Many of first-generation drugs act as antagonists at muscarinic receptors that are normally activated by acetylcholine. This leads to typical anti-cholinergic effects such as blurred vision, dry mouth, tachycardia, urinary retention, and constipation.

In addition to blocking dopamine and muscarinic receptors, many first-generation antipsychotic drugs act as antagonists at α_1-adrenergic receptors. These receptors are found on smooth muscle cells that contract

Fig. 11.18 Potential receptor interactions of the second-generation drugs used in the treatment of psychosis. Note that drug interaction with the D_2 and $5\text{-}HT_2$ receptors is necessary for symptomatic relief, but it can also result in unpleasant or dangerous side effects. While these drugs are relatively selective for D_2 and $5\text{-}HT_2$ receptors, they still interact with a number of other receptors. These non-selective interactions are often the source of additional side effects. Also note that use of most of these drugs will result in only a limited number of the potential side effects illustrated here. (**Sources:** Lehne, R. A. [2001]. *Pharmacology for nursing care* [4th ed.]. Philadelphia: Saunders; Varcarolis, E. [2002]. *Foundations of psychiatric mental health nursing* [4th ed.]. Philadelphia: WB Saunders; and Keltner, N. L., & Folks, D. G. [2001]. *Psychotropic drugs* [3rd ed.]. St. Louis: Mosby.)

in response to norepinephrine released from sympathetic nervous system neurons. In blood vessels, for example, antagonism of these receptors can bring about vasodilation and a consequent drop in blood pressure and provoke orthostatic hypotension.

α_1-Adrenergic receptors are also found on the vas deferens and are responsible for the propulsive contractions leading to ejaculation. Antagonism of these receptors can lead to a failure to ejaculate. Finally, many of these first-generation antipsychotic drugs, as well as a variety of other psychiatric drugs, block the histamine H_1 receptors. The two most significant adverse effects of blocking these receptors are sedation and substantial weight gain. The sedation may be beneficial in severely agitated patients.

It is believed that patient adherence is negatively affected due to the numerous and sometimes severe adverse effects of the first-generation drugs used in the treatment of psychosis. A quest for efficacious drugs to treat psychosis with fewer adverse effects led to the development of the second generation of antipsychotic drugs.

Second-Generation Antipsychotic Drugs

Introduced in the 1990s, second-generation antipsychotic drugs (or *atypicals*) used to treat psychosis target both the positive and possibly the negative symptoms of schizophrenia (see Chapter 15) and may produce fewer EPS. They are thought to differ from the first generation of drugs because of a difference in their pharmacological profile. While, like the first-generation drugs, they act as dopamine D_2 receptor antagonists, they also act as antagonists at a type of serotonin receptor that can regulate neurotransmitter release. This interaction may alleviate the negative symptoms, as well as the cognitive and memory effects of schizophrenia. In addition, it is the antagonism of these receptors that is believed to result in fewer EPS (Li et al., 2016). These newer drugs are often chosen as first-line treatment over the first generation of antipsychotic drugs because of a lower risk of EPS (Leucht et al., 2009).

However, several of the available second-generation drugs can increase the risk for a metabolic syndrome, resulting in increased weight, elevated blood glucose, and elevated levels of triglycerides. This is, again, due in part to the fact that while selective for their therapeutic targets, these drugs will still interact with other neurotransmitter receptors. The simultaneous blockade of muscarinic, 5-HT, and H_1 receptors is associated with weight gain due to increased appetite stimulation via the hypothalamic eating centres. Strong anti-muscarinic properties on pancreatic beta cells may cause insulin resistance, leading to hyperglycemia. The mechanism leading to elevated triglycerides is currently unknown (Stahl, 2013). Clozapine and olanzapine use has a high risk of causing metabolic syndrome, whereas aripiprazole and ziprasidone use has a lower risk (De Hert et al., 2012).

Clozapine. Clozapine (Clozaril), the first of the second-generation drugs to be developed, is relatively free of extrapyramidal motor disturbances. It is thought that clozapine preferentially blocks the dopamine receptors in the mesolimbic system, rather than those in the nigrostriatal area. This pattern of selectivity allows clozapine to exert an antipsychotic action while minimizing EPS. In addition, clozapine is an antagonist at serotonin $5-HT_{2A}$ receptors. Although people who take clozapine are more likely to adhere to their medication regimen than those who are taking other antipsychotic drugs, it has the potential to suppress bone marrow and induce agranulocytosis. Because any deficiency in white blood cells renders a person prone to serious infection, regular measurement of white blood cell count is required. As a result of these risks, all patients taking clozapine must have cell counts weekly for the first 6 months, every other week for the next 6 months, and monthly thereafter. To ensure that these blood tests are completed, clozapine is dispensed at these same intervals. Due to the significant risk of agranulocytosis and seizure (in 5% of patients) associated with its use, clozapine should be limited to patients with treatment-resistant schizophrenia who are non-responsive to, or intolerant of, other antipsychotic drugs.

Caution should be used when introducing other drugs that can increase the concentration of clozapine. There is also a potential for myocarditis that should be monitored, and for fever, but the most common adverse effects of clozapine are drowsiness and sedation, hypersalivation, reflex tachycardia, constipation, and dizziness and vertigo.

Risperidone. Risperidone (Risperdal) acts at D_2 receptors and is also a potent antagonist at $5-HT_{2A}$ receptors. This drug has a low potential for inducing agranulocytosis or convulsions. However, high therapeutic doses (greater than 6 mg/day) may lead to motor-related complications. It has the highest risk of EPS among the second-generation antipsychotic drugs and may increase prolactin release, which may lead to sexual dysfunction. Risperidone can cause orthostatic hypotension that can lead to falls, a serious problem among older persons. Weight gain, sedation, and sexual dysfunction are adverse effects that may affect adherence to the medication regimen and should be discussed with patients. It is notable that risperidone is the first of the second-generation antipsychotic drugs available as a long-acting depot injection. Risperdal Consta, administered every 2 weeks, provides an alternative to the depot injection of first-generation antipsychotic drugs. A rare but serious adverse effect is an increased risk of stroke and transient ischemic attacks in older persons with dementia who are being treated for agitation (Lee et al., 2004).

Quetiapine. Quetiapine (Seroquel) has a broad receptor-binding profile. Along with its ability to act as an antagonist at D_2 receptors, it is a potent antagonist of both $5-HT_{1A}$ and $5-HT_{2A}$ receptors. Its strong antagonism of H_1 receptors accounts for its ability to induce sedation. The combination of H_1 and serotonin receptor antagonism leads to the weight gain associated with use of this drug and also to a moderate risk for metabolic syndrome. Due to its antagonism of α_1-adrenergic receptors, it can cause orthostatic hypotension, dizziness, and syncope. Patients taking quetiapine have a low risk for EPS or prolactin elevation. Studies investigating how quetiapine interacts with D_2 receptors show that it dissociates rapidly and therefore does not occupy the binding site for dopamine for long periods of time. This characteristic is thought to be the reason why quetiapine tends to produce few EPS and prolactin-related adverse effects.

Other second-generation antipsychotic drugs.

- Olanzapine (Zyprexa) is similar to clozapine in chemical structure. Adverse effects include sedation, weight gain, hyperglycemia with new-onset type 2 diabetes, and higher risk for metabolic syndrome.
- Ziprasidone (Zeldox) binds to a variety of dopamine and 5-HT receptors and is also an SNRI. The main adverse effects are dizziness and moderate sedation. Ziprasidone is contraindicated in patients with a known history of QT interval prolongation, recent acute myocardial infarction, or uncompensated heart failure.
- Aripiprazole (Abilify) is a unique antipsychotic drug known as a *dopamine system stabilizer*. Its unique profile is thought to be due to the fact that, rather than acting as a D_2 antagonist, this drug is actually a partial agonist. This means that at low dopamine levels, the drug will partially activate D_2 receptors. However, at high levels, the drug will prevent excess dopamine from activating the receptor but still provide some degree of receptor activation itself. In this way it tends to prevent extreme fluctuations in D_2 receptor activation that may occur with other drugs that are antagonists. It induces little sedation or weight gain. Adverse effects include insomnia and akathisia.
- Paliperidone (Invega) is the major active metabolite of risperidone. It has similar adverse effects to risperidone, such as EPS and prolactin elevation. Additional adverse effects are orthostasis and sedation. It is also available as a prolonged-release injectable suspension.

- Lurasidone (Latuda) has high affinity for $5\text{-}HT_{2A}$ and D_2 receptors in addition to other serotonergic receptors such as $5\text{-}HT_{1A}$. Lurasidone has similar pharmacological properties to the tetracyclic antidepressant mirtazapine. Lurasidone has high affinity for serotonergic (such as $5\text{-}HT_{2A}$ and $5\text{-}HT_{2C}$), noradrenergic, and dopaminergic receptors (D_3 and D_4). There is minimal muscarinic receptor antagonism.
- Asenapine (Saphris) is unique among antipsychotic drugs as being administered in a sublingual formulation. Thus it avoids much of the hepatic metabolism that restricts its availability when administered orally. Bioavailability of asenapine is reduced from 35% with sub-lingual administration to less than 2% with oral administration. Patients should avoid food and water for 10 minutes after sublingual administration (Zacher & Holmes, 2012). It has a higher affinity for $5\text{-}HT_{2A}$ receptors than D_2 receptors. It also has antagonistic activity at α_1-adrenergic receptors, which accounts for the orthostatic hypotension, and H_1 antagonistic activity, which causes sedation.

Traditionally, the drugs that are used to treat psychosis have been grouped together based on the order in which they were introduced into clinical practice (first or second generation) or by comparison of effects between groups (typical vs. atypical). However, given the often overlapping range of pharmacological targets and adverse effect profiles of the members of these groups, the usefulness of such categorization is limited. Consideration of each drug on an individual basis would seem to be a more informative way of assessing the suitability of a drug (Leucht et al., 2013).

The antipsychotic drugs are discussed in detail in Chapter 15, including the indications for use, adverse effects, nursing implications, and patient and family teaching.

Drug Treatment for Attention-Deficit/Hyperactivity Disorder

Children and adults with attention-deficit/hyperactivity disorder (ADHD) show symptoms of short attention span, impulsivity, and overactivity. Paradoxically, the mainstay of treatment for this condition in children, and increasingly in adults, is the administration of psychostimulant drugs. Both methylphenidate (Biphentin, Concerta, Ritalin) and amphetamines such as amphetamine (Adderall XR) seem to show efficacy in treating these conditions. They block the reuptake of norepinephrine and dopamine into the presynaptic neuron and increase the concentration of these monoamines in the synaptic cleft. Thus they potentiate the signalling pathways of these neurotransmitters. How this translates into clinical efficacy is far from understood, but it is thought that the monoamines may inhibit an overactive part of the limbic system to prolong periods of concentration and focus on tasks.

Among many concerns with the use of these drugs are the adverse effects of agitation, exacerbation of psychotic thought processes, hypertension, and long-term growth suppression, as well as their potential for misuse and abuse. One medication that is not classified as a stimulant and is available for the treatment of ADHD is atomoxetine (Strattera), a selective norepinephrine reuptake inhibitor approved for use in children 6 years and older, adolescents, and adults. Common adverse effects include decreased appetite and weight loss, fatigue, and dizziness. Refer to Chapter 27 for more details on these drugs.

Drug Treatment for Alzheimer's Disease

The insidious and progressive loss of memory and other higher executive brain functions brought about by Alzheimer's disease is a tremendous individual, family, and social tragedy. Because the disease seems to involve progressive structural degeneration of the brain, there are two major pharmacological directions in its treatment. The first is to attempt to prevent or slow the structural degeneration. Although actively pursued, this approach has been unsuccessful so far. The second is to attempt to maintain normal brain function for as long as possible.

Much of the memory loss in this disease has been attributed to dysfunction of neurons that use acetylcholine as a neurotransmitter. The anti-cholinesterase drugs (also called *cholinesterase inhibitors*) show some efficacy in slowing the rate of memory loss and, in some patients, may even improve memory. The drugs work by interfering with the action of acetylcholinesterase, an enzyme that normally degrades acetylcholine. Inhibition of this enzyme leads to reduced breakdown of acetylcholine and therefore to a higher concentration in the synapse. Three of the four drugs approved for the treatment of mild to moderate Alzheimer's disease in Canada are acetylcholinesterase inhibitors: donepezil (Aricept), galantamine (generic only), and rivastigmine (Exelon). The fourth drug is memantine (Ebixa), an NMDA receptor antagonist. The glutamatergic neurotransmitter system plays an important role in memory formation. Amyloid plaques in the brain that form during the course of the disease can lead to glutamatergic dysfunction. When glutamate binds to NMDA receptors in a healthy brain, it opens calcium channels and calcium flows into the neurons. Excessive stimulation of these receptors by high concentrations of glutamate can lead to something called excitotoxicity. This is a phenomenon whereby too much calcium enters a neuron and may lead to neuronal damage and death. Memantine acts to prevent glutamate from binding to the NMDA receptor and activating the calcium channel. Memantine is used in treatment of moderate to severe Alzheimer's disease.

Refer to Chapter 17 for a more detailed discussion of these drugs, as well as their nursing considerations and patient and family teaching.

Natural Health Products

The growing interest in natural health products is driven by a variety of factors. Many people think that these products are safer either because they are "natural" or because they believe they have fewer adverse effects than conventional medications.

Natural health products, such as kava kava and St. John's wort, have been studied in clinical trials to determine safety and clinical efficacy (Sarris & Kavanagh, 2009). Some natural health products have been found to lack any therapeutic efficacy (Leach & Page, 2015), while others have been shown to potentially be deadly if taken over long periods of time or in combination with other chemical substances and prescription drugs (Brown, 2017; Gurley et al., 2012). For example, the risk of bleeding may be increased in patients taking the natural product ginkgo biloba in combination with warfarin (a drug that inhibits blood clotting), and taking the natural product kava kava by itself may increase the risk of hepatotoxicity at doses over 240 mg/day.

Among the major concerns of health care providers are the potential long-term effects of some natural health products (nerve, kidney, and liver damage) and the possibility of adverse chemical reactions when natural health products are taken in conjunction with other substances, especially conventional medications (Gurley et al., 2012).

St. John's wort can have serious interactions with a number of conventional medications (Hoffman et al., 2015). For example, St. John's wort when taken with other serotonergic drugs (e.g., SSRIs, triptans) can cause serotonin syndrome. This is a potentially life-threatening reaction that occurs when there is excessive 5-HT neurotransmission in the CNS. Symptoms include agitation, overactive reflexes (hyperreflexia), tremors, excessive sweating, racing heart, rapid changes in blood pressure, nausea, and loss of coordination (ataxia). St. John's wort may also reduce the effectiveness of other medications by increasing their rate of metabolism and reducing blood levels of these medications. This is because St. John's wort is a CYP3A4 enzyme inducer. The levels of any medications that are metabolized by CYP3A4 (e.g., hormonal contraceptives, human immunodeficiency virus [HIV] protease inhibitors, HIV non-nucleoside reverse transcriptase inhibitors, the immunosuppressant drugs cyclosporine and tacrolimus, the antineoplastic drugs irinotecan and imatinib) may drop to subtherapeutic levels, as their metabolism will be increased (Alpert, 2016). Drugs with a narrow therapeutic index should be monitored more closely when St. John's wort is added or discontinued or when its dosage is changed.

Another key concern regarding the use of natural health products is how they are regulated. Health Canada provides information on natural health products via the Licensed Natural Health Products Database. Any product authorized by Health Canada carries an eight-digit number. This means that it has been authorized for sale in Canada and meets the safety and efficacy guidelines of Health Canada (Health Canada, 2017a). Health care providers, especially nurses, need to stay current, using unbiased sources of product information and passing this information to patients who are contemplating using alternative remedies. Recalls and warnings to stop use of certain brands are available at MedEffect Canada (Health Canada, 2017b). It should be noted that there is often little to no substantive scientific evidence that natural health products are therapeutically effective. It is important that nurses and other health care providers explore the patient's use of natural health products in a non-judgemental manner by asking, "What over-the-counter medications or natural health products do you take to help your symptoms? Do they help? How much are you taking? How long have you been taking them?" Individuals taking medications or other natural health products should be made aware of drug or substance interactions and product safety. Such discussion should be part of the initial and ongoing interviews with patients. Complementary and integrative therapies are covered in more detail in Chapter 35.

> ⚡ **SAFETY TIP**
>
> As you know, all medications have potential therapeutic effects, adverse effects, and drug interactions. Even natural herbal remedies, vitamins, and minerals may block the action or increase the potency of medications used to treat mental health or other medical problems.
> Further, an important risk of pursuing a complementary or integrative therapy is the possible delay of other well-established treatments.

KEY POINTS TO REMEMBER

- All actions of the brain, sensory, motor, and intellectual, are carried out physiologically through the interactions of neurons. These interactions involve impulse conduction, neurotransmitter release, and receptor activation and response. Alterations in these basic processes can lead to mental disturbances and physical manifestations.
- In particular, it seems that overactivity of dopamine-related signalling pathways underlies the thought disturbances of schizophrenia, and that deficiencies in pathways involving norepinephrine, serotonin, or both underlie depression and anxiety. Insufficient GABA-related signalling may play a role in anxiety.
- Pharmacological treatment of mental health disturbances is directed at suspected neurotransmitter–receptor problems. Antipsychotic drugs ameliorate dopamine signalling; anti-depressant drugs alter neurotransmission by norepinephrine, serotonin, or both; and anti-anxiety drugs enhance the actions of GABA, 5-HT, norepinephrine, or all three.
- Because the immediate target activity of a drug can result in many downstream alterations in neuronal activity, drugs with a variety of chemical actions may show efficacy in treating the same clinical condition. Thus newer drugs with novel mechanisms of action are being used in the treatment of schizophrenia, depression, and anxiety.

- Unfortunately, drugs used to treat mental health disease can cause various undesired effects. Prominent among these can be sedation or excitement, motor disturbances, anti-cholinergic effects, α_1-adrenergic receptor antagonism, sexual dysfunction, and weight gain. There is a continuing effort to develop new drugs that are effective, safe, and well tolerated.

CRITICAL THINKING

1. No matter where you practise psychiatric mental health nursing, individuals under your care will be taking psychotropic drugs. Consider the importance of understanding normal brain structure and function as they relate to mental disturbances and psychotropic drugs by answering the following questions:
    a. How can you use the knowledge of normal brain function (control of peripheral nerves, skeletal muscles, the autonomic nervous system, hormones, and circadian rhythms) to better understand how a patient can be affected by psychotropic drugs or psychiatric illness?
    b. What information from the various brain imaging techniques can you use to understand and treat patients with mental health disorders and to provide support to their families? How might you use that information for patient and family teaching?
2. Based on your understanding of symptoms that may occur when the following components of neurotransmission are altered, what specific information would you include in medication teaching?
    a. Dopamine D_2 (as with use of antipsychotic drugs)
    b. Muscarinic receptors (as with use of phenothiazines and other drugs)
    c. α_1-Adrenergic receptors (as with use of phenothiazines and other drugs)
    d. Histamine receptors (as with use of phenothiazines and other drugs)
    e. Monoamine oxidase (MAO) (as with use of a monoamine oxidase inhibitor [MAOI])
    f. Gamma-aminobutyric acid (GABA) (as with use of benzodiazepines)
    g. Serotonin (as with use of selective serotonin reuptake inhibitors [SSRIs] and other drugs)
    h. Norepinephrine (as with use of serotonin–norepinephrine reuptake inhibitors [SNRIs])

CHAPTER REVIEW

1. Alterations in the activity of which neurotransmitters are important in drug treatment of depression?
    a. Acetylcholine and histamine
    b. GABA and glycine
    c. Dopamine and glutamate
    d. Serotonin and norepinephrine
2. Which of the following medication orders would the nurse question?
    a. Buspirone—take in the morning
    b. Temazepam—take at bedtime
    c. Zopiclone—take early in the morning
    d. Flurazepam—take at bedtime
3. Which patient statement would require the nurse to provide further teaching?
    a. "I should report any unusual bleeding when I take gingko biloba."
    b. "I should not take St. John's wort with sertraline hydrochloride."
    c. "Natural health products are safe because they are made with all-natural ingredients."
    d. "I will tell my doctor that I am taking a natural health product."

4. The nurse is caring for a patient who is taking lithium. Which adverse effect would the nurse anticipate?
   a. Oliguria
   b. Confusion
   c. Constipation
   d. Hyperthyroidism
5. The nurse understands that norepinephrine is involved with the stimulation of which bodily process?
   a. The fight-or-flight response to stress
   b. The hypothalamus to release hormones
   c. Involvement in the inflammatory response
   d. The parasympathetic nervous system

http://evolve.elsevier.com/Canada/Varcarolis/psychiatric/

REFERENCES

Alpert, J. E., et al. (2016). Drug–drug interactions in psychopharmacology. In T. A. Stern, J. F. Rosenbaum, & M. Fava et al. (Eds.), *Comprehensive clinical psychiatry* (pp. 552–566). Philadelphia: Elsevier.

Amstadter, A. B., Myers, J. M., & Kendler, K. S. (2014). Psychiatric resilience: Longitudinal twin study. *The British Journal of Psychiatry, 205*(4), 275–280.

Brent, D. A. (2016). Antidepressants and suicidality. *Psychiatric Clinics of North America, 39*, 503–512.

Brown, A. C. (2017). Liver toxicity related to herbs and dietary supplements: Online table of case reports: Part 3 of 6. *Food and Chemical Toxicology. An International Journal Published for the British Industrial Biological Research Association, 107*(Pt A), 472–501. https://doi.org/10.1016/j.fct.2016.07.001

Castren, E., & Kojima, M. (2017). Brain-derived neurotrophic factor in mood disorders and antidepressant treatments. *Neurobiology of Disease, 97*, 119–126.

Cipriani, A., Furukawa, T. A., Salanti, G., Chaimani, A., Atkinson, L. Z., Ogawa, Y., Leucht, S., Ruhe, H. G., Turner, E. H., Higgins, J. P. T., Egger, M., Takeshima, N., Hayasaka, Y., Imai, H., Shinohara, K., Tajika, A., Ioannidis, J. P. A., & Geddes, J. R. (2018). Comparative efficacy and acceptability of 21 antidepressant drugs for the acute treatment of adults with major depressive disorder: A systematic review and network meta-analysis. *Lancet, 391*(10128), 1357–1366. https://doi.org/10.1016/S0140-6736(17)32802-7

Corrado, A. C., & Walsh, J. P. (2016). Mechanisms underlying the benefits of anticonvulsants over lithium in the treatment of bipolar disorder. *Neuroreport, 27*(3), 131–135. https://doi.org/10.1097/WNR.0000000000000510

Curtis, J., Andrews, L., Davis, M., Smits, J., & Hofmann, S. G. (2017). A meta-analysis of pharmacotherapy for social anxiety disorder: An examination of efficacy, moderators, and mediators. *Expert Opinion on Pharmacotherapy, 18*, 243–251.

De Hert, M., Detraux, J., van Winkel, R., Yu, W., & Correll, C. U. (2012). Metabolic and cardiovascular adverse effects associated with antipsychotic drugs *Nature Reviews Endocrinology, 8*(2), 114–126.

Dubicka, B., Cole-King, A., Reynolds, S., & Ramchandani, P. (2016). Paper on suicidality and aggression during antidepressant treatment was flawed and the press release was misleading. *British Medical Journal, 352*, i911. https://doi.org/10.1136/bmj.i911

Duman, R. S. (2018). The dazzling promise of ketamine. *Cerebrum, 2018*. PMID: 30746033; PMCID: PMC6353120

Forlenza, O. V., De-Paula, V. J. R., & Diniz, B. S. O. (2014). Neuroprotective effects of lithium: Implications for the treatment of Alzheimer's disease and related neurodegenerative disorders. *ACS Chemical Neuroscience, 5*(6), 443–450. https://doi.org/10.1021/cn5000309

Fu, C. H., & Costafreda, S. G. (2013). Neuroimaging-based biomarkers in psychiatry: Clinical opportunities of a paradigm shift. *Canadian Journal of Psychiatry, 58*(9), 499–508.

Garland, E. J., Kutcher, S., Virani, A., & Elbe, D. (2016). Update on the use of SSRIs and SNRIs with children and adolescents in clinical practice. *Journal of the Canadian Academy of Child and Adolescent Psychiatry, 25*(1), 4–10.

Gurley, B. J., Fifer, E. K., & Gardner, Z. (2012). Pharmacokinetic herb-drug interactions (part 2): Drug interactions involving popular botanical dietary supplements and their clinical relevance. *Planta Medica, 78*(13), 1490–1514.

Hashimoto K. (2020). Molecular mechanisms of the rapid-acting and long-lasting antidepressant actions of (R)-ketamine. *Biochemical Pharmacology, 177*, 113935. https://doi.org/10.1016/j.bcp.2020.113935

Health Canada. (2017a). *Licensed Natural Health Database (LNHPD)*. http://www.hc-sc.gc.ca/dhp-mps/prodnatur/applications/licen-prod/lnhpd-bdpsnh-eng.php

Health Canada. (2017b). *MedEffect Canada: Adverse reaction reporting*. http://www.hc-sc.gc.ca/dhp-mps/medeff/report-declaration/index-eng.php

Ho, S. C., Chong, H. Y., Chaiyakunapruk, N., Tangiisuran, B., & Jacob, S. A. (2016). Clinical and economic impact of non-adherence to antidepressants in major depressive disorder: A systematic review. *Journal of Affective Disorders, 193*, 1–10.

Hoffman, R. S., Howland, M. A., Lewin, N. A., Nelson, L. S., & Goldfrank, L. R. (2015). *Goldfrank's toxicologic emergencies* (10th ed.). Toronto: McGraw Hill.

Leach, M. J., & Page, A. T. (2015). Herbal medicine for insomnia: A systematic review and meta-analysis. *Sleep Medicine Reviews, 24*, 1–12. https://doi.org/10.1016/j.smrv.2014.12.003

Lee, P. E., Gill, S. S., Freedman, M., Bronskill, S. E., Hillmer, M. P., & Rochon, P. A. (2004). Atypical antipsychotic drugs in the treatment of behavioural and psychological symptoms of dementia: Systematic review. *British Medical Journal, 329*, 75. https://doi.org/10.1136/bmj.38125.465579.55

Leucht, S., Cipriani, A., Spineli, L., Mavridis, D., Orey, D., Richter, F., Samara, M., Barbui, C., Engel, R. R., Geddes, J. R., Kissling, W., Stapf, M. P., Lässig, B., Salanti, G., & Davis, J. M. (2013). Comparative efficacy and tolerability of 15 antipsychotic drugs in schizophrenia: A multiple-treatment meta-analysis. *Lancet, 382*, 951–962.

Leucht, S., Corves, C., Arbter, D., Engel, R. R., Li, C., & Davis, J. M. (2009). Second-generation versus first-generation antipsychotic drugs for schizophrenia: A meta-analysis. *Lancet, 373*(9657), 31–41.

Li, P., Snyder, G., & Vanover, K. E. (2016). Dopamine targeting drugs for the treatment of schizophrenia: Past, present and future. *Current Topics in Medicinal Chemistry, 16*(29), 3385–3403.

Lui, S. L., Zhou, X. J., Sweeney, J. A., & Gong, Q. (2016). Psychoradiology: The frontier of neuroimaging in psychiatry. *Radiology, 281*(2), 357–372.

Malhi, G. S., & Outhred, T. (2016). Therapeutic mechanisms of lithium in bipolar disorder: Recent advances and current understanding. *CNS Drugs, 30*(1), 931–949. https://doi.org/10.1007/s40263-016-0380-1

Palix Foundation. (2022). *The foundations of lifelong health: The brain story*. https://www.albertafamilywellness.org/what-we-know/the-brain-story

Prabhavalkar, K. S., Poovanpallil, N. B., & Bhatt, L. K. (2015). Management of bipolar depression with lamotrigine: An antiepileptic mood stabilizer. *Frontiers in Pharmacology, 6*, 242. https://doi.org/10.3389/fphar.2015.00242

Preston, J. D., O'Neal, J. H., & Talaga, M. C. (2013). *Handbook of clinical psychopharmacology for therapists* (7th ed.). Oakland: New Harbinger.

Rang, H. P., Ritter, J. M., Flower, R. J., & Henderson, G. (2016). *Rang and Dales's pharmacology* (8th ed.). London: Churchill Livingstone.

Sadock, B. J., Sadock, V. A., & Ruiz, P. (2015). *Kaplan and Sadock's synopsis of psychiatry: Behavioral science/clinical psychiatry* (11th ed.). Kingston upon Thames: Wolters Kluwer.

Sarris, J., & Kavanagh, D. J. (2009). Kava and St. John's wort: Current evidence for use in mood and anxiety disorders. *Journal of Alternative & Complementary Medicine, 15*(8), 827–836.

Sendt, K., Tracy, D. K., & Bhattacharyya, S. (2015). A systematic review of factors influencing adherence to antipsychotic medication in schizophrenia-spectrum disorders. *Psychiatry Research, 225*, 14–30.

Sharma, T., Guski, L. S., Freund, N., & Gøtzsche, P. C. (2016). Suicidality and aggression during antidepressant treatment: Systematic review and meta-analyses based on clinical study reports. *British Medical Journal, 352*, i65. https://doi.org/10.1136/bmj.i65

Stahl, S. W. (2013). *Stahl's essential psychopharmacology: Neuroscientific basis and practical applications* (4th ed.). New York: Cambridge University Press.

Wei, Y., Chang, L., & Hashimoto, K. (2020). A historical review of antidepressant effects of ketamine and its enantiomers. *Pharmacology, Biochemistry and Behaviour, 190*, 172870–172878.

Wilner, P., Scheel-Kruger, J., & Belzung, C. (2013). The neurobiology of depression and antidepressant action. *Neuroscience and Biobehavioral Reviews, 37*, 2331–2371.

Yatham, L. N., Kennedy, S. H., Parikh, S. V., Schaffer, A., Bond, D. J., Frey, B. N., Sharma, V., Goldstein, B. I., Rej, S., Beaulieu, S., Alda, M., MacQueen, G., Milev, R. V., Ravindran, A., O'Donovan, C., McIntosh, D., Lam, R. W., Vazquez, G., Kapczinski, F., … Berk, M. (2018). Canadian Network for Mood and Anxiety Treatments (CANMAT) and International Society for Bipolar Disorders (ISBD) 2018 guidelines for the management of patients with bipolar disorder. *Bipolar Disorders, 20*(2), 97–170. https://doi.org/10.1111/bdi.12609

Zacher, J. L., & Holmes, J. C. (2012). Second-generation antipsychotics: A review of recently-approved agents and drugs in the pipeline. *Formulary (Cleveland, Ohio), 47*, 106–121.

Zanos, P., & Gould, T. D. (2018). Mechanisms of ketamine action as an antidepressant. *Molecular Psychiatry, 23*(4), 801–811.

UNIT 4

Psychobiological Disorders

12. Anxiety and Related Disorders

13. Depressive Disorders

14. Bipolar Disorders

15. Schizophrenia Spectrum and Other Psychotic Disorders

16. Eating and Feeding Disorders

17. Neurocognitive Disorders

18. Psychoactive Substance Use and Treatment

19. Personality Disorders

20. Sleep–Wake Disorders

12

Anxiety and Related Disorders

Cheryl L. Pollard
Originating US chapter by Margaret Jordan Halter

 https://evolve.elsevier.com/Canada/Varcarolis/psychiatric/

OBJECTIVES

1. Compare and contrast the four levels of anxiety in relation to perceptual field, ability to learn, and physical and other defining characteristics.
2. Identify defence mechanisms and consider one adaptive and one maladaptive use of each.
3. Compare and contrast foundational characteristics of anxiety, obsessive-compulsive, post-traumatic stress, somatic symptom, and dissociative disorders.
4. Identify genetic, biological, psychological, and cultural factors that may contribute to anxiety and related disorders.
5. Describe feelings that may be experienced by nurses caring for patients with anxiety disorders.
6. Identify essential assessment components for anxiety, somatic symptom, and dissociative disorders.
7. Formulate four appropriate nursing diagnoses that can be used in providing care to a person with an anxiety or related disorder.
8. Propose realistic outcome criteria for a patient with (1) generalized anxiety disorder, (2) panic disorder, and (3) post-traumatic stress disorder.
9. Identify nursing interventions for patients with anxiety, obsessive-compulsive, post-traumatic stress, somatic symptom, and dissociative disorders.
10. Discuss three classes of medications appropriate for the treatment of anxiety and related disorders.
11. Describe basic-level and advanced-practice interventions for anxiety and related disorders.

KEY TERMS AND CONCEPTS

acute stress disorder
agoraphobia
alternate personality (alter)
anxiety
compulsions
conversion disorder
dissociative amnesia
dissociative disorders
dissociative fugue
dissociative identity disorder
fear

flashbacks
generalized anxiety disorder
illness anxiety disorder
la belle indifférence
mild anxiety
moderate anxiety
normal anxiety
obsessions
panic
panic attack
panic disorder

post-traumatic stress disorder
secondary gains
selective inattention
severe anxiety
social phobia
somatic symptom disorders
specific phobias
subpersonality
substance-induced anxiety disorder

For most people, stress and anxiety are an everyday part of life: "I was really stressed when I couldn't find a parking space just before my final exam. I think I would have done better without that worry." For some people, however, anxiety-related symptoms become severely debilitating and interfere with normal functioning: "Today I was so worried that I wouldn't find a parking space before the final exam, I stayed home." Imagine being so incapacitated by anxiety, you live in dread of germs to the point that handwashing has become the focal point of your day (obsessive-compulsive disorder [OCD]). Consider repeatedly feeling the immediate terror of emotionally reliving a horrific event in your life, such as hydroplaning on the highway and finding yourself facing oncoming traffic in the wrong lane. You may refuse to drive when it rains (post-traumatic stress disorder [PTSD]). Or when you get into a car, it seems as if your surroundings are foggy, dreamlike: visually distorted (depersonalization/derealization disorder). Anxiety can also affect individuals through physical symptoms, such as fatigue, pain, or numbness. Imagine thinking about your somatic symptoms all the time. This causes you significant distress, and you try to talk with your doctor and the nurse every day. If the doctor is away, you will go to the hospital emergency department. You are unable to maintain friendships because there is no time left after you have attended all your appointments, and you have spent most of your money on various therapies that are not covered by your health plan (somatic symptom disorder [SSD]).

This chapter examines disorders with a common phenomenology of fear and anxiety. The concept of anxiety and defences against anxiety are described. A brief overview of anxiety disorders, OCDs, dissociative disorders, and SSDs is provided. There are many commonalities in treatment approaches and associated nursing care strategies for these illnesses that may be used by nurses who work in either a psychiatric or a medical setting.

❤ HOW A NURSE HELPED ME

I Am Not the Only One

I am in my mid-fifties now, but when I was a young girl, I lived a secret life. I was always a quiet girl, preferring to play dolls by myself or with Judy, my best and only friend, rather than with a group of girls. I was especially uncomfortable with the boys. I don't know what it was; I just didn't feel comfortable with them. I often felt as though others were judging me and making comments about me. I never told anyone how being around a group of people made me feel: I felt embarrassed and stupid. My parents called me "the quiet one" of the family, and I lived up to that label. I struggled through school, constantly feeling on edge, and worrying that a teacher would ask me a question.

I know it seems silly, but one of my greatest fears was having to introduce myself in a group. I would start sweating, my heart pounded, I felt like I was going to die, and I was petrified that I might stutter. I became good at managing this situation by always volunteering to go first. You see, if I introduced myself first, then I could relax. I was very pleased with myself when I made this discovery. But other situations that caused even greater anxiety began to crop up. When I had to do a presentation in front of the class, I would pretend that I was ill, and my mother would let me stay home. I found that when I was extremely anxious, I would have difficulty breathing. This led to another strategy for getting out of embarrassing situations: I was diagnosed with childhood asthma, and I very quickly learned how to bring on an asthma attack to get out of going to school. My fear of being found out was always present, and I hated lying to my parents, but I was too ashamed to tell them that I was afraid of sweating, dying, or stuttering in public.

When I went on to university, I would force myself to step out of my comfort zone. I always had a sense of doom and a fear that I was going to die of embarrassment. It was not so much the situation that caused me anxiety; it was more the fear of doing something to embarrass myself that caused me anxiety. It was as if I feared the fear.

My adult years have been lonely. I wanted to talk with people and have fun, but I couldn't get over my anxiety. Then, 5 years ago, I met a nurse who works in psychiatry. He asked me how long I had been struggling with social anxiety disorder (social phobia). "You mean the way I feel is a disorder? I am not the only one?" He arranged for me to see a psychiatrist, who ordered a low dose of medication and enrolled me in 20 cognitive behavioural therapy classes (in a group, of course). The change in me has been remarkable. I still get anxious in some situations, but I am able to reframe my thoughts and move on. I no longer feel as if I am going to die of embarrassment.

A therapist could be many things, but the following points describe the nurse who was able to help me with my anxiety disorder:

1. Was kind, compassionate, and easy to talk to
2. Conversed with me to get a feel for how strong or resilient my character is
3. Was able to "walk a mile in my shoes," so to speak
4. Was willing to research the problem on the Internet and in books, as needed
5. Considered my feelings and offered constructive yet gentle criticism
6. Suggested tangible ways that I could try to advance my position and rectify my problem one step at a time
7. Offered positive self-esteem–enhancing comments during the process as, more than likely, these were lacking in my life
8. Encouraged me to be proud of myself for my accomplishments
9. Challenged me occasionally so that I could continue to move forward
10. Realized when I was emotionally and physically well or exhausted or overwhelmed and in need of rest
11. Helped me recognize coping strategies for relapse prevention or maintenance of my current level of coping
12. Helped me better understand my illness and the types of evidence-informed treatments available
13. Helped to educate me about my medication and to monitor for adverse effects
14. Unmasked the real problem in my core before attempting to rectify the manifestation of my condition, which is probably very obvious
15. Took time during appointments to "read between the lines" of what I say
16. Was available if I really needed to speak with him
17. Asked questions, especially if he was unsure of what I meant
18. Gave me some homework
19. Kept the therapy on point for both of us
20. Engaged in a truly well-rounded therapeutic relationship with me
21. Learned from me as I learned from him

Being positive and being interested—it is a tall order!

Source: Holly, a patient with an anxiety disorder.

ANXIETY

Anxiety is a universal human experience and is the most basic of emotions. It can be defined as a feeling of apprehension, uneasiness, uncertainty, or dread resulting from a real or perceived threat. Whereas anxiety is a vague sense of dread related to an unspecified or unknown danger, fear is a reaction to a real or perceived specific danger. Another important distinction between anxiety and fear is that anxiety affects us at a deeper level: it invades the central core of the personality and erodes feelings of self-esteem and personal worth. Physiologically, however, the body reacts to anxiety and fear in similar ways. In 2020 there was a significant rise in numbers of Canadians experiencing anxiety. This rise in numbers has a direct relationship to the impact COVID-19 has had on the lives of every Canadian. Based on data from an online questionnaire of 46 000 Canadians, Statistics Canada (2020) reports that 88% of respondents had at least one symptom of anxiety in the last 2 weeks. The most frequently reported symptom was "feeling nervous, anxious or on edge." The highest anxiety was experienced by people who had been financially impacted by COVID-19. Even before the impact of the pandemic was felt in Canada, on any given day, approximately 500 000 people were unable to attend work because of mental health challenges (Benjamin & Boyer, 2019). Pre-pandemic, the yearly costs for disability claims due to anxiety-related disorders was nearly $17 billion (Benjamin & Boyer, 2019).

Normal anxiety is a healthy reaction necessary for survival. It provides us with energy to carry out everyday tasks and strive toward goals; motivates us to make and survive change; and prompts constructive behaviours, such as studying for an examination, being on time for a job interview, preparing for a presentation, and working toward making an individual change, such as a move, or advocating for social change, for instance, concerning what Usher and colleagues refer to as eco-anxiety (Usher, Durkin & Bhullar, 2019).

An understanding of the levels of anxiety and the defensive patterns used in response to anxiety is fundamental to psychiatric mental health nursing care. With this understanding and practice, you will become skilled at identifying levels of anxiety, recognizing the defences used to alleviate anxiety, evaluating the possible stressors that contribute to increased anxiety, and planning interventions to lower anxiety levels (including one's own) effectively.

People with anxiety-related disorders will often use rigid and ineffective behaviours repetitively to try to control their anxiety. The common element of such disorders is that those affected experience a degree of anxiety so high that it interferes with personal, occupational, or social functioning. Recent studies also suggest that the presence of chronic anxiety disorders may increase the number of cardiovascular system–related deaths (Chauvet-Gelinier & Bonin, 2017). All anxiety-related disorders tend to be persistent and are often disabling.

Levels of Anxiety

As di1scussed in Chapter 4, Hildegard Peplau had a profound role in shaping the specialty of psychiatric mental health nursing. She identified anxiety as one of the most important concepts and developed an anxiety model that consists of four levels: mild, moderate, severe, and **panic** (Peplau, 1968). The boundaries between these levels are not distinct, and the behaviours and characteristics of individuals experiencing anxiety can and often do overlap. Identification of a patient's specific level of anxiety is essential because interventions are based on the degree of the anxiety.

Mild Anxiety

Mild anxiety, which occurs in the normal experience of everyday living, allows an individual to perceive reality in sharp focus. A person experiencing a mild level of anxiety sees, hears, and grasps more information, and problem solving becomes more effective. Physical symptoms may include slight discomfort, restlessness, irritability, or mild tension-relieving behaviours (e.g., nail biting, foot or finger tapping, fidgeting, wringing of hands).

Moderate Anxiety

As anxiety increases, the perceptual field narrows, and some details are excluded from observation. The person experiencing **moderate anxiety** sees, hears, and grasps less information and may demonstrate **selective inattention**, in which only certain things in the environment are seen or heard unless they are pointed out. While the person's ability to think clearly is hampered, learning and problem solving can still take place, although not at an optimal level. Physical symptoms of moderate anxiety include tension, pounding heart, increased pulse and respiratory rate, perspiration, and mild somatic symptoms (gastric discomfort, headache, urinary urgency). Voice tremors and shaking may be noticed. Mild or moderate anxiety levels can be constructive because anxiety may signal that something in the person's life needs attention or is dangerous.

Severe Anxiety

The perceptual field of a person experiencing **severe anxiety** is greatly reduced. A person with severe anxiety may focus on one particular detail or many scattered details and has difficulty noticing their environment, even when it is pointed out by another. Learning and problem solving are not possible at this level, and the person may be dazed and confused. Behaviour becomes automatic (e.g., wringing hands, pacing) and is aimed at reducing or relieving anxiety. Somatic symptoms such as headache, nausea, dizziness, and insomnia often increase; trembling and a pounding heart are common; and the person may hyperventilate and experience a sense of impending doom or dread (see Case Study and Nursing Care Plan 12.1).

Panic

Panic, the most extreme level of anxiety, results in noticeably disturbed behaviour. Someone in a state of panic is unable to process what is going

---

CASE STUDY AND NURSING CARE PLAN 12.1
Severe Level of Anxiety

The following case study describes a man experiencing a severe level of acute anxiety. See if you can match his signs and symptoms with those in Table 12.1.

Ted Silvestri, a 63-year-old man, comes into the emergency department (ED) with his wife, Julie. She has taken an overdose of sleeping pills and antidepressant medications. Ten years earlier, Julie's mother died, and since that time Julie has suffered several episodes of severe depression with suicide attempts. She has needed hospitalization during these episodes. Julie had been released from the hospital 2 weeks earlier after treatment for depression and threatened suicide.

Ted has a long-established routine of giving his wife her antidepressant medications in the morning and her sleeping medication at night and keeping the bottles hidden when he is not at home. Today he had forgotten to hide the medications before he went to work. His wife had taken the remaining pills from both bottles with large quantities of alcohol. When Ted returned home for lunch, Julie was comatose. In the ED Julie suffers cardiac arrest and is taken to the critical care unit (CCU).

Ted appears very jittery. He moves about the room aimlessly. He drops his hat, a medication card, and his keys. His hands are trembling, and he looks around the room, bewildered. He appears unable to focus on any one thing. He says over and over, in a loud, high-pitched voice, "Why didn't I hide the bottles?" He is wringing his hands and begins stomping his feet, saying, "It's all my fault. Everything is falling apart."

Other people in the waiting room appear distracted and alarmed by his behaviour. Ted seems to be oblivious to his surroundings.

Assessment

Jean Gautier, the psychiatric nurse working in the ED, comes into the waiting room and assesses Ted's behaviour as indicative of a severe anxiety level. After talking with Ted briefly, Jean believes that nursing intervention is indicated, based on the following assessment of the patient:

Objective Data	Subjective Data
Unable to focus on anything	"Everything is falling apart."
Engaging in purposeless activity (walking around aimlessly)	"Why didn't I hide the bottles?"
Oblivious to his surroundings	"It's all my fault."
Showing unproductive relief behaviour (stomping, wringing hands, dropping things)	

Diagnosis

1. Anxiety (severe) related to the patient's perception of responsibility for his wife's coma and possible death

Supporting Data

- Inability to focus
- Confusion
- The feeling that "everything is falling apart"

CASE STUDY AND NURSING CARE PLAN 12.1—cont'd
Severe Level of Anxiety

Outcomes Identification
Patient will demonstrate effective coping strategies.

Planning
Jean thinks that if he can lower Ted's anxiety to a moderate level, he can work with Ted to get a clear picture of his situation and place the events in a more realistic perspective. He also thinks Ted needs to talk to someone and share some of his pain and confusion to help sort out his feelings. Jean identifies two short-term goals:
1. Patient's anxiety will decrease from severe to moderate by 1600 hours.
2. Patient will verbalize his feelings and a need for assistance by 1600 hours.

Implementation
Jean takes Ted to a quiet room in the back of the ED. He introduces himself and comments that he notices that Ted is upset. He says, "I will stay with you." At first, Ted finds it difficult to sit down and continues pacing around the room. Jean sits quietly and calmly while listening to Ted's self-recriminations. He attends carefully to what Ted is saying—and what he is not saying—to identify themes.

After a while, Ted becomes calmer and is able to sit next to Jean. Jean offers him orange juice, which he accepts and holds tightly.

Jean speaks calmly, using simple, clear statements. He uses communication tools that are helpful to Ted in sorting out his feelings and naming them.

Dialogue	Therapeutic Tool or Comment
Ted: "Yes … yes … I forgot to hide the bottles. She usually tells me when she feels bad. Why didn't she tell me?"	
Nurse: "You think that if she had told you she wanted to kill herself, you would have hidden the pills?"	Jean asks for clarification of Ted's thinking.
Ted: "Yes, if I had only known, this wouldn't have happened."	
Nurse: "It sounds as if you believe you should have known what your wife was thinking without her telling you."	Here, Jean clarifies Ted's expectations that he should be able to read his wife's mind.
Ted: "Well, yes … when you put it that way … I just don't know what I'll do if she dies."	

When Jean thinks that Ted has discussed his feelings of guilt sufficiently, he asks Ted to clarify his thinking about his wife's behaviour. Ted is able to place his feelings of guilt in a more realistic perspective. Next, Jean brings up another issue—the question of whether Ted's wife will live or die.

Dialogue	Therapeutic Tool or Comment
Nurse: "You said that if your wife dies, you don't know what you will do."	Jean reflects Ted's feelings back to him.
Ted: "Oh, God" (he begins to cry) "I can't live without her. She's all I have in the world."	
Silence	
Nurse: "She means a great deal to you."	Jean reflects Ted's feelings back to him.
Ted: "Everything. Since her mother died, we are each other's only family."	
Nurse: "What would it mean to you if your wife died?"	Jean asks Ted to evaluate his feelings about his wife.
Ted: "I couldn't live by myself, alone. I couldn't stand it." (Starts to cry again.)	
Nurse: "It sounds as if being alone is very frightening to you."	Jean restates in clear terms Ted's experience and feelings.
Ted: "Yes, I don't know how I'd manage by myself."	
Nurse: "A change like that could take time to adjust to."	Jean validates that Ted's wife dying would be very painful for Ted. At the same time, he implies hope that Ted could work through the death in time.
Ted: "Yes … it would be very hard."	

Again, Jean gives Ted a chance to sort out his feelings and fears. Jean helps him focus on the reality that his wife may die and encourages him to express fears related to her possible death. After a while, Jean offers to go to the CCU with Ted to see how his wife is doing. When they arrive, they learn that although Julie is still comatose her condition has stabilized and she is breathing on her own.

After his arrival at the CCU, Ted starts to worry about whether he remembered to lock the door at home. Jean suggests that he call neighbours and ask them to check the door. Ted is now able to focus on everyday things. Jean makes arrangements to see Ted the next day when he comes in to visit his wife.

The next day, Julie has regained consciousness. She is discharged 1 week later. At the time of her discharge, Ted and Julie Silvestri are considering family therapy once a week with a nurse in the outpatient psychiatry department.

Evaluation
The first short-term goal is to lower Ted's anxiety level from severe to moderate. Jean can see that Ted has become more visibly calm: his trembling, wringing of hands, and stomping of feet have ceased, and he is able to focus on his thoughts and feelings with Jean's help.

The second short-term goal established for Ted is that he will verbalize his feelings and his need for assistance. Ted is able to identify and discuss with Jean his feelings of guilt and fear of being left alone in the world if his wife should die. Both of these feelings are overwhelming him. He is also able to state that he needs assistance in coping with these feelings in order to make tentative plans for the future.

on in the environment and may lose touch with reality, even experiencing hallucinations, or false sensory perceptions (e.g., seeing people or objects not really there). Physical manifestations may include pacing, running, shouting, screaming, or withdrawal, and actions may become erratic, uncoordinated, and impulsive. These sorts of automatic behaviours are used to reduce or relieve anxiety, although such efforts may be ineffective. Acute panic may lead to exhaustion.

Table 12.1 distinguishes among the levels of anxiety in regard to their (1) effects on perceptual field, (2) effects on the ability to learn, and (3) physical and other defining characteristics.

Defences Against Anxiety

Dysfunctional behaviour (e.g., compulsions, stress headaches, detachment) is a result of *defence mechanisms* (automatic coping styles that protect people from anxiety and maintain self-image by blocking feelings, conflicts, and memories). When behaviour is recognized as dysfunctional, nurses can initiate interventions to reduce anxiety. As anxiety decreases, dysfunctional behaviour will frequently decrease, although initially, as dysfunctional behaviour decreases, anxiety may actually increase until the individual learns to cognitively restructure thoughts. Therefore nurses must be available to help support alternative coping strategies as the individual learns to restructure their thinking patterns.

Sigmund Freud and his daughter, Anna Freud, outlined most of the defence mechanisms we recognize today. Although they operate all the time, defence mechanisms are not always apparent to the individual using them. The *adaptive use* of defence mechanisms helps people lower their anxiety to achieve goals in acceptable ways. The excessive application of defence mechanisms, however, results in their *maladaptive use* and is particularly problematic when immature defences are called upon. Figure 12.1 operationally defines anxiety and illustrates how defences come into play.

TABLE 12.1 Levels of Anxiety.

Mild	Moderate	Severe	Panic
Perceptual Field			
May have heightened perceptual field	Has narrow perceptual field	Has greatly reduced perceptual field	Is unable to focus on the environment
	Grasps less of what is going on	Focuses on details or one specific detail	
		Attention is scattered	
Is alert and can see, hear, and grasp what is happening in the environment	Can attend to more if pointed out by another (selective inattention)	May not be able to attend to events in environment even when pointed out by another	Experiences the utmost state of terror and emotional paralysis
			Feels he or she "ceases to exist"
Can identify things that are disturbing and are producing anxiety		Completely absorbed with self	May have hallucinations or delusions that take the place of reality
		In severe to panic levels of anxiety, the environment is blocked out. It is as if these events are not occurring.	
Ability to Learn			
Able to work effectively toward a goal and examine alternatives	Able to solve problems but not at optimal ability	Unable to see connections between events or details	May be mute or have extreme psychomotor agitation, leading to exhaustion
	Benefits from guidance of others	Has distorted perceptions	Shows disorganized or irrational reasoning
Mild and moderate levels of anxiety can alert the person that something is wrong and can stimulate appropriate action.		*Severe and panic levels prevent problem solving and discovery of effective solutions. Unproductive relief behaviours are called into play, thus perpetuating a vicious cycle.*	
Physical or Other Characteristics			
Slight discomfort	Voice tremors	Feelings of dread	Feeling of terror
Attention-seeking behaviours	Change in voice pitch	Ineffective functioning	Immobility or severe hyperactivity, fight-or-flight or freeze
Restlessness, irritability, or impatience	Difficulty concentrating	Confusion	Dilated pupils
Mild tension-relieving behaviour (e.g., foot or finger tapping, lip chewing, fidgeting)	Shakiness	Purposeless activity	Unintelligible communication or inability to speak
	Repetitive questioning	Sense of impending doom	
	Somatic complaints (e.g., urinary frequency and urgency, headache, backache, insomnia)	More intense somatic complaints (e.g., dizziness, nausea, headache, sleeplessness)	Severe shakiness
			Sleeplessness
	Increased respiration rate	Hyperventilation	Severe withdrawal
	Increased pulse rate	Tachycardia	Hallucinations or delusions—likely out of touch with reality
	Increased muscle tension	Withdrawal	
	More extreme tension-relieving behaviour (e.g., pacing, banging hands on table)	Loud and rapid speech	
		Threats and demands	

Fig. 12.1 Anxiety operationally defined.

With the exception of sublimation and altruism, which are always healthy coping mechanisms, all defence mechanisms can be used in both healthy and unhealthy ways. Most people use a variety of defence mechanisms but not always at the same level. Keep in mind that evaluating whether the use of defence mechanisms is adaptive or maladaptive is determined, for the most part, by their frequency, intensity, duration of use, and effect on relationships. Table 12.2 describes defence mechanisms and their adaptive and maladaptive uses.

Clinical Picture

Anxiety exerts a powerful influence on the mind and body. The experience of anxiety is an underlying factor in several disorders, including:

- Acute stress disorder
- Anxiety disorder not otherwise specified
- Anxiety due to medical conditions
- Depersonalization/derealization disorder
- Generalized anxiety disorder (GAD)
- OCD and related disorders
- Panic disorders (PDs)
- Phobias
- PTSD
- SSD
- Substance-induced anxiety disorder

Anxiety Disorders

The following disorders share symptoms related to excessive fear and anxiety that result in behavioural changes or disturbances. Fear is a response to an imminent threat. Anxiety is related to the perception of a future threat.

Panic Disorder

Panic disorder is an anxiety disorder characterized by recurring severe **panic attacks**. It may also effect significant behavioural changes lasting at least a month and ongoing worry about having other attacks. A panic attack is the sudden onset of extreme apprehension or fear, usually associated with feelings of impending doom. The feelings of terror present during a panic attack are so severe that normal function is suspended, the perceptual field is extremely limited, severe personality disorganization is evident, and misinterpretation of reality may occur. The following vignette gives an example of a patient with signs and symptoms of a panic attack.

> **Vignette**
> Sophia, a 30-year-old pharmacist, began to experience tension, irritability, and sleep disturbances after her mother's death from heart disease. On several occasions, Sophia has awakened gasping for breath. Her heart pounds and she feels a tight sensation like a band around her chest. Her pulse typically increases to more than 110 beats per minute, and she experiences dizziness. She fears that she is going to die. The symptoms come on within 10 minutes (sudden onset) and then dissipate. On these occasions, Sophia telephones a friend to come over. The friend typically finds Sophia wringing her hands, moaning, and appearing totally disorganized. In each instance, the friend takes Sophia to the emergency department, where Sophia remains overnight for observation and tests. All diagnostic test results are normal. Because the physician finds no apparent organic basis for the episodes, she suggests that they are likely panic attacks.

People experiencing panic attacks may believe that they are losing their minds or having a heart attack since the attacks are often accompanied by highly uncomfortable physical symptoms such as palpitations, chest pain, breathing difficulties, nausea, a choking feeling, chills, and hot flashes. Typically, panic attacks occur within 10 minutes "out of the blue" (i.e., suddenly, and not necessarily in response to stress), are extremely intense, last a matter of minutes, and then subside. Table 12.3 outlines a generic nursing care plan for PD (see also Case Study and Nursing Care Plan 12.1).

Agoraphobia. When individuals actively avoid situations from which escape might be difficult or embarrassing or in which help might not be available if panic-like symptoms were to occur, they may be diagnosed with **agoraphobia**. Agoraphobia without a history of panic attacks occurs only rarely and early in the patient's history. Over time, panic attacks usually develop over the course of this

TABLE 12.2 Adaptive and Maladaptive Uses of Defence Mechanisms

Defence Mechanism	Adaptive Use	Maladaptive Use
Altruism is dedicating oneself to meeting the needs of others as a means of diffusing potentially anxious situations.	A person who is worried that their boss is angry at them will go out of his way and try to be helpful.	*The use of altruism is always constructive.*
Compensation is used to make up for perceived deficiencies and to cover up shortcomings related to these deficiencies to protect the conscious mind from recognizing them.	A shorter-than-average person becomes assertively verbal and excels in business.	An individual drinks alcohol when self-esteem is low to temporarily diffuse discomfort.
Conversion is the unconscious transformation of anxiety into a physical symptom with no organic cause. Often the symptom functions to gain attention or to provide an excuse.	A student is unable to take a final examination because of a terrible headache.	A person becomes blind after seeing their spouse flirt with other people.
Denial involves escaping unpleasant, anxiety-causing thoughts, feelings, wishes, or needs by ignoring their existence.	A person reacts to news of the death of a loved one by saying, "No, I don't believe you. The doctor said they were fine."	A person whose spouse died 3 years earlier still keeps their clothes in the closet and talks about them in the present tense.
Displacement is the transference of emotions associated with a particular person, object, or situation to another nonthreatening person, object, or situation.	A patient criticizes a nurse after their family fails to visit.	A child who is unable to acknowledge fear of their father becomes fearful of animals.
Dissociation is a disruption in the usually integrated functions of consciousness, memory, identity, or perception of the environment. It may result in a separation between feeling and thought. Dissociation can also be manifested by compartmentalizing uncomfortable or unpleasant aspects of oneself.	A nursing student is able to mentally separate themselves from the noisy environment in the gymnasium as they writes their final exam.	As the result of an abusive childhood and the need to separate from its realities, a patient finds themselves perpetually in a world where they feel disconnected from reality. They feel like an outside observer to their thoughts, feelings, and body sensations.
Identification is attributing to oneself the characteristics of another person or group, which may be done consciously or unconsciously.	An 8-year-old dresses up like their teacher and puts together a pretend classroom for their friends.	A young child thinks a neighbourhood gang leader with money and drugs is someone to look up to.
Intellectualization is the process of analyzing events based on remote, cold facts (i.e., without passion), rather than incorporating feeling into the processing.	Despite the fact that a patient has lost their farm to a tornado, they analyzes their options and leads their child to safety.	A patient responds to the death of their spouse by focusing on the details of day care and operating the household, rather than processing the grief with their children.
Introjection is the process by which the outside world is incorporated or absorbed into a person's view of the self.	After their wife's death, a patient has transient complaints of chest pains and difficulty breathing—the symptoms their wife had before she died.	A patient whose parents overcriticized and belittled them as a child grows up thinking they are no good. They have taken on their parents' evaluation of them as part of their self-image.
Projection refers to the unconscious rejection of emotionally unacceptable features and the transfer of them onto other people, objects, or situations. You can remember this defence through the childhood retort of "What you say is what you are."	A person who is unconsciously attracted to other people teases his partner about being attracted to other people.	A patient who has repressed an attraction toward people of the same sex refuses to socialize. They have fears another same-sex person will make homosexual advances toward them.
Rationalization consists of justifying illogical or unreasonable ideas, actions, or feelings by developing acceptable explanations that satisfy the teller as well as the listener.	An employee says, "I didn't get the raise because the boss doesn't like me."	A patient who thinks his child was the product of a suspected affair between his wife and best friend excuses his malicious treatment of the child by saying, "They are lazy and disobedient," when that is not the case.
Reaction formation occurs when unacceptable feelings or behaviours are controlled and kept outside of awareness by developing the opposite behaviour or emotion.	A patient in recovery from substance use disorder constantly preaches about the evils of drinking alcohol.	A patient who has an unconscious hostility toward their child is overprotective and hovers over them to protect them from harm, interfering with their normal growth and development.
Regression is the reversion to an earlier, more primitive, and childlike pattern of behaviour that may or may not have been previously exhibited.	A 4-year-old with a new baby sibling starts sucking their thumb and wanting a bottle.	A patient who loses a promotion starts complaining to others, hands in sloppy work, misses appointments, and comes in late for meetings.
Repression is a first-line psychological defence against anxiety. It is the unconscious temporary or long-term exclusion of unpleasant or unwanted experiences, emotions, or ideas from conscious awareness.	An individual forgets their partner's birthday after a verbal disagreement.	A patient is unable to enjoy sex after having pushed out of awareness a traumatic sexual incident from childhood.

TABLE 12.2 Adaptive and Maladaptive Uses of Defence Mechanisms—cont'd

Defence Mechanism	Adaptive Use	Maladaptive Use
Splitting is the inability to integrate the positive and negative qualities of oneself or others into a cohesive image. Aspects of the self and of others tend to alternate between opposite poles—for example, either good, loving, worthy, and nurturing, or bad, hateful, destructive, rejecting, and worthless.	A toddler views their parents as superhuman and wants to be like them.	A 26-year-old patient has difficulty maintaining close relationships. Although they can initially find many positive qualities about new acquaintances, eventually they become disillusioned when the people they are attracted to, inevitably turn out to be flawed.
Sublimation is an unconscious process of substituting mature, constructive, and socially acceptable activity for immature, destructive, and unacceptable impulses. Often these impulses are sexual or aggressive.	A patient who is angry with their boss writes a short story about a heroic character.	*The use of sublimation is always constructive.*
Suppression is the conscious denial of a disturbing situation or feeling.	An individual who is preparing to make an important speech later in the day is told by their partner that morning that they want a divorce. Although visibly upset, the patient puts the incident aside until after their speech, so they can give the matter their total concentration.	A patient who feels a lump in their breast shortly before leaving for a 3-week vacation puts the information in the back of their mind until after returning from the vacation.
Undoing, most commonly seen in children, is atoning for an act or communication.	After flirting with their assistant, a patient brings their spouse tickets to a concert they want to see.	A patient with rigid, moralistic beliefs and repressed sexuality is driven to wash their hands to gain composure when around people they find attractive.

TABLE 12.3 Generic Care Plan for Panic Disorder

Short-Term Goal	Intervention	Rationale
1. Patient's anxiety will decrease to moderate by (date).	1a. If hyperventilation occurs, encourage patient to take slow, deep breaths. Breathing with the patient may be helpful.	1a. Focus is shifted away from distressing symptoms. Slow, deep breathing triggers a relaxation response.
	1b. Keep expectations minimal and simple.	1b. Anxiety limits ability to attend to complex tasks.
2. Patient will gain mastery over panic episodes by (date).	2a. Help patient connect feelings before attack with onset of attack: "What were you thinking about just before the attack?" "Can you identify what you were feeling just before the attack?"	2a. Physiological symptoms of anxiety usually appear first as the result of a stressor. They are immediately followed by automatic thoughts, such as "I'm dying" or "I'm going crazy," which are distorted assessments.
	2b. Help patient recognize symptoms as resulting from anxiety, not from a catastrophic physical problem. Examples: Explain physical symptoms of anxiety. Discuss the fact that anxiety causes sensations similar to those of physical events, such as a heart attack.	2b. Factual information and alternative interpretations can help patient recognize distortions in thought.
	2c. Identify effective therapies for panic episodes.	2c. Cognitive behavioural treatment is highly effective. Antianxiety medication is appropriate.
	2d. Teach patient abdominal breathing.	2d. Breathing breaks the cycle of escalating symptoms of anxiety.
	2e. Teach patient to reframe anxiety by using positive self-talk, such as "I can control my anxiety."	2e. Cognitive restructuring is an effective way to replace negative self-talk.
	2f. Teach patient and family about any medication ordered for patient's panic attacks.	2f. Patient and family need to know what the medication can do, the adverse effects and toxic effects, and when to offer medication to the patient.

Nursing diagnosis: *Anxiety* as evidenced by sudden onset of fear or sense of impending doom, increased pulse and respirations, shortness of breath, possible chest pain, dizziness, abdominal distress, and panic attacks.

Outcome: Panic attacks will become less intense, and time between episodes will lengthen so that patient can function comfortably at the usual level.

illness. Situations that are commonly avoided by people with agoraphobia include being outside alone; waiting in line at a grocery store; travelling in a car, bus, or airplane; being on a bridge; riding in an elevator; or going to a movie theatre. These types of feared places are avoided in an effort to control anxiety. Avoidance behaviours, however, can be debilitating and life constricting. Consider the effect on a father whose agoraphobia renders him unable to leave home and prevents him from seeing his child's high school graduation, or on the businesswoman whose avoidance of flying prevents her from attending distant business conferences.

> **Vignette**
> Dmitri is a 28-year-old man who suffers from panic attacks with agoraphobia. He once lived a very active life, often participating in thrill-seeking activities like bungee jumping and skydiving. Dmitri's father, who had severe cardiovascular disease, died 2 years previously on his way to work one day. Since then, Dmitri has become increasingly fearful of the outdoors. He has gradually stopped leaving the family home because he experiences panic attacks, fearing he will die if he goes out.

Phobias

A *phobia* is a persistent, irrational fear of a specific object, activity, or situation that leads to a desire for avoidance or to actual avoidance of the object, activity, or situation despite the awareness and reassurance that it is not dangerous. **Specific phobias**, which are more intense, cause impaired daily functioning and last at least half a year. They are characterized by the experience of high levels of anxiety or fear in response to specific objects or situations, such as dogs, spiders, heights, storms, water, blood, closed spaces, tunnels, and bridges. Specific phobias are common and usually do not cause sufferers much difficulty because they can contrive to avoid the feared object. See Table 12.4 for clinical names for common phobias.

> **Vignette**
> Abdi developed a morbid fear of elevators after being trapped in one for 3 hours during a power outage. As his fear and anxiety intensified, it became necessary for him to use only stairs or escalators. Abdi even became anxious if he had to enter closets or small storage rooms. He had developed claustrophobia, a fear of closed spaces.

Social phobia, also called *social anxiety disorder (SAD)*, is characterized by severe anxiety or fear provoked by exposure to a social or performance situation (e.g., fear of being scrutinized, saying something that sounds foolish in public, not being able to answer questions in a classroom, eating in public, performing on stage). Fear of public speaking is the most common social phobia.

Characteristically, phobic individuals experience overwhelming and crippling anxiety when faced with the object or situation provoking the phobia. Phobic people go to great lengths to avoid the feared object or situation. A phobic person may not be able to think about or visualize the object or situation without becoming severely anxious. The life of a phobic person becomes increasingly restricted as activities are given up in order to avoid the phobic object. All too frequently, complications ensue when people try to decrease anxiety through self-medication with alcohol or drugs.

TABLE 12.4 Clinical Names for Common Phobias

Clinical Name	Feared Object or Situation
Acrophobia	Heights
Agoraphobia	Open spaces
Apiphobia	Bees
Astraphobia	Electrical storms
Claustrophobia	Closed spaces
Glossophobia	Public speaking
Hematophobia	Blood
Hydrophobia	Water
Monophobia	Being alone
Mysophobia	Germs or dirt
Nyctophobia	Darkness
Pyrophobia	Fire
Social phobia	Fear of a social or performance situation
Triskaidekaphobia	Fear of the number 13
Zoophobia	Animals

> **Vignette**
> David, a 22-year-old musical theatre major, has developed a fear of performing on stage. He suffers severe anxiety attacks whenever he is scheduled to appear in a student production. Recently, he has become severely anxious when faced with giving classroom readings or singing solo in music class. He is thinking about changing his major.

Generalized Anxiety Disorder

Generalized anxiety disorder is an anxiety reaction characterized by persistent and exaggerated apprehension and tension. Worry is the major concern in GAD. The individual's beliefs about worry are then linked to beliefs about themself, such as having the inability to control anxiety and fear, that if they worry significantly about an upcoming issue it will be prevented, or that worrying is a valued part of their personal identity (Macaulay et al., 2017). The individual with GAD also displays many of the following symptoms:

- Restlessness
- Fatigue
- Poor concentration
- Irritability
- Tension
- Sleep disturbance

The individual's anxiety is out of proportion to the true impact of the event or situation about which they worry. Examples of concerns typical of GAD include inadequacy in interpersonal relationships, job responsibilities, finances, the health of family members, household chores, and lateness for appointments. Sleep disturbance is common because the individual pores over the day's events and real or imagined mistakes, reviews past problems, and anticipates future difficulties. Decision making becomes difficult, owing to poor concentration and dread of making a mistake. Refer to Table 12.5 for a generic care plan for GAD.

TABLE 12.5 Generic Care Plan for Generalized Anxiety Disorder

Short-Term Goal	Intervention	Rationale
1. Patient will state that immediate distress is decreased by end of session.	1a. Stay with patient.	1a. Conveys acceptance and ability to give help.
	1b. Speak slowly and calmly.	1b. Conveys calm and promotes security.
	1c. Use short, simple sentences.	1c. Promotes comprehension.
	1d. Assure patient that you are in control and can assist them.	1d. Counters feeling of loss of control that accompanies severe anxiety.
	1e. Give brief directions.	1e. Reduces indecision; conveys belief that patient can respond in a healthy manner.
	1f. Decrease excessive stimuli; provide quiet environment.	1f. Reduces need to focus on diverse stimuli; promotes ability to concentrate.
	1g. After assessing level of anxiety, administer appropriate dose of anxiolytic agent if warranted.	1g. Reduces anxiety and allows patient to use coping skills.
	1h. Monitor and control own feelings.	1h. Avoids transmission of anxiety (which is transmissible); displays of negative emotion can cause patient anxiety.
2. Patient will be able to identify source of anxiety by (date).	2a. Encourage patient to discuss preceding events.	2a. Promotes future change through identification of stressors.
	2b. Link patient's behaviour to feelings.	2b. Promotes self-awareness.
	2c. Teach cognitive therapy principles: • Anxiety is the result of a dysfunctional appraisal of a situation. • Anxiety is the result of automatic thinking.	2c. Provides a basis for behavioural change.
	2d. Ask questions that clarify and dispute illogical thinking: • "What evidence do you have?" • "Explain the logic in that." • "Are you basing that conclusion on fact or feeling?" • "What's the worst thing that could happen?"	2d. Helps promote accurate cognition.
	2e. Have patient give an alternative interpretation.	2e. Broadens perspective; helps patient think in a new way about problem or symptom.
3. Patient will identify strengths and coping skills by (date).	3a. Have patient identify what has provided relief in the past.	3a. Provides awareness of self as individual with some ability to cope.
	3b. Have patient write assessment of strengths.	3b. Increases self-acceptance.
	3c. Reframe situation in ways that are positive.	3c. Provides a new perspective and converts distorted thinking.

Nursing diagnosis: *Ineffective coping* related to persistent anxiety as evidenced by fatigue and irritability.
Outcome: Patient will maintain role performance.

Vignette

Jane is a 49-year-old legal secretary. She comes to the clinic complaining of feeling "so anxious I could jump out of my skin." She is shaky and diaphoretic; she has dilated pupils, an elevated pulse, and a quivering voice. She tells the nurse, "It was probably foolish to come here. Nobody understands me." Jane's only daughter is expecting her first child. Although the pregnancy is going well, Jane worries that something is wrong with the baby. "What if it's premature? What if it's deformed?"

Jane describes herself as tense and irritable. She has difficulty initiating sleep and cannot concentrate at her job. She worries about making mistakes at work, about being fired from her position, and about the financial problems that could result. She often says, "I just can't cope." Her daughter has begun calling several times a day to reassure her that all is well with the pregnancy and to try to decrease Jane's worry over other matters. The daughter has also begun shopping and housecleaning for Jane "to help her get some rest."

Substance-Induced Anxiety Disorder

Substance-induced anxiety disorder is characterized by symptoms of anxiety, panic attacks, **obsessions**, and compulsions that develop with the use of a substance or within a month of discontinuing use of the substance.

Anxiety Due to Nonpsychiatric Medical Conditions

In anxiety due to a medical condition, the individual's symptoms of anxiety are a direct physiological result of a medical condition, such as hyperthyroidism, pulmonary embolism, or cardiac dysrhythmias. Central nervous system involvement in COVID-19 and other viral infections is thought to contribute to anxiety (Speth et al., 2020). Determining such a source of anxiety symptoms requires a careful and comprehensive assessment of multiple factors. Once again, evidence must be present in the history, physical examination, or laboratory findings for a diagnosis of anxiety due to a medical condition. Table 12.6 lists medical disorders that may contribute to anxiety symptoms.

TABLE 12.6 Common Nonpsychiatric Medical Causes of Anxiety

System	Disorders
Respiratory	Chronic obstructive pulmonary disease
	Pulmonary embolism
	Asthma
	Hypoxia
	Pulmonary edema
Cardiovascular	Angina pectoris
	Arrhythmias
	Congestive heart failure
	Hypertension
	Hypotension
	Mitral valve prolapse
Endocrine	Hyperthyroidism
	Hypoglycemia
	Pheochromocytoma
	Carcinoid syndrome
	Hypercortisolism
Neurological	Delirium
	Essential tremor
	Complex partial seizures
	Parkinson disease
	Akathisia
	Otoneurological disorders
	Postconcussion syndrome
Metabolic	Hypercalcemia
	Hyperkalemia
	Hyponatremia
	Porphyria

Epidemiology

Anxiety disorders are one of the most common forms of psychiatric disorders in Canada. In 2020 Mental Health Research Canada reported approximately 17% of Canadians reported symptoms of an anxiety disorder in the previous 12 months (Dozois & Mental Health Research Canada, 2020). *Report from the Canadian Chronic Disease Surveillance System: Mood and Anxiety Disorders in Canada, 2016* indicates that the prevalence of these disorders is increasing in children and youth. The highest relative increase in prevalence was seen among those aged 5 to 10 years.

Comorbidity

Clinicians and researchers have clearly demonstrated that anxiety disorders frequently co-occur with other psychiatric problems (Alonzi et al., 2020). Anxiety-related disorders occur so frequently with depressive disorders that the treatments for both disorders are similar due to shared neurobiology, symptom similarities, and abnormalities of emotional processing.

SOMATIC SYMPTOM AND RELATED DISORDERS

In contrast to nonpsychiatric medical conditions causing anxiety, somatic symptoms may also cause anxiety, fear, and worry. This may occur in patients who are living with chronic diseases. For example, someone who has the fear of cancer reoccurrence or that they have a genetic disorder. Lebel et al. (2020) refer to these experiences as health anxiety. COVID-19 has amplified health anxiety in the population in ways that are only beginning to be understood (Tyrer, 2020). Health anxiety is experienced on a continuum from mild transient worries to severe and debilitating worry. There is no "normal" amount of worry that people with chronic illness experience. Worrying only becomes problematic when it interferes with a person's day to day ability to function. SSD manifests itself through distress or a significant disruption in quality of life related to physical symptoms or health concerns that are disproportionate to the seriousness of the symptoms. Included in the most common symptoms that prompt visits to primary care providers are chest pain, fatigue, dizziness, headache, swelling, back pain, shortness of breath, insomnia, abdominal pain, and numbness. Health-related quality of life is frequently severely impaired, and patients appraise their body symptoms as unduly troublesome, threatening, or harmful, often fearing the worst about their health. Some patients feel that their medical assessment and treatment have been inadequate. Often the patient has a comorbid psychiatric disorder such as depression, anxiety, or a personality disorder.

Somatic symptom disorders (*soma* is the Greek word for "body") are a complex spectrum of physical and emotional signs and symptoms. Health care providers working in traditional medical settings are more likely to see individuals experiencing a psychiatric illness with predominantly somatic symptoms than are those working within a psychiatric setting. Individuals with these disorders will have physical symptoms and abnormal alterations in thoughts, feelings, and behaviours directly related to the physical symptoms experienced. There may, or may not be, a nonpsychiatric medical diagnosis made related solely to the physical symptoms. These illnesses are often misunderstood and mislabelled. For example, in the Middle Ages, a person who exhibited physical symptoms for no known cause was said to have a "disease of the soul." It was often women who had these "diseases," and many believed they were bewitched or possessed by the devil (Soltis-Jarrett, 2010, p. 183). Freud later used the term *hysteria*, the Greek term meaning "uterus," to refer to somatic and "histrionic" behaviours, behaviours that were attention seeking, emotionally over-reactive, and often inappropriately seductive.

Somatization, the expression of psychological stress through physical symptoms, can affect people of all ages and genders. Anxiety, depression, and trauma exert a powerful influence on the mind and may lead to a variety of clinical conditions, both mental and physical. When psychiatric disorders are present along with general medical conditions, increased health care costs and lengths of stay may result. They also can negatively affect outcomes and increase morbidity and mortality (Burton et al., 2020). Patient personality can contribute to an inadequate workup: for example, a "difficult" patient may receive a somatic diagnosis more readily than a "pleasant" patient. In fact, studies show that the strongest predictor of misdiagnosing somatic disorders is the primary care provider's dissatisfaction with the clinical encounter (Falanga & Pillot, 2019) (see Case Study and Nursing Care Plan 12.2). Chapter 30 is a further resource on how to nurse the psychological needs of patients with medical conditions.

Clinical Picture

The somatic disorders include:
- SSD
- Illness anxiety disorder (previously *hypochondriasis*)
- Conversion disorder (also called *functional neurological symptom disorder*)
- Psychological factors affecting medical condition
- Factitious disorder

CASE STUDY AND NURSING CARE PLAN 12.2
Somatic Symptom Disorder

Cara, age 49, a recently divorced mother of twin teenage daughters, works as a copy editor for a local newspaper and has been trying to sell her house in order to downsize after her daughters graduate from high school next year. She has a 2-year history of numerous physical complaints—insomnia, fatigue, muscle aches, irritable bowel syndrome, and occasional paroxysmal atrial tachycardia (PAT); she feels "nervous most of the time"; and she leaves the house only to go to work or to do grocery shopping. She attends work regularly but has no real social life, as she is often "too tired to go out."

She has been referred to a variety of specialists, but there continues to be no evidence of organic origins of her ailments. Today, she presented in the local emergency department with tachycardia and shortness of breath. All diagnostic tests were normal.

Cara agreed to attend an outpatient mental health intensive outpatient program (IOP) three mornings each week. After attending IOP for 2 days, she has not made much progress and states concern about a possible job loss if she does not return to work as soon as possible. She says that she feels happy at times when at home but is very frustrated that her fatigue and physical symptoms are continuing. She says that nothing seems to help her, that she is not sure what she is doing here, and that her future looks bleak. Most staff members have reported frustration that Cara is helpful with other patients but not actively engaged in working on any of her own issues and that she continually states that her mood is fine but her body is a "major problem."

Assessment
Self-Assessment
Ms. Silverthorn, a registered nurse, has 3 years of experience in this IOP. She recognizes that she has mixed feelings toward Cara. On the one hand, the patient is interesting, talkative, and charming as she discusses her happy childhood. On the other, she refuses to identify any psychological concerns and consistently prods staff to see if she can "graduate" from this program and go back to work. Staff members feel that Cara negates all of their suggestions. Ms. Silverthorn realizes that she has to carefully monitor her emotional reactions to Cara and adopt a persistent matter-of-fact approach to encourage the patient to be more assertive, self-aware, and independent. Ms. Silverthorn plans to actively support Cara in creating her discharge plan.

Objective Data	Subjective Data
Results of all diagnostic tests are negative.	"I don't know what I'm doing here."
Onset of symptoms coincides with her divorce and impending loss of daughters as their high school graduations are approaching.	She says her mood is fine, but her body is a "major problem."
There is no prior history of somatic or psychiatric disorders.	

Diagnosis
1. *Complicated grieving* related to loss of significant other (spouse) and anticipatory losses of children and home

Supporting Data
1. *Social isolation* related to fatigue and pain
   - Patient has difficulty communicating needs or emotions.
   - Patient reports recent and impending losses with lack of emotion or concern.

Supporting Data
- Patient has minimal support system.
- Patient reports frequent fatigue and loss of social interests.

Outcomes Identification
Long-term goal: Patient will identify and express emotions without physical symptoms.

Planning
The initial plan is to encourage Cara to explore feelings related to recent and impending losses and develop a support system.

Implementation
The personalized plan for Cara is:

Short-Term Goal	Intervention	Rationale	Evaluation
1. Patient will identify levels of anxiety in at least three situations and encounters with other patients and staff.	1. Develop a relationship with the patient that includes a mutually agreed-upon contract that details expected changes in behaviours.	1. A contract provides a concrete means to keep track of patient's actions and enhances self-direction and independent actions.	1. After spending 3 weeks in the intensive outpatient mental health program, Cara developed a trusting relationship with one staff member and two patients.

Continued

CASE STUDY AND NURSING CARE PLAN 12.2—cont'd
Somatic Symptom Disorder

Short-Term Goal	Intervention	Rationale	Evaluation
2. Patient will seek support from staff and patients when feelings of anxiety become difficult to handle or physical symptoms increase.	2. Educate the patient about sharing feelings of loss with staff, friends, and family members.	2. Communication and expression of feelings with family and friends help alters may also behave as individuals to alleviate stress and often provides a more supportive environment.	2a. Ms. Silverthorn made several attempts to engage Cara in discussion of feelings, losses, and conflicts to no avail until she arranged for a family meeting with Cara, her daughters, and her former husband. Cara was able to express her anxiety and occasional anger about the loss of her role as wife and the impending loss of her daughters when they attend university away from home. 2b. Cara also became more active in expressing her grief, particularly in the assertiveness and anger-management classes, and actively sought out Ms. Silverthorn on three occasions to discuss her feelings.
3. Patient will make a list with contacts and phone numberswof community resources of interest to her and make plans to attend a community event within a week.	3. Identify available support systems.	3. Patients are more successful handling stressful life events if they have adequate support.	3. Cara decided to take piano lessons and also enrolled in some of her town's adult-education classes.
4. Patient will remain free of injury throughout the hospitalization.	4. Assess for suicidal ideation.	4. Suicidal ideation may occur in response to depression or hopelessness over medical conditions.	4. Cara made no attempts to self-injure while in the hospital.

Evaluation
Many of Cara's symptoms have decreased; in particular, there have been no further episodes of tachycardia. However, Cara states that she is still hindered by some fatigue and muscle pain but much less so than previously. She admits she has not fully adhered to her exercise and healthy-eating plan, and occasionally she still feels furious with herself for not coping as well as she would like in social situations. Cara feels that the assertiveness training was particularly helpful to her, as she has realized how her passivity and bottled-up anger could have contributed to her physical symptoms and distress. Cara will continue to see her nurse therapist weekly to work on assertiveness skills, identification of and expression of feelings, and living a healthier lifestyle.

Illness Anxiety Disorder

Previously known as *hypochondriasis*, illness anxiety disorder results in the misinterpretation of physical sensations as evidence of a serious illness. Illness anxiety can be quite obsessive as thoughts about illness may be intrusive and hard to dismiss even when patients realize that their fears are unrealistic (Lebel et al., 2020). People with this disorder experience extreme worry and fear about the possibility of having a disease. Even normal body changes, such as a change in heart rate or abdominal cramps, can be seen as red flags for serious illness and imminent death.

In response to a patient's symptoms, primary care providers may suggest a consultation with a mental health professional, but the suggestion typically is refused. The course of the illness is chronic and relapsing, with symptoms becoming amplified during times of increased stress. Furthermore, depressive symptoms may be a catalyst for the diagnosis of illness anxiety (Alonzi et al., 2020).

Conversion Disorder

Conversion disorder (also known as *functional neurological symptom disorder*) manifests itself as neurological symptoms in the absence of a neurological diagnosis (Miller et al., 2020). Conversion disorder is marked by the presence of deficits in voluntary motor or sensory functions, including paralysis, blindness, movement disorder, gait disorder, numbness, paresthesia (tingling or burning sensations), loss of hearing, or seizures resembling epilepsy.

Conversion disorder is a clinical problem that requires the application of multiple perspectives, namely, biological, psychological, and social, to fully understand the symptoms of individual patients. Experiences of childhood physical or sexual abuse are common among patients with conversion disorder, and comorbid psychiatric conditions include depression, anxiety, PTSD, other somatic disorders, and personality disorders. Patients with conversion disorder symptoms may be found to have "no neurological disorder" by the neurologist and "no psychiatric disorder" by the psychiatrist, thus adding to the complexity of treatment planning (Yakobov et al., 2017).

Conversion disorder is attributed to the channelling of emotional conflicts or stressors into physical symptoms; however, some magnetic resonance imaging (MRI) studies suggest that patients with conversion disorder have an abnormal pattern of cerebral activation (Miller et al., 2020). While some patients become quite distressed about their symptoms, many show a lack of emotional concern about them (*la belle indifférence*). Imagine someone casually discussing sudden blindness. Care providers should assume an organic cause for the symptoms until physical pathology has been ruled out. Patients truly believe in the presence of the symptoms; they are not fabricated or under voluntary control. The course of the disorder is related to its acuity and the length of symptom durations. In cases of acute onset during stressful events, remission rate is high; in cases of a more gradual onset, the disorder is not as readily treatable (Yakobov et al., 2017).

> **Vignette**
>
> Gerald is a 63-year-old, married real estate agent who was recently hospitalized for heart failure. Because of insomnia, lack of appetite, and some anger problems toward his wife, his primary care provider has referred him for a mental health consultation. During this consultation, Gerald complains of waking up at night obsessing about possibly losing his job, his lack of retirement savings, and providing for his wife in case he dies. He states, "I am very scared, and I worry about my health and being forced to retire. I don't know where I would get the money to live. I am too old to start another career." These observations were reported to the nurse practitioner. After a thorough assessment and medical workup, it is determined that Gerald is experiencing depression and severe anxiety, which precipitated increased symptoms of heart failure. Gerald has responded well to couples therapy and a men's support group. His blood pressure has decreased, and his mood is improved. Gerald has been able to return to work.

Epidemiology

Specific prevalence rates for SSD in the general population are unknown. Instead, the literature describes their occurrence in the population of individuals who seek medical care but do not have an underlying physiological cause for their symptoms. In the latest edition of the *Diagnostic and Statistical Manual of Mental Disorders (DSM)* the requirement for no underlying psychological cause for their symptoms was removed. As a result, there is very limited current information on the prevalence of this disorder based on the new diagnostic criteria.

Comorbidity

A thorough psychosocial history is also required to confirm a SSD diagnosis, as well as any comorbid psychiatric disorders. People with this type of illness will also have a depressive, psychotic, or anxiety disorder.

Both the medical and the mental health communities recognize the interrelationships between psychiatric and medical illnesses (Alonzi et al., 2020). This relationship was first introduced by Hans Selye (1956). Selye's description of the *general adaptation syndrome* (see Chapter 5) and Cannon's 1914 identification of the *fight-or-flight response* (see Chapter 23) provided insight into the biological and molecular reactions to stressors in the sympathetic nervous system, the hypothalamic–pituitary–adrenocortical axis, and the immune system. Extensive studies have left little doubt that psychosocial stress affects the course and severity of illness (Table 12.7). Psychological factors may present a risk for a medical disease, or they may magnify or adversely affect a nonpsychiatric medical condition. For example, researchers are consistently providing evidence demonstrating links between mental disorders and cardiovascular disease (Kehler et al., 2019) and cancer (Deimling et al., 2017).

OBSESSIVE-COMPULSIVE DISORDERS

Obsessions are defined as thoughts, impulses, or images that persist and recur and cannot be dismissed from the mind. Obsessions often seem senseless to the individual who experiences them (*ego-dystonic*), and their presence causes severe anxiety.

Compulsions are ritualistic behaviours or thoughts an individual feels compelled to perform in an attempt to reduce anxiety. Performing the compulsive act temporarily reduces high levels of anxiety. Primary gain is achieved by compulsive rituals, but because the relief is only temporary, the compulsive act must be repeated again and again until it feels "just right" (Haase, 2002).

Although obsessions and compulsions can exist independently of each other, they most often occur together (Table 12.8). Common types of obsessions include losing control, harm, contamination, perfectionism, sexual, and religious. There are also common categories of compulsions: washing and cleaning, checking, repeating, and mental compulsions. Obsessive-compulsive behaviour exists along a continuum. "Normal" individuals may experience mildly obsessive-compulsive behaviour. For example, nearly everyone has had the experience of having a tune run persistently through the mind despite attempts to push it away. Many people have had nagging doubts as to whether a door is locked or not. These doubts may require people to go back to check the door once, but then they can carry on with their day. Compulsive superstitions such as touching a lucky charm or avoiding a black cat are not harmful, and mild compulsions about timeliness, orderliness, and reliability are, in fact, valued traits in Canadian society.

At the pathological end of the continuum are obsessive-compulsive symptoms that typically involve issues of contamination, fear of losing control, need for symmetry, unwanted thoughts of a sexual nature, and recurrent feelings of doubt. Pathological obsessions or compulsions cause marked distress to individuals, who often feel humiliation and shame for these behaviours. The rituals are time consuming and interfere with normal routines, social activities, and relationships with others. Severe OCD consumes so much of the individual's mental processes that the performance of cognitive tasks may be impaired.

The fifth edition of the *Diagnostic and Statistical Manual of Mental Disorders (DSM-5)* (American Psychiatric Association, 2013) includes a new chapter on obsessive-compulsive and related disorders to reflect the increasing evidence of these disorders' relatedness to one another and their distinction from other anxiety disorders, as well as to help clinicians better identify and treat individuals suffering from these disorders. Disorders in this chapter of *DSM-5* include OCD, body dysmorphic disorder, and trichotillomania (hair-pulling disorder), as well as two new disorders: hoarding disorder and excoriation (skin-picking) disorder. For further patient information, visit https://www.psychiatry.org/patients-families/ocd.

> **Vignette**
>
> Scott is a 23-year-old university student who is having difficulty handing in assignments on time, and his marks are suffering because of it. He is spending hours on assignments. Each page needs to be perfect. When the assignments are handwritten there needs to be no erasure marks, no cross-outs, and no white-out; all the ink needs to be exactly the same shade; and all margins need to be exactly 4 cm. If he hasn't stayed up all night to complete an assignment, he tries to sleep, but only after his bedtime rituals of checking all electrical appliances for fear that he had started a fire, all faucets for fear that he had left them running, and all door locks for fear that he had left them open. These checks are done three times before he can retire to bed. These checks require approximately 2 hours to complete.

TABLE 12.7 Common Medical Conditions Negatively Affected by Stress

Medical Condition	Incidence	Genetic and Biological Correlates	Common Precipitating Factors	Potential Holistic Therapies Used in Addition to Medical Management
Cardiovascular disease (e.g., coronary heart disease)	Rates higher in White males until age 60 years	Risk factors: family history of cardiac disease, hypertension, increased serum lipid levels, obesity, sedentary lifestyle, cigarette smoking Psychosocial risk factors: stress, depression, loneliness High anxiety risk in patient with prior cardiac events	Sudden stress preceded by a period of losses, frustration, and disappointments (often resulting in myocardial infarction)	Relaxation training, stress management, group social support, and psychosocial intervention Support groups for type A personalities
Peptic ulcer (caused by *Helicobacter pylori* infection)	Occurs in 12% of men, 6% of women (more prevalent in industrialized societies)	Infection with *H. pylori* is associated with 95%–99% of peptic ulcers Both peptic and duodenal ulcers cluster in families, but separately from each other	Periods of social tension and increased life stress Losses Postmenopause	Biofeedback to alter gastric acidity Cognitive behavioural approaches to reduce stress (stress management)
Cancer	Men: most common in lung, prostate, colon, and rectum Women: most common in breast, uterus, colon, and rectum Death rate higher in men than in women	Genetic evidence suggesting dysfunction of cellular proliferation Familial patterns of breast cancer, colorectal cancer, stomach cancer, melanoma	Prolonged and intensive stress Stressful life events (e.g., separation from or loss of significant other 2 years before diagnosis) Feelings of hopelessness, helplessness, and despair (depression)	Relaxation (e.g., meditation, autogenic training, self-hypnosis) Visualization Psychological counselling Support groups Massage therapy Stress management
Tension headache	Occurs in 80% of population when under stress Begins at end of workday or early evening		Associated with anxiety and depression	Psychotherapy for chronic tension headaches Learning to cope or avoiding tension-creating situations or people Relaxation and stress-management techniques Cognitive restructuring techniques
Essential hypertension	Rates higher in males until age 60 years	Risk factors: family history of cardiac disease and hypertension	Life changes and traumatic life events Stressful job (e.g., air traffic controller)	Behavioural feedback, stress reduction techniques, meditation, yoga, hypnosis *Note:* Pharmacological treatment considered primary for treatment of hypertension

Epidemiology

OCD is the fourth most common psychiatric illness. Everyone on occasion will obsess about something. However, only 1 to 3% of people will spend more than an hour a day having obsessive thoughts. The typical age of onset is bimodal (10 years and 21 years) (Sinopoli et al., 2019). Males generally will have an earlier onset than females. Childhood OCD is diagnosed almost three times as frequently in boys than in girls. However, by adulthood OCD occurs with approximately equal frequency in women and men.

Comorbidity

Other psychiatric conditions with common symptoms of rumination (mood disorder) and worry (anxiety disorder) commonly occur with OCD. Psychotic disorders may also occur, however; people with only OCD are able to recognize that their thoughts are irrational but that they cannot control them.

TABLE 12.8 Common Obsessions and Compulsions

Type of Obsession	Example	Accompanying Compulsion
Losing control	Fear of acting on an impulse to harm oneself	Praying to prevent harm to oneself
	Fear of violent or horrific images in one's mind	Thinks about something else when horrific images come to mind
		Praying to get rid of the images
Harm	Fear of being responsible for something terrible happening	Checking that nothing terrible happened
		Checking that you did not make a mistake
	Fear of harming others because of not being careful enough (e.g., dropping something on the ground will cause another person to fall and break an arm)	Praying to prevent harm to prevent terrible consequences.
		Checking that you did not or will not harm others
Perfectionism	Need for symmetry—concern about evenness	Rereading or rewriting
		Putting things in order or arranging things until it "feels right"
	Inability to decide whether to keep or discard things	Collecting items that results in significant clutter in the home (hoarding)
Contamination	Environmental contaminants (radiation, oil, or lead)	Cleaning household items in a certain way to remove contaminants
	Germs or viruses	Washing hands excessively
Unwanted sexual thoughts	Forbidden or perverse sexual thoughts or images	Telling, asking, or confessing to get reassurance
	Obsessions about aggressive sexual behaviour toward others	Avoiding situations that might trigger your obsessions
Religious obsessions	Concern with offending God	Praying to seek forgiveness
		Repeatedly touching or kissing religious objects
	Excessive concern with morality	Replaying interactions with others and repeatedly reviewing every remark to determine if you said anything wrong
Other obsessions	Concern about getting a disease, such as cancer, colitis, or diabetes	Checking some parts of your physical condition or body
	Superstitious ideas	Repeating activities in "multiples" (e.g., doing a task three times because three is a "good," "right," or "safe" number)

RESEARCH HIGHLIGHT

"On My Own, but Not Alone"—Adolescents' Experiences of Internet-Delivered Cognitive Behavioural Therapy for Obsessive-Compulsive Disorder

Problem
Obsessive-compulsive disorder (OCD) can effectively be treated with cognitive behavioural therapy (CBT). However, many people with this illness do not have access to a health provider who is experienced in delivering this treatment.

Purpose of Study
The purpose of this study was to describe the experience of adolescents with OCD who had received Internet-provided CBT. This treatment was delivered via a secure Internet platform that enabled age-appropriate presentation of different treatment content to pediatric patients.

Methods
Participants in this study were a subset of participants who were in a research project that evaluated the effectiveness and efficiency of Internet-provided CBT to adolescents. The Internet-provided CBT content is presented in chapters, much like chapters in a self-help book.

The chapters contain psychoeducative texts, films, and CBT exercises, such as exposure exercises and cognitive interventions. Patients have regular contact with an experienced clinician via messages that can be sent inside the treatment platform (resembling email). The clinician can also directly comment on exercises that the patient has been working on and can therefore give specific feedback and support and motivate the patient. In this way a patient usually has contact with their treating clinician several times a week.

Key Findings
The effectiveness and efficiency portion of this research program indicated that the Internet could be used effectively and efficiently to provide CBT to adolescents. In this study, participants described the ability to work independently with the treatment material and, through that, have some degree of control over the therapy process. In addition, several participants also reported advantages of being able to choose when and where to work. Participants were willing to communicate information about themselves, such as thoughts, feelings, doubts, failures, successes, and fears, and at the same time felt secure about doing so.

Implications for Nursing Practice
Service accessibility is an issue for many people in Canada. This study supports the use of alternate delivery formats as a means of supporting patient recovery. This type of alternate service delivery model allowed for a relationship to develop between the patient and service provider in a manner that promoted patient autonomy.

Source: Lenhard, F., Vigerland, S., Engberg, H., et al. (2016). "On my own, but not alone"—Adolescents' experiences of internet-delivered cognitive behavior therapy for obsessive-compulsive disorder. *PLoS ONE, 11*(10), e0164311. https://doi.org/10.1371/journal.pone.0164311

TRAUMA- AND STRESSOR-RELATED DISORDERS

Acute Stress Disorder

Acute stress disorder occurs within 1 month of a highly traumatic event, such as those that precipitate PTSD. To be diagnosed with acute stress disorder, the individual must display at least three dissociative symptoms either during or after the traumatic event, including a subjective sense of numbing, detachment, or absence of emotional responsiveness; a reduction in awareness of surroundings; derealization (a sense of unreality related to the environment); depersonalization (a sense of unreality or self-estrangement); or dissociative amnesia (loss of memory) (Wawer et al., 2020). By definition, acute stress disorder resolves within 4 weeks.

> **Vignette**
>
> Olivia, a 22-year-old university student, is sexually assaulted by a family friend. In the emergency department she describes feeling detached from her body and being unaware of her surroundings during the assault, "as though it took place in a vacuum." She displays virtually no affect (i.e., she does not cry or appear anxious, angry, or sad). Olivia finds it difficult to concentrate on the examiner's questions. Three days later, Olivia still feels as though her mind is detached from her body; she reports having difficulty sleeping, not being able to concentrate, and startling whenever anyone touches her. When she sees the nurse 4 weeks after the event, Olivia expresses feelings of anger and sadness over the assault, displays the ability to concentrate, and states that she no longer feels as though her mind and body are detached. She reports being able to sleep better and not being so jittery and easily startled.

Post-Traumatic Stress Disorder

Post-traumatic stress disorder is included in a new chapter in the *DSM-5* on trauma- and stressor-related disorders. PTSD is an acute emotional response to a traumatic event or situation involving severe environmental stress. The following is an introduction to how trauma and anxiety are related. Refer to Chapters 21, 22, 23, 24, and 25 for more detailed information about trauma and relevant interventions. Chapter 29 will discuss recovery, survivorship, and public mental approaches.

The individual with PTSD persistently re-experiences a traumatic event that involved threatened or actual death or serious injury to self or others, and to which the person responded with intense fear, helplessness, or horror. PTSD may present after any traumatic event that is outside the range of usual experience, such as military combat, detention as a prisoner of war, natural disasters (e.g., floods, tornadoes, earthquakes), human disasters (e.g., plane and train accidents), crime-related events (e.g., sexual abuse, bombing, assault, mugging, rape, being taken hostage), or diagnosis of a life-threatening illness.

Due to the traumatic events faced by members of the Canadian Armed Forces, it has been estimated that nearly 20% of Canadian Armed Forces veterans have an operational stress injury (OSI) such as PTSD, addiction, or another mental health problem (Pearson et al., 2014). PTSD symptoms often begin within 3 months of the trauma, but a delay of several months or years is not uncommon.

The major features of PTSD are:

- Persistent re-experiencing of the trauma through recurrent intrusive recollections of the event, dreams about the event, and flashbacks—dissociative experiences during which the event is relived (i.e., the person behaves as though they are experiencing the event in the present)
- Persistent avoidance of stimuli associated with the trauma, causing the individual to avoid talking about the trauma or avoid activities, people, or places that rouse memories of the trauma
- Persistent numbing of general responsiveness, as evidenced by the individual's feeling empty inside or feeling disconnected from others
- Persistent symptoms of increased arousal, as evidenced by irritability, difficulty sleeping, difficulty concentrating, hypervigilance, or exaggerated startle response

Difficulty with interpersonal, social, or occupational relationships nearly always accompanies PTSD, and trust is a common issue of concern. Child and spousal abuse may be associated with hypervigilance and irritability, and chemical abuse may begin as an attempt to self-medicate to relieve anxiety (see Case Study and Nursing Care Plan 12.3).

CASE STUDY AND NURSING CARE PLAN 12.3
Post-Traumatic Stress Disorder

Mr. Charbonneau, age 46, is brought to the emergency department by his distraught wife after she finds him writing a suicide note and planning to shoot himself in the woods with a handgun. He had written: "I don't deserve to live. I should have died with the others." Mr. Charbonneau is subdued and shows minimal affect, and his breath has the distinct odour of alcohol. When asked about suicidal thoughts, he states that he is worthless and that his wife and family would be better off if he were dead. The decision is made to hospitalize him to protect him from danger to himself.

Mr. Charbonneau's wife gives further history. Her husband is a construction contractor who served in the Canadian Armed Forces during the War in Afghanistan. He lost half of his squad in a roadside bombing. He walks with a permanent limp due to a leg injury acquired during this attack. Upon returning home, he showed no signs of anxiety and refused offers of crisis treatment, stating, "I was in a war—I can handle stress." But 6 months later, Mrs. Charbonneau noticed that her husband had trouble sleeping, his mood was irritable or withdrawn, he avoided news reports on television, and he started drinking alcohol daily. He complained of nightmares but would not talk to her about his fears. He agreed to go to the psychiatrist only to request sleeping medication.

Mr. Charbonneau was admitted to the psychiatric unit and his care was assigned to Ms. Dawson, a dually educated (general and psychiatric) nurse. She observes that, as he is oriented to the unit, Mr. Charbonneau is quiet and passive but that he looks around vigilantly and is easily startled by sounds on the unit.

Assessment

Self-Assessment

Ms. Dawson initially feels sympathy for Mr. Charbonneau, and he reminds her of her uncle James, who served in World War II. She is concerned because his suicide plan was lethal and he is guarded in his speech, not revealing his thoughts or feelings. She realizes that as she implements suicide precautions, she must demonstrate an attitude of hope and acceptance to encourage him to develop trust. Also, she must stay neutral and not convey pity or sympathy.

CASE STUDY AND NURSING CARE PLAN 12.3—cont'd
Post-Traumatic Stress Disorder

Objective Data	Subjective Data
Sleep difficulty, nightmares	"I don't deserve to live. I should have died with the others."
Hypervigilance	
Alcohol use	
Irritability	
Withdrawn mood	
Constricted range of affect	
Feels estranged from wife and children	
Avoidance of news coverage with potential for emergency reports	
Refusal of treatment and safety contract	
Plan for suicide	

Diagnosis
1. *Risk for suicide* related to anger and hopelessness due to severe trauma, as evidenced by suicidal plan and verbalization of intent.

Supporting Data
- Lethal plan with weapon.
- Refusal to agree to a safety plan—that is, to speak to staff when experiencing suicidal ideation.
- Emotional withdrawal from wife, as evidenced by his refusal to talk to her about his fears.

Outcomes Identification
Patient will consistently refrain from attempting suicide.

Planning
The initial plan is to maintain safety for Mr. Charbonneau while encouraging him to express feelings and recognize that his situation is not hopeless.

Implementation
Mr. Charbonneau's plan of care is personalized as follows:

Short-Term Goal	Intervention	Rationale	Evaluation
1. Patient will speak to staff whenever experiencing self-destructive thoughts.	1a. Administer medications with mouth checks.	1a. Addresses risk of hiding medications.	**Goal Met** After 8 hours, patient agrees to safety plan every shift and starts to discuss feelings of self-harm.
	1b. Provide ongoing surveillance of patient and environment.	1b. Provides one-to-one monitoring for safety.	
	1c. Agrees to safety plan, to talk with staff when experiencing suicidal ideation.	1c. Encourages increased self-control.	
	1d. Use direct, nonjudgemental approach in discussing suicide.	1d. Shows acceptance of patient's situation with respect.	
	1e. Provide teaching about post-traumatic stress disorder.	1e. Offers reality of treatment.	
2. Patient will express feelings by the third day of hospitalization.	2a. Interact with patient at regular intervals to convey caring and openness and to provide an opportunity to talk.	2a. Encourages development of trust.	**Goal Met** By second day, patient occasionally answers questions about feelings and admits to anger and grief.
	2b. Use silence and listening to encourage expression of feelings.	2b. Shows positive expectation that patient will respond.	
	2c. Be open to expressions of loneliness and powerlessness.	2c. Allows patient to voice these uncomfortable feelings.	
	2d. Share observations or thoughts about patient's behaviour or response.	2d. Directs attention to here-and-now treatment situation.	

Continued

CASE STUDY AND NURSING CARE PLAN 12.3—cont'd
Post-Traumatic Stress Disorder

Short-Term Goal	Intervention	Rationale	Evaluation
3. Patient will express will to live by discharge from unit.	3a. Listen to expressions of grief.	3a. Supports patient and communicates that such feelings are natural.	**Goal Met** By fifth day, patient becomes tearful and states that he does not want to hurt his wife and daughter.
	3b. Encourage patient to identify own strengths and abilities.	3b. Affirms patient's worth and potential to survive.	
	3c. Explore with patient previous methods of dealing with life problems.	3c. Reinforces patient's past coping skills and ability to problem-solve now.	
	3d. Assist in identifying available support systems.	3d. Addresses fact that anxiety has narrowed patient's perspective, distorting reality about loved ones.	
	3e. Refer patient to spiritual advisor of his choice.	3e. Allows patient opportunity to explore spiritual values and self-worth.	

Evaluation
See individual outcomes and evaluation within the care plan.

DISSOCIATIVE DISORDERS

Dissociative disorders are a group of disorders precipitated by significant adverse experiences or traumas and resulting in the unconscious altering of mind–body connections. Dissociation is an unconscious defence mechanism that protects the individual against overwhelming anxiety and stress through an emotional separation; however, this separation results in disturbances in memory, consciousness, self-identity, and perception.

Patients with dissociative disorders are able to assess a situation realistically, rather than for what they want it to be or fear that it might be. They do not have hallucinations or delusions (meaning that they have "intact reality testing"), but they may have flashbacks or see images that are triggered by current events that are related to the past trauma. Mild, fleeting dissociative experiences are relatively common to all of us; for example, we may be listening to someone and suddenly realize that we have not heard part or all of what was said. These common experiences are distinctly different from the processes of pathological dissociation.

Pathological dissociation is involuntary and results in failure of control over one's mental processes and the integration of conscious awareness (Brand et al., 2019). With pathological dissociation, pieces of a memory become fragmented. For example, normally, when people remember an experience, they can recall the people who were there, maybe a significant smell (like cooking turkey), maybe singing, and maybe an uncle who wore a bright red suit. However, when memories become fragmented, as in pathological dissociation, a person may recall a sound or smell but not be able to link these sensations to the actual event, instead feeling as though there is something familiar about the smell or sound but not knowing why. If the pieces of memory are associated with a traumatic experience, the fragments can leave the person fearful, confused, or both. If the memory was very traumatic, the fragments may cause the person to re-enact, as well as re-experience, trauma without consciously knowing why.

Symptoms of dissociation may be either *positive* or *negative*. Positive symptoms refer to unwanted additions to mental activity, such as flashbacks; negative symptoms refer to deficits, such as memory problems or the inability to sense or control different parts of the body. It is thought that dissociation decreases the immediate subjective distress of the trauma (a self-protective mechanism) and also continues to protect the individual from full awareness of the disturbing event. Continued dissociative symptoms, however, can interfere with activities of daily living and relationships.

In the case of abused or neglected children dissociation can be interpreted as somewhat protective, allowing the child to continue to be attached to abusive or neglectful caretakers. This instinctive mechanism highlights the importance of attachments and relationships in allowing the child to grow socially, intellectually, and cognitively. If abuse or neglect has occurred, memories of it become compartmentalized and often do not intrude into awareness until later in life during a stressful situation or in trying to develop another significant relationship.

All of the dissociative disorders affect both the patient and the patient's family. For example, people with depersonalization disorder are often fearful that others may perceive their appearance as distorted and may avoid being seen in public. If they exhibit consistently high levels of anxiety, the family is likely to find it difficult to keep relationships stable. By comparison, people who experience fugue states often function adequately in their new identities by choosing simple, undemanding occupations, and having few intimate social interactions. Patients with amnesia, in contrast to those with fugue, may be more dysfunctional. Their perplexity often renders them unable to work, and their memory loss impairs normal relationships. Families often direct considerable attention toward the patient but may exhibit concern over having to assume roles that were once assigned to the patient. Finally, patients with **dissociative identity disorder** (DID) often have both family and work problems. Families find it difficult to accept the seemingly erratic behaviours of the patient. Employers dislike the lost time that may occur when alternate identities are in control.

Clinical Picture

Dissociative disorders include (1) depersonalization/derealization disorder, (2) dissociative amnesia, and (3) DID.

Depersonalization/Derealization Disorder

Depersonalization/derealization disorder may cause a person to feel mechanical, dreamy, or detached from the body. Some people suffer episodes of these problems that come and go, while others have episodes that begin with stressors and eventually become constant. People with this disorder may experience episodes of depersonalization or derealization or both. When experiencing depersonalization, individuals feel as though they are observers of their own body or mental processes—there is an internal feeling of disconnect. Similarly, with derealization, there is a recurring feeling that one's surroundings are unreal or distant—an external or outside feeling of disconnect. These feelings are not consciously controlled by the patients with dissociative disorders and are reported to be very distressing to those who experience them.

> **Vignette**
> Marguerite describes becoming very troubled by perceived changes in her appearance when she looks in a mirror. She thinks that her image looks wavy and indistinct. Soon after, she describes feeling as though she is floating in a fog, with her feet not actually touching the ground. Questioning reveals that Marguerite's son has recently confided to her that he tested positive for human immunodeficiency virus (HIV) and that she is extremely worried about him.

Dissociative Amnesia

Dissociative amnesia is marked by the inability to recall important autobiographical information, often of a traumatic or stressful nature, that is too pervasive to be explained by ordinary forgetfulness. While autobiographical memory is available (i.e., stored within the brain), the information is not accessible (i.e., the memory cannot be retrieved). When memories are stored, information about the situation (*retrieval cues*) is also stored. This additional information can be about the environment (smell, place, colour) or about a feeling (happy, sad, mad) or about an activity at the time (walking, crying, sitting, studying). Seeing or thinking about these retrieval cues helps us recall the memory. For example, have you ever got up from watching television and gone into the kitchen to do something but then forgotten what you were going to do once you got to the kitchen? But then you go back and sit down in front of the television and you remember? You have just accessed a memory using a retrieval cue.

In contrast, a patient with generalized amnesia is unable to recall information about their entire lifetime. The generalized amnesia may be *localized* (the patient is unable to remember all events in a certain period) or *selective* (the patient is able to recall some but not all events in a certain period). For the person with generalized amnesia, the information is neither available nor accessible, contrary to dissociative amnesia.

A subtype of dissociative amnesia, also usually precipitated by a traumatic event, is dissociative fugue. This disorder is characterized by sudden, unexpected travel away from the customary locale and an inability to recall one's identity and information about some or all of the past. The word *fugue* comes from the Latin word for *flight*. In rare cases, an individual with dissociative fugue assumes a whole new identity. During a fugue state (individuals are in a different location, unable to recall personal information about themselves or their past), individuals show no signs of illness and tend to lead rather simple lives, rarely calling attention to themselves. Only the memories tied to their identities are lost. If the person experiencing the fugue state knows how to drive, use the computer, make meals, and use a public transit system, they retain that knowledge. After a few weeks to a few months, the person may become confused about their identity or remember the former identity and then become amnesic for the time spent in the fugue state.

Dissociative Identity Disorder

The essential feature of DID is the presence of two or more distinct personality states that alternately and recurrently take control of behaviour. It is believed that severe sexual, physical, or psychological trauma in childhood predisposes an individual to the development of DID. Each alternate personality (alter), or subpersonality, has its own pattern of perceiving, relating to, and thinking about the self and the environment. Each alter is a complex unit with its own memories, behaviour patterns, and social relationships that dictate how the person acts when that personality is dominant. If the original or primary personality is religious and moralistic, the subpersonality or subpersonalities are often pleasure seeking and nonconforming. The alters may also behave as individuals of a different sex, race, or religion.

DID appears to be associated with two dissociative identity states (alternate personalities): (1) a state in which the individual blocks access and responses to traumatic memories so as to be able to function daily and (2) a state fixated on traumatic memories. The primary personality, or *host*, is usually not aware of the subpersonalities and is perplexed by lost time and unexplained events. Experiences such as finding unfamiliar clothing in the closet, being called a different name by a stranger, and not having childhood memories are characteristic of DID. Subpersonalities are often aware of the existence of each other to some degree. Transition from one personality to another occurs during times of stress and may range from a dramatic to a barely noticeable event. Some patients experience the transition when awakening. Shifts may last from minutes to months, although shorter periods are more common.

Epidemiology

Although mental health care providers in Canada believe that dissociative disorders are rare, depersonalization disorder prevalence rates range from about 1% to 3%, which is comparable to disorders such as schizophrenia, bipolar disorder, and OCD (Spiegel et al., 2011). More recently the international general population prevalence rates are estimated to be between 9% and 18% (Brand et al., 2019).

Comorbidity

Psychiatric comorbidities are extremely common for people with dissociative disorders. Patients with dissociative disorders usually seek treatment for another problem such as anxiety, mood dysregulation, or substance use issues.

ETIOLOGY OF ANXIETY-RELATED DISORDERS

There is no longer any doubt that biological factors predispose some individuals to develop pathological emotional and mental states (e.g., generalized anxiety, phobias, panic attacks, dissociation, somatization). However, traumatic life events, psychological factors, and sociocultural factors are also etiologically significant for all the disorders identified in this chapter. Regardless of the age at which symptoms start, their purpose is to reduce disturbing feelings and protect the person from the effects of the trauma.

Biological Factors
Genetic

Numerous studies substantiate that anxiety disorders tend to cluster in families. Twin studies demonstrate the existence of a genetic component to anxiety disorders (Torvick et al., 2019). First-degree biological relatives of those with OCD or phobias have a higher frequency of these disorders than exists in the general population, and relatives of people with a SSD are more likely to have persistent pain, depressive disorder, and alcohol dependence. Although genetic variability is thought to play a role in stress reactivity, dissociation is thought to be largely due to extreme stress or environmental factors.

Neurobiological

Certain anatomical pathways in the midbrain (the limbic system) provide the transmission structure for the electrical impulses that occur when anxiety-related responses are sent or received. Neurons release chemicals (neurotransmitters) that convey these messages. The neurochemicals that regulate anxiety-related disorders include epinephrine, norepinephrine, dopamine, serotonin, gamma-aminobutyric acid (GABA), and endogenous opioids. Repeated trauma or stress not only alters the release of neurotransmitters but also changes the anatomy of the brain. Animal studies show that early, prolonged emotional detachment from the caretaker negatively affects the development of the limbic system, which is where traumatic memories are processed; therefore trauma negatively interferes with the normal development of the limbic system. Patients with PTSD have a malfunctioning hypothalamic–pituitary–adrenal system. Individuals with dissociative disorders have increased activation of the orbital frontal cortex, which inhibits activation of the amygdala and insular cortex as well as the hippocampal areas, where traumatic memories are stored (Spiegel et al., 2011). Any abnormality in the structure of the brain or the function of the neurotransmitters can lead to a misinterpretation of ordinary events. For example, the brain may misunderstand (or amplify the significance of) a stimulus, such as identifying a minor gas pain as a serious abdominal injury (somatization). The brain may also over-react in its analysis of the stimulus, deciding that the same minor gas pain is a sign of colon cancer (illness anxiety) and then hoping that death comes quickly.

Psychological Factors
Psychodynamic Theories

Psychodynamic theories about the development of anxiety disorders centre on the idea that unconscious childhood conflicts are the basis for symptom development. Sigmund Freud suggested that anxiety results from the threatened breakthrough of repressed ideas or emotions from the unconscious into consciousness. Freud also suggested that the individual uses ego defence mechanisms to keep anxiety at manageable levels (see Chapter 4). The use of defence mechanisms results in behaviour that is not wholly adaptive because of its rigidity and repetitive nature.

Harry Stack Sullivan (1953) believed that anxiety is linked to the emotional distress caused when early needs go unmet or disapproval is experienced (interpersonal theory). He also suggested that anxiety is "contagious," being transmitted to the infant from the mother or caregiver. Thus the anxiety experienced early in life becomes the prototype for anxiety experienced when unpleasant events occur later in life.

Since the late nineteenth century, psychoanalytic theory has dominated medical thinking about conversion disorder. Nurses using this approach to guide treatment modalities frame the psychosomatic complaints of pain, illness, or loss of physical function within the context of the individual repressing a conflict or unwelcome experiences (usually of an aggressive or sexual nature) and that the transformation of anxiety into a physical symptom is symbolically related to the conflict. For example, in conversion disorder, conversion symptoms permit the individual to communicate a need for special treatment or consideration from others.

There are two primary schools of thought that guide the treatment of illness anxiety disorder. The first has psychodynamic origins. Nurses using this perspective will view anger, aggression, or hostility as an expression of a need for help as a result of past losses or disappointments. Those nurses who work with a psychoanalytic worldview will see illness anxiety as a defence against guilt or low self-esteem. Patients may themselves interpret their somatic symptoms as a form of punishment.

Behavioural Theory

Behavioural theories suggest that anxiety is a learned response to specific environmental stimuli (*classical conditioning*). Anxiety may also be learnt through the modelling of parents or peers. For example, a mother who is fearful of thunder and lightning and hides in closets during storms may transmit her anxiety to her children, who adopt her behaviour into adulthood. Such individuals can unlearn this behaviour by observing others who react normally to a storm, perhaps by lighting candles and telling stories.

Behaviourists suggest that people with somatic symptoms learn methods of communicating helplessness. These "helpless" behaviours are used to get their needs met. The symptoms become more intense when they are reinforced by attention from others. Behaviourists also identify potential **secondary gains** from many disorders. Secondary gains are those benefits derived from the symptoms alone; for example, in the sick role, the patient is not able to perform the usual family, work, and social functions and receives extra attention from loved ones. Other potential benefits include avoiding activities the individual considers distasteful, obtaining financial benefit, and gaining some advantage in interpersonal relationships due to the symptom.

Cognitive Theory

Cognitive theorists believe that anxiety disorders are caused by distortions in an individual's thoughts and perceptions. Because individuals with such distortions may believe that any mistake will have catastrophic results, they experience acute anxiety. In contrast, patients with somatic symptoms focus on body sensations, misinterpret their meaning, and then become excessively alarmed by them.

Learning Theory

Dissociation is one of the most primitive ego defence mechanisms. The pattern of avoidance occurs when an individual deals with an unpleasant event by consciously deciding not to think about it. The more anxiety provoking the event is, the greater is the need to avoid thinking about it. As the individual increasingly depends on this coping strategy, dissociation becomes easier, and it becomes more likely that this defence mechanism will be the individual's predominant means of reacting to stress. Thus learning theory suggests that dissociative disorders can be explained as learned methods for avoiding stress and anxiety.

Environmental Factors

The environmental factors related to a person developing an anxiety-related disorder are exposures to traumatic events, including any experience that is overwhelming to the person, such as a motor vehicle accident, combat experience, emotional or verbal abuse, incest, neglectful or abusive caregivers, and imprisonment. Experiencing adverse childhood events can result in lifelong problems, including PTSD, anxiety disorders, dissociative disorders, and somatic disorders. The Adverse Childhood Experiences (ACE) Study (Fuller-Thomson et al., 2011) surveyed more than 16 000 adults and discovered that childhood trauma exposure accounted for negative outcomes across a variety of diagnoses in later life, including multiple somatic symptoms of diabetes, heart disease, cancer, gastrointestinal conditions, and immune functioning.

Sociocultural Factors

Reliable data on the incidence of anxiety disorders are sparse, but sociocultural variation in symptoms of anxiety disorders has been noted. In some cultures most individuals express anxiety through somatic symptoms, whereas in other cultures, cognitive symptoms predominate. Panic attacks in Latin Americans and Northern Europeans often involve sensations of choking, smothering, numbness, or tingling, as well as fear of dying. In some other cultural groups panic attacks involve fear of magic or witchcraft. Physical symptoms are believed to result from the casting of spells. Spellbound individuals often seek the help of traditional healers in addition to modern medical staff. The medical health care provider may diagnose a non–life-threatening SSD, whereas the traditional healer may offer an entirely different explanation and prognosis. The individual might not show improvement until the traditional healer removes the spell.

The type and frequency of psychosomatic symptoms vary across cultures as well (Brown & Lewis-Fernandez, 2011). The sensation of burning hands and feet, worms in the head, or ants under the skin is more common in Africa and southern Asia than in North America. Fainting is a symptom commonly associated with culture-specific religious and healing rituals.

SSD, which is rarely seen in men in North America, is often reported in Greek and Puerto Rican men, suggesting that cultural customs permit these men to somatize as an acceptable approach to dealing with life stress. Somatization related to post-traumatic stress and depression was the most prevalent psychiatric symptom in North Korean defectors to South Korea (Kim et al., 2011). West Indians (Caribbean) attribute somatic symptoms to chronic overwork and the irregularity of daily living, citing symptoms such as dizziness, fatigue, joint pain, and muscle tension. For more specific information on cultural implications for psychiatric mental health nursing refer to Chapter 8.

Culture-Bound Syndromes

Up to 175 culture-bound syndromes have been identified. Culture-bound syndromes express distress about a range of personal and social problems in a culture and do not necessarily indicate psychopathology (e.g., heat in the head, heart-squeezed, bored). Some, such as trance, possession states, and fainting or seizure-like episodes, may in Western thinking be assessed as pathological (e.g., delusions or hallucinations) but are accepted expressions of distress in other cultures. In addition, cultural idioms of distress encompass explanatory mechanisms for behaviours or symptoms (e.g., evil eye, witchcraft, extreme emotion that upsets hot–cold balance) (Flaskerud, 2009).

Rather than listing various culture-bound syndromes, the *DSM-5* provides a cultural formulation interview guide to help mental health practitioners assess information about the cultural features of an individual's mental health, history, and social context. Nurses need to show acceptance of and respect for culture-bound syndromes. However, showing acceptance and respect does not mean that the patient is not offered antipsychotics or other medications. Depending on the results of a thorough assessment, medication may be used to help alleviate a patient's distress. The Considering Culture box discusses factors relevant to the intersection of cultural adaptation of the implementation of evidence-based practices. Review Chapter 8 for more discussion of cultural issues.

> ### ⊕ CONSIDERING CULTURE
> *Evidence-Based Practice and Cultural Adaptations*
>
> When delivering treatment for anxiety guided by an evidence-based practice guideline, the clinician must become aware of the cultural assumptions of the research on which the guidelines have been developed. Usually, implementing an evidence-based practice guideline is an opportunity to improve the effectiveness and efficiency of nursing care. However, most evidence-based practice guidelines are developed from research using data collected from the dominant cultural group. This results in shortfalls in understanding the responsiveness of interventions within minority cultural groups. The guidelines identify the determinants of effective treatment. However, is it reasonable to assume that all cultural groups define effective treatment for anxiety in the same way? As a result, clinicians need to question the universal applicability of evidence-based practice guidelines and determine whether sociocultural differences necessitate different forms of interventions and how cultural factors affect the impact of the guideline. Once it is determined whether a guideline requires cultural adaptation, the dimensions of language—metaphors, symbols, and sayings—the language of the intervention, cultural values of the community, and unique context of the individual are reviewed prior to treatment initiation.

> ### ⚡ SAFETY TIP
> Understanding culture is not as easy as it sounds. Cultural safety begins with respect for others, humility, and self awareness. Ask yourself: what are my personal beliefs, values, and biases. We all have biases. Some that we are aware of and others to which we are blinded.
> - Think about the assumptions you make about your friends, peers, people you work with, and strangers. What assumptions do you make?
> - Be curious and open-minded about other cultures. Do some research; check out on-line resources, attend local food and cultural festivals, or maybe reach out and connect with an international pen pal.
> - Be open to cultural experiences. If you have an opportunity to travel, this is a means of opening yourself up to new cultures. You could also virtually travel and participate in virtual tours. The Smithsonian has a number of virtual travel experiences that can be accessed from https://www.smithsonianmag.com/travel/virtual-travel-180974440/
>
> Learning about someone's culture allows you to complete a more accurate assessment and recognize when they are becoming distressed.

APPLICATION OF THE NURSING PROCESS

Assessment

General Assessment

People with anxiety disorders rarely need hospitalization unless they are in extreme distress, suicidal, or have **compulsions** that cause injury (e.g., cutting self, banging a body part). When assessing any patient, it is essential that all aspects of patient safety are considered. Most patients prone to anxiety disorders are encountered in non–mental health settings. A common example is someone taken to an emergency department to rule out a heart attack when, in fact, the individual is experiencing a panic attack. It is essential for clinicians to determine whether the anxiety is secondary to another source (medical condition or substance) or is the primary problem, as in an anxiety disorder.

Rating Scales

The Hamilton Anxiety Rating Scale is a popular tool for measuring anxiety (Table 12.9). High scores may indicate GAD or PD, although it is important to note that high anxiety scores may also be a symptom of major depressive disorder. Keep in mind that although the Hamilton Anxiety Rating Scale highlights important areas in the assessment of anxiety, it is intended for use by experienced clinicians as a guide for planning care and not as a method of self-diagnosis.

TABLE 12.9 Hamilton Anxiety Rating Scale

Item	Symptoms	Rating
1. Anxious mood	Worry, anticipation of the worst, fearful anticipation, irritability	_____
2. Tension	Feelings of tension, fatigability, startle response, moved to tears easily, trembling, feelings of restlessness, inability to relax	_____
3. Fear	Fearful of dark, strangers, being left alone, animals, traffic, crowds	_____
4. Insomnia	Difficulty in falling asleep, broken sleep, unsatisfying sleep and fatigue on waking, dreams, nightmares, night terrors	_____
5. Intellectual (cognitive) manifestations	Difficulty in concentrating, poor memory	_____
6. Depressed mood swings	Loss of interest, lack of pleasure in hobbies, depression, early waking, diurnal	_____
7. Somatic (sensory) symptoms	Tinnitus, blurring of vision, hot and cold flushes, feelings of weakness, skin picking urges	_____
8. Somatic (muscular) symptoms	Pains and aches, twitching, stiffness, myoclonic jerks, grinding of teeth, unsteady voice, increased muscular tone	_____
9. Cardiovascular symptoms	Tachycardia, palpitations, skipped beats, pain in chest, throbbing of vessels, fainting feelings	_____
10. Respiratory symptoms	Pressure of constriction in chest, choking feelings, sighing, dyspnea	_____
11. Gastrointestinal symptoms	Difficulty in swallowing, flatulence, abdominal pain, burning sensations, abdominal fullness, nausea, vomiting, borborygmi, looseness of bowels, loss of weight, constipation	_____
12. Genitourinary symptoms	Frequency of urination, urgency of urination, amenorrhea, menorrhagia, development of frigidity, premature ejaculation, loss of libido, impotence	_____
13. Autonomic symptoms	Dry mouth, flushing, pallor, tendency to sweat, giddiness, tension headache, raising of hair	_____
14. Behaviour at interview	Fidgeting, restlessness or pacing, tremor of hands, furrowed brow, strained face, sighing or rapid respiration, facial pallor, swallowing, belching, brisk tendon jerks, dilated pupils, exophthalmos	_____

Source: Adapted from Hamilton, M. (1959). The assessment of anxiety states by rating. *British Journal of Medical Psychology, 32,* 50–55. https://doi.org/10.1111/j.2044-8341.1959.tb00467.x. Copyright © 2011, John Wiley and Sons.
Scoring: 14–17 = mild anxiety; 18–24 = moderate anxiety; 25–30 = severe anxiety.
The symptom inventory provides scaled information that classifies anxiety behaviours and assists the clinician in targeting behaviours and achieving outcome measures. Provide a rating for each indicator based on the following scale: 0 = none; 1 = mild; 2 = moderate; 3 = disabling; 4 = severe, grossly disabling.

ASSESSMENT GUIDELINES
Anxiety Disorders

1. Ensure that a sound physical and neurological examination is performed to help determine whether the anxiety is primary or secondary to another psychiatric disorder, medical condition, or substance use.
2. Assess for substance use (i.e., prescription and nonprescription medication, alcohol consumption, nicotine and caffeine consumption).
3. Determine current level of anxiety (mild, moderate, severe, or panic).
4. Assess for potential for self-harm and suicide; people suffering from high levels of intractable anxiety may become desperate and attempt suicide.
5. Perform a psychosocial assessment. Always ask the person, "What is going on in your life that may be contributing to your anxiety?" The patient may identify a problem that should be addressed by counselling (e.g., stressful marriage, recent loss, stressful job or school situation).
6. Remember that culture can affect how anxiety is manifested.

Goodman et al. (1989) developed the Yale-Brown Obsessive Compulsive Scale (YBOCS). To review this scale, you may access it at https://psychology-tools.com/yale-brown-obsessive-compulsive-scale/. The YBOCS has become the preferred measurement tool for OCD. It is important to note that the YBOCS is not a diagnostic tool. Rather, it is a scale used to gauge the severity and nature of OCD symptoms. Foa and colleagues (1998) developed the Obsessive-Compulsive Inventory (OCI) with the following subscales: washing, checking, doubting, ordering, obsessions, hoarding, and neutralizing. The Panic Disorder Severity Scale (PDSS) is a clinician-administered questionnaire developed to measure the severity of panic disorder and to monitor treatment outcome (Shear et al., 1997). The PDSS consists of seven items: panic frequency, distress during panic, panic-focused anticipatory anxiety, phobic avoidance of situations, phobic avoidance of physical sensations, impairment in work functioning, and impairment in social functioning.

A useful assessment tool to understand the degree of somatization is the Patient Health Questionnaire–15 (PHQ), a somatic symptom severity scale for the purpose of diagnosis (Figure 12.2). The questionnaire inquires about 15 somatic symptoms (stomach pain, back pain, headache, chest pain, dizziness, fainting, palpitations, shortness of breath, bowel complaints, nausea, fatigue, sleep problems, pain in joints or limbs, menstrual pain, and problems during sexual intercourse) that account for more than 90% of physical complaints reported in the primary care setting by asking patients to rate the severity of symptoms during the previous 4 weeks on a three-point scale (Korber et al., 2011). In addition, information should be sought about the patient's ability to meet their own basic needs. Rest, comfort, activity, and hygiene needs may be altered as a result of patient problems such as fatigue, weakness, insomnia, muscle tension, pain, and avoidance of diversional activities (hobbies). Safety and security needs may be threatened by patient experiences of blindness, deafness, loss of balance, and anaesthesia of various parts of the body. During assessment, it is important to determine whether symptoms are under the patient's voluntary control. Somatic symptoms *are not* under the individual's voluntary control. Although the relationship between symptoms and interpersonal conflicts may be obvious to others, the patient is not aware of it.

During the past four (4) days how much have you been bothered by . . .		Not bothered at all	Bothered a little	Bothered a lot
1.	Stomach pain	0	1	2
2.	Back pain	0	1	2
3.	Pain in your arms, legs, or joints	0	1	2
4.	Menstrual cramps or other problems with your periods (women)	0	1	2
5.	Headaches	0	1	2
6.	Chest pain	0	1	2
7.	Dizziness	0	1	2
8.	Fainting spells	0	1	2
9.	Feeling your heart pound or race	0	1	2
10.	Shortness of breath	0	1	2
11.	Pain or problems during sexual intercourse	0	1	2
12.	Constipation, loose bowels, or diarrhea	0	1	2
13.	Nausea, gas, or indigestion	0	1	2
14.	Feeling tired or having no energy	0	1	2
15.	Trouble sleeping	0	1	2

Scores of 5 or less indicate mild somatization, 10 or less are moderate somatization, and 15 or more are considered severe indications of somatization.

Fig. 12.2 Patient Health Questionnaire Somatic Symptom—Short Form (PHQ-SSS). (**Source:** Adapted from Kroenke, K., Spitzer, R. L., Williams, J. B. W., et al. (2010). The patient health questionnaire somatic, anxiety, and depressive symptom scales: A systematic review. *General Hospital Psychiatry, 32*(4), 345–359. https://doi.org/10.1016/j.genhosppsych.2010.03.006. Copyright © 2010, with permission from Elsevier.)

ASSESSMENT GUIDELINES
Somatic Symptom Disorders

1. Assess for nature, location, onset, characteristics, and duration of the symptom(s).
2. Assess the patient's ability to meet basic needs.
3. Assess risks to the safety and security needs of the patient as a result of the symptom(s).
4. Determine whether the symptoms are under the patient's voluntary control.
5. Identify any secondary gains the patient is experiencing from symptom(s).
6. Explore the patient's cognitive style and ability to communicate feelings and needs.
7. Assess the type and amount of medication the patient is using.

Several scales have been developed to assess dissociation, including the Dissociative Experiences Scale (DES) (Bernstein & Putnam, 1986), the Structured Clinical Interview for Dissociative Disorders (SCID-D) (Schlozman & Nonacs, 2008), the Somatoform Dissociation Questionnaire (SDQ) (http://www.enijenhuis.nl/sdq/), and the Dissociative Disorders Interview Schedule (DDIS) (http://www.rossinst.com/downloads/DDIS-DSM-5.pdf). For a diagnosis of a dissociative disorder to be made, other medical and neurological illnesses, substance use, and other coexisting (comorbid) psychiatric disorders must be ruled out as the cause of the patient's symptoms. Specific information about identity, memory, consciousness, life events, mood, suicide risk, and the impact of the disorder on the patient and the family is important to assess. The assessment should include objective data from physical examination, electroencephalography, imaging studies, and specific questions to identify dissociative symptoms. Assessment tools are important because a psychiatric interview will often miss the presence of dissociation because the individual does not know what they do not know; that is, by definition, dissociative periods involve lapses of memory of which the person may not even be aware.

ASSESSMENT GUIDELINES
Dissociative Disorders

1. Assess identity and memory.
   a. Assess for signs of dissociation.
      - Can you remember recent and past events?
      - Is your memory clear and complete or partial and fuzzy?
      - Are you aware of gaps in memory (e.g., lack of memory for events such as a graduation or a wedding)?

- Do your memories place you with a family, in school, or in an occupation?
- Do you ever lose time or have blackouts?
- Do you find yourself in places with no idea how you got there?

b. Assess for a history of a similar episode in the past with benign outcomes.
- Have you ever found yourself wearing clothes you cannot remember buying?
- Have you ever had strange people greet and talk to you as though they were old friends?
- Does your ability to engage in things such as athletics, artistic activities, or mechanical tasks seem to change?
- Do you have differing sets of memories about childhood?

2. Determine if there are comorbid medical conditions.
   - Have you sustained a recent injury, such as a concussion?
   - Do you have a history of epilepsy, especially temporal lobe epilepsy?
3. Establish whether the person suffered abuse, trauma, or loss as a child.
4. Evaluate mood and level of anxiety.
5. Identify support systems through a psychosocial assessment.
6. Identify relevant psychosocial distress issues by performing a basic psychosocial assessment.
7. Assess for safety of self and others.

Psychosocial Factors

Psychosocial factors are relevant to anxiety-related symptoms, and the way a patient thinks and feels can have a profound effect on recovery. For example, strong emotions such as fear, anger, sadness, confusion, and guilt can affect a patient's physical, emotional, and spiritual recovery. Patients may feel overwhelmed and alone, and friends and family members may feel helpless and at a loss emotionally. Thus the nurse must complete a psychosocial assessment in tandem with a thorough physical workup and mental status examination (Table 12.10).

Coping skills. Assessing how a patient has dealt with adversity in the past provides information about the availability of coping skills. Health care workers can also support the patient in gaining additional coping skills that may help them better manage.

Spirituality and religion. Nurses and other health care workers are becoming increasingly aware of the role spirituality or religion plays in many patients' lives and its importance as a source of peace. Support from a priest, pastor, rabbi, imam, or other religious leader may be indicated, especially in a case of spiritual distress. Religious beliefs and practices are forces that can promote resilience. Practising healthy coping depends on the capacity to create meaning from life experiences.

Secondary gains. The nurse should try to identify secondary gains the patient may be receiving from the symptoms. If a patient derives personal benefit from the symptoms, giving up the symptoms is more difficult unless the patient can achieve the same benefits through healthier avenues, such as learning to communicate more adaptively and to connect with others; skills the clinician can help the patient learn. One approach to identifying the presence of secondary gains is to ask the patient questions such as:

- What are you unable to do now that you used to be able to do?
- How has this problem affected your life?

Self-Assessment

As a nurse working with an individual with an anxiety-related disorder, you may experience uncomfortable personal reactions. You may have feelings of frustration or anger while working with a patient, especially if the symptoms seem to be a matter of choice or under personal control. For example, the rituals of the patient with OCD may hinder

TABLE 12.10 Psychosocial Assessment of Patients

Areas to Assess	Specific Questions to Ask
Social Supports and Cultural Issues	
Family	What were the effects of the patient's illness, treatments, and recovery on the family in the past?
Friends	Who can the patient share painful feelings with?
	Does the patient have friends to joke and laugh with?
	Are there people the patient believes would stand by them?
Religious or spiritual beliefs	Does the patient find comfort and support in spiritual practices? Is the patient a member of a spiritual or religious group in the community (e.g., church, temple, other place of worship)? Does the patient find inner peace and strength in religious or spiritual practices? *The following statements may be used in performing a spiritual assessment of a patient:* • I (often/sometimes/seldom) believe that life has value, meaning, and direction. • I (often/sometimes/seldom) feel a connection with the universe. • I (often/sometimes/seldom) believe in a power greater than myself. • I (often/sometimes/seldom) believe that my actions make a difference. • I (often/sometimes/seldom) believe that my actions express my true self.
Cultural beliefs	Does the patient use specific culture-oriented treatments or remedies for their condition?
	Do the patient's cultural beliefs allow for adequate treatment by Western medical standards?
Work	Are there colleagues at work that the patient can count on for support?
	Have there been any work-related changes or sudden stressful events or occurrences?
Coexisting Physical Conditions Affecting Psychosocial Well-Being	
Physical pain	Is the patient in pain?
	How does the patient cope with the pain?
	Is the pain disabling?
	Are there pain-reducing techniques that might help?

TABLE 12.10	Psychosocial Assessment of Patients—cont'd
Areas to Assess	Specific Questions to Ask
Major illness	Does the patient have a co-occurring major illness that will negatively affect their current condition?
	Is the patient undergoing treatments that are affecting daily life more than expected?
	Are there interventions that would help the patient better cope with the sequelae of the illness and treatments?
	Has the patient been hospitalized in the past?
	How many times?
	For what?
	How did the patient cope?
Addictions and mental health	Does the patient have a co-occurring mental health problem (e.g., depression, anxiety, compulsions)?
	Has the patient suffered a mental illness in the past?
	Does the patient participate in any compulsive behaviour (e.g., smoking, overworking, excessive spending, gambling, cybersex)?
	Does the patient use substances (e.g., alcohol, drugs [illicit, over-the-counter, prescription])?

your ability to accomplish certain nursing tasks within the usual time. Communicating with such patients can be difficult since patients with a phobia may acknowledge that the fear is exaggerated and unrealistic yet continue to practise avoidant behaviour, which may bewilder the nurse.

It is natural for nurses to experience feelings of scepticism while caring for patients who are diagnosed with dissociative disorders. Believing in the authenticity of the symptoms the patient is displaying can be difficult and feeling confused and bewildered by the presence of dissociative symptoms is not unusual. Some nurses even experience feelings of fascination and get caught up in the intrigue of caring for a patient with dissociative symptoms.

Unlike the patient who just needs a dressing changed several times a week, the patient with an anxiety-related disorder requires "emotional bandaging" much more often, and behavioural change is often accomplished slowly. When rapid progress is not made, nurses can become impatient. Most people with dissociative disorders have experienced a significant trauma or have been in relationships in which trust was betrayed. As a result, developing a therapeutic relationship with these patients can be a slower process than with patients who have other mental illnesses. Nurses may therefore feel inadequate and frustrated by their efforts. At the very least, they are likely to experience increased tension and fatigue from mental strain. They may also feel anger or frustration and, as a consequence, may withdraw from the patient emotionally and physically. Such negative feelings are easily transmitted to the patient, who then feels increasingly anxious and may also withdraw.

Therefore patience, the ability to provide clear structure, and empathy are important assets when working with patients with anxiety and related disorders. Staging outcomes in small, attainable steps can help prevent the nurse from feeling overwhelmed by the patient's slow progress and help the patient gain a sense of control.

By having a clear understanding of the emotional pitfalls of working with patients who have anxiety and related disorders, a nurse is better prepared to minimize and avoid the guilt associated with strong negative feelings. It is important, then, to examine your personal feelings so you can better understand their origin and respond objectively and constructively.

Diagnosis

Many nursing diagnoses can be considered for patients experiencing anxiety and anxiety-related disorders. The "related to" component will vary with the individual patient. Table 12.11 identifies potential nursing diagnoses for the patient experiencing anxiety, Table 12.12 for patients experiencing SSD, Table 12.13 for patients experiencing dissociative disorders, and signs and symptoms that might be found upon assessment to support the diagnosis are included.

Outcomes Identification

The *Nursing Outcomes Classification (NOC)* identifies desired outcomes for patients with anxiety or anxiety-related disorders (Moorhead et al., 2018). Each outcome contains a definition and rating scale to measure the severity of the symptom or the frequency of the desired response. This rating scale enables you to evaluate outcomes in the nursing care plan. Some of the *NOC*-recommended outcomes related to anxiety include *Anxiety self-control, Anxiety level, Stress level, Coping, Social interaction skills,* and *Symptom control*. Refer to Table 12.14 for examples of intermediate and short-term indicators related to *NOC* outcomes.

Because shared decision making promotes goal attainment, patients should participate in identifying desired outcomes. Outcome criteria must be realistic and attainable. Structuring outcomes in small steps helps the patient and the nurse see concrete evidence of progress. The following are examples of possible outcomes for a patient with a SSD (Ackley et al., 2017):

- Patient will exhibit sensitivity to self-needs and needs of others.
- Patient will resume performance of work, family, and social role behaviours.
- Patient will identify ineffective coping patterns.
- Patient will make realistic appraisal of strengths and weaknesses.
- Patient will assertively verbalize feelings such as anger, shame, or guilt.

Planning

Planning for the delivery of specific nursing care is influenced by both the setting (community or inpatients) and the presenting problem. A top priority stated in the report *Changing Directions, Changing Lives: The Mental Health Strategy for Canada* (Mental Health Commission of Canada, 2012) is to identify and integrate mental health needs into primary care settings. Anxiety disorders are encountered in all health care settings. Nurses care for people with co-existing anxiety disorders in medical–surgical units, as well as in homes, day programs, and clinics. Patients with anxiety disorders usually do not require admission to inpatient psychiatric units, so planning for their care may involve selecting interventions that can be implemented in a community setting.

TABLE 12.11 Potential Diagnoses for Anxiety Disorders

Signs and Symptoms	Nursing Diagnoses
Concern that a panic attack will occur	Anxiety (moderate, severe, panic)
Exposure to phobic object or situation	Fear
Presence of obsessive thoughts	
Recurrent memories of traumatic event	
Fear of panic attacks	
High levels of anxiety that interfere with the ability to work, disrupt relationships, and change ability to interact with others	Inadequate coping
	Reduced diversional activity
Avoidance behaviours (phobia, agoraphobia)	Social isolation
Hypervigilance after a traumatic event	Inadequate role performance
Inordinate time taken for obsession and compulsions	
Difficulty with concentration	Inadequate health maintenance
Preoccupation with obsessive thoughts	
Disorganization associated with exposure to phobic object	
Intrusive thoughts and memories of traumatic event	Post-trauma syndrome
Excessive use of reason and logic associated with overcautiousness and fear of making a mistake	Decisional conflict
Disruption in sleep related to intrusive thoughts, worrying, replaying of a traumatic event, hypervigilance, fear	Insomnia
	Sleep deprivation
	Fatigue
Feelings of hopelessness, inability to control one's life, low self-esteem related to inability to have some control in one's life	Hopelessness
	Chronic low self-esteem
	Spiritual distress
Inability to perform self-care related to rituals	Self-care deficit
Skin excoriation related to rituals of excessive washing or excessive picking at the skin	Reduced skin integrity
Inability to eat because of constant ritual performance	Imbalanced nutrition: less than body requirements
Feeling of anxiety or excessive worrying that overrides appetite and the need to eat	
Excessive overeating to appease intense worrying or high anxiety levels	Imbalanced nutrition: more than body requirements

TABLE 12.12 Potential Nursing Diagnoses for Somatic Symptom Disorders

Signs and Symptoms	Nursing Diagnoses
Inability to meet occupational, family, or social responsibilities because of symptoms	Inadequate coping
Inability to participate in usual community activities or friendships because of psychogenic symptoms	Inadequate role performance
	Reduced social interaction
Dependence on pain relievers	Powerlessness
Distortion of body functions and symptoms	Disturbed body image
Presence of secondary gains by adoption of sick role	Pain, acute or chronic
Inability to meet family role function and need for family to assume role function of the somatic individual	Interrupted family processes
	Inadequate sexuality pattern
Assumption of some of the roles of the somatic parent by the children	Inadequate parenting
Shifting of the sexual partner's role to that of caregiver or parent and the patient's role to that of recipient of care	Risk for caregiver role strain
Feeling of inability to control symptoms or understand why they cannot find help	Chronic low self-esteem
Development of negative self-evaluation related to losing body function, feeling useless, or not feeling valued by significant others	Spiritual distress
Inability to take care of basic self-care needs related to conversion symptoms (paralysis, seizures, pain, fatigue)	Self-care deficit
Inability to sleep due to psychogenic pain	Disturbed sleep pattern

Whenever possible, the patient should be encouraged to participate actively in planning. By including the patient in decision making, you increase the likelihood of positive outcomes. Shared planning is especially appropriate for someone with mild or moderate anxiety. When experiencing severe levels of anxiety, a patient may be unable to participate in planning, and the nurse may be required to take a more directive role.

One of the many advantages of integrating mental health services into primary health care settings is less stigmatization of treatment for mental illness and of people with mental health disorders. Because primary health care services are not associated with any specific health conditions, this level of care seems far more "acceptable," and therefore accessible, for most users and families. Many primary care centres have psychiatric mental health nurses as part of the regular treatment team, as these nurses can bring a strong perspective in terms of managing both physical and mental health needs in integrated care settings.

Establishing a therapeutic relationship is the first step in delivering effective nursing care. The following strategies can be used to build an effective therapeutic relationship.

1. Provide frequent, brief, and regular office visits.
2. Avoid making disparaging comments such as "Your symptoms are all in your head."
3. Set reasonable therapeutic goals such as maintaining function despite ongoing pain.

A phase-oriented treatment model is recommended for individuals with a dissociative disorder for any setting and includes (International Society for the Study of Trauma and Dissociation, 2012):

Phase 1: Establishing safety, stabilization, and symptom reduction
Phase 2: Confronting, working through, and integrating traumatic memories
Phase 3: Integrating identity and rehabilitating

The nurse will most often encounter the patient in times of crisis (i.e., when the patient is suicidal or expressing homicidal behaviour), and in times of crisis the care plan will focus on Phase 1 strategies to ensure safety and crisis intervention. Basic nursing interventions should be implemented. Phases 2 and 3 are advanced interventions, so clinicians using these interventions require special training.

Implementation

Determining Levels of Distress

When working with patients with anxiety disorders, you must first determine what level of distress they are experiencing. A general framework for anxiety interventions can then be built on a solid foundation of understanding.

TABLE 12.13 Potential Nursing Diagnoses for Dissociative Disorders

Signs and Symptoms	Nursing Diagnoses
Amnesia or fugue related to a traumatic event	Disturbed personal identity
Symptoms of depersonalization; feelings of unreality or body-image distortions	Disturbed body image
Alterations in consciousness, memory, or identity	Inadequate coping
Use of substances related to dissociation	Inadequate role performance
Disorganization or dysfunction in usual patterns of behaviour (absence from work, withdrawal from relationships, changes in role function)	
Disturbances in memory and identity	Interrupted family processes
Interrupted family processes related to amnesia or erratic and changing behaviour	Inadequate parenting
Feeling of being out of control of memory, behaviours, and awareness	Anxiety Spiritual distress
Inability to explain actions or behaviours when in altered state	Potential for other-directed violence Potential for self-directed violence

TABLE 12.14 *NOC* Outcomes for Anxiety Disorders

Nursing Outcome and Definition	Intermediate Indicators	Short-Term Indicators
Anxiety self-control: Personal actions to eliminate or reduce feelings of apprehension, tension, or uneasiness from an unidentifiable source	Controls anxiety response Maintains role performance	Monitors intensity of anxiety Uses relaxation techniques to decrease anxiety Decreases environmental stimuli when anxious Maintains adequate sleep
Coping: Personal actions to manage stressors that tax an individual's resources	Identifies multiple coping strategies Modifies lifestyle as needed	Reports decrease in physical symptoms of stress Identifies ineffective coping patterns Verbalizes need for assistance Seeks information concerning illness and treatment
Self-esteem: Personal judgement of self-worth	Describes pride in self Describes success in social groups	Maintains eye contact Maintains grooming and hygiene Accepts self-limitations Accepts compliments from others
Knowledge: Disease process: Extent of understanding conveyed about a specific disease process	Describes usual disease course	Describes signs and symptoms Describes cause or contributing factors Describes signs and symptoms of complications Describes precautions to prevent complications

Source: Moorhead, S., Johnson, M., Maas, M., et al. (2018). *Nursing outcomes classification (NOC)* (6th ed.) Measurement of Health Outcomes. St. Louis: Mosby. *NOC,* Nursing Outcomes Classification.

Mild to moderate levels of anxiety. A person experiencing a mild to moderate level of anxiety is still able to solve problems; however, the ability to concentrate decreases as anxiety increases. A patient can be helped to focus and solve problems when you use specific nursing communication techniques, such as asking open-ended questions, giving broad openings, and exploring and seeking clarification. Closing off topics of communication and bringing up irrelevant topics can increase a person's anxiety, making the nurse, but not the patient, feel better.

Reducing the patient's anxiety level and preventing escalation to more distressing levels can be aided by providing a calm presence, recognizing the anxious person's distress, and being willing to listen. Evaluation of effective past coping mechanisms is also useful. Often you can help the patient consider alternatives to problematic situations and offer activities that may temporarily relieve feelings of inner tension. Table 12.15 identifies interventions useful in assisting people experiencing mild to moderate levels of anxiety.

Severe to panic levels of anxiety. A person experiencing a severe to panic level of anxiety is unable to solve problems and may have a poor grasp of what is happening in the environment. Unproductive relief behaviours may take over, and the person may not be in control of their actions. Extreme regression and aimless running about are behavioural manifestations of a person's intense psychic pain.

Appropriate nursing interventions are to provide for the safety of the patient and others and to meet physical needs (e.g., fluids, rest) to prevent exhaustion. Anxiety reduction measures may take the form of removing the person to a quiet environment (seclusion room) with minimal stimulation and providing gross motor activities to drain some of the tension. The use of medications may have to be considered, but both medications and a seclusion room should be used only after other more personal and less restrictive interventions have failed to decrease anxiety to safer levels. Although a patient's communication may be scattered and disjointed, feeling understood can reduce anxiety and decrease the overwhelming sense of isolation.

Because individuals experiencing severe to panic levels of anxiety are unable to solve problems, the techniques suggested for communicating with people with mild to moderate levels of anxiety may not be effective at more severe levels. These patients are out of control, so they need to know they are safe from their own impulses. Firm, short, and simple statements are useful. Reinforcing what is observable in the environment (e.g., the door, the painting) and pointing out reality when there are distortions can also be useful interventions for severely anxious people. Table 12.16 suggests some basic nursing interventions for patients with severe to panic levels of anxiety.

Anxiety management and reduction are primary concerns when working with patients who have anxiety disorders, but these patients may have a variety of other needs as well. When developing a plan of care, psychiatric mental health nurses can refer to the appropriate standards of practice for their governing body. The *Nursing Interventions Classification (NIC)* offers pertinent interventions in the behavioural and safety domains (Butcher et al., 2019) (Box 12.1).

The following are basic nursing interventions:

1. Identify community resources that can offer the patient specialized, effective treatment.
2. Identify community support groups for people with specific anxiety disorders and their families.
3. Use counselling, milieu therapy, promotion of self-care activities, and psychobiological and health teaching interventions as appropriate.

TABLE 12.15 Interventions for Mild to Moderate Levels of Anxiety

Intervention	Rationale
Help the patient identify anxiety: "Are you comfortable right now?"	It is important to validate observations with the patient, name the anxiety, and start to work with the patient to lower anxiety.
Anticipate anxiety-provoking situations.	Escalation of anxiety to a more disorganizing level is prevented.
Use nonverbal language to demonstrate interest (e.g., lean forward, maintain eye contact, nod your head).	Verbal and nonverbal messages should be consistent. The presence of an interested person provides a stabilizing focus.
Encourage the patient to talk about their feelings and concerns.	When concerns are stated aloud, problems can be discussed, and feelings of isolation decreased.
Avoid closing off avenues of communication that are important for the patient. Focus on the patient's concerns.	When staff anxiety increases, changing the topic or offering advice is a common temptation, but this action isolates the patient.
Ask questions to clarify what is being said: "I'm not sure what you mean. Give me an example."	Increased anxiety results in scattering of thoughts. Clarifying helps the patient identify thoughts and feelings.
Help the patient identify thoughts or feelings before the onset of anxiety. "What were you thinking right before you started to feel anxious?"	The patient is assisted in identifying thoughts and feelings, and problem solving is facilitated.
Encourage problem solving with the patient.[a]	Encouraging patients to explore alternatives increases sense of control and decreases anxiety.
Assist in developing alternative solutions to a problem through role-play or modelling behaviours.	The patient is encouraged to try out alternative behaviours and solutions.
Explore behaviours that have worked to relieve anxiety in the past.	The patient is encouraged to mobilize successful coping mechanisms and strengths.
Provide outlets for working off excess energy (e.g., walking, playing Ping-Pong, dancing, exercising).	Physical activity can provide relief of built-up tension, increase muscle tone, and increase endorphin levels.

[a]Patients experiencing mild to moderate anxiety levels can problem-solve.

Nursing diagnosis: *Anxiety (moderate)* related to situational event or psychological stress, as evidenced by increase in vital signs, moderate discomfort, narrowing of perceptual field, and selective inattention

TABLE 12.16 Interventions for Severe to Panic Levels of Anxiety

Intervention	Rationale
Maintain a calm manner.	Anxiety is communicated interpersonally. The quiet calmness of the nurse can serve to calm the patient. The presence of anxiety can escalate anxiety in the patient.
Always remain with the person experiencing an acute severe to panic level of anxiety.	Alone with immense anxiety, a person feels abandoned. A caring face may be the patient's only contact with reality when confusion becomes overwhelming.
Minimize environmental stimuli. Move to a quieter setting and stay with the patient.	A quieter setting helps minimize further escalation of anxiety.
Use clear and simple statements and repetition.	A person experiencing a severe to panic level of anxiety has difficulty concentrating and processing information.
Use a low-pitched voice; speak slowly.	A high-pitched voice can convey anxiety. A low pitch can decrease anxiety.
Reinforce reality if distortions occur (e.g., seeing objects that are not there or hearing voices when no one is present).	Anxiety can be reduced by focusing on and validating what is going on in the environment.
Listen for themes in communication.	In severe to panic levels of anxiety, verbal communication themes may be the only indication of the patient's thoughts or feelings.
Attend to physical and safety needs (e.g., warmth, fluids, elimination, pain relief, family contact) when necessary.	High levels of anxiety may obscure the patient's awareness of physical needs.
Because safety is an overall goal, physical limits may need to be set. Speak in a firm, authoritative voice: "You may not hit anyone here. If you can't control yourself, we will help you."	A person who is out of control is often terrorized. Staff must offer the patient and others protection from destructive and self-destructive impulses.
Provide opportunities for exercise (e.g., walk with nurse, punching bag, Ping-Pong game).	Physical activity helps channel and dissipate tension and may temporarily lower anxiety.
When a person is constantly moving or pacing, offer high-calorie fluids.	Dehydration and exhaustion must be prevented.
Assess need for medication or seclusion after other interventions have been tried but have not been successful.	Exhaustion and physical harm to self and others must be prevented.

Nursing diagnosis: *Anxiety (severe, panic)* related to severe threat (biochemical, environmental, psychosocial), as evidenced by verbal or physical acting out, extreme immobility, sense of impending doom, inability to differentiate reality (possible hallucinations or delusions), and inability to problem solve.

BOX 12.1 *NIC* INTERVENTIONS FOR ANXIETY DISORDERS

Coping Enhancement

Definition of coping enhancement: Assistance provided to a patient in adapting to perceived stressors, changes, or threats that interfere with meeting life demands and roles.

Activities[a]
- Provide an atmosphere of acceptance.
- Encourage verbalization of feelings, perceptions, and fears.
- Acknowledge the patient's spiritual or cultural background.
- Discourage decision making when the patient is under severe stress.

Hope Inspiration

Definition of hope inspiration: Enhancement of the belief in one's capacity to initiate and sustain actions.

Activities[a]
- Assist the patient to identify areas of hope in life.
- Demonstrate hope by recognizing the patient's intrinsic worth and viewing the patient's illness as only one facet of the individual.
- Avoid masking the truth.
- Help the patient expand the spiritual self.

Self-Esteem Enhancement

Definition of self-esteem enhancement: Assistance provided to a patient in increasing their personal judgement of self-worth.

Activities[a]
- Make positive statements about the patient.
- Monitor frequency of self-negating verbalizations.
- Explore previous achievements.
- Explore reasons for self-criticism or guilt.

Relaxation Therapy

Definition of relaxation therapy: The use of techniques to encourage and elicit relaxation for the purpose of decreasing undesirable signs and symptoms such as pain, muscle tension, or anxiety.

Activities[a]
- Demonstrate and practise the relaxation technique with the patient.
- Provide written information about preparing and engaging in relaxation techniques.
- Anticipate the need for the use of relaxation.
- Evaluate and document the response to relaxation therapy.

[a]Partial list.
NIC, Nursing Interventions Classification.
Source: Butcher, H. K., Bulechek, G. M., McCloskey Dochtermanm J. M., & Wagner, C. (2019). *Nursing Interventions Classification (NIC)* (7th ed.). Toronto: Elsevier.

Psychosocial Interventions

People who have distressing symptoms are vulnerable to a variety of psychosocial stresses. How they cope with these stresses may make the difference between living with an acceptable quality of life and experiencing despair, withdrawal, helplessness, hopelessness, and suicidal ideation. Nurses are in a position to assess and understand patients' psychosocial stressors, identify needed coping skills, and teach stress-management techniques. Nurses can play an important role not only in managing patients' immediate care but also in helping patients improve their ability to cope and increase their quality of life during the course of their illness.

Effective coping skills that can be taught are many and varied (e.g., assertiveness training, cognitive reframing, problem-solving skills, social supports). A nurse is in a key position to assess, educate, or provide referrals to a patient to enable healthier ways of looking at and dealing with illness. Consider referring the patient for instruction in relaxation techniques such as reiki, meditation, guided imagery, breathing exercises, and others, or teach the patient some techniques yourself. Behavioural techniques, such as progressive muscle relaxation and biofeedback (which nurses can get special training to perform), are also useful. Relaxation techniques, stress-management skills, and supportive education should be part of patient care, regardless of the comorbid conditions.

The following interventions have all been shown to positively affect a patient's recovery:
- Educating the patient about specific treatments
- Referring the patient to community support groups (or systems)
- Teaching patients more effective coping skills that take into consideration patients' values, preferences, and lifestyle
- Focusing on a patient's strengths and reinforcing coping skills that work (e.g., prayerfulness, participation in hobbies, relaxation techniques)

To be successful, therapeutic interventions must address patient needs. The primary goal is to help patients identify ways to get their needs met without using harmful defence mechanisms or having pathological behaviour reinforced. The secondary gains derived from illness behaviours become less important to the patient when underlying needs can be met directly. Table 12.17 provides basic-level interventions for SSD. *Reattribution treatment*, an advanced nursing treatment approach also used with the treatment of somatization (Box 12.2), helps toward this goal.

Refer to Table 12.18 for examples of basic-level interventions for individuals experiencing a dissociative disorder.

Counselling

Psychiatric mental health nurses use counselling to reduce anxiety, enhance coping and communication skills, and intervene in crises. From a behaviourist perspective, when appropriate, relaxation training would occur during the counselling session. The training would include teaching relaxation exercises used to relax breathing or muscle groups. The relaxation response is the opposite of the stress response and results in a reduced heart rate, slower breathing, and relaxed muscles. Refer to Chapter 5 for a description of different approaches to relaxation training. When psychiatric mental health nurses begin to practise from a cognitive therapy perspective, they will help patients identify that what they think is linked with what they feel.

Health Teaching and Health Promotion

Health teaching is a significant nursing intervention for patients with anxiety disorders. Patients may conceal symptoms for years before seeking treatment and often come to the attention of health care

TABLE 12.17 Basic-Level Interventions for Somatic Symptom Disorders

Intervention	Rationale
Offer explanations and support during diagnostic testing.	Reduces anxiety while ruling out organic illness.
After physical complaints have been investigated, avoid further reinforcement (e.g., do not take vital signs each time patient complains of palpitations).	Directs focus away from physical symptoms.
Spend time with patient at times other than when patient summons nurse to voice physical complaint.	Rewards non–illness-related behaviours and encourages repetition of desired behaviour.
Observe and record frequency and intensity of somatic symptoms. (Patient or family can give information.)	Establishes a baseline and later enables evaluation of effectiveness of interventions.
Do not imply that symptoms are not real.	Acknowledges that psychogenic symptoms are real to the patient.
Shift focus from somatic complaints to feelings or to neutral topics.	Conveys interest in patient as a person rather than in patient's symptoms; reduces need to gain attention via symptoms.
Assess secondary gains "physical illness" provides for patient (e.g., attention, increased dependency, distraction from another problem).	Allows these needs to be met in healthier ways and thus minimizes secondary gains.
Use matter-of-fact approach to patient exhibiting resistance or covert anger.	Avoids power struggles; demonstrates acceptance of anger and permits discussion of angry feelings.
Have patient direct all requests to primary nurse.	Reduces manipulation.
Help patient look at effect of illness behaviour on others.	Encourages insight; can help improve family relationships.
Show concern for patient while avoiding fostering dependency needs.	Shows respect for patient's feelings while minimizing secondary gains from "illness."
Reinforce patient's strengths and problem-solving abilities.	Contributes to positive self-esteem; helps patient realize that needs can be met without resorting to somatic symptoms.
Teach assertive communication.	Provides patient with a positive means of getting needs met; reduces feelings of helplessness and need for manipulation.
Teach patient stress-reduction techniques, such as meditation, relaxation, and mild physical exercise.	Provides alternative coping strategies; reduces need for medication.

TABLE 12.18 Nursing Interventions for Dissociative Disorders

Intervention	Rationale
Ensure patient safety by providing safe, protected environment and frequent observation.	Patient's sense of bewilderment may lead to inattention to safety needs
Provide undemanding, simple routine.	Reduces anxiety
Confirm identity of patient and orientation to time and place.	Supports reality and promotes ego integrity
Encourage patient to do things for self and make decisions about routine tasks.	Enhances self-esteem by reducing sense of powerlessness and reduces secondary gain associated with dependence
Assist with other decision making until memory returns.	Lowers stress and prevents patient from having to live with the consequences of unwise decisions
Support patient during exploration of feelings surrounding the stressful event.	Helps lower the defence of dissociation used by patient to block awareness of the stressful event
Do not flood patient with data regarding past events.	Memory loss serves the purpose of preventing severe to panic levels of anxiety from overtaking and disorganizing the individual
Allow patient to progress at own pace as memory is recovered.	Prevents undue anxiety and resistance
Provide support during disclosure of painful experiences. Do not force the patient to disclose.	Can be healing, while minimizing feelings of isolation. Forced disclosure can retraumatize the patient
Help patients see consequences of using dissociation to cope with stress.	Increases insight and helps patient understand own role in choosing behaviours
Accept patient's expression of negative feelings.	Conveys permission to have negative or unacceptable feelings
Teach stress-reduction methods.	Provides alternatives for anxiety relief
If patient does not remember significant others, work with involved parties to re-establish relationships.	Helps patient experience satisfaction and relieves sense of isolation

BOX 12.2 Reattribution Treatment to Link Physical Complaints and Psychological Distress: An Example of an Advanced-Level Intervention

Reattribution treatment is a structured intervention designed to provide a simple explanation of somatic symptoms to patients. Health care providers with reattribution skills help patients feel understood and help them make the link between physical complaints and psychological distress.

Reattribution has four stages:

Stage 1: Feeling Understood
The health care provider uses empathetic listening skills in taking the history of physical, emotional, spiritual, and social factors of the presenting symptoms, including patient beliefs about and perceptions of the cause of illness, times when it is worse, and what helps improve symptoms. This stage includes a brief, focused physical examination.

Stage 2: Broadening the Agenda
The health care provider gives feedback of assessment findings, discusses the implications of the findings, and acknowledges the patient's distress.

Stage 3: Making the Link
The health care provider uses empowering explanations for symptoms—for example, "You may have a heightened sensitivity to particular stressors that is affected by genetics, your personal experiences, and the environment." This comment is patient centred and does not blame the patient for the symptoms (Fuller-Thomson et al., 2011).

Stage 4: Negotiating Further Treatment
The health care provider and the patient collaboratively create a treatment plan that includes regular follow-up visits and short-term and long-term goals.

Source: Adapted from Walters, P., Tylee, A., Fisher, J., et al. (2007). Teaching junior doctors to manage patients who somatise: Is it possible in an afternoon? *Medical Education, 41*, 995–1001. https://doi.org/10.1111/j.1365-2923.2007.02833.x. Copyright © 2007, John Wiley and Sons.

providers because of a co-occurring problem. Three out of every five individuals with an anxiety disorder do not consult a health care provider about their disorder (Public Health Agency of Canada, 2016). And those who do often wait years before getting medical attention.

Teaching about the specific disorder and available effective treatments is a major step toward improving the quality of life for those with anxiety disorders. Whether in a community or hospital setting, nurses can teach patients about signs and symptoms of anxiety disorders, presumed causes or risk factors (especially substance use), medications, the use of relaxation techniques, and the benefits of psychotherapy. When patients request or prefer to use integrative therapies, the nurse performs assessment and teaching as appropriate.

Some patients who somatize as a way of coping with anxiety may benefit from education about body functions. The type and depth of teaching is determined by the information the patient already understands. Others may know extensively about their physical body. In these situations, the teaching would focus on accurately assessing and interpreting the body's responses to digestion, stress, fatigue, and excitement.

Stress management and coping skills are important areas of health education for people with dissociative disorders. Normalizing experiences by explaining that symptoms are adaptive responses to past overwhelming events is important. Often the victim of childhood trauma feels as if they are a bad person and grows up with the false negative belief that the abuse was deserved punishment.

Another important intervention strategy is to teach grounding techniques that help the person focus on the present and help to counter dissociative symptoms. Examples of grounding techniques include stomping one's feet on the ground, taking a shower, holding an ice cube, exercising, breathing deeply, counting beads, and touching fabric or upholstery on a chair. Patients can also be taught to keep a daily journal to increase their awareness of feelings and to identify triggers of their dissociative symptoms. If a patient has never written a journal, the nurse should suggest beginning with 5 to 10 minutes of daily writing.

Milieu Therapy

As mentioned earlier, most patients with anxiety disorders can be treated successfully as outpatients. Hospital admission is necessary only if severe anxiety or symptoms interfere with the individual's health or if the individual is suicidal. When hospitalization is necessary, providing a safe environment is fundamental. Other characteristics of a therapeutic milieu that can be especially helpful to the patient are:

- Structuring the daily routine to offer physical safety and predictability, thus reducing anxiety over the unknown
- Providing daily activities to promote sharing and cooperation
- Providing therapeutic interactions, including one-on-one nursing care and behaviour contracts
- Including the patient in decisions about their own care

Promotion of Self-Care Activities

Patients with anxiety disorders are usually able to meet their own basic physical needs. Individuals with a SSD may require more assistance with self-care activities due to the physical limitations of their illness. Self-care activities that are most likely to be affected are discussed in the following sections.

Nutrition and fluid intake. Patients who engage in ritualistic behaviours may be too involved with their rituals to take time to eat and drink. Some phobic patients may be so afraid of germs, they cannot eat. In general, nutritious diets with snacks should be provided. Adequate intake should be firmly encouraged, but a power struggle should be avoided. Weighing patients frequently (e.g., three times a week) is useful in assessing whether nutrition needs are being met.

Personal hygiene and grooming. Some patients, especially those with OCD and phobias, may be excessively neat and engage in time-consuming rituals associated with bathing and dressing. Hygiene, dressing, and grooming may take several hours. Maintenance of skin integrity may become a problem when the rituals involve excessive washing and skin becomes excoriated and infected.

Some patients are indecisive about bathing or about what clothing should be worn. For the latter, limiting choices to two outfits is helpful. In the event of severe indecisiveness, simply presenting the patient with the clothing to be worn may be necessary. You may also need to remain with the patient to give simple directions: "Put on your shirt. Now put on your slacks." Matter-of-fact support is effective in assisting patients to perform as much of a task as possible independently. Encourage patients to express thoughts and feelings about self-care. This communication can provide a basis for later health teaching or for ongoing dialogue about the patient's abilities.

Elimination. Patients with OCD may be so involved with the performance of rituals that they may suppress the urge to void and defecate, sometimes resulting in constipation or urinary tract infections. Interventions may include creating a regular schedule for taking the patient to the bathroom.

Sleep. Patients experiencing anxiety frequently have difficulty sleeping. They may perform rituals to the exclusion of resting and sleeping, causing physical exhaustion. Those with GAD, PTSD, and acute stress disorder often experience sleep disturbance from nightmares. Teaching patients ways to promote sleep (e.g., warm bath, warm milk, relaxing music) and monitoring sleep through a sleep record are useful interventions. Chapter 20 offers an in-depth discussion of sleep disturbances.

Pharmacological Interventions

Several classes of medications have been found to be effective in the treatment of anxiety disorders. The Drug Treatment box identifies medications approved by Health Canada for the treatment of anxiety, as well as medications that do not have specific approval but are commonly used "off-label" for anxiety-related disorders. Review Chapter 11 for more detailed explanations of the actions of psychotropic medications.

Researchers are currently investigating the effectiveness of medications for the treatment of SSDs. Medication trials with antidepressants (including serotonin–norepinephrine reuptake inhibitors [SNRIs], such as venlafaxine [Effexor XR] and duloxetine [Cymbalta], and a noradrenergic and specific serotonergic antidepressant, such as mirtazapine [Remeron], have been effective in reducing the somatic symptoms, but further controlled trials are needed to determine the most effective antidepressants (Garcia-Martin et al., 2012). Patients may also benefit from short-term use of antianxiety medication, which must be monitored carefully because of the risk for dependence.

There are no specific medications used to treat patients with dissociative disorders, but medications are often prescribed for the presenting symptoms (International Society for the Study of Trauma and Dissociation, 2012). In the acute care setting intravenous benzodiazepines may be used to decrease intense anxiety; subsequently, the nurse may witness dramatic memory retrieval in patients with dissociative amnesia or fugue. Other medications sometimes prescribed are antidepressants, anxiolytics, and antipsychotics. As is the case whenever medications are prescribed, substance use disorders and potential suicidal risk must be assessed carefully prior to selecting a safe and appropriate medication.

DRUG TREATMENT OF PATIENTS WITH ANXIETY DISORDERS

Generic (Trade)	Health Canada–Approved Uses	Off-Label Uses
Antidepressants		
Selective serotonin reuptake inhibitors		
Citalopram hydrobromide (Celexa)		Panic disorder
		Social anxiety disorder
		Obsessive-compulsive disorder
		Generalized anxiety disorder
		Post-traumatic stress disorder
Escitalopram oxalate (Cipralex)	Generalized anxiety disorder	Panic disorder
		Social anxiety disorder
		Obsessive-compulsive disorder
		Post-traumatic stress disorder
Fluoxetine hydrochloride (Prozac)	Obsessive-compulsive disorder	Social anxiety disorder
		Generalized anxiety disorder
		Panic disorder
		Post-traumatic stress disorder

DRUG TREATMENT OF PATIENTS WITH ANXIETY DISORDERS

Generic (Trade)	Health Canada–Approved Uses	Off-Label Uses
Fluvoxamine maleate (Luvox)	Obsessive-compulsive disorder	Panic disorder Generalized anxiety disorder Post-traumatic stress disorder
Paroxetine hydrochloride (Paxil)	Social anxiety disorder Panic disorder Social anxiety disorder Obsessive-compulsive disorder Generalized anxiety disorder Post-traumatic stress disorder	
Sertraline hydrochloride (Zoloft)	Panic disorder Social anxiety disorder Obsessive-compulsive disorder Post-traumatic stress disorder	Generalized anxiety disorder
Selective serotonin–norepinephrine reuptake inhibitors		
Duloxetine hydrochloride (Cymbalta)	Panic disorder Generalized anxiety disorder	Obsessive-compulsive disorder Post-traumatic stress disorder
Venlafaxine hydrochloride (Effexor XR)	Generalized anxiety disorder Social anxiety disorder Panic disorder	Obsessive-compulsive disorder Post-traumatic stress disorder
Tricyclics		
Amitriptyline hydrochloride (Elavil)		Panic disorder Generalized anxiety disorder Post-traumatic stress disorder
Clomipramine hydrochloride (Anafranil)	Obsessive-compulsive disorder	Panic disorder Generalized anxiety disorder Post-traumatic stress disorder
Desipramine hydrochloride (Norpramin)		Panic disorder Generalized anxiety disorder Post-traumatic stress disorder
Doxepin hydrochloride (Adapin, Sinequan)		Panic disorder Generalized anxiety disorder Post-traumatic stress disorder
Imipramine hydrochloride (Tofranil)		Panic disorder Generalized anxiety disorder Post-traumatic stress disorder
Nortriptyline hydrochloride (Aventyl, Norventyl)		Panic disorder Generalized anxiety disorder Post-traumatic stress disorder
Monoamine oxidase inhibitors		
Phenelzine sulphate (Nardil)		Panic disorder Social anxiety disorder Generalized anxiety disorder Post-traumatic stress disorder
Tranylcypromine sulphate (Parnate)		Panic disorder Social anxiety disorder Generalized anxiety disorder Post-traumatic stress disorder
Antianxiety Agents *Benzodiazepines*		
Alprazolam (Xanax)	Panic disorder Generalized anxiety disorder	Social anxiety disorder
Chlordiazepoxide hydrochloride (Librax)		Panic disorder Social anxiety disorder Generalized anxiety disorder
Clonazepam (Rivotril)	Panic disorder	Generalized anxiety disorder Social anxiety disorder

DRUG TREATMENT OF PATIENTS WITH ANXIETY DISORDERS

Generic (Trade)	Health Canada–Approved Uses	Off-Label Uses
Diazepam (Valium)	Generalized anxiety disorder	Panic disorder
		Social anxiety disorder
Lorazepam (Ativan)		Panic disorder
		Social anxiety disorder
		Generalized anxiety disorder
Oxazepam (Serax)		Panic disorder
		Social anxiety disorder
		Generalized anxiety disorder
Nonbenzodiazepines		
Buspirone hydrochloride (Bustab)	Generalized anxiety disorder	Social anxiety disorder
		Obsessive-compulsive disorder
Other Classes		
Antihistamines		
Hydroxyzine hydrochloride (Atarax)		Generalized anxiety disorder
Hydroxyzine pamoate (Vistaril)		Generalized anxiety disorder
Beta blockers		
Atenolol (Tenormin)		Social anxiety disorder
Propranolol (Inderal)		Social anxiety disorder
Anticonvulsants		
Carbamazepine (Tegretol)		Post-traumatic stress disorder
		Panic disorder
Gabapentin (Neurontin)		Panic disorder
		Social anxiety disorder
		Generalized anxiety disorder
		Post-traumatic stress disorder
Valproic acid (Depakote)		Panic disorder
		Social anxiety disorder
		Generalized anxiety disorder
		Post-traumatic stress disorder

Sources: Health Canada. (2016). *Drug product database (DPD)*.https://www.hc-sc.gc.ca/dhp-mps/index-eng.php; and Schatzberg, A. F. (2017). *Textbook of psychopharmacology* (*DSM-5* ed.). Arlington: American Psychiatric Association Publishing.

Antidepressants. Antidepressants prescribed for anxiety have the secondary benefit of treating comorbid depressive disorders. Selective serotonin reuptake inhibitors (SSRIs) are the first-line treatment for acute stress disorders and PTSD (Schatzberg, 2017). Some of the SSRIs, however, exert more of an "activating" effect than others and therefore may increase anxiety. Sertraline (Zoloft) and paroxetine (Paxil) seem to have a more calming effect than do other SSRIs. SSRIs are preferable to the tricyclic antidepressants (TCAs) because they have a more rapid onset of action and fewer problematic adverse effects.

Monoamine oxidase inhibitors (MAOIs) are reserved for treatment-resistant conditions because of the risk for life-threatening hypertensive crisis in patients who do not follow dietary restrictions (e.g., to not eat foods containing tyramine). The risk for hypertensive crisis also makes the use of MAOIs contraindicated in patients with comorbid substance use.

Antianxiety drugs. Antianxiety drugs (also called anxiolytics) are often used to treat the somatic and psychological symptoms of anxiety disorders (Schatzberg, 2017). When moderate or severe anxiety is reduced, patients are better able to participate in treatment of any underlying problems. Benzodiazepines are most commonly used because they have a quick onset of action. However, due to the potential for dependence, these medications ideally should be used for short periods, only until other medications or treatments reduce symptoms. An important nursing intervention is to monitor for adverse effects of the benzodiazepines, including sedation, ataxia, and decreased cognitive function. Benzodiazepines are not recommended for patients with a known substance use problem and should not be given during pregnancy or lactation. Other important information for patients and their families is outlined in the Patient and Family Teaching box.

PATIENT AND FAMILY TEACHING

Antianxiety Medications

1. Caution the patient:
   - Not to increase dose or frequency of ingestion without prior approval of doctor
   - That these medications reduce the ability to handle mechanical equipment (e.g., cars, machinery)
   - Not to drink alcoholic beverages or take other antianxiety drugs, because depressant effects of both would be potentiated
   - To avoid drinking beverages containing caffeine, because they decrease the desired effects of the drug
2. Recommend that the patient taking benzodiazepines avoid becoming pregnant because these drugs increase the risk of congenital anomalies.
3. Advise the patient not to breastfeed while taking benzodiazepines because these drugs are excreted in the milk and would have adverse effects on the infant.

4. Teach a patient who is taking monoamine oxidase inhibitors the details of a tyramine-restricted diet.
5. Teach the patient that:
   - Cessation of benzodiazepines after 3 to 4 months of daily use may cause withdrawal symptoms such as insomnia, irritability, nervousness, dry mouth, tremors, convulsions, and confusion.
   - Medications should be taken with or shortly after meals or snacks to reduce gastrointestinal discomfort.
   - Drug interactions can occur: antacids may delay absorption; cimetidine interferes with metabolism of benzodiazepines, causing increased sedation; central nervous system depressants, such as alcohol and barbiturates, cause increased sedation; serum phenytoin concentration may build up because of decreased metabolism.

Buspirone (BuSpar) is an alternative antianxiety medication that does not cause dependence, but 2 to 4 weeks are required for it to reach full effect. The drug may be used for long-term treatment and should be taken regularly.

Other classes of medications. Other classes of medications sometimes used to treat anxiety disorders include beta blockers, antihistamines, and anticonvulsants. These agents are often added if the first course of treatment is ineffective. Beta blockers block the nerves that stimulate the heart to beat faster and have been used to treat SAD. Anticonvulsants have shown some benefit in the management of GAD, PD, PTSD, and SAD (Schatzberg, 2017). Antihistamines are a safe, nonaddictive alternative to benzodiazepines to lower anxiety levels, and again are helpful in treating patients with substance use problems.

Another therapeutic strategy may come in a most unusual form: D-cycloserine, an antibiotic used to treat tuberculosis, has also been demonstrated to enhance learning. D-cycloserine binds with *N*-methyl-D-aspartate (NMDA) receptors in the amygdala, the area of the brain that mediates fears and phobic responses, and may help patients unlearn fear responses more quickly. Administering this drug to a patient undergoing cognitive behavioural therapy (CBT) actually promotes fear extinction, not just fear conditioning, in phobic individuals. It has also been useful when combined with extinction-based exposure therapy in the treatment of OCD and SAD (Rodrigues et al., 2014).

Integrative Therapy

Chapter 35 identifies a number of complementary practices or integrative therapies that people use to cope with stress in their lives. Herbal and complementary therapy is popular in Canada; however, herbs and dietary supplements are not subject to the same rigorous testing as prescription medications. Also, herbs and dietary supplements are not required to be uniform, and there is no guaranteed bioequivalence of the active compound among preparations.

Problems that can occur with the use of psychotropic herbs include toxic adverse effects and herb–drug interactions. Nurses and other health care providers do well to improve their knowledge of these products so that discussions with their patients provide informed and reliable information. The Integrative Therapy box discusses kava kava, an herb often used for its sedative and antianxiety effects.

🌿 INTEGRATIVE THERAPY
Kava Kava

Kava kava is prepared from a South Pacific plant (*Piper methysticum*) and is marketed as an herbal sedative with antianxiety effects. Prior to seeking psychiatric treatment, patients with anxiety disorders may try kava kava in the belief that herbs are safer than medications, but it may have a darker side.

Kava kava is known to dramatically inhibit a liver enzyme (P450) necessary for the metabolism of many medications. This inhibition could result in liver failure, especially when taken along with alcohol or other medications such as central nervous system depressants (antianxiety agents fall into this category). This potentially dangerous interaction highlights the need for the nurse to ask about all medications the patient is taking, both prescribed and over-the-counter, before administering medications to those with anxiety disorders. Several countries have actually taken kava kava off the market, but some researchers believe that the benefits of this herb may outweigh the risks, compared to other medications used to treat anxiety.

The bottom line is that kava kava is considered to be beneficial for short-term use for mild to moderate anxiety. However, as with any drug, it should be used carefully.

Source: Chua, H. C., Christensen, E. T., Hoestgaard-Jensen, K., et al. (2016). Kavain, the major constituent of the anxiolytic kava extract, potentiates GABA$_A$ receptors: Functional characteristics and molecular mechanism. *PLoS ONE, 11*(6), e0157700. https://doi.org/10.1371/journal.pone.0157700

Advanced Interventions

Advanced-practice nurses may use various types of psychotherapy or provide consultation to primary care providers who treat patients with anxiety and related disorders. Because nursing has as a major focus viewing the patient in a holistic way, the advanced-practice nurse can lead the health care team in assessing each patient's unique biological, environmental, psychological, spiritual, and sociocultural needs to develop the most comprehensive, individualized plan of care to alleviate the distress of symptoms. Advanced-practice nurses build on basic nursing interventions and use more complex cognitive and behavioural treatment strategies, including modelling, systematic desensitization, flooding, response prevention, and thought stopping.

Managing both psychiatric and physical symptoms can be a challenge for general medical nurses. Psychiatric liaison nurses, a subspecialty of psychiatric mental health nursing initiated in the early 1960s, can bridge that gap. Usually, the psychiatric liaison nurse has a master's degree and a background in psychiatric and medical–surgical nursing. they function as a consultant assisting other nurses in managing psychiatric symptoms and as a clinician working directly to help the patient deal more effectively with physical and emotional problems. The psychiatric liaison nurse first meets with the nurse who initiated the consultation and then reviews the patient's medical records, talks with the physicians, and interviews the patient. After the patient interview, the liaison nurse discusses the assessment and suggestions with the referring nurse. If a psychiatric consultation is warranted, the psychiatric liaison nurse initiates the consultation by contacting the patient's physician. The liaison nurse will support general practice nurses to learn how to deliver more advanced intervention. A case conference is sometimes needed to enhance communication and consistency in the care of a particular patient.

Behavioural therapy. Beyond basic interventions, there are several forms of behavioural therapy currently used to decrease anxious or avoidant behaviour:

- **Modelling**—The therapist or significant other acts as a role model to demonstrate appropriate behaviour in a feared situation, and then the patient imitates it. For example, the role model rides in an elevator with a claustrophobic patient.
- **Systematic desensitization**—The patient is gradually introduced to a feared object or experience through a series of steps, from the least frightening to the most frightening (graduated exposure). The

patient is taught to use a relaxation technique at each step when anxiety becomes overwhelming. For example, a patient with agoraphobia would start with opening the door to the house to go out on the steps and advance to attending a movie in a theatre. The therapist may start with imagined situations in the office before moving on to in vivo (real-life) exposures.

- **Flooding**—Unlike systematic desensitization, flooding exposes the patient to a large amount of an undesirable stimulus in an effort to extinguish the anxiety response. The patient learns through prolonged exposure that survival is possible and that anxiety diminishes spontaneously. For example, an obsessive patient who usually touches objects with a paper towel may be forced to touch objects with a bare hand for 1 hour. By the end of that period, the anxiety level is lower.
- **Response prevention**—Patients with compulsive behaviour are not allowed to perform the compulsive ritual (e.g., handwashing), and the patient learns that anxiety subsides even when the ritual is not completed. After trying this activity in the office, the patient learns to set time limits at home to gradually lengthen the time between rituals until the urge fades away.
- **Thought stopping**—With this technique, a negative thought or obsession is interrupted. The patient may be instructed to say "Stop!" out loud when the idea comes to mind or to snap a rubber band worn on the wrist. This distraction briefly blocks the automatic undesirable thought and cues the patient to select an alternative, more positive idea. (After learning the exercise, the patient gives the command silently.)

Cognitive therapy. Advanced forms of cognitive therapy will build on the basic intervention of establishing that our thoughts have a link to our emotions. For example, "I have to be perfect or my boyfriend will not love me." Through a process called *cognitive restructuring*, the therapist helps the patient to (1) identify automatic negative beliefs that cause anxiety, (2) explore the basis for these thoughts, (3) re-evaluate the situation realistically, and (4) replace negative self-talk with supportive ideas.

Cognitive behavioural therapy. CBT is the most consistently supported treatment for the full spectrum of anxiety and related disorders. CBT combines cognitive therapy with specific behavioural therapies to reduce the anxiety responses and distress. CBT includes a combination of cognitive restructuring, psychoeducation, breathing, muscle relaxation, teaching of self-monitoring for symptoms, and in vivo (real-life) exposure to feared objects or situations. Refer to Chapter 4 for a more complete explanation of CBT. More information about CBT can be found in Chapters 4, 13, 16, 20, 27, and 33.

Somatic therapy. Verbal and body psychotherapies are seen as complementary interventions. A specific type of somatic psychotherapy, sensorimotor psychotherapy, combines talking therapy with body-centred interventions and movement to address the dissociative symptoms inherent in trauma (Ogden & Fisher, 2015). This type of therapy is integrated into phase-oriented trauma treatment to facilitate symptom reduction and stability, to integrate the traumatic memory, and to restore the person's ability to stay in the present moment. This therapy is based on the premise that the body, mind, emotions, and spirit are interrelated, and that a change at one level results in changes at the others. Being aware, focusing on the present, and recognizing touch as a means of communicating are some of the principles of this therapy. During psychotherapy sessions, the patient is asked to describe physical sensations they are experiencing. The goal is to safely disarm the pathological defence mechanism of dissociation and replace it with other resources, especially body awareness and mindfulness.

Evaluation

Evaluation of patients with anxiety-related disorders is a simple process when measurable behavioural outcomes have been written clearly and realistically. Each *NOC* outcome has a built-in rating scale that helps the nurse measure improvement. In general, evaluation of outcomes for patients with anxiety disorders deals with questions such as:

- Has patient safety been maintained?
- Is the patient experiencing a reduced level of anxiety or distress?
- Does the patient recognize symptoms as anxiety related?
- Does the patient continue to display obsessions, compulsions, phobias, worrying, or other symptoms of anxiety disorders? If still present, are they more or less frequent? More or less intense?
- Is the patient able to use newly learned behaviours to manage their symptoms?
- Can the patient adequately perform self-care activities?
- Can the patient maintain satisfying interpersonal relations?
- Can the patient assume usual roles?

KEY POINTS TO REMEMBER

- Anxiety has an unknown or unrecognized source, whereas fear is a reaction to a specific threat.
- Peplau operationally defined four levels of anxiety: mild, moderate, severe, and panic. The patient's perceptual field, ability to learn, and physical and other characteristics are different at each level (see Table 12.1).
- Defences against anxiety can be adaptive or maladaptive. Table 12.2 provides adaptive and maladaptive examples of the more common defence mechanisms.
- Anxiety, somatic symptom, or dissociative disorders frequently co-occur with mood disorders or substance use and addictive disorders.
- Research has identified genetic and biological factors in the etiology of anxiety and related disorders.
- Psychological theories and cultural influences are also pertinent to the understanding of anxiety and related disorders.
- People with anxiety disorders suffer from panic attacks, irrational fears, excessive worrying, uncontrollable rituals, or severe reactions to stress.
- Dissociative disorders involve a disruption in consciousness with a significant impairment in memory, identity, or perceptions of self.
- Nursing interventions include counselling, milieu therapy, promotion of self-care activities, psychobiological intervention, health teaching, and behavioural and cognitive behavioural therapies.
- Because these patients may not seek psychiatric treatment, the nurse does not usually see them in the acute psychiatric setting, except during a period of crisis such as suicidal risk.
- The nursing assessment is especially important to clarify the history and course of past symptoms, as well as to obtain a complete picture of the current physical and mental status.
- Although these patients do respond to crisis intervention, they usually require referral for longer-term treatment to attain sustained improvement in level of functioning.

CRITICAL THINKING

1. Ethan is in his final year of university and is taking his examinations for an engineering course. The professor catches him copying from the examination of his willing partner, Jessica, and takes his exam away. Ethan's heart immediately begins to pound, his pulse and respiration rates increase, and he has to wipe perspiration from his hands and face several times. He feels as if he needs to vomit

and has a throbbing in his head. When talking with the professor after the examination, he initially has difficulty focusing; when he starts to speak, his voice trembles. Ethan says that Jessica convinced him that cheating was done all the time, in fact, it was her idea. Ethan goes on to say that this "silly little exam" does not mean anything anyway, that he already passed the important courses. He tells the professor, "I thought you were the greatest, and now I see that you're a fool." The professor remains calm and explains that regardless of Ethan's thoughts on this matter, Ethan was caught cheating, he will have to take responsibility for his actions, and the choice to cheat was his. The professor will have Ethan go before the disciplinary board, which is the well-known procedure when one is caught cheating. When Ethan realizes that this incident could affect his graduating on time, he begins to yell at the professor and call him offensive names. Another professor walking past the classroom witnesses this encounter.
   a. Identify the level of anxiety Ethan was experiencing once he was caught cheating, and describe the signs and symptoms that helped you determine this level.
   b. Identify and define five defence mechanisms Ethan used to lessen his anxiety.
   c. Given the circumstances, once Ethan was caught, how could he have reacted using healthier coping defences in a manner that would have reflected more self-responsibility?
2. Ms. Halevy, a patient with OCD, washes her hands until they are cracked and bleeding. Your nursing goal is to promote healing of her hands. What interventions will you plan?
3. A patient with suspected somatic symptom disorder has been admitted to the medical–surgical unit after an episode of chest pain with possible electrocardiographic changes. She frequently complains of palpitations, asks the nurse to check her vital signs, and begs staff to stay with her. Some nurses take her pulse and blood pressure when she asks. Others evade her requests. Most staff members try to avoid spending time with her.
   a. How would you feel as a nurse in this situation? Consider why staff might wish to avoid her.
   b. Design interventions to cope with the patient's behaviours. Give rationales for your interventions.
4. How would you assess for anxiety in an adolescent who has repeated attacks of asthma prior to examinations at school?

CHAPTER REVIEW

1. Since learning that he will have a trial pass to a new group home tomorrow, Bill's behaviour has changed. He has started to pace rapidly, has become very distracted, and is breathing rapidly. He has trouble focusing on anything other than the group home issue and complains that he suddenly feels very nauseated. Which initial nursing response is most appropriate for Bill's level of anxiety?
   a. "You seem anxious. Would you like to talk about how you are feeling?"
   b. "If you do not calm down, I will have to give you medicine to calm you."
   c. "Bill, slow down. Listen to me. You are safe. Take a nice, deep breath."
   d. "We can delay the visit to the group home if that would help you calm down."
2. A patient who seems to be angry when his family again fails to visit as promised tells the nurse that he is fine and that the visit was not important to him anyway. When the nurse suggests that perhaps he might be disappointed or even a little angry that the family has again let him down, the patient responds that it is his family who is angry, not him, or else they would have visited. Which of the following defence mechanisms is this patient using to deal with his feelings?
   a. Rationalization.
   b. Introjection.
   c. Regression.
   d. Dissociation.
3. John, a construction worker, is on duty when a wall under construction suddenly falls, crushing a number of co-workers. Shaken initially, he seems to be coping well with the tragedy but later begins to experience tremors, nightmares, and periods during which he feels numb or detached from his environment. He finds himself frequently thinking about the tragedy and feeling guilty that he was spared while many others died. Which statement about this situation is most accurate?
   a. John is experiencing post-traumatic stress disorder (PTSD) and requires therapy.
   b. John has acute stress disorder and should be treated with antianxiety medications.
   c. John is experiencing anxiety and grief and should be monitored for PTSD symptoms.
   d. John is experiencing mild anxiety and a normal grief reaction; no intervention is needed.
4. A patient states that she has been ill for several months with stomach pain, headache, and dizziness. A review of her records shows that she has been tested repeatedly for various conditions. She has been diagnosed with dyspepsia and vertigo. She states that her pain is "10 out of 10" on a scale of 1 to 10. She has been treated in the past for anxiety and depression. Which condition should the nurse anticipate?
   a. Illness anxiety disorder.
   b. Somatic symptom disorder.
   c. Dissociation disorder.
   d. Generalized anxiety disorder.
5. An older person in the outpatient internal medicine clinic complains of feeling a sense of dread and fearfulness without apparent cause. It has been growing steadily worse and is to the point that it is interfering with the patient's sleep and volunteer work. After a brief interview and cursory physical exam, the nurse diagnoses the patient with generalized anxiety disorder and suggests a referral to the mental health clinic. Which responses by the medical clinic nurse would be the priority response?
   a. Complete the referral to the mental health clinic.
   b. Meet with the patient's family to discuss treatment options for generalized anxiety disorder.
   c. Instruct the patient in deep-breathing and basic cognitive behavioural techniques for coping with worry.
   d. Suggest that a battery of blood tests, including a complete blood count (CBC), be ordered and reviewed.

REFERENCES

Ackley, B., Ladwig, G., & Makic, B. F. (2017). *Nursing diagnosis handbook: An evidence-based guide to planning care* (11th ed.). St. Louis: Mosby/Elsevier.

Alonzi, S., La Torre, A., & Silverstein, M. W. (2020). The psychological impact of preexisting mental and physical health conditions during the COVID-19 pandemic. *Psychological Trauma: Theory, Research, Practice and Policy, 12*(S1), S236–S238. https://doi.org/10.1037/tra0000840

American Psychiatric Association. (2013). *Diagnostic and statistical manual of mental disorders* (5th ed.). Arlington: Author.

Benjamin, B., & Boyer, C. (2019). Canada's mental health agenda should address mental health in the workplace. *The Hill Times*. https://www.hilltimes.com/2019/10/07/canadas-mental-health-agenda-should-address-mental-health-in-the-workplace/217852

Bernstein, E. M., & Putnam, F. W. (1986). Development, reliability, and validity of a dissociation scale. *Journal of Nervous and Mental Disorders, 174*(12), 727–735. https://doi.org/10.1097/00005053-198612000-00004

Brand, B. L., Schielke, H. J., Putnam, K. T., et al. (2019). An online educational program for individuals with dissociative disorders and their clinicians: 1-year and 2-year follow-up. *Journal of Traumatic Stress, 32*(1), 156–166. https://doi.org/10.1002/jts.22370

Brown, R. J., & Lewis-Fernandez, R. (2011). Culture and conversion disorder: Implications for *DSM-5*. *Psychiatry: Interpersonal & Biological Processes, 74*(3), 187–206. https://doi.org/10.1521/psyc.2011.74.3.187

Burton, C., Fink, P., & Henningsen, P. EURONET-SOMA Group. (2020). Functional somatic disorders: Discussion paper for a new common classification for research and clinical use. *BMC Medicine, 18*(1), 1–7. https://doi-org.ezproxy.macewan.ca/10.1186/s12916-020-1505-4

Butcher, H. K., Bulechek, G. M., Dochterman, J. M., et al. (2019). *Nursing interventions classification (NIC)* (7th ed.). Toronto: Elsevier.

Chauvet-Gelinier, J., & Bonin, B. (2017). Stress, anxiety and depression in heart disease patients: A major challenge for cardiac rehabilitation. *Annals of Physical and Rehabilitation Medicine, 60*(1), 6–12. https://doi.org/10.1016/j.rehab.2016.09.002

Deimling, G. T., Albitz, C., Monnin, K., et al. (2017). Personality and psychological distress among older adult, long-term cancer survivors. *Journal of Psychosocial Oncology, 35*(1), 17–31. https://doi.org/10.1080/07347332.2016.1225145

Dozois, D. J. A. Mental Health Research Canada. (2020). Anxiety and depression in Canada during the COVID-19 pandemic: A national survey. *Canadian Psychology/Psychologie canadienne, 62*(1), 136–142. https://doi.org/10.1037/cap0000251

Falanga, R., & Pillot, L. (2019). Co-presence of a family doctor and psychologist in the management of patients with psychosocial and somatic symptom disorders. *Medical Science Pulse, 13*(4), 11–16. https://doi.org/10.5604/01.3001.0013.6016

Flaskerud, J. H. (2009). What do we need to know about culture-bound syndromes? *Issues in Mental Health Nursing, 30*, 406–407. https://doi.org/10.1080/01612840902812947

Foa, E. B., Kozak, M. J., Salkovskis, P. M., et al. (1998). The validation of a new obsessive compulsive disorder scale: The Obsessive Compulsive Inventory (OCI). *Psychological Assessment, 10*, 206–214.

Fuller-Thomson, E., Sulman, J., Brennenstuhl, S., et al. (2011). Functional somatic syndromes and childhood physical abuse in women: Data from a representative community-based sample. *Journal of Aggression, Maltreatment and Trauma, 20*, 445–469.

Garcia-Martin, I., Miranda-Vicario, E. M., & Soutullo, C. A. (2012). Duloxetine in the treatment of adolescents with somatoform disorders: A report of two cases. *Actas Espanolas de Psiquiatra, 20*(3), 165–168.

Goodman, W. K., Price, L. H., & Rasmussen, S. A. (1989). The Yale-Brown Obsessive Compulsive Scale. *Archives of General Psychiatry, 46*, 1006–1011.

Haase, M. (2002). Uncommon experiences: Living with obsessive compulsive disorder. In M. van Manen (Ed.), *Writing in the dark: Phenomenological studies in interpretive inquiry* (pp. 62–83). London: Althouse Press.

Hamilton, M. A. X. (1959). The assessment of anxiety states by rating. *British Journal of Medical Psychology, 32*(1), 50-55.

International Society for the Study of Trauma and Dissociation. (2012). Guidelines for treating dissociative identity disorder in adults (3rd rev.). *Journal of Trauma and Dissociation, 12*(2), 115–187. https://doi.org/10.1080/15299732.2011.537247

Kehler, D. S., Stammers, A. N., Horne, D., et al. (2019). Impact of preoperative physical activity and depressive symptoms on post-cardiac surgical outcomes. *PLoS ONE, 14*(2), 1–13. https://doi.org/10.1371/journal.pone.0213324

Kim, H. H., Lee, Y. J., Kim, H. K., et al. (2011). Prevalence and correlates of psychiatric symptoms in North Korean defectors. *Psychiatry Investigation, 8*(3), 179–185.

Korber, S., Frieser, D., Steinbrecher, N., et al. (2011). Classification characteristics of Patient Health Questionnaire-15 Screening for somatoform disorders in a primary care setting. *Journal of Psychosomatic Research, 71*, 142–147.

Lebel, S., Mutsaers, B., Tomei, C., et al. (2020). Health anxiety and illness-related fears across diverse chronic illnesses: A systematic review on conceptualization, measurement, prevalence, course, and correlates. *PLoS ONE, 15*(7), e0234124. https://doi.org/10.1371/journal.pone.0234124

Macaulay, C., Angus, L., Khattra, J., et al. (2017). Client retrospective accounts of corrective experience in motivational interviewing integrated with cognitive behavioral therapy for generalized anxiety disorder. *Journal of Clinical Psychology, 73*(2), 168–181. https://doi.org/10.1002/jclp.22430

Mental Health Commission of Canada. (2012). Changing directions, changing lives: The mental health strategy for Canada. strategy.mentalhealthcommission.ca/pdf/strategy-images-en.pdf.

Miller, L., Archer, R. L., & Kapoor, N. (2020). Conversion disorder: Early diagnosis and personalized therapy plan is the key. *Case Reports in Neurological Medicine, 2020*, 1967581. https://doi.org/10.1155/2020/1967581

Moorhead, S., Johnson, M., Maas, M., et al. (2018). *Nursing Outcomes Classification (NOC)* (6th ed.). St. Louis: Mosby.

Ogden, P., & Fisher, J. (2015). *Sensorimotor psychotherapy: Interventions for trauma and attachment*. New York: Norton Professional Books.

Pearson, C., Zamorski, M., & Janz, T. (2014). *Health at a glance: Mental health of the Canadian Armed Forces*. Ottawa: Statistics Canada.

Peplau, H. E. (1968). A working definition of anxiety. In S. F. Burd, & M. A. Marshall (Eds.), *Some clinical approaches to psychiatric nursing* (pp. 323–327). New York: Macmillan.

Public Health Agency of Canada. (2016). Report summary: Mood and anxiety disorders in Canada, 2016. https://www.canada.ca/content/dam/phac-aspc/migration/phac-aspc/publicat/hpcdp-pspmc/36-12/assets/pdf/ar-05-eng.pdf

Rodrigues, H., Figueira, I., Lopes, A., et al. (2014). Does D-cycloserine enhance exposure therapy for anxiety disorders in humans? A meta-analysis. *PLoS ONE, 9*(7), e93519. https://doi.org/10.1371/journal.pone.0093519

Schatzberg, A. F. (2017). *Textbook of psychopharmacology (DSM-5 ed.)*. Arlington: American Psychiatric Association Publishing.

Schlozman, S. C., Nonacs, R. M., et al. (2008). Dissociative disorders. In T. A. Stern, J. F. Rosenbaum, & M. Fava et al (Eds.), *Massachusetts General Hospital comprehensive clinical psychiatry* (pp. 481–486). St. Louis: Mosby.

Selye, H. (1956). What is stress?. *Metabolism: Clinical and Experimental, 5*(5), 525–530.

Shear, M. K., Brown, T. A., Barlow, D. H., et al. (1997). Multicenter collaborative panic disorder severity scale. *American Journal of Psychiatry, 154*(11), 1571–1575. https://doi.org/10.1176/ajp.154.11.1571

Sinopoli, V. M., Erdman, L., Burton, C. L., et al. (2019). Serotonin system genes and obsessive-compulsive trait dimensions in a population-based, pediatric sample: A genetic association study. *Journal of Child Psychology & Psychiatry, 60*(12), 1289–1299. https://doi.org/10.1111/jcpp.13079

Soltis-Jarrett, V. M. (2010). His-story or her-story: Deconstruction of the concepts of somatization towards a new approach in advanced nursing practice care. *Perspectives in Psychiatric Care, 47*(4), 183–193. https://doi.org/10.1111/j.1744-6163.2010.00288.x

Spiegel, D., Loewenstein, R., Lewis-Fernandez, R., et al. (2011). Dissociative disorders in *DSM-5*. *Depression and Anxiety, 28*, 824–852. https://doi.org/10.1002/da.20874

Statistics Canada. (2020). Canadians' mental health during the COVID-19 pandemic. *The Daily*. https://www150.statcan.gc.ca/n1/daily-quotidien/200527/dq200527b-eng.htm

Sullivan, H. S. (1953). *The interpersonal theory of psychiatry*. New York: W. W. Norton.

Torvik, Rosenström, T. H., Gustavson, K., Ystrom, E., Kendler, K. S., Bramness, J. G., Czajkowski, N., & Reichborn-Kjennerud, T. (2019). Explaining the association between anxiety disorders and alcohol use disorder: A twin study. *Depression and Anxiety, 36*(6), 522–532. https://doi.org/10.1002/da.22886

Tyrer, P. (2020). COVID-19 health anxiety. *World Psychiatry, 19*(3), 307–308. https://doi.org/10.1002/wps.20798

Usher, K., Durkin, J., & Bhullar, N. (2019). Eco-anxiety: How thinking about climate change-related environmental decline is affecting our mental health. *International Journal of Mental Health Nursing, 28*(6), 1233–1234. https://doi.org/10.1111/inm.12673

Wawer, E., Viprey, M., Floccard, B., et al. (2020). Early detection of patients at risk of developing a post-traumatic stress disorder after an ICU stay. *Critical Care Medicine, 48*(11), 1572–1579. https://doi.org/10.1097/CCM.0000000000004551

Yakobov, E., Jurcik, T., Sullivan, M. L., et al. (2017). Conversion disorder. In M. A. Budd, S. Hough, S. T. Wegener et al. (Eds.), *Practical psychology in medical rehabilitation* (pp. 277–285). Cham: Springer International Publishing.

13
Depressive Disorders

Cheryl L. Pollard
Originating US chapter by Margaret Jordan Halter

 https://evolve.elsevier.com/Canada/Varcarolis/psychiatric/

OBJECTIVES

1. Compare and contrast major depressive disorder and persistent depressive disorder (dysthymia).
2. Discuss the origins of depression.
3. Assess behaviours in a patient with depression with regard to each of the following areas: (1) affect, (2) thought processes, (3) feelings, (4) physical behaviour, and (5) communication.
4. Formulate five nursing diagnoses for a patient with depression, and include outcome criteria.
5. Name unrealistic expectations a nurse may have while working with a patient with depression, and compare them to your own personal thoughts.
6. Demonstrate six principles of communication useful in working with patients with depression.
7. Identify major classifications of antidepressants and general advantages and disadvantages of each.
8. Develop a medication teaching plan for a patient taking an antidepressant, including adverse effects, toxic reactions, and other drugs or foods that can trigger an adverse reaction.
9. Write a nursing care plan incorporating the recovery model of mental health.
10. Discuss non-pharmaceutical interventions for major depressive disorder such as electroconvulsive therapy (ECT).

KEY TERMS AND CONCEPTS

affect
anergia
anger
anhedonia
Beck's cognitive triad
depressive disorder due to another medical condition
diathesis–stress model of depression
disruptive mood dysregulation disorder
electroconvulsive therapy
hypersomnia
learned helplessness
light therapy
major depressive disorder
mood disorders
persistent depressive disorder
premenstrual dysphoric disorder
psychomotor agitation
psychomotor retardation
serotonin syndrome
substance/medication-induced depressive disorder
suicidal ideation
transcranial magnetic stimulation
vagus nerve stimulation
vegetative signs of depression

No textbook chapter can adequately convey the personal pain and suffering experienced by the individual with depression, not to mention the pain, helplessness, and frustration felt by the affected individual's friends and loved ones. However, it is essential for nursing students to gain a fundamental understanding of mood disorders. **Mood disorders** (also called affective disorders) are a group of psychiatric disorders including depression and bipolar disorder. People of all ethnicities, cultures, ages, socioeconomic groups, education levels, and geographic areas are susceptible to depressive episodes, but some individuals are more susceptible than others. Virtually all nurses will come into contact with patients with depression or whose primary needs are complicated by depression. This chapter includes basic information and therapeutic tools that will facilitate the care of patients with depression.

CLINICAL PICTURE

Major depressive disorder (MDD) is one of the most common psychiatric disorders. Women experience depression approximately two times more often than men (Government of Canada, 2016) and approximately one in eight adults (12.6%) have identified symptoms that met the criteria for a

 HOW A NURSE HELPED ME
Diagnosed but Not Forgotten

After months of my not having any interest in doing anything and withdrawing from friends and family, my husband took me to the hospital emergency department, where I was admitted to the hospital's mental health unit and diagnosed with major depressive disorder (MDD). While major depression is common, I believed that this diagnosis would change my life. During my 2 weeks in hospital, psychiatric nurses helped me to understand the distorted beliefs I had about myself and others. Outside of the one-on-one time with the nurses, they taught me how to incorporate yoga and exercise in my treatment plan. Initially, because of my fear of gaining weight, I wanted to stop taking my venlafaxine (Effexor XR), but the nurses taught me about the importance of taking my medications even once I was feeling better. The nurses also helped me to identify a support system. My husband and girlfriend help me along when I want to give up. I also attend a monthly depression group, and if I feel as though I am slipping back into a depression, I know I can call the mental health clinic or speak to the psychiatric nurse in the emergency department. It has been 10 years since I was diagnosed with major depression, and there are still times when I need help; however, I know that my life has changed and is not over.

mood disorder at some point during their lifetime. Depression is the leading cause of disability worldwide (Jakobsen et al., 2020). MDD, or major depression, is characterized by a persistently depressed mood lasting for a minimum of 2 weeks. The length of a depressive episode may vary. About 20% of cases become chronic (i.e., lasting more than 2 years). While depression begins with a single occurrence, most people experience recurrent episodes. People experience a recurrence within the first year about 50% of the time and within a lifetime up to 85% of the time. The full criteria for MDD are listed in *Diagnostic and Statistical Manual of Mental Disorders, fifth edition (DSM-5)*: Diagnostic Criteria for Major Depressive Disorder.

The diagnosis for MDD may include one of the following specifiers to describe the most recent episode of depression:

- **Psychotic features.** Indicates the presence of disorganized thinking, delusions (e.g., delusions of guilt or of being punished for sins, somatic delusions of horrible disease or body rotting, delusions of poverty or going bankrupt), or hallucinations (usually auditory, voices berating person for sins).
- **Melancholic features.** This outdated term indicates a severe form of endogenous depression (not attributable to environmental stressors) characterized by severe apathy, weight loss, profound guilt, symptoms that are worse in the morning, early morning awakening, and often suicidal ideation.
- **Atypical features.** Refers to dominant vegetative symptoms (e.g., overeating, oversleeping). Onset is younger, psychomotor activities are slow, and anxiety is often an accompanying problem, which may cause misdiagnosis.
- **Catatonic features.** Marked by non-responsiveness, extreme psychomotor retardation (may seem paralyzed), withdrawal, and negativity.
- **Postpartum onset.** Indicates onset within 4 weeks after childbirth. It is common for psychotic features to accompany this depression. Severe ruminations or delusional thoughts about the infant signify increased risk of harm to the infant.
- **Seasonal features (seasonal affective disorder [SAD]).** Indicates that episodes mostly begin in fall or winter and remit in spring. These patients have reduced cerebral metabolic activity. SAD is characterized by anergia (lack of energy or passivity), hypersomnia (excessive daytime sleep), overeating, weight gain, and a craving for carbohydrates; it responds to light therapy.

While the focus in this chapter is MDD, you should also be aware of several other depressive disorders:

- Disruptive mood dysregulation disorder
- Persistent depressive disorder (dysthymia)
- Pre-menstrual dysphoric disorder
- Substance/medication-induced depressive disorder
- Depressive disorder due to another medical condition

Disruptive Mood Dysregulation Disorder

Disruptive mood dysregulation disorder is a disorder characterized by severe and recurrent temper outbursts that are inconsistent with developmental level. This disorder was introduced in 2013 in response to an alarming number of children and adolescents being diagnosed with bipolar disorder. A bipolar diagnosis resulted in exposure to powerful medications that probably were not helping and a lifelong label of serious mental illness. Perhaps the most compelling reason to change this diagnostic practice was that most of the young people who received a diagnosis of bipolar disorder did not go on to exhibit classic bipolar symptoms as adults. In fact, most children and adolescents once diagnosed with bipolar disorder actually converted to MDD or an anxiety disorder in adulthood.

The basic symptoms of disruptive mood dysregulation disorder are constant and severe irritability and anger in individuals between the ages of 6 and 18. Onset is before age 10. Temper tantrums with verbal or behavioural outbursts out of proportion to the situation occur at least three times a week. Sometimes children and adolescents with this

---

DSM-5
Diagnostic Criteria for Major Depressive Disorder

A. Five (or more) of the following symptoms have been present during the same 2-week period and represent a change from previous functioning; at least one of the symptoms is either (1) depressed mood or (2) loss of interest of pleasure.
   Note: Do not include symptoms that are clearly attributable to another medical condition.
   1. Depressed mood most of the day, nearly every day, as indicated by either subjective report (e.g., feels sad, empty, hopeless) or observation made by others (e.g., appears tearful). (**Note:** In children and adolescents it can be irritable mood.)
   2. Markedly diminished interest or pleasure in all, or almost all, activities most of the day, nearly every day (as indicated by either subjective account or observation).
   3. Significant weight loss when not dieting or weight gain (e.g., a change of more than 5% of body weight in a month) or decrease or increase in appetite nearly every day. (**Note:** In children consider failure to make expected weight gain.)
   4. Insomnia or hypersomnia nearly every day.
   5. Psychomotor agitation or retardation nearly every day (observable by others, not merely subjective feelings of restlessness or being slowed down).
   6. Fatigue or loss of energy nearly every day.
   7. Feelings of worthlessness or excessive or inappropriate guilt (which may be delusional) nearly every day (not merely self-reproach or guilt about being sick).
   8. Diminished ability to think or concentrate or indecisiveness nearly every day (either by subjective account or as observed by others).
   9. Recurrent thoughts of death (not just fear of dying), recurrent suicidal ideation without a specific plan, or a suicide attempt or a specific plan for suicide.

B. The symptoms cause clinically significant distress or impairment in social, occupational, or other important areas of functioning.

C. The episode is not attributable to the physiological effects of a substance or to another medical condition.
   Note: Criteria A through C represent a major depressive episode.
   Note: Responses to a significant loss (bereavement, financial ruin, losses from a natural disaster, a serious medical illness or disability) may include the feelings of intense sadness, rumination about the loss, insomnia, poor appetite, and weight loss as noted in Criterion A, which may resemble a depressive episode. Although such symptoms may be understandable or considered appropriate to the loss, the presence of a major depressive episode in addition to the normal response to a significant loss should also be carefully considered. This decision inevitably requires the exercise of clinical judgment based on the individual's history and the cultural norms for the expression of distress in the context of loss.

D. The occurrence of the major depressive episode is not better explained by schizoaffective disorder, schizophrenia, schizophreniform disorder, delusional disorder, or other specified and unspecified schizophrenia spectrum and other psychotic disorders.

E. There has never been a manic or a hypomanic episode.
   Note: This exclusion does not apply to all of the manic-like or hypomanic-like episodes that are substance induced or are attributable to the physiological effects of another medical condition.

Source: American Psychiatric Association. (2013). *Diagnostic and statistical manual of mental disorders* (5th ed.). Arlington: Author.

problem can maintain control in certain settings such as school. To be diagnosed with disruptive mood dysregulation disorder, individuals need to exhibit the irritability, anger, and temper tantrums in at least two of these settings: home, school, and with peers.

The prevalence rate for disruptive mood dysregulation disorder is believed to fall in the range of 2% to 5%. It is more common in males than females, and it is more common in children than adolescents.

There is little information available on the treatment of disruptive mood dysregulation disorder. Boland (2021) suggests a symptom-based approach. If the disorder resembles major depression, antidepressants may be considered. If the disorder is accompanied by attention-deficit/hyperactivity disorder (ADHD), medications for that condition could be tried. Antidepressants may be used to address irritability. The second-generation antipsychotics risperidone (Risperdal) and aripiprazole (Abilify) have approval from Health Canada for irritability in autism and are sometimes used for disruptive mood dysregulation disorder.

Psychosocial interventions such as cognitive behavioural therapy (CBT) are essential considering the degree of turmoil this disorder brings about. Parent training helps parents to interact with a child in such a way as to predict and reduce aggression and irritability through consistency and rewarding appropriate behaviour. There is some evidence that these young people may be misperceiving others' facial expressions as angry. Computer-based training can help them become more aware of the meaning of facial expressions.

Persistent Depressive Disorder

Persistent depressive disorder (dysthymia) is diagnosed when feelings of depression occur most of the day, for the majority of days. These low-level depressive feelings last at least 2 years in adults and 1 year in children and adolescents. In addition to depressed mood, individuals with this disorder have at least two of the following: decreased appetite or overeating, insomnia or hypersomnia, low energy, poor self-esteem, difficulty thinking, and hopelessness.

The symptoms are difficult for the patient to live with and bring about social and occupational distress, but they are usually not severe enough to require hospitalization. Because the onset of persistent depressive disorder usually occurs in teenage years, patients frequently express that they have "always felt this way" and that being depressed seems like a normal way of functioning. It is not uncommon for people with this low-level depression to also have periods of full-blown major depressive episodes.

The one year prevalence of persistent depressive disorder in the Canadian population ranges from 0.5% to 1.5%. The problem tends to have an early onset and, as the name suggests, it is a chronic illness.

Treatment for this disorder is similar to that for MDD, which we discuss in more depth later in this chapter. Psychotherapy, particularly CBT, is quite useful in managing symptoms. Antidepressants such as selective serotonin reuptake inhibitors (SSRIs), serotonin–norepinephrine reuptake inhibitors (SNRIs), and tricyclics are the other main treatments.

Premenstrual Dysphoric Disorder

Premenstrual dysphoric disorder is a relatively new addition to the diagnostic system for psychiatry. It refers to a cluster of symptoms that occur in the last week before the onset of a menstrual period. Premenstrual dysphoric disorder causes problems severe enough to interfere with the ability to work or interact with others. Symptoms include mood swings, irritability, depression, anxiety, feeling overwhelmed, and difficulty concentrating. Other physical manifestations include lack of energy, overeating, hypersomnia or insomnia, breast tenderness, aching, bloating, and weight gain. Symptoms decrease significantly or disappear with the onset of menstruation.

The prevalence of premenstrual dysphoric disorder is about 2% to 6% of menstruating people. Symptoms cease after menopause, although they may return with hormone replacement therapy.

Treatment for this disorder includes regular exercise, particularly aerobic exercise. Other recommendations include eating food rich in complex carbohydrates and getting sufficient sleep. Acupuncture, light therapy, and relaxation therapy have also been used to reduce symptoms.

Several drugs have Health Canada approval for treatment of this disorder. A drospirenone and ethinyl estradiol combination (Yaz) is a contraceptive that improves symptoms. Fluoxetine (Prozac), sertraline (Zoloft), and controlled-release paroxetine (Paxil CR) have been used successfully. Diuretics may be useful in reducing bloating and weight gain brought on by water retention.

Substance/Medication-Induced Depressive Disorder

Substance/medication-induced depressive disorder is a depressive disorder, such as MDD, that is a result of prolonged use of or withdrawal from drugs and alcohol. The depressive symptoms last longer than the expected length of physiological effects, intoxication, or withdrawal of the substance. The person with this diagnosis would not experience depressive symptoms in the absence of drug or alcohol use or withdrawal. Symptoms appear within 1 month of use. Once the substance is removed, depressive symptoms usually remit within a few days to several weeks.

The lifetime prevalence rate is fairly low, about 0.25%. Medications associated with depressive symptoms include antiviral agents, cardiovascular drugs, retinoic acid derivatives, antidepressants, anticonvulsants, antimigraine agents, antipsychotics, hormonal agents, smoking cessation agents, and immunological agents.

Depressive Disorder due to Another Medical Condition

Depressive disorder due to another medical condition may be caused by disorders that affect the body's systems or from long-term illnesses that cause ongoing pain. The depressive symptoms are the same as the diagnostic criteria for the depressive disorders. It is important to review medications being used for the medical condition to rule out them being the causative agents.

There are clear associations, along with neuroanatomical changes, with some disease states. The prevalence rate of depression in people who have suffered a cerebrovascular accident (stroke) is high, 20% to 50%, in the first year (Lanctot et al., 2020). Parkinson's disease, Huntington's disease, Alzheimer's disease, and traumatic brain injury are also clearly associated with depressive disorders. Neuroendocrine conditions such as Cushing's disease and hypothyroidism are also commonly accompanied by depression. Arthritis, back pain, metabolic conditions (e.g., vitamin B_{12} deficiency), human immunodeficiency virus (HIV), diabetes, infection (including COVID-19), cancer, and autoimmune problems may also contribute to depressions. Table 13.1 summarizes medical problems and substances that are associated with major depression.

Depression and Grieving

People who experience a significant loss can exhibit feelings and behaviours similar to depression. They may cry, feel hopeless about the future, have disruptions in eating and sleeping, and lose pleasure in everyday activities. They may even experience a lack interest in caring for themselves and neglect normal hygiene. At what point does grief become pathological? This is a controversial question and one that is not easily answered.

Until recently, clinicians were advised against diagnosing a person with depression in the first 2 months following a significant loss. This was called the bereavement exclusion. The rationale for avoiding a psychiatric diagnosis follows:

TABLE 13.1 Medical Conditions and Substances or Medications Associated With Major Depressive Disorder

Substances or Medication	
Central nervous system depressants	Alcohol, barbiturates, benzodiazepines, clonidine
Central nervous system medications	Amantadine, bromocriptine, levodopa, phenothiazines, phenytoin
Psychostimulants	Amphetamines
Systemic medications	Corticosteroids, digoxin, diltiazem, enalapril, ethionamide, isotretinoin, mefloquine, methyldopa, metoclopramide, quinolones, reserpine, statins, thiazides, vincristine
Medical Conditions	
Neurological	Epilepsy, Parkinson's disease, multiple sclerosis, Alzheimer's disease, Huntington's disease, traumatic brain injury, cerebrovascular accident
Infectious or inflammatory	Neurosyphilis, human immunodeficiency virus (HIV)
Cardiac disorders	Ischemic heart disease, cardiac failure, cardiomyopathies
Endocrine	Hypothyroidism, diabetes mellitus, vitamin deficiencies, parathyroid disorders
Inflammatory disorders	Collagen vascular diseases, irritable bowel syndrome, chronic liver disorders
Neoplastic disorders	Central nervous system tumours, paraneoplastic syndromes

1. Normal mourning could be labelled pathological.
2. A psychiatric diagnosis could result in a lifelong label.
3. Unnecessary medications might be prescribed.

Although controversial, a diagnosis of depression can now be given in the first 2 months following death of a loved one or other loss. The reason for the change is that grief, like other stressors, can result in depression. For some people, waiting 2 months for an official diagnosis of major depression may delay treatment and adversely affect prognosis. Further research about grief may clarify diagnostic categories and prevent overdiagnosis of depression in the presence of grief. See Chapter 31 for more on mental health and illness in grief and loss.

CONSIDERING CULTURE

Suicide and Suicide Prevention Among Inuit in Canada

Inuit in Canada have among the highest suicide rates in the world, and suicide occurs primarily among their youth. Risk factors include known ones such as depression, substance use, a history of abuse, and knowing others who have made attempts or have killed themselves; however, of importance are the negative effects of colonialism. Multiple generations are affected by historical trauma. The origins of this trauma took place for Inuit primarily during the government era starting in the 1950s, when Inuit were moved from their family-based land camps to crowded settlements run by White men, and children were removed from their parents and placed in residential or day schools. This caused more disorganization than reorganization within their family-based collectivist culture. The most negative effect of this rapid culture change brought about by colonialism and imperialism for Inuit has been on their relationships. There have been changes in parenting practices, domestic violence rates, and language loss. Many Inuit youth feel alone and rejected. Their relational bond, ungajuk, or sense of belonging, ilagijauttiarniq, has been disrupted.

Suicide prevention programs that include the involvement of elders and connecting with the land through family-focused activities have been the most successful. Connecting with their family members and friends has been identified as an important factor in building resilience among Inuit youth. Western suicide prevention programs, when used without integrating Indigenous knowledge, have not been effective, as suicide rates continued to rise when these programs were used. Canada's National Aboriginal Youth Suicide Prevention Strategy, which was developed in partnership with Indigenous organizations, has supported the Indigenous reclamation of control over their lives.

Mental health factors for Indigenous peoples are often cultural. It is recommended that health care practitioners work with the community and with Indigenous organizations. Empowered communities can be healing through identifying individual responsibility and acknowledging historical and current injustices.

Source: Kral, M. J. (2016). Suicide and suicide prevention among Inuit in Canada. *The Canadian Journal of Psychiatry, 61*(11), 688–695. https://doi.org/10.1177/0706743716661329

EPIDEMIOLOGY

Depression is the leading cause of disability in the world. The lifetime prevalence of a major depressive episode or the total number of adults in Canada who will experience the disorder within their lifetime is 11.3% (Jakobsen et al., 2020). The average age of MDD onset is between 15 and 45 years of age. Studies find that mood disorders are more common in women than men (Jakobsen et al., 2020). See Figure 13.1 for rates of depression in Canada. Several Canadian studies found that MDD tends to have higher prevalence rates in lower-income or unemployed populations and unmarried or divorced people.

Children and Adolescents

Children as young as 3 years of age have been diagnosed with depression; however, the prevalence is relatively low, with little difference between boys and girls. Levels rise in the early teen years, more sharply among girls than boys (Scaini et al., 2020). This is especially troubling since a youth onset carries a high recurrence rate, setting the stage for lifelong periods of depression. In the last edition of the *Diagnostic and Statistical Manual of Mental Disorders (DSM-5)*, disruptive mood dysregulation disorder was added to represent the presentation of irritability and frequent episodes of uncontrolled behaviour in an attempt to deal with the potential of children being misdiagnosed with schizophrenia, a personality disorder, or bipolar disorder (American Psychiatric Association, 2013).

Older Persons

Although depression in older persons is common, it is *not* a normal result of aging. The risk for depression in the elderly increases as health deteriorates. About 1% to 5% of older persons who live in the community have depression. This statistic rises to 11.5% for hospitalized older persons and 13.5% for those requiring home care (Mood Disorders Society of Canada, 2019). A disproportionate number of older persons with depression are likely to die by suicide.

Many older persons suffer from *subsyndromal depression* in which they experience many, but not all, of the symptoms of a major depressive episode. These individuals have an increased risk of eventually developing major depression. Sometimes the psychomotor slowing and cognitive effects of depression lead others to believe that the older

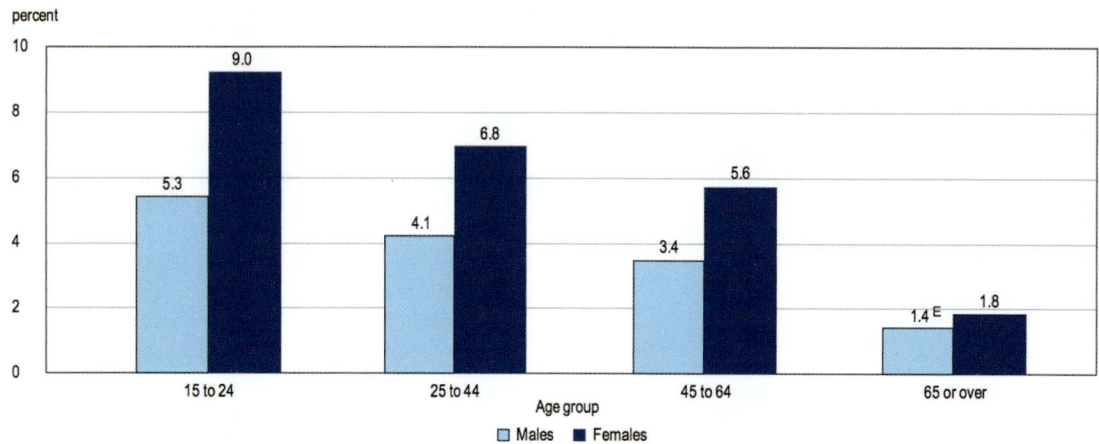

Fig. 13.1 Rates of depression, 12-month, by age and sex, Canada, household population 15 and older, 2012 use with caution (these data have a coefficient variation from 1.6.6% to 33.3%). Respondents were classified with depression if they met the criteria for this condition in the 12 months prior to the survey. (**Source:** Statistics Canada. [2013]. *Canadian Community Health Survey: Mental health, 2012.* Ottawa: Author.)

person is developing a neurocognitive disorder such as Alzheimer's disease. This condition is referred to as pseudodementia, a problem that can be reversed when the underlying depression is treated and eliminated.

COMORBIDITY

A depressive syndrome frequently accompanies other psychiatric disorders, such as anxiety disorders, schizophrenia, substance use, eating disorders, and schizoaffective disorder. People with anxiety disorders (e.g., panic disorder, generalized anxiety disorder, obsessive-compulsive disorder) commonly present with depression, as do people with personality disorders (particularly borderline personality disorder), adjustment disorder, and brief depressive reactions.

The combination of anxiety and depression is perhaps one of the most common psychiatric presentations. Symptoms of anxiety occur in an average of 70% of cases of major depression. Some clinicians believe that mixed anxiety and depression should be a stand-alone diagnosis and be treated as a distinct entity.

ETIOLOGY

Although many theories attempt to explain the cause of depression, many psychological, biological, and cultural variables make identification of any one cause difficult; furthermore, it is unlikely that there is a single cause of depression. The high variability in symptoms, response to treatment, and course of the illness support the supposition that depression results from a complex interaction of causes. For example, genetic predisposition to the illness combined with childhood stress may lead to significant changes in the central nervous system (CNS) that result in depression. However, there seem to be several common risk factors for depression, listed in Box 13.1.

Biological Factors
Genetic
Twin studies consistently show that genetic factors play a role in the development of depressive disorders. The concordance rate for MDD among monozygotic (identical) twins is nearly 50%. That is, if one twin is affected, the second has about a 50% chance of being affected as well. It is likely that multiple genes are involved, each one having a small but

> **BOX 13.1 Risk Factors for Depression**
>
> - Female gender
> - Early childhood trauma
> - Stressful life events
> - Family history of depression, especially in first-degree relatives
> - High levels of neuroticism (a negative personality trait characterized by anxiety, fear, moodiness, worry, envy, frustration, jealousy, and loneliness)
> - Other disorders such as substance use, anxiety, and personality disorders
> - Chronic or disabling medical conditions

substantial role in the development and severity of depression. For instance, certain genetic markers seem to be related to depression when accompanied by early childhood maltreatment or a history of stressful life events. In this case there is no gene directly related to the development of the mood disorder; however, there is a genetic marker associated with depression in the context of stressful life events.

One of the more important aspects of understanding the role of genetics in relation to mental illness such as major depression may be in pharmacological treatments. Understanding genetic influences on the role of the transport of certain neurotransmitters, such as serotonin, across synapses will make it much easier to prescribe effective medical treatment of depression based on individual genetic patterns.

Biochemical
The brain is a highly complex organ that contains billions of neurons. There is much evidence to support the concept that many CNS neurotransmitter abnormalities may cause clinical depression. These neurotransmitter abnormalities may be the result of genetic or environmental factors or other medical conditions, such as cerebral infarction, Parkinson's disease, hypothyroidism, acquired immunodeficiency syndrome (AIDS), or drug use.

Two of the main neurotransmitters involved in mood are serotonin (5-hydroxytryptamine [5-HT]) and norepinephrine. Serotonin is an important regulator of sleep, appetite, and libido. Therefore serotonin circuit dysfunction can result in sleep disturbances, decreased appetite, low sex drive, poor impulse control, and irritability. Norepinephrine modulates attention and behaviour. It is stimulated by stressful situations, which may result in overuse and a deficiency of norepinephrine. A deficiency, an imbalance as compared with other neurotransmitters, or an impaired ability to use available norepinephrine can result in apathy, reduced responsiveness, or slowed psychomotor activity.

Research suggests that depression results from the dysregulation of a number of neurotransmitter systems beyond serotonin and norepinephrine. For example, glutamate is a common neurotransmitter that increases the ability of a nerve fibre to transmit information. A deficit in glutamate can interfere with normal neuron transmission in the areas of the brain that affect mood, attention, and cognition.

Stressful life events, especially losses, seem to be a significant factor in the development of depression. Norepinephrine, serotonin, and acetylcholine play a role in stress regulation. When these neurotransmitters become overtaxed through stressful events, neurotransmitter depletion may occur. Research indicates that stress is associated with a reduction in neurogenesis, which is the ability of the brain to produce new brain cells.

At this time, no single mechanism of depressant action has been found. The relationships among the serotonin, norepinephrine, dopamine, acetylcholine, gamma-aminobutyric acid (GABA), and glutamate systems are complex and need further assessment and study. However, treatment with medication that helps regulate these neurotransmitters has proven to be empirically successful in the treatment of many patients. Figure 13.2 shows a positron emission tomography (PET) scan of the brain of a woman with depression before and after taking medication.

Hormonal

The neuroendocrine characteristic most widely studied in relation to depression has been hyperactivity of the hypothalamic–pituitary–adrenal axis. People with major depression have increased urine cortisol levels and elevated levels of corticotrophin-releasing hormone. Dexamethasone, an exogenous steroid that suppresses cortisol, is used in the dexamethasone suppression test (DST) for depression. Results of this test are abnormal in about 50% of people with depression, which indicates hyperactivity of the hypothalamic–pituitary–adrenal axis.

Depression rates are almost equal for males and females in the years preceding puberty and in older persons. The lifetime rate of depression is 2 times greater in women with child-bearing potential than in men (Mood Disorders Society of Canada, 2019). As the relationships between sex hormones such as estrogen in women and testosterone in males are better understood, more effective therapies may be developed.

Inflammation

Inflammation is the body's natural defence to physical injury. There is growing evidence that inflammation may be the result of psychological injury as well. Researchers have focused on two important blood components related to inflammation, C-reactive protein and interleukin-6. In young females with a history of adversity depression is accompanied by elevations in these blood components, but this elevation does not occur in children without a history of adversity (Rodriguez, 2018). Adversity in life may compromise resilience and place children at risk for depression and other disorders.

While we do not believe that inflammation causes depression, research indicates that it does play a role (Doney et al., 2021). Support for this belief includes the finding that about a third of people with major depression have elevated inflammatory biomarkers in the absence of a physical illness. Also, people who have inflammatory diseases have increased risk for major depression. Finally, people treated with cytokines to enhance immunity during cancer treatment develop major depression at a high rate.

Diathesis–Stress Model

The diathesis–stress model of depression takes into account the interplay of biology and life events in the development of depressive disorders. It is believed that psychosocial stressors and interpersonal events trigger neurophysical and neurochemical changes in the brain. Early life trauma may result in long-term hyperactivity of the CNS corticotropin-releasing factor (CRF), which releases the cortisol hormone, and norepinephrine systems, with a consequent neurotoxic effect on the hippocampus, which leads to overall neuronal loss. These changes could cause sensitization of the CRF circuits to even mild stress in adulthood, leading to an exaggerated stress response (Lemos & Alvarez, 2020).

Some people may be born with a predisposition toward depression, which is then triggered by a stressful life event. The experience of depression further alters the neurological connections in the brain, further increasing the predisposition toward depression. The result is a

Fig. 13.2 Positron Emission Tomography (PET) Scans of a 45-Year-Old Woman With Recurrent Depression. The scan on the *left* was taken when the patient was on no medication and very depressed. The scan on the *right* was taken several months later when the patient was well after she had been treated with medication for her depression. Note that her entire brain, particularly the left prefrontal cortex, is more active when she is well. (**Source**: Courtesy Mark George, MD, Biological Psychiatry Branch, National Institute of Mental Health.)

vicious cycle of recurrent depressive disorder. Early, effective treatment is needed to break the cycle.

Psychological Factors

Cognitive Theory

In cognitive theory the underlying assumption is that a person's thoughts will result in emotions. If a person looks at their life in a positive way, the person will experience positive emotions, but negative interpretation of life events can result in sorrow, anger, and hopelessness. Cognitive theorists believe that people may acquire a psychological predisposition to depression due to early life experiences. These experiences contribute to negative, illogical, and irrational thought processes that may remain dormant until they are activated during times of stress (Beck & Rush, 1995). Beck and Rush (1995) found that people with depression process information in negative ways, even in the midst of positive factors. They believed that automatic, negative, repetitive, unintended, and not readily controllable thoughts perpetuate depression. Three thoughts constitute **Beck's cognitive triad:**

1. A negative, self-deprecating view of self
2. A pessimistic view of the world
3. The belief that negative reinforcement (or no validation for the self) will continue in the future

Realizing that one has an ability to interpret life events in positive ways provides an element of control over emotions and, therefore, over depression.

Learned Helplessness

An older but still plausible theory of depression is that of **learned helplessness**. Seligman (1973) stated that although anxiety is the initial response to a stressful situation, it is replaced by depression if the person feels no control over the outcome of a situation. A person who believes that an undesired event is their fault and that nothing can be done to change it is prone to depression. The theory of learned helplessness has been used to explain the development of depression in certain social groups, such as older persons, people living in impoverished areas, and women.

APPLICATION OF THE NURSING PROCESS

Assessment

MDD often goes unrecognized and underdiagnosed, yet early treatment can result in improved outcomes. Nurses at both the generalist and advanced-practice level are frequently in the position to screen and assess for signs of depression, thereby facilitating early and appropriate treatment.

General Assessment

Assessment tools. Numerous standardized depression screening tools that help assess the type of depression are available, including the Beck Depression Inventory, the Hamilton Depression Rating Scale, the Zung Self-Rating Depression Scale, and the Geriatric Depression Scale. A sample of the Hamilton Depression Rating Scale is provided in Box 13.2.

The Patient Health Questionnaire–9 (PHQ-9), a short inventory that highlights predominant symptoms of depression, is presented here because of its ease of use (Figure 13.3). Many clinicians also use the mnemonic SIGECAPS (sleep, interest, guilt, energy, concentration, appetite, psychomotor activity, and suicidal thoughts) to guide their assessment.

The website https://heretohelp.bc.ca/screening/online/, sponsored by the BC Partners for Mental Health and Addictions Information,

---

BOX 13.2 HAMILTON DEPRESSION RATING SCALE

The Hamilton Depression Rating Scale (HDRS) was originally developed for hospital inpatients, thus the emphasis on melancholic and physical symptoms of depression. A limitation of the HDRS is that atypical symptoms of depression (e.g., hypersomnia, hyperphagia) are not assessed.

Scoring
The method of scoring varies by version. A score of 0 to 7 is generally accepted to be within a normal range. A score of 20 or higher is suggestive of a moderately severe depression.

Instructions
Items on this scale should be used to generate questions within the context of a therapeutic assessment. Ask the patient to select the one "cue" which best characterizes the patient. Be sure to record the answers in the appropriate spaces (positions 0 through 4).

DEPRESSED MOOD (sadness, hopeless, helpless, worthless)
0 [ ] Absent.
1 [ ] These feeling states indicated only on questioning.
2 [ ] These feeling states spontaneously reported verbally.
3 [ ] communicates feeling states non-verbally, i.e. through facial expression, posture, voice, and tendency to weep.
4 [ ] Patient reports virtually only these feeling states in his/her spontaneous verbal and non-verbal communication.

FEELINGS OF GUILT
0 [ ] Absent.
1 [ ] Self reproach, feels he/she has let people down.
2 [ ] Ideas of guilt or rumination over past errors or sinful deeds.
3 [ ] Present illness is a punishment. Delusions of guilt.
4 [ ] Hears accusatory or denunciatory voices and/or experiences threatening visual hallucinations.

SUICIDE
0 [ ] Absent.
1 [ ] Feels life is not worth living.
2 [ ] Wishes he/she were dead or any thoughts of possible death to self.
3 [ ] Ideas or gestures of suicide.
4 [ ] Attempts at suicide or a serious attempt.

SOMATIC SYMPTOMS GASTROINTESTINAL
0 [ ] None.
1 [ ] Loss of appetite. Eating with own volition. Heavy feelings in abdomen.
2 [ ] Difficulty eating without consistent encouragement and urging. Or requests or requires laxatives or medication for bowels or medication for gastrointestinal symptoms.

LOSS OF WEIGHT (rate either column A or B)

A	B
0 [ ] No weight loss.	0 [ ] Less than 0.45 kg weight loss in a week.
1 [ ] Probable weight loss associated with present illness.	1 [ ] Greater than 0.45 kg weight loss in a week.
2 [ ] Definite (according to patient) weight loss.	2 [ ] Greater than 0.9 kg weight loss in a week
3 [ ] Not assessed.	3 [ ] Not assessed

BOX 13.2 HAMILTON DEPRESSION RATING SCALE—cont'd

GENERAL SOMATIC SYMPTOMS
0 [ ] None.
1 [ ] Heaviness in limbs, back, or head. Backaches, headaches, muscle aches. Loss of energy and fatigability.
2 [ ] Specific symptom (any).

REPRODUCTIVE SYMPTOMS (symptoms such as loss of libido, menstrual disturbances)
0 [ ] Absent.
1 [ ] Mild.
2 [ ] Severe.

ILLNESS ANXIETY
0 [ ] Not present.
1 [ ] Preoccupation with health.
2 [ ] Preoccupation with illness.
3 [ ] Frequent concerns, visits to health care provider, etc.
4 [ ] Altered body perceptions.

MOTOR (slowness of thought and speech, impaired ability to concentrate, decreased motor activity)
0 [ ] Normal speech and thought.
1 [ ] Slight slowing during the interview.
2 [ ] Obvious retardation during the interview.
3 [ ] Interview difficult.

AGITATION
0 [ ] None.
1 [ ] Fidgetiness.
2 [ ] Playing with hands, hair, etc.
3 [ ] Moving about, can't sit still.
4 [ ] Hand wringing, nail biting, hair-pulling, biting of lips.
5 [ ] Complete stupor.

ANXIETY PSYCHIC
0 [ ] No difficulty.
1 [ ] Subjective tension and irritability.
2 [ ] Worrying about minor matters.
3 [ ] Apprehensive attitude apparent in face or speech.
4 [ ] Fears expressed without questioning.

ANXIETY SOMATIC (physiological experiences of anxiety)
gastrointestinal—dry mouth, indigestion, diarrhea, gas, cramps, belching
cardiovascular—palpitations, headaches
respiratory—hyperventilation, sighing
urinary – frequency
autonomic nervous system – sweating
0 [ ] Absent.
1 [ ] Mild.
2 [ ] Moderate.
3 [ ] Severe.
4 [ ] Incapacitating.

INSOMNIA: EARLY IN THE NIGHT
0 [ ] No difficulty falling asleep.
1 [ ] Complains of occasional difficulty falling asleep, i.e., more than 0.5 hour.
2 [ ] Complains of nightly difficulty falling asleep.

INSOMNIA: MIDDLE OF THE NIGHT
0 [ ] No difficulty.
1 [ ] Patient complains of being restless and disturbed during the night.
2 [ ] Repeated waking during the night or any single episode of getting out of bed rates (except for purposes of elimination).

INSOMNIA: EARLY HOURS OF THE MORNING
0 [ ] No difficulty.
1 [ ] Waking in early hours of the morning but goes back to sleep.
2 [ ] Unable to fall asleep again if he/she gets out of bed.
Add the numbers to the right of the selected answers. Total score: []

WORK AND ACTIVITIES
0 [ ] No difficulty.
1 [ ] Thoughts and feelings of incapacity, fatigue, or weakness related to activities, work, or hobbies.
2 [ ] Loss of interest in activity, hobbies, or work – either directly reported by the patient or indirect in listlessness, indecision, and vacillation (feels he/she has to push self to work or activities).
3 [ ] Decrease in actual time spent in activities, decrease in productivity or the patient spends less than three hours a day in activities, work, or hobbies.
4 [ ] Stopped working because of present illness, or the patient does not engage in any activities except for minimal routines, or is unable to complete chores unassisted.

INSIGHT
0 [ ] Acknowledges being depressed and ill.
1 [ ] Acknowledges illness but attributes cause to bad food, climate, overwork, virus, need for rest, etc.
2 [ ] Denies being ill at all.
This scale is in the public domain.

---

enables people to take an online confidential screening test for depression and anxiety and find reliable information on the illness.

Assessment of Suicide Potential

Suicidal ideation. The most dangerous aspect of MDD is a preoccupation with death. A patient may fantasize about their funeral or experience recurring dreams about death. Beyond these passive fantasies are thoughts of wanting to die. As a whole, all of these nihilistic thoughts are referred to as suicidal ideation. These thoughts may be relatively mild and fleeting, or persistent and involve a plan. Suicidal ideation, especially that in which the patient has a plan for suicide and the means to carry the plan out, represents an emergency requiring immediate intervention (refer to Chapter 22). Suicidal thoughts are a major reason for hospitalization for patients with major depression.

Patients diagnosed with MDD should always be evaluated for suicidal ideation. Risk for suicide is increased when depression is accompanied by hopelessness, substance use problems, a recent loss or separation, a history of past suicide attempts, or acute suicidal ideation. The following statements and questions help set the stage for assessing suicide potential:

- You have said you are depressed. Tell me what that is like for you.
- When you feel depressed, what thoughts go through your mind?
- Have you gone so far as to think about taking your own life?
- Do you have a suicide plan?
- Do you have the means to carry out your plan?
- Is there anything that would prevent you from carrying out your plan?

Refer to Chapter 22 for a detailed discussion of suicide, critical risk factors, warning signs, and strategies for suicide prevention. Also see Case Study and Nursing Care Plan 13.1.

PATIENT HEALTH QUESTIONNAIRE-9 (PHQ-9)

Over the last 2 weeks, how often have you been bothered by any of the following problems?	Not at all	Several days	More than half the days	Nearly every day
1. Little interest or pleasure in doing things	0	1	2	3
2. Feeling down, depressed, or hopeless	0	1	2	3
3. Trouble falling or staying asleep, or sleeping too much	0	1	2	3
4. Feeling tired or having little energy	0	1	2	3
5. Poor appetite or overeating	0	1	2	3
6. Feeling bad about yourself — or that you are a failure or have let yourself or your family down	0	1	2	3
7. Trouble concentrating on things, such as reading the newspaper or watching television	0	1	2	3
8. Moving or speaking so slowly that other people could have noticed? Or the opposite — being so fidgety or restless that you have been moving around a lot more than usual	0	1	2	3
9. Thoughts that you would be better off dead or of hurting yourself in some way	0	1	2	3

_0_ + _____ + _____ + _____

= Total score: _____

If you checked off any problems, how difficult have these problems made it for you to do your work, take care of things at home, or get along with other people?

- Not difficult at all ☐
- Somewhat difficult ☐
- Very difficult ☐
- Extremely difficult ☐

I confirm this information is accurate. | Patient's/Subject's initials: | Date:

A

B

Fig. 13.3 (A) Patient Health Questionnaire–9 (PHQ-9). (B) Scoring the PHQ-9. (**Source:** © 2005 Pfizer, Inc. Developed by Drs. Robert L. Spitzer, Janet B. Williams, Kurt Kroenke, and colleagues.)

Key Assessment Findings

A depressed mood and **anhedonia** (loss of ability to experience joy or pleasure in living) are the key symptoms of depression. Almost 97% of people with depression have anhedonia. Anxiety, a common symptom in depression, is seen in about 60% to 90% of patients with depression. **Psychomotor agitation** may be evidenced by constant pacing and wringing of hands. The slowed movements of **psychomotor retardation**, however, are more common. Somatic complaints (e.g., headaches, malaise, backaches) are also common. **Vegetative signs of depression**, alterations in those activities necessary to support physical life and growth (e.g., change in bowel movements and eating habits, sleep disturbances, lack of interest in sex), are universally present.

Areas to Assess

Affect. **Affect** is the outward presentation of a person's internal state of being. It is reported as an objective finding based on the nurse's assessment. A person who has depression sees the world through grey-coloured glasses. Posture is poor, and the patient may look older than their stated age. Facial expressions convey sadness and dejection, and the patient may have frequent bouts of weeping. Conversely, the patient may say that they are unable to cry. Feelings of worthlessness, guilt, anger, helplessness, hopelessness, and despair are readily reflected in the person's affect. For example, the patient may not make eye contact, may speak in a monotone, may show little or no facial expression (flat affect), and may make only "yes" or "no" responses. Some individuals can be very depressed yet present as the "smiling depressed."

Thought processes. During a depressive episode, the person's ability to solve problems and think clearly is negatively affected. Judgement is poor, and indecisiveness is common, largely because thinking is slow and memory and concentration are poor. People with depression also dwell on and exaggerate their perceived faults and failures and are unable to focus on their strengths and successes. They may experience delusions of being punished for doing bad deeds or being a terrible person. Common statements of delusional thinking are "I have committed unpardonable sins," "God wants me dead," and "I am wicked and should die."

Mood. Mood is the patient's subjective experience of sustained emotions or feelings. People, when asked to describe their mood, will describe how they are feeling. Should a patient describe a feeling when asked about their mood, the clinician needs to follow up with a question asking about how long they have felt this way. Mood is about feelings that last over several days, weeks, or months.

Feelings. Feelings frequently reported by those with depression include worthlessness, guilt, helplessness, hopelessness, and anger. Feelings of worthlessness range from feeling inadequate to having an unrealistically negative evaluation of self-worth. These feelings reflect the low self-esteem that is a painful partner to depression. Statements such as "I am no good" or "I'll never amount to anything" are common. Anhedonia (*an* "without" + *hedone* "pleasure" = inability to feel happy) refers to the absence of happiness or pleasure in aspects of life that once made the patient happy.

Guilt is a nearly universal accompaniment to depression. A person may ruminate over present or past failings: "I was never a good parent," or "it's my fault that project at work failed." These thoughts tend to occur again and again and are difficult for the patient to stop. These negative ruminations fill in the hours of lost sleep.

Cognitive changes. Helplessness is demonstrated by a person's inability to solve problems in response to common concerns. In severe situations helplessness may be evidenced by the inability to carry out the simplest tasks (e.g., grooming, doing housework, working, caring for children) because they seem too difficult to accomplish. With feelings of helplessness come feelings of hopelessness, which are particularly correlated with suicidality. Even though most depressive episodes are time limited, people experiencing them believe that things will never change. This feeling of utter hopelessness can lead people to view suicide as a way out of constant mental pain. Hopelessness includes the following attributes:

- Negative expectations for the future
- Loss of control over future outcomes
- Passive acceptance of the futility of planning to achieve goals
- Emotional negativism, as expressed in despair, despondency, or depression

Anger is a strong feeling of displeasure or hostility. It is a natural outcome of profound feelings of helplessness. Anger in depression is often expressed inappropriately through hurtful verbal attacks, physical aggression toward others, or destruction of property, and anger may be directed toward the self in the form of suicidal or otherwise self-destructive behaviours (e.g., alcohol abuse, substance use, overeating, smoking). These behaviours often reinforce feelings of low self-esteem and worthlessness.

Physical behaviour. Lethargy and fatigue may result in psychomotor retardation, in which movements are extremely slow, facial expressions are decreased, and the gaze is fixed. The continuum of psychomotor retardation may range from slowed and difficult movements to complete inactivity and incontinence. Psychomotor agitation, in which patients constantly pace, bite their nails, smoke, tap their fingers, or engage in some other tension-relieving activity, may also be observed. At these times, patients commonly feel fidgety and unable to relax.

Vegetative signs of depression refer to alterations in those activities necessary to support physical life and growth (e.g., eating, sleeping, elimination, sex). Appetite changes vary in individuals experiencing depression. Appetite loss is common, and sometimes patients can lose up to 5% of their body weight in less than a month. Other patients find they eat more often and complain of weight gain.

Change in sleep pattern is a cardinal sign of depression. Often people experience insomnia, wake frequently, and have a total reduction in sleep, especially deep-stage sleep. Waking at 3 or 4 a.m. and then staying awake is common, as is sleeping for short periods only. The light sleep of a person with depression tends to prolong the agony of depression over a 24-hour period. For some, sleep is increased (hypersomnia) and provides an escape from painful feelings. In any event sleep is rarely restful or refreshing.

Grooming, dressing, and personal hygiene may be markedly neglected. People who usually take pride in their appearance and dress may allow themselves to look shabby and unkempt. They may neglect to bathe, change clothes, or engage in other basic self-care activities.

Sexual interest declines (loss of libido) during depression. Some men experience impotence, and a declining interest in sex often occurs among both men and women, which can further complicate marital and social relationships.

Changes in bowel habits are common. Constipation is seen most frequently in patients with psychomotor retardation. Diarrhea occurs less frequently, often in conjunction with psychomotor agitation or anxiety.

Communication. A person with depression may speak and comprehend very slowly. The lack of an immediate response by the patient to a remark does not necessarily mean the patient has not heard or chooses not to reply; the patient may need more time to comprehend what was said and then compose a reply. In extreme depression however, a person may become mute.

Religious beliefs and spirituality. Many studies have found a negative correlation between relational spiritual factors and depression. Specifically, it seems to be spiritual instability and a disappointment in a higher power that are predictors of depression (Paine & Sandage, 2017). In addressing spirituality nurses must assess patients' spiritual strengths, whether peace focused, meaning, or religious. Addressing spiritual issues is not the domain of one discipline. Encouraging a connection with religious or spiritual practices that have brought the patient comfort in the past may be therapeutic.

Age Considerations

Assessment of children and adolescents. As children grow and develop, they may display a wide range of mood and behaviour, making it easy to overlook signs of depression. The core symptoms of depression in children and adolescents are the same as for adults, which are sadness and loss of pleasure. What differs is how these symptoms are displayed. For example, a very young child may cry, a school-aged child might withdraw, and a teenager may become irritable in response to feeling sad or hopeless. Younger children may suddenly refuse to go to school while adolescents may engage in substance use or sexual promiscuity and be preoccupied with death or suicide.

Assessment of older persons. Because older persons are more likely to complain of physical illness than emotional concerns, depression might be overlooked. Older patients actually do have comorbid physical problems, and it is difficult to determine whether fatigue, pain, and weakness are the result of an illness or depression. The Geriatric Depression Scale is a 30-item tool that is both valid and reliable in screening for depression in the older person (Sheikh & Yesavage, 1986). Its "yes" or "no" format makes this scale easier to administer to patients with cognitive deficits. It can be helpful in determining suicidality in this population.

Self-Assessment

Patients with depression often reject the advice, encouragement, and understanding of the nurse and others, and they often appear not to respond to nursing interventions and seem resistant to change. When this occurs, the nurse may experience feelings of frustration, hopelessness, and annoyance. These problematic responses can be altered in the following ways:

- Recognizing any unrealistic expectations for yourself or the patient
- Identifying feelings that originate with the patient
- Understanding the roles that biology and genetics play in the precipitation and maintenance of a depressed mood

Unrealistic expectations of self. Nursing students and others new to caring for individuals with depression may have unrealistic expectations of themselves and their patients, and problems result when these expectations are not met. Unmet expectations usually result in a nurse feeling anxious, hurt, angry, helpless, or incompetent. Unrealistic expectations of self and others may be held even by experienced health care workers, a phenomenon that contributes to staff burnout. Many of your nursing expectations may not be conscious, but when these expectations are made conscious and are worked through with peers and more experienced clinicians (supervisors), more realistic expectations can be formed and attainable outcomes identified. Realistic expectations of self and the patient can decrease feelings of helplessness and increase a nurse's self-esteem and therapeutic potential.

> **SAFETY TIP**
>
> Unrealistic expectations of yourself can lead to moral distress, and for some it is the start of intensive self-questioning and doubt. For some nurses it can even lead to leaving the profession. In order to protect your own personal sense of self and self-worth, it is important to build a support network with colleagues, peers, and friends. Recognizing that the system we work in is complicated and not every problem has an answer or a solution that will "feel good" to us, but understanding that it is the best that could happen in a bad situation is an important aspect to building moral resilience

Feeling what the patient is feeling. It is not uncommon for nurses and other health care providers to experience intense anxiety, frustration, annoyance, hopelessness, and helplessness while caring for individuals with depression; nurses empathically sense what the patient is feeling. Novice nurses may interpret these emotions as personal reactions to the patient with whom they are working. However, these feelings can be important diagnostic clues to the patient's experience. You can discuss feelings of annoyance, hopelessness, and helplessness with peers and supervisors to separate personal feelings from those originating with the patient. If personal feelings are not recognized, named, and examined, the nurse is likely to withdraw.

People instinctively avoid situations and other people that arouse feelings of frustration, annoyance, or intimidation. If the nurse also has

---

⚡ RESEARCH HIGHLIGHT
Describing the Population Health Burden of Depression

Problem
Few studies have evaluated the impact of depression in terms of losses to both premature mortality and health-related quality of life (HRQOL) on the overall population.

Purpose of Study
The objective of the study was to estimate period life expectancy (LE) and health-adjusted life expectancy (HALE) of Canadian adults (ages 20 years and older) according to depression status. HALE is a summary measure of population health that combines both morbidity and mortality into a single summary statistic that describes the current health status of a population.

Methods
National Population Health Survey (NPHS) participants 20 years and older (n = 12 373) were followed for mortality outcomes from 1994 to 2009, based on depression status. Depression was defined as having likely experienced a major depressive episode in the previous year as measured by the Composite International Diagnostic Interview Short Form. LE was estimated by building period abridged life tables by sex and depression status using the relative risks of mortality from the NPHS and mortality data from the Canadian Chronic Disease Surveillance System (2007 to 2009). The Canadian Community Health Survey (2009/10) provided estimates of depression prevalence, and the Health Utilities Index was used as a measure of HRQOL. Using the combined mortality, depression prevalence, and HRQOL estimates, HALE was estimated for the adult population according to depression status and by sex.

Key Findings
- Men and women in Canada who have depression live a substantially higher proportion of their life in an unhealthy state compared to their counterparts without depression.
- This gap in healthy LE between Canadians with and without depression is primarily associated with losses in quality of life.
- Emotional state, cognitive state, and pain are the key attributes associated with losses in quality of life for Canadians experiencing a recent major depressive episode.
- Based on observations from past studies of the Canadian household population, the burden of depression on healthy LE at a population level appears to be greater than that associated with other chronic conditions such as diabetes, hypertension, and obesity.

Implications for Nursing Practice
The population of adult men and women with depression in Canada has a substantially lower healthy LE than those without depression. Reducing hopelessness and increasing positive future anticipation are factors associated with improving quality of life for people who experience depression. Nurses will need to consider using a future-directed therapy.

Source: Steensma, C., Loukine, L., Orpana, H., et al. (2016). Describing the population health burden of depression: Health-adjusted life expectancy by depression status in Canada. *Maladies Chroniques et Blessures au Canada, 36*(10), 205–213. Retrieved from https://www.phac-aspc.gc.ca/publicat/hpcdp-pspmc/index-fra.php

VIGNETTE

Velma is working with Aleks, a patient with depression who is living at a homeless shelter after losing his job and being evicted from his apartment. Aleks expresses a lot of hopelessness about his future and believes that he will never get another job or be able to live on his own. During clinical conference, Velma states that she is feeling threatened and frustrated because Aleks rejects her suggestions and her attempts to help. She confesses that she thinks Aleks is not trying to feel better or improve his situation. Velma spends time reviewing the illness of depression, common behaviours, and patient needs. She also reviews the recovery model of mental illness. In subsequent visits she refocuses on Aleks and stops giving him suggestions. After 4 weeks, Aleks has worked out a plan to live with relatives while he undergoes vocational training. He thanks Velma for listening and not making him "feel like a failure."

ASSESSMENT GUIDELINES
Depression

1. Always evaluate the patient's risk for harm to self or others. Overt hostility is highly correlated with suicide (see Chapter 22).
2. Depression is a mood disorder that can be secondary to a host of medical or other psychiatric disorders, as well as to medications. A thorough medical and neurological examination helps determine if the depression is primary or secondary to another disorder. Essentially, evaluate whether:
   - The patient is psychotic
   - The patient has taken drugs or alcohol
   - Medical conditions are present
   - The patient has a history of a comorbid psychiatric syndrome (eating disorder, borderline or anxiety disorder)
3. Assess the patient's past history of depression, what past treatments worked and did not work, and any events that may have triggered this episode of depression.
4. Assess support systems, family, significant others, and the need for information and referrals.

unresolved feelings of anger and depression, the complexity of the situation is compounded. There is no substitute for competent and supportive supervision to facilitate growth, both professionally and personally. Being supervised by a more experienced clinician and sharing with peers help minimize feelings of confusion, frustration, and isolation and can increase your therapeutic potential and self-esteem while you care for individuals with depression.

DIAGNOSIS

Depression is a complex disorder, and individuals with depression have a variety of needs; therefore nursing diagnoses are many. However, a high priority for the nurse is determining the risk for suicide, and the nursing diagnosis of *Risk for suicide* is always considered. Refer to Chapter 22 for assessment guidelines and interventions for suicidal individuals. Other key targets for nursing interventions are represented by the diagnoses of *Hopelessness, Ineffective coping, Social isolation, Spiritual distress,* and *Self-care deficit* (bathing, dressing, feeding, toileting). Table 13.2 identifies signs and symptoms commonly experienced in depression and offers potential nursing diagnoses.

TABLE 13.2 Potential Nursing Diagnoses for Depression

Signs and Symptoms	Potential Nursing Diagnoses
Previous suicide attempts, putting affairs in order, giving away prized possessions, suicidal ideation (has plan, ability to carry it out), overt or covert statements regarding killing self, feelings of worthlessness, hopelessness, helplessness	Risk for suicide Risk for self-mutilation Risk for self-harm
Lack of judgement, memory difficulty, poor concentration, inaccurate interpretation of environment, negative ruminations, cognitive distortions	Altered thought processes
Difficulty with simple tasks, inability to function at previous level, poor problem solving, poor cognitive functioning, verbalizations of inability to cope	Ineffective coping Interrupted family processes Risk for impaired attachment Ineffective role performance
Difficulty making decisions, poor concentration, inability to take action	Decisional conflict
Feelings of helplessness, hopelessness, powerlessness	Hopelessness Powerlessness
Questioning the meaning of life and own existence, inability to participate in usual religious practices, conflict over spiritual beliefs, anger toward spiritual deity or religious representatives	Spiritual distress Impaired religiosity Risk for impaired religiosity
Feelings of worthlessness, poor self-image, negative sense of self, self-negating verbalizations, feeling of being a failure, expressions of shame or guilt, hypersensitivity to slights or criticism	Chronic low self-esteem Situational low self-esteem
Withdrawal, non-communicativeness, monosyllabic speech, avoidance of contact with others	Impaired social interaction Social isolation Risk for loneliness
Vegetative signs of depression: changes in sleeping, eating, grooming and hygiene, elimination, sexual patterns	Self-care deficit (bathing, dressing, feeding, toileting) Imbalanced nutrition: less than body requirements Disturbed sleep pattern Constipation Sexual dysfunction

OUTCOMES IDENTIFICATION

The Recovery Model

In 1993 Dr. William Anthony changed the focus of mental health to recovery from mental illness rather than treatment of it. The recovery model emphasizes that individuals with mental illnesses, including depression, can learn to live with their disease. It is individuals who define who they are, not their diseases. Recovery is attained through partnership with health care providers who focus on the patient's strengths. Treatment goals are mutually developed based on the patient's personal needs and values, and interventions are evidence informed. The recovery model is consistent with the focus on patient-centred care, which is a key component of safe, quality health care.

Remember that MDD can be a recurrent and chronic illness. Care should be directed not only at the resolution of the acute phase but also at long-term management. The nurse and the patient identify realistic outcome criteria and formulate concrete, measurable short-term and intermediate indicators. Each patient is a unique individual, and indicators should be selected according to individual needs.

Table 13.3 presents some outcome criteria from the *Nursing Outcomes Classification (NOC)* (Moorhead et al., 2018). Indicators for the outcomes of the vegetative or physical signs of depression (e.g., reports adequate sleep) are formulated to show, for example, evidence of weight gain, return to normal bowel activity, sleep duration of 6 to 8 hours per night, or return of sexual desire.

PLANNING

The planning of care for patients with depression is geared toward the patient's phase of depression, particular symptoms, and personal goals. At all times during the care of a person with depression, nurses and members of the health care team must be cognizant of the potential for suicide; therefore assessment of risk for self-harm (or harm to others) is ongoing. A combination of therapy (cognitive, behavioural, and interpersonal) and psychopharmacology is an effective approach to the treatment of depression across all age groups.

Be aware that the vegetative signs of depression (e.g., changes in eating, sleeping, and sexual satisfaction), as well as changes in concentration, activity level, social interaction, care for personal appearance, and so on, often need targeting. The planning of care for a patient with depression is based on the individual's symptoms and goals, and it attempts to encompass a variety of areas in the person's life. Safety is always the highest priority.

IMPLEMENTATION

There are three phases in the treatment of and recovery from major depression:

1. The *acute phase* (6 to 12 weeks) is directed at reduction of depressive symptoms and restoration of psychosocial and work function. Hospitalization may be required.
2. The *continuation phase* (4 to 9 months) is directed at prevention of relapse through pharmacotherapy, education, and depression-specific psychotherapy.
3. The *maintenance phase* (1 year or more) of treatment is directed at prevention of reoccurrences of depression.

It is important to keep in mind that the primary goal of both the continuation and the maintenance phases is keeping the patient a functional and contributing member of the community after recovery from the acute phase.

Counselling and Communication Techniques

Some patients with depression may be so withdrawn that they are unwilling or unable to speak. Nurses often experience some difficulty communicating with patients without talking; just sitting with them in silence may seem like a waste of time or be uncomfortable. As anxiety increases, the nurse may start daydreaming, feel bored, remember something that "must be done now," and so on. It is important to be aware, however, that this time can be meaningful, especially for the nurse who has a genuine interest in learning about the patient with depression.

Determining when a withdrawn patient will be able to respond is difficult. However, certain techniques are known to be useful in guiding effective nursing interventions. Some communication techniques to use with a severely withdrawn patient are listed in Guidelines for Communication: Communicating With Severely Withdrawn People. Counselling guidelines for use with patients with depression are offered in Guidelines for Communication: Counselling People With Depression.

Health Teaching and Health Promotion

One basic premise of the recovery model of mental illness is that each person controls their own treatment based on individual goals. Within this model, health teaching is especially important because it allows patients to make informed choices. Health teaching is also an avenue for providing hope to the patient and should include the following information:

- Depression is an illness that is beyond a person's voluntary control.
- Although it is beyond voluntary control, depression can be managed through medication and lifestyle.
- Illness management depends in large part on understanding personal signs and symptoms of relapse.
- Illness management depends on understanding the role of medication and possible adverse effects of medication.
- Long-term management is best assured if the patient undergoes psychotherapy along with taking medication.

TABLE 13.3 NOC Outcomes Related to Depression

Nursing Outcome and Definition	Intermediate Indicators	Short-Term Indicators
Depression self-control: Personal actions to minimize melancholy and maintain interest in life events	Reports improved mood	Monitors intensity of depression
	Adheres to therapy schedule	Identifies precursors of depression
	Takes medication as prescribed	Plans strategies to reduce effects of precursors
	Follows treatment plan	Reports changes in symptoms to health care provider

Source: Moorhead, S., Johnson, M., Maas, M., et al. (2012). *Nursing Outcomes Classification (NOC)* (5th ed.). St. Louis: Mosby.

GUIDELINES FOR COMMUNICATION
Communicating With Severely Withdrawn People

Intervention	Rationale
When a patient is mute, use the technique of making observations: "There are many new pictures on your wall." "You are wearing your new shoes." "You ate some of your breakfast."	When a patient is not ready to talk, direct questions can raise the patient's anxiety level and frustrate the nurse. Pointing to commonalities in the environment draws the patient into and reinforces reality.
Use simple, concrete words.	Slowed thinking and difficulty concentrating impair comprehension.
Allow time for the patient to respond.	Slowed thinking necessitates time to formulate a response.
Listen for covert messages and ask about suicide plans.	People often experience relief and a decrease in feelings of isolation when they share thoughts of suicide.
Avoid platitudes such as "Things will look up," "Everyone gets down once in a while," or "Tomorrow will be better."	Platitudes tend to minimize the patient's feelings and can increase feelings of guilt and worthlessness, because the patient cannot "look up" or "snap out of it."

GUIDELINES FOR COMMUNICATION
Counselling People With Depression

Intervention	Rationale
Help the patient question underlying assumptions and beliefs and consider alternative explanations for problems.	Reconstructing a healthier and more hopeful attitude about the future can alter depressed mood.
Work with the patient to identify cognitive distortions that encourage negative self-appraisal. For example: a. Overgeneralizations b. Self-blame c. Mind reading d. Discounting of positive attributes	Cognitive distortions reinforce a negative, inaccurate perception of self and world. a. The patient takes one fact or event and makes a general rule out of it ("He always..."; "I never..."). b. The patient consistently blames self for everything perceived as negative. c. The patient assumes others do not like them without any real evidence that assumptions are correct. d. The patient focuses on the negative.
Encourage activities that can raise self-esteem. Identify need for (1) problem-solving skills, (2) coping skills, and (3) assertiveness skills.	Many people with depression, especially women, are not taught a range of problem-solving and coping skills. Increasing social, family, and job skills can change negative self-assessment.
Encourage exercise, such as running or weight lifting.	Exercise can improve self-concept and potentially shift neurochemical balance.
Encourage formation of supportive relationships, such as through support groups, therapy, and peer support.	Such relationships reduce social isolation and enable the patient to work on personal goals and relationship needs.
Provide information referrals, when needed, for religious or spiritual information (e.g., readings, programs, tapes, community resources).	Spiritual and existential issues may be heightened during depressive episodes; many people find strength and comfort in spirituality or religion.

- Identifying and coping with the stress of interpersonal relationships, whether they are familial, social, or occupational, is a key to illness management.
- Including the family in discharge planning is also important and helps the patient in the following ways:
  - Increases the family's understanding and acceptance of the family member and helps family recognize the importance of medication adherence during the aftercare period.
  - Increases the patient's use of aftercare facilities in the community.
  - Contributes to higher overall adjustment in the patient after discharge.

Promotion of Self-Care Activities

In addition to feelings of hopelessness, despair, and physical discomfort, signs of physical neglect may be apparent, in which case nursing measures for improving physical well-being and promoting adequate self-care are initiated. Some effective interventions targeting physical needs are listed in Table 13.4. Nurses in the community can work with family members to encourage a family member with depression to perform and maintain their self-care activities.

Milieu Management: Teamwork and Safety

Safe, quality inpatient care requires the skills of a well-coordinated team. Treating a patient with depression requires the skills of nurses and prescribers. Other members of the team include mental health technicians, pharmacists, dietitians, social workers, and the patient's significant others.

Safety becomes the most important issue facing a team that cares for people with depression who may be at high risk for suicide. Suicide precautions are usually instituted and include the removal of all harmful objects such as "sharps" (e.g., razors, scissors, nail files), strangulation risks (e.g., belts), and medication that can be used to overdose. Some patients with severe depression may need to have someone check on them frequently, perhaps every 15 minutes, or even have one-to-one observation.

TABLE 13.4 Interventions Targeting the Vegetative Signs of Depression

Intervention	Rationale
Nutrition—Anorexia	
Offer small, high-calorie and high-protein snacks frequently throughout the day and evening.	Low weight and poor nutrition render the patient susceptible to illness. Small, frequent snacks are more easily tolerated than large plates of food when the patient is anorexic.
Offer high-protein and high-calorie fluids frequently throughout the day and evening.	These fluids prevent dehydration and can minimize constipation.
When possible, encourage family or friends to remain with the patient during meals.	This strategy reinforces the idea that someone cares, can raise the patient's self-esteem, and can serve as an incentive to eat.
Ask the patient which foods or drinks they like. Offer choices. Involve the dietitian.	The patient is more likely to eat the foods provided.
Weigh the patient weekly and observe the patient's eating patterns.	Monitoring the patient's status gives the information needed for revision of the intervention.
Sleep—Insomnia	
Provide periods of rest after activities.	Fatigue can intensify feelings of depression.
Encourage the patient to get up and dress and to stay out of bed during the day.	Minimizing sleep during the day increases the likelihood of sleep at night.
Encourage the use of relaxation measures in the evening (e.g., tepid bath, warm milk).	These measures induce relaxation and sleep.
Reduce environmental and physical stimulants in the evening—provide decaffeinated coffee, soft lights, soft music, and quiet activities.	Decreasing caffeine and epinephrine levels increases the possibility of sleep.
Self-Care Deficits	
Encourage the use of toothbrush, washcloth, soap, makeup, shaving equipment, and so forth.	Being clean and well groomed can temporarily increase self-esteem.
When appropriate, give step-by-step reminders such as "Wash the right side of your face; now the left."	Slowed thinking and difficulty concentrating make organizing simple tasks difficult.
Elimination—Constipation	
Monitor intake and output, especially bowel movements.	Many patients with depression are constipated. If the condition is not checked, fecal impaction can occur.
Offer foods high in fibre, and provide periods of exercise.	Roughage and exercise stimulate peristalsis and help evacuation of fecal material.
Encourage the intake of fluids.	Fluids help prevent constipation.
Evaluate the need for laxatives and enemas.	These measures prevent fecal impaction.

Pharmacological Interventions

At the cellular level, mood disorders are caused by problems with neurotransmitters. It follows that medications that alter brain chemistry are an important component in their treatment. Refer to Figure 13.4 for a brief description of the neurobiology of depression. Antidepressant therapy is an effective strategy for most cases of MDD, particularly in severe cases. A combination of psychotherapies and antidepressant therapy is superior to either psychotherapy or psychopharmacological treatment alone (de Roten et al., 2017).

Antidepressant Drugs

Antidepressant drugs can positively alter poor self-concept, degree of withdrawal, vegetative signs of depression, and activity level. Target symptoms include:
- Sleep disturbance
- Appetite disturbance (decreased or increased)
- Fatigue
- Decreased sex drive
- Psychomotor retardation or agitation
- Diurnal variations in mood (often worse in the morning)
- Impaired concentration or forgetfulness
- Anhedonia

A drawback of antidepressant drugs is that improvement in mood may take 1 to 3 weeks or longer. If a patient is acutely suicidal, electroconvulsive therapy (discussed in detail later in this chapter) can be a reliable and effective alternative.

The goal of antidepressant therapy is the complete remission of symptoms. Often the first antidepressant prescribed is not the one that will ultimately bring about remission; aggressive treatment helps in finding the proper treatment. An adequate trial for the treatment of depression is 3 months. Individuals experiencing their first depressive episode are maintained on antidepressants for 6 to 9 months after symptoms of depression remit. Some people may have multiple episodes of depression or may have a chronic form (similar to the chronicity of diabetes) and benefit from indefinite antidepressant therapy.

Neurobiology of Depression and the Effect of Antidepressants

The imbalance of certain neurotransmitters (serotonin and norepinephrine) contributes to depression in certain parts of the brain.
Prefrontal cortex: regulates role in executive functions and emotional control and memory.

Limbic system: regulates activities such as emotions, physical and sexual drives, and the stress response, as well as processing, learning, and memory (amygdala, hypothalamus, hippocampus).

Anterior cingulate cortex: regulates heart rate and blood pressure. Other functions include decision making, emotional regulation, error detection, preparation for tasks, and executive functions.

Various Parts of the Brain Along the Noradrenergic Pathway
The axons of these neurons project upward through the forebrain to the cerebral cortex, the limbic system, the thalamus, and the hippocampus.

Norepinephrine (NE) and the Noradrenergic System: plays a major role in mood and emotional behaviour as well as energy, drive, anxiety, focus, and metabolism.

Various Parts of the Brain Along the Serotonergic Pathway
The axons of serotonergic neurons originate in the raphe nuclei of the brainstem and project to the cerebral cortex, the limbic system, cerebellum, and spinal cord.

Serotonin (5-HT) and the Serotonergic System: involved in the regulation of pain, depression, pleasure, anxiety, panic arousal, sleep cycle, carbohydrate craving, and premenstrual syndrome.

Medications for Depression
Medications for depression include the selective serotonin reuptake inhibitors (**SSRIs**), serotonin–norepinephrine reuptake inhibitors (**SNRIs**), serotonin antagonist and reuptake inhibitors (**SARIs**), norepinephrine–dopamine reuptake inhibitor (**NDRI**), noradrenergic and specific serotonergic antidepressants (**NaSSAs**), tricyclic antidepressants (**TCAs**), and monoamine oxidase inhibitors (**MAOIs**).
They all work equally well and are chosen by their safety profile and side effects.* All have a delayed response, a discontinuation syndrome, and a Black Box Warning for suicide.

Patient's Problem*	Side-Effect Profile*	Example of Drug*
Fatigue	Stimulates the CNS	Fluoxetine (SSRI)
Insomnia	Substantial sedation	Mirtazapine (NaSSA)
Sexual dysfunction	Enhances libido	Bupropion (NDRI)
Chronic pain	Relieves pain	TCAs or duloxetine (SNRI)

*Adapted from Burchum, J. R., & Rosenthal, L. D. (2016). *Lehne's pharmacology for nursing care* (9th ed.). St. Louis: Elsevier.

Fig. 13.4 Neurobiology of depression.

Antidepressants may precipitate a psychotic episode in a person with schizophrenia or a manic episode in a patient with bipolar disorder. Patients with bipolar disorder often receive a mood-stabilizing drug along with an antidepressant.

Choosing an antidepressant. All antidepressants work to increase the availability of one or more of the neurotransmitters, serotonin, norepinephrine, or dopamine. All antidepressants work equally well; however, a variety of antidepressants or a combination of antidepressants may need to be tried before the most effective regimen is found for an individual patient. Each of the antidepressants has different adverse effects, costs, safety issues, and maintenance considerations. Selection of the appropriate antidepressant is based on the following considerations:

- Adverse-effect profile (e.g., sexual dysfunction, weight gain)
- Ease of administration
- History of past response
- Safety and medical considerations

Drug Treatment of Patients with Major Depression provides an overview of antidepressants used in Canada.

DRUG TREATMENT OF PATIENTS WITH MAJOR DEPRESSION

Generic (Trade)	Action	Notes	Adverse Effects	Warnings
Selective Serotonin Reuptake Inhibitors (SSRIs)				
Citalopram (Celexa) Fluoxetine (Prozac) Fluvoxamine (Luvox) Paroxetine (Paxil) Sertraline (Zoloft) Escitalopram (Cipralex)	Blocks the reuptake of serotonin	First-line treatment for major depression. Some SSRIs activate and others sedate; choice depends on patient symptoms. Risk of lethal overdose minimized with SSRIs	Agitation, insomnia, headache, nausea and vomiting, sexual dysfunction, hyponatremia	Discontinuation syndrome—dizziness, insomnia, nervousness, irritability, nausea, and agitation—may occur with abrupt withdrawal (depending on half-life); taper slowly. Contraindicated in people taking MAOIs
Serotonin–Norepinephrine Reuptake Inhibitors (SNRIs)				
Venlafaxine (Effexor) Duloxetine (Cymbalta)	Blocks the reuptake of serotonin and norepinephrine	Effexor is a popular next-step strategy after trying SSRIs. Cymbalta has the advantage of decreasing neuropathic pain	Hypertension (venlafaxine), nausea, insomnia, dry mouth, sweating, agitation, headache, sexual dysfunction	Monitor blood pressure with Effexor, especially at higher doses and with a history of hypertension. Hypertension may be particularly noted in the diastolic measurement. Discontinuation syndrome (see SSRIs above). Contraindicated in people taking MAOIs
Norepinephrine Reuptake Inhibitors (NRIs)				
Venlafaxine (Effexor XR) Duloxetine (Cymbalta)	Blocks the reuptake of norepinephrine and enhances its transmission	Antidepressant effects similar to SSRIs and TCAs. Useful with severe depression and impaired social functioning	Insomnia, sweating, dizziness, dry mouth, constipation, urinary hesitancy, tachycardia, decreased libido	Contraindicated in people taking MAOIs
Norepinephrine–Dopamine Reuptake Inhibitors (NDRIs)				
Bupropion (Wellbutrin)	Blocks the reuptake of norepinephrine and dopamine. Not indicated for patients under 18 years of age	Stimulant action may reduce appetite. May increase sexual desire. Used as an aid to quit smoking	Agitation, insomnia, headache, nausea and vomiting, seizures (0.4%)	Contraindicated in people taking MAOIs. High doses increase seizure risk, especially in people who are predisposed to seizures
Serotonin–Norepinephrine Disinhibitors (SNDIs)				
Mirtazapine (Remeron)	Blocks α_1-adrenergic receptors that normally inhibit norepinephrine and serotonin	Antidepressant effects equal SSRIs and may occur faster	Weight gain, sedation, dizziness, headache; sexual dysfunction is rare	Drug-induced somnolence exaggerated by alcohol, benzodiazepines, and other CNS depressants. Contraindicated in people taking MAOIs

DRUG TREATMENT OF PATIENTS WITH MAJOR DEPRESSION—cont'd

Generic (Trade)	Action	Notes	Adverse Effects	Warnings
Tricyclic Antidepressants (TCAs)				
Amitriptyline (Elavil) Clomipramine (Anafranil) Nortriptyline (Aventyl)	Inhibits the reuptake of serotonin and norepinephrine Antagonizes adrenergic, histaminergic, and muscarinic receptors	Therapeutic effects similar to SSRIs, but adverse effects are more prominent May work better in melancholic depression TCAs can worsen many cardiac and other medical conditions	Dry mouth, constipation, urinary retention, blurred vision, orthostatic hypotension, cardiac toxicity, sedation	Lethal in overdose Use cautiously in older persons and those with cardiac disorders, elevated intraocular pressure, urinary retention, hyperthyroidism, seizure disorders, or liver or kidney dysfunction Contraindicated in people taking MAOIs
Monoamine Oxidase Inhibitors (MAOIs)				
Phenelzine (Nardil) Tranylcypromine (Parnate)	Inhibits the enzyme monoamine oxidase, which normally breaks down neurotransmitters, including serotonin and norepinephrine	Efficacy similar to other antidepressants, but dietary restrictions and potential drug interactions make this drug type less desirable	Insomnia, nausea, agitation, confusion Potential for hypertensive crisis or serotonin syndrome with concurrent use of other antidepressants	Contraindicated in people taking other antidepressants Tyramine-rich food could bring about a hypertensive crisis Many other drug interactions
Moclobemide (Manerix)	Acts on serotonin, norepinephrine, and dopamine	MDD and social anxiety	Nausea and dizziness	Contraindicated if known hypersensitivity to moclobemide

CNS, Central nervous system.
Sources: Canadian Pharmacists Association & Canadian Pharmaceutical Association. (2020). *Compendium of pharmaceuticals and specialties: Canada's trusted drug reference*. Toronto: Canadian Pharmaceutical Association; Burchum, J., & Rosenthal, L. (2019). *Lehne's pharmacology for nursing care* (10th ed.). St. Louis: Elsevier.

Selective serotonin reuptake inhibitors. The SSRIs are recommended as first-line therapy for most types of depression. Essentially, the SSRIs selectively block the neuronal uptake of serotonin (e.g., 5-HT, 5-HT$_1$ receptors), which increases the availability of serotonin in the synaptic cleft. Refer to Chapter 11 for a more detailed discussion of how the SSRIs work.

SSRI antidepressant drugs have a relatively low adverse-effect profile compared with the older antidepressants (tricyclics—discussed later in this chapter); blurred vision, or urinary retention, making it easier for patients to take these medications as prescribed. Adherence to the medication regimen is a crucial step toward recovery or remission of symptoms. The SSRIs are effective in depression with anxiety features and in depression with psychomotor agitation.

Because the SSRIs cause relatively few adverse effects and have low cardiotoxicity, they are less dangerous than older antidepressants when taken in overdose. The SSRIs, SNRIs, and atypical antidepressants have a low lethality risk in suicide attempts, whereas the tricyclic antidepressants (TCAs) have a very high potential for lethality with overdose.

Indications. The SSRIs have a broad base of clinical use. In addition to their use in treating depressive disorders, the SSRIs have been prescribed with success to treat some anxiety disorders, in particular, obsessive-compulsive disorder and panic disorder (see Chapter 12). Fluoxetine has been found to be effective in treating some women who suffer from late luteal phase dysphoric disorder and bulimia nervosa.

Common adverse reactions. Drugs that selectively enhance synaptic serotonin within the CNS may induce agitation, anxiety, sleep disturbance, tremor, sexual dysfunction (primarily anorgasmia), or tension headache. The effect of the SSRIs on sexual performance may be the most significant undesirable outcome reported by patients. Autonomic reactions (e.g., dry mouth, sweating, weight change, mild nausea, loose bowel movements) may also be experienced with the SSRIs.

Potential toxic effects. One rare and life-threatening event associated with SSRIs is serotonin syndrome. This syndrome is thought to be related to overactivation of the central serotonin receptors, caused by either too high a dose or interaction with other drugs, including non-prescription medication like St. John's wort. Symptoms include abdominal pain, diarrhea, sweating, fever, tachycardia, elevated blood pressure, altered mental state (delirium), myoclonus (muscle spasms), increased motor activity, irritability, hostility, and mood change. Severe manifestations can induce hyperpyrexia (excessively high fever), cardiovascular shock, or death.

The risk of this syndrome seems to be greatest when an SSRI is administered in combination with a second serotonin-enhancing agent, such as a monoamine oxidase inhibitor (MAOI). A patient should discontinue all SSRIs for 2 to 5 weeks before starting an MAOI. Box 13.3 lists the signs and symptoms of serotonin syndrome and gives emergency treatment guidelines. Patient and Family Teaching: Selective Serotonin Reuptake Inhibitors (SSRIs) is a useful tool for teaching the patient and family about the SSRIs.

Serotonin–norepinephrine reuptake inhibitors. The SNRIs inhibit the reuptake of both serotonin and norepinephrine. Pharmacological adverse effects are similar to those of the SSRIs, although the SSRIs may be tolerated better. The SNRIs are indicated for MDD.

Other newer antidepressants. Several other classifications of antidepressants have been introduced and have provided people with depression and prescribers with more options. The name of the classification describes the action of the antidepressants. They are the serotonin antagonist and reuptake inhibitors (SARIs), a norepinephrine–dopamine

BOX 13.3 Serotonin Syndrome: Symptoms and Interventions

Symptoms
- Hyperactivity or restlessness
- Tachycardia → cardiovascular shock
- Fever → hyperpyrexia
- Elevated blood pressure
- Altered mental states (delirium)
- Irrationality, mood swings, hostility
- Seizures → status epilepticus
- Myoclonus, incoordination, tonic rigidity
- Abdominal pain, diarrhea, bloating
- Apnea → death

Interventions
- Remove offending agents
- Initiate symptomatic treatment:
  - Serotonin receptor blockade with cyproheptadine, methysergide, propranolol
  - Cooling blankets, chlorpromazine for hyperthermia
  - Dantrolene, diazepam for muscle rigidity or rigours
  - Anticonvulsants
  - Artificial ventilation
  - Paralysis

PATIENT AND FAMILY TEACHING

Selective Serotonin Reuptake Inhibitors (SSRIs)
- May cause sexual dysfunction or lack of sex drive. Inform nurse or primary care provider if this occurs.
- May cause insomnia, anxiety, and nervousness. Inform nurse or primary care provider if this occurs.
- May interact with other medications. Tell primary care provider about other medications patient is taking (digoxin, warfarin). SSRIs should not be taken within 14 days of the last dose of a MAOI.
- No over-the-counter drug should be taken without first notifying primary care provider.
- Common adverse effects include fatigue, nausea, diarrhea, dry mouth, dizziness, tremor, and sexual dysfunction or lack of sex drive.
- Because of the potential for drowsiness and dizziness, patient should not drive or operate machinery until these adverse effects are ruled out.
- Alcohol should be avoided.
- Liver and renal function tests should be performed and blood counts checked periodically.
- Medication should not be discontinued abruptly. If adverse effects become bothersome, patient should ask primary care provider about changing to a different drug. Abrupt cessation can lead to serotonin withdrawal.
- Any of the following symptoms should be reported to the primary care provider immediately:
  - Increase in depression or suicidal thoughts
  - Rash or hives
  - Rapid heartbeat
  - Sore throat
  - Difficulty urinating
  - Fever, malaise
  - Anorexia and weight loss
  - Unusual bleeding
  - Initiation of hyperactive behaviour
  - Severe headache

reuptake inhibitor (NDRI), and a noradrenergic and specific serotonergic antidepressant (NaSSA). Chapter 11 provides more detail about these drug classifications.

Tricyclic antidepressants. The TCAs inhibit the reuptake of norepinephrine and serotonin by the presynaptic neurons in the CNS, increasing the amount of time norepinephrine and serotonin are available to the postsynaptic receptors. This increase in norepinephrine and serotonin in the brain is believed to be responsible for mood elevations.

Indications. The sedative effects of the TCAs are attributed to the blockage of histamine receptors (Burchum & Rosenthal, 2019). Patients must take therapeutic doses of TCAs for 10 to 14 days or longer before they begin to work; full effects may not be seen for 4 to 8 weeks, but an effect on some symptoms of depression, such as insomnia and anorexia, may be noted earlier. Choosing a TCA for a patient is based on what has worked for the patient or a family member in the past and the drug's adverse effects for that patient.

A stimulating TCA, such as desipramine (Desipramine), may be best for a patient who is lethargic and fatigued. If a more sedating effect is needed for agitation or restlessness, drugs such as amitriptyline (Elavil) and doxepin (Sinequan) may be more appropriate choices. Regardless of which TCA is given, the initial dose should always be low and increased gradually.

Common adverse reactions. The chemical structure of the TCAs closely resembles that of antipsychotic medications, and the anticholinergic actions are similar (e.g., dry mouth, blurred vision, tachycardia, constipation, urinary retention, esophageal reflux). These adverse effects are more common and more severe in patients taking antidepressants than in patients taking antipsychotic medications. They usually are not serious and are often transitory, but urinary retention and severe constipation warrant immediate medical attention. Weight gain is also a common complaint among people taking TCAs.

The α-adrenergic blockade of the TCAs can produce postural-orthostatic hypotension and tachycardia. Postural hypotension can lead to dizziness and increase the risk for falls.

Administering the total daily dose of TCA at night is beneficial for two reasons: (1) most TCAs have sedative effects and thereby aid sleep, and (2) the minor adverse effects occur while the individual is sleeping, which increases adherence to drug therapy.

Potential toxic effects. The most serious effects of the TCAs are cardiovascular: dysrhythmias, tachycardia, myocardial infarction, and heart block have been reported. Because the cardiac adverse effects are so serious, TCA use is considered a risk in older persons and patients with cardiac disease. Patients should have a thorough cardiac workup before beginning TCA therapy.

Adverse drug interactions. A few of the more common medications usually not given while TCAs are being used are MAOIs, phenothiazines, barbiturates, disulfiram, oral contraceptives (or other estrogen preparations), anticoagulants, some antihypertensives, benzodiazepines, and alcohol. A patient who is taking any of these medications along with a TCA should have medical clearance because some of the reactions can be fatal.

Contraindications. People who have recently had a myocardial infarction (or other cardiovascular problems), those with narrow-angle glaucoma or a history of seizures, and women who are pregnant should not be treated with TCAs, except with extreme caution and careful monitoring.

Patient and family teaching. Topics for the nurse to discuss when teaching patients and their families about TCA therapy are presented in Patient and Family Teaching: Tricyclic Antidepressants (TCAs).

PATIENT AND FAMILY TEACHING
Tricyclic Antidepressants (TCAs)

- The patient and family should be told that mood elevation may take from 7 to 28 days. Up to 6 to 8 weeks may be required for the full effect to be reached and for major depressive symptoms to subside.
- The family should reinforce this information frequently to the family member with depression, who may have trouble remembering and may respond to ongoing reassurance.
- The patient should be reassured that drowsiness, dizziness, and hypotension usually subside after the first few weeks.
- The patient should be cautioned to be careful when working around machines, driving cars, and crossing streets because of possible altered reflexes, drowsiness, or dizziness.
- Alcohol can block the effects of antidepressants. The patient should be told to refrain from drinking.
- If possible, the patient should take the full dose at bedtime to reduce the experience of adverse effects during the day.
- If the bedtime dose (or the once-a-day dose) is missed, the patient should take the dose within 3 hours; otherwise, the patient should wait until the usual medication time on the next day. The patient should not double the dose.
- Suddenly stopping TCAs can cause nausea, altered heartbeat, nightmares, and cold sweats within 2 to 4 days. The patient should call the primary care provider or take one dose of the TCA until the primary care provider can be contacted.

Monoamine oxidase inhibitors. The enzyme monoamine oxidase is responsible for inactivating, or breaking down, certain monoamine neurotransmitters in the brain, such as norepinephrine, serotonin, dopamine, and tyramine. When a person ingests an MAOI, these amines do not get inactivated, and there is an increase of neurotransmitters available for synaptic release in the brain. The increase in norepinephrine, serotonin, and dopamine is the desired effect because it results in mood elevation. The increase in tyramine, on the other hand, poses a problem. When the level of tyramine increases, and it is not inactivated by monoamine oxidase, high blood pressure, hypertensive crisis, and eventually cerebrovascular accident can occur. Therefore people taking these drugs must reduce or eliminate their intake of foods and drugs that contain high amounts of tyramine (Box 13.4; Table 13.5).

BOX 13.4 Drugs That Can Interact With Monoamine Oxidase Inhibitors (MAOIs)

- Over-the-counter medications for colds, allergies, or congestion (any product containing ephedrine or phenylpropanolamine)
- Tricyclic antidepressants (imipramine, amitriptyline)
- Narcotics
- Antihypertensives (methyldopa, spironolactone)
- Amine precursors (levodopa, L-tryptophan)
- Sedatives (alcohol, barbiturates, benzodiazepines)
- General anesthetics
- Stimulants (amphetamines, cocaine)

TABLE 13.5 Foods That Can Interact With Monoamine Oxidase Inhibitors (MAOIs)

Foods That Contain Tyramine

Category	Unsafe Foods (High Tyramine Content)	Safe Foods (Little or No Tyramine)
Vegetables	Avocados, especially if over-ripe; fermented bean curd; fermented soybean; soybean paste	Most vegetables
Fruits	Figs, especially if over-ripe; bananas, in large amounts	Most fruits
Meats	Meats that are fermented, smoked, or otherwise aged; spoiled meats; liver, unless very fresh	Meats that are known to be fresh (exercise caution in restaurants; meats may not be fresh)
Sausages	Fermented varieties; bologna, pepperoni, salami, others	Non-fermented varieties
Fish	Dried or cured fish; fish that is fermented, smoked, or otherwise aged; spoiled fish	Fish that is known to be fresh; vacuum-packed fish, if eaten promptly or refrigerated only briefly after opening
Milk, milk products	Practically all cheeses	Milk, yogurt, cottage cheese, cream cheese
Foods with yeast	Yeast extract (e.g., Marmite, Bovril)	Baked goods that contain yeast
Beer, wine	Some imported beers, Chianti wines	Major domestic brands of beer; most wines
Other foods	Protein dietary supplements; soups (may contain protein extract); shrimp paste; soy sauce	

Foods That Contain Other Vasopressors

Food	Comments
Chocolate	Contains phenylethylamine, a pressor agent; large amounts can cause a reaction.
Fava beans	Contain dopamine, a pressor agent; reactions are most likely with over-ripe beans.
Ginseng	Headache, tremulousness, and mania-like reactions have occurred.
Caffeinated beverages	Caffeine is a weak pressor agent; large amounts may cause a reaction.

Source: Burchum, J., & Rosenthal, L. (2019). *Lehne's pharmacology for nursing care* (10th ed.). St. Louis: Elsevier.

Because people with depression are often lethargic, confused, and apathetic, adherence to strict dietary limitations may not be realistic. That is why MAOIs, although highly effective, are not often given as a first-line treatment.

Indications. MAOIs are particularly effective for people with atypical depression (characterized by mood reactivity, oversleeping, and overeating), along with panic disorder, social phobia, generalized anxiety disorder, obsessive-compulsive disorder, post-traumatic stress disorder, and bulimia. The MAOIs commonly used in Canada at present are phenelzine (Nardil) and tranylcypromine sulphate (Parnate).

Common adverse reactions. Some common and troublesome long-term adverse effects of the MAOIs are orthostatic hypotension, weight gain, edema, change in cardiac rate and rhythm, constipation, urinary hesitancy, sexual dysfunction, vertigo, overactivity, muscle twitching, hypomanic and manic behaviour, insomnia, weakness, and fatigue.

Potential toxic effects. The most serious reaction to the MAOIs is an increase in blood pressure, with the possible development of intracranial hemorrhage, hyperpyrexia, convulsions, coma, and death. Therefore routine monitoring of blood pressure, especially during the first 6 weeks of treatment, is necessary.

Because many drugs, foods, and beverages can cause an increase in blood pressure in patients taking MAOIs, hypertensive crisis is a constant concern. The hypertensive crisis usually occurs within 15 to 90 minutes of ingestion of the contraindicated substance. Early symptoms include irritability, anxiety, flushing, sweating, and a severe headache. The patient then becomes anxious, restless, and develops a fever. Eventually the fever becomes severe, seizures ensue, and coma or death is possible.

When a hypertensive crisis is suspected, immediate medical attention is crucial. If ingestion is recent, gastric lavage and charcoal may be helpful. Pyrexia is treated with hypothermic blankets or ice packs. Fluid therapy is essential, particularly with hyperthermia. A short-acting antihypertensive agent such as nitroprusside, nitroglycerine, or phentolamine may be used. Intravenous benzodiazepines are useful for agitation and seizure control.

Table 13.6 identifies common adverse effects and toxic effects of the MAOIs, and Patient and Family Teaching: Monoamine Oxidase Inhibitors (MAOIs) can be used as an MAOI teaching guide for patients and their families.

PATIENT AND FAMILY TEACHING
Monoamine Oxidase Inhibitors (MAOIs)

- Educate and provide details to the patient and family to avoid certain foods and all medications (especially cold remedies) unless prescribed by and discussed with the patient's primary care provider (see Table 13.5 and Box 13.4 for specific food and drug restrictions).
- Give the patient a wallet card describing the MAOI regimen.
- Instruct the patient to avoid Chinese restaurants (sherry, brewer's yeast, and other contraindicated products may be used).
- Advise the patient to go to the emergency department immediately if they have a severe headache.
- Ideally, blood pressure should be monitored during the first 6 weeks of treatment (for both hypotensive and hypertensive effects).
- After the MAOI is stopped, instruct the patient that dietary and drug restrictions should be maintained for 14 days.

Contraindications. The use of MAOIs may be contraindicated with each of the following:
- Cerebrovascular disease
- Hypertension and congestive heart failure
- Liver disease
- Consumption of foods containing tyramine, tryptophan, and dopamine (see Table 13.5)
- Use of certain medications (see Box 13.3)
- Recurrent or severe headaches
- Surgery in the previous 10 to 14 days
- Age younger than 16 years

Use of antidepressants by pregnant people. The risk of depression in pregnancy may be as high as 20% (Olivier et al., 2015). There is evidence that depression has a negative effect on birth outcomes. Preeclampsia, diabetes, and hypertension have all been associated with maternal depression. Low birth weight, preterm birth, and small size for gestational age have been noted effects in infants born to maternal depression. It is known that antidepressants cross the placenta. Treatment of severe depression, particularly with suicidal ideation, must weigh out the risks versus the benefits.

TABLE 13.6 Adverse Reactions to and Toxic Effects of Monoamine Oxidase Inhibitors (MAOIs)

Adverse Reactions	Comments
Hypotension	Hypotension is a normal adverse effect of MAOIs.
Insomnia	Orthostatic blood pressures should be taken—first lying down, then sitting or standing after 1–2 minutes. Hypotension may be a dangerous adverse effect, especially in older persons who may fall and sustain injuries as a result of dizziness from the blood pressure drop.
Changes in cardiac rhythm	
Anorgasmia or sexual impotence	
Urinary hesitancy or constipation	
Weight gain	

Toxic Effects	Comments
Hypertensive crisis: • Severe headache • Tachycardia, palpitations • Hypertension • Nausea and vomiting	Patient should go to local emergency department immediately—blood pressure should be checked. One of the following may be given to lower blood pressure: • 5 mg intravenous phentolamine • Sublingual nifedipine to promote vasodilation Patients may be prescribed a 10 mg nifedipine capsule to carry in case of emergency.

Sources: Data from Canadian Pharmacists Association & Canadian Pharmaceutical Association. (2016). *Compendium of pharmaceuticals and specialties: Canada's trusted drug reference*. Toronto: Canadian Pharmaceutical Association; Burchum, J., & Rosenthal, L. (2019). *Lehne's pharmacology for nursing care* (10th ed.). St. Louis: Elsevier.

Use of antidepressants by children and adolescents. There are very few antidepressants that are approved by Health Canada for use in children and youth. In 2005 Health Canada issued a Black Box Warning for all antidepressants, alerting the public to the increased risk for suicidal thinking or suicide attempts in children or adolescents under the age of 18 who are taking antidepressants. Following the Black Box Warning, the number of prescriptions written for SSRIs for children and young adults decreased, but the rates of suicide in those age groups actually increased (Mood Disorders Society of Canada, 2019). Dudley and colleagues concluded that the risk for suicide is greater in children and adolescents with depression who do not take antidepressants. To minimize the risk for suicide in people taking antidepressants, close monitoring by health care providers and patient and caregiver education are essential. Chapter 22 has a more detailed discussion of suicide risk factors and warning signs.

Use of antidepressants by older persons. Polypharmacy and the normal process of aging contribute to concerns about prescribing antidepressants for older persons. SSRIs are a first-line treatment for older persons, but they have the potential for aggravated adverse effects. Starting doses are recommended to be half the lowest adult dose, with dose adjustments occurring no more frequently than every 7 days.

TCAs and MAOIs have adverse-effect profiles that are more dangerous for older persons, specifically cardiotoxicity with TCAs and hypotension with both classes. Any medication with an adverse effect of hypotension or sedation in older persons increases the risk for falls. Older persons should be cautioned against abrupt discontinuation of antidepressants because of the possibility of discontinuation syndrome, which causes anxiety, dysphoria, flulike symptoms, dizziness, excessive sweating, and insomnia.

Biological Interventions
Electroconvulsive Therapy

Electroconvulsive therapy (ECT) is a procedure in which electrical currents are passed through the brain, intentionally triggering a brief seizure. ECT seems to cause changes in brain chemistry that can quickly reverse symptoms of certain mental illnesses. It often works when other treatments are unsuccessful. However, despite being a highly effective somatic (physical) treatment for psychiatric disorders, ECT has a bad reputation. This may be due to media portrayals of patients being restrained on a gurney while having a full-blown seizure induced. Given the current sophistication of anesthetic and paralytic agents, ECT is actually not dramatic at all.

Indications. ECT is an effective acute treatment for non-responsive depression (Van de Velde et al., 2020). Psychotic illnesses are the second most common indication for ECT. For drug-resistant patients with psychosis, a combination of ECT and antipsychotic medication has resulted in sustained improvement about 80% of the time. Depression associated with bipolar disorder remits in about 50% of the cases after ECT.

While medication is generally the first line of treatment, ECT may be a primary treatment in the following cases:
- When a patient is experiencing intense suicidal ideation, and there is a need for a rapid, definitive response
- When a patient is severely malnourished, exhausted, and dehydrated due to lengthy depression (after rehydration)
- If previous medication trials have not successfully treated the illness
- If the patient chooses
- When there is marked agitation, marked vegetative symptoms, or catatonia
- For major depression with psychotic features
- In pregnant people
- For people with rapid cycling mood swings (four or more in one year)

ECT is not effective, however, in patients with dysthymia, atypical depression, personality disorders, drug dependence, or depression secondary to situational or social difficulties.

Risk factors. Using ECT requires clinicians to weigh the risk of using this method versus the risk of suicide, quality of life, and potential complications. Several conditions pose risks and require careful assessment and management. For example, because the heart can be stressed at the onset of the seizure and for up to 10 minutes after, careful assessment and management of hypertension, congestive heart failure, cardiac arrhythmias, and other cardiac conditions is warranted (Van de Velde et al., 2020). ECT also stresses the brain as a result of increased cerebral oxygen, blood flow, and intracranial pressure. Conditions such as brain tumours and subdural hematomas may increase the risk of using ECT. Providers of care and patients need to weigh the risk of continued disability or potential suicide from depression against ECT treatment risks.

Procedure. The usual course of ECT for a patient with depression is two or three treatments per week to a total of 6 to 12 treatments. The procedure is explained to the patient, and informed consent is obtained from the patient or the patient's substitute decision maker. The patient is usually given a general anesthetic to induce sleep and a muscle-paralyzing agent to prevent muscle distress and fractures. These medications have revolutionized the comfort and safety of ECT.

Patients should have a pre-ECT assessment, including a chest X-ray, electrocardiogram (ECG), urinalysis, complete blood count, blood urea nitrogen, and electrolyte panel. Benzodiazepines should be discontinued, as they will interfere with the seizure process.

An electroencephalogram (EEG) monitors brain waves, and an ECG monitors cardiac responses. Brief seizures (30 to 60-plus seconds) are deliberately induced by an electrical current (as brief as 1 second) transmitted through electrodes attached to one or both sides of the head (Figure 13.5). To ensure that patients experience a seizure over the entire brain, a blood pressure cuff may be inflated on the lower arm or leg before administration of the paralytic agent. In that way the convulsion can be visualized in the unparalyzed extremity.

Adverse reactions. Patients wake about 15 minutes after the procedure. The patient is often confused and disoriented for several hours. The nurse and family may need to orient the patient frequently during the course of treatment. Most people experience what is called retrograde amnesia, which is a loss of memory of events leading up to and including the treatment itself.

Fig. 13.5 Electroconvulsive therapy. (**Source:** Illustration from National Institute of Mental Health.)

Fig. 13.6 Transcranial magnetic stimulation. (**Source:** Photo courtesy Neuronetics.)

Transcranial Magnetic Stimulation

Transcranial magnetic stimulation (TMS) is a non-invasive treatment modality that uses magnetic resonance imaging (MRI)–strength magnetic pulses to stimulate focal areas of the cerebral cortex (Figure 13.6).

Indications. In 2002 Canada approved the use of TMS for patients who have been unresponsive to at least one antidepressant. Researchers suggest that TMS be used to enhance cognitive function in healthy, non-depressed individuals (Clark & Parasuraman, 2013).

Risk factors. The only absolute contraindication to this procedure is the presence of metal in the area of stimulation. Cochlear implants, brain stimulators, or medication pumps are examples of metals that could interfere with the procedures (Camprodon et al., 2016).

Procedure. Outpatient treatment with TMS takes about 30 minutes and is typically ordered for 5 days a week for 4 to 6 weeks. Patients are awake and alert during the procedure. An electromagnet is placed on the patient's scalp, and short, magnetic pulses pass into the prefrontal cortex of the brain (see Figure 13.6). These pulses are similar to those used by MRI scanners but are more focused. The pulses cause electrical charges to flow and induce neurons to fire or become active. During TMS, patients feel a slight tapping or knocking in the head, contraction of the scalp, and tightening of the jaw.

Potential adverse reactions. After the procedure, patients may experience a headache and lightheadedness. No neurological deficits or memory problems have been noted. Seizures are a rare complication of TMS. Most of the common adverse effects of TMS are mild and include scalp tingling and discomfort at the administration site.

Nerve Stimulation

The use of vagus nerve stimulation (VNS) originated as a treatment for epilepsy. VNS is approved in Canada for treatment-resistant depression (TRD). Clinicians noted that while VNS decreased seizures, it also appeared to improve mood in a population that normally experiences increased rates of depression. The theory behind VNS relates to the action of the vagus nerve, the longest cranial nerve, which extends from the brainstem to organs in the neck, chest, and abdomen. Researchers believe that electrical stimulation of the vagus nerve results in boosting the level of neurotransmitters, thereby improving mood and also improving the action of antidepressants.

Indications. Nearly a decade after VNS was approved for use in Europe, in 2001 Health Canada granted approval for VNS use for TRD. The cost of the stimulation unit is between $15 000 and $25 000, which is generally not covered by provincial health plans. The efficacy of VNS in treating depression is still being established. Other potential applications of VNS include anxiety, obesity, and pain.

Procedure. The surgery to implant VNS is typically an outpatient procedure. A pacemaker-like device is implanted surgically into the left chest wall. The device is connected to a thin, flexible wire that is threaded upward and wrapped around the vagus nerve on the left side of the neck (Figure 13.7). After surgery, an infrared magnetic wand is held against the chest while a personal computer or personal digital assistant is used to program the frequency of pulses. Pulses are usually delivered for 30 seconds, every 5 minutes, 24 hours a day. Antidepressant action usually occurs in several weeks.

Non-surgical methods of VNS include deep diaphragmatic breathing, "om" chanting, and collecting saliva in your mouth and then submerging your tongue in the saliva pool.

Potential adverse reactions. The implantation of VNS (see Figure 13.7) is a surgical procedure, carrying with it the risks inherent in any surgical procedure (e.g., pain, infection, sensitivity to anesthesia). Adverse effects of active VNS therapy are due to the position of the lead on the vagus nerve, which is close to the laryngeal and pharyngeal branches of the left vagus nerve. Voice alteration occurs in more than half of patients. Other adverse effects include neck pain, cough, paresthesia, and dyspnea, which tend to decrease with time. The device can be temporarily turned off at any time by placing a special magnet over the implant. This may be especially helpful when engaging in public speaking or heavy exercise.

Advanced-Practice Interventions

Nurses and nurse practitioners are qualified to provide counselling, social skills training, and group therapy (Canadian Nurses Association, 2019). In some provinces nurse practitioners who have met appropriate educational standards may also be certified to prescribe medication to treat depression.

Psychological interventions

Psychotherapy. CBT, interpersonal therapy (IPT), time-limited focused psychotherapy, and behavioural therapy all are considered especially effective in the treatment of mild to moderate depression.

Fig. 13.7 Vagus nerve stimulation. (**Source:** Image courtesy Cyberonics, Inc.)

INTEGRATIVE THERAPY

Complementary, Alternative, and Integrative Approaches

There is a vast array of complementary, alternative, and integrative approaches in the treatment of depression, including the use of dietary supplements, acupuncture, aromatherapy, meditation, light therapy, homeopathy, and yoga. Herbal products and supplements for depression have become a multi-million dollar industry; however, the long-term effects of these products are not yet clear. The approaches briefly discussed here are light therapy, use of St. John's wort, and exercise.

Light Therapy

Light therapy has been researched for nearly 20 years and is accepted as a first-line treatment for SAD. In the *DSM-5* (American Psychiatric Association, 2013) SAD is considered a subtype of MDD and listed as "with seasonal pattern." People with SAD often live in regions in which there are marked seasonal differences in the amount of daylight.

Light therapy's effectiveness is thought to be the influence of light on melatonin. Melatonin is secreted by the pineal gland and is necessary for maintaining and shifting biological rhythms. Exposure to light suppresses the nocturnal secretion of melatonin, which seems to have a therapeutic effect on people with SAD.

Ideal treatment consists of 30 to 45 minutes of exposure daily to a 10 000-lux light source. Morning exposure is best. However, success has been reported when exposure occurs at other times of the day or in divided doses. Anecdotal reports suggest that increasing the available light by adding additional light sources may also help to elevate mood. For those affected by SAD, light therapy has been found to be as effective in reducing depressive symptoms as medications. Negative adverse effects include headache and jitteriness.

St. John's Wort

St. John's wort (*Hypericum perforatum*) is a flower that can be processed into tea or tablets. This herb may increase the amount of serotonin, norepinephrine, and dopamine in the brain, resulting in antidepressant effects. Studies of St. John's wort used in the treatment of depression provide mixed evaluations. It has generally been found to be as effective as antidepressants in the treatment of mild to moderate depression, but usefulness in severe depression has not been established (Ghosh, 2020). Because St. John's wort is not regulated in Canada, concentrations of the active ingredients may vary from preparation to preparation, an inconsistency that may account for some variation in research results. St. John's wort has the potential for adverse reactions when taken with other medications, and safety has not been established for use during pregnancy or use in children. For example, when taken with prescribed antidepressants, there is an increased risk of patients experiencing serotonin syndrome.

Exercise

Exercise has biological, social, and psychological effects on symptoms of depression. Research shows that exercise increases the availability of serotonin in the brain. It has also been demonstrated to dampen the activity of the hypothalamic–pituitary–adrenal axis, which is believed to be overly active in depression. People with depression who exercise regularly report feeling an elevated mood and greater happiness, and they become more socially involved. Additional benefits of exercise are that it is more easily accessed, less expensive, and results in fewer adverse effects than antidepressants.

Source: Ghosh, D. (2020). *Nutraceuticals in brain health and beyond* (1st ed.). Philadelphia: Elsevier Academic Press.

However, only CBT and IPT were shown to demonstrate superiority in the maintenance phase. CBT helps people change their negative thought patterns and behaviours, whereas IPT focuses on working through personal relationships that may contribute to depression.

Group therapy. Group therapy is a widespread modality for the treatment of depression; it increases the number of people who can receive treatment at a decreased cost per individual. Another advantage is that groups offer patients an opportunity to socialize and share common feelings and concerns, which decreases feelings of isolation, hopelessness, helplessness, and alienation. Therapy groups also provide a controlled environment in which patients can explore their patterns of interaction and response to others, which may contribute to or exacerbate their depression.

Future of Treatment

Many Canadians continue to have their quality of life negatively affected by depression. As a result, their sense of meaning, fulfillment, and relational connections are affected. To reduce these sequelae, earlier detection, earlier intervention, prevention of progression, achievement of remission, and further integration of neuroscience and behavioural science in the treatment of depression are needed. Priority areas for further development and research are:
- Improving screening for high-risk ages and groups, including:
  - Individuals in late adolescence and early adulthood
  - Women in reproductive years
  - Adults and older persons with medical problems (e.g., pain)
  - People with a family history of depression
- Increasing education, particularly about the link between physical symptoms and depression
- Integrating psychopharmacological treatment augmented with psychological and other non-pharmacological therapies
- Inclusion of more self-care strategies, such as:
  - Promotion of sleep hygiene
  - Increase in exercise
  - Better overall health care

EVALUATION

Short-term indicators and outcome criteria are frequently evaluated during the course of treatment for depression. For example, if the patient with depression came into the unit with suicidal thoughts, the nurse evaluates whether suicidal thoughts are still present, the patient is able to state alternatives to suicidal impulses in the future, the patient is able to explore thoughts and feelings that precede suicidal impulses, and so forth. Outcomes relating to thought processes, self-esteem, and social interactions are frequently formulated, because these areas are often problematic in people with depression.

Physical needs warrant nursing or medical attention. If a patient has lost weight because of anorexia, is the appetite returning? If the patient was constipated, are the bowels now functioning normally? If the patient was suffering from insomnia, are they now sleeping 6 to 8 hours per night? If indicators have not been met, an analysis of the data, nursing diagnoses, goals, and planned nursing interventions is made. The care plan is reassessed and reformulated as necessary.

CASE STUDY AND NURSING CARE PLAN 13.1

Depression

Ms. Glessner is a 35-year-old executive secretary. She has been divorced for 3 years and has two sons, 11 and 13 years of age. She is brought into the emergency department (ED) by her neighbour. She has some slashes on her wrists and is bleeding. The neighbour states that both of Ms. Glessner's sons are visiting their father for the summer. Ms. Glessner has become more and more despondent since terminating a 2-year relationship with a married man 4 weeks previously. According to the neighbour, for 3 years after her divorce, Ms. Glessner talked constantly about not being pretty or good enough and doubted that anyone could really love her. The neighbour states that Ms. Glessner has been withdrawn for at least 3 years. After the relationship with her boyfriend ended, she became even more withdrawn and sullen. Ms. Glessner is about 10 kg overweight, and her neighbour states that Ms. Glessner often stays awake late into the night, drinking by herself and watching television. She sleeps through most of the day on the weekends.

After receiving treatment in the ED, Ms. Glessner is seen by a psychiatrist. The initial diagnosis is persistent depressive disorder with suicidal ideation. A decision is made to hospitalize her briefly for suicide observation and evaluation for appropriate treatment.

The nurse, Ms. Ward, admits Ms. Glessner to the unit from the ED.

Nurse: "Hello, Ms. Glessner. I'm Marcia Ward. I'll be your primary nurse."

Ms. Glessner: "Yeah, I don't need a nurse, a doctor, or anyone else. I just want to get away from this pain."

Nurse: "You want to get away from your pain?"

Ms. Glessner: "I just said that, didn't I? Oh, what's the use? No one understands."

Nurse: "I would like to understand, Ms. Glessner."

Ms. Glessner: "Look at me. I'm fat ... ugly ... and no good to anyone. No one wants me."

Nurse: "Who doesn't want you?"

Ms. Glessner: "My husband didn't want me, and now Jerry has left me to go back to his wife."

Nurse: "You think because Jerry went back to his wife that no one else could care for you?"

Ms. Glessner: "Well, he doesn't anyway."

Nurse: "Because he doesn't care, you believe that no one else cares about you?"

Ms. Glessner: "Yes ...."

Nurse: "Who do you care about?"

Ms. Glessner: "No one ... except my sons. I do love my sons, even though I don't often show it."

Nurse: "Tell me more about your sons."

Ms. Ward continues to speak with Ms. Glessner. Ms. Glessner talks about her sons with some affect and apparent affection; however, she continues to state that she does not think of herself as worthwhile.

Assessment

Self-Assessment

Ms. Ward is aware that when patients have depression, they can be negative, think life is hopeless, and be hostile toward those who want to help. When Ms. Ward was new to the unit, she withdrew from patients with depression and sought out patients who appeared more hopeful and appreciative of her efforts. The unit coordinator was very supportive of Ms. Ward when she was first on the unit. Ms. Ward, along with other staff, was sent to clinical education sessions on working with patients with depression and was encouraged to speak up in staff meetings about the feelings that many of these patients evoked in her. As a primary nurse, she was assigned a variety of patients. She found that as time went on, with the support of her peers and the opportunity to speak up at staff meetings, she was able to take what patients said less personally and not feel so responsible when patients did not respond as fast as she would like.

After 2 years, she had had the experience of seeing many patients who seemed hopeless and despondent on admission respond well to nursing and medical interventions and go on to lead full and satisfying lives. This also made it easier for Ms. Ward to understand that even though the patient with depression may think life is hopeless and may believe there is nothing in life to live for, change is always possible.

Objective Data	Subjective Data
Slashed her wrists	"No one wants me."
Recently broke up with boyfriend	"I just want to get rid of this pain."
Has thought poorly of herself for 3 years, since divorce	"I'm fat ... ugly ... and no good to anyone."
Has two sons she cares about	"I do love my sons, even though I don't often show it."
Is 10 kg overweight	
Stays awake late at night, drinking by herself	
Has been withdrawn since divorce	

Diagnosis

The nurse evaluates Ms. Glessner's strengths and weaknesses and decides to concentrate on two initial nursing diagnoses that seem to have the highest priority:

1. *Risk for suicide* related to separation from 2-year relationship, as evidenced by actual suicide attempt

Supporting Data

- Slashed her wrists
- Recently broke up with boyfriend
- Drinks at night by herself
- Withdrawn for 3 years since divorce

2. *Situational low self-esteem* related to divorce and recent termination of love relationship, as evidenced by derogatory statements about self

CASE STUDY AND NURSING CARE PLAN 13.1—cont'd
Depression

Supporting Data
- "No one wants me."
- "I'm fat ... ugly ... and no good to anyone."
- "I do love my sons, even though I don't often show it."

Outcomes Identification
Patient refrains from attempting suicide.

Planning
Because Ms. Glessner is discharged after 48 hours, the issue of disturbance in self-esteem continues to be addressed in her therapy after discharge. Ms. Ward later reviews the goals for her work with Ms. Glessner in the community.

Implementation
Ms. Glessner's plan of care is personalized as follows:

Short-Term Goal	Intervention	Rationale	Evaluation
1. Patient expresses at least one reason to live, apparent by the second day of hospitalization.	1a. Observe patient every 15 minutes while she is suicidal.	1a, b. Patient safety is ensured. The risk for impulsive self-harmful behaviour is minimized.	**Goal Met** By the end of the second day, Ms. Glessner states that she really did not want to die; she just couldn't stand the loneliness in her life. She states that she loves her sons and would never want to hurt them.
	1b. Remove all dangerous objects from patient.		
	1c. Obtain a "no self-harm" contract with patient for a specific period of time, to be renegotiated (Note: some provinces no longer use contracting).	1c. Contract may help patient gain a sense of control and a feeling of responsibility.	
	1d. Spend regularly scheduled periods of time with patient throughout the day.	1d. This interaction reinforces that the patient is worthwhile and builds her experience in relating better to the nurse on a one-to-one basis.	
	1e. Assist patient in evaluating both positive and negative aspects of her life.	1e. A person with depression is often unable to acknowledge any positive aspects of life unless they are pointed out by others.	
	1f. Encourage appropriate expression of angry feelings.	1f. Providing for expression of pent-up hostility in a safe environment can reinforce more adaptive methods of releasing tension and may minimize need to act out self-directed anger.	
	1g. Accept patient's negativism.	1g. Acceptance enhances feelings of self-worth.	
2. Patient will identify two outside supports she can call on if she feels suicidal in the future.	2a. Explore usual coping behaviours.	2a. Behaviours that need reinforcing and new coping skills that need to be introduced can be identified.	**Goal Met** By discharge, Ms. Glessner states that she is definitely going to try cognitive behavioural therapy. She also discusses joining a women's support group that meets once a week in a neighbouring town.
	2b. Assist patient in identifying members of her support system.	2b. Strengths and weaknesses in her available support systems can be evaluated.	
	2c. Suggest a number of community-based support groups she might wish to discuss or visit (e.g., hotlines, support groups, women's groups).	2c. Patient needs to be aware of community supports to use them.	

Continued

CASE STUDY AND NURSING CARE PLAN 13.1—cont'd
Depression

Short-Term Goal	Intervention	Rationale	Evaluation
	2d. Assist patient in identifying realistic alternatives she is willing to use.	2d. Unless patient agrees with any plan, she will be unable or unwilling to follow through in a crisis.	

Evaluation

During the course of her work with Ms. Ward, Ms. Glessner decides to go to some meetings of Parents Without Partners. She states that she is looking forward to getting back to work and feels much more hopeful about her life. She has also lost 1.5 kg while attending Weight Watchers. She states, "I need to get back into the world." Although Ms. Glessner still has negative thoughts about herself, she admits to feeling more hopeful and better about herself, and she has learned important tools to deal with her negative thoughts.

KEY POINTS TO REMEMBER

- There are a number of subtypes of depression and depressive clinical phenomena. The two primary depressive disorders are major depressive disorder (MDD) and persistent depressive disorder (dysthymia).
- The symptoms of major depression are usually severe enough to interfere with a person's social or occupational functioning. A person with MDD may or may not have psychotic symptoms, and the symptoms usually exhibited during an episode of major depression are different from the characteristics of the normal personality prior to the onset of MDD.
- The symptoms of persistent depressive disorder are often chronic (lasting at least 2 years) and are considered mild to moderate. Usually, a person's social or occupational functioning is not greatly impaired. The symptoms in persistent depressive disorder are often congruent with the person's usual pattern of functioning.
- Many theories exist about the cause of depression. The most accepted is biological (genetic and biochemical) factors; however, cognitive theory, learned helplessness theory, and the diathesis–stress theory help explain triggers to depression and maintenance of depressive thoughts and feelings.
- Nursing assessment includes the evaluation of affect, thought processes (especially suicidal thoughts), mood, feelings, physical behaviour, communication, and religious beliefs and spirituality. The nurse also must be aware of the symptoms that may mask depression.
- Nursing diagnoses can be numerous. Individuals with depression are always evaluated for risk for suicide. Some other common nursing diagnoses are *Disturbed thought processes*, *Chronic low self-esteem*, *Imbalanced nutrition*, *Constipation*, *Disturbed sleep pattern*, *Ineffective coping*, and *Interrupted family processes*.
- Working with people who have depression can evoke intense feelings of hopelessness and frustration in health care workers. Nurses must clarify expectations of themselves and their patients and sort personal feelings from those communicated by the patient via empathy. Peer supervision and individual supervision by an experienced nurse clinician, psychiatric social worker, or psychologist are useful in increasing therapeutic potential.
- Interventions for patients who have depression involve several approaches. Basic-level interventions include using specific principles of communication, planning activities of daily living, administering or participating in psychopharmacological therapy, maintaining a therapeutic environment, and teaching patients about the biochemical aspects of depression.
- Advanced-practice interventions may include several short-term psychotherapies that are effective in the treatment of depression, including interpersonal therapy (IPT), cognitive behavioural therapy (CBT), skills training (assertiveness and social skills), and some forms of group therapy.
- Depression is often overlooked in children, adolescents, and older persons because symptoms of depression are often mistaken for signs of normal development.
- Children and adolescents with disruptive mood dysregulation disorder had previously been diagnosed with bipolar disorder. Usually people with this disorder grow up and are diagnosed with MDD or an anxiety disorder.
- Planning and interventions for patients with depression are based on the recovery model, which involves a therapeutic alliance with health care providers in order to achieve outcomes based on individual patient needs and values.
- Evaluation is ongoing throughout the nursing process, and patients' outcomes are compared with the stated outcome criteria and short-term and intermediate indicators. The care plan is revised when indicators are not being met.

CRITICAL THINKING

1. You are spending time with Mr. Plotsky, who is undergoing a workup for depression. He hardly makes eye contact, slouches in his seat, and wears a blank but sad expression. Mr. Plotsky has had numerous bouts of major depression in the past and says to you, "This will be my last depression. I will never go through this again."
    a. Since safety is the first concern, what are the appropriate questions to ask Mr. Plotsky at this time?
    b. In terms of behaviours, thought processes, activities of daily living, and ability to function at work and home, give examples of the kinds of signs and symptoms you might find when assessing a patient with depression.
    c. Mr. Plotsky tells you that he has been on every medication there is, but none has worked. He asks you about the herb St. John's wort. What should you tell him about its effectiveness for severe depression, interactions with other antidepressants, and regulatory status?
    d. What might be some somatic options for a person who is resistant to antidepressant medications?
    e. Mr. Plotsky asks what causes depression. In simple terms how might you respond to his query?
    f. Mr. Plotsky tells you that he has never tried therapy because he thinks it is for weaklings. What information could you give him about various therapeutic modalities that have proven effective for other patients with depression?

2. You are working with Ms. Fok, a 28-year-old with MDD on long-term antidepressant therapy. She asks you about the possibility of pregnancy while taking her SSRIs.
   a. What are some of the things Ms. Fok might want to consider about taking antidepressants if she plans to get pregnant?
   b. If she decides to stop taking her antidepressants, what are some things she might do to help manage her depression?
3. You are working with Mrs. Burton, who has recently been diagnosed with chronic heart failure. In caring for Mrs. Burton, what are two key areas of assessment?
4. What are some of the key areas to consider when working with an older person considering ECT for depression?

CHAPTER REVIEW

1. The nurse is caring for a patient who exhibits disorganized thinking and delusions. The patient repeatedly states, "I hear voices of aliens trying to contact me." The nurse should recognize this presentation as which type of major depressive disorder (MDD)?
   a. Catatonic
   b. Atypical
   c. Melancholic
   d. Psychotic
2. Which patient statement indicates learned helplessness?
   a. "I am a horrible person."
   b. "Everyone in the world is just out to get me."
   c. "It's all my fault that my husband left me for another woman."
   d. "I hate myself."
3. The nurse is planning care for a patient with depression who will be discharged to home soon. What aspect of teaching should be the priority on the nurse's discharge plan of care?
   a. Pharmacological teaching
   b. Safety risk
   c. Awareness of symptoms of increasing depression
   d. The need for interpersonal contact
4. The nurse is reviewing orders given for a patient with depression. Which order should the nurse question?
   a. A low starting dose of a tricyclic antidepressant
   b. An SSRI given initially with an MAOI
   c. Electroconvulsive therapy to treat suicidal thoughts
   d. Elavil to address the patient's agitation
5. Which of the following are considered vegetative signs of depression?
   a. Hallucinations and delusions
   b. Expressions of guilt and worthlessness
   c. Feelings of helplessness and hopelessness
   d. Changes in physiological functioning such as appetite and sleep disturbances
6. Which assessment question asked by the nurse demonstrates an understanding of comorbid mental health conditions associated with major depressive disorder? **Select all that apply**.
   a. "Do rules apply to you?"
   b. "What do you do to manage anxiety?"
   c. "Do you have a history of disordered eating?"
   d. "Do you think that you drink too much?"
   e. "Have you ever been arrested for committing a crime?"
7. Which chronic medical condition is a common trigger for major depressive disorder?
   a. Pain
   b. Hypertension
   c. Hypothyroidism
   d. Crohn's disease

 http://evolve.elsevier.com/Canada/Varcarolis/psychiatric/

REFERENCES

American Psychiatric Association. (2013). *Diagnostic and statistical manual of mental disorders* (5th ed.). Arlington: Author.

Beck, A. T., & Rush, A. J. (1995). Cognitive therapy. In H. I. Kaplan, & B. J. Sadock (Eds.), *Comprehensive textbook of psychiatry/VI* (Vol. 2, pp. 1847–1856). Baltimore: Williams & Wilkins.

Boland, R. (2021). *Kaplan and Sadock's synopsis of psychiatry* (12th ed.). Philadelphia: Wolters Kluwer.

Burchum, J., & Rosenthal, L. (2019). *Lehne's pharmacology for nursing care* (10th ed.). St Louis: Elsevier.

Camprodon, J. A., Kaur, N., Rauch, S. L., et al. (2016). Neurotherapeutics. In T. Stern, M. Fava, & T. E. Wilens et al (Eds.), *Massachusetts General Hospital handbook of general hospital psychiatry* (2nd ed.). Philadelphia: Elsevier.

Canadian Nurses Association. (2019). *Advanced nursing practice: A pan-Canadian framework*. Ottawa: Author.

Clark, V. P., & Parasuraman, R. (2013). Neuroenhancement: Enhancing brain and mind in health and disease. *Neuroimage, 85*, 889–894.

de Roten, Y., Ambresin, G., Herrera, F., et al. (2017). Efficacy of adjunctive brief psychodynamic psychotherapy to usual inpatient treatment of depression: Results of a randomized controlled trial. *Journal of Affective Disorders, 209*(2017), 105–113. https://doi.org/10.1016/j.jad.2016.11.013

Doney, E., Cadoret, A., Dion-Albert, L., Lebel, M., & Menard, C. (2021). Inflammation-driven brain and gut barrier dysfunction in stress and mood disorders. *The European Journal of Neuroscience*, 1–44. https://doi.org/10.1111/ejn.15239

Ghosh, D. (2020). *Nutraceuticals in brain health and beyond* (1st ed.). Philadelphia: Elsevier Academic Press.

Government of Canada. (2016). *What is depression?*. Ottawa: Author.

Jakobsen, J. C., Gluud, C., & Kirsch, I. (2020). Should antidepressants be used for major depressive disorder?. *BMJ Evidence-Based Medicine, 25*(4), 130–136. https://doi.org/10.1136/bmjebm-2019-111238

Lanctot, K. L., Patrice Lindsay, M., Smith, E. E., et al. (2020). Canadian Stroke Best Practice Recommendations: Mood, cognition and fatigue following stroke, 6th edition update 2019. *International Journal of Stroke, 15*(6), 668–688. https://doi.org/10.1177/1747493019847334

Lemos, J. C., & Alvarez, V. A. (2020). The upside of stress: A mechanism for the positive motivational role of corticotropin releasing factor. *Neuropsychopharmacol, 45*, 219–220. https://doi.org/10.1038/s41386-019-0510-9

Mood Disorders Society of Canada. (2019). *Quick facts: Mental health & addictions in Canada*. Bellville: Author.

Moorhead, S., Johnson, M., Maas, M., et al. (2018). *Nursing Outcomes Classification (NOC)* (6th ed.). St. Louis: Mosby.

Olivier, J. D. A., Akerud, H., & Promomaa, I. S. (2015). Antenatal depression and antidepressants during pregnancy. *European Journal of Pharmacology, 753*, 257–262.

Paine, D. R., & Sandage, S. J. (2017). Religious involvement and depression: The mediating effect of relational spirituality. *Journal of Religion and Health, 56*(1), 269–283. https://doi.org/10.1007/s10943-016-0282-z

Rodriguez, T. (2018). Exploring the link between persistent infection, inflammation, and mood disorders. *Psychiatry Advisor*. Retrieved May 25 from https://www.psychiatryadvisor.com/home/bipolar-disorder-advisor/exploring-the-link-between-persistent-infection-inflammation-and-mood-disorders/

Scaini, S., Centorame, G., Lissandrello, F., et al. (2020). The role of genetic and environmental factors in covariation between anxiety and anger in childhood. *European Child & Adolescent Psychiatry, 30*(4), 607–617. https://doi.org/10.1007/s00787-020-01543-2

Seligman, M. E. (1973). Fall into hopelessness. *Psychology Today, 7*(1), 43–48.

Sheikh, J., & Yesavage, J. (1986). Geriatric depression scale (GDS): Recent evidence and development of a shorter version. *Clinical Gerontologist, 5*(1–2), 165–173.

Van de Velde, N., Kappen, M., Koster, E. H. W., et al. (2020). Cognitive remediation following electroconvulsive therapy in patients with treatment resistant depression: Randomized controlled trial of an intervention for relapse prevention—study protocol. *BMC Psychiatry, 20*(453). https://doi.org/10.1186/s12888-020-02856-x

14

Bipolar Disorders

Cheryl L. Pollard

Originating US chapter by Margaret Jordan Halter

 https://evolve.elsevier.com/Canada/Varcarolis/psychiatric/

OBJECTIVES

1. Assess a person experiencing mania for (1) mood, (2) behaviour, and (3) thought processes, and be alert to possible dysfunction.
2. Describe the signs and symptoms of bipolar I, bipolar II, and cyclothymic disorder.
3. Distinguish between mania and hypomania.
4. Formulate three nursing diagnoses appropriate for a person with mania, and include supporting data.
5. Explain the rationales behind five methods of communication that may be used with a person experiencing mania.
6. Distinguish the focus of treatment for a person in the acute manic phase from the focus of treatment for a person in the continuation or maintenance phase.
7. Describe common medications used for bipolar disorders.
8. Distinguish between signs of early and severe lithium toxicity.
9. Write a medication care plan specifying five areas of teaching regarding lithium carbonate.
10. Evaluate specific indications for the use of seclusion for a person experiencing mania.
11. Review at least three of the items presented in the patient and family teaching plan (see Patient and Family Teaching: Bipolar Disorder) with a person with bipolar disorder.

KEY TERMS AND CONCEPTS

acute phase
anticonvulsant drugs
bipolar I disorder
bipolar II disorder
clang associations
continuation phase
cyclothymic disorder
euphoric mood
flight of ideas
grandiosity
hypomania
maintenance phase
mania
manic episode
rapid cycling
seclusion protocol

Once commonly known as *manic depression*, bipolar disorder is a chronic, recurrent illness that must be carefully managed throughout a person's life. Bipolar disorder frequently goes unrecognized, and people suffer for years before receiving a proper diagnosis and treatment. Bipolar disorder is marked by shifts in mood, energy, and ability to function. The course of the illness is variable, and symptoms range from **mania**, an exaggerated euphoria or irritability, to depression (Figure 14.1). Periods of normal functioning may alternate with periods of illness (highs, lows, or a combination of both). However, many individuals continue to experience chronic interpersonal or occupational difficulties even during remission. According to the Mood Disorders Society of Canada (2019), approximately 1% of Canadians will experience bipolar disorder. The mortality rate among individuals with bipolar disorder is two to three times greater than that of the general population. Suicide accounts for 5% of deaths among women and 10% of deaths among men with bipolar disorder compared with 1 and 2%, respectively, in the general population.

CLINICAL PICTURE

The three types of bipolar and related disorders that we discuss in this chapter are bipolar I, bipolar II, and cyclothymic disorder.

Bipolar I Disorder

Bipolar I disorder is marked by severe shifts in mood, energy, and inability to function. Periods of normal functioning may alternate with periods of illness (highs, lows, or a combination of both). Many individuals continue to experience chronic interpersonal or occupational difficulties even during remission.

Individuals with bipolar I disorder have experienced at least one manic episode. Mania is a period of intense mood disturbance with persistent elevation, expansiveness, irritability, and extreme goal-directed activity or energy. These periods last at least 1 week for most of the day, every day. Symptoms of mania are so severe that this state is a psychiatric emergency. Manic episodes usually alternate with depression or a mixed state of anxiety and depression (refer to Chapter 13 for a full discussion of depression).

Initially, individuals experiencing a **manic episode** feel euphoric and energized, they don't sleep or eat, and they are in perpetual motion. They often take significant risks and engage in hazardous activities. Unfortunately, the person with mania does not recognize the behaviours as being problematic and will usually resist treatment.

As the mania intensifies, individuals may become psychotic and experience hallucinations, delusions, and dramatically disturbed thoughts and behaviour. Hallucinations tend to be auditory, and individuals may

249

Fig. 14.1 Continuum of bipolar symptoms.

❤ HOW A NURSE HELPED ME
Support and Care for My Brother and Me

Life was always different in our house; there were good days and bad days, but there really wasn't a dull day. To my brother and me, Mom was normal, we knew no differently. But to my friends, Mom was strange and "crazy" sometimes. My brother and I often moved around, from relative to relative and from place to place. When I was 17, my mom had another episode and was in hospital once again, and I was left to raise my little brother. Mom was discharged from hospital after 2 months of care, a little longer than usual, but I thought nothing of this as Mom had been in and out of hospital throughout my childhood. Everything was settled for the next couple of months, but I noticed Mom giving away household items as well as buying a lot of new things for the house, this time really quickly. This was a sign, I had learned over the years, that Mom was becoming unwell again. She had bought a new mobile home and airline tickets for an overseas holiday, something we never actually used. Mom had been admitted to hospital again to stabilize, as the nurses always explained to me. This hospital stay was different, as she stayed in for only 2 weeks and was provided with a case manager to follow up with her at home. The case manager was a nurse who was invaluable to Mom's care, but the nurse was also a wealth of help and care to my brother and me. Mom's case manager came over regularly, talked to Mom about her medications and about her signs and symptoms of becoming unwell but, more importantly, about her ongoing care. The nurse also helped my brother and me understand and watch for signs and symptoms of Mom's bipolar disorder. Mom was stable for a little while, and although she had no money left after the extravagant holiday she'd booked and the new mobile home in our yard, life was more stable, until Mom asked me to join her and the nurse case manager for a chat. I was to find out that Mom had cancer. She'd had it for a while, and the future was not positive. Mom died 2 months after that chat, and life was yet again upside down for my brother and me. It was the nurse who helped us move forward. We all thought that, since Mom had died, there would be no reason for the nurse to visit, but this was not the case. Not only did she make Mom's last days with us comfortable and some of the most stable times we'd had with Mom, but she continued to visit my brother and me, provide support for us both, and help link us with various community supports. The nurse supported my mom but also my brother and me, and without this caring nurse and the continued support after Mom died, my brother and I would not have had the happy memories we have of Mom today. It is the nurse we thank not only for teaching us about bipolar disorder but also for bringing us to an understanding and appreciation of what a good mom we had, even during the rough times, and to the realization that there is support for people who are in the same position as my mom.

begin to hear voices, sometimes the voice of God. They may believe that they are a person of extreme influence and power.

The initial euphoria of mania gives way to agitation and irritability. Utter exhaustion eventually happens, and many people ultimately collapse into depression. Depression and the agitated state of mania is a dangerous combination that can lead to extreme behaviours such as violence or suicide.

People may be at equal risk for developing anxiety as depression after an episode of mania (Olfson et al., 2017). They may even experience a major depressive disorder and generalized anxiety disorder simultaneously after a manic event. If clinicians adopted a broader definition of bipolar disorder that includes anxiety as an alternating symptom, we possibly would be able to identify bipolar disorder earlier and develop different treatment approaches. Individuals whose main symptom is anxiety should be assessed for a history of mania before being treated for anxiety (see *DSM-5*: Diagnostic Criteria for Bipolar I Disorder box).

Bipolar II Disorder

Individuals with **bipolar II disorder** have experienced at least one hypomanic episode and at least one major depressive episode. **Hypomania** refers to a lower-level and less dramatic mania. However, this level of mania still causes significant issues in relationships and occupational functioning. Like mania, hypomania is accompanied by excessive activity and energy for at least 4 days and involves at least three of the behaviours listed under Criterion B in the *Diagnostic and Statistical Manual of Mental Disorders, fifth edition (DSM-5)*. Unlike mania, psychosis is never present with hypomania. Psychotic symptoms may, however, accompany the depressive side of the disorder. Hospitalization is rare. However, the depressive symptoms can be quite profound and may put those who suffer from it at particular risk for suicide.

Among adults, bipolar II disorder is believed to be underdiagnosed and is often mistaken for major depression or personality disorders,

> **DSM-5**
> *Diagnostic Criteria for Bipolar I Disorder*
>
> For a diagnosis of bipolar I disorder, it is necessary to meet the following criteria for a manic episode. The manic episode may have been preceded by and may be followed by hypomanic or major depressive episodes.
>
> **Manic Episode**
> A. A distinct period of abnormally and persistently elevated, expansive, or irritable mood and abnormally and persistently increased goal-directed activity or energy, lasting at least 1 week and present most of the day, nearly every day (or any duration if hospitalization is necessary).
> B. During the period of mood disturbance and increased energy or activity, three (or more) of the following symptoms (four if the mood is only irritable) are present to a significant degree and represent a noticeable change from usual behaviour:
>   1. Inflated self-esteem or grandiosity.
>   2. Decreased need for sleep (e.g., feels rested after only 3 hours of sleep).
>   3. More talkative than usual or pressure to keep talking.
>   4. Flight of ideas or subjective experience that thoughts are racing.
>   5. Distractibility (i.e., attention too easily drawn to unimportant or irrelevant external stimuli), as reported or observed.
>   6. Increase in goal-directed activity (either socially, at work or school, or sexually) or psychomotor agitation (i.e., purposeless non–goal-directed activity).
>   7. Excessive involvement in activities that have a high potential for painful consequences (e.g., engaging in unrestrained buying sprees, sexual indiscretions, or foolish business investments).
> C. The mood disturbance is sufficiently severe to cause marked impairment in social or occupational functioning or to necessitate hospitalization to prevent harm to self or others, or there are psychotic features.
> D. The episode is not attributable to the physiological effects of a substance (e.g., a drug of abuse, a medication, other treatment) or to another medical condition.
>
> **Hypomanic episode**
> A. The mood change must be accompanied by persistently increased energy or activity levels.
> B. Same criteria as manic episode except:
>   - shorter duration (may last only 4 days)
>   - does not cause significant impairment (without psychotic features or requiring hospitalization)
>
> **Depressive episode**
> A. 5 or more of the following symptoms (at least one of which is 1 or 2)
>   1. depressed mood
>   2. diminished interest in activities
>   3. significant weight loss or gain
>   4. insomnia or hypersomnia
>   5. psychomotor agitation or retardation
>   6. fatigue/loss of energy
>   7. feelings of worthlessness or guilt
>   8. decreased concentration/indecisiveness
>   9. suicidal ideation/attempt
>
> **Note:** A full manic episode that emerges during antidepressant treatment (e.g., medication, electroconvulsive therapy) but persists at a fully syndromal level beyond the physiological effect of that treatment is sufficient evidence for a manic episode and, therefore, a bipolar I diagnosis.
>
> **Note:** Criteria A through D constitute a manic episode. At least one lifetime manic episode is required for the diagnosis of bipolar I disorder.

Source: American Psychiatric Association. (2013). *Diagnostic and statistical manual of mental disorders* (5th ed.). Arlington: Author.

when it actually may be the most common form of bipolar disorder. Clinicians may downplay bipolar II and consider it to simply be the milder version of bipolar disorders. However, it is a source of significant morbidity and mortality, particularly due to the occurrence of severe depression. Anyone with major depression should be assessed for symptoms of hypomania because these symptoms are frequently associated with a progression to bipolar disorder.

Cyclothymic Disorder

Cyclothymic disorder has symptoms of hypomania alternating with symptoms of mild to moderate depression for at least 2 years in adults and 1 year in children. Hypomanic and depressive symptoms do not meet the criteria for either bipolar II or major depression, yet the symptoms are disturbing enough to cause social and occupational impairment.

As part of the spectrum of bipolar disorders, cyclothymic disorder may be difficult to distinguish from bipolar II disorder. Individuals with cyclothymic disorder tend to have irritable hypomanic episodes. Children with cyclothymic disorder experience irritability and sleep disturbance.

Some people experience **rapid cycling** and may have at least four changes in mood episodes in a 12-month period. The cycling can also occur within the course of a month or even a 24-hour period. Rapid cycling is associated with more severe symptoms, such as poorer global functioning, high recurrence risk, and resistance to conventional somatic treatments.

Other Bipolar Disorders

Several other bipolar and related disorders are included in the *DSM-5*. They include:

- Substance/Medication-Induced Bipolar and Related Disorder
- Bipolar and Related Disorder Due to Another Medical Condition
- Other Specified Bipolar and Related Disorder
- Unspecified Bipolar and Related Disorder

EPIDEMIOLOGY

The lifetime risk, or the percentage of the population that will ever have a bipolar I or bipolar II disorder, is nearly 4% (Olfson et al., 2017). Table 14.1 provides a snapshot of statistics regarding the bipolar disorders in adults and adolescents 13 to 18 years of age.

Men and women have nearly equal rates of bipolar disorders, yet they respond somewhat differently to their conditions. Men with a bipolar disorder are more likely to have legal problems and commit acts of violence. Women with a bipolar disorder are more likely to abuse alcohol, commit suicide, and develop thyroid disease.

Women who experience a severe postpartum psychosis within 2 weeks of giving birth have a four times greater chance of subsequent

TABLE 14.1 Statistics Related to Bipolar I and II Disorders in Adults and Adolescents

	Bipolar I	Bipolar II
Lifetime prevalence: adult	1.0%	1.1%
Lifetime prevalence: adolescent	2.5%	
12-month prevalence: adult	0.6%	0.8%
12-month prevalence: adolescent	2.2%	
Mean age of onset	18 years	20 years

Source: American Psychiatric Association. (2013). *Diagnostic and statistical manual of mental disorders* (5th ed.). Washington, DC: Author.

conversion to bipolar disorder (Perry et al., 2020). Giving birth may act as a trigger for the first symptoms of bipolar disorder. The precipitant may be hormonal changes and sleep deprivation.

Children and Adolescents

The existence of bipolar disorder in non-adults has been the subject of controversy. At the beginning of the twenty-first century, there was an alarming increase in the number of children and adolescents being diagnosed with bipolar disorder. This diagnosis was given to young people who had chronic irritability and anger along with frequent verbal or behavioural outbursts that were an overreaction to the situation. A bipolar diagnosis for this troubled population provided for additional support from the health care and social systems, an answer for bewildered parents, and an established treatment pathway.

However, clinicians and parents alike had concerns over the trend of diagnosing bipolar disorder in children. The most fundamental issue was that these children and adolescents did not usually go on to have bipolar disorder as adults. More commonly, they would eventually be diagnosed with major depression. Unfortunately, a bipolar diagnosis is a lifelong label, one that is stigmatized more than depression. This diagnosis also results in exposure to powerful medications during crucial growth periods. In 2013 the American Psychiatric Association developed a new diagnosis to reverse this troubling diagnostic problem, disruptive mood dysregulation disorder. Chapter 13 discusses this new disorder in more detail.

Bipolar disorder in adolescence, particularly late adolescence, is a serious problem. The prevalence rate in this age group mirrors that of adults (Olfson et al., 2017). Researchers estimate that one in five young people with mania plus depression will attempt suicide. Also, these young people experience nearly 2 months per year of role impairment. This impairment has significant implications for individuals who are positioning themselves for a lifetime and a career, as well as developing relationship patterns.

Cyclothymic Disorder

Cyclothymic disorder usually begins in adolescence or early adulthood. There is a 15% to 50% risk that an individual with this disorder will subsequently develop bipolar I or bipolar II disorder. A major risk factor for developing cyclothymic disorder is having a first-degree relative, parent, sibling, or child, with bipolar I disorder.

COMORBIDITY

Bipolar I Disorder

About 75% of people with bipolar I disorder also experience an anxiety disorder. These individuals may experience panic attacks, social anxiety disorder, and specific phobias.

Other challenging disorders may also complicate the clinical presentation and management of the often dramatic bipolar I disorder. They include attention-deficit/hyperactivity disorder and all of the disruptive, impulse control, or conduct disorders. A substance use disorder is present in more than half of individuals with bipolar I, perhaps in an attempt to self-medicate or as a symptom related to increased risk taking. More than 50% of individuals have an alcohol use disorder, which in turn elevates the risk for suicide.

Further complicating treatment is a higher than normal rate of serious medical conditions. Migraines are more common. Metabolic syndrome, a cluster of problems such as high blood pressure, high blood glucose, excess body fat around the waist, and abnormal cholesterol levels, may lead to pre-mature death due to heart disease, stroke, and diabetes.

Bipolar II Disorder

As with bipolar I, about 75% of individuals with bipolar II disorder have a comorbid anxiety disorder. Typically, the anxiety disorders come about before the hypomania and depressive symptoms. Substance use disorders are also common and affect about 37% of people with bipolar II. Anxiety and eating disorders seem to be associated with the depressive side of bipolar II, while substance use disorder symptoms arise along with hypomanic symptoms. Eating disorders, particularly binge eating disorder, affects about 14% of this population.

Cyclothymic Disorder

As with the bipolar disorders, substance use disorders are common with cyclothymic disorder. This may be due to efforts to self-medicate and subdue the bipolar symptoms. Sleep disorders where people have difficulty going to sleep and staying asleep are often present in this disorder. Attention-deficit/hyperactivity disorder is more common among children with cyclothymic disorder than those with other mental health conditions.

ETIOLOGY

Bipolar disorders are thought to be distinctly different from one another; for example, bipolar I disorder, bipolar II disorder, and cyclothymia have different characteristics. Episodes of depression in bipolar disorders are different from unipolar depression (i.e., depression without episodes of mania, see Chapter 13). Depressive episodes in bipolar disorder affect younger people, produce more episodes of illness, and require more frequent hospitalization. They are also characterized by higher rates of divorce and marital conflict.

Theories of the development and onset of bipolar disorders focus on biological, psychological, and environmental factors. Most likely, multiple variables contribute to the occurrence of bipolar disorder. For this reason, a biopsychosocial approach will likely be the most successful approach to treatment.

Biological Factors
Genetic

Bipolar illnesses tend to run in families, and the lifetime risk for individuals with an affected parent is 15% to 30% greater (Perry et al., 2020). Recent research suggests that there may be an overlap between rare genetic variations linked to bipolar disorder and those implicated in schizophrenia and autism (Johansson et al., 2019).

The concordance rate among identical twins is around 70%. This means that if one twin has the disorder, 70% of the time the other one will, too. Despite the high concordance rate in identical twins, it is uncommon for clinicians to find a positive family history for bipolar disorder in these twins' families (Johansson et al., 2019). This finding probably means that the disease is polygenic or that a number of genes contribute to its expression.

Some evidence suggests that bipolar disorders are more prevalent in adults who had high intelligence quotients (IQs), and who were particularly verbal, as children (Smith et al., 2015). People with bipolar disorders appear to achieve higher levels of education and higher occupational status than individuals with unipolar depression. Also, the proportion of patients with bipolar disorders among creative writers, artists, highly educated men and women, and professionals is higher than in the general population.

Neurobiological

Neurotransmitters (norepinephrine, dopamine, and serotonin) have been studied since the 1960s as causal factors in mania and depression. One simple explanation is that having too few of these chemical messengers will result in depression and having an oversupply will cause mania. However, proportions of neurotransmitters in relation to one another may be more important. Receptor site insensitivity could also be at the root of the problem, even if there is enough of a certain neurotransmitter, it may not be going where it needs to go.

Additional research has found that the interrelationships in the neurotransmitter system are complex, and more elaborate theories have been developed since the amine hypotheses were originally proposed. Mood disorders are most likely a result of interactions among various chemicals, including neurotransmitters and hormones.

Brain Structure and Function

Structural neuroimaging techniques (e.g., computed tomography [CT] and magnetic resonance imaging [MRI]) provide still pictures of the scalp, skull, and brain. Structural imaging is useful in viewing bones, tissues, blood vessels, tumours, infection, damage, or bleeding. *Functional* neuroimaging techniques (e.g., positron emission tomography [PET], functional MRI [fMRI], and magnetoencephalography [MEG]) provide measures related to brain activity. Functional imaging reveals activity and chemistry by measuring the rate of blood flow, chemical activity, and electrical impulses in the brain during specific tasks.

With bipolar disorder, functional imaging techniques reveal dysfunction in the prefrontal cortical region, the region associated with executive decision making, personality expression, and social behaviour (Phillips & Swartz, 2014). Dysfunction is also evident in the hippocampus, which is primarily associated with memory, and the amygdala, which is associated with memory, decision making, and emotion. Dysregulation in these areas results in the characteristic emotional lability, heightened reward sensitivity, and emotional dysregulation of bipolar disorder. These abnormalities may be due to grey matter loss in these areas.

Neuroendocrine

The hypothalamic–pituitary–thyroid–adrenal (HPTA) axis has been the object of significant research in bipolar disorder. In fact, hypothyroidism is one of the most common physical abnormalities associated with bipolar disorder. Typically, the thyroid dysfunction is not dramatic and the problem is often undetected.

In both manic and depressive states peripheral inflammation is increased. This inflammation tends to decrease between episodes (Fries et al., 2019). These findings are consistent with changes in the HPTA axis, which are known to drive inflammatory activation.

The role of estrogen in bipolar disorder is also under review. Childbirth is known to be associated with the onset of mood and anxiety disorders. Estrogen studies have shown that people with postpartum psychosis have very low levels of estrogen and improve after estrogen replacement therapy (Meinhard et al., 2014). Selective estrogen receptor modulators (e.g., tamoxifen) have also been shown to produce antimanic effects. Further research in this area is required.

Environmental Factors

Bipolar disorder is a worldwide problem that generally affects all races and ethnic groups equally, but some evidence suggests that bipolar disorders may be more prevalent in upper socioeconomic classes. The exact reason for this finding is unclear; however, people with bipolar disorders appear to achieve higher levels of education and higher occupational status than individuals with unipolar depression. The educational levels of individuals with unipolar depressive disorders, on the other hand, appear to be no different from those of individuals with no symptoms of depression within the same socioeconomic class.

Children who have a genetic and biological risk of developing bipolar disorder are most vulnerable when their social determinants

CONSIDERING CULTURE
Influence of Religion and Supernatural Beliefs in Patients With Bipolar Disorder

Background
Religious and supernatural beliefs influence help-seeking and treatment practices in bipolar disorder, but these are rarely explored by clinicians. This study aimed to understand religiousness, magico-religious beliefs, prevalence of religious and supernatural psychopathology, and treatment practices among patients with bipolar disorder in euthymic state.

Methodology
A total of 185 patients with bipolar disorder currently in remission were assessed cross-sectionally for their clinical profile and their current clinical status on the Hamilton Depression Rating Scale (HDRS), Young Mania Rating Scale (YMRS), and Global Assessment of Functioning (GAF). A semistructured instrument for magico-religious beliefs, etiological models, treatment seeking, and treatment practices was administered.

Results
More than a third of patients (37.8%) had psychopathology with either religious or supernatural content, or both, in their lifetime. Almost half of patients (45.4%) believed in a supernatural or religious causation for their illness. Among the specific causes, planetary influences (13.5%) and God's will (30.8%) were the most common supernatural and religious cause, respectively. Almost half of patients (44.3%) had first treatment contact with religious or supernatural treatment providers. More than 90% of patients reported a belief in God, yet about 70% reported that their doctors did not ask them sufficient questions to understand their religiosity.

Conclusion
Magico-religious beliefs are common among those with bipolar disorder, and a large number of patients attribute these as etiological factors for their illness. Consequently, they tend to seek treatment from traditional practitioners prior to approaching medical practitioners and may continue treatment with them alongside medical management.

Source: Grover, S., Hazari, N., Aaneja, J., et al. (2016). Influence of religion and supernatural beliefs on clinical manifestation and treatment practices in patients with bipolar disorder. *Nordic Journal of Psychiatry, 70*(6), 442–449. Retrieved from https://www.tandfonline.com/doi/abs/10.3109/08039488.2016.1151930. Copyright © 2016 by Taylor & Francis. Reprinted by Permission of Taylor & Francis.

of health are compromised. Stressful family life and adverse life events may result in a more severe course of illness in these individuals. Stress is also a common trigger for mania and depression in adults.

Psychological Factors

With the advent of improved neuroimaging techniques and treatment advances, psychological theories are largely dismissed. Mania was once thought to be a defence against underlying anxiety and depression. Mania was also thought to help individuals tolerate loss or tragedy, such as the death of a loved one. Psychodynamic theorists believed that a faulty ego uses mania when it is overwhelmed by pleasurable impulses such as sex or feared impulses such as aggression. An overactive and critical superego being replaced with the euphoria of mania has also been suggested as the cause.

Psychological factors may present differently among individuals of different cultures. Refer to Chapter 8 for information about cultural implications for psychiatric nursing care.

MOOD DISORDER QUESTIONNAIRE

Instructions: Please answer each question as best you can.

	Yes	No
1. Has there ever been a period of time when you were not your usual self and...		
you felt so good or so hyper that other people thought you were not your normal self or you were so hyper that you got into trouble?	☐	☐
you were so irritable that you shouted at people or started fights or arguments?	☐	☐
you felt much more self-confident than usual?	☐	☐
you got much less sleep than usual and found you didn't really miss it?	☐	☐
you were much more talkative or spoke much faster than usual?	☐	☐
thoughts raced through your head or you couldn't slow down your mind?	☐	☐
you were so easily distracted by things around you that you had trouble concentrating or staying on track?	☐	☐
you had much more energy than usual?	☐	☐
you were much more active or did many more things than usual?	☐	☐
you were much more social or outgoing than usual; for example, you telephoned friends in the middle of the night?	☐	☐
you were much more interested in sex than usual?	☐	☐
you did things that were unusual for you or that other people might have thought were excessive, foolish, or risky?	☐	☐
spending money got you or your family into trouble?	☐	☐
2. If you answered "Yes" to more than one of the above, have several of these ever happened during the same period of time?	☐	☐
3. How much of a problem did any of these cause you — like being unable to work; having family, money, or legal troubles; or getting into arguments or fights? Please select one response only.		

☐ No problem   ☐ Minor problem   ☐ Moderate problem   ☐ Serious problem

	Yes	No
4. Have any of your blood relatives (children, siblings, parents, grandparents, aunts, uncles) had manic-depressive illness or bipolar disorder?	☐	☐
5. Has a health care professional ever told you that you have manic-depressive illness or bipolar disorder?	☐	☐

Criteria for Results: Answering "Yes" to 7 or more of the events in question 1, answering "Yes" to question 2, and answering "Moderate problem" or "Serious problem" to question 3 is considered a positive screen result for bipolar disorder.

Fig. 14.2 The Mood Disorder Questionnaire (MDQ). (**Source:** Hirschfeld, R., Williams, J., Spitzer, R., et al. (2000). Development and validation of a screening instrument for bipolar spectrum disorder: The Mood Disorder Questionnaire. *American Journal of Psychiatry, 157*(11), 1873–1875. Copyright © 2004, Eli Lilly and Company.)

APPLICATION OF THE NURSING PROCESS

Assessment

Individuals with bipolar disorder are often misdiagnosed or underdiagnosed. Early diagnosis and proper treatment can help people avoid:
- Suicide attempts
- Alcohol or substance use
- Marital or work problems
- Development of medical comorbidity

Figure 14.2 presents the Mood Disorder Questionnaire (MDQ). This diagnostic test, while not definitive, is a helpful initial screening device.

General Assessment

Individuals with bipolar disorder tend to spend more time in a depressed state than in a manic state. For a complete discussion of nursing care for the depressive aspects of bipolar disorder, refer to Chapter 13. In this chapter we focus on nursing care for individuals experiencing mania.

The characteristics of mania discussed in the following sections are (1) mood, (2) behaviour, (3) thought processes and speech patterns, and (4) cognitive function.

Mood. The euphoric mood associated with mania is unstable. During euphoria, patients may state that they are experiencing an intense feeling of well-being, are "cheerful in a beautiful world," or are becoming "one with God." The overly joyous mood may seem out of proportion to what is going on, and cheerfulness may be inappropriate for the circumstances, considering that patients are full of energy with little or no sleep. Their mood may change quickly to irritation and anger when they are thwarted. The irritability and belligerence may be short-lived, or it may become the prominent feature of the manic phase of bipolar disorder.

People experiencing a manic state may laugh, joke, and talk in a continuous stream, with uninhibited familiarity. They often demonstrate boundless enthusiasm, treat others with confidential friendliness, and incorporate everyone into their plans and activities. They know no strangers, and energy and self-confidence seem boundless.

To people experiencing mania, no aspirations are too high, and no distances are too far, no boundaries exist to curtail them. Often during impulsive, intrusive, and demanding behaviours, they can become easily angered and show a shift in mood at anyone attempting to stop them or set limits.

As the clinical course progresses from hypomania to mania, sociability and euphoria are replaced by a stage of hostility, irritability, and paranoia. The following is a patient's description of the painful transition from hypomania to mania:

> At first when I'm high, it's tremendous ... ideas are fast ... like shooting stars you follow until brighter ones appear ... all shyness disappears, the right words and gestures are suddenly there ... uninteresting people, things become intensely interesting. Sensuality is pervasive; the desire to seduce and be seduced is irresistible. Your marrow is infused with unbelievable feelings of ease, power, well-being, omnipotence, euphoria ... you can do anything ... but somewhere this changes.... The fast ideas become too fast and there are far too many ... overwhelming confusion replaces clarity ... you stop keeping up with it—memory goes. Infectious humour ceases to amuse—your friends become frightened ... everything now is against the grain ... you are irritable, angry, frightened, uncontrollable, and trapped in the blackest caves of the mind—caves you never knew were there. It will never end. Madness carves its own reality. (Jamison, 1995, p. 70)

Behaviour. When people experience hypomania, they have appetites for social engagement, spending, and activity, even indiscriminate sex. The increased activity and a reduced need for sleep prevent proper rest. Although short periods of sleep are possible, some patients may not sleep for several days in a row. This non-stop physical activity and the lack of sleep and food can lead to physical exhaustion and worsening of mania.

When in full-blown mania, a person constantly goes from one activity, place, or project to another. Many projects may be started, but few, if any, are completed. Inactivity is impossible, even for the shortest period of time. Hyperactivity may range from mild, constant motion to frenetic, wild activity. Flowery and lengthy letters are written,

> ### SAFETY TIP
> Individuals experiencing the symptoms of mania are disinhibited. The nurse may become a source of irritation, flirtation, or another type of pre-occupation. These types of patient reactions are more related to the patient's illness/disease than the qualities of the nurse or other healthcare provider. The nurse needs to interpret the patient's comments through the lens of the patient's illness. Ask yourself, how do the symptoms of mania contribute to the patient's current behaviours? How am I going to react to these behaviours, so I don't contribute to further disinhibited behaviours? Some suggestions include: setting empathetic therapeutic boundaries, keeping conversations simple, focus on the tasks that need to be accomplished, try not to take what the patient says to you personally, neither the positive feedback nor the negative criticisms.

RESEARCH HIGHLIGHT

What Youth With Bipolar Disorder Want When Seeking Health Information Online

Problem

People are increasingly using the Internet to search for health-related information. There was no reported research on how best to help youth with bipolar disorder access online mental health information.

Purpose of Study

The purpose of this study was to examine: (1) how Bipolar Youth Action Project participants currently seek mental health information online, and (2) youth preferences and desires for future developments in the arena of online mental health information provision.

Methods

A multi-disciplinary collaborative research team that included an academic researcher, health care providers, and community members was established. The work of the research team was guided by the belief that collaborating with those with direct involvement and knowledge about the issues will result in relevant findings. As a result, significant community input was sought throughout the research proves. Focus groups were conducted to gather answers to the following question: What are the best methods for sharing information on self-management strategies with other youth, their families, and the wider community?

Key Findings

- Stigma was a significant barrier to accessing information online. Participants described fears related to posting information and being judged.
- Platforms with more anonymity allowed the participants to participate in a more "faceless" manner. However, this did not result in less stigma or less distressing content.
- Finding credible, high-quality online content was a significant barrier.

Implications for Nursing Practice

Many individuals access information online prior to seeking support and guidance from a health professional. Creating credible online mental health information is critical. Providing online mental health services is also increasing. Nursing competencies related to information management and technology will play a larger part in our future practice.

Source: Noack, K., Elliott, N. B., Canas, E., et al. (2016). Credible, centralized, safe, and stigma-free: What youth with bipolar disorder want when seeking health information online. *University of British Columbia Medical Journal, 8*(1), 27–30. Retrieved from https://ojs.library.ubc.ca/index.php/ubcmj/article/view/188033

and excessive phone calls are made. Individuals become involved in pleasurable activities that can have painful consequences, for example, spending large sums of money on frivolous items, giving money away indiscriminately, throwing lavish parties, visiting expensive night clubs and restaurants, or making foolish business investments that can leave an individual or family penniless. Sexual indiscretion can dissolve relationships and marriages and lead to sexually transmitted infections. Religious pre-occupation is a common symptom of mania.

Individuals experiencing mania may be manipulative, profane, fault finding, and adept at exploiting others' vulnerabilities. They constantly push limits. These behaviours often alienate family, friends, employers, health care providers, and others.

Modes of dress often reflect the person's grandiose yet tenuous grasp of reality. Dress may be described as outlandish, bizarre, colourful, and noticeably inappropriate. Makeup may be garish and overdone. People with mania are highly distractible. Concentration is poor, and individuals with mania go from one activity to another without completing anything. Judgement is poor. Impulsive marriages and divorces can take place.

People often emerge from a manic state startled and confused by the shambles of their lives. The following description conveys one patient's experience:

> *Now there are only others' recollections of your behaviour—your bizarre, frenetic, aimless behaviour—at least mania has the grace to dim memories of itself … now it's over, but is it? … Incredible feelings to sort through … Who is being too polite? Who knows what? What did I do? Why? And most hauntingly, will it—when will it—happen again? Medication to take—to resist, to resent, to forget, but always to take. Credit cards revoked … explanations at work … bad cheques and apologies overdue … memory flashes of vague men (what did I do?) … friendships gone, a marriage ruined. (Jamison, 1995, p. 86)*

Thought processes and speech patterns. **Flight of ideas** is a nearly continuous flow of accelerated speech with abrupt changes from topic to topic that are usually based on understandable associations or plays on words. At times, the attentive listener can keep up with the flow of words, even though the direction changes from moment to moment. Speech is rapid, verbose, and circumstantial (including minute and unnecessary details). When the condition is severe, speech may be disorganized and incoherent. The incessant talking often includes joking, puns, and teasing: "How are you doing, kid? No kidding around, I'm going home … home sweet home … home is where the heart is, the heart of the matter is I want out, and that ain't hay … hey, Doc … get me out of this place."

The content of speech is often sexually explicit and ranges from grossly inappropriate to vulgar. Themes in the communication of the individual with mania may revolve around extraordinary sexual prowess, brilliant business ability, or unparalleled artistic talents (e.g., writing, painting, dancing). The person may actually have only average ability in these areas.

Speech is not only profuse but also loud, bellowing, or even screaming. One can hear the force and energy behind the rapid words. As mania escalates, flight of ideas may give way to clang associations. **Clang associations** are the stringing together of words because of their rhyming sounds, without regard to their meaning: "Cinema I and II, last row. Row, row, row your boat. Don't be a cutthroat. Cut your throat. Get your goat. Go out and vote. And so I wrote."

Grandiosity (inflated self-regard) is apparent in both the ideas expressed and the person's behaviour. People with mania may exaggerate their achievements or importance, state that they know famous people, or believe that they have great powers. They boast of exceptional powers, and status can take delusional proportions during mania. Grandiose persecutory delusions are common. For example, people may think that God is speaking to them or that authorities are out to stop them from saving the world. Sensory perceptions may become altered as the mania escalates, and hallucinations may occur. However, no evidence of delusions or hallucinations is present during hypomania.

Cognitive function. The onset of bipolar disorder is often preceded by comparatively high cognitive function. However, there is growing evidence that about one-third of patients with bipolar disorder display significant and persistent cognitive problems and difficulties in psychosocial areas. Cognitive deficits in bipolar disorder are milder but similar to those in patients with schizophrenia. Cognitive impairments are greater in bipolar I but are also present in bipolar II.

The potential cognitive dysfunction among many people with bipolar disorder has specific clinical implications:
- Cognitive function affects overall function.
- Cognitive deficits correlate with a greater number of manic episodes, history of psychosis, chronicity of illness, and poor functional outcome.
- Early diagnosis and treatment are crucial to prevent illness progression, cognitive deficits, and poor outcome.
- Medication selection should consider not only the efficacy of the drug in reducing mood symptoms but also the cognitive impact of the drug on the patient.

Self-Assessment

The person experiencing mania (who is often out of control and resists being controlled) can elicit numerous intense emotions in a nurse. The person may use humour, manipulation, power struggles, or demanding behaviour to prevent or minimize the staff's ability to set limits on and control dangerous behaviour. People with mania have the ability to "staff split," or divide the staff into the "good guys" and the "bad guys": "The nurse on the day shift is always late with my medication and never talks with me. You are the only one who seems to care." This divisive tactic may pit one staff member or group against another, undermining a unified front and consistent plan of care. Frequent team meetings to deal with the behaviours of the person and the nurses' responses to these behaviours can help minimize staff splitting and feelings of anger and isolation. Limit setting (e.g., lights out after 2300 hours) is the main theme in treating a person with mania. Consistency among staff is imperative if the limit setting is to be carried out effectively.

The person can become aggressively demanding, which often triggers frustration, worry, and exasperation in health care providers. The behaviour of a person experiencing mania is often aimed at decreasing the effectiveness of staff control, which could be accomplished by staff members getting involved in power plays. For example, the person might taunt the staff by pointing out faults or oversights and drawing negative attention to one or more staff members. Usually this taunting is done in a loud and disruptive manner, which provokes staff to become defensive and thereby escalates the environmental tension and the person's degree of mania.

If you are working with a person experiencing mania, you may find yourself feeling helplessness, confusion, or even anger. Understanding, acknowledging, and sharing these responses and counter-transference reactions will enhance your professional ability to care for the person and perhaps promote your personal development as well. Collaborating with the interprofessional team, accessing the supervision (as a nursing student) of your nursing faculty member, and sharing your experience with peers in post-conference may be helpful, perhaps essential.

Nursing Diagnosis

Nursing diagnoses vary among people experiencing mania. A primary consideration for a person in acute mania is the prevention of exhaustion

ASSESSMENT GUIDELINES
Bipolar Disorder

1. Assess whether the person is a danger to self or others:
   - People experiencing mania can exhaust themselves to the point of death.
   - People experiencing mania may not eat or sleep, often for days at a time.
   - Poor impulse control may result in harm to others or self.
   - Uncontrolled spending may occur.
2. Assess the need for protection from uninhibited behaviours. External control may be needed to protect the person from such things as bankruptcy because people experiencing mania may give away all of their money or possessions.
3. Assess the need for hospitalization to safeguard and stabilize the person.
4. Assess medical status. A thorough medical examination helps to determine whether mania is primary (a mood disorder, bipolar disorder or cyclothymia) or secondary to another condition.
   - Mania may be secondary to a general medical condition.
   - Mania may be substance induced (caused by use or abuse of a drug or substance or by toxin exposure).
5. Assess for any coexisting medical condition or other situation that warrants special intervention (e.g., substance use, anxiety disorder, legal or financial crises).
6. Assess the person's and family's understanding of bipolar disorder, knowledge of medications, and knowledge of support groups and organizations that provide information on bipolar disorder.

and death from cardiac collapse. Because of the person's poor judgement, excessive and constant motor activity, probable dehydration, and difficulty evaluating reality, *Risk for injury* is a likely and appropriate diagnosis. Table 14.2 lists potential nursing diagnoses for bipolar disorders.

Outcomes Identification

Outcome criteria will be based on which of the three phases of the illness the patient is experiencing. The *Nursing Outcomes Classification (NOC)* (Moorhead et al., 2018) provides useful outcomes for each phase.

Acute Phase

The acute phase occurs during an intense manic, hypomanic or depressive episode. The overall outcome of the **acute phase** is injury prevention. The person may be hospitalized during this phase. Outcomes in the acute phase reflect both physiological and psychiatric issues. For example, the patient will:

- Be well hydrated
- Maintain stable cardiac status
- Maintain and obtain tissue integrity
- Get sufficient sleep and rest
- Demonstrate thought self-control
- Make no attempt at self-harm

Relevant *NOC* outcomes for this phase include *Hydration, Cardiac pump effectiveness, Tissue integrity: Skin and mucous membranes, Sleep, Distorted thought self-control,* and *Suicide self-restraint*. Refer to Chapter 13 for outcomes that also relate to the depressive phase of bipolar disorders.

TABLE 14.2 Potential Nursing Diagnoses for Bipolar Disorders

Signs and Symptoms	Nursing Diagnoses
Excessive and constant motor activity	Risk for injury
Poor judgement	Risk for self-neglect
Lack of rest and sleep	
Poor nutritional intake (excessive or relentless mix of above behaviours can lead to cardiac collapse)	
Loud, profane, hostile, combative, aggressive, demanding behaviours	Risk for other-directed violence
	Risk for self-directed violence
	Risk for suicide
Intrusive and taunting behaviours	Ineffective coping
Inability to control behaviour	Self-neglect
Rage reaction	
Manipulative, angry, or hostile verbal and physical behaviours	Defensive coping
Impulsive speech and actions	Ineffective coping
Property destruction or lashing out at others in a rage reaction	Ineffective impulse control
Racing thoughts, grandiosity, poor judgement	Ineffective coping
	Ineffective impulse control
Giving away of valuables, neglect of family, impulsive major life changes (divorce, career changes)	Interrupted family processes
	Caregiver role strain
Continuous pressured speech, jumping from topic to topic (flight of ideas)	Impaired verbal communication
Constant motor activity, going from one person or event to another	Impaired social interaction
Annoyance or taunting of others, loud and crass speech	Risk for ineffective relationships
Provocative behaviours	
Failure to eat, groom, bathe, or dress self because person is too distracted, agitated, and disorganized	Imbalanced nutrition: less than body requirements
	Deficient fluid volume
	Self-care deficit (bathing, dressing, feeding, toileting)
Inability to sleep because patient is too frantic and hyperactive (sleep deprivation can lead to exhaustion and death)	Disturbed sleep pattern

Continuation Phase

During this stage the presenting symptoms are being controlled but the individual's mental health is still quite fragile. The continuation phase lasts for 4 to 9 months. Although the overall outcome of this phase is relapse prevention, many other outcomes must be accomplished to achieve relapse prevention. These outcomes include:

- Psychoeducational classes for the patient and family related to:
  - Knowledge of disease process
  - Knowledge of medication
  - Consequences of substance addictions for predicting future relapse
  - Knowledge of early signs and symptoms of relapse
- Support groups or therapy (cognitive behavioural, interpersonal)
- Communication and problem-solving skills training

Relevant NOC outcomes for this phase include *Adherence behaviour*, *Knowledge: Disease process*, *Social support*, and *Substance addiction consequences*.

Maintenance Phase

The overall outcomes for the maintenance phase continue to focus on prevention of relapse and limitation of the severity and duration of future episodes. Relevant *NOC* outcomes include *Knowledge: Disease process*, *Adherence behaviour*, and *Family support during treatment*. Additional outcomes include:

- Participation in learning interpersonal strategies related to work, interpersonal, and family problems
- Participation in psychotherapy, group, or other ongoing supportive therapy modality

Planning

Planning care for an individual with bipolar disorder is usually geared toward the particular phase of mania the person is in (acute, continuation, or maintenance), as well as any other co-occurring issues identified in the assessment (e.g., risk for suicide, risk for violence to person or property, family crisis, legal crises, substance use, risk-taking behaviours).

Acute Phase

During the acute phase, planning focuses on medically stabilizing the person while maintaining safety. Therefore the hospital is usually the safest environment for accomplishing this stabilization (see Case Study and Nursing Care Plan 14.1). Nursing care is geared toward managing medications, decreasing physical activity, increasing food and fluid intake, ensuring at least 4 to 6 hours of sleep per night, alleviating any bowel or bladder problems, and intervening to see that self-care needs are met. Some patients may require seclusion or even electroconvulsive therapy (ECT) to assist with stabilization.

Continuation Phase

During the continuation phase, planning focuses on maintaining adherence to the medication regimen and prevention of relapse. Interventions are planned in accordance with the assessment data regarding the person's interpersonal and stress-reduction skills, cognitive functioning, employment status, substance-related problems, and social support systems. During this time, psychoeducational teaching is necessary for the patient and family. The need for referrals to community programs, groups, and support for any co-occurring disorders or problems (e.g., substance use, family problems, legal issues, financial crises) is evaluated.

Evaluation of the need for communication skills training and problem-solving skills training is also an important consideration. People with bipolar disorders often have interpersonal and emotional problems that affect their work, family, and social lives. Residual problems resulting from reckless, violent, withdrawn, or bizarre behaviour that may have occurred during a manic episode often leave lives shattered and family and friends hurt and distant. For some patients, cognitive behavioural therapy (CBT) (in addition to medication management) is useful to address these issues, although the focus of psychotherapeutic treatment will vary over time for each individual.

Maintenance Phase

During the maintenance phase, planning focuses on preventing relapse and limiting the severity and duration of future episodes. Patients with bipolar disorders require medications over long periods of time or even an entire lifetime. Psychotherapy, support groups, psychoeducational groups, and periodic evaluations help patients maintain their family, social, and occupational lives.

Implementation

The younger the age of onset of symptoms associated with bipolar disorders is a predictor of delays in receiving treatment (Pinto et al., 2020). Patients may minimize the destructive consequences of their behaviours or deny the seriousness of the disease, and some are reluctant to give up the increased energy, euphoria, and heightened sense of self-esteem of hypomania. Unfortunately, non-adherence to the regimen of mood-stabilizing medication is a major cause of relapse, so establishing a therapeutic alliance with the individual with bipolar disorder is crucial. Another reason for the delay of adequate treatment is that individuals often present to health care providers requesting assistance with their depression and have not yet had a manic episode.

Acute Phase

Depressive episodes. Depressive episodes of bipolar disorder have the same symptoms and risks as those of major depression (see Chapter 13 for appropriate interventions during the depressive phase of the illness). Hospitalization may be required if suicidal ideation, psychosis, or catatonia is present. Pharmacological treatment is affected by concerns of bringing on a manic phase. A discussion of medication therapy is included in this chapter.

Manic episodes

Acute phase. Hospitalization provides safety for a person experiencing acute mania (bipolar I disorder), imposes external controls on destructive behaviours, and provides for medication stabilization. There are unique approaches to communicating with and maintaining the safety of the person during the hospitalization period (Table 14.3). Staff members continuously set limits in a firm, non-threatening, and neutral manner to prevent further escalation of mania and provide safe boundaries for the person and others.

Continuation phase. The continuation phase is crucial for patients and their families. The outcome for this phase is prevention of relapse, and community resources are chosen based on the needs of the person, the appropriateness of the referral, and the availability of resources. Frequently, a case manager evaluates appropriate follow-up care for patients and their families.

Medication adherence during this phase is perhaps the most important treatment outcome. Often, this follow-up is handled in a community mental health clinic. However, adherence to the medication regimen is also addressed in outpatient clinics and psychiatric home care visits. Patients who are not too excitable and are able to tolerate a certain level of stimuli may attend an outpatient clinic. In addition to medication management, community mental health clinics offer structure, decrease social isolation, and help patients channel their time and energy. If a person is homebound, community psychiatric home care is the appropriate modality for follow-up care.

TABLE 14.3 Interventions for the Patient Experiencing Acute Mania

Intervention	Rationale
Communication	
Use firm and calm approach: "John, come with me. Please eat this sandwich."	Structure and control are provided for the person who is out of control. Feelings of security can result: "Someone is in control."
Use short and concise explanations or statements.	Short attention span limits comprehension to small bits of information.
Remain neutral; avoid power struggles and value judgements.	Person can use inconsistencies and value judgements as justification for arguing and escalating mania.
Be consistent in approach and expectations.	Consistent limits and expectations minimize potential for person's manipulation of staff.
Have frequent staff meetings to plan consistent approaches and set agreed-on limits.	Consistency of all staff is needed to maintain controls and minimize manipulation by patient.
With other staff, decide on limits, and communicate these with the person in simple, concrete terms with consequences. Example: "John, do not yell at or hit Peter. If you cannot control yourself, we will help you." Or, "The seclusion room will help you feel less out of control and prevent harm to yourself and others."	Clear expectations help the person experience outside controls, as well as understand reasons for medication, seclusion, or restraints (if they are not able to control behaviours).
Hear and act on legitimate complaints.	Underlying feelings of helplessness are reduced, and acting-out behaviours are minimized.
Firmly redirect energy into more appropriate and constructive channels.	Distractibility is the nurse's most effective tool with the person experiencing mania.
Structure in a Safe Milieu	
Maintain low level of stimuli in patient's environment (e.g., away from bright lights, loud noises, people).	Escalation of anxiety can be decreased.
Provide structured solitary activities with nurse or aide.	Structure provides security and focus.
Provide frequent high-calorie fluids.	Serious dehydration is prevented.
Provide frequent rest periods.	Exhaustion is prevented.
Redirect violent behaviour.	Physical exercise can decrease tension and provide focus.
When warranted in acute mania, use phenothiazines and seclusion to minimize physical harm.	Exhaustion and death can result from dehydration, lack of sleep, and constant physical activity.
Observe for signs of lithium toxicity.	There is a small margin of safety between therapeutic and toxic doses.
Prevent person from giving away money and possessions. Hold valuables in hospital safe until rational judgement returns.	Person's "generosity" is a manic defence that is consistent with irrational, grandiose thinking.
Physiological Safety: Self-Care Needs	
Nutrition	
Monitor intake, output, and vital signs.	Adequate fluid and caloric intake are ensured; development of dehydration and cardiac collapse are minimized.
Offer frequent, high-calorie, protein drinks and finger foods (e.g., sandwiches, fruits, milkshakes).	Constant fluid and calorie replacement are needed. Person may be too active to sit at meals. Finger foods allow "eating on the run."
Frequently remind person to eat. "Tom, finish your milkshake." "Sally, eat this banana."	The person experiencing mania is unaware of bodily needs and is easily distracted. Needs supervision to eat.
Sleep	
Encourage frequent rest periods during the day.	Lack of sleep can lead to exhaustion and death.
Keep person in areas of low stimulation.	Relaxation is promoted, and manic behaviour is minimized.
At night, provide warm baths, soothing music, and medication when indicated. Avoid giving person caffeine.	Relaxation, rest, and sleep are promoted.
Hygiene	
Supervise choice of clothes; minimize flamboyant and bizarre dress (e.g., garish stripes or plaids and loud, unmatching colours).	The potential is decreased for ridicule, which lowers self-esteem and increases the need for manic defence. The person is helped to maintain dignity.
Give simple, step-by-step reminders for hygiene and dress. "Here is your razor. Here are your toothbrush and toothpaste."	Distractibility and poor concentration are countered through simple, concrete instructions.
Elimination	
Monitor bowel habits; offer fluids and foods that are high in fibre. Evaluate need for laxative. Monitor input and output.	Fecal impaction resulting from dehydration and decreased peristalsis is prevented.

Maintenance phase. The goal of the maintenance phase is to prevent recurrence of an episode of bipolar disorder. The community resources cited earlier are helpful, and patients and their families often greatly benefit from mutual support and self-help groups, which are discussed later in this chapter.

Pharmacological Interventions

The recommendations for the management of acute mania remain mostly unchanged for the continuation and maintenance phases. Lithium carbonate, valproic acid (Depakene), and several atypical antipsychotics continue to be first-line treatments for acute mania. Tamoxifen is occasionally used as a third-line augmentation option because of the link to altered estrogen levels. Combining olanzapine (Zyprexa) and carbamazepine (Tegretol) is not recommended, as both affect hepatic CYP1A2 metabolism, thereby decreasing the effectiveness of both medications. For the management of bipolar depression, lithium, divalproex, lamotrigine (Lamictal), and quetiapine (Seroquel) are used for a monotherapy therapy approach. Olanzapine plus a selective serotonin reuptake inhibitor (SSRI) (except paroxetine), or lithium or valproic acid plus an SSRI or bupropion (Wellbutrin) are used as first-line options when combination therapy is required (Goldberg, 2019).

There may be times when a benzodiazepine antianxiety medication can help reduce agitation or anxiety. Due to the concern of dependency, use of benzodiazepines is usually short term until the mania subsides. The high-potency antianxiety benzodiazepines clonazepam and lorazepam are useful in the treatment of acute mania. They may calm agitation and reduce insomnia, aggression, and panic.

Mood Stabilization

Mood stabilizers refer to classes of drugs used to treat symptoms associated with bipolar disorder. The original intent of the term *mood stabilizers* was to indicate that these drugs were effective in the treatment of both mania and depression. This is not precisely true. While all of the medications in this category are effective in treating mania, not all of them do as well in treating depression.

Lithium carbonate. Lithium carbonate ($LiCO_3$ or Li^+) is effective in the treatment of bipolar I acute and recurrent manic and depressive episodes. Onset of action is usually within 10 to 21 days. Because the onset of action is so slow, it is usually supplemented in the early phases of treatment by atypical antipsychotics, anticonvulsants, or antianxiety medications.

The clinical benefits of lithium can be incredible. However, newer medications have been introduced and approved that carry lower toxicity, have fewer adverse effects, and require less frequent laboratory testing. The use of these newer medications has resulted in a decline in lithium use.

Before lithium is administered, a medical evaluation is performed to assess the person's ability to tolerate the medication. In particular, baseline physical and laboratory examinations should include assessment of renal function; determination of thyroid status, including levels of thyroxine and thyroid-stimulating hormone; and evaluation for dementia or neurological disorders, which presage a poor response to lithium. Other clinical and laboratory assessments, including an electrocardiogram, are performed as needed, depending on the individual's physical condition.

Indications. Lithium is particularly effective in reducing:
- Elation, grandiosity, and expansiveness
- Flight of ideas
- Irritability and manipulation
- Anxiety

To a lesser extent, lithium controls:
- Insomnia
- Psychomotor agitation
- Threatening or assaultive behaviour
- Distractibility
- Hypersexuality
- Paranoia

In the acute manic phase lithium is usually started at 600 to 1200 mg a day in two or three divided doses. It is then increased every few days by 300 mg a day with a maximum dose of 1800 mg a day. Lithium must reach therapeutic levels in the patient's blood to be effective. Reaching this level usually takes 7 to 14 days, or longer for some patients. Older adults appear to be more susceptible to adverse effects and may experience a higher incidence of neurotoxicity at lithium concentrations considered therapeutic for younger adults.

During the acute phase of the illness, an antipsychotic or a benzodiazepine can be used to prevent exhaustion, coronary collapse, and death until lithium reaches therapeutic levels. Antipsychotics act promptly to slow speech, inhibit aggression, and decrease psychomotor activity. As lithium becomes effective in reducing manic behaviour, the antipsychotic medications are usually discontinued.

Margaret Trudeau (former wife of the late prime minister Pierre Trudeau and mother to current prime minister Justin Trudeau) struggled with undiagnosed bipolar disorder for more than 30 years. In 2001 after overcoming the stigma and admitting herself to the Royal Ottawa Mental Health Centre, she was finally diagnosed with bipolar depression. In her book *Changing My Mind* she describes bipolar disorder as a heavy cross to bear, and one she will carry for the rest of her life. She wrote: "[my] contentment, you should know is not solely drug induced. I take a mild dose of mood stabilizer, and will likely for the rest of my days. Family, friends, meaningful work, exercise, diet, meditation, yoga, nature, gardening, lessons, cooking, music and art all play a role these days in keeping my demons at bay" (Trudeau, 2010, p. 12).

Therapeutic and toxic levels. There is a small window between the therapeutic and toxic levels of lithium. Lithium must reach therapeutic blood levels to be effective. This usually takes 7 to 14 days, or longer for some patients. Blood serum levels should reach 0.6 to 1.2 mEq/L (Burchum & Rosenthal, 2019). Lithium levels should not exceed 1.5 mEq/L to avoid serious toxicity. Table 14.4 details expected adverse effects, signs of toxicity, and interventions for both.

Lithium levels should be measured at least 5 days after beginning lithium therapy and after any dosage change, until the therapeutic level has been reached. Blood levels are determined every month. After 6 months to a year of stability, it is common to measure blood levels every 3 months. Blood should be drawn in the morning, 10 to 12 hours after the last dose of lithium is taken. For older adult patients, the principle of start low and go slow still applies.

Maintenance therapy. Although lithium is an effective intervention for treating the acute manic phase of bipolar disorder, it is not a cure. Some clinicians suggest that patients with bipolar disorder need to be given lithium for 9 to 12 months, and some patients may need lifelong lithium maintenance to prevent further relapses. Individuals receive lithium for maintenance indefinitely and experience manic and depressive episodes if the medication is discontinued. Many patients respond well to lower dosages during maintenance or prophylactic lithium therapy.

Complete suppression occurs in only 50% of patients or fewer, even with adherence to the maintenance therapy regimen. Therefore the patient and family should be given careful instructions about (1) the purpose and requirements of lithium therapy, (2) its adverse effects, (3) its toxic effects and complications, and (4) situations in which the physician should be contacted. The patient and family should also be advised that suddenly stopping lithium can lead to relapse and recurrence of mania. Health care providers must stress to patients and their families the importance of discontinuing maintenance therapy gradually.

TABLE 14.4 Lithium Adverse Effects and Signs of Lithium Toxicity

Level	Signs and Symptoms	Interventions
Expected Adverse Effects		
<0.4–1.2 mEq/L (therapeutic level)	Fine hand tremor, polyuria, mild thirst, mild nausea and general discomfort, weight gain	Symptoms may persist throughout therapy. Symptoms often subside during treatment. Weight gain may be helped with diet, exercise, and nutritional management.
Early Signs of Toxicity		
<1.5 mEq/L	Nausea, vomiting, diarrhea, thirst, polyuria, lethargy, slurred speech, muscle weakness, and fine hand tremor	Medication should be withheld, blood lithium levels measured, and dosage re-evaluated. Dehydration, if present, should be addressed.
Advanced Signs of Toxicity		
1.5–2.0 mEq/L	Coarse hand tremor, persistent gastrointestinal upset, mental confusion, muscle hyperirritability, electroencephalographic changes, incoordination, sedation	Interventions outlined above or below should be used, depending on severity of circumstances.
Severe Toxicity		
2.0–2.5 mEq/L	Ataxia, confusion, large output of dilute urine, serious electroencephalographic changes, blurred vision, clonic movements, seizures, stupor, severe hypotension, coma; death is usually secondary to pulmonary complications	Hospitalization is indicated. The drug is stopped, and excretion is hastened. If patient is alert, an emetic is administered.
>2.5 mEq/L	Convulsions, oliguria; death can occur	In addition to the interventions above, hemodialysis may be used in severe cases.

Source: Data from Burchum, J., & Rosenthal, L. (2019). *Lehne's pharmacology for nursing care* (10th ed.). St. Louis: Elsevier; and Boland, R. (2021). *Kaplan and Sadock's synopsis of psychiatry* (12th ed.). Philadelphia: Wolters Kluwer.

Patient and Family Teaching: Lithium Therapy outlines teaching regarding lithium therapy for the patient and family.

People taking lithium need to know that two major long-term risks of lithium therapy are hypothyroidism and impairment of the kidneys' ability to concentrate urine. Therefore a person receiving lithium therapy must have periodic follow-ups to assess thyroid and renal function. Health Canada (2014) has also issued warnings that taking lithium carries a high risk of hypercalcemia and hyperparathyroidism. Symptoms of hypercalcemia and hyperparathyroidism can include fatigue, depression, mental confusion, nausea, vomiting, excessive thirst, appetite loss, abdominal pain, frequent urination, muscle and joint aches, and muscle weakness. In the most serious situations, these conditions lead to coma and death.

Contraindications. Lithium therapy is generally contraindicated in patients with cardiovascular disease, brain damage, renal disease, thyroid disease, or myasthenia gravis. Whenever possible, lithium is not given to people who are pregnant because it may harm the fetus. The fear of becoming pregnant and the wish to become pregnant are both major concerns for many patients taking lithium. Lithium use is also contraindicated in breastfeeding people and in children younger than 12 years of age.

PATIENT AND FAMILY TEACHING
Lithium Therapy

The patient and the patient's family should be given the following information, be encouraged to ask questions, and be given the material in written form as well.

1. Lithium treats your current emotional problem and also helps prevent relapse. Therefore it is important to continue taking the medication after the current episode is over.
2. Because therapeutic and toxic dosage ranges are so close, it is important to monitor lithium blood levels very closely, more frequently at first and then once every several months after that.
3. Lithium is not addictive.
4. It is important to eat a normal diet, with normal salt and fluid intake (1500 to 3000 mL or six 350-mL glasses of fluid). Lithium decreases sodium reabsorption in the kidneys, which could lead to a deficiency of sodium. A low sodium intake leads to a relative increase in lithium retention, which could produce toxicity.
5. You should stop taking lithium if you have excessive diarrhea, vomiting, or sweating. All of these symptoms can lead to dehydration. Dehydration can raise lithium levels in the blood to toxic levels. Inform your physician if you have any of these problems.
6. Do not take diuretics (water pills) while you are taking lithium.
7. Lithium is irritating to the lining of your stomach. Take lithium with meals.
8. It is important to have your kidneys and thyroid checked periodically, especially if you are taking lithium over a long period. Talk to your doctor about this follow-up.
9. Do not take any over-the-counter medicines without checking first with your doctor.
10. If you find that you are gaining a lot of weight, you may need to talk this change over with your doctor or dietitian.
11. Many self-help groups are available to provide support for people with bipolar disorder and their families. The local self-help group is (give name and telephone number).
12. You can find out more information by calling (give name and telephone number).
13. Keep a list of adverse effects and toxic effects handy, along with the name and number of a person to contact if these effects occur (see Table 14.4).
14. If lithium is to be discontinued, your dosage will be tapered gradually to minimize the risk of relapse.

Anticonvulsant drugs. In the 1980s researchers hypothesized that mood instability could be viewed much the same as epilepsy and that a chain reaction of sensitivity, or *kindling*, was responsible for the worsening of bipolar symptoms over time (Shapero et al., 2017). This hypothesis led to the use of anticonvulsant drugs, such as carbamazepine (Tegretol), valproic acid (Depakene), and lamotrigine (Lamictal), as a treatment for mania that has been refractory to lithium therapy. They also proved useful in treating people who need rapid de-escalation and who do not respond to other treatment approaches. Subsequent research did not support the kindling theory, however, suggesting that symptom improvement for bipolar disorder is based on another mechanism of action of these anticonvulsant drugs and not on their seizure prevention mechanism.

Anticonvulsant drugs are thought to be:
- Superior for continuously cycling patients
- More effective when there is no family history of bipolar disorder
- Effective at dampening affective swings in schizoaffective patients
- Effective at diminishing impulsive and aggressive behaviour in some non-psychotic patients
- Helpful in cases of alcohol and benzodiazepine withdrawal
- Beneficial in controlling mania (within 2 weeks) and depression (within 3 weeks or longer)

Valproate

Divalproex sodium (Epival). Valproate (available as divalproex sodium [Epival] and valproic acid [Depakene]) has surpassed lithium in treating acute mania. Valproate is also helpful in preventing future manic episodes. Although serious complications are rare, it is important to monitor liver function and platelet count periodically. Divalproex doses can cause drowsiness and dizziness and increase thoughts of suicide; therefore mood, ideations, and behaviour should be monitored on a regular basis. Therapeutic serum levels that range from 50 to 100 mcg/mL and 50 to 125 mcg/mL for mania should be monitored to prevent toxicity and overdose (Burchum & Rosenthal, 2019). Symptoms of central nervous system toxicity can include confusion, fatigue, dizziness, hallucinations, headache, and ataxia.

Carbamazepine. Some patients with treatment-resistant bipolar disorder improve after taking carbamazepine (Tegretol) and lithium, or carbamazepine and an antipsychotic. Carbamazepine seems to work better in patients with rapid cycling and in severely paranoid, angry patients experiencing manias rather than in euphoric, overactive, overly friendly patients experiencing manias. It is thought to also be more effective in dysphoric patients experiencing manias.

Liver enzymes should be monitored at least weekly for the first 8 weeks of treatment because the drug can increase levels of liver enzymes that can speed its own metabolism. In some instances this can cause bone marrow suppression and liver inflammation. Complete blood counts should also be done periodically since carbamazepine is known to cause leukopenia and aplastic anemia.

Lamotrigine. Lamotrigine (Lamictal) is a first-line treatment for bipolar depression and is approved for acute and maintenance therapy. Lamotrigine is generally well tolerated but has one serious, though rare, dermatological reaction: a potentially life-threatening rash. Patients should be instructed to seek immediate medical attention if a rash appears, although most are likely benign.

Adverse drug reactions (ADRs), as indicated by the Canadian Network for Mood and Anxiety Treatments (CANMAT), that require patient safety monitoring are:
- Both valproic acid and carbamazepine may cause blood dyscrasias, hepatotoxicity, and teratogenicity.
- Carbamazepine has also been linked to hyponatremia and serious dermatological adverse effects.
- Valproic acid has been associated with polycystic ovary syndrome, weight gain, acute pancreatitis, and hyperammonemic encephalopathy.
- The severe ADRs associated with lamotrigine are dermatological, namely Stevens–Johnson syndrome.
- Drug interactions such as lamotrigine–valproic acid and carbamazepine–hormonal contraceptives are also important to be aware of.

Antianxiety drugs. Diazepam (Valium), clonazepam (Rivotril), and lorazepam (Ativan) are antianxiety (anxiolytic) drugs useful in the treatment of acute mania in some patients who are resistant to other treatments. These drugs are also effective in managing the psychomotor agitation seen in mania. They should be avoided, however, in patients with a history of substance use.

Atypical antipsychotics. Many of the second-generation antipsychotics are approved for acute mania. In addition to showing sedative properties during the early phase of treatment (help with insomnia, anxiety, agitation), the second-generation antipsychotics seem to have mood-stabilizing properties. Most evidence supports the use of olanzapine (Zyprexa) or risperidone (Risperdal).

This classification of drugs may bring about serious adverse effects that stem from a tendency toward weight gain that may lead to insulin resistance, diabetes, dyslipidemia, and cardiovascular impairment.

The Drug Treatment box provides an overview of drugs used to treat bipolar disorder that are approved by Health Canada and the *Canadian Food and Drugs Act*.

Electroconvulsive Therapy

ECT is used to subdue severe manic behaviour, especially in patients with treatment-resistant mania and in those with rapid cycling (i.e., those who experience four or more episodes of illness per year).

ECT seems to be far more effective than medication-based therapy for treatment-resistant bipolar depression (Fornaro et al., 2020). Depressive episodes, particularly those with severe, catatonic, or treatment-resistant depression, are an indication for this treatment.

Milieu Management

Control of hyperactive behaviour during the acute phase almost always includes immediate treatment with an antipsychotic medication. However, when a person is dangerously out of control, use of a seclusion room or restraints may also be required. A seclusion room provides comfort and relief to many patients who are unable to control their own behaviour. Seclusion serves the following purposes:
- Reduces overwhelming environmental stimuli
- Protects a person from injuring themself or others, including staff
- Prevents destruction of personal property or property of others

Seclusion is warranted when documented data collected by the nursing and medical staff reflect the following points:
- Substantial risk of harm to others or self is clear.
- The person is unable to control their actions.
- Problematic behaviour has been sustained (continues or escalates despite other measures).
- Other measures have failed (e.g., setting limits beginning with verbal de-escalation or using chemical restraints).

The use of seclusion or restraints is associated with complex therapeutic, ethical, and legal issues. Most provincial and territorial laws prohibit the use of unnecessary physical restraint or isolation. Barring an emergency, the use of seclusion and restraints requires consent. Therefore most hospitals have well-defined protocols for treatment with seclusion. Seclusion protocol includes a proper reporting procedure, through the appropriate channels, when a person is to be secluded. For example, the use of seclusion and restraint is permitted only on the written order of a physician and must be reviewed and rewritten every 24 hours. The order must include the type of restraint to be used.

DRUG TREATMENT OF PATIENTS WITH BIPOLAR DISORDER

Generic (Trade)	Health Canada–Approved	Off-Label Uses	CANMAT Recommendations
Lithium carbonate	Acute mania	Depression	First-line treatment for bipolar depression
	Maintenance		Recommended for acute mania
	Mood stabilizer		Treatment and prevention of manic episodes
Anticonvulsants			
Valproic acid (Depakene)	Acute mania	Depression	Recommended for acute mania
Divalproex sodium (Epival)		Maintenance	First-line maintenance treatment for bipolar disorder
Carbamazepine (Tegretol)	Acute mania	Depression	Recommended for maintenance treatment of bipolar disorder, mood-stabilizing effect
		Maintenance	
Lamotrigine (Lamictal)	Maintenance	Depression (can worsen mania)	First-line treatment for bipolar depression
			Recommended for maintenance treatment of bipolar disorder
Gabapentin (Neurontin) and topiramate (Topamax)		Acute mania	Recommended for maintenance treatment of bipolar disorder
		Maintenance	
Atypical Antipsychotics			
Aripiprazole (Abilify)	Mania	Depression	
	Maintenance		
Olanzapine (Zyprexa)	Mania	Depression	Recommended for acute mania
	Maintenance		
Quetiapine fumarate (Seroquel)	Depression		
	Mania		
	Maintenance		
Risperidone (Risperdal)	Mania	Depression	First-line treatment for severe mania
		Maintenance	
Ziprasidone (Zeldox)	Acute mania		Acute mania
	Mixed features		

Sources: Data from Yatham, L. N., Kennedy, S. H., Parikh, S. V., et al. (2018). Canadian Network for Mood and Anxiety Treatments (CANMAT) and International Society for Bipolar Disorders (ISBD) 2018 guidelines for the management of patients with bipolar disorder. *Bipolar Disorders, 20*(2), 97–170. https://doi.org/10.1111/bdi.12609

INTEGRATIVE THERAPY

Omega-3 Fatty Acids as a Treatment for Bipolar Disorder

A few generations ago, children resisted a nightly dose of cod liver oil that mothers swore by as constipation prevention. While the foul-tasting, evil-smelling liquid undoubtedly helped win that particular battle, cod liver oil may have had other benefits as well. It is rich in omega-3 fatty acids, which have drawn increasing attention as being important in mood regulation. Fish oil is the target of this attention. It contains two omega-3 fatty acids, eicosapentaenoic acid and docosahexaenoic acid, which are important in central nervous system functioning.

The interest in these particular fatty acids developed as research began to suggest that people who live in areas with low seafood consumption, especially of cold water seafood, exhibited higher rates of depression and bipolar disorder. This led researchers to explore the influence of omega-3 fatty acids as protective for bipolar disorder.

In 2020 Knopf conducted a small randomized control trial to compare monotherapy with fish oil to a placebo. She concluded that there is no evidence to support the use of omega-3 in treating adolescents with a family history of bipolar I disorder.

Source: Knopf, A. (2020). Fish oil no better than placebo for depression in teens at risk for BPD. *Brown University Child & Adolescent Psychopharmacology Update, 22*(10), 1–3. https://doi.org/10.1002/cpu.30525

Seclusion and observation levels and care protocols must be carefully adhered to as per individual hospital or employer policy.

Seclusion protocols also identify specific nursing responsibilities, such as how often the patient's behaviour is to be observed and documented (e.g., every 15 minutes), how often the patient is to be offered food and fluids (e.g., every 30 to 60 minutes), and how often the patient is to be toileted (e.g., every 1 to 2 hours). Medication is often administered to patients in seclusion; therefore vital signs should be measured frequently, as per hospital policy.

Careful and precise documentation is a legal necessity. The nurse documents the following:

- The behaviour leading up to the seclusion or restraint
- The actions taken to provide the least restrictive alternative
- The time the patient was placed in seclusion
- Every 15 minutes, the patient's behaviour, needs, nursing care, and vital signs
- The time and type of medications given and their effects on the patient

When a patient requires seclusion to prevent self-harm or violence toward others, it is ideal for one nurse on each shift to work with the patient on a continuous basis. Communication with a patient in seclusion is concrete and direct but also empathic and limited to brief instructions. Patients need reassurance that seclusion is only a temporary measure and that they will be returned to the unit when their behaviour is more controlled and they demonstrate the ability to safely be around others.

Frequent staff meetings regarding personal feelings are necessary to prevent using seclusion as a form of punishment or leaving a patient in seclusion for long periods of time without proper supervision. Restraints and seclusion are never to be used as punishment or for the convenience of the staff. Refer to Chapter 7 for a more detailed discussion of the legal implications of seclusion and restraints. Chapter 4 provides more information on milieu therapy.

Support Groups

Patients with bipolar disorder, as well as their friends and families, benefit from forming mutual support groups. Often these are coordinated by organizations such as the Mood Disorders Society of Canada and the Canadian Mental Health Association. Chapter 29 further explores a variety of recovery, survivorship, and public health approaches.

Health Teaching and Health Promotion

Patients and families need information about bipolar disorder, with particular emphasis on its chronic and highly recurrent nature. In addition, patients and families need to be taught the warning signs and symptoms of impending episodes. For example, changes in sleep patterns are especially important because they usually precede, accompany, or precipitate mania. Even a single night of unexplainable sleep loss can be taken as an early warning of impending mania. Health teaching stresses the importance of establishing regularity in sleep patterns, meals, exercise, and other activities. Patient and Family Teaching: Bipolar Disorder lists health-teaching guidelines for patients with bipolar disorder and their families.

PATIENT AND FAMILY TEACHING

Bipolar Disorder

1. Patients with bipolar disorder and their families need to know:
   - The chronic and episodic nature of bipolar disorder
   - The fact that bipolar disorder is long term. Treatment will require that one or more mood-stabilizing medications be taken for a long time
   - The expected side effects and toxic effects of the prescribed medication, as well as who to call and where to go in case of an adverse reaction
   - The signs and symptoms of relapse that may "come out of the blue"
   - The role of family members and others in preventing a full relapse
   - The phone numbers of emergency contact people, which should be kept in an easily accessed place
2. The use of alcohol, drugs of abuse, caffeine (particularly in energy drinks), and over-the-counter medications can cause a relapse.
3. Good sleep hygiene is critical to stability. Frequently, the early symptom of a manic episode is lack of sleep. In some cases, mania may be averted by the use of sleep medications.
4. Coping strategies are important for dealing with work, interpersonal, and family problems to lower stress, to enhance a sense of personal control, and to increase community functioning.
5. Group and individual therapy are valuable for gaining insight and skills in relapse prevention, providing social support, increasing coping skills in interpersonal relations, improving adherence to the medication regimen, reducing functional morbidity, and decreasing need for hospitalization.

Most of the medications used to treat bipolar disorder may cause weight gain and other metabolic disturbances such as altered metabolism of lipids and glucose. These alterations increase the risk for diabetes, high blood pressure, dyslipidemia, cardiac problems, or all of these in combination (metabolic syndrome). Not only do these disturbances impair quality of life and lifespan, they are also a major reason for nonadherence. Teaching aimed at weight reduction and management is essential to keep patients physically healthy and emotionally stable.

Recovery concepts are particularly important for patients with bipolar disorder, who often have issues with adherence to treatment. The best method of addressing this problem is to follow a collaborative care model in which responsibilities for treatment adherence are shared. In this model patients are responsible for making it to appointments and openly communicating information, and the health care provider is responsible for keeping current on treatment methods and listening carefully as patients share perceptions. Through this sharing, treatment adherence becomes a self-managed responsibility.

Psychotherapy

Pharmacotherapy and psychiatric mental health care and management are essential in the treatment of acute manic attacks and during the continuation and maintenance phases of bipolar disorder. Individuals with bipolar disorder must deal with the psychosocial consequences of their past episodes and their vulnerability to experiencing future episodes. They also have to face the burden of long-term treatments that may involve unpleasant adverse effects. Many patients have strained interpersonal relationships, marital and family problems, academic and occupational problems, and legal or other social difficulties. Psychotherapy can help them work through these difficulties, decrease some of the psychic distress, and increase self-esteem. Psychotherapeutic treatments can also help patients improve their functioning between episodes and attempt to decrease the frequency of future episodes.

Often the patients receiving medication and therapy place more value on psychotherapy than clinicians do. Kay Redfield Jamison is an American clinical psychologist and mood disorder researcher who has suffered from bipolar disorder since her early adulthood. She describes her feelings about drug therapy and psychotherapy as follows:

> I cannot imagine leading a normal life without lithium. From startings and stoppings of it, I now know it is an essential part of my sanity. Lithium prevents my seductive but disastrous highs, diminishes my depressions, clears out the weaving of my disordered thinking, slows me, gentles me out, keeps me in my relationships, in my career, out of a hospital, and in psychotherapy. It keeps me alive, too. But psychotherapy heals, it makes some sense of the confusion, it reins in the terrifying thoughts and feelings, it brings back hope and the possibility of learning from it all. Pills cannot, do not, ease one back into reality. They bring you back headlong, careening, and faster than can be endured at times. Psychotherapy is a sanctuary, it is a battleground, and it is where I have come to believe that someday I may be able to contend with all of this. No pill can help me deal with the problem of not wanting to take pills, but no amount of therapy alone can prevent my manias and depressions. I need both. (Jamison, 1995, p. 139)

Advanced-Practice Interventions

Many advanced-practice registered nurses are able to diagnose and prescribe medications for treating bipolar disorder. In addition, they may use psychotherapy to help the patient cope more adaptively to stresses in the environment and decrease the risk of relapse. Specific approaches to psychotherapy include CBT, interpersonal and social rhythm therapy, and family-focused therapy.

Cognitive behavioural therapy. CBT is typically used as an adjunct to pharmacotherapy in many psychiatric disorders. It involves identifying maladaptive thoughts ("I am always going to be a loser") and behaviours ("I might as well drink") that may be barriers to a person's recovery and ongoing mood stability.

CBT focuses on adherence to the medication regimen, early detection and intervention for manic or depressive episodes, stress and lifestyle management, and the treatment of depression and comorbid conditions. Some research demonstrates that patients treated with cognitive therapy are more likely to take their medications as prescribed than are patients who do not participate in therapy, and psychotherapy results in greater adherence to the medication regimen.

Interpersonal and social rhythm therapy. Depression and manic-type states impair a person's ability to interact with others. Even in between episodes, relationships have been so damaged it may seem impossible to correct the problems. The advanced-practice nurses can use a specialized approach, interpersonal and social rhythm therapy. This approach aims to regulate social routines and stabilize interpersonal relationships to improve depression and prevent relapse. Psychoeducation is a major component of this therapy and includes symptom recognition, adherence with medication and sleep routines, stress management, and maintenance of social supports.

Family-focused therapy. Family-focused therapy helps improve communication among family members. During depressive and manic episodes, family life can become a challenge or even intolerable. Negative patterns of communicating develop and become part of the fabric of the family. Advanced-practice nurses can help people recognize and reduce negative expressed emotion and stressors that provoke episodes.

EVALUATION

Outcome criteria often dictate the frequency of evaluation of short-term and intermediate indicators. Are the person's vital signs stable? Are they well hydrated? Is the person able to control personal behaviour or respond to external controls? Is the person able to sleep for 4 or 5 hours a night or take frequent, short rest periods during the day? Does the family have a clear understanding of the patient's disorder and need for medication? Do the patient and family know which community agencies might help them?

If outcomes or related indicators are not achieved satisfactorily, the preventing factors are analyzed. Were the data incorrect or insufficient? Were nursing diagnoses inappropriate or outcomes unrealistic? Was intervention poorly planned? After the outcomes and care plan are reassessed, the plan is revised, if indicated. Longer-term outcomes include adherence to the medication regimen; resumption of functioning in the community; achievement of stability in family, work, and social relationships and in mood; and improved coping skills for reducing stress.

CASE STUDY AND NURSING CARE PLAN 14.1
Mania

Hannah is brought to the emergency department after being found on the highway shortly after her car broke down. She is dressed in a long red dress, a blue and orange scarf, many long chains, and a pair of yellow shoes. The police report that when they came to her aid, she told them she was "driving to fame and fortune." She appeared overly cheerful and was constantly talking, laughing, and making jokes. At the same time, she paced up and down beside the car, sometimes tweaking the cheek of one of the policemen. She was coy and flirtatious with the police officers, saying at one point, "Boys in blue are fun to do."

When she reached into the car and started drinking from an open bottle of vodka, the police decided that her behaviour and general condition might result in harm to herself or others. When they explained to Hannah that they wanted to take her to the hospital for a general checkup, her jovial mood turned to anger and rage, yet 2 minutes after getting into the police car, she was singing "Jailhouse Rock."

On admission to the emergency department, Hannah is seen by a psychiatrist, and her sister is called. The sister states that Hannah stopped taking her lithium about 5 weeks ago and has been becoming more and more agitated and out of control. She reports that Hannah has not eaten in 2 days, has stayed up all night calling friends and strangers all over the province, and finally fled the house when the sister called an ambulance to take her to the hospital. The psychiatrist contacts Hannah's regular physician, and her previous history and medical management are discussed. It is decided that she should be hospitalized during the acute manic phase and restarted on lithium therapy. It is hoped that medications and a controlled environment will prevent further escalation of the manic state and prevent possible exhaustion and cardiac collapse.

Assessment

Self-Assessment

Jake has worked as a nurse on the psychiatric unit for 2 years. He has learned to deal with many of the challenging behaviours associated with the manic defence. For example, he no longer takes most of the verbal insults personally, even when the remarks are cutting and hit close to home. He is also better able to recognize and set limits on some of the tactics used by the person experiencing mania to split the staff. The staff on this unit work closely with one another, making the atmosphere positive and supportive; therefore communication is good among staff. Frequent and effective communication is needed to prevent staff splitting, maximize external controls, and maintain consistency in nursing care.

The only aspects of Hannah's behaviour Jake thinks he may have difficulty with are the sexual advances and loud sexual comments she makes toward him. He knows that these behaviours could make him anxious, and his concern is that Hannah might pick up on his anxiety. When he discusses this concern with the senior nurse, they decide that two nurses should provide care for Hannah. A female nurse will spend time with her in her room, and Jake will spend time with her in quiet areas on the unit. It is decided that neither Jake nor any male staff member will be alone with Hannah in her room at any time. Jake will ask for relief if Hannah's sexual remarks and acting-out behaviours make him anxious.

Continued

CASE STUDY AND NURSING CARE PLAN 14.1—cont'd
Mania

Objective Data	Subjective Data
Little if anything to eat for days	"Driving to fame and fortune."
Little if any sleep for days	"Boys in blue are fun to do."
History of mania	
History of lithium maintenance	
Very loud and distracting to others	
Anger when wishes are denied	
Flight of ideas	
Loud and inappropriate dress	
Sexually suggestive remarks and actions	
Remarks that suggest grandiose thinking	
Poor judgement	

Diagnosis

1. *Risk for injury* related to dehydration and faulty judgement, as evidenced by inability to meet own physiological needs and set limits on own behaviour

Supporting Data

- Has not slept for days
- Has not consumed food or fluids for days

2. *Defensive coping* related to biochemical changes, as evidenced by change in usual communication patterns

Supporting Data

- Remarks suggest sexual themes
- Remarks suggesting grandiose thinking
- Flight of ideas
- Constantly talking, laughing, and making jokes

Outcomes Identification

Physical status will remain stable during manic phase.

Planning

The nurse plans interventions that will help de-escalate Hannah's activity to minimize potential physical injury (dehydration, cardiac instability) through the use of medication and provision of a non-stimulating environment.

Implementation

Jake makes the following nursing care plan:

Short-Term Goal	Intervention	Rationale	Evaluation
1. Person will be well hydrated, as evidenced by good skin turgor and normal urinary output and specific gravity, within 24 hours.	1a. Give olanzapine (Zyprexa) intramuscularly immediately and as ordered. 1b. Check vital signs frequently (every 1–2 hours). 1c. Place person in private or quiet room (whenever possible). 1d. Stay with person and divert person away from stimulating situations. 1e. Offer high-calorie, high-protein drink (250 mL) every hour in quiet area. 1f. Frequently remind person to drink: "Take two more sips."	1a. Continuous physical activity and lack of fluids can eventually lead to cardiac collapse and death. 1b. Cardiac status is monitored. 1c. Environmental stimuli are reduced—escalation of mania and distractibility are minimized. 1d. Nurse's presence provides support. Ability to interact with others is temporarily impaired. 1e. Proper hydration is mandatory for maintenance of cardiac status. 1f. Person's concentration is poor; she is easily distracted.	**Goal Met** After 3 hours, person takes small amounts of fluid (60–120 mL per hour). After 5 hours, patient starts taking 250 mL per hour with a lot of reminding and encouragement. After 24 hours, urine specific gravity is within normal limits.

CASE STUDY AND NURSING CARE PLAN 14.1—cont'd

Mania

Short-Term Goal	Intervention	Rationale	Evaluation
	1g. Offer finger food frequently, in quiet area.	1g. Person is unable to sit; snacks she can eat while pacing are more likely to be consumed.	
	1h. Maintain record of intake and output.	1h. Such a record allows staff to make accurate nutritional assessment for person's safety.	
	1i. Weigh person daily.	1i. Monitoring of nutritional status is necessary.	
1. Person will sleep or rest 3 hours during the first night in the hospital with aid of medication and nursing interventions.	2a. Continue to direct person to areas of minimal activity.	2a. Lower levels of stimulation can decrease excitability.	Person is awake most of the first night. Sleeps for 2 hours from 0400 to 0600 hours.
	2b. When possible, try to direct energy into productive and calming activities (e.g., pacing to slow, soft music; slow exercise; drawing alone; writing in quiet area).	2b. Directing patient to paced, non-stimulating activities can help minimize excitability.	Person is able to rest on the second day for short periods and engage in quiet activities for short periods (5–10 minutes).
	2c. Encourage short rest periods throughout the day (e.g., 3–5 minutes every hour) when possible.	2c. Person may be unaware of feelings of fatigue. Can collapse from exhaustion if hyperactivity continues without periods of rest.	
	2d. Drinks such as coffee, tea, and colas should be decaffeinated only.	2d. Caffeine is a central nervous system stimulant that inhibits needed rest or sleep.	
	2e. Provide nursing measures at bedtime that promote sleep (e.g., warm milk, soft music).	2e. Such measures promote non-stimulating and relaxing mood.	
1. Person's blood pressure (BP) and pulse (P) will be within normal limits within 24 hours, with the aid of medication and nursing interventions.	3a. Continue to monitor BP and P frequently throughout the day (every 30 minutes).	3a. Physical condition is presently a great strain on patient's heart.	**Goal Met** Baseline measures on unit are not obtained because of hyperactive behaviour. Information from family physician states that baseline BP is 130/90 mm Hg and baseline P is 88 beats per minute.
	3b. Keep staff informed, by verbal and written reports, of baseline vital signs and patient progress.	3b. Alerting all staff regarding person's status can increase medical intervention if a change in status occurs.	BP at end of 24 hours is 130/70 mm Hg; P is 80 beats per minute.

Evaluation

After 2 days, the medical staff feel that Hannah's physical status is stable. Her vital signs are within normal limits, she is consuming sufficient fluids, and her urinary output is normal. Although her hyperactivity persists, it does so to a lesser degree; she is able to get periods of rest during the day and is sleeping 3 to 4 hours during the night.

Hannah's hyperactivity continues to be a challenge to the nurses; however, she is able to participate in some activities that require gross motor movement. These activities are useful in channelling some of her aggressive energy. Shortly after her arrival on the unit, Hannah starts a fight with another patient, but seclusion is avoided because she is able to refrain from further violent episodes as a result of medication and nursing interventions. She can be directed toward solitary activities, which channel some of her energies, at least for short periods.

As the effect of the medications progresses, Hannah's activity level decreases, and by discharge, she is able to discuss issues of concern with the nurse and make some useful decisions about her future. She is to come for follow-up at the community centre and agrees to join a family psychoeducational group for patients with bipolar disorder and their families, which she will attend with her sister.

KEY POINTS TO REMEMBER

- Bipolar I disorder is characterized by the presence or history of at least one manic episode, whereas bipolar II disorder is characterized by the presence or history of at least one hypomanic episode.
- Cyclothymia is a bipolar-related disorder with symptoms of hypomania and symptoms of mild to moderate depression.
- Genetics plays a strong role in the risk for the bipolar disorders.
- Neurotransmitter (norepinephrine, dopamine, serotonin) excess and imbalance are also related to bipolar mood swings, supporting the existence of neurobiological influences. Neuroendocrine and neuroanatomical findings provide strong evidence for biological influences.
- Early detection of bipolar disorder can help diminish comorbid substance use, suicide, and decline in social and personal relationships and may help promote more positive outcomes.
- Bipolar disorder often goes unrecognized.
- The nurse assesses the person's level of mood (hypomania, acute mania), behaviour, and thought processes and is alert to cognitive dysfunction.
- Analyzing the objective and subjective data helps the nurse formulate appropriate nursing diagnoses. Some of the nursing diagnoses appropriate for patients with mania are *Risk for violence, Defensive coping, Ineffective coping, Disturbed thought processes,* and *Situational low self-esteem.*
- During the acute phase of mania, physical needs often take priority and demand nursing interventions. Therefore *Deficient fluid volume, Imbalanced nutrition, Imbalanced elimination,* and *Disturbed sleep pattern* are usually addressed in the nursing plan.
- The diagnosis of *Interrupted family processes* is vital. Support groups, psychoeducation, and guidance for the family can greatly affect the person's adherence to the medication regimen.
- Planning involves identifying the specific needs of the patient and family during the three phases of mania (acute, continuation, and maintenance). Can the patient benefit from communication skills training, improvement in coping skills, legal or financial counselling, or further psychoeducation? What community resources does the person need at this time?
- Health care workers, family, and friends often feel angry and frustrated by the person's disruptive behaviours. When these feelings are not examined and shared with others, the therapeutic potential of the staff is reduced, and feelings of confusion and helplessness remain.
- Mood stabilizers are usually the first line of defence for bipolar disorder and include lithium and several anticonvulsants.
- Lithium is approved for treating acute mania and maintenance. Blood levels, kidney function, and thyroid function should be assessed regularly.
- Most anticonvulsant drugs are approved for acute mania. Lamotrigine is approved for maintenance.
- Antipsychotic medications, particularly the second-generation antipsychotics, are used for their sedating and mood-stabilizing properties. Screening for metabolic problems (e.g., diabetes) is essential in this population.
- For some patients, ECT may be an appropriate medical treatment.
- Patient and family teaching takes many forms and is most important in encouraging adherence to the medication regimen and reducing the risk of relapse.
- Evaluation includes examining the effectiveness of the nursing interventions, changing the outcomes as needed, and reassessing the nursing diagnoses. Evaluation is an ongoing process and is part of each of the other steps in the nursing process.

CRITICAL THINKING

1. Jian has been diagnosed with bipolar disorder and has been taking lithium for 4 months. During a clinic visit, he tells you that he does not think he will be taking his lithium anymore because he feels fine and misses his old "intensity." He says he is able to function well at his job and at home with his family and that his wife agrees that he "has this thing licked."
    a. What are Jian's needs in terms of teaching?
    b. What are the needs of his family?
    c. Write a teaching plan for Jian, or use an already constructed plan that includes the following teaching topics with sound rationales:
        1. Use of alcohol, drugs, caffeine, and over-the-counter medications
        2. Need for sleep and hygiene
        3. Types of community resources available
        4. Signs and symptoms of relapse
2. How would you explain the importance of a normal sleep–wake cycle to a patient with bipolar disorder?
    a. Research has shown that a faulty circadian rhythm may be to blame for sleep disruption in the mania phase of bipolar disorder. Therefore it is important to maintain a normal sleep–wake cycle for mood stabilization because sleep disruptions can trigger mania.

CHAPTER REVIEW

1. Which behaviour exhibited by a person with mania should the nurse choose to address first?
    a. Indiscriminate sexual relations
    b. Excessive spending of money
    c. Declaration of "being at one with the world"
    d. Demonstration of flight of ideas
2. The nurse is caring for a person experiencing mania. Which is the most appropriate nursing intervention?
    a. Provide consistency among staff members when working with the person
    b. Negotiate limits so the person has a voice in the plan of care
    c. Allow only certain staff members to interact with the person
    d. Attempt to control the person's emotions
3. The nurse is planning care for a person experiencing the acute phase of mania. Which is the priority intervention?
    a. Prevent injury
    b. Maintain stable cardiac status
    c. Get the person to demonstrate thought self-control
    d. Ensure that the person gets sufficient sleep and rest
4. What critical information should the nurse provide about the use of lithium?
    a. "You will still have hypersexual tendencies, so be certain to use protection when engaging in intercourse."
    b. "Lithium will help you to feel only the euphoria of mania but not the anxiety."
    c. "It will take 1 to 2 weeks and maybe longer for this medication to start working fully."
    d. "This medication is a cure for bipolar disorder."
5. The nurse has provided education for a person in the continuation phase, after discharge from the hospital. What indicates that the plan of care has been successful? Select all that apply.
    a. Person identifies three signs and symptoms of relapse.
    b. Person states, "My wife doesn't mind if I still drink a little."
    c. Person reports that medication has been helpful but he is ready to stop.
    d. Person states, "I no longer have a disease."

6. Luc's family comes home one evening to find him extremely agitated and they suspect in a full manic episode. The family calls emergency medical services. While one medic is talking with Luc and his family, the other medic is counting something on his desk. What is the medic most likely counting?
   a. Hypodermic needles
   b. Fast food wrappers
   c. Empty soda cans
   d. Energy drink containers
7. Which nursing responses demonstrate accurate information that should be discussed with the female patient diagnosed with bipolar disorder and her support system? **Select all that apply.**
   a. "Remember that alcohol and caffeine can trigger a relapse of your symptoms."
   b. "Due to the risk of a manic episode, you should not take birth control pills."
   c. "It's critical to let your health care provider know immediately if you aren't sleeping well."
   d. "Is your family prepared to be actively involved in helping you manage this disorder?"
   e. "The physical symptoms tend to come and go, so you need to be able to recognize the early signs."

https://evolve.elsevier.com/Canada/Varcarolis/psychiatric/

REFERENCES

American Psychiatric Association. (2013). *Diagnostic and statistical manual of mental disorders* (5th ed.). Arlington: Author.

Burchum, J., & Rosenthal, L. (2019). *Lehne's pharmacology for nursing care* (10th ed.). St Louis: Elsevier.

Fornaro, M., Carvalho, A. F., Fusco, A., et al. (2020). The concept and management of acute episodes of treatment-resistant bipolar disorder: A systematic review and exploratory meta-analysis of randomized controlled trials. *Journal of Affective Disorders, 276*, 970–983. https://doi.org/10.1016/j.jad.2020.07.109

Fries, G. R., Walss-Bass, C., Bauer, M. E., & Teixeira, A. L. (2019). Revisiting inflammation in bipolar disorder. *Pharmacology, Biochemistry and Behavior, 177*, 12–19. https://doi.org/10.1016/j.pbb.2018.12.006

Goldberg, J. F. (2019). Complex combination pharmacotherapy for bipolar disorder: Knowing when less Is more or more is better. *Focus: The Journal of Lifelong Learning in Psychiatry, 17(3)*: 218–231. Retrieved from https://focus.psychiatryonline.org/doi/epdf/10.1176/appi.focus.20190008

Health Canada. (2014). Health professional and consumer advisories. *Canadian Adverse Reaction Newsletter, 24*(2), 5. Retrieved from https://www.hc-sc.gc.ca/index-eng.php

Jamison, K. R. (1995). *An unquiet mind.* New York: Knopf.

Johansson, V., Hultman, C. M., Kizling, I., et al. (2019). The schizophrenia and bipolar twin study in Sweden (STAR). *Schizophrenia Research, 204*, 183–192. https://doi.org/10.1016/j.schres.2018.08.001

Meinhard, N., Kessing, L. V., & Vinberg, M. (2014). The role of estrogen in bipolar disorder: A review. *Nordic Journal of Psychiatry, 68*(2), 81–87. https://doi.org/10.3109/08039488.2013.775341

Mood Disorders Society of Canada. (2019). *Quick facts: Mental health & addictions in Canada.* Bellville: Author.

Moorhead, S., Johnson, M., Maas, M., et al. (2018). *Nursing Outcomes Classification (NOC)* (6th ed.). St. Louis: Mosby.

Olfson, M., Mojtabai, R., Merikangas, K. R., et al. (2017). Reexamining associations between mania, depression, anxiety and substance use disorders: Results from a prospective national cohort. *Molecular Psychiatry, 22*(2), 235–241. https://doi.org/10.1038/mp.2016.64

Perry, A., Gordon-Smith, K., Di Florio, A., et al. (2020). Adverse childhood experiences and postpartum depression in bipolar disorder. *Journal of Affective Disorders, 263*, 661–666. https://doi.org/10.1016/j.jad.2019.11.042

Phillips, M. L., & Swartz, H. A. (2014). A critical appraisal of neuroimaging studies of bipolar disorder: Toward a new conceptualization of underlying neural circuitry and roadmap for future research. *American Journal of Psychiatry, 171*(8), 829–843. https://doi.org/10.1176/appi.ajp.2014.13081008

Pinto, J. V., Saraf, G., Kozicky, J., et al. (2020). Remission and recurrence in bipolar disorder: The data from Health Outcomes and Patient Evaluations in Bipolar Disorder (HOPE-BD) study. *Journal of Affective Disorders, 268*, 150–157. https://doi.org/10.1016/j.jad.2020.03.018

Shapero, B. G., Weiss, R. B., Burke, T. A., et al. (2017). Kindling of life stress in bipolar disorder: Effects of early adversity. *Behavior Therapy, 48*(3), 322–334. https://doi.org/10.1016/j.beth.2016.12.003

Smith, D. J., Anderson, J., Zammit, S., et al. (2015). Childhood IQ and risk of bipolar disorder in adulthood: Prospective birth cohort study. *British Journal of Psychiatry Open, 1*, 74–80.

Trudeau, M. (2010). *Changing my mind.* Toronto: Harper Collins Publishers Ltd.

15

Schizophrenia Spectrum and Other Psychotic Disorders

Lisa-Marie Forcier, Eric MacMullin
Originating US chapter by Edward A. Herzog

 https://evolve.elsevier.com/Canada/Varcarolis/psychiatric/

OBJECTIVES

1. Describe the progression of symptoms, focus of care, and intervention needs for the pre-psychotic through maintenance phases of schizophrenia.
2. Discuss at least three of the neurobiological, anatomical, and genetic findings that indicate that schizophrenia is a brain disorder.
3. Differentiate among the positive and negative symptoms of schizophrenia in terms of psychopharmacological treatment and effect on the quality of life.
4. Discuss the concept of recovery for people living with schizophrenia.
5. Discuss how to deal with common reactions the nurse may experience while working with a person with schizophrenia.
6. Develop teaching plans for people taking conventional antipsychotic medications (e.g., haloperidol [Haldol]) and atypical antipsychotic medications (e.g., risperidone [Risperdal]).
7. Compare and contrast the conventional antipsychotic medications with atypical antipsychotic medication.
8. Identify nonpharmacological interventions that may be used to address symptoms of schizophrenia.
9. Create a nursing care plan that incorporates evidence-informed interventions for key areas of dysfunction in schizophrenia, including hallucinations, delusions, paranoia, cognitive disorganization, anosognosia, and impaired self-care.
10. Role-play intervening with a person who is hallucinating, delusional, and exhibiting disorganized thinking.

KEY TERMS AND CONCEPTS

abnormal motor behaviour
acute dystonia
affective symptoms
agranulocytosis
akathisia
anosognosia
anticholinergic-induced delirium
associative looseness
automatic obedience
boundary impairment
catatonia
circumstantiality
clang association
cognitive symptoms
command hallucinations
concrete thinking
delusions
depersonalization
derealization
disorganized thinking
echolalia
echopraxia
extrapyramidal side effects
hallucinations
ideas of reference
illusions
impaired impulse control
negative symptoms
negativism
neologisms
neuroleptic malignant syndrome
paranoia
positive symptoms
pseudoparkinsonism
psychomotor agitation
psychomotor retardation
psychosis
reality testing
recovery model
stereotyped behaviours
tangentiality
tardive dyskinesia
waxy flexibility
word salad

Schizophrenia spectrum and other psychotic disorders are complex disorders that affect a person's thinking, language, emotions, social behaviour, and ability to perceive reality accurately. These disorders are characterized by **psychosis**, which refers to altered cognition, altered perception, and/or an impaired ability to determine what is or is not real (an ability known as reality testing). Psychosis itself is a symptom and not classified as a mental illness (Schizophrenia Society of Canada, 2020).

The most severe disorder defined by the presence of psychosis is *schizophrenia*, which is the major focus of this chapter. Schizophrenia affects 1 in every 100 people in Canada, with 56% of people diagnosed being male and 44% being female (Government of Canada, 2020; Health Quality Ontario, 2018; Schizophrenia Society of Canada, 2018). Psychosis affects 3% of the population at any given time (Schizophrenia Society of Canada, 2018). "Schizophrenia is one of the most widely misunderstood and feared illnesses in society. The lingering stigma and myths associated with this illness often result in discrimination and, consequently, a reluctance to seek appropriate help" (Schizophrenia Society of Canada, 2018, p. 4). Negative attitudes toward people living with schizophrenia can interfere with recovery and impair their quality of life (Gaebel et al., 2017; Walker et al., 2016). For example, many mistakenly believe that people living with schizophrenia are likely to be violent or that offenders are likely to have been "psychotic" preceding episodes of violence. In fact, the rate of psychosis before violence is low even among high-risk offenders (Mental Health Commission of Canada, 2021; Skeem et al., 2015). Among those with severe forms of mental illness, such as schizophrenia, incidents of violence against strangers is extremely rare—one incident of homicide per 14.3 million people per year—and usually occurs in combination with substance use and psychosis (Nielssen & Large, 2010). Overall, people who experience mental illness are much more likely to be victims of crime, hate, and discrimination then to be the perpetrators of them (Hodgins & Klein, 2017; Mental Health Commission of Canada, 2017). Violence directed to oneself is a greater likelihood, with high levels of self-harm and suicide attempts reported in individuals with psychosis (Sanchez SanSegundo et al., 2018). Self-harm in these cases was associated with younger age of onset, female gender, comorbid depressive episode, comorbid alcohol abuse or dependence, current suicidality, awareness of illness, and low adherence to prescribed medication (Mork et al., 2012). According to Sanchez SanSegundo et al. (2018, para. 2), between 4% and 5% of patients with schizophrenia and other psychoses complete suicide, between 40% and 79% report suicidal ideation, and between 20% and 40% of these individuals make suicide attempts during the course of illness. In a recent study the suicide rate for people living with schizophrenia spectrum disorders was found to be 20 times higher than the general population (Centre for Addiction and Mental Health, 2020; Zaheer et al., 2020).

Practices that concentrate on building trusting therapeutic relationships are practical ways to counter discrimination and promote recovery in the care of those experiencing psychosis and schizophrenia (Mental Health Commission of Canada, 2016). The *How a Nurse Helped Me* story demonstrates the four elements of the LEAP approach (Amador, 2021), which is based on the belief that trusting relationships are key to healing partnerships:

- **L**isten—Both nurses listened with compassion and genuineness.
- **E**mpathize—It is clear that both nurses were able to convey that they cared about understanding what Tammy was feeling.
- **A**gree—Both nurses believed in Tammy, affirmed that she was indeed worried and struggling. They supported her in her goals, never looking down on her or judging her but helping her on her own road to recovery.
- **P**artner—Clearly, both nurses respected Tammy and worked with her as partners for recovery.

LEAP is described as a technique; however, inherent in that description is the risk of seeing it only technically. The LEAP approach must be underpinned by genuineness and caring. Cynthia and Rhonda invited Tammy into a trusting and therapeutic relationship. They did not apply these components as "techniques"; instead, it appears that the LEAP principles flowed naturally out of genuine caring. As genuine understanding, empathy, and respect for Tammy's point of view was communicated, common ground on which the nurses could partner with Tammy followed. Through this process, the professional opinions and support of her "team" started to matter to Tammy. Without this approach, suspicious and delusional ideas can be challenging to understand and manage. Tammy's story demonstrates how empowering and therapeutic it is to experience being truly listened to, empathized with, and collaborated with in all relationships, and particularly with managing psychosis.

CLINICAL PICTURE

There are five key features associated with psychotic disorders:

1. **Delusions:** Alterations in *thought content* (what a person thinks about). Delusions are false fixed beliefs that cannot be corrected by reasoning or evidence to the contrary. Beliefs maintained by one's culture or subculture are not delusions.
2. **Hallucinations:** Perception of a sensory experience for which no external stimulus exists (e.g., hearing a voice when no one is speaking).

HOW A NURSE HELPED ME

They Listen With Compassion and Dignity: I Know I Am Not Alone

I live with schizoaffective disorder. I am 30 now, and I was diagnosed with a mental illness when I was 15. I experience both the symptoms of psychosis often present in schizophrenia and a mood disorder, often in the form of rapid cycling of moods from depression to extreme highs. For the first 5 to 10 years of coping with my mental illness, the hospital was like a revolving door for me. It took me numerous years to find the right medications and therapies.

I have been able to overcome my intense symptoms by finding balance in my chaotic moods and a decrease in my delusional symptoms and paranoia. Nurses like Cynthia and Rhonda help me to find that balance when it is lost. Cynthia, who works in the hospital, is a nurse who goes out of her way to be there for her patients. I first met Cynthia 10 years ago on my first admission. She has had such a positive impact on my life because she believes in me even when I don't trust and believe in myself. She brings cheerfulness to the ward that is scary and full of strangeness when you are admitted. If you are depressed or not feeling well, she is most often able to cheer you up. (That is no matter how bad you feel or how painful your day has been.) She has truly listened to me—when I have been really unwell and hospitalized. At those times I am just so scared. I even wonder about the special meaning in the numbers or letter that could be anywhere—even on the menu ordering my food on the ward! It can freak me out a little, but Cynthia listens and talks me through it. Even if I am not cured in that instant, I am comforted and can carry on. Her dedication to finding ways to work through even my worst suspicions has never wavered. Cynthia is one of a kind.

Rhonda, the community mental health nurse who I work with as an outpatient, is one of the most dedicated and compassionate nurses I have ever met. She has also had a tremendous influence on my life. She often works after-hours to offer full support to her patients. Sometimes I have called her past 6:00 in the evening, thinking I would leave a message, yet to my surprise she is still there, and she works with me on my schedule and needs. She, too, listens to my fears and worries. She treats me with dignity and respect, and I know truly wants me to be successful in the world. I have never felt like I have been looked down upon or judged—even if what I bring up to her must seem totally weird or off track sometimes! One of my fears is that I must look stupid when I am fearful of things, but Rhonda has an open mind, and her compassion has supported me through many rough and painful times. Rhonda has always believed in me, and this has helped me on my road to recovery. I look forward to appointments with Rhonda because she always allows me to see life situations from a realistic and positive perspective. She provides me with ongoing encouragement. I have been successful at working at the bank now for 3 years and have managed to keep up my friendships and have not scared my boyfriend away. I know I owe Rhonda for much of that success. Through it all, I know that I am not alone, and with this help I can figure my way out of even the worst thoughts or worries.

Source: Story inspired by Tammy L. (shared with her permission).

3. **Disorganized thinking:** The loosening of associations, manifested as jumbled and illogical speech and impaired reasoning.
4. **Abnormal motor behaviour:** Alterations in behaviour, including bizarre and agitated behaviours (e.g., stilted, rigid demeanor; eccentric dress, grooming, and rituals). Grossly disorganized behaviours may include mutism, stupor, or catatonic excitement.
5. **Negative symptoms:** The absence of something that should be present but is not, for example, the ability to make decisions or to follow through on a plan. Negative symptoms contribute to poor social functioning and social withdrawal.

While this chapter concentrates on assessment and treatment of schizophrenia, other psychotic disorders (e.g., schizophreniform, schizoaffective, brief psychotic disorders) are described in Box 15.1.

Adding to observations made by Emil Kraepelin (1856–1926), Eugen Bleuler (1857–1939) coined the term *schizophrenia*. He first proposed that schizophrenia was not one illness but a heterogeneous group of illnesses with different characteristics and clinical courses. Clinicians in Canada use the criteria of the *Diagnostic and Statistical Manual of Mental Disorders*, fifth edition (American Psychiatric Association, 2013), for the diagnosis of schizophrenia spectrum and other psychotic disorders. All those diagnosed with schizophrenia exhibit at least one psychotic symptom, such as delusions; hallucinations; or disorganized thinking, speech, or behaviour. The person experiences extreme difficulty with or an inability to function in family, social, or occupational realms and frequently neglects basic needs such as nutrition or hygiene. Over a period of 6 months, there may be times when the symptoms of psychosis are absent, and in their place the person may experience apathy or depression. It is important to note, the course of illness is unique in all individuals and each presentation may be different.

EPIDEMIOLOGY

The lifetime prevalence of schizophrenia is 1% worldwide; anyone can develop schizophrenia, it affects people of all races and cultures (Schizophrenia Society of Canada, 2020). It is more common among persons growing up in urban areas (Health Quality Ontario, 2018). Onset in males is usually between the ages of 15 and 25 years and is associated with poorer functioning and more structural abnormality in the brain. The onset tends to be somewhat later in women (ages 25 to 35 years), who tend to have a better prognosis and experience fewer structural changes in the brain (Dean et al., 2016). People who are diagnosed later in life with schizophrenia often experience an earlier prodromal phase during which some milder symptoms of the disorder develop, often months or years before the disorder becomes fully apparent (Miller, 2016). Childhood schizophrenia, although rare, does exist, occurring in 1 out of 40 000 children. Early onset occurs more often in males and is associated with poor functioning before onset and increased levels of apathy. Individuals with a later onset are more likely to be female, have less structural brain abnormality, and have better outcomes.

COMORBIDITY

Substance use disorders (particularly alcohol and marijuana related) have a greater prevalence for individuals living with schizophrenia and other psychotic disorders (Cookey et al., 2020; Crockford & Addington, 2017; Hodgins & Klein, 2017; Schizophrenia Society of Canada, 2020). A large epidemiologic survey suggests that the prevalence of substance use disorders (excluding nicotine and caffeine use disorders) in persons living with schizophrenia is 47%, respectively (Crockford & Addington, 2017, p. 624). Evidence suggests people may use substances, or alcohol in an attempt to quiet voices, calm thoughts that are disordered, cope with stresses and/or trauma (Schizophrenia Society of Canada, 2020). Approximately 21% of people living with schizophrenia are diagnosed with alcohol use disorder in their lifetime and 27% are diagnosed with cannabis use disorder (Cookey et al., 2020). Cannabis and stimulant use in particular are associated with the development of symptoms of psychosis (Cookey et al., 2020; Crockford & Addington, 2017). Regular cannabis use in adolescence appears to significantly increase the risk of developing symptoms of psychosis (Crockford & Addington, 2017).

BOX 15.1 Psychotic Disorders Other Than Schizophrenia

Schizophreniform Disorder
The features of schizophreniform disorder are similar to schizophrenia, but the total duration of the illness is less than 6 months. This disorder may or may not develop into schizophrenia.

Brief Psychotic Disorder
This disorder involves a sudden onset of psychosis or grossly disorganized or catatonic behaviour lasting less than 1 month. It is often precipitated by extreme stressors and is followed by a return to premorbid functioning.

Schizoaffective Disorder
Schizoaffective disorder is a subgroup of psychoses in which affective symptoms and symptoms of schizophrenia are prominent simultaneously. The symptoms are not due to any substance use or to a medical condition and present with either bipolar or depressive affective symptoms alongside psychosis.

Delusional Disorder
Delusional disorder is characterized by nonbizarre delusions (i.e., situations that could occur in real life, such as being followed, being deceived by a spouse, or having a disease). The person's ability to function is not markedly impaired nor is behaviour otherwise odd or psychotic. A related disorder, Capgras syndrome, involves a delusion about a significant other (e.g., family member, pet) being replaced by an imposter; this disorder may be a result of psychiatric or organic brain disease (Salvatore et al., 2014).

Substance- or Medication-Induced Psychotic Disorder
Psychosis may be induced by substances such as drugs of abuse, alcohol, or medications. (Schizophrenia Society of Canada, 2020).

Psychosis or Catatonia Associated With Another Medical Condition or Another Mental Disorder
Psychoses may also be caused by a medical condition (delirium, neurological or metabolic conditions, hepatic or renal diseases, and many others) as well as by mental illness such as post-traumatic stress disorder (Alsawy et al., 2015) or depression, particularly with co-existing victimization from sexual violence or bullying (Nam et al., 2016). Medical conditions and substance use must always be ruled out before a diagnosis of schizophrenia or other psychotic disorder can be made.

Sources: Alsawy, S., Wood, L., Taylor, P. J., et al. (2015). Psychotic experiences and PTSD: Exploring associations in a population survey. *Psychological Medicine, 45*(13), 2849. https://doi.org/10.1017/S003329171500080X; Nam, B., Hilimire, M., Schiffman, J., et al. (2016). Psychotic experiences in the context of depression: The cumulative role of victimization. *Journal of Psychiatric Research, 82*, 136–140. https://doi.org/10.1016/j.jpsychires.2016.07.023; Salvatore, P., Bhuvaneswar, C., Tohen, M., et al. (2014). Capgras' syndrome in first-episode psychotic disorders. *Psychopathology, 47*(4), 261. https://doi.org/10.1159/000357813; Schizophrenia Society of Canada. (2020). *Hope & recovery–Your guide to living with and beyond schizophrenia.* https://schizophrenia.ca/wp-content/uploads/2020/05/Hope-and-Recovery-Guide.pdf

Nicotine use is reported in 60% to 90% of people living with schizophrenia (Crockford & Addington, 2017) this can contribute to an increased incidence of cardiovascular and respiratory disorders and double the risk for cancers (Akbarian & Kundakovic, 2015).

Anxiety, depression, and suicide co-occur frequently in schizophrenia. Anxiety may be a response to symptoms (e.g., hallucinations) or circumstances (e.g., isolation, overstimulation) and may worsen schizophrenia symptoms and prognosis. Physical illnesses overall are more common among people living with schizophrenia than in the general population. Studies have indicated that people living with schizophrenia are at risk for premature death with the average life expectancy being approximately 15 to 20 years less than the general population (Health Quality Ontario, 2018). "The all-cause mortality rate in people diagnosed with schizophrenia is 2.8 times higher than those without" (Government of Canada, 2020). These significantly higher death rates reflect a combination of (1) higher risk factors for many chronic diseases and some types of cancer; (2) the iatrogenic effects of some psychiatric medications; (3) higher rates of suicide, accidental, and violent death; and (4) disparities in health care access and use (Correll et al., 2015; Thornicroft, 2011). Communication problems or difficulties with informed consent may be part of the issue of health care access (Pelletier et al., 2015). Despite having more contact with family physicians than the general population, persons with psychiatric disorders are less likely to be assessed and treated for conditions such as hypertension or to receive preventive care such as smoking cessation (Pelletier et al., 2015).

Incentives and barriers to engaging people with severe mental illness in lifestyle interventions have not been extensively studied, though there is some evidence that these interventions can be effective (Happell et al., 2013). Barriers that are reported in the literature include illness symptoms, treatment effects, lack of support, and negative staff attitudes; incentives include peer and staff support, staff participation, reduction of symptoms, knowledge, and personal attributes (Happell et al., 2013).

ETIOLOGY

Schizophrenia is a complicated disorder. In fact, what we call *schizophrenia* is a group of different illnesses with common but varying features and multiple, overlapping etiologies (Schizophrenia Society of Canada, 2020). What is known is that brain chemistry, structure, and activity are different in a person with schizophrenia from those in a person who does not have the disorder.

While there is not one specific cause of schizophrenia, the scientific consensus is that schizophrenia occurs when multiple inherited gene abnormalities combine with nongenetic factors (viral infections, birth injuries, pre-natal malnutrition) and are influenced by environmental and social factors. These alter the structures of the brain, affecting the brain's neurotransmitter systems, injuring the brain directly, or doing all three. This effect is called the *diathesis–stress model of schizophrenia* (Berry & Cirulli, 2016).

Biological Factors
Genetic Factors
Evidence suggests that multiple genes on different chromosomes interact with each other in complex ways to create vulnerability for schizophrenia. About 80% of the risk of schizophrenia comes from genetic and epigenetic factors (factors such as toxins or psychological trauma that affect the expression of genes). More than 100 loci in the human genome are associated with an increased risk for schizophrenia (Castellani et al., 2015). While no one particular gene is identified as causal, schizophrenia is said to be inherited, and compared to the usual 1% risk in the general population, having a first-degree relative with schizophrenia increases the risk to 10%. Further, a variability of expression of schizophrenia has been identified, and it depends on environmental factors; schizoaffective disorder and cluster A personality disorders are more common in relatives of people living with schizophrenia. Concordance rates (i.e., how often one twin will have the disorder when the other twin has it) are about 50% for identical twins and about 15% for fraternal twins.

Neurobiological Factors
Dopamine theory. The dopamine theory of schizophrenia is derived from the study of the action of the first antipsychotic medications, collectively known as *conventional* (or *first-generation*) *antipsychotic medication* (e.g., haloperidol and chlorpromazine). These medications block the activity of dopamine D_2 receptors in the brain, limiting the activity of dopamine and reducing some of the symptoms of schizophrenia. However, because the dopamine-blocking medications do not alleviate all symptoms of schizophrenia, it is recognized that other neurochemicals are involved in generating the symptoms of schizophrenia. Amphetamines, cocaine, methylphenidate (Ritalin), and levodopa increase the activity of dopamine in the brain and, in biologically susceptible people, may precipitate the onset of schizophrenia. If schizophrenia is already present, these substances may also exacerbate its symptoms. Almost any drug of abuse, particularly marijuana, can increase the risk for schizophrenia in biologically vulnerable individuals (Morgan et al., 2016).

Other neurochemical hypotheses. A newer class of medications, collectively known as *atypical* (or *second-generation*) *antipsychotic medications*, block serotonin as well as dopamine, which suggests that serotonin may play a role in schizophrenia as well. A better understanding of how atypical medications modulate the expression and targeting of 5-hydroxytryptamine 2A (5-HT2A) and its receptors would likely lead to a better understanding of schizophrenia.

Researchers have long been aware that phenylcyclohexyl piperidine (PCP) induces a state closely resembling schizophrenia. This observation led to interest in the *N*-methyl-D-aspartate (NMDA) receptor complex and the possible role of glutamate in the pathophysiology of schizophrenia.

Glutamate, dopamine, and serotonin act synergistically in neurotransmission, and thus glutamate may also play a role in causing psychosis (Andreou et al., 2015). Neurotransmission by another calming neurotransmitter, gamma-aminobutyric acid (GABA), is also impaired in schizophrenia (Frankle et al., 2015). Kesby et al. (2018) suggest, "excessive dopamine signalling in the associative striatum may directly lead to symptoms of psychosis by compromising the integration of cortical inputs" (p. 4).

Brain Structure Abnormalities
Disruptions in communication pathways in the brain are thought to be severe in schizophrenia. Therefore it is conceivable that structural abnormalities cause disruption of the brain's functioning. Structural differences may be due to errors in neurodevelopment or errors in the normal pruning of neuronal tissue that happens in late adolescence and early adulthood. Inflammation or neurotoxic effects from factors such as oxidative stress, infection, or autoimmune dysfunction may also alter the brain's structure (Sekar et al., 2016).

Using brain imaging techniques—computed tomography (CT), magnetic resonance imaging (MRI), functional MRI (fMRI), and positron emission tomography (PET)—researchers (Dean et al., 2016) have demonstrated structural brain abnormalities, including:
- Reduced volume in the right anterior insula (may contribute to negative symptoms)
- Reduced volume and changes in the shape of the hippocampus

- Accelerated age-related decline in cortical thickness
- Grey matter deficits in the dorsolateral prefrontal cortex area, thalamus, and anterior cingulate cortex, as well as in the frontotemporal, thalamocortical, and subcortical-limbic circuits
- Reduced connectivity among various brain regions
- Neuronal overgrowth in some areas, possibly due to inflammation or inadequate neural pruning
- Widespread white matter abnormalities (e.g., in the corpus callosum)

In addition, MRI and CT scans demonstrate lower brain volume and more cerebrospinal fluid in people living with schizophrenia. PET scans also show a lowered rate of blood flow and glucose metabolism in the frontal lobes, which govern planning, abstract thinking, social adjustment, and decision making, all of which are affected in schizophrenia. (Figure 11.5 in Chapter 11 shows a PET scan demonstrating reduced brain activity in the frontal lobe of a person with schizophrenia.) Such structural changes may worsen as the disorder continues. Postmortem studies on individuals with schizophrenia reveal a reduced volume of grey matter in the brain, especially in the temporal and frontal lobes; those with the most tissue loss had the worst symptoms (e.g., hallucinations, delusions, bizarre thoughts, depression).

Psychological, Social, and Environmental Factors

Several psychosocial and environmental stressors, particularly those occurring during vulnerable periods of neurological development, are believed to combine with genetic vulnerabilities which could cause schizophrenia. Reducing such stressors is believed to have the potential to reduce the severity of the disorder or even prevent it (Schifani et al., 2018).

Pre-natal Stressors

A history of pregnancy or birth complications is associated with an increased risk for schizophrenia. According to Hodgins and Klein (2017), the abnormal neural development in schizophrenia begins *in utero* as environmental factors interact with specific genotypes (p. 90). Pre-natal risk factors include viral infection, poor nutrition, hypoxia or poor neural development, and exposure to toxins. Infection during pregnancy increases the risk for mental illness in the child. Pre-natal infections in the mother also increase the risk for infection in the child after birth, and those infections in the children also can make them more vulnerable to mental illness (Blomström et al., 2016). Weiser et al. (2020) found in a recent study that advanced paternal age at birth of the first offspring does not predict increased risk for schizophrenia. Psychological trauma and increased stress during pregnancy can also contribute to the development of schizophrenia (Lipner et al., 2019).

Psychological Stressors

Although there is no evidence that stress alone causes schizophrenia, psychological and physical stress increase cortisol levels, impeding hypothalamic development and causing other changes that may precipitate the illness in vulnerable individuals. Schizophrenia often manifests at times of developmental and social stress, such as beginning university or moving away from one's family. Social, psychological, and physical stressors may also play a significant role in both the severity and course of the disorder and the person's quality of life.

Other risk factors include childhood sexual abuse, exposure to social adversity (e.g., chronic poverty), migration to or growing up in a foreign culture, and exposure to psychological trauma or social defeat (Hodgins & Klein, 2017; Howes & McCutcheon, 2017). These factors may cause structural changes in the brain via epigenetic changes to the genome. Even psychological trauma in a parent or grandparent may cause epigenetic changes that increase vulnerability, and this increased risk can be passed on to one's descendants. It has also been discovered that elevated dopaminergic function places recent immigrants at risk of developing psychosis (Egerton et al., 2017).

Environmental Stressors

Environmental factors such as toxins, including the solvent tetrachloroethylene (used in dry cleaning and to line water pipes, and sometimes found in drinking water), are also believed to contribute to the development of schizophrenia in vulnerable people (Aschengrau et al., 2012). Living in urban areas or high-crime environments is also believed to increase the risk for schizophrenia (Haddad et al., 2015).

Environmental factors within broader social environments are also believed to contribute to the development of schizophrenia in vulnerable people. These include exposure to social adversity (e.g., living in chronic poverty) and migration to or growing up in a foreign culture (Egerton et al., 2017).

CONSIDERING CULTURE
The Stigma of Schizophrenia

Mrs. Chou, a 25-year-old woman, left China for North America 6 months ago to join her husband. In China she lived with her parents and had learned English. She was shy and looked to her parents, and later to her husband, for guidance and support. Shortly after arrival in her new country, her mother developed pneumonia and died. Mrs. Chou later told her husband that if she had stayed in China, her mother would not have become ill, and that evil would now come to their 1-year-old child because Mrs. Chou had not taken proper care of her mother.

Mrs. Chou became increasingly lethargic, staring into space and mumbling to herself. When Mr. Chou asked who she was talking to, she answered, "My mother."

Mr. Chou realized that something was terribly wrong with his wife, yet he was reluctant to ask either relatives or professionals for assistance since mental illness is strongly stigmatized in the Chinese culture (Xu et al., 2017). In fact, mental illness may be believed to be a punishment for personal failings.

Mrs. Chou was finally admitted to a psychiatric unit when Mr. Chou noticed she had quit eating and taking care of herself and was certainly unable to care for their child. During her admission assessment, she sat motionless and mute. Mr. Nolan, her primary nurse, noticed that after he checked her pulse, her arm remained in midair until he lowered it for her. Mrs. Chou was unkempt and pale, and her skin turgor was poor.

Mr. Nolan also spoke with Mr. Chou, who was visibly distressed by his wife's condition. He discovered that Mr. Chou blamed himself for his wife's illness because his relocation prevented her from caring for her ailing mother. He agreed with his wife that their mutual failings placed their child at risk of retribution. He conceded that coming to the hospital had been very difficult, owing to embarrassment about both his wife's mental illness and his own belief that he should not burden others with the care of himself and his wife. Mr. Nolan helped Mr. Chou recognize that in North American culture, family members shared caregiving burdens, professional help was more available, and stigmatization was less intense.

Gradually, Mr. Chou's distress lessened as he came to appreciate that he would not have to carry the level of burden he had anticipated. As Mrs. Chou's psychosis subsided, both she and Mr. Chou came to ascribe more culpability for the illness to fate, reducing their burden of self-blame. They agreed to meet with a case manager, who helped them integrate the beliefs of their culture and resources, with the treatment and medications that assisted Mrs. Chou. By doing this they reported, it reduced their guilt and distress and led to an understanding of mental illness.

Source: Wong, D. F. K., Tsui, H. K. P., Pearson, V., et al. (2004). Family burdens, Chinese health beliefs, and the mental health of Chinese caregivers in Hong Kong. *Transcultural Psychiatry, 4*, 497–513.

Course of the Disorder

The onset of symptoms or forewarning (prodromal) symptoms may appear a month to a year before the first psychotic break or full-blown manifestations of the illness; such symptoms represent a clear deterioration in previous functioning. The course of the disorder thereafter typically includes recurrent exacerbations separated by periods of reduced or dormant symptoms. Some people will have a single episode of schizophrenia without recurrences or have several episodes and none thereafter. A study of more than 2000 persons found four patterns of the course of the illness. Although the course of schizophrenia varied, all showed an initial deterioration followed by improvement (Levine et al., 2011). Remission and recovery are increasingly common outcomes with early detection, appropriate treatment, and social support (Walker et al., 2016).

In the prodromal phase complaints about anxiety, phobias, obsessions, dissociative features, and compulsions may be noted. As anxiety increases, indications of a thought disorder become evident. Concentration, memory, and completion of school- or job-related work deteriorate. Intrusive thoughts, "mind wandering," and the need to devote more time to maintaining one's thoughts are reported.

The person may feel that something "strange" or "wrong" is happening. Events are misinterpreted, and mystical or symbolic meanings may be given to ordinary events. For example, the person may think that certain colours have special powers or that a song on the radio is a message from a higher being. Reducing misunderstandings and fear of schizophrenia can reduce stigma and support individuals living with this illness (Government of Canada, 2020).

Phases of Schizophrenia

Schizophrenia usually progresses through predictable phases, although the presenting symptoms during a given phase and the length of the phase can vary widely. The phases of schizophrenia are (Chung et al., 2008):

- **Phase I—Acute:** Onset or exacerbation of florid, disruptive symptoms (hallucinations, delusions, apathy, withdrawal) with resultant loss of functional abilities; increased care or hospitalization may be required.
- **Phase II—Stabilization:** Symptoms are diminishing, and there is movement toward one's previous level of functioning (baseline); day hospitalization or care in a residential crisis centre or a supervised group home may be needed.
- **Phase III—Maintenance:** The person is at or nearing baseline (or premorbid) functioning; symptoms are absent or diminished; level of functioning allows the person to live in the community. Ideally, recovery with few or no residual symptoms has occurred. Most people in this phase live in their own residences. Although this phase has been termed *maintenance*, current literature shows a trend toward reframing it with a greater emphasis on recovery.

Prognosis

An abrupt onset of symptoms is usually a favourable prognostic sign, and those with good premorbid social, sexual, and occupational functioning have a greater chance for a good remission or a complete recovery (Sandler et al., 2011).

Some patients may require repeated or lengthy inpatient care or institutionalization as part of their treatment. Factors associated with a less positive prognosis include a slow onset (e.g., more than 2 to 3 years), younger age at onset, longer duration between first symptoms and first treatment, longer periods of untreated illness, and more negative symptoms. A childhood history of withdrawn, reclusive, eccentric, and tense behaviour is also an unfavourable diagnostic sign, as is a preponderance of negative symptoms (Freudenreich, 2020a). Reducing the frequency, intensity, and duration of relapse (when previously controlled symptoms return) is believed to improve the long-term prognosis. While there is no cure for schizophrenia (Government of Canada, 2020), schizophrenia is treatable (Addington et al., 2017a; Government of Canada, 2020; Schizophrenia Society of Canada, 2020). Successful treatment of schizophrenia requires an organized, recovery-oriented, mental health system with coordinated services (Addington et al., 2017a, p. 663).

According to Addington et al. (2017a), "in Canada, mental health services are delivered through provincially funded services. The organization, funding and delivery of mental health services vary from province to province; there are no national standards for service delivery, although there is a National Strategy. In Canada, the Mental Health Strategy identifies supporting recovery as a core value for mental health services" (pp. 662–663).

Early Detection

Some clinicians suggest that there is an earlier prodromal (or pre-psychotic) phase, in which subtle symptoms or deficits associated with schizophrenia are present. Detection and treatment programs in most major Canadian cities aim to detect psychosis in the prodromal phase and prevent acute episodes of schizophrenia. Strategies of health promotion to improve outcomes, include reducing the duration of untreated psychosis, reducing delay in treatment, and providing early and appropriate interventions adapted for younger people (adolescents) and their families during the early course of the illness (Abidi et al., 2017; Srihari et al., 2012). A list of Canadian programs can be found on the website of IEPA Early Intervention in Mental Health at https://iepa.org.au

There is, however, controversy as to whether the benefits of early intervention can be maintained over time. A study at the Prevention and Early Intervention Program for Psychoses (PEPP) in London, Ontario, found symptom improvement was not only maintained at the 5-year follow-up but increased for an additional 2 to 5 years (Norman et al., 2011). This program provides continuity of care for 5 years, with more intense intervention in the initial 2 years and a gradual, individualized transfer to usual services. When compared to programs that provide only 2 years of treatment, the PEPP approach demonstrates better durability of benefit (Srihari et al., 2012). A large longitudinal study in the United Kingdom found that treatment within an early intervention psychosis service was associated with better health and social outcomes and reduced costs (Tsiachristas et al., 2016). Family involvement in early intervention has been found to be an important component of treatment, the most functional and adaptive family coping approaches being those that involve planning, seeking social support, positive reinterpretation, acceptance and turning to religion, and rare use of "avoidant" coping strategies (e.g., denial or disengagement, use of alcohol and non-prescription medications) (Gerson et al., 2011). A systematic review of family interventions for psychosis established that such interventions improved patient functioning and reduced the likelihood of relapse. Symptoms of psychosis were significantly reduced in the longer term; however, caregiver well-being did not sustain the same benefit over time (Fornells-Ambrojo et al., 2017).

APPLICATION OF THE NURSING PROCESS

Assessment

Nursing assessment of people who have or may have a psychotic disorder focuses largely on symptoms, coping, functioning, and safety. Assessment involves interviewing the person and observing behaviour and other outward manifestations of the disorder. It also should include mental status and spiritual assessments, cultural assessments, biological, psychological, social, and environmental elements. Further, reviews of medical records and history taken from other sources (e.g., family) are critical (Addington et al., 2017b). Sound therapeutic communication skills, an understanding of the disorder and the ways in which the person may be experiencing the world, and the establishment of trust and a therapeutic nurse–patient relationship all strengthen the assessment (see Chapter 10 for more on communication and the clinical interview). Indeed, as discussed in Chapter 9, the therapeutic relationship is of critical importance. A helping partnership between the nurse and the person with schizophrenia facilitates recovery (Chester et al., 2016).

One effective approach to developing this trusting relationship for patients with psychosis is the LEAP approach described by Amador (2021) and referenced at the beginning of this chapter. It consists of four steps: (1) listen—try to put yourself in the other person's shoes to gain a clear idea of their experience; (2) empathize—seriously consider and empathize with the other person's point of view; (3) agree—find common ground and identify facts you can both agree on; (4) partner—collaborate on accomplishing the agreed-upon goals (Amador, 2021). In this way, trust can be gained, and an alliance can be formed.

During the Pre-psychotic Phase

Experts believe that detection and treatment of symptoms that may warn of schizophrenia's onset lessen the risk of developing the disorder or decrease the severity of the disorder if it does develop. Early and appropriate interventions can improve symptoms since one-third of all adults with schizophrenia have their onset before the age of 18 (Abidi et al., 2017). Further, recommendations for children and young people experiencing first episode psychosis, include offering antipsychotic medication in conjunction with psychological/psychosocial interventions (Abidi et al., 2017).

Therefore early assessment plays a key role in improving the prognosis for persons living with schizophrenia (Lieberman et al., 2019). This form of primary prevention involves monitoring those at high risk (e.g., children of parents diagnosed with schizophrenia) for symptoms such as abnormal social development and cognitive dysfunction. Intervening to reduce stressors (i.e., reduce or avoid exposure to triggers), enhancing social and coping skills (e.g., building resilience), and administering prophylactic antipsychotic medication may also be of benefit.

Similarly, in people who have already developed the disorder, minimizing the onset and duration of relapses is believed to improve the prognosis. Research suggests that with each relapse of psychosis, there is an increase in residual dysfunction and deterioration. Recognition and personal tracking of the individual early warning signs of relapse, such as reduced sleep and concentration, are important to prevention of relapse. Limiting stress in work, relationships, and social or environmental domains, as well as enlisting the support of friends or loved ones and increasing the frequency of professional supports for monitoring and intensification of treatment, are essential. For this reason, for some, adherence to a medication regimen of antipsychotic medication can be more important than the risk of adverse effects because most adverse effects are reversible, whereas the consequences of relapse may not be (Brown & Gray, 2015).

General Assessment

Not all people living with schizophrenia have the same symptoms, and some of the symptoms of schizophrenia are also found in other disorders such as schizoaffective disorder, delusional disorder, brief psychotic disorder, postpartum psychosis, and substance-induced psychotic disorder. Figure 15.1 describes the four main symptom groups of schizophrenia:

1. **Positive symptoms:** the presence of something that is not normally present
2. **Negative symptoms:** the absence of something that should be present but is not
3. **Cognitive symptoms:** abnormalities in how a person thinks
4. **Affective symptoms:** symptoms involving emotions and their expression

Positive symptoms. Positive symptoms usually appear early in the person's illness and can precipitate hospitalization. These symptoms can cause misunderstanding, fear, and stigmatization. It is, important to reduce misunderstanding and fear, which can reduce stigma and support people living with schizophrenia (Government of Canada, 2020). Positive symptoms usually respond to antipsychotic medication. Positive symptoms are associated with:

- Acute onset
- Normal premorbid functioning
- Normal social functioning during remissions
- Normal CT findings
- Normal neuropsychological test results
- Favourable response to antipsychotic medication

The positive symptoms presented here are categorized as alterations in *thinking*, *speech*, *perception*, and *behaviour*.

Alterations in thinking. All people experience occasional and momentary errors in thinking (e.g., "Why are all these lights turning red when I'm already late? Someone must be trying *to slow me down!*"), but most can catch and correct the error by using intact **reality testing**—the ability to determine accurately whether an experience is based in reality. People with impaired reality testing, however, maintain the error, which contributes to delusions, or alterations in *thought* content. A person experiencing delusions is convinced that what they believe to be real *is* real. Table 15.1 provides definitions and examples of frequent types of delusions.

Approximately 75% of people living with schizophrenia experience delusions at some time during the course of illness. The most common delusions are persecutory or grandiose or those involving religious or hypochondriacal ideas. A delusion may be a response to anxiety or may reflect areas of concern for a person; for example, someone with poor self-esteem may believe they are Beethoven or a prophet, allowing them to feel more powerful or important. Looking for and addressing such underlying themes or needs can be a key nursing intervention. At times, delusions can hold some truth. For example, a patient was convinced that staff were poisoning them and refusing all food unless sealed. Later, staff found out that family members were concealing medication in the patient's food.

Concrete thinking refers to an impaired ability to think abstractly. The person interprets statements literally. For example, the nurse might ask what brought the person to the hospital, and the person might answer, concretely, "a bus" (rather than explaining that they had been hearing voices). Traditionally, concreteness has been assessed through the patient's interpretation of proverbs. However, this assessment is not accurate if the person is from another culture or is otherwise unfamiliar with the proverb (Haynes & Resnick, 1993). It is preferable to use the *similarities test*, which involves asking the person to explain how two things are similar—for example, an orange and an apple, a chair and a table, or a child and an adult. A description of physical characteristics ("apples and oranges are both round") would be a concrete answer, whereas an abstract answer recognizes ideas such as classifications ("apples and oranges are fruit"). Concreteness reduces one's ability to understand and address abstract concepts such as love or the passage of time or to reality-test delusions or other symptoms. Educational strategies need to take into account a person's ability to think abstractly.

Alterations in speech. Alterations in speech demonstrate difficulties with *thought process* (how a person thinks). *Associations* are the threads that tie one thought logically to another. In **associative looseness** these threads are interrupted or illogically connected; thinking becomes haphazard, illogical, and difficult to follow:

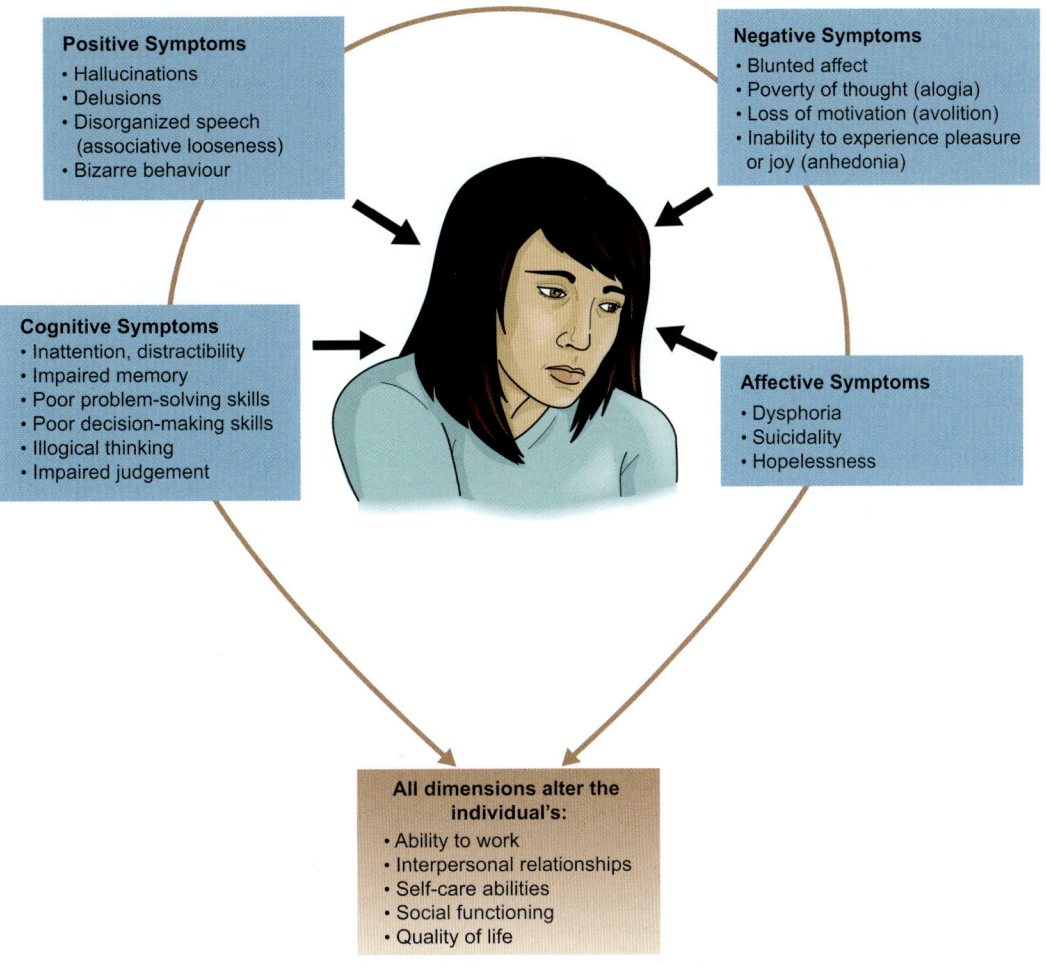

Fig. 15.1 The four main symptom groups of schizophrenia.

TABLE 15.1	Summary of Delusions	
Delusion	**Definition**	**Example**
Thought insertion	Believing that another person, group of people, or external force controls thoughts	Bruce explains he always wears a hat so that aliens don't insert thoughts into his brain.
Thought withdrawal	Believing that others are taking thoughts out of a person's mind	Bernadette explains she covers her windows with foil so the police can't empty her mind.
Thought broadcasting	Believing that one's thoughts are being involuntarily broadcasted to others	Marcel was convinced that everyone could hear what he was thinking at all times.
Ideas of reference	Giving personal significance to trivial events; perceiving events as relating to you when they do not	When Maria noticed staff talking, she believed they were plotting against her.
Ideas of influence	Believing that you have somehow influenced events that are, in fact, out of your control	Jean Pierre is convinced they caused the flooding in Manitoba.
Persecution	Believing that one is being singled out for harm by others; this belief often takes the form of a plot by people in power	Saied believed that the Royal Canadian Mounted Police were planning to kill him by poisoning his food. Therefore he would eat only food he bought from machines.
Grandeur	Believing that one is a very powerful or important person	Sam believed they were a famous playwright and tennis pro.
Somatic	Believing that the body is changing in an unusual way (e.g., rotting inside)	David told the physician that his heart had stopped, and his insides were rotting away.
Erotomanic	Believing that another person desires you romantically	Although she barely knew her, Millie insisted that Justine would marry her if only her current wife would stop interfering.
Jealousy	Believing that one's mate is unfaithful	Harry wrongly accused his girlfriend of going out with other men. His proof was that she came home from work late twice that week, even though the girlfriend's boss explained that everyone had worked late.

Nurse: "Are you going to the picnic today?"
Patient: "I'm not an elephant hunter; no tiger teeth for me."

At times, the nurse may be able to decipher or decode the patient's messages and begin to understand the patient's feelings and needs. Any exchange in which a person feels understood is useful. Therefore the nurse might respond to the patient in this way:

Nurse: "Are you saying that you're afraid to go out with the others today?"
Patient: "Yeah, no tiger getting me today."

Sometimes it is not possible to understand the person's meaning because their speech is too fragmented. For example:

Patient: "I sang out for my mother … for this to school I went. These little hills hop aboard, share the Christmas mice spread … the elephant will be washed away."

If the nurse does not understand what the patient is saying, it is important that they let the patient know this. Clear messages, communication, trust, and honesty are a vital part of working effectively in psychiatric mental health nursing. An honest response lets the person know that the nurse does not understand, would like to understand, and can be trusted to be honest.

Other alterations in speech that can make communication challenging are *circumstantiality, tangentiality, neologisms, echolalia, clang association,* and *word salad*:

- **Circumstantiality** refers to the inclusion of unnecessary and often tedious details in one's conversation (e.g., describing attending group therapy when asked how the day is).
- **Tangentiality** is a departure from the main topic to talk about less important information; the patient goes off on tangents in a way that takes the conversation off-topic.
- **Neologisms** are made-up words (or idiosyncratic uses of existing words) that have meaning for the person but a different or nonexistent meaning to others (e.g., "*I was going to tell him the mannerologies of his hospitality won't do*"). This eccentric use of words represents disorganized thinking and interferes with communication.
- **Echolalia** is the pathological repeating of another's words and is often seen in catatonia.
  Nurse: "*Rowan, come get your medication.*"
  Rowan: "*Come get your medication.*"
- **Clang association** is the choosing of words based on their sound rather than their meaning, often rhyming and sometimes having a similar beginning sound (e.g., "*On the track, have a Big Mac,*" "*Click, clack, clutch, close*"). Clanging may also be seen in neurological disorders.
- **Word salad** is a jumble of words that is meaningless to the listener—and perhaps to the speaker as well—because of an extreme level of disorganization.

Alterations in perception. Alterations in perception are errors in one's view of reality. The most common form of altered perception in psychosis are hallucinations, but depersonalization, derealization, and boundary impairment are sometimes experienced as well:

- **Depersonalization** is a nonspecific feeling that a person has lost their identity and that the self is different or unreal. People may feel that body parts do not belong to them or may sense that their body has drastically changed. For example, a person may see their fingers as snakes or arms as rotting wood.
- **Derealization** is the false perception that the environment has changed. For example, everything seems bigger or smaller, or familiar surroundings have become somehow strange and unfamiliar. Both depersonalization and derealization can be interpreted as *loss of ego boundaries* (sometimes called *loose ego boundaries*).
- **Boundary impairment** is an impaired ability to sense where one's self ends and others' selves begin. For example, a person might drink another's beverage, believing that because it is in their vicinity, it is theirs.
- **Hallucinations** result from perceiving a sensory experience for which no external stimulus exists (e.g., hearing a voice when no one is speaking).
- Hallucinations differ from **illusions** in that illusions are misperceptions or misinterpretations of a real experience; for example, a person sees their coat on a coat rack and believes it is a bear about to attack. They see something real but misinterprets what it is.

Causes of hallucinations include psychiatric disorders, substance use, medications, organic disorders, hyperthermia, toxicity (e.g., digitalis), and other conditions. Hallucinations can involve any of the five body senses. Table 15.2 provides definitions and examples of these types of hallucinations.

Auditory hallucinations are experienced by 5% to 28% of the general population, and in 75% of people living with schizophrenia (Thakur & Gupta, 2021). Auditory hallucinations are sensory perceptions of hearing sounds without an external stimulus, which activates the auditory processing areas of the brain when they are heard by a person (Thakur & Gupta, 2021). Another theory is "voices" are a misperception of one's internally generated conversation (Hoffman & Varanko, 2006). John Nash (n.d.), the world-renowned mathematician portrayed in the 2001 film *A Beautiful Mind*, described the voices he heard during the acute phase of his illness: "*I thought of the voices as … something a little different from aliens. I thought of them more like angels. … It's really my subconscious talking, it was really that. … I know that now.*"

People can describe voices as people familiar or unknown, single, or multiple. They may be perceived as supportive and pleasant or derogatory and frightening. Voices commenting on the person's behaviour or conversing with the person are most common. A person who hears

TABLE 15.2 Summary of Hallucinations

Hallucination	Definition	Example
Auditory	Hearing voices or sounds that do not exist in the environment	Juan is alone in his room and is heard yelling. When staff arrive in his room, Juan tells them that he is hearing an angry voice.
Visual	Seeing a person, object, animal, colours, or visual patterns that do not exist in the environment	Antonia became frightened and screamed, "*There are rats coming at me!*"
Olfactory	Smelling odours that do not exist in the environment	Theresa "smells" their insides rotting.
Gustatory	Tasting sensations that do not exist	Simon will not eat his food because he "tastes" the poison they are putting in it.
Tactile	Feeling strange sensations on the skin where no external objects stimulate such feelings; *common in delirium tremens* (DTs)	Jack "feels" bugs on/under skin.

voices when no one is present often struggles to understand the experience, sometimes developing related delusions to explain the voices (e.g., the person may believe the voices are from a higher being, spirits, or deceased relatives). In a study by Docherty et al. (2015) patients with internal hallucinations did not differ from those with external-only hallucinations in severity of positive, negative, general, or overall symptoms, but they were more depressed, and reported that their hallucinations were more emotionally negative, distressing, and disruptive (p. 6). Further, they reported their hallucinations lasted longer and were less controllable, they were more likely to experience voices commenting and voices conversing, as well as persecutory voices and commands to harm or kill others, and their hallucinations were less likely to have remitted over time (p. 7). Of note, patients were more likely to have insight into the self-generated nature of their voices (Docherty et al., 2015, p. 7).

Command hallucinations are "voices" that direct the person to take an action. All hallucinations must be assessed and monitored carefully because the voices may command the person to hurt self or others. For example, voices might command a person to "*use a weapon or method to harm themselves*" or "*use a weapon or method to harm someone else*." Command hallucinations are often terrifying and may herald a psychiatric emergency.

> ⚡ **SAFETY TIP**
> In all cases it is essential to assess what the person hears, the person's ability to recognize the hallucination as real or not real, and the person's ability to resist any commands.

A person may falsely deny hallucinations, requiring behavioural assessment to support (validate) or refute the person's report. Outward indications of possible hallucinations include turning or tilting the head as if to listen to someone, suddenly stopping current activity as if interrupted, and moving the lips silently.

Visual hallucinations occur less frequently in schizophrenia and are more likely to occur in organic disorders such as acute alcohol withdrawal or dementia. Olfactory, tactile, or gustatory hallucinations are unusual; when present, other physical causes should be investigated (Sadock et al., 2017).

Alterations in behaviour. Alterations in behaviour include bizarre and agitated behaviours involving such things as stilted, rigid demeanor or eccentric dress, grooming, and rituals. Other behavioural changes seen in schizophrenia include:

- **Catatonia**, a pronounced increase or decrease in the rate and amount of movement. The most common form is stuporous behaviour, in which the person moves little or not at all.
- **Psychomotor retardation**, a pronounced slowing of movement. It is important to differentiate the slowed movements secondary to schizophrenia from those seen in depression; careful assessment of thought content and thought processes is essential for making this determination.
- **Psychomotor agitation**, excited behaviour such as running or pacing rapidly, often in response to internal or external stimuli. Psychomotor agitation can pose a risk to others and to the person, who is at risk for exhaustion, collapse, and even death.
- **Stereotyped behaviours**, repeated motor behaviours that do not presently serve a logical purpose.
- **Automatic obedience**, the performance by a catatonic person of all simple commands in a robot-like fashion.
- **Waxy flexibility**, the extended maintenance of posture usually seen in catatonia. For example, the nurse raises the person's arm, and the person retains this position in a statue-like manner.
- **Negativism**, akin to resistance but may not be intentional. In *active negativism* the person does the opposite of what they are told to do; *passive negativism* is a failure to do what is requested.
- **Impaired impulse control**, a reduced ability to resist one's impulses. Examples include performing socially inappropriate behaviours such as grabbing another's cigarette, throwing food on the floor, and changing TV channels while others are watching.
- **Echopraxia**, the mimicking of the movements of another. It is also seen in catatonia.

Negative symptoms. Negative symptoms develop slowly and are those that most interfere with a person's adjustment and ability to cope. They tend to be persistent and crippling because they render the person inert and *unmotivated*. Negative symptoms impede one's ability to:
- Initiate and maintain conversations and relationships
- Obtain and maintain a job
- Make decisions and follow through on plans
- Maintain adequate hygiene and grooming

Negative symptoms contribute to poor social functioning and social withdrawal. During the *acute phase*, they are difficult to assess because positive symptoms (such as delusions and hallucinations) dominate. Selected negative symptoms are outlined in Table 15.3.

In schizophrenia affect, the external manifestation of feeling or emotion that is manifested in facial expression, tone of voice, and body language, may not always coincide with inner emotions. Affect in schizophrenia can usually be categorized in one of four ways:
- **Flat**—immobile or blank facial expression
- **Blunted**—reduced or minimal emotional response
- **Inappropriate**—emotional response incongruent with the tone or circumstances of the situation (e.g., a patient laughs when told a family member has died)
- **Bizarre**—odd, illogical, emotional state that is grossly inappropriate or unfounded; especially prominent in disorganized schizophrenia and includes grimacing and giggling

Cognitive symptoms. Cognitive symptoms represent the third symptom group and are evident in most people living with schizophrenia. They include difficulty with attention, memory, information processing, cognitive flexibility, and executive functions (e.g., decision making, judgement, planning, problem solving) (Carbon & Correll, 2014). Cognitive symptoms include:

TABLE 15.3 Selected Negative Symptoms of Schizophrenia

Negative Symptom	Description
Affective blunting	A reduction in the expression, range, and intensity of affect (in *flat affect*, no facial expression is present)
Anergia	Lack of energy; passivity or lack of persistence at work or school; may also be a symptom of depression, so needs careful evaluation
Anhedonia	Inability to experience pleasure in activities that usually produce it; result of profound emotional barrenness
Avolition	Reduced motivation; inability to initiate tasks such as social contacts, grooming, and other activities of daily living (ADLs)
Poverty of content of speech	While adequate in amount, speech conveys little information because of vagueness or superficiality
Poverty of speech (alogia)	Reduced amount of speech—responses range from brief to one-word answers

- *Concrete thinking* is an impaired ability to think abstractly, resulting in interpreting or perceiving things in a literal manner. For example, a nurse might ask how the patient found the relaxation class, and the patient answers *"by walking down the hall"* rather than describing their experience of the class. An abstract interpretation of *"The grass is always greener on the other side of the fence"* is that it always seems we would be happier given other circumstances. A concrete interpretation could be *"That side gets more sun, so it's greener there."* Concreteness reduces one's ability to understand and respond to concepts requiring abstract reasoning, such as love or humour.

  Concreteness, especially when combined with an impaired ability to recognize variations in affect or tone of voice, can also make it difficult to recognize social cues such as sarcasm. For example, a patient who had forgotten their wallet asked a store clerk if they could pay later for a bag of chips. When the clerk sarcastically replied, *"Oh sure, we let our customers pay whenever they want,"* the patient took this literally. The patient was distressed when they were arrested for theft despite their protests that they had permission not to pay.

- *Impaired memory* affects short-term memory and the ability to learn. Repetition and verbal or visual cues may help the patient to learn and recall needed information (e.g., a picture of a toothbrush on the patient's wall and/or mirror as a reminder to brush their teeth).

- *Impaired information processing* can lead to problems such as delayed responses, misperceptions, or difficulty understanding others. Patients may lose the ability to screen out insignificant stimuli such as background sounds or objects in one's peripheral vision. This can lead to overstimulation.

- *Impaired executive functioning* includes difficulty with reasoning, setting priorities, comparing options, placing things in logical order or groups, anticipation and planning, and inhibiting undesirable impulses or actions. Impaired executive functioning interferes with problem solving and can contribute to inappropriateness in social situations.

These impairments have a considerable impact on longer-term functioning and can leave the person unable to manage personal health care, hold a job, initiate or maintain a support system, or live alone. Some psychosocial treatments, including cognitive behavioural therapy (CBT), cognitive remediation, social skills training, and computer-assisted training programs, have shown therapeutic benefits and should be offered in conjunction with antipsychotic medications (Carbon & Correll, 2014).

Affective symptoms. Affective symptoms, the fourth symptom group, are common and increase a person's suffering. These involve the experience and expression of emotions. Mood may be unstable, erratic, labile (changing rapidly and easily), or incongruent (not what would be expected for the circumstances).

A serious affective change often seen in schizophrenia is depression. Depression may occur as part of a shared inflammatory reaction affecting the brain or may simply be a reaction to the stress and despair that can come from living with a chronic illness. Assessment for depression is crucial because it may indicate an impending relapse, further impair functioning, and increase risk for substance use disorders. It may also be necessary to assess for a more prolonged and marked affective aspect of the illness, indicating schizoaffective disorder. Most importantly, depression puts people at increased risk for suicide.

This assessment can be done by inquiring into mood and the presence of depressive thoughts or suicidal ideation (see also Chapters 13 and 22).

Self-Assessment

Working with individuals with schizophrenia produces strong emotional reactions in most health care practitioners. The acutely ill person's intensely anxious, lonely, dependent, and distrustful presentation evokes similarly intense, uncomfortable, and frightening emotions in others. The chronicity, repeated exacerbations, and slow response to treatment that many people experience can lead to feelings of helplessness and powerlessness in staff. Some behaviour (especially violent behaviour) can produce strong emotional responses (called *countertransference*) such as fear or anger (see Chapter 9).

Ironically, knowledge that schizophrenia is a disease of the mind may contribute to stigmatizing attitudes and feelings of hopelessness. When public education and nursing practice focus on illness without including personal contact or information about recovery, stigma actually increases or becomes entrenched (Morera et al., 2017). Inpatient nurses, in particular, witness people who are acutely unwell and not able to attend to activities of daily living (ADLs). It is important for them to build recovery into their nursing care while such care remains primarily focused on stabilization and symptom relief (Waldemar et al., 2016). The importance of hope in the nursing care for people living with schizophrenia and their families is well documented, and being hopeful is an essential characteristic of mental health providers in this field (Koehn & Cutliffe, 2007). It is important to set realistic, achievable goals; and to acknowledge and celebrate small steps/gains. Negative symptoms can be particularly slow to resolve. It may also take a long time to gain trust in the therapeutic relationship, so the nurse can expect the orientation phase of the helping relationship to be prolonged.

Clinical mentoring is important for nurses. Without support and the opportunity and willingness to explore feelings with more experienced staff, the nurse is at risk to develop nontherapeutic behaviours and communication, denial, withdrawal, avoidance, and anger, most commonly. These behaviours and communications effect the patient's progress and undermine the nurse's self-esteem. Comments such as *"I don't see any hope"* and *"I feel like all I do is babysit people"* are indications of unrecognized or unresolved counter-transference that, if left uncorrected, create hostility, negative therapeutic relationships, and interfere with both treatment and work satisfaction. The experience of stress and burnout of mental health staff is particularly problematic compared to staff in other clinical areas. It has effects on individual well-being, productivity, and patient care (Johnson et al., 2018). Building personal resilience has been identified as an essential strategy for coping with work-related stress and responding to and overcoming experiences of workplace adversity (Davey et al., 2020).

People living with schizophrenia may experience fear, self-stigma, or shame related to their mental illness, leading them to conceal some aspects of their experience. Negativism and alogia (reduced verbalization) can also limit the person's responses. Many people living with schizophrenia can experience **anosognosia**, an inability to realize that they are ill, which is caused by the illness itself. The resulting lack of insight can make assessment (and treatment) challenging, delaying completion of a full assessment, and requiring additional skills on the part of the nurse. Selected techniques that may help you overcome these challenges can be found in Table 15.4.

The Unpleasant Voices Scale has been designed for assessment of the risk of harm related to command hallucinations and can be used in conjunction with the *Harm Command Safety Protocol* (Gerlock et al., 2010). The items in these assessment tools are found in Figs. 15.2 and 15.3.

TABLE 15.4 Interventions for Overcoming Obstacles to Assessment

Intervention	Rationale	Example
Use empathic comments and observations to prompt the patient to provide information.	Empathy conveys understanding and builds trust and rapport.	**Nurse:** "It must be difficult to be admitted to a psychiatric unit. We are here to help and keep you safe." **Patient:** "Yes … it has been difficult, I am scared of being away from home, and I worry that people are going to harm me"
Minimize questioning, especially closed-ended questioning. Seek data conversationally, using prompts and open-ended questions.	Extended questioning can increase suspiciousness, whereas closed-ended questions elicit minimal information. Both become wearying and off-putting.	"Could you please tell me more about … ?" "Tell me what life has been like for you lately."
Use short, simple sentences and introduce only one idea at a time. Allow time for responses to questions.	Long sentences or rambling questions can confuse a person who has difficulty processing auditory information or is actively hallucinating. Also, a person with alogia requires more time to respond to questions.	**Therapeutic:** "Would you like to join us for a basketball game?" **Nontherapeutic:** "Would you like to join us for a basketball game? Sports can be very good for you, you know, and you seem very lonely, so it would help you a lot. I really hope you will come play a game."
Directly but supportively seek the needed information, explaining the reasons for the assessment.	Being direct but supportive conveys genuineness, builds rapport, and helps reduce anxiety.	"I have noticed that you are not participating in group therapy or socializing with your peers like you have been previously. Has something happened? I am here to support you."
Judiciously use indirect, supportive (therapeutic) confrontation. Seek other data to support (validate) the person's report (obtain further history from third parties, past medical records, and other treatment providers when possible), preferably with the person's permission.	Blunt contradiction or premature confrontation increases resistance. Patients may be unable or unwilling to provide information fully and reliably. Validating their reports ensures the validity of the assessment.	"I realize that admitting to hearing voices might be difficult to do. I notice you talking as if to others when no one is there." "Your brother reports that he works at a factory. Is that your understanding?"
Prioritize the data you seek, and avoid seeking nonessential data.	Patients may have limited tolerance for the assessment interview and answer only a limited number of inquiries. Seeking nonessential information does not benefit the person or assessment.	**Patient:** "Sometimes when I feel anxious, I take extra medication to fall asleep." **Nurse: (less therapeutic)** "Why do you take extra medication?" **Nurse: (more therapeutic)** "Can you tell me more about taking extra medication when you are anxious." (Paraphrasing prompts elaboration and confirmation or refutation of the comment.)

1. Please rate your unpleasant "voices" during the past 24 hours by circling one of the following numbers:

   0   1   2   3   4   5   6   7   8   9   10

   No voices heard   Hardly unpleasant at all   The most unpleasant your voices could be

2. Please rate your unpleasant "voices" over the past week by circling one of the following numbers:

   0   1   2   3   4   5   6   7   8   9   10

   No voices heard   Hardly unpleasant at all   The most unpleasant your voices could be

3. Do you ever hear pleasant voices? Please circle one	Yes	No
4. Are your voices commanding you to harm yourself?	Yes*	No
5. Do you intend to harm yourself?	Yes*	No
6. Are your voices commanding you to harm someone else?	Yes*	No
7. Do you intend to harm someone else?	Yes*	No

* If you answered "yes", please stay after and speak to one of the group leaders. Thank you.

FIG. 15.2 Unpleasant Voices Scale. (**Source:** Gerlock, A. A., Buccheri, R., Buffum, M. D., et al. (2010). Responding to command hallucinations to harm self and others: The Unpleasant Voices Scale and Harm Command Safety Protocol. *Journal of Psychosocial Nursing and Mental Health Services, 48*(5), 26–33. https://doi.org/10.3928/02793695-20100304-03)

ASSESSMENT GUIDELINES
Schizophrenia and Other Psychotic Disorders

1. Assess for risk to self or others.
2. Assess for suicide risk (see Chapter 22).
3. Assess for command hallucinations (e.g., voices telling the patient to harm self or others). If present, ask the person:
   - *Do you recognize the voices?*
4. *Do you believe the voices are real? Do you plan to follow the command?* (A positive response to any of these questions suggests an increased risk that the person will act on the commands). Assess for ability to ensure self-safety, addressing:
   - Adequacy of food and fluid intake
   - Hygiene and self-care
   - Handling of potentially hazardous activities, such as smoking and cooking
   - Ability to transport self safely
   - Impulse control and judgement
   - Appropriate dress for weather conditions. Assess whether the person abuses or is dependent on alcohol or substances. Assess the patient's belief system. Is it fragmented or poorly organized? Is it systematized? Are the beliefs or content delusions? If yes, then ask:
   - *Do you feel that you or your loved ones are being threatened or are in danger?*
   - *Do you feel the need to act against a person or organization to protect or avenge yourself or your loved ones?* (A positive response to either of these questions suggests an increased risk of danger to others.)
5. Assess for the presence and severity of *positive* and *negative* symptoms. Complete a mental status examination, noting which symptoms are present, how they affect functioning, and how the patient is managing them.
6. Assess the patient's insight, knowledge of the illness, relationships and support systems, other coping resources, and strengths.
7. Determine if the patient has had a medical workup. Are there any indications of physical and/or medical problems that might mimic psychosis (e.g., digitalis or anticholinergic [ACh] toxicity, brain trauma, drug intoxication, delirium, fever)?
8. Assess for coexisting disorders:
   - Depression
   - Anxiety
   - Mood disorders
   - Substance use disorders or dependency
   - Medical disorders (especially brain trauma, toxicity, delirium, cardiovascular disease, obesity, and diabetes)
9. Assess medications the patient has been prescribed, whether and how the patient is taking the medications, and what factors (e.g., costs, mistrust of staff, adverse effects) are affecting adherence.
10. Assess the family's knowledge of and response to the patient's illness and its symptoms. Are family members overprotective? Hostile? Anxious? Are they familiar with family support groups and respite resources?

Intent to Harm Self:

When a patient responds yes to question 5 on the Unpleasant Voices Scale ("...intent to harm self"), determine whether there is a need for the patient to be assessed for hospitalization. This will be especially important if the patient also indicates the voices are loud and distressing, and the patient does not feel that he or she has much control over the voices (questions on the Characteristics of Auditory Hallucinations Questionnaire—CAHQ; Buccheri et al., 2004).

After class or group, talk privately with the patient and use this script to determine the need for further assessment:

- "You marked here that the voices are commanding you to harm yourself. It can be very scary to hear voices telling you to harm yourself."
- "What is (are) the voice(s) commanding you to do to yourself?"
- "Do you plan to carry this out?"
- "Do you have the *means* to carry this out?" (Credible?)
- "Has (have) the voice(s) ever commanded you to do this before?"
- "Have you ever harmed yourself as the voice(s) said to do?"
- "How long ago?"

If the patient indicates that he or she has attempted suicide before (because of the voices), has the means and intent, is distressed, and does not feel much control over the voices, then refer the patient for an evaluation for hospitalization.

- "We (I) would like to get some extra help with this today, and would like you to wait with us (me) until the psychiatrist/crisis team (insert whatever is appropriate for your setting) is able to see you?"

Risk Assessment Checklist*

	YES	NO
Has the means to kill/harm self (credible threat)		
Tried to kill/harm self previously		
Outcome today (who notified):		

* If yes to intent to harm self

Continue to monitor for change under these conditions: patient has chronic suicidal command hallucinations, has never acted on them, does not have the means, has no intent, is not distressed, and feels in control.

FIG. 15.3 Harm Command Safety Protocol. (**Source:** Gerlock, A. A., Buccheri, R., Buffum, M. D., et al. (2010). Responding to command hallucinations to harm self and others: The Unpleasant Voices Scale and Harm Command Safety Protocol. *Journal of Psychosocial Nursing and Mental Health Services, 48*(5), 26–33. https://doi.org/10.3928/02793695-20100304-03)

The Inventory of Voice Experiences, a nursing tool developed in Canada, is another assessment tool for perceptual disturbances that offers increased accuracy of assessment of voices (England, 2007).

DIAGNOSIS

People living with schizophrenia have multiple disturbing and disabling symptoms that require a multifaceted approach to care and treatment of both the patient and the family. Table 15.5 lists potential nursing diagnoses for a person with schizophrenia.

OUTCOMES IDENTIFICATION

Desired outcomes vary with the phase of the illness. *Nursing Outcomes Classification (NOC)* (Moorhead et al., 2018) is a useful guide. Ideally, outcomes should focus on enhancing strengths and minimizing the effects of the patient's deficits and symptoms. Outcomes should be consistent with the recovery model (see Chapter 29), which stresses hope, living a full and productive life, and eventual recovery rather than focusing on controlling symptoms and adapting to disability.

Phase I—Acute

During the acute phase, the overall goal is the person's safety and medical stabilization. Therefore if the person is at risk for violence to self or others, initial outcome criteria address safety issues (e.g., *Person refrains from self-harm*). Table 15.6 gives selected short-term and intermediate indicators for the outcome *Distorted thought self-control*.

Phase II—Stabilization

Outcome criteria during phase II focus on helping the patient adhere to treatment, become stabilized on medications, and control or cope with symptoms. The outcomes target the negative symptoms and may include ability to succeed in social, vocational, or self-care activities.

Phase III—Maintenance

Outcome criteria for phase III focus on maintaining achievement, preventing relapse, and achieving independence and a satisfactory quality of life.

PLANNING

The planning of appropriate interventions is guided by the phase of the illness and the strengths and needs of the patient. It is influenced by cultural considerations, available resources, and the patient's preferences.

Phase I—Acute

Hospitalization is indicated if the patient is considered a danger to self or others, refuses to eat or drink, or is too disorganized or otherwise impaired to function safely in the community without supervision. The planning process focuses on the best strategies to ensure the person's safety and provide symptom stabilization. In addition, during the patient's hospitalization, this process includes discharge planning.

In discharge planning the patient and interprofessional treatment team identify aftercare needs for follow-up and support. Discharge

TABLE 15.5 Potential Areas That Will Require Nursing Intervention for People Living With Schizophrenia

Symptom	Potential Areas Requiring Nursing Intervention
Positive Symptoms	
Hears voices that others do not *(auditory hallucinations)*	Auditory perceptions
Hears voices telling them to hurt self or others *(command hallucinations)*	Self-directed violence
	Other-directed violence
Delusions	Thought processes
Shows loose association of ideas *(associative looseness)*	Thought processes
Conversation is derailed by unnecessary and tedious details *(circumstantiality)*	Verbal communication
Negative Symptoms	
Uncommunicative, withdrawn	Social isolation
Expresses feelings of rejection or aloneness (lies in bed all day, positions back to door)	Social interaction
	Loneliness
Talks about self as "bad" or "no good"	Low self-esteem
Feels guilty because of "bad thoughts"; extremely sensitive to real or perceived slights	Self-directed violence
Shows lack of energy *(anergia)*	Ineffective coping
Shows lack of motivation *(avolition)*, unable to initiate tasks (social contact, grooming, and other aspects of daily living)	Self-care (bathing, dressing, feeding, toileting)
	Constipation
Other	
Families and significant others become confused or overwhelmed, lack knowledge about disorder or treatment, feel powerless in coping with the patient	Family coping
	Caregiver role strain
	Health literacy
Stops taking medication (because of anosognosia, adverse medication effects, medication costs, mistrust of staff), stops going to therapy, is not supported in treatment by significant others	Decision-making

TABLE 15.6 NOC Outcomes Related to Distorted Thought Self-Control

Nursing Outcome and Definition	Intermediate Indicators	Short-Term Indicators
Distorted thought self-control: Self-restraint of disruptions in perception, thought processes, and thought content	Maintains affect consistent with mood	Recognizes that hallucinations or delusions are occurring
	Interacts appropriately	Refrains from attending to and responding to hallucinations or delusions
	Perceives environment and the ideas of others accurately	Describes content of hallucinations or delusions
	Exhibits logical thought flow patterns	Reports decrease in hallucinations or delusions
	Exhibits reality-based thinking	Asks for validation of reality
	Exhibits appropriate thought content	

Source: Moorhead, S., Swanson, E., Johnson, M., & Maas, M. L. (Eds.). (2018). *Nursing Outcomes Classification (NOC): Measurement of health outcomes* (6th ed.). St. Louis: Elsevier.

planning considers not only external factors, such as the person's living arrangements, economic resources, social supports, and family relationships, but also internal factors, such as resilience and repertoire of coping skills. Because relapse can be devastating to the person's circumstances (resulting in loss of employment, housing, and relationships) and worsen the long-term prognosis, vigorous efforts are made to connect the person and family with (and not simply refer them to) community resources that provide therapeutic programming and social, financial, and other needed support.

Phase II—Stabilization and Phase III—Maintenance

Planning during the stabilization and maintenance phases includes providing individual and family education and skills training (psychosocial education). Relapse prevention skills are vital. Planning identifies interpersonal, coping, health care, and vocational needs and addresses how and where these needs can best be met within the community.

IMPLEMENTATION

Interventions are geared toward the phase of schizophrenia the person is experiencing. For example, during the acute phase, the clinical focus is on crisis intervention, medication for symptom stabilization, and safety. Interventions are often hospital based; however, people in the acute stage are increasingly being treated in the community.

Phase I—Acute
Settings
A number of factors affect the choice of treatment setting, including:
- Level of care and restrictiveness needed to protect the person from harm to self or others
- Person's need for external structure and support
- Person's ability to cooperate with treatment
- Need for a particular treatment available only in particular settings
- Need for treatment of a coexisting medical condition
- Availability of supportive others who can provide critical information and treatment history to staff and permit stabilization in less restrictive settings

The use of less restrictive and more cost-effective alternatives to hospitalization that work for many people include:
- **Partial hospitalization:** Patients sleep at home and attend treatment sessions (similar to what they would receive if admitted) during the day or evening.
- **Residential crisis centres:** Patients who are unable to remain in the community but do not require full in-person services can be admitted (usually for 1 to 14 days) to receive increased supervision, guidance, and medication stabilization.
- **Group homes:** Patients live in the community with a group of other people, sharing expenses and responsibilities. Staff are present in the house 24 hours a day, 7 days a week to provide supervision and therapeutic activities.
- **Day treatment programs:** Patients reside in the community and attend structured programming during the day.

These programs may include group and individual therapy, supervised activities, and specialized skill training. It is vital that staff be aware of these and other community resources and make this information available to discharged people and their families, ideally by directly connecting them with these resources. Patients and family members should be given telephone numbers and addresses of local support groups such as their provincial *Schizophrenia Society*. Northern and rural communities, however, may not have local support groups. It is critical for staff in these areas to review services that are available for patients and/or advocate for increased services. Other community resources include community mental health centres (usually providing medication services, day treatment, access to 24-hour emergency services, psychotherapy, psychoeducation, and case management); home health services; supported employment programs, offering services from job training to on-site coaches, who help people learn to succeed in the work environment, often via peer-led services (e.g., drop-in centres, sometimes called "clubhouses," that offer social contact, constructive activities, and sometimes employment opportunities); family educational and skills groups (e.g., Schizophrenia Society of Canada's "*Strengthening Families Together*" program); and respite care for caregivers.

Interventions

Acute phase interventions include:
- Psychiatric, medical, and neurological evaluation
- Psychopharmacological treatment
- Support, psychoeducation, and guidance
- Supervision and limit setting in the milieu

Due to a shortage of inpatient beds, there is pressure to keep the length of hospitalization short. This situation may create an ethical dilemma for treatment teams, as short initial hospital stays have been found to be related to high rates of readmission and shorter intervals between hospitalizations. According to the Canadian Institute for Health Information (CIHI, 2021), 1 in 11 patients are readmitted within a month of leaving the hospital. Further, one in eight patients living with mental illnesses have at least three hospital stays per year (CIHI, 2021). Typically, as soon as the acute symptoms are adequately stabilized, the patient is discharged to the community, where appropriate treatment can be continued during the stabilization and maintenance phases. However, in some cases, discharge may be delayed while appropriate housing and supports are sought.

Phase II—Stabilization and Phase III—Maintenance

Effective long-term care of an individual with schizophrenia relies on a three-pronged approach: medication administration and adherence, nursing intervention, and community support. Family psychoeducation, a key role of the nurse, is an essential intervention. All interventions and strategies are geared to the patient's strengths, culture, personal preferences, and needs.

Milieu Management

Effective hospital care provides (1) protection from stressful or disruptive environments and (2) structure. People in the acute phase of schizophrenia show greater improvement in a structured milieu rather than on an open unit that allows for increased stimulation. A therapeutic milieu is consciously designed to maximize safety, opportunities for learning skills, therapeutic activities, and access to resources. The milieu also provides guidance, supportive staff and peer contact, and opportunities for practicing conflict resolution, stress-reduction techniques, and dealing with symptoms.

Activities and Groups

Participation in activities and groups appropriate to the patient's level of functioning may decrease withdrawal, enhance motivation, modify unacceptable behaviours, develop friendships, and increase social competence. Activities such as drawing, reading poetry, and listening to music may be used to focus conversation and promote the recognition and expression of feelings. Self-esteem is enhanced as patients experience successful task completion. Recreational activities such as picnics and outings to stores and restaurants are not simply diversions; they teach constructive leisure skills, increase social comfort, facilitate growth in social concern and interactional skills, and enhance the ability to develop boundaries and set limits on self and others. After discharge, group therapy can provide necessary structure within the patient's community milieu.

Safety

A small percentage of people living with schizophrenia, especially during the acute phase, may exhibit a risk for physical violence. Several interrelated risk factors, including demographics (i.e., age, marital status, gender) and social factors (i.e., homelessness, limited education, history of maltreatment or criminality), presence of persecutory delusions or command hallucinations, comorbid antisocial personality pathology, concurrent substance use, inadequate insight, treatment nonadherence, and physiological factors, increase the risk for violence in patients with psychosis. Nonadherence to treatment is a key risk factor predicting violence in patients with psychosis (Lamsma & Harte, 2015).

 SAFETY TIP
When the potential for violence exists, measures to protect the patient, staff, and others become the priority.

Interventions include assessing for risk, increasing staff supervision, reducing stimulation (e.g., noise, crowds), addressing paranoia and other contributing symptoms, providing constructive diversion and outlets for physical energy, teaching and practicing coping skills, implementing cognitive behavioural approaches (to correct unrealistic expectations or selectively extinguish aggression), de-escalating tension verbally, and, when necessary, using seclusion and chemical (i.e., medication) or physical restraints. *The Harm Command Safety Protocol* provides guidelines for how to respond when a person indicates intent to harm someone else (Gerlock et al., 2010). Refer to Chapter 24 for more detailed discussions of caring for the aggressive person, seclusion, and restraints.

Counselling and Communication Techniques

Therapeutic communication techniques for patients with schizophrenia aim to lower the person's anxiety, build trust, encourage clear communication, decrease defensiveness, encourage interaction, enhance self-esteem, and reinforce skills such as reality testing and assertiveness. It is important to remember that people living with schizophrenia may have memory impairment and require repetition. They may also have limited tolerance for interaction, owing to the stimulation it creates. Therefore shorter (<30 minutes) but more frequent interactions may be more therapeutic. Interventions for paranoia and other selected presentations are discussed later in this chapter.

Hallucinations

When a patient is experiencing a hallucination, the nursing focus is on understanding the person's experiences and responses. Suicidal or homicidal themes or commands necessitate appropriate safety measures. For example, "voices" that tell a patient a particular individual plans to harm them may lead to aggressive actions against that person; one-to-one supervision of the patient or transfer of the potential victim to another unit is often essential.

> **GUIDELINES FOR COMMUNICATION**
> *Helping Patients Who Are Experiencing Hallucinations*
>
> **Nursing Care**
> 1. Observe the patient for hallucinating cues such as eyes tracking an unheard speaker, garbled words under breath or talking to self, appearing distracted, suddenly stopping conversing as if interrupted, or intently watching a vacant area of the room.
> 2. Ask the patient about the content of the hallucinations and how they are reacting to it. Assess for command hallucinations and whether the hallucinations are causing fear, distress, or upset for the patient.
> 3. Avoid referring to hallucinations as if they are real. Do not ask, "*What are the voices saying to you?*" Rather, ask, "*What are you hearing?*"
> 4. Be aware of and continue to assess for signs of anxiety, which may indicate that hallucinations are intensifying or that they are of a command type.
> 5. Do not negate the patient's experience but offer your own perceptions and convey empathy. "*I don't hear the angry voices that you are hearing right now, they must be very frightening for you.*"
> 6. Focus on reality-based "here-and-now" activities such as conversations or simple projects. "*The voice you are hearing in your mind sounds very real, it is part of your illness, and it cannot harm you. You are safe. Focus on my voice and what you can see around you.*"
> 7. Address any underlying emotion, need, or theme that seems to be indicated by the hallucination, such as fear with menacing voices or guilt with accusing voices.
> 8. Promote and guide reality testing. If the patient has frightening hallucinations, guide them to scan the area to see if others are frightened; if they are not frightened, encourage the patient to consider that these might be hallucinations.
> 9. As the patient begins to develop insight, guide them to interpret the hallucinations as a symptom of the illness.

Sources: Buccheri, R., Trygstad, L., Buffum, M., et al. (2013). Self-management of unpleasant auditory hallucinations: A tested practice model. *Journal of Psychosocial Nursing and Mental Health Services, 51*(11), 26–34. https://doi.org/10.3928/02793695-20130731-02; Herzog, E. (2014). *Caring for the hallucinating patient: Non-pharmacological interventions*. Presentation at the 28th annual conference of the American Psychiatric Nurses Association, Indianapolis, IN.

Hallucinations are real to the patient who is experiencing them and may be distracting during nurse–patient interactions. Call the person by name, speak simply but in a louder voice than usual, approach the person in a non-threatening and non-judgemental manner, maintain eye contact, and redirect the person's focus to the conversation as needed (Farhall et al., 2007). Guidelines for Communication: Helping Patients Who Are Experiencing Hallucinations lists other techniques for communicating with patients experiencing hallucinations.

Delusions

Delusions may be the patient's attempts to understand confusion and distorted experiences. They reflect the misperception of one's circumstances, which go uncorrected in schizophrenia due to impaired reality testing. When, as a nurse, you attempt to see the world through the eyes of the patient, it is easier to understand their experience. For example:

Patient: *"You people are all alike ... all in on the RCMP plot to destroy me."*

Nurse: *"Quinn, I am a nurse, I am not going to harm you, you are safe with me. Thinking that people are plotting to destroy you must be very frightening."*

In this example the nurse acknowledges the patient's experience, conveys empathy about the patient's fearfulness, and avoids focusing on the content of the delusion, but identifies the patient's feelings so they can be explored, as tolerated. Note that talking about the feelings is helpful, but extended focus on delusional material is not.

It is *never* useful to debate or attempt to dissuade the patient regarding the delusion. Doing so can intensify the patient's retention of irrational beliefs and cause them to view you as rejecting or oppositional. However, it *is* helpful to clarify misinterpretations of the environment and gently suggest, as tolerated, a more reality-based perspective. For example:

Patient: *"I see the doctor is here; he is out to destroy me."*

Nurse: *"It is true the doctor is here. He does patient rounds every morning at 9:00 a.m. He will talk to you about how you are feeling and your treatment. Would you feel more comfortable talking to him in the day room?"*

Focusing on specific reality-based activities and events in the environment helps to minimize the focus on delusional thoughts. The more time the patient spends engaged in activities or with people, the more opportunities there are to receive feedback about and become comfortable with reality.

Work with the patient to find out which coping strategies succeed and how the patient can make the best use of them. Guidelines for Communication: People Experiencing Delusions lists techniques for communicating with people experiencing delusions, and Patient and Family Teaching: Coping With Auditory Hallucinations or Delusions presents patient and family teaching topics for coping with hallucinations and delusions.

Associative Looseness

Associative looseness often mirrors the person's abnormal thoughts and reflects poorly organized thinking. An increase in associative looseness often indicates that the person is feeling increased anxiety or is overwhelmed by internal and external stimuli. The person's speech may also produce confusion and frustration in the nurse. The following guidelines are useful for intervention with a patient whose speech is confused and disorganized:

- Do *not* pretend you understand the patient's words or meaning when you do not; tell the person you are having difficulty understanding.

GUIDELINES FOR COMMUNICATION
People Experiencing Delusions

- To build trust, be open, honest, and reliable.
- Respond to suspicions in a matter of fact, empathic, supportive, and calm manner.
- Ask the person to describe the delusions. Example: *"Tell me more about someone trying to hurt you."*
- Avoid debating the delusional content but interject doubt where appropriate.
- Focus on the feelings that underlie or flow from the delusions. Example: *"You seem to wish you could be more powerful"* or *"It must feel frightening to think others want to hurt you."*
- Once it is understood and addressed, do not dwell further on the delusion. Instead, focus on more reality-based topics. If the person obsesses about delusions, set firm limits on the amount of time you will talk about them, and explain your reason for these limits.
- Observe for events that trigger delusions. If possible, help the person find ways to reduce or manage them.
- Validate a part of the delusion that is real. Example: *"Yes, there was someone at the nurses' station, they were not speaking about you."*

Source: Data from Farhall, J., Greenwood, K. M., & Jackson, H. J. (2007). Coping with hallucinated voices in schizophrenia: A review of self-initiated strategies and therapeutic interventions. *Clinical Psychology Review, 27*, 476–493. https://doi.org/10.1016/j.cpr.2006.12.002

PATIENT AND FAMILY TEACHING
Coping With Auditory Hallucinations or Delusions

Prevention and Stress Management
- Avoid loud or stressful places or activities.
- Avoid negative or critical people and seek out supportive people.
- Learn assertive communication skills so you can tell others *"no"* if they pressure or upset you.
- When faced with increased stress, slow and deepen your breathing. Count slowly from one to four as you inhale, hold the breath, and exhale.
- Gently tense and then relax your muscles, one area of the body at a time, starting at your head (e.g., closing your eyes and then opening them, clenching your teeth and then relaxing your jaw) and working your way down to your hands and feet.
- Discover other ways that help you manage stress (e.g., going for a walk, meditation, taking a hot bath, reading or listening to music, imagining yourself in a less stressful situation [sometimes called a *mental vacation*]).

Distraction
- Listening to music
- Reading (aloud may help more)
- Counting backwards from 100
- Watching television

Interaction
- Talking with another person
- Group therapy
- Cognitive behavioural therapy or dialectical behavioural therapy

Activity
- Walking
- Cleaning the house
- Having a relaxing bath

- Playing the guitar or singing
- Going to the gym (or any place you enjoy being, where others will be present)

Talking to Yourself
- Telling the voices or thoughts to go away
- Telling yourself that the voices and thoughts are symptoms and not real
- Telling yourself that no matter what you hear, voices can be safely ignored

Social Action
- Talking to a trusted friend or member of the family
- Calling a help line/crisis line/ support line or going to a drop-in centre
- Visiting a favourite place or a comfortable public place

Physical Action
- Taking as-needed medication as prescribed, or following up with physician to review medication
- Meditation
- Mindfulness

Sources: Buccheri, R., Trygstad, L., Buffum, M., et al. (2013). Self-management of unpleasant auditory hallucinations: A tested practice model. *Journal of Psychosocial Nursing and Mental Health Services, 51*(11), 26–34. https://doi.org/10.3928/02793695-20130731-02; Farhall, J., Greenwood, K. M., & Jackson, H. J. (2007). Coping with hallucinated voices in schizophrenia: A review of self-initiated strategies and therapeutic interventions. *Clinical Psychology Review, 27*, 476–493. https://doi.org/10.1016/j.cpr.2006.12.002

- Place the difficulty in understanding on yourself, *not* on the patient. Example: "I'm having trouble following what you are saying," *not* "You're not making any sense."
- Look for recurring topics and themes in the patient's communications, and tie these to events and timelines. Example: *"You've mentioned trouble with your family several times, usually after visits. Can you tell me about your family and your visits with them?"*
- Summarize or paraphrase the patient's communications to role-model more effective ways of making their point and to give the person a chance to correct anything you may have misunderstood.
- Reduce stimuli in the vicinity, and speak concisely, clearly, and concretely.
- Tell the person what you *do* understand, and reinforce clear communication and accurate expression of needs, feelings, and thoughts.

Health Teaching and Health Promotion

Education is an essential strategy and includes teaching the patient and family about illness, including possible causes, treatment plans, medications and medication adverse effects, coping strategies, what to expect, and prevention of relapse. Understanding these things helps the patient and family to recognize the impact of stress, enhances their understanding of the importance of treatment to a good outcome, encourages involvement in (and support of) therapeutic activities, and identifies resources for consultation and ongoing support throughout the illness.

Including family members in any strategies aimed at reducing symptoms of psychosis reduces family anxiety and distress and enables the family to reinforce the healthcare providers' efforts. The family plays an important role in the stability of the patient. The patient who returns to a warm, concerned, and supportive environment is less likely to experience relapse. An environment in which people are critical or their involvement in the patient's life is intrusive is associated with relapse and poorer outcomes.

Lack of understanding of the disease and its symptoms can lead others to misinterpret the patient's apathy and lack of drive as *"laziness,"* fostering a potential hostile response by family members, caregivers, or community. Thus, public education/health teaching about the symptoms of schizophrenia can reduce tensions in families, as well as in communities. The most effective education occurs over time and is available when the family is most receptive (Brady et al., 2017). Patient and Family Teaching: Schizophrenia offers guidelines for patient and family teaching about schizophrenia.

PATIENT AND FAMILY TEACHING
Schizophrenia

1. Learn all you can about the illness.
   - Attend psychoeducational and support groups.
   - Join the National Network for Mental Health (https://nnmh.ca/).
   - Contact your provincial/regional Schizophrenia Society.
2. Develop a relapse prevention plan.
   - Know the early warning signs of relapse (e.g., isolation, difficulty sleeping, troubling/intrusive thoughts).
   - Know who to call, what to do, and where to go when early signs of relapse appear. Make a list and keep it with you.
   - Understand that relapse is part of illness, not a sign of failure.
3. Take advantage of all psychoeducational tools.
   - Participate in family, group, and individual therapy.
   - Learn new ways to act and coping skills to help handle family, work, and social stress. Get information from your nurse, case manager, physician, self-help group, community mental health group, or hospital.
   - Have a documented plan, of what to do to cope during stressful times.
   - Recognize that everyone needs a place to address their fears and losses and to learn new ways of coping.
4. Adhere to treatment.
   - People who adhere to treatment that works for them do the best in coping with the disorder.
   - Engaging in struggles over adherence does not help but tying adherence to the patient's own goals does. (*"Staying in treatment will help you keep your job and avoid trouble with the police."*)
   - Share any medication side effects or concerns (e.g., sexual problems, weight gain, "feeling funny") with your nurse, case manager, physician, or social worker; most side effects can be helped.
   - Discontinuing medication treatment suddenly can be dangerous and symptoms can re-emerge.
5. Avoid alcohol and illicit substances; they can act on the brain and cause a relapse.
6. Keep in touch with supportive people—those with shared patient and family experiences and others.
7. Maintain healthy lifestyle and balance.
   - Taking care of one's diet, health, and hygiene helps prevent medical illnesses.
   - Maintain a regular sleep pattern.
   - Keep active (hobbies, friends, groups, sports, job, special interests).
   - Nurture yourself, and practice stress-reduction activities daily.
   - Mindfulness

Further information on facilitating family support is available through Schizophrenia Society of Canada's third edition of *Strengthening Families Together: Helping Canadians Live With Mental Illness*, http://www.schizophrenia.ca/docs/SFT3_facilitator.pdf, or via the Your Recovery Journey website (Schizophrenia Society of Canada), https://www.your-recovery-journey.ca/

> ### 🌿 INTEGRATIVE THERAPY
>
> #### Mindfulness as an Adjunctive Treatment for Schizophrenia
>
> Mindfulness interventions are gaining popularity as a complementary and integrative practice for people with a number of emotional and psychological concerns. Research illustrating how to adapt mindfulness groups for people with current psychosis has shown mindfulness for psychosis is both safe and therapeutic (Chadwick, 2019). These therapies employ elements of acceptance and compassion in addition to mindfulness.
>
> Research finds key benefits of mindfulness therapies included improved insight, medium to larger improvement in mood, trends toward improvement in quality of life, and significant improvements in positive and negative symptoms of schizophrenia. No significant improvement in anxiety was found as a result of the mindfulness therapies. Certain therapies were examined to meet particular needs most effectively; for example, group mindfulness therapy for psychosis was found to improve clinical functioning and enhance mindful response to stressful thoughts. There is also reasonable evidence from one large trial that Internet-based, self-help mindfulness therapy effects moderate reductions in depressive symptoms and symptoms of obsessive-compulsive disorder in outpatients with psychosis.
>
> The review concluded that mindfulness therapies can be safely used with people with psychosis and that they provide a number of therapeutic benefits compared with routine care and, in some cases, other interventions.

Source: Aust, J., & Bradshaw, T. (2017). Mindfulness interventions for psychosis: A systematic review of the literature. *Journal of Psychiatric and Mental Health Nursing, 24*(1), 69–83. https://doi.org/10.1111/jpm.12357

Pharmacological Interventions

The psychotropic medications used to treat psychotic disorders are primarily *antipsychotic medications*. They first became available in the 1950s. Before that time, the available medications provided only sedation, not treatment of the disorder itself. Until the 1960s, people who had even one episode of schizophrenia usually spent months or years in provincial mental health hospitals. Episodes of psychosis resulted in great emotional burdens to families and people living with schizophrenia. The advent of antipsychotic medications at last provided symptom control and allowed people to live in the community.

Two groups of antipsychotic medications exist: conventional antipsychotic medications (traditional dopamine antagonists [dopamine D_2 receptor antagonists]), also known as *typical* or *first-generation antipsychotic medications*, and atypical antipsychotic medications (serotonin–dopamine antagonists [5-HT_{2A} receptor antagonists]), also known as *second-generation antipsychotic medications*. A "third generation" of medications (aripiprazole and brexpiprazole [Rexulti]) give hope for enhanced effectiveness and adverse-effect reduction (Howland, 2015). Other medications, such as *anticonvulsants* and *antiparkinsoninal* medications, are also used to augment antipsychotic medications.

Antipsychotic medications are effective for *most* exacerbations of schizophrenia and for reduction or mitigation of relapse. Conventional antipsychotic medications primarily affect the positive symptoms of schizophrenia (e.g., hallucinations, delusions, disordered thinking). Atypical antipsychotic medications can improve negative symptoms (e.g., asociality, blunted affect, lack of motivation) as well. The choice of antipsychotic medication should be made by both the patient and physician together, after the review of benefits and adverse effects (Remington et al., 2017).

Evidence suggests medications should be trialed between 4 and 6 weeks for efficacy (Remington et al., 2017). Only about 10% of people living with schizophrenia fail to respond to antipsychotic medications.

It is not unusual for patients to be prescribed a combination of antipsychotic medications, sometimes both oral and depot (long-acting injectable [LAI]) or both typical and atypical. These individuals may also be taking antiparkinson medications and other medications to combat adverse effects. It is important in these cases to have the medication regimen carefully and regularly reviewed by both the physician and a pharmacist and to monitor closely for adverse effects. These patients would be at high risk for ACh toxicity, a potentially life-threatening situation (see Table 15.8).

Antipsychotic medications are not addictive. However, they should be discontinued gradually to minimize a discontinuation syndrome that can include dizziness, nausea, tremors, insomnia, electric shock–like pains, and anxiety. Patients taking antipsychotic medications are at increased risk of falls due to orthostatic (postural) hypotension, sedation, and gait impairment (Wynaden et al., 2015).

Additional Medication Administration Issues

Liquid or fast-dissolving forms, available for selected antipsychotic medications, can make it difficult for a patient to "*cheek*" or "*palm*" medication (*hiding it in their cheek or placing in palm and later dispose of it*).

Some antipsychotic medications are also available in short-acting injectable form, used primarily for treatment of agitation, behavioural emergencies (imminent harm to self or others), or when patients refuse court-mandated oral antipsychotic medications. Adverse effects can be intensified and less easily managed when medication is administered directly into the system intramuscularly (IM).

In addition, some medications are available in LAI formulations that need to be administered only every 2 to 4 weeks (*some examples: aripiprazole [Abilify Maintena], paliperidone [Invega Sustenna], risperidone [Risperdal Consta]*) or, in one case, every 3 months (*paliperidone [Invega Trinza]*). These may be referred to as "depot" medications. Some require special administration protocols. By requiring less frequent medication administration, adherence is improved and conflict about taking medications is reduced. The downside is a lack of dosing flexibility, and patients may feel as if they have less control.

Atypical Antipsychotic Medication

Atypical antipsychotic medication first emerged in the early 1990s with clozapine (Clozaril). When patients whose illness was previously treatment resistant were started on clozapine, they showed response rates between 30 and 60% (Remington et al., 2017). Unfortunately, clozapine produces agranulocytosis in 0.8% to 1% of those who take it and also increases the risk for seizures. Due to the risk for agranulocytosis, people taking clozapine must have weekly white blood cell counts for the first 6 months, then frequent monitoring thereafter, to obtain the medication. As a result of nonadherence, clozapine use is declining.

Atypical medications are often discussed with patients as a potential first choice because they treat both the positive and the negative symptoms of schizophrenia. Furthermore, they produce minimal to no extrapyramidal side effects (EPSs) or tardive dyskinesia (TD) in most people, although these effects may still occur for some patients. Adverse effects tend to be significantly less, resulting in greater adherence to treatment.

Atypical antipsychotic medications include risperidone (Risperdal), lurasidone (Latuda), olanzapine (Zyprexa), paliperidone (Invega), quetiapine (Seroquel), ziprasidone (Zeldox).

A subset of the atypical antipsychotic medications are those medications referred to as third generation antipsychotic medications. These medications include aripiprazole (Abilify) and brexpiprazole (Rexulti). They can be described as dopamine system stabilizers that act by reducing dopamine activity in some brain regions while increasing it in others. Aripiprazole and brexpiprazole act as D_2 partial agonists (meaning that they attach to the D_2 receptor without fully activating it, reducing the effective level of dopamine activity).

One significant disadvantage of the atypical medication, with the exception of ziprasidone and aripiprazole, is metabolic syndrome, which includes weight gain, dyslipidemia, and altered glucose metabolism, a significant concern due to increased risk for diabetes, hypertension, and atherosclerotic heart disease (McDaid & Smyth, 2015). An additional disadvantage of atypical antipsychotic medications is cost: they are more expensive than conventional antipsychotic medication. Table 15.7 lists the classifications, routes, and adverse-effect profiles of the antipsychotic medications.

Conventional Antipsychotic Medication

Conventional antipsychotic medication are antagonists at the dopamine D_2 receptor site in both the limbic and the motor centres. This blockage of dopamine D_2 receptor sites in the motor areas causes **extrapyramidal side effects**, which include akathisia, acute dystonias, pseudo-parkinsonism, and TD. The symptoms of EPS are debilitating, can interfere with social functioning and communication, motor tasks, and ADLs (D'Souza & Hooten, 2020). EPS is often associated with poor quality of life and adherence to medication, which may result in disease relapse and rehospitalization (D'Souza & Hooten, 2020). Other adverse reactions include ACh effects, orthostasis, photosensitivity, and lowered seizure threshold.

Conventional antipsychotic medications are becoming less common in the treatment of schizophrenia because of their minimal impact on negative symptoms and their adverse effects. However, conventional antipsychotic medications are effective in treating positive symptoms, are much less expensive than atypical medications, and come in a depot (long-acting) injectable form. (*Note:* Risperidone, an atypical antipsychotic medication, is also available in a depot form [Risperdal Consta].) For people who respond to them and can tolerate their adverse effects, conventional antipsychotic medications can remain an appropriate choice (CAMH, 2021), especially when metabolic syndrome or cost is a concern.

The conventional antipsychotic medications are often divided into low-potency and high-potency medications on the basis of their ACh adverse effects, EPSs, and sedative profiles:

TABLE 15.7 Antipsychotic Medications: Classification, Route, and Adverse-Effect Profile

Generic (Brand)	Route	EPSs	Sedation	Orthostatic Hypotension	Anticholinergic	Weight Gain	Diabetes
Atypical Antipsychotic Medication—Treat Positive and Negative Symptoms							
Aripiprazole (Abilify)	PO	Very low	Low	Low	None	Low	Low
Clozapine (Clozaril)	PO	Very low	High	Moderate	High	High	High
Olanzapine (Zyprexa)	PO, IM	Very low	High	Moderate	High	High	High
Paliperidone (Invega)	PO	Moderate	Low	Low	None	Moderate	a
Quetiapine (Seroquel)	PO	Very low	Moderate	Moderate	None	Moderate	Moderate
Risperidone (Risperdal)	PO, IM	Very low	Low	Low	None	Moderate	Moderate
Ziprasidone (Zeldox)	PO, IM	Moderate	Moderate	Moderate	None	Low	Low
Conventional Antipsychotic Medication—Treat Positive Symptoms							
Low Potency							
Chlorpromazine (generic only)	PO, IM, IV, R	Moderate	High	High	Moderate	Moderate	—
Medium Potency							
Loxapine (Loxapac)	PO	Moderate	Moderate	Low	Low	Low	—
Perphenazine (generic only)	PO	Moderate	Moderate	Low	Low	—	—
High Potency							
Thiothixene (generic only)	PO	High	Low	Moderate	Low	Moderate	—
Fluphenazine (generic only)	PO, IM	High	Low	Low	Low	—	—
Haloperidol (Haldol)	PO, IM	High	Low	Low	Low	Moderate	—
Pimozide (Orap)	PO	High	Moderate	Low	Moderate	—	—
Conventional Antipsychotic Medication for Which Limited Data Are Available							
Flupentixol (Fluanxol, Fluanxol Depot)	PO, IM	High	Low	Moderate	Low	—	—
Zuclopenthixol (Clopixol, Clopixol Depot, Clopixol Acuphase)	PO, IM	—	—	—	May potentiate ACh adverse effects of other medications	—	—

ACh, Anticholinergic; *EPSs*, extrapyramidal side effects; *IM*, intramuscular; *IV*, intravenous; *PO*, oral; *R*, rectal.
aData unavailable.
Sources: Centre for Addiction and Mental Health. (2020). *Understanding psychiatric medications: Antipsychotic medication.* https://www.camh.ca/en/education/about/camh_publications/Documents/Flat_PDFs/upm_antipsychotic medication.pdf; Burchum, J., & Rosenthal, L. (2016). *Lehne's pharmacology for nursing care* (9th ed.). St. Louis: Elsevier; Freudenreich, O. (2020). Antipscyhotics: Clinical effectiveness. In O. Freudenreich (Ed.), *Psychotic disorders: A practical guide* (2nd ed., pp. 215–230). Cham: Springer.

Low potency = high sedation + high ACh + low EPSs
High potency = low sedation + low ACh + high EPSs

Conventional antipsychotic medication must be used cautiously in people with seizure disorders, as they can lower the seizure threshold. Three of the more common EPSs are **acute dystonia** (acute sustained contraction of muscles, usually of the head and neck), **akathisia** (psychomotor restlessness evident as pacing or fidgeting, sometimes pronounced and very distressing to patients), and **pseudo-parkinsonism** (a medication-induced, temporary constellation of symptoms associated with Parkinson's disease: tremor, reduced accessory movements, impaired gait, and stiffening of muscles).

EPSs can usually be minimized by lowering dosages of antipsychotic medications or adding antiparkinson medication, especially centrally acting ACh medications such as trihexyphenidyl and benztropine mesylate. Diphenhydramine hydrochloride (Benadryl) is also useful. Lorazepam, a benzodiazepine, may be helpful in reducing akathisia.

Unfortunately, antiparkinson medications can cause significant ACh adverse effects and worsen the ACh adverse effects of conventional antipsychotic medication and other ACh medications. These adverse effects include ACh syndrome, which is seen in the peripheral nervous system (tachycardia, hyperthermia, hypertension, dry skin, urinary retention, functional ileus) and central nervous system (mydriasis, hallucinations, delirium, seizures, and, in some cases, coma) (Wilson et al., 2017). Other troubling adverse effects of conventional antipsychotic medications include sexual dysfunction, endocrine disturbances (e.g., galactorrhea), drooling, and tardive dyskinesia, discussed next. Impotence and sexual dysfunction are occasionally reported (but frequently experienced) by men and may also necessitate a medication change.

Table 15.8 identifies common adverse effects of the conventional antipsychotic medications, their usual times of onset, and related nursing and medical interventions.

Tardive dyskinesia (TD) is a persistent EPS that usually appears after prolonged treatment and persists even after the medication has been discontinued. TD is evidenced by involuntary tonic muscular contractions that typically involve the tongue, fingers, toes, neck, trunk, or pelvis. This potentially serious EPS is most frequently seen in women and older persons and affects up to 50% of individuals receiving long-term, high-dose therapy. TD varies from mild to moderate and can be disfiguring or incapacitating; a common presentation is a "guppy like" mouth movement sometimes accompanied by tongue protrusion. Its appearance can contribute to the stigmatization of people with mental illness and antipsychotic medications.

Early symptoms of TD are fasciculations of the tongue (described as looking like a bag of worms) or constant smacking of the lips. These symptoms can progress into uncontrollable biting, chewing, or sucking motions; an open mouth; and lateral movements of the jaw. No reliable treatment exists for TD. The National Institute of Mental Health developed the *Abnormal Involuntary Movement Scale (AIMS)*, a 12-item clinician-rated scale to assess severity of dyskinesias (specifically, orofacial movements and extremity and truncal movements) in patients taking neuroleptic medications. Additional items assess the overall severity, incapacitation, and the patient's level of awareness of the movements, and distress associated with them (Guy, 1976) (Figure 15.4). It examines facial, oral, extremity, and trunk movement.

Potentially Dangerous Responses to Antipsychotic Medication

Nurses need to know about some rare, but serious and potentially fatal, effects of antipsychotic medications, including neuroleptic malignant syndrome, agranulocytosis, liver impairment, and ACh-induced delirium.

Neuroleptic malignant syndrome (NMS) occurs in about 0.2% to 1% of people who have taken conventional antipsychotic medications, although it can occur with atypical medication as well. Acute reduction in brain dopamine activity plays a role in its development. NMS is a life-threatening medical emergency and is fatal in about 10% of cases. It can occur any time during treatment.

NMS is characterized by reduced consciousness, increased muscle tone (muscular rigidity), and autonomic dysfunction, including hyperpyrexia, labile hypertension, tachycardia, tachypnea, diaphoresis, and drooling. Treatment consists of early detection, discontinuation of the antipsychotic, management of fluid balance, temperature reduction, and monitoring for complications. Mild cases of NMS may be treated with benzodiazepines, vitamins E and B_6, or bromocriptine.

Agranulocytosis is a serious, potentially fatal, adverse effect. Liver impairment may also occur (see Table 15.8).

> ⚡ **SAFETY TIP**
> Nurses need to be aware of the prodromal signs and symptoms of these adverse effects and teach them to patients and their families.

Anticholinergic-induced delirium is a potentially life-threatening adverse effect usually seen in older persons, although it can occur in younger people as well. It is also seen in patients taking multiple antipsychotic medications. See Table 15.8 for symptoms and treatment of this serious adverse effect.

Adjuncts to Antipsychotic Medication Therapy

Antidepressants are recommended along with antipsychotic medication for the treatment of depression, which is common in schizophrenia. Refer to Chapter 13 for a more detailed discussion of depression and antidepressant medications.

Antimanic (mood-stabilizing) medications have been helpful in enhancing the effectiveness of antipsychotic medication. Divalproex sodium/valproic acid (Epival, Depakene) are used during acute exacerbations of psychosis to hasten response to antipsychotic medication (Freudenreich, 2020b). Lamotrigine may be given along with clozapine to improve therapeutic effects.

Augmentation with benzodiazepines (e.g., clonazepam) can reduce anxiety and agitation and contribute to improvement in positive and negative symptoms (Wilson et al., 2017).

When to Change an Antipsychotic Regimen

The following circumstances suggest a need to adjust or change the antipsychotic medication or add supplemental medications (e.g., lithium, carbamazepine, valproate):

- Inadequate improvement in target symptoms despite an adequate trial of the medication
- Persistence of dangerous or intolerable adverse effects

Specific Interventions for Paranoia, Catatonia, and Disorganization

The following sections discuss paranoia, catatonia, and disorganization in psychoses and identify pertinent communication guidelines, self-care needs, and milieu needs.

Paranoia

Any intense and strongly defended irrational suspicion can be regarded as **paranoia**. Paranoia is evident, at least intermittently, in many people without psychotic disorders but is verified as irrational and discarded by the reality-testing process. This process fails in people experiencing

TABLE 15.8 Adverse Effects of Conventional Antipsychotic Medication and Related Nursing Interventions

Adverse Effect	Nursing Interventions
Dry mouth	Provide frequent sips of water, ice chips, and sugarless candy or gum; if severe, provide moisture spray (Important note: monitor patient's fluid intake for potential water intoxication).
Urinary retention and hesitancy	Check voiding Try warm towel on abdomen, and consider catheterization if no result. Review medication to ensure not a potential side effect.
Constipation	Usually short term May use stool softener Ensure adequate fluid intake Increase fibre intake Use dietary laxatives (e.g., prune juice)
Blurred vision	Usually abates in 1–2 weeks May require use of reading or magnifying glasses If intolerable, consider consult regarding change in medication
Photosensitivity	Encourage person to wear sunglasses, sunscreen, and sun-blocking clothing Limit exposure to sunlight
Dry eyes	Use artificial tears
Inhibition of ejaculation or impotence in men	Consult prescriber: person may need alternative medication
Anticholinergic-induced delirium: dry mucous membranes; reduced or absent peristalsis; mydriasis; nonreactive pupils; hot, dry, red skin; hyperpyrexia without diaphoresis; tachycardia; agitation; unstable vital signs; worsening of symptoms of psychosis; delirium; urinary retention; seizure; repetitive motor movements	***Potentially life-threatening medical emergency*** Consult physician immediately Hold all medications Implement emergency cooling measures as ordered (cooling blanket, alcohol, or ice bath) Implement urinary catheterization as needed Administer benzodiazepines or other sedation as ordered Physostigmine may be ordered as a special access toxicology antidote
Pseudo-parkinsonism: mask-like facies, stiff and stooped posture, shuffling gait, drooling, tremor, "pill-rolling" phenomenon *Onset:* 5 hours–30 days	Consult physician, administer as needed antiparkinson medication (e.g., trihexyphenidyl or benztropine) Consult physician regarding medication change Provide towel or handkerchief to wipe excess saliva
Acute dystonic reactions: acute contractions of tongue, face, neck, and back (usually tongue and jaw first) Opisthotonos: tetanic heightening of entire body, head and belly up Oculogyric crisis: eyes locked upward Laryngeal dystonia: could threaten airway (rare) Cogwheel rigidity: stiffness and clicking in elbow joints felt by the examiner during passive range of motion (early indicator of acute dystonia) *Onset:* 1–5 days	Consult physician immediately Administer anti-parkinson medication as above—give IM for more rapid effect and because of swallowing difficulty Also consider diphenhydramine hydrochloride (Benadryl) 25–50 mg IM or IV Relief usually occurs in 5–15 minutes Prevent further dystonias with antiparkinson medication (see Table 15.8) Experience can be frightening, and person may fear choking Accompany to quiet area to provide comfort and support Assist person to understand the event and avert distortion or mistrust of medications Monitor airway
Akathisia: motor inner-driven restlessness (e.g., tapping foot incessantly, rocking forward and backward in chair, shifting weight from side to side) *Onset:* 2 hours–60 days	Consult physician regarding possible medication change Give antiparkinson medication Tolerance to akathisia does not develop, but akathisia disappears when neuroleptic is discontinued Propranolol (Inderal), lorazepam (Ativan), or diazepam (Valium) may be used (Important note: In severe cases may cause great distress and contribute to potential suicidality, physician must be aware)

Continued

TABLE 15.8 Adverse Effects of Conventional Antipsychotic Medication and Related Nursing Interventions—cont'd

Adverse Effect	Nursing Interventions
Tardive dyskinesia (TD): *Face:* protruding and rolling tongue, blowing, smacking, licking, spastic facial distortion, smacking movements *Limbs:* Choreic: rapid, purposeless, and irregular movements Athetoid: slow, complex, and serpentine movements *Trunk:* neck and shoulder movements, dramatic hip jerks and rocking, twisting pelvic thrusts *Onset:* Months to years	No known treatment Discontinuing the medication rarely relieves symptoms Possibly 20% of people taking these medications for >2 years may develop TD Nurses and physicians should encourage people to be screened for TD at least every 3 months Onset may merit reconsideration of medications Changes in appearance may contribute to stigmatizing response Teach patient actions to conceal involuntary movements (purposeful muscle contraction overrides involuntary tardive movements)
Hypotension and postural hypotension	Check blood pressure before giving medication: a systolic pressure of 80 mm Hg when standing is indication not to give the current dose Advise person to rise slowly to prevent dizziness and hold on to railings or furniture while rising to reduce falls Effect usually subsides when medication is stabilized in 1–2 weeks Elastic bandages may prevent pooling If any abnormal reading of blood pressure, consult physician immediately regarding medication change, volume expanders, or pressure medications
Tachycardia	Always evaluate patients with existing cardiac problems before antipsychotic medications are administered Haloperidol (Haldol) is usually the preferred medication because of its low ACh effects
Agranulocytosis (a rare occurrence, but a possibility the nurse should be aware of): symptoms include sore throat, fever, malaise, and mouth sores; any flulike symptoms should be carefully evaluated *Onset:* During the first 12 weeks of therapy, occurs suddenly	**A potentially dangerous blood dyscrasia** Blood work usually done every week for 6 months, then every 2 months Physician may order blood work to determine presence of leukopenia or agranulocytosis If test results are positive, the medication is discontinued, and reverse isolation may be initiated Mortality is high if the medication is not ceased and if treatment is not initiated Teach person to observe for signs of infection
Cholestatic jaundice: rare, reversible, and usually benign if caught in time; prodromal symptoms are fever, malaise, nausea, and abdominal pain; jaundice appears 1 week later	Consult physician regarding possible medication change Bed rest and high-protein, high-carbohydrate diet if ordered Liver function tests should be performed every 6 months
Neuroleptic malignant syndrome (NMS): rare, potentially fatal *Severe extrapyramidal:* severe muscle rigidity, oculogyric crisis, dysphasia, flexor-extensor posturing, cogwheeling *Hyperpyrexia:* elevated temperature (over 39°C or 103°F) *Autonomic dysfunction:* hypertension, tachycardia, diaphoresis, incontinence *Delirium, stupor, coma* *Onset:* variable, progresses rapidly over 2–3 days *Risk factors:* concomitant use of psychotropics, older age, female, presence of a mood disorder, and rapid dose titration (increase)	**Acute, life-threatening medical emergency** Consult physician immediately Stop neuroleptic Transfer stat to medical unit Bromocriptine can relieve muscle rigidity and reduce fever Cool body to reduce fever (cooling blankets, alcohol, cool water, or ice bath as ordered) Maintain hydration with oral and IV fluids; correct electrolyte imbalance Arrhythmias should be treated Small doses of heparin may decrease possibility of pulmonary emboli Early detection increases patient's chance of survival

Ach, Anticholinergic; *IM,* intramuscular; *IV,* intravenous.
Source: Kemmerer, D. A. (2007). Anticholinergic syndrome. *Journal of Emergency Nursing, 33,* 76–78. https://doi.org/10.1016/j.jen.2006.10.013

ABNORMAL INVOLUNTARY MOVEMENT SCALE (AIMS)

Public Health Service
Alcohol, Drug Abuse, and Mental Health Administration
National Institute of Mental Health

Name: _____
Date: _____
Prescribing Practitioner: _____

Code:
- 0 = None
- 1 = Minimal, may be extreme normal
- 2 = Mild
- 3 = Moderate
- 4 = Severe

Instructions: Complete Examination Procedure before making ratings.

	Movement ratings: Rate highest severity observed. Rate movements that occur upon activation one *less* than those observed spontaneously. Circle movement as well as code number that applies.	Rater Date	Rater Date	Rater Date	Rater Date
Facial and Oral Movements	1. **Muscles of facial expression** (e.g., movements of forehead, eyebrows, periorbital area, cheeks, including frowning, blinking, smiling, grimacing)	0 1 2 3 4	0 1 2 3 4	0 1 2 3 4	0 1 2 3 4
	2. **Lips and perioral area** (e.g., puckering, pouting, smacking)	0 1 2 3 4	0 1 2 3 4	0 1 2 3 4	0 1 2 3 4
	3. **Jaw** (e.g., biting, clenching, chewing, mouth opening, lateral movement)	0 1 2 3 4	0 1 2 3 4	0 1 2 3 4	0 1 2 3 4
	4. **Tongue:** Rate only increases in movement both in and out of mouth — *not* inability to sustain movement. Darting in and out of mouth.	0 1 2 3 4	0 1 2 3 4	0 1 2 3 4	0 1 2 3 4
Extremity Movements	5. **Upper (arms, wrists, hands, fingers):** Include choreic movements (i.e., rapid, objectively purposeless, irregular, spontaneous) and athetoid movements (i.e., slow, irregular, complex, serpentine). *Do not include tremor* (i.e., repetitive, regular, rhythmic).	0 1 2 3 4	0 1 2 3 4	0 1 2 3 4	0 1 2 3 4
	6. **Lower (legs, knees, ankles, toes)** (e.g., lateral knee movement, foot tapping, heel dropping, foot squirming, inversion and eversion of foot)	0 1 2 3 4	0 1 2 3 4	0 1 2 3 4	0 1 2 3 4
Trunk Movements	7. **Neck, shoulder, hips** (e.g., rocking, twisting, squirming, pelvic gyrations)	0 1 2 3 4	0 1 2 3 4	0 1 2 3 4	0 1 2 3 4
Global Judgments	8. **Severity of abnormal movements overall**	0 1 2 3 4	0 1 2 3 4	0 1 2 3 4	0 1 2 3 4
	9. **Incapacitation due to abnormal movements**	0 1 2 3 4	0 1 2 3 4	0 1 2 3 4	0 1 2 3 4
	10. **Patient's awareness of abnormal movements:** Rate only patient's report. No awareness 0 Aware, no distress 1 Aware, mild distress 2 Aware, moderate distress 3 Aware, severe distress 4	0 1 2 3 4	0 1 2 3 4	0 1 2 3 4	0 1 2 3 4
Dental Status	11. **Current problems with teeth and/or dentures**	No Yes	No Yes	No Yes	No Yes
	12. **Are dentures usually worn?**	No Yes	No Yes	No Yes	No Yes
	13. **Edentia**	No Yes	No Yes	No Yes	No Yes
	14. **Do movements disappear in sleep?**	No Yes	No Yes	No Yes	No Yes

Fig. 15.4 Abnormal Involuntary Movement Scale (AIMS).

paranoia concomitant with psychotic disorders. For them, paranoid ideas cannot be corrected by experiences or modified by facts or reality. *Projection* is the most common defence mechanism used in paranoia: when individuals with paranoia feel angry (or self-critical), they project the feeling onto others and believe that others are angry with (or harshly critical toward) them, as if to say, *"I'm not angry—you are!"*

Schizophrenia with predominantly paranoid symptoms usually has a later age of onset (late twenties to thirties), develops rapidly in individuals with good premorbid functioning, tends to be intermittent during the first 5 years of the illness, and, in some cases, is associated with a good outcome or complete recovery. People with paranoia are usually frightened and may behave defensively. The paranoia is often

AIMS Examination Procedure
Either before or after completing the Examination Procedure, observe the patient unobtrusively, at rest (e.g., in waiting room).

The chair to be used in this examination should be a hard, firm one without arms.

1. Ask patient to remove shoes and socks.
2. Ask patient whether there is anything in his or her mouth (e.g., gum, candy) and, if there is, to remove it.
3. Ask patient about the *current* condition of his or her teeth. Ask patient if he or she wears dentures. Do teeth or dentures bother the patient *now*?
4. Ask patient whether he or she notices any movements in mouth, face, hands, or feet. If yes, ask to describe and to what extent they *currently* bother patient or interfere with his or her activities.
5. Have patient sit in chair with hands on knees, legs slightly apart, and feet flat on floor. Look at entire body movements while in this position.
6. Ask patient to sit with hands hanging unsupported: if male, between legs; if female and wearing a dress, hanging over knees. Observe hands and other body areas.
7. Ask patient to open mouth. Observe tongue at rest within mouth. Do this twice.
8. Ask patient to protrude tongue. Observe abnormalities of tongue movement. Do this twice.
9. Ask patient to tap thumb, with each finger, as rapidly as possible for 10 to 15 seconds, separately with right hand, then with left hand. Observe each facial and leg movement.
10. Flex and extend patient's left and right arms (one at a time). Note any rigidity.
11. Ask patient to stand up. Observe in profile. Observe all body areas again, hips included.
12. Ask patient to extend both arms outstretched in front with palms down. Observe trunk, legs, and mouth.
13. Have patient walk a few paces, turn, and walk back to chair. Observe hands and gait. Do this twice.

Fig. 15.4 cont'd.

a defense against painful feelings of loneliness, despair, helplessness, and fear of abandonment. Useful nursing strategies are outlined in the following sections.

Communication guidelines. People with paranoia can have difficulty trusting those around them, and may be guarded, tense, and/or reserved. To ensure interpersonal distance, they may adopt a superior, aloof, hostile, or sarcastic attitude, disparaging and dwelling on the shortcomings of others to maintain their self-esteem. Although they may shun interpersonal contact, functional impairment other than paranoia may be minimal. These people frequently misinterpret the intent or actions of others, perceiving oversights as personal rejection. They also may personalize unrelated events (**ideas of reference**, or *referentiality*). For example, a patient might see a nurse talking to the psychiatrist and believe that the two are talking about them.

During care, a patient suffering from paranoia may make offensive yet accurate criticisms of staff and unit policies. It is important that responses focus on reducing the patient's anxiety and fear and not be defensive reactions or rejections of the patient. Staff conferences and clinical supervision help maintain objectivity and a therapeutic perspective about the patient's motivation and behaviour, increasing professional effectiveness.

Self-care needs. People with paranoia usually have stronger ego resources than do individuals in whom other symptoms predominate; this is particularly evident in occupational functioning and capacity for independent living. Grooming, dress, and self-care may not be problems and may, in fact, be meticulous. Nutrition, however, may be affected by a delusion, such as that the food is poisoned. Providing foods in commercially sealed packaging, for example, peanut butter and crackers or nutritional drinks in cartons, can improve nutrition. If people worry that others will harm them when they are asleep, they may be fearful of going to sleep, a problem that impairs restorative rest and warrants nursing intervention.

Milieu needs. A person with paranoia may become physically aggressive in response to paranoid hallucinations or delusions. The person projects hostile drives onto others and then acts on these drives.

An environment that provides a sense of security and safety minimizes anxiety and environmental distortions. Activities that distract the patient from ruminating on paranoid themes also decrease anxiety.

Case Study and Nursing Care Plan 15.1 discusses a person with paranoia.

Catatonia: Withdrawn Phase

The essential feature of catatonia is abnormal levels of motor behaviour, either *extreme motor agitation* or *extreme motor retardation*. Other associated behaviours include posturing, waxy flexibility (described later), stereotyped behaviour, muteness, extreme negativism or automatic obedience, echolalia, and echopraxia (discussed earlier in this chapter). The onset of catatonia is usually abrupt, and the prognosis favourable. With pharmacotherapy and improved individual management, severe catatonic symptoms are rarely seen today. Useful nursing strategies for intervening in catatonia are discussed in the following sections.

Communication guidelines. People with catatonia can be so withdrawn they appear stuporous or comatose. They can be mute and may remain so for hours, days, or even weeks or months if untreated. Although such patients may not appear to pay attention to events going on around them, they are acutely aware of the environment and may accurately remember events at a later date. Developing skill and confidence in working with withdrawn patients takes practice. The person's inability or refusal to cooperate or participate in activities challenges staff to work to remain objective and avert frustration and anger.

Self-care needs. In extreme withdrawal a person may need to be hand- or tube-fed to maintain adequate nutritional status. Aspiration is a risk. Normal control over bladder and bowel functions may be interrupted, so the assessment and management of urinary or bowel retention or incontinence is essential. When physical movements are minimal or absent, range-of-motion exercises can reduce muscular atrophy, calcium depletion, and contractures. Dressing and grooming usually require direct assistance.

Milieu needs. The catatonic person's appearance may range from decreased spontaneous movement to complete stupor. Waxy flexibility is often seen; for example, if the patient raises arms over the head, they may maintain that position for hours or longer. Caution is advised because, even after holding a single posture for long periods, the patient may suddenly and without provocation show brief outbursts of gross motor activity in response to inner hallucinations, delusions, and changes in neurotransmitter levels.

Catatonia: Excited Phase

Communication guidelines. During the excited stage of catatonia, the patient is in a state of greatly increased motor activity. They may talk or shout continually and incoherently, requiring the nurse's communication to be clear, direct, and loud (enough to focus the patient's attention on the nurse) and to reflect concern for the safety of the patient and others.

Self-care needs. A person who is constantly and intensely hyperactive can become completely exhausted and be at risk of death if medical attention is not available. Patients with co-existing medical conditions (e.g., congestive heart failure) are most at risk. Intramuscular administration of a sedating antipsychotic is often required to reduce psychomotor agitation to a safer level. During heightened physical activity, the patient requires stimulation reduction and additional fluids, calories, and rest. It is not unusual for the agitated person to be destructive or aggressive to others in response to hallucinations or delusions or inner distress. Many of the concerns and interventions are the same as those for mania. See Chapter 14 for more information about bipolar disorders.

Disorganization

A person with disorganization may have marked associative looseness, grossly inappropriate affect, bizarre mannerisms, and incoherence of speech and may display extreme social withdrawal. Delusions and hallucinations are fragmentary and poorly organized. Behaviour may be considered odd, and a giggling or grimacing response to internal stimuli is common.

Disorganization has an earlier age of onset (early to middle teens), often develops insidiously, is associated with poor premorbid functioning and a significant family history of psychiatric disorders, and carries a poor prognosis. Often people reside in long-term care facilities and can live safely in the community only in a structured, well-supervised setting or with intensive follow-up such as a PACT (Program for Assertive Community Treatment) service. Families of patients living at home need significant community support, respite care, and access to day hospital services. Unfortunately, individuals experiencing disorganization can experience housing instability, which further adds to stressors that contribute to psychosis and difficulties with access to mental health services as well as adherence to antipsychotic prescription (Rezansoff et al., 2016). See the Case Study and Nursing Care Plan for Disorganized Thinking on the Evolve website.

Communication guidelines. People with disorganization experience persistent and severe perceptual and communication problems. Communication should be concise, clear, and concrete. Tasks should be broken into discrete tasks that are performed one at a time. Repeated refocusing may be needed to keep the patient on topic or to allow task completion. This repetition can be frustrating to the nurse and others, requiring special effort to identify and correct counter-transference and nontherapeutic responses.

Self-care needs. In people with disorganization grooming is neglected; hair is often unkempt and matted, and clothes are unclean and often inappropriate for the weather (presenting a risk to self). Cognition, memory, and executive function are grossly impaired, and the person is frequently too disorganized to carry out simple ADLs. Areas of nursing focus include encouraging optimal levels of functioning, preventing further regression, and offering alternatives for inappropriate behaviours whenever possible. Significant direct assistance for ADLs is also needed.

Milieu needs. People with disorganization need assistance with their behaviour and social expectations. Creating a care plan is important to assist patients with structure, initiation of ADLs, increased supervision, and offering alternatives for inappropriate behaviours. Equally important is modifying the care plan as the patient develops more organization in thoughts and behaviours. Nurses must provide for the patient's privacy needs. A sense of safety and decreased stimulation is of utmost importance. Peer education about the disorder may reduce peer frustration and acting out.

> **VIGNETTE**
>
> Martin, a 36-year-old man, is accompanied to the mental health centre by his mother. Antoine, Martin's nurse, obtains background information from his mother. According to her, he had been in a long-term care facility for treatment of schizophrenia for 3 months and, after his discharge, had been doing well at home until recently. His only employment history was 5 months as a janitor after high school graduation. His mother states that, as a teenager, Martin was an excellent athlete and received average grades. At age 17, he had his first "psychotic break," when he took various illicit substances. His behaviour became markedly bizarre (e.g., eating cat food and swallowing a rubber-soled heel, which precipitated an emergency laparotomy).
>
> Antoine meets with Martin. During assessment, Antoine notes the following: Martin is unshaven and dishevelled. He is wearing a headband that holds Popsicle sticks and paper scraps. He chain-smokes, paces, and frequently changes position. He reports that he is Alice from Alice in the Underground and that people from space hurt him with needles. His speech is marked by associative looseness and occasional blocking, and he often stops in the middle of a phrase and giggles to himself.
>
> He starts to giggle, and when Antoine asks what he is thinking about, Martin states, "You interrupted me." He then begins to shake his head while repeating in a singsong voice, "Shake them tigers ... shake them tigers ..." He denies suicidal or homicidal ideation. Antoine notes that Martin has great difficulty accurately perceiving what is going on around him. He exhibits regressed social behaviours (e.g., eating with his hands and picking his nose in public). He has no insight into his mental illness, telling Antoine that his biggest current problem is the people in space.

Advanced-Practice Interventions

Services that may be provided by specifically trained nurses and advanced-practice nurses include psychotherapy, CBT, group therapy, medication administration, social skills training, cognitive remediation, and family therapy. Family therapy is one of the most important interventions implemented for the patient living with schizophrenia.

Family Therapy

Family therapy is a service usually delivered by healthcare providers with specific education in this area, including advanced-practice nurses, master's-prepared social workers, and registered marriage and family therapists. The field of family therapy was originally developed as a treatment for schizophrenia. Families of people living with schizophrenia, particularly direct caregivers, often endure considerable hardships while coping with the psychotic and residual symptoms of the illness. The patient and family may become isolated from other relatives, communities, and support systems. In fact, until the 1970s, families were often blamed for causing schizophrenia in the affected family member.

Family education and family therapy improve the quality of life for the person living with schizophrenia and reduce the relapse rate for many.

Programs that provide support, education, coping skills training, and social network development are extremely effective. This psychoeducational

> ## RESEARCH HIGHLIGHT
> ### Family Psychoeducation Interventions for Psychosis and Schizophrenia
>
> **Problem**
> Family psychoeducation seeks to engage family members as more sophisticated partners, complementing interventions by clinicians with specialized interactions and coping skills that counter the neurological deficits inherent to the disorder.
>
> Although the scientific evidence is increasingly strong that the major psychotic disorders are based on genetic, neurochemical, inflammatory, and/or neurodevelopmental defects involving brain function and structure, there is also abundant evidence that the first onset, progression, and relapse of psychotic or severe mood symptoms are the result of psychosocial stress. Family psychoeducation is a structured method for incorporating a patient's family members, other caregivers, and friends into acute and ongoing treatment and rehabilitation. Based on a family–patient–professional partnership, the approach differs from family therapy, as the family is not the object of therapy but rather the collaborative implementer of therapy. The most common models are essentially cognitive behavioral therapy with consistent inclusion of family members as collaborators.
>
> **Purpose of Study**
> This study sought to understand particular mechanisms of efficacy of family psychoeducation.
>
> **Methods**
> This study method was a comprehensive scientific, theoretical, and clinical review of the evidence spanning four decades.
>
> **Key Findings**
> Family psychoeducation has proved to be one of the most consistently effective treatments available. Reports on outcome studies now number more than 100, while meta-analyses put relapse rate reduction at 50% to 60% over treatment as usual. The most recent application in first episode and prodromal psychosis, combined with other evidence-based interventions, is yielding some of the most promising results yet achieved, substantial return of functioning and avoidance of psychosis altogether. Patients who experience frequent hospitalizations or prolonged unemployment benefit substantially and often dramatically, as do families who are especially exasperated or confused about the illness or even hostile toward the patient.
>
> **Implications for Nursing Practice**
> Family psychoeducation has been deemed an evidence-based practice and has been included in various treatment guidelines for schizophrenia and other serious mental illnesses. Family intervention is particularly beneficial in the early years of the course of a mental illness, when improvements can have a dramatic and long-term effect and while family members are still involved and open to participation, change in attitude, and interaction with the patient.
>
> **Source:** McFarlane, W. R. (2016). Family interventions for schizophrenia and the psychoses: A review. Family Process, 55(3), 460–482. https://doi.org/10.1111/famp.12235

approach brings educational and behavioural approaches into family treatment and does not blame families for illness. In family therapy sessions, fears, faulty communication patterns, and distortions are identified; problem-solving skills are taught; healthier alternatives to conflict are explored; and guilt and anxiety can be lessened.

EVALUATION

Evaluation is especially important in planning care for people who have psychotic disorders. Outcome expectations that are unrealistic discourage the patient and staff alike. It is critical for staff to remember that change is a process that occurs over time. For a person with schizophrenia, progress may occur erratically, and gains may be difficult to discern in the short term.

Chronically ill people must be reassessed regularly so that new data can be considered and treatment adjusted when needed. Questions to be asked include:
- Is the patient not progressing because a more important need is not being met?
- Are the staff making the best use of the patient's strengths and interests to promote treatment and achieve desired outcomes?
- Are any other possible interventions being overlooked?
- Are new or better interventions/treatments available?
- How is the patient responding to existing or recently changed medications or other treatments?
- Is the patient becoming discouraged, anxious, or depressed?
- Is the patient participating in treatment? Are adverse medication effects controlled or troubling?
- Is functioning improving or regressing?
- What is the patient's quality of life, and is it improving?
- Is the family involved, supportive, and knowledgeable regarding the patient's disorder and treatment?

Active staff involvement and interest in the patient's progress communicate concern and caring, help the patient to maximize progress, promote participation in treatment, and reduce staff feelings of helplessness and burnout. Input from the patient can offer valuable information about why a certain desired outcome has not occurred.

CASE STUDY AND NURSING CARE PLAN 15.1
Paranoia in Schizophrenia

> Tom, a 34-year-old man, is an inpatient at a Veterans Affairs Canada hospital. He has been separated from his wife and four children for 3 years. His records state that he has been in and out of hospitals for 13 years. Tom is a former master seaman who first "heard voices" at the age of 21 while he was serving as a peacekeeper in Afghanistan. He subsequently received a medical discharge.
>
> The hospitalization was precipitated by an exacerbation of auditory hallucinations. "I thought people were following me. I hear voices, usually a woman's voice, and she's tormenting me. People say that it happens because I don't take my medications. The medications make me tired, and I can't have sex." Tom also uses marijuana, which he knows increases his paranoia. "It makes me feel good, and not much else does." Tom finished 11 years of school but did not graduate. He says he has no close friends. He spent 5 years in prison for manslaughter and was abusing alcohol and illicit drugs when the crime occurred. Drug use has also been a contributing factor to Tom's psychiatric hospitalizations.
>
> Jodie is Tom's nurse. Tom is dressed in a T-shirt and jeans, his hygiene is good, and he is well nourished. He reports that "the voices get worse at night, and I can't sleep." Jodie notes in Tom's medical record that he has had two episodes of suicidal ideation, during which the voices were telling him to jump "off rooftops" and "in

CASE STUDY AND NURSING CARE PLAN 15.1—cont'd
Paranoia in Schizophrenia

front of trains." During the first interview, Tom rarely makes eye contact and speaks in a low monotone. At times, he glances about the room as if distracted, mumbles to himself, and appears upset.

Nurse: "Tom, my name is Jodie. I will be your nurse today and every day that I am here. If it is okay with you, we will meet every day for 30 minutes at 10 in the morning. We can talk about areas of concern to you."
Tom: "Well, don't believe what they say about me. I want to start. … Are you married?"
Nurse: "This time is for you to talk about your concerns."
Tom: "Oh …" (Looks furtively around the room, then lowers his eyes) "I think someone is trying to kill me. …"
Nurse: "You seem to be focusing on something other than our conversation."
Tom: "The voices tell me things … I can't say …"
Nurse: "It seems like the voices are upsetting to you. I can't hear them. What kinds of things are they saying?"
Tom: "The voices tell me bad things."

Jodie stays with Tom and encourages him to communicate with her. As Tom focuses more on the conversation, his anxiety appears to lessen. His thoughts become more connected, he is able to concentrate more, and he mumbles to himself less.

Assessment
Self-Assessment
On the first day of admission, Tom assaults another male patient, stating that the other person looked at him the wrong way.

Tom's difficulty with impulse control frightens Jodie. She has concerns regarding Tom's ability to curb his impulses and the possibility of Tom's striking out at her, especially when Tom is hallucinating and highly delusional. Jodie mentions her concerns to the nursing coordinator, who suggests that Jodie meet with Tom in the day room until he demonstrates more control and less suspicion of others. After 5 days, Tom is "less excitable," and the sessions are moved to a room reserved for private interviews. Jodie also speaks with a senior staff nurse regarding her fears. By talking to the senior nurse and understanding more clearly her own fear, Jodie is able to manage her fear and identify interventions to help Tom regain a better sense of control.

Objective Data	Subjective Data
Speaks in low monotone	"I hear voices."
Makes poor eye contact	"I think someone is trying to kill me. …"
Weight appropriate for height	"I don't take my medications. [They] make me tired, and I can't have sex."
Clean, bathed, clothes match	"The voices get worse at night and I can't sleep."
Impaired reality testing	"[Marijuana] makes me feel good, and not much else does."
Has a history of drug use (marijuana), which appears to contribute to relapses	Voices have told him to jump "off rooftops" and "in front of trains."
Has no close friends, separated from wife and children	
Was first hospitalized at age 21 and has not worked since that time	
Has had suicidal impulses twice, both associated with command hallucinations	
Was imprisoned for 5 years for violence (manslaughter) and assaulted a peer in the hospital	
Thoughts scattered when anxious	

Diagnosis
1. *Disturbed thought processes* related to alteration in neurological function, as evidenced by persecutory hallucinations and paranoia

Supporting Data
- Voices have told him to jump "off rooftops" and "in front of trains."
- "I think someone is trying to kill me."
- Abuses marijuana (although it increases paranoia) because "it makes me feel good."

2. *Nonadherence to medication regimen* related to adverse effects of therapy, as evidenced by verbalization of nonadherence and persistence of symptoms

Supporting Data
- Failure to take prescribed medications because "they make me tired, and I can't have sex."
- Chronic history of relapse of symptoms

Outcomes Identification
1. Tom consistently refrains from acting on his "voices" and suspicions.
2. Tom consistently adheres to treatment regimen.

Planning
The nurse plans interventions that will (1) help Tom deal with his disturbing thoughts and (2) minimize drug use and adverse effects of medication to increase adherence and decrease the potential for relapse and violence.

Implementation
1. Nursing diagnosis: *Disturbed thought processes*
   Outcome: Tom consistently refrains from acting on his "voices" and suspicions when they occur.

Continued

CASE STUDY AND NURSING CARE PLAN 15.1—cont'd
Paranoia in Schizophrenia

Short-Term Goal	Intervention	Rationale	Evaluation
1. By the end of the first week, Tom will recognize the presence of hallucinations and identify one or more contributing factors, as evidenced by telling his nurse when they occur and what preceded them.	1a. Meet with Tom each day for 30 minutes to establish trust and rapport. 1b. Explore those times when voices are most threatening and disturbing, noting the circumstances that precede them. 1c. Provide noncompetitive activities that focus on the here and now.	1a. Short, consistent meetings help decrease anxiety and establish trust. 1b. Identifying events that increase anxiety and trigger "voices" and then learning to manage triggers, hallucinations can be reduced. 1c. Increased time spent in reality-based activities decreases focus on hallucinations.	**Goal Met** By the end of the first week, Tom tells the nurse when he is experiencing hallucinations.
2. By the end of the first week, Tom will recognize hallucinations as "not real" and ascribe them to his illness.	2a. Explore content of hallucinations with Tom. 2b. Educate Tom about the nature of hallucinations and ways to determine if "voices" are real.	2a. Exploring hallucinations identifies suicidal or aggressive themes or command hallucinations. 2b. Education improves Tom's reality testing and helps him begin to attribute his experiences to schizophrenia.	**Goal Met** Tom identifies that the voices tell him he is a loser and he needs to be careful "because someone is after me." He identifies that the voices are worse at nighttime. He notes that others do not seem to hear what he hears and also states that smoking marijuana produces very threatening voices.
3. By discharge, Tom will consistently report a decrease in hallucinations.	3. Explore with Tom possible actions that can minimize anxiety and reduce hallucinations, such as whistling or reading aloud.	3. Such activities offer alternatives while anxiety level is relatively low.	**Goal Met** Tom states that he is hearing voices less often, and they are less threatening to him. Tom identifies that if he whistles or sings, he stays calm and can control the voices.

2. Nursing diagnosis: Nonadherence to medication regimen
Outcome: Tom consistently adheres to medication regimen.

Short-Term Goal	Intervention	Rationale	Evaluation
1. By the end of week 1, Tom will discuss his concerns about medication with staff.	1a. Evaluate medication response and adverse-effect issues. 1b. Initiate medication change to olanzapine (Zyprexa). Administer a large dose at bedtime to increase sleep and a small dose during the day to decrease fatigue. 1c. Educate Tom regarding adverse effects—how long they last and what actions can be taken.	1a. Such evaluation identifies medications and dosages that have increased therapeutic value and decreased adverse effects. 1b. Olanzapine causes no known sexual difficulties. 1c. This knowledge can give an increased sense of control over symptoms.	**Goal Met** Tom identifies the reasons for stopping his medication. He agrees to try olanzapine because he trusts staff's assurances that the adverse effects will be reduced. Tom states that he sleeps better at night but is still tired during the day.
2. By the end of week 2, Tom will describe two ways to reduce or cope with adverse effects and two ways the medications help him meet his goals (e.g., avoiding jail, reducing fear).	2. Connect Tom with the local Schizophrenia Society support group.	2. Being part of a group provides peer support and a chance to hear from others (further along in recovery) how medications can be helpful and adverse effects can be managed. The peer group can also offer suggestions for dealing with his loneliness and other problems.	**Goal Met** Week 1: Tom attends meeting. Week 2: He speaks in the group about "not feeling good." Several group members say they understand and try to help him figure out why he is not feeling good. Peers tell him how taking medication has helped them feel better.

Evaluation
By discharge, Tom expresses hope that the medications will help him feel better and avoid problems like jail. He has a better understanding of his medications and what to do for adverse effects. He knows that marijuana increases his symptoms and explains that when he gets lonely, he now has ideas of things other than marijuana he can do to "feel good." Tom continues with the support group and outpatient counselling, stating that his reason for doing so is "because Jodie really cared about me"; her empathy and caring made him want to get better and led him to trust what staff told him. He reports sleeping much better and says that he has more energy during the day.

CHAPTER 15 Schizophrenia Spectrum and Other Psychotic Disorders

KEY POINTS TO REMEMBER

- Schizophrenia is a complex disorder of the brain. It is not one disorder but a group of disorders with overlapping symptoms and treatments.
- Recovery is possible with early identification, new treatments, and adequate social supports.
- The primary differences among subtypes involve the spectrum of symptoms that dominate their severity, the impairment in affect and cognition, and the impact on social and other areas of functioning.
- Symptoms of psychosis are often more pronounced and obvious than are symptoms found in other disorders, making psychosis and schizophrenia more likely to be apparent to others and increasing the risk of stigmatization.
- Neurochemical (catecholamines and serotonin), genetic, and neuroanatomical findings help explain the symptoms of schizophrenia. However, no one theory accounts fully for the complexities of schizophrenia.
- There are four categories of symptoms of schizophrenia: positive, negative, cognitive, and affective. Symptoms vary considerably among people and fluctuate over time.
- The positive symptoms of schizophrenia (e.g., hallucinations, delusions, associative looseness) are more pronounced and respond best to antipsychotic medication therapy.
- The negative symptoms of schizophrenia (e.g., social withdrawal and dysfunction, lack of motivation, reduced affect) respond less well to antipsychotic therapy and tend to be more debilitating.
- The degree of cognitive impairment (cognitive symptom) warrants careful assessment and active intervention to increase the patient's ability to adapt, function, and maximize their quality of life.
- Coexisting depression (affective symptom) must be identified and treated to reduce potential risk for suicide, substance use, nonadherence, and relapse.
- Some applicable nursing diagnoses include *Disturbed sensory perception, Disturbed thought processes, Impaired communication, Ineffective coping, Risk for self-directed or other-directed violence,* and *Impaired family coping.*
- Outcomes are chosen based on the type and phase of schizophrenia and the person's individual needs, strengths, and level of functioning. Short-term and intermediate indicators are also developed to better track the incremental progress typical of schizophrenia.
- Interventions for people living with schizophrenia include trust building, therapeutic communication techniques, support, assistance with self-care, promotion of independence, stress management, promotion of socialization, psychoeducation to promote understanding and adaptation, milieu management, cognitive behavioural interventions, cognitive enhancement or remediation techniques, and medication administration.
- Because antipsychotic medications are essential in the care of people living with schizophrenia, the nurse must understand the properties, adverse and toxic effects, and dosages of conventional and atypical antipsychotic medication and other medications used to treat schizophrenia. The nurse helps the patient and family understand and appreciate the importance of medication to recovery.
- Schizophrenia can produce counter-transference responses in staff; clinical supervision and self-assessment help the nurse remain objective and therapeutic.
- Hope is closely tied to recovery; it is essential for nurses to hold hope for people living with schizophrenia.

CRITICAL THINKING

1. Jasmine, a 24-year-old woman, is hospitalized after an abrupt onset of psychosis and is diagnosed with paranoid schizophrenia. Jasmine is recently divorced and works as a legal secretary. Her work had become erratic, and her suspiciousness was attracting negative responses. Jasmine is being discharged in 2 days to her mother's care until she is able to resume her job. Jasmine's mother is overwhelmed and asks the nurse how she is going to cope. She says, "I can hardly say anything to Jasmine without her getting upset. She is still mad at me because I called 911 and had her admitted. She says there is nothing wrong with her, and I'm worried she'll stop her medication once she is home. What am I going to do?"
   a. Explain Jasmine's behaviour and symptoms to a classmate as you would to Jasmine's mother.
   b. How would you respond to the mother's immediate concerns?
   c. What are some of the priority concerns the nurse should address before discharge?
   d. Identify interventions that are based on the concepts of the recovery model.
   e. What are some community resources that can help support this family? Describe how each could be helpful to this family.
   f. What do you think of the prognosis for Jasmine? Support your position with data regarding Jasmine's diagnosis and the treatment you have planned.

CHAPTER REVIEW

1. Which characteristic in an adolescent female is sometimes associated with the prodromal phase of schizophrenia?
   a. Always afraid another student will steal her belongings.
   b. An unusual interest in numbers and specific topics.
   c. Demonstrates no interest in athletics or organized sports.
   d. Appears more comfortable among males.
2. Which nursing intervention is particularly well chosen for addressing a population at high risk for developing schizophrenia?
   a. Screening a group of males between the ages of 15 and 25 for early symptoms.
   b. Forming a support group for females ages 25 to 35 who are diagnosed with substance use issues.
   c. Providing a group for patients between the ages of 45 and 55 with information on coping skills that have proven to be effective.
   d. Educating the parents of a group of developmentally delayed 5- to 6-year-olds on the importance of early intervention.
3. To provide effective care for the patient diagnosed with schizophrenia, the nurse should frequently assess for which associated conditions? **Select all that apply.**
   a. Alcohol use disorder.
   b. Major depressive disorder.
   c. Stomach cancer.
   d. Polydipsia.
   e. Metabolic syndrome.
4. A female patient diagnosed with schizophrenia has been prescribed a first-generation antipsychotic medication. What information should the nurse provide to the patient regarding her signs and symptoms?
   a. Her memory problems will likely decrease.
   b. Depressive episodes should be less severe.
   c. She will probably enjoy social interactions more.
   d. She should experience a reduction in hallucinations.

5. Which characteristic presents the greatest risk for injury to others by the patient diagnosed with schizophrenia?
   a. Depersonalization.
   b. Pressured speech.
   c. Negative symptoms.
   d. Paranoia.
6. Gilbert, age 19, is described by his parents as a "moody child" with an onset of odd behaviour at about age 14, which caused Gilbert to suffer academically and socially. Gilbert has lost the ability to complete household chores, is reluctant to leave the house, and is obsessed with the locks on the windows and doors. Due to Gilbert's early and slow onset of what is now recognized as schizophrenia, his prognosis is considered:
   a. Favourable with medication.
   b. In the relapse stage.
   c. Improvable with psychosocial interventions.
   d. To have a less positive outcome.
7. Which therapeutic communication statement might a psychiatric mental health registered nurse use when a patient's nursing diagnosis is *Altered thought processes*?
   a. "It must be difficult to hear voices like that, though I cannot hear them."
   b. "Stop listening to the voices, they are NOT real."
   c. "You say you hear voices; what are they telling you?"
   d. "Just tell the voices to leave you alone for now."
8. When patients diagnosed with schizophrenia suffer from anosognosia, they often refuse medication, believing that:
   a. Medications provided are ineffective.
   b. Nurses are trying to control their minds.
   c. The medications will make them sick.
   d. They are not actually ill.
9. Kyle, a patient with schizophrenia, began to take the first-generation antipsychotic haloperidol (Haldol) last week. One day you find him sitting very stiffly and not moving. He is diaphoretic, and when you ask if he is okay, he seems unable to respond verbally. His vital signs are BP 170/100, P 110, T 40.1°C/104.2°F. What is the priority nursing intervention?
   a. Hold his medication and contact his prescriber.
   b. Wipe him with a washcloth wet with cold water or alcohol.
   c. Administer a medication such as benztropine IM to correct this dystonic reaction.
   d. Reassure him that although there is no treatment for his tardive dyskinesia, it will pass.
   e. Hold his medication for now and consult his prescriber when he comes to the unit later today.
10. Tomas is a 21-year-old male with a recent diagnosis of schizophrenia. Tomas's nurse recognizes that self-medicating with excessive alcohol is common in this disease and can co-occur along with:
    a. Generally good health despite the mental illness.
    b. An aversion to drinking fluids.
    c. Anxiety and depression.
    d. The ability to express his needs.

http://evolve.elsevier.com/Canada/Varcarolis/psychiatric/

REFERENCES

Abidi, S., Mian, I., Garcia-Ortega, I., et al. (2017). Canadian guidelines for the pharmacological treatment of schizophrenia spectrum and other psychotic disorders in children and youth. *The Canadian Journal of Psychiatry, 62*(9), 635–647.

Addington, D., Anderson, E., Kelly, M., et al. (2017a). Canadian practice guidelines for comprehensive community treatment for schizophrenia and schizophrenia spectrum disorders. *The Canadian Journal of Psychiatry, 62*(9), 662–672.

Addington, D., Abidi, S., Garcia-Ortega, I., et al. (2017b). Canadian guidelines for the assessment and diagnosis of patients with schizophrenia spectrum and other psychotic disorders. *The Canadian Journal of Psychiatry, 62*(9), 594–603.

Akbarian, S., & Kundakovic, M. (2015). CHRNA7 and CHRFAM7A: Psychosis and smoking? Blame the neighbors. *The American Journal of Psychiatry, 172*(11), 1054.

Amador, H. (2021). Henry Amador, Center on Anosognosia. https://hacenter.org/about-leap

American Psychiatric Association. (2013). *Diagnostic and statistical manual of mental disorders* (5th ed.). Washington, DC: Author.

Andreou, D., Söderman, E., Axelsson, T., et al. (2015). Cerebrospinal fluid monoamine metabolite concentrations as intermediate phenotypes between glutamate-related genes and psychosis. *Psychiatry Research, 229*(1–2), 497–504. https://doi.org/10.1016/j.psychres.2015.06.023

Aschengrau, A., Weinberg, J., Janulewicz, P., et al. (2012). Occurrence of mental illness following prenatal and early childhood exposure to tetrachloroethylene (PCE)-contaminated drinking water: A retrospective cohort study. *Environmental Health: A Global Access Science Source, 11*(1), 1–12.

Berry, A., & Cirulli, F. (2016). Toward a diathesis-stress model of schizophrenia in a neurodevelopmental perspective. In V. Mikhail, & J. L. Waddington (Eds.), *Handbook of behavioral neuroscience* (pp. 209–224). St. Louis: Elsevier.

Blomström, A., Karlsson, H., Gardner, R., et al. (2016). Associations between maternal infection during pregnancy, childhood infections, and the risk of subsequent psychotic disorder—A Swedish cohort study of nearly 2 million individuals. *Schizophrenia Bulletin, 42*(1), 125–133. https://doi.org/10.1093/schbul/sbv112

Brady, P., Kangas, M., & McGill, K. (2017). "Family matters": A systematic review of the evidence for family psychoeducation for major depressive disorder. *Journal of Marital and Family Therapy, 43*(2), 245–263. https://doi.org/10.1111/jmft.12204

Brown, E., & Gray, R. (2015). Tackling medication non-adherence in severe mental illness: Where are we going wrong? *Journal of Psychiatric and Mental Health Nursing, 22*(3), 192–198. https://doi.org/10.1111/jpm.12186

Buccheri, R. K., Trygstad, L. N., Buffum, M. D., et al. (2013). Self-management of unpleasant auditory hallucinations: A tested practice model. *Journal of Psychosocial Nursing and Mental Health Services, 51*(11), 26. https://doi.org/10.3928/02793695-20130731-02

Canadian Institute for Health Information (CIHI). 2021. *Quality of care*. https://yourhealthsystem.cihi.ca/hsp/inbrief?lang=en#!/themes/002/quality-of-care

Carbon, M., & Correll, C. U. (2014). Thinking and acting beyond the positive: The role of the cognitive and negative symptoms in schizophrenia. *CNS Spectrums, 19*(Suppl. 1), 38–53. https://doi.org/10.1017/S1092852914000601

Castellani, C., Melka, M., Gui, J., et al. (2015). Integration of DNA sequence and DNA methylation changes in monozygotic twin pairs discordant for schizophrenia. *Schizophrenia Research, 169*(1–3), 433–440. https://doi.org/10.1016/j.schres.2015.09.021

Centre for Addiction and Mental Health. (2020). *Suicide rate for people with schizophrenia spectrum disorders over 20 times higher than the general population*. https://www.camh.ca/en/camh-news-and-stories/suicide-rate-for-people-with-schizophrenia-spectrum-disorders#:~:text=June%2018%2C%202020%20%28Toronto%29%20%E2%80%93%20The%20suicide%20 rate,Research%2C%20a%20figure%20the%20authors%20call%20%E2%80%9Ctragically%20high.%E2%80%9D

Centre for Addiction and Mental Health (CAMH). (2021). *Antipsychotic medications.* https://www.camh.ca/en/health-info/mental-illness-and-addiction-index/antipsychotic-medication/

Chadwick, P. (2019). Mindfulness for psychosis: A humanizing therapeutic process. *Current Opinion in Psychology, 28*, 317–320.

Chester, P., Ehrlich, C., Warburton, L., et al. (2016). What is the work of recovery oriented practice? A systematic literature review. *International Journal of Mental Health Nursing, 25*(4), 270–285. https://doi.org/10.1111/inm.12241

Chung, Y. S., Kang, D., Shin, N. Y., et al. (2008). Deficit of theory of mind in individuals at ultra-high risk for schizophrenia. *Schizophrenia Research, 99*, 111–118.

Correll, C. U., Detraux, J., De Lepeleire, J., et al. (2015). Effects of antipsychotics, antidepressants and mood stabilizers on risk for physical diseases in people with schizophrenia, depression and bipolar disorder. *World Psychiatry, 14*(2), 119–136.

Cookey, J., McGavin, J., Crocker, C. E., et al. (2020). A retrospective study of the clinical characteristics associated with alcohol and cannabis use in early phase psychosis. *The Canadian Journal of Psychiatry, 65*(6), 426–435.

Crockford, D., & Addington, D. (2017). Canadian schizophrenia guidelines: Schizophrenia and other psychotic disorders with coexisting substance use disorders. *The Canadian Journal of Psychiatry, 62*(9), 624–634.

Davey, Z., Jackson, D., & Henshall, C. (2020). The value of nurse mentoring relationships: Lessons learnt from a work-based resilience enhancement programme for nurses working in the forensic setting. *International Journal of Mental Health Nursing, 29*(5), 992–1001.

Dean, D., Orr, J., Bernard, J., et al. (2016). Hippocampal shape abnormalities predict symptom progression in neuroleptic-free youth at ultrahigh risk for psychosis. *Schizophrenia Bulletin, 42*(1), 161–169. https://doi.org/10.1093/schbul/sbv086

Docherty, N. M., Dinzeo, T. J., McCleery, A., et al. (2015). Internal versus external auditory hallucinations in schizophrenia: Symptom and course correlates. *Cognitive Neuropsychiatry, 20*(3), 187–197.

D'Souza, R. S, & Hooten, W. M. (2020). Extrapyramidal symptoms. In *StatPearls* [Internet]. Treasure Island: StatPearls Publishing. https://www.ncbi.nlm.nih.gov/books/NBK534115/

Egerton, A., Howes, O. D., Houle, S., et al. (2017). Elevated striatal dopamine function in immigrants and their children: A risk mechanism for psychosis. *Schizophrenia Bulletin, 43*(2), 293–301. https://doi.org/10.1093/schbul/sbw181

England, M. (2007). Accuracy of nurses' perceptions of voice hearing and psychiatric symptoms. *Journal of Advanced Nursing, 58*(2), 130–139. https://doi.org/10.1111/j.1365-2648.2006.04162.x

Farhall, J., Greenwood, K. M., & Jackson, H. J. (2007). Coping with hallucinated voices: A review of self-initiated strategies and therapeutic interventions. *Clinical Psychology Review, 27*, 476–493. https://doi.org/10.1016/j.cpr.2006.12.002

Fornells-Ambrojo, M., Claxton, M., & Onwumere, J. (2017). Do family interventions improve outcomes in early psychosis? A systematic review and meta-analysis. *Frontiers in Psychology, 8*, 371. https://doi.org/10.3389/fpsyg.2017.00371

Frankle, W. G., Cho, R. Y., Prasad, K. M., et al. (2015). In vivo measurement of GABA transmission in healthy subjects and schizophrenia patients. *American Journal of Psychiatry, 172*, 1148–1159.

Freudenreich, O. (2020a). Natural history of schizophrenia. In O. Freudenreich (Ed.), *Psychotic disorders: A practical guide* (2nd ed., pp. 87–100). Cham: Springer.

Freudenreich, O. (2020b). Adjunctive medications. In O. Freudenreich (Ed.), *Psychotic disorders: A practical guide.* (2nd ed., pp. 263–275). Cham: Springer.

Gaebel, W., Rössler, W., & Sartorius, N. (2017). *The stigma of mental illness: End of the story?* Cham: Springer.

Gerlock, A. A., Buccheri, R., Buffum, M. D., et al. (2010). Responding to command hallucinations to harm self and others: The Unpleasant Voices Scale and Harm Command Safety Protocol. *Journal of Psychosocial Nursing and Mental Health Services, 48*(5), 26–33. https://doi.org/10.3928/02793695-20100304-03

Gerson, R., Wong, C., Davidson, L., et al. (2011). Self-reported coping strategies in families of patients in early stages of psychotic disorder: An exploratory study: Coping by families in early psychosis. *Early Intervention in Psychiatry, 5*(1), 76–80. https://doi.org/10.1111/j.1751-7893.2010.00251.x

Government of Canada. (2020). *Schizophrenia in Canada.* https://www.canada.ca/en/public-health/services/publications/diseases-conditions/schizophrenia-canada.html

Guy, W. (1976). *ECDEU Assessment manual for psychopharmacology: Revised* (DHEW publication number ADM 76-338) (pp. 534–537). Rockville: US Department of Health, Education and Welfare, Public Health Service, Alcohol, Drug Abuse and Mental Health Administration, NIMH Psychopharmacology Research Branch, Division of Extramural Research Programs.

Haddad, L., Schäfer, A., Streit, F., et al. (2015). Brain structure correlates of urban upbringing, an environmental risk factor. *Schizophrenia Bulletin, 41*(1), 115–122. https://doi.org/10.1093/schbul/sbu072

Happell, B., Platania-Phung, C., & Scott, D. (2013). Mental health nurse incentive program: Facilitating physical health care for people with mental illness?. *International Journal of Mental Health Nursing, 22*(5), 399–408. https://doi.org/10.1111/inm.12006

Haynes, R. M., & Resnick, P. J. (1993). Proverb familiarity and the mental status exam. *Bulletin of the Menninger Clinic, 57*(4), 523–529.

Health Quality Ontario. (2018). *Quality Standards—Schizophrenia care in the community for adults.* https://hqontario.ca/Portals/0/documents/evidence/quality-standards/qs-schizophrenia-community-clinician-guide-en.pdf

Hodgins, S., & Klein, S. (2017). New clinically relevant findings about violence by people with schizophrenia. *The Canadian Journal of Psychiatry, 62*(2), 86–93.

Hoffman, R. E., & Varanko, M. (2006). Seeing voices: Fused visual/auditory verbal hallucinations reported by three persons with schizophrenia-spectrum disorder. *Acta Psychiatrica Scandinavica, 114*, 290–293.

Howes, O. D., & McCutcheon, R. (2017). Inflammation and the neural diathesis–stress hypothesis of schizophrenia: A reconceptualization. *Translational Psychiatry, 7*(2), e1024. https://doi.org/10.1038/tp.2016.278 [Electronic Resource].

Howland, R. H. (2015). Brexpiprazole: Another multipurpose antipsychotic drug?. *Journal of Psychosocial Nursing and Mental Health Services, 53*(4), 23–25. https://doi.org/10.3928/02793695-20150323-01

Johnson, J., Hall, L. H., Berzons, K., et al. (2018). Mental healthcare staff well-being and burnout: A narrative review of trends, causes, implications, and recommendations for future interventions. *International Journal of Mental Health Nursing, 27*(1), 20–32.

Kesby, J. P., Eyles, D. W., McGrath, J. J., et al. (2018). Dopamine, psychosis and schizophrenia: The widening gap between basic and clinical neuroscience. *Translational Psychiatry, 8.* https://www.nature.com/articles/s41398-017-0071-9

Koehn, C. V., & Cutliffe, J. R. (2007). Hope and interpersonal psychiatric/mental health nursing: A systematic review of the literature: Part one. *Journal of Psychiatric and Mental Health Nursing, 14*, 134–140. https://doi.org/10.1111/j.1365-2850.2007.01054.x

Lamsma, J., & Harte, J. M. (2015). Violence in psychosis: Conceptualizing its causal relationship with risk factors. *Aggression and Violent Behavior, 24*, 75–82. https://doi.org/10.1016/j.avb.2015.05.003

Levine, S. Z., Lurie, I., Kohn, R., et al. (2011). Trajectories of the course of schizophrenia: From progressive deterioration to amelioration over three decades. *Schizophrenia Research, 126*, 184–191. https://doi.org/10.1016/j.schres.2010.10.026

Lieberman, J. A., Small, S. A., & Girgis, R. R. (2019). Early detection and preventive intervention in schizophrenia: From fantasy to reality. *American Journal of Psychiatry, 176*(10), 794–810. https://doi.org/10.1176/appi.ajp.2019.19080865

Lipner, E., Murphy, S. K., & Ellman, L. M. (2019). Prenatal maternal stress and the cascade of risk to schizophrenia spectrum disorders in offspring. *Reproductive Psychiatry and Women's Health, 21*, 99.

McDaid, T. M., & Smyth, S. (2015). Metabolic abnormalities among people diagnosed with schizophrenia: A literature review and implications for mental health nurses. *Journal of Psychiatric and Mental Health Nursing, 22*(3), 157–170. https://doi.org/10.1111/jpm.12185

Mental Health Commission of Canada. (2016). *Guidelines for recovery-oriented practice: Hope, dignity, inclusion.* http://www.mentalhealthcommission.ca/sites/default/files/2016-07/MHCC_Recovery_Guidelines_2016_ENG.PDF

Mental Health Commission of Canada. (2021). The mental health needs of justice-involved persons. A rapid scoping. *Review of the Literature.* https://mentalhealthcommission.ca/wp-content/uploads/2021/05/Justice_Scoping_Review_eng.pdf

Mental Health Commission of Canada. (2022). *Stigma and discrimination.* https://mentalhealthcommission.ca/what-we-do/stigma-and-discrimination/

Miller, B. (2016). Neuroinflammation marker may foretell psychosis. *Psychiatric Times.* https://www.psychiatrictimes.com/schizophrenia/neuroinflammation-marker-may-foretell-psychosis

Moorhead, S., Swanson, E., Johnson, M., & Maas, M. L. (Eds.). (2018). *Nursing Outcomes Classification (NOC): Measurement of health outcomes* (6th ed.). St. Louis: Elsevier.

Morera, T., Pratt, D., & Bucci, S. (2017). Staff views about psychosocial aspects of recovery in psychosis: A systematic review. *Psychology and Psychotherapy, 90*(1), 1–24. https://doi.org/10.1111/papt.12092

Morgan, C., Freeman, T., Powell, J., et al. (2016). AKT1 genotype moderates the acute psychotomimetic effects of naturalistically smoked cannabis in young cannabis smokers. *Translational Psychiatry, 6*, e738. https://doi.org/10.1038/tp.2015.219

Mork, E., Mehlum, L., Barrett, E. A., et al. (2012). Self-harm in patients with schizophrenia spectrum disorders. *Archives of Suicide Research, 16*(2), 111–123. https://doi.org/10.1080/13811118.2012.667328

Nash, J. (n. d.). Nash: Film no white wash. In CBC News, David Kohn, March 14, 2002. https://www.cbsnews.com/news/nash-film-no-whitewash/

Nielssen, O., & Large, M. (2010). Rates of homicide during the first episode of psychosis and a systematic review and meta-analysis. *Schizophrenia Bulletin, 36*(4), 702–712. https://doi.org/10.1093/schbul/sbn144

Norman, R. M., Manchanda, R., Malia, A. K., et al. (2011). Symptom and functional outcomes for a 5-year early intervention program for psychoses. *Schizophrenia Research, 129*(2–3), 111–115. https://doi.org/10.1016/j.schres.2011.04.006

Pelletier, J., Lesage, A., Boisvert, C., et al. (2015). Feasibility and acceptability of patient partnership to improve access to primary care for the physical health of patients with severe mental illnesses: An interactive guide. *International Journal for Equity in Health, 14*, 78. https://doi.org/10.1186/s12939-015-0200-0

Remington, G., Addington, D., Honer, W., et al. (2017). Guidelines for the pharmacotherapy of schizophrenia in adults. *The Canadian Journal of Psychiatry, 62*(9), 604–616.

Rezansoff, S. N., Moniruzzaman, A., Fazel, S., et al. (2016). Adherence to antipsychotic medication among homeless adults in Vancouver, Canada: A 15-year retrospective cohort study. *Social Psychiatry and Psychiatric Epidemiology, 51*(12), 1623–1632. https://doi.org/10.1007/s00127-016-1259

Sadock, B. J., Sadock, V. A., & Ruiz, P. (2017). *Concise textbook of clinical psychiatry* (4th ed.). Philadelphia: Lippincott Williams & Wilkins.

Sanchez SanSegundo, M., Ferrer-Cascales, R., Bellido, J. H., et al. (2018). Prediction of violence, suicide behaviors and suicide ideation in a sample of institutionalized offenders with schizophrenia and other psychosis. *Frontiers in Psychology, 9*, 1–10. https://doi.org/10.3389/fpsyg.2018.01385

Sandler, J., Kotov, R., & Bromet, E. (2011). Predictors of trajectories of illness course over 10 years in schizophrenia. *Comprehensive Psychiatry, 52*(6), e14. https://doi.org/10.1016/j.comppsych.2011.04.044

Schifani, C., Tseng, H-H., Kenk, M., et al. (2018). Cortical stress regulation is disrupted in schizophrenia but not in clinical high risk for psychosis. *Brain, 141*(7), 2213.

Schizophrenia Society of Canada. (2018). *Hope support and care—Annual Report 2017–2018.* https://schizophrenia.ca/wp-content/uploads/2020/05/SSC-and-SSCF-Annual-Report-2017-2018.pdf

Schizophrenia Society of Canada. (2020). *Hope & recovery—Your guide to living with and beyond schizophrenia.* https://schizophrenia.ca/wp-content/uploads/2020/05/Hope-and-Recovery-Guide.pdf

Sekar, A., Bialas, A., de Rivera, H., et al. (2016). Schizophrenia risk from complex variation of complement component 4. *Nature, 530*(7589), 177–183. https://doi.org/10.1038/nature16549.

Skeem, J., Kennealy, P., Monahan, J., et al. (2015). Psychosis uncommonly and inconsistently precedes violence among high-risk individuals. *Clinical Psychological Science, 4*, 40–49. https://doi.org/10.1177/2167702615575879

Srihari, V. H., Shah, J., & Keshavan, M. S. (2012). Is early intervention for psychosis feasible and effective?. *The Psychiatric Clinics of North America, 35*(3), 613–631. https://doi.org/10.1016/j.psc.2012.06.004

Thakur, T, & Gupta, V. (2021). Auditory hallucinations. In *Stat Pearls [Internet].* Treasure Island: StatPearls Publishing. PMID: 32491565.

Thornicroft, G. (2011). Physical health disparities and mental illness: The scandal of premature mortality. *The British Journal of Psychiatry: The Journal of Mental Science, 199*(6), 441–442. https://doi.org/10.1192/bjp.bp.111.092718

Tsiachristas, A., Thomas, T., Leal, J., et al. (2016). Economic impact of early intervention in psychosis services: Results from a longitudinal retrospective controlled study in England. *BMJ Open, 6*(10), e012611. https://doi.org/10.1136/bmjopen-2016-012611

Waldemar, A. K., Arnfred, S. M., Petersen, L., et al. (2016). Recovery-oriented practice in mental health inpatient settings: A literature review. *Psychiatric Services, 67*(6), 596–602. https://doi.org/10.1176/appi.ps.201400469

Walker, A. K., Arnfred, S. M., Petersen, L., et al. (2016). Recovery-oriented practice in mental health inpatient settings: A literature review. *Psychiatric Services, 67*(6), 596–602. https://doi.org/10.1176/appi.ps.201400469

Weiser, M., Fenchel, D., Fruchter, E., et al. (2020). Understanding the association between advanced paternal age and schizophrenia and bipolar disorder. *Psychological Medicine, 50*(3), 431–437. https://doi.org/10.1017/S0033291719000242

Wilson, B. A., Shannon, M. T., & Sheilds, K. (2017). *Pearson nurse's drug guide 2017*. Upper Saddle River: Pearson/Prentice Hall.

Wynaden, D., Tohotoa, J., Heslop, K., et al. (2015). Recognizing falls risk in older adult mental health patients and acknowledging the difference from the general older adult population. *Collegian (Royal College of Nursing, Australia), 23*(1), 97–102. https://dx.doi.org/10.1016/j.colegn.2014.12.002

Xu, X., Li, X. M., Zhang, J., et al. (2017). Mental health-related stigma in China. *Issues in Mental Health Nursing, 38*(2), 126–134.

Zaheer, J., Olfson, M., Mallia, E., et al. (2020). Predictors of suicide at time of diagnosis in schizophrenia spectrum disorder: A 20-year total population study in Ontario Canada. *Schizophrenia Research, 222*, 382–388.

16

Eating and Feeding Disorders

Bonnie Fournier
Originating US chapter by Rachel M. Childs, Carissa R. Enright

 https://evolve.elsevier.com/Canada/Varcarolis/psychiatric/

OBJECTIVES

1. Discuss four theories of eating disorders.
2. Compare and contrast the signs and symptoms (clinical picture) of anorexia nervosa and bulimia nervosa.
3. Identify three life-threatening conditions, stated in terms of nursing diagnoses, for a patient with an eating disorder.
4. Identify three realistic outcome criteria for (1) a patient with anorexia nervosa and (2) a patient with bulimia nervosa.
5. Describe therapeutic interventions appropriate for anorexia nervosa and bulimia nervosa in the acute phase and long-term phase of treatment.
6. Explain the basic premise of cognitive behavioural therapy in the treatment of eating disorders.
7. Differentiate between the long-term prognoses of anorexia nervosa, bulimia nervosa, and binge eating disorder.

KEY TERMS AND CONCEPTS

anorexia nervosa
binge eating disorder
bulimia nervosa
feeding disorder
ideal body weight

Of all the psychiatric disorders, eating disorders may be the most perplexing. Food, like water and air give us life. The eating and sharing of food are usually pleasurable and culturally important. It is difficult for many of us to understand how people could starve themselves or induce vomiting and seem to have little regard for how it affects them physically and socially. Cases of anorexia nervosa are documented in ancient writings; however, bulimia and binge eating necessitate an abundance of food and therefore may be more modern-age eating disorders. Many theories of the etiology of these disorders have been postulated, but to date the reasons behind the behaviour are still a mystery that drives research. In this chapter we focus on the three main types of eating disorders, anorexia nervosa, bulimia nervosa, and binge eating disorder, and introduce feeding disorders (American Psychiatric Association, 2013) with a brief description.

CLINICAL PICTURE

There is not one eating disorder but rather several subtypes, predominantly identified as anorexia nervosa, bulimia nervosa, binge eating disorder, and eating disorder not otherwise specified (NOS). All types of disordered eating have both cognitive and behavioural components (Morris & Anderson, 2021). Psychiatric classifications such as the *Diagnostic and Statistical Manual of Mental Disorders (DSM-5)* (American Psychiatric Association, 2013) and *International Classification of Diseases (ICD-11)* (World Health Organization, 2018) are reliant on symptoms and treatment is tied to existing categorization of each eating disorder. It is important to keep in mind that not meeting all the listed criteria does not automatically exclude an eating disorder and an individuals' diagnosis may drift across categories during the course of illness.

 HOW A NURSE HELPED ME
A Patient's Challenges

> When I was 10 years old, I began overeating. It was at that time that my best friend moved away; I had other friends, but they were not the same. I am not exactly sure why, but eating helped me relax. The food demanded nothing of me, it did not judge me; it did not need me to do anything; it allowed me just to be.
>
> Fortunately, as soon as I finished university, I had no problem finding my first teaching job. It was in a town approximately 300 kilometres away. Moving away was hard for me, but that was where the work was. I was still eating when I felt stressed, and I certainly felt stressed with the new job, in a new town, and with no friends. I was also starting to feel depressed. It was at that point that I went to the local community mental health centre for help. I knew I was smart, as I was successful at school and university, but this was one area I just couldn't seem to get a handle on. I met with a nurse who asked me a number of questions related to my mood, thoughts, feelings, and energy. The nurse helped me change my relationship with food by helping me understand how my thoughts and experiences affected how much I ate. She taught me how to use a journal to record my thoughts and experiences. It helped me identify my thoughts and feelings about food, eating, and not eating. I always hated counting calories and was worried that I would have to do that; to my surprise, we talked about my daily intake of food in relationship to the nutrients my body needed. I was counting food groups and portion sizes, but not calories. Another trick she taught me to manage my stress-related food consumption was to plan ahead for the times and places where I would be eating. This really helped because, when I felt stress, I knew just when I would be eating again, so I did not panic and binge-eat. The nurse did not judge me or criticize me because I was overweight; she listened and took me seriously.

Individuals with **anorexia nervosa** refuse to maintain a minimally normal weight for their height and express an intense fear of gaining weight. The term *anorexia* is a misnomer because it literally means a loss of appetite, which is not specifically the case. Rather, in anorexia nervosa the clinical condition is a behavioural restriction of food intake or, for others, involves binge eating and purging.

Anorexia nervosa is a chronic illness that waxes and wanes. The 1-year relapse rate approaches 50%, and long-term studies show that up to 40% of patients continue to meet some criteria for anorexia nervosa after 4 years (Harrington et al., 2015). Recovery is evaluated as a stage in the process rather than a fixed event. Factors that influence the stage of recovery include percentage of ideal body weight that has been achieved, the extent to which self-worth is defined by shape and weight, and the amount of disruption existing in the patient's personal life.

Individuals with **bulimia nervosa** engage in repeated episodes of binge eating followed by compensatory behaviours, such as self-induced vomiting; misuse of laxatives, diuretics, or other medications; fasting; or excessive exercise. This disorder is characterized by a significant disturbance in the perception of body shape and weight.

Individuals with **binge eating disorder** engage in repeated episodes of binge eating, after which they experience significant distress; they do not regularly use compensatory behaviours, such as those seen in patients with bulimia nervosa. Many individuals have combinations of eating disorder symptoms that are not sufficient for a specific diagnosis of anorexia nervosa, bulimia nervosa, or binge eating disorder; these individuals are therefore diagnosed as having an eating disorder NOS. While distinct, there are a number of both cognitive and behavioural similarities among eating problems, the defining characteristics of which are highlighted in Box 16.1.

Other problems related to eating are identified as **feeding disorders**, where the patient experiences an inability to or difficulty in eating or drinking sufficient quantities to maintain optimal nutritional status. These disorders have a typical onset in childhood and continue into adulthood. They include avoidant/restrictive food intake disorder, pica, and rumination disorder.

Avoidant/Restrictive Food Intake Disorder

Up to 40% of all toddlers will experience mealtime difficulties that resolve spontaneously with or without caregiver support and education. About 5% to 20% of children without other disorders may have feeding disorders. Pre-maturity, failure to thrive, autism, and genetic syndromes result in ranges of 40% to 80% with feeding disorders (Romano, 2015). There are no unifying etiologies for food refusal. Lack of interest in eating or food may result in weight loss, growth delay, and nutritional deficiency. It most commonly begins in infancy or early childhood and may continue into adulthood. Anxiety and family anxiety are risk factors.

The primary treatment modality is some form of behavioural modification to increase regular food consumption. Families caring for a child with a feeding disorder often need support and education in specific behavioural techniques, but family therapy is not usually necessary. Treating anxiety and depressive symptoms may be helpful in some cases.

Pica

Pica is the persistent eating of substances such as dirt, chalk, yarn, glue, or paint that have no nutritional value. In institutionalized children the rate of this disorder may be as high as 26%. Pica usually begins in early childhood and lasts for a few months. Eating non-food items may interfere with eating nutritional items. Eating non-food items can also be dangerous. Paint may contain lead and result in brain damage. Objects that cannot be digested, such as stones, can result in intestinal blockage. Sharp objects such as paper clips can result in intestinal damage or laceration. Bacteria from dirt or other soiled objects can result in serious infection. Tooth decay may result from stomach acids. Monitoring the child's eating behaviour is obviously an essential aspect of treating this problem. Behavioural interventions such as rewarding appropriate eating are helpful.

Rumination Disorder

Rumination disorder is characterized by undigested food being returned to the mouth. It is then rechewed, reswallowed, or spit out. It may be diagnosed after 1 month of symptoms. Rumination symptoms can occur at any age, and the onset in infants is between 3 and 12 months. Intellectual development disorder is associated with rumination. Neglect is a predisposing factor to the development of this disorder. The symptoms frequently remit spontaneously but may become habitual and result in severe malnutrition and even death.

Interventions include repositioning infants and small children during feeding. Improving the interaction between caregiver and child and making mealtimes a pleasant experience often reduce rumination. Distracting the child when the behaviour starts is also helpful. Family therapy may be required.

EPIDEMIOLOGY

It is extremely difficult to determine the specific number of people afflicted with eating disorders, as fewer than half seek health care for their illness. Many people with disordered eating patterns do not meet full *DSM-5* criteria and are not included in the statistics gathered in epidemiological reports. It is estimated that 725 800 to 1 088 700 Canadians meet the diagnostic criteria for an eating disorder at any given time (National Initiative for Eating Disorders, 2017). However, it is important to keep in mind that any reported statistics are likely grossly underestimated given that shame and secrecy are associated with eating disorders. The COVID-19 pandemic has exacerbated the burden of eating disorders world wide (Zipfel et al., 2022). Self-reports, misdiagnosis or under diagnosis may all play a role in limiting our understanding of the prevalence of eating disorders.

BOX 16.1 CHARACTERISTICS OF EATING PROBLEMS

Anorexia Nervosa	Bulimia Nervosa	Binge Eating
• Intense fear of weight gain • Distorted body image • Restricted calories with significantly low body mass index (BMI) • Subtypes: • Restricting (no consistent bulimic features) • Binge eating/purging type (primarily restriction, some bulimic behaviours)	• Recurrent episodes of uncontrollable binging • Inappropriate compensatory behaviours: vomiting, laxatives, diuretics, or exercise • Self-image largely influenced by body image and external validation	• Recurrent episodes of uncontrollable binging without compensatory behaviours • Binging episodes induce guilt, depression, embarrassment, or disgust and are often preceded by emotional distress with poor coping

Female sex, younger age, sexual and physical abuse, participation in esthetic or weight-oriented sports, and heritability are found to be most consistently associated with higher eating disorder prevalence and incidence (Dahlgren et al., 2017; Santomauro et al., 2021). Most eating disorders begin in the early teens to mid-twenties, commonly following puberty, although bulimia generally occurs in later adolescence. Anorexia nervosa may start early (between ages 7 and 12), but bulimia nervosa is rarely seen in children younger than 12 years. For women, the lifetime incidence of anorexia nervosa is 0.9%, and the lifetime incidence for men is 0.24% (Rosenvinge & Petterson, 2015). The 12-month prevalence of bulimia nervosa among young women is 1% to 1.5%. The lifetime incidence of bulimia nervosa for women is 2.3%, and the lifetime incidence for men is 0.5% (Rosenvinge & Petterson, 2015). Bulimia commonly begins in later adolescence, when the prevalence peaks up to young adulthood. Onset of bulimia nervosa is rare in children younger than 12 and adults older than 40 years of age.

Binge eating disorder is the most common eating disorder. For women, the lifetime incidence of binge eating disorder is 3.6%, and the lifetime incidence for men is 2.1% (Rosenvinge & Petterson, 2015). Gender differences have been examined, with men being more likely to report overeating; women being significantly more likely than men to report body checking and avoidance, binge eating, and self-induced vomiting (Smith et al., 2021). The presence of binge eating disorder is higher in overweight populations (3%) than in the general population (2%).

Eating disorders among middle-aged women seem to be common, with a greater number of diagnoses of binge eating disorder and eating disorder NOS as compared to the "classical" diagnoses of anorexia and bulimia nervosa. Middle-aged women are seeking treatment for chronic, recurrent, or late onset eating disorders but may be overlooked as a diagnosis by health care providers (Samuels et al., 2019). Eating disturbances also appear to be underassessed and underdiagnosed among older men (those ages 40 to 75 years of age), though extreme dietary and exercise behaviours, more common in this population, represent an under-recognized form of purging behaviour (Mangweth-Matzek et al., 2016).

Patterns of eating disorders, and implications for psychiatric mental health nursing practice, are also prevalent among university and elite sports athletes, as well as among dance and theatre performers. A substantial amount of evidence suggests that collegiate and elite athletes involved in weight-sensitive sports are at particular risk of developing eating disorders (Karrer et al., 2020; Wells et al., 2020), as are those involved in aesthetic performance work (Francisco, 2018).

Comparing eating disorders across cultures is often complicated and contradictory. The majority of eating disorder assessment, screening, and diagnostic tools have been developed among White female populations. However, as new tools are being developed, trends are showing that while there is a stabilization of the incidence of anorexia nervosa and possibly lower incidence rates of bulimia nervosa in White North American and Northern European groups; an increase in rates are appearing in Arab (Melisse et al., 2020) and Asian countries (Nakai et al., 2018). Middle Eastern and North African regions continue to develop and undergo epidemiologic transition and cultural change, the burden of eating disorders in these countries is rising (Erskine et al., 2016). Additionally, there are increasing rates of binge eating and bulimia nervosa in Hispanic and Black American minority groups in North America (Galmiche et al., 2019).

Recent eating disorder trends are also emerging regarding individuals who identify as LGBTQ2 (lesbian, gay, bisexual, transgender, queer, and two-spirit), Black and racialized people, people with disabilities, and non-binary communities. In a systematic review LGBTQ2 populations generally demonstrate higher rates of disordered eating with an elevated risk for disordered eating pathology among transgender or ethnic minorities (Calzo et al., 2017), which may be attributed to increased stress from stigma and prejudice (Parker & Harringer, 2020). However, further research in this area is needed as there is an absence of data examining eating disorders by sexual orientation among individuals of diverse gender identities.

Although patients with eating disorders are at risk for medical complications that may result in death, the major cause of death among those affected by eating disorders is suicide. Adolescents diagnosed with anorexia nervosa or bulimia nervosa have a suicide rate that is more than six times greater than the norm for their age group. Overall, among all ages, people with bulimia nervosa make more suicide attempts, and there is a higher incidence of completion in those with anorexia nervosa (Cliffe et al., 2020).

Self-injurious behaviours are also frequent in people with eating disorders, with higher rates among those whose disorders include binge and purge behaviours and an overall lifetime prevalence of 27.3% in patients with eating disorders (Cucchi et al., 2016). Self-injurious behaviours, which may or may not include suicidal intent, are especially high among adolescents with eating disorders. Overexercising, often considered a self-injurious behaviour among individuals with eating disorders, may also pose additional risk beyond the physical consequence of the activity itself, contributing to a higher risk for suicide (Anderson et al., 2017). These alarming rates highlight the need for ongoing safety assessment and evaluation for suicidal ideation and self-injurious behaviours in persons with eating disorders and for routinely taking a family psychiatric history for all patients. This complex and emerging epidemiological landscape underscores the public mental health significance of all types of eating disorders.

RESEARCH HIGHLIGHT

Effects of Yoga on Eating Disorders: A Systematic Review

Issue

Yoga practice can be relaxing and have a positive influence on body image. However, individuals with eating disorders may turn to yoga to burn calories or to suppress hunger.

Purpose of Study

The aim of the review was to systematically assess the effectiveness and safety of yoga in patients with eating disorders and other individuals with disordered eating and/or body dissatisfaction.

Methods

The Preferred Reporting Items for Systematic Reviews and Meta-Analyses guidelines and recommendations of the Cochrane Collaboration were used for the reporting structure of this review. Randomized controlled trials, non-randomized controlled clinical trials, and longitudinal observational studies were eligible. No language restrictions were applied. Studies were eligible only if they were published as full paper. Studies on adults, children, and adolescents with a diagnosed eating disorder, including but not limited to anorexia nervosa, bulimia, binge-eating disorder, were eligible. Studies involving participants with disordered eating and/or body dissatisfaction but without a formal diagnosis of an eating disorder were also eligible for inclusion as were studies involving participants with comorbid physical or mental health disorders. Twelve studies involving a total of 495 participants met the inclusion criteria and were included in the qualitative analysis

Key Findings

The review found that no strong recommendation can be made for or against yoga for patients with eating disorders. Yoga can however be preliminarily considered as an additional treatment option in multi-modal psychiatric treatment programs. Excessive yoga practice by patients with eating disorders should be prevented and safety of the intervention should be closely monitored.

Implications for Nursing Practice
Nurses are often responsible for developing and implementing health promotion and prevention programs. Being aware of the benefits and drawbacks for individuals with eating disorders is important when designing and suggesting interventions.

Source: Ostermann, T., Vogel, H., Boehm, K., et al. (2019). Effects of yoga on eating disorders—A systematic review. *Complementary Therapies in Medicine, 46,* 73–80. https://doi.org/10.1016/j.ctim.2019.07.021

COMORBIDITY

Depression and anxiety are common comorbid conditions in people with all types of eating disorders. The estimated lifetime prevalence of mood disorders in anorexia nervosa ranges from 31% to 89%, and in bulimia nervosa ranges from 24% to 90%. The fact that depressive symptoms accompany any type of starvation makes determining an exact prevalence difficult.

The incidence of obsessive-compulsive disorder (OCD) has been reported to be as high as 25% in patients with anorexia nervosa. The OCD symptoms centre on food pre-occupation and may be manifested in collecting cookbooks, preparing elaborate meals for others, and hoarding food. Anxiety disorders, particularly social phobia, are also common. In addition, significant associations have been found between risk for an eating disorder and alcohol dependence, as well as the lifetime abuse of and dependence on illicit drugs (Bahji et al., 2019).

People with eating disorders who are also living with depression, a substance use disorder, or difficulty with impulse control are at greater risk for relapse. There is some evidence that the younger the person is when anorexic symptoms begin, the better the chance for positive outcomes is (Lindstedt et al., 2017).

Personality disorders may occur in 42% to 75% of people with eating disorders. There is a high rate of avoidant personality disorders with all eating disorders. Avoidance fits the clinical picture of being overly concerned with acceptance and approval and fearing criticism or rejection. Patients with anorexia nervosa are more likely to have a Cluster C personality disorder (avoidant, dependent, obsessive-compulsive, or passive-aggressive) (Gárriz et al., 2021). Obsessive-compulsive and dependent personality disorders are also common in patients with bulimia. Borderline personality disorder is common in patients with binge eating disorder. See Chapter 19 for more information on personality disorders.

There have been several significant conclusions in the research literature examining the relationship between trauma and eating disorders. Associated traumas now include not only childhood sexual abuse but also other forms of abuse and neglect and are more common in eating disorders involving bingeing and purging behaviours. Also, the research findings have been extended to boys and men with eating disorders.

ETIOLOGY

The eating disorders, anorexia nervosa, bulimia nervosa, binge eating disorder, and eating disorder NOS, are actually entities or syndromes and are not considered to be discrete diseases. Experts tend to agree that there is no single cause of eating disorders. Eating disorders often result from an attempt to regulate mood, especially anxiety and depression. There is a complex and dynamic interplay between biological or genetic predispositions, psychological factors, environmental factors, and sociocultural influences that are involved in the development of an eating disorder (Mayhew et al., 2018). A number of theories attempt to explain eating disorders.

Biological Factors
Genetic
There is a strong genetic link to eating disorders. A review of relevant studies has suggested that the heritability of anorexia nervosa is 60% (Yilmaz et al., 2015). A genetic vulnerability may lead to poor affect and impulse control or to an underlying neurotransmitter dysfunction, but researchers have not discovered any single causative gene to date. It is likely that a gene–environment interaction may predispose a person to have symptoms of eating disorders and even confer a risk for developing full-blown eating disorders (Yilmaz et al., 2015).

Neurobiological
Research demonstrates that altered brain serotonin function contributes to dysregulation of appetite, mood, and impulse control in the eating disorders. Patients with eating disorders consistently exhibit personality traits of perfectionism, obsessive-compulsiveness, and dysphoric mood, all of which are modulated through serotonin pathways in the brain. Because these traits appear to begin in childhood, before the onset of actual eating disorder symptoms, and persist into recovery, experts believe that they contribute to a vulnerability to disordered eating (Kappou et al., 2021).

Tryptophan, an amino acid essential to serotonin synthesis, is available only through diet. A normal diet boosts serotonin in the brain and regulates mood. Temporary drops in dietary tryptophan may actually relieve symptoms of anxiety and dysphoria and provide a reward for caloric restriction. Restricting food intake in this way becomes powerfully reinforcing because it provides a temporary respite from dysphoric mood, setting up a feedback loop that further establishes the disordered eating behaviour (Kappou et al., 2021). The dietary need for tryptophan may account for the fact that antidepressants that boost serotonin do not improve mood symptoms until after an underweight patient has been restored to 90% of optimal weight.

Newer brain imaging capabilities allow for better understanding of the etiological factors of anorexia nervosa. There is a consistent finding that patients with eating disorders who are acutely ill and those who have recovered show differences in the frontal, cingulated, temporal, or parietal regions of the brain, or in a combination of these regions, in comparison to controls. Relative to other psychiatric disorders, however, there are few brain scanning studies of the eating disorders, so conclusions are tentative. This is, however, a promising area of research that may contribute to the diagnosis and treatment of this difficult disease. Studies so far suggest that there is a difference in the reward and executive function parts of the brains of people with anorexia nervosa (Kappou et al., 2021).

Psychological Factors
Because anorexia nervosa was observed primarily in girls approaching puberty, early psychoanalytic theories linked the symptoms to an unconscious aversion to sexuality. By maintaining a child-like body, the patient avoids the anxiety associated with developing into a mature sexual being. Throughout the 1900s, many authors examined the family dynamics of these patients and concluded that a failure to separate from parents and a rebellion against the maternal bond explained the disordered eating behaviours. Further work by Bruch (1978) explored the symptoms as a defence against overwhelming feelings of ineffectiveness and powerlessness. Even with further insight into the intrapsychic

origin of the behaviour, the process of psychoanalysis, with the goal of making unconscious processes conscious, failed to effect a cure for these syndromes (Vrabel & Zeigler-Hill, 2020).

Family theorists maintain that eating disorders are a problem of the whole family, and often the symptoms in the child serve to take the attention away from a distressed marriage. Families with a child who has anorexia are often described as enmeshed and perfectionistic; the child feels smothered by protectiveness and at the same time abandoned. The literature gives empirical support for family therapy methods in the treatment of children and adolescents with eating disorders (Haworth-Hoeppner, 2017).

Currently, cognitive behavioural theorists suggest that eating disorders are based on learned behaviour that has positive reinforcement. For example, a mildly overweight 14-year-old has the flu and loses a little weight. She returns to school, and her friends say, "Wow, you look great," and when people say, "Wow, you look really skinny," she still hears, "Wow, you look great." Now she purposefully strives to lose weight. Her behaviour is powerfully reinforced by these comments despite the fact that her health is at risk. Emotional disregulation has been found to be associated with the cognitive (rather than the behavioural) symptoms of those with all types of eating disorders (Pisetsky et al., 2017).

Psychological trauma appears to be strongly associated with eating disorders of all types. There is an increased prevalence of sexual trauma for individuals with eating disorders. Recent evidence suggests that sexual trauma precedes and contributes to the development of eating disorders, however further research is needed to assess the potential causal role that sexual trauma may play in the etiology of eating disorders (Pop et al., 2020).

Environmental Factors

The Western cultural ideal that equates feminine beauty with tall, thin models has received much attention in the media as an etiology for eating disorders. Studies have shown that culture influences the development of self-concept and satisfaction with body size. Further, culture and political support of corporate agencies shape the food regulation and marketing industries. In this context a 2016 Senate report revealed that almost two-thirds of Canadian adults are now considered either overweight or obese. Canada ranks third among 46 countries for obesity prevalence, measured at 25.8% of adults (Organisation for Economic Co-operation and Development [OECD], 2017). Obesity rates among children are also dangerously high, with nearly 13% of children between the ages of 5 and 17 being obese and another 20% being overweight. These numbers reflect at least a twofold increase in the proportion of obese adults and a threefold increase in the proportion of obese children since 1980, a trend that is alarming, has a number of health and social implications, and has prompted a concerted effort to address the complex issues at a social level of intervention (Canadian Senate, 2016).

Record numbers of men and women are on diets to reduce body weight, but no study has been able to explain why only an estimated 0.3 to 3% of the population develops an eating disorder. Although a causal link between cultural norms or the social ideal of thinness portrayed in the media and eating disorders has not been proven (Doris et al., 2015), all patients with eating disorders have low self-esteem that is negatively affected by their inability to conform to an impossible cultural standard of beauty (Uchôa et al., 2019).

Disordered forms of eating behaviour have emerged in the broader society and transnationally, in settings and cultures where eating disorders were not previously identified. Cultural transitions in response to societal changes, as well as the necessity to adapt to changing cultural norms, can produce distress that manifests in some as disordered eating.

CONSIDERING CULTURE
Weight Bias/Weight Stigma

Although cultural beliefs about physical beauty do not cause eating disorders, they influence self-esteem and set the standard of beauty for men and women. An unhealthy cultural ideal therefore can pose health risks if not addressed.

For centuries, body weight was an indicator of wealth and the availability of food, so the ideal was to achieve a large body. However, in many countries thinness is equated with beauty. Eating disorders are on the rise in non-Western societies. Fear of weight gain can drive eating behaviors that end up actually causing weight gain. Weight bias also known as weight stigma, refers to negative attitudes, beliefs, and behaviors toward individuals on judging their weight (Cheng et al., 2018). Weight stigma may cause overeating. Studies have shown that the more a person feels stigmatized, the more severe binge eating symptoms they experience. In Asian countries eating disorders and weight bias have also been found to be pervasive, and specifically in Hong Kong, similar to that of the West (Cheng et al., 2018).

Nurses must be aware of weight bias when planning care for individuals with eating disorders. Nurses may endorse strong beliefs that weight lies solely under an individual's control without taking into consideration how the social determinants play a role. Nurses' unconscious beliefs may lead to discriminatory behaviours towards individuals with eating disorders. These behaviours can be subtle or overt such as being subjected to unsolicited weight loss advice and commentary when recording an individual's weight.

Source: Cheng, M. Y., Wang, S. M., Lam, Y. Y., et al. (2018). The relationships between weight bias, perceived weight stigma, eating behavior, and psychological distress among undergraduate students in Hong Kong. *The Journal of nervous and mental disease, 206*(9), 705–710.

ANOREXIA NERVOSA

Anorexia nervosa and bulimia nervosa are two separate syndromes that present two clinical pictures on assessment. Box 16.2 lists several thoughts and behaviours associated with anorexia nervosa, and Table 16.1 identifies clinical signs and symptoms of anorexia nervosa found on assessment, together with their causes.

APPLICATION OF THE NURSING PROCESS

Assessment

Eating disorders are serious and, in extreme cases, can lead to death. Box 16.3 identifies a number of medical complications that can occur in individuals with anorexia nervosa and the laboratory findings that may result. Because the eating behaviours in these conditions are so extreme, hospitalization may become necessary. Box 16.4 identifies

BOX 16.2 Thoughts and Behaviours Associated With Anorexia Nervosa

- Terror of gaining weight
- Pre-occupation with food
- View of self as fat even when emaciated
- Peculiar handling of food:
  - Cutting food into small bits
  - Pushing pieces of food around plate
- Possible development of rigorous exercise regimen
- Possible self-induced vomiting, use of laxatives and diuretics
- Cognition so disturbed that individual judges self-worth by their weight

TABLE 16.1 Possible Signs and Symptoms of Anorexia Nervosa

Clinical Presentation	Cause
Low weight	Caloric restriction, excessive exercising
Amenorrhea	Low weight
Yellow skin	Hypercarotenemia
Lanugo	Starvation
Cold extremities	Starvation
Peripheral edema	Hypoalbuminemia and refeeding
Muscle weakening	Starvation, electrolyte imbalance
Constipation	Starvation
Abnormal laboratory values (low triiodothyronine, thyroxine levels)	Starvation
Abnormal computed tomography (CT) scans, electroencephalography (EEG) changes	Starvation
Cardiovascular abnormalities (hypotension, bradycardia, heart failure)	Starvation, dehydration; Electrolyte imbalance
Impaired renal function	Dehydration
Hypokalemia (low potassium)	Starvation
Anemic pancytopenia	Starvation
Decreased bone density	Estrogen deficiency, low calcium intake

BOX 16.3 Medical Complications of Anorexia Nervosa

- Bradycardia
- Orthostatic changes in pulse or blood pressure
- Cardiac arrhythmias
- Prolonged QT interval and ST-T wave abnormalities
- Peripheral neuropathy
- Acrocyanosis
- Symptomatic hypotension
- Leukopenia
- Lymphocytosis
- Carotenemia (elevated carotene levels in blood), which produces skin with yellow pallor
- Hypokalemic alkalosis (with self-induced vomiting or use of laxatives and diuretics)
- Elevated serum bicarbonate levels, hypochloremia, and hypokalemia
- Electrolyte imbalances, which lead to fatigue, weakness, and lethargy
- Osteoporosis, indicated by decrease in bone density
- Fatty degeneration of liver, indicated by elevation of serum enzyme levels
- Elevated cholesterol levels
- Amenorrhea
- Abnormal thyroid functioning
- Hematuria
- Proteinuria

Source: Data from Mitchell, J. E., & Wonderlich, S. A. (2014). Feeding and eating disorders. In R. E. Hales, S. C. Yudofsky, & L. Weiss Roberts (Eds.), *Textbook of psychiatry* (6th ed., pp. 557–587). Washington, DC: American Psychiatric Publishing.

BOX 16.4 Criteria for Hospital Admission of Patients With Eating Disorders

Physical Criteria
- Weight loss, <85% below ideal
- Rapid decline in weight with food refusal even if not <85% below ideal
- Inability to gain weight with outpatient treatment
- Temperature <36°C or <97°F
- Heart rate <40 beats per minute
- Systolic blood pressure <90/60 mm Hg
- Severe dehydration
- Hypokalemia (serum potassium <3 mEq/L) or other electrolyte imbalance
- Glucose <60 mg/dL; poorly controlled diabetes
- Hepatic, renal, or cardiovascular organ compromise requiring acute treatment

Psychiatric Criteria
- Risk for suicide
- Failure to adhere to treatment contract
- Severe depression or other psychiatric disorder that would require hospitalization
- Family crisis or dysfunction

Source: American Psychiatric Association (APA). (2006). *Practice guideline for the treatment of patients with eating disorders* (3rd ed.). Washington, DC: Author.

physical and psychiatric criteria for hospitalization of an individual with an eating disorder. Fundamental to the care of individuals with eating disorders is establishing and maintaining a therapeutic alliance. Developing this partnership will take both time and diplomacy on the part of the nurse. In treating patients who have been sexually abused or who have otherwise been victims of boundary violations it is critical that the nurse and other health care workers respect the impact of the patient's history of trauma and associated complex eating disorder (Rodgers et al., 2019). Establishing therapeutic boundaries and practising with a trauma-informed care approach will facilitate the helping relationship and enhance outcomes (see Unit 5 for more on trauma interventions).

General Assessment

Individuals with the binge–purge type of anorexia nervosa may present with severe electrolyte imbalance (as a result of purging) and enter the health care system through admission to an intensive care unit. The patient with anorexia will be severely underweight and may have growth of fine, downy hair (lanugo) on the face and back. The patient will also have mottled, cool skin on the extremities and low blood pressure, pulse, and temperature readings, consistent with a malnourished, dehydrated state (see Table 16.1).

As with any comprehensive psychiatric nursing assessment, a complete evaluation of biopsychosocial function is mandatory. The areas to be covered include the patient's:

- Perception of the problem
- Eating habits
- History of dieting
- Methods used to achieve weight control (restricting, purging, exercising)
- Value attached to a specific shape and weight
- Interpersonal and social functioning
- Mental status and physiological parameters

INTEGRATIVE THERAPY

Ma Huang

In an attempt to lose weight and fight hunger many patients with eating disorders turn to weight-loss products that contain herbs, such as Ma Huang, the Chinese name for the *Ephedra sinica* plant. Health Canada has issued several health advisories warning consumers not to use unauthorized products that contain ephedrine or ephedra in combination with caffeine or other stimulants due to the risk of serious adverse effects. Canadian retailers have also been reminded not to sell unauthorized products containing these ingredients; however, they may still be contained in natural products sold over the Internet. In a small study of patients with eating disorders 42% of patients who actually experienced adverse effects while using ephedra products decided to continue taking the herb.

Source: Steffen, K. J., Roerig, J. L., Mitchell, J. E., et al. (2006). A survey of herbal and alternative medication use among participants with eating-disorder symptoms. *International Journal of Eating Disorders, 39*, 741–746. https://doi.org/10.1002/eat.20233

Self-Assessment

When caring for the patient with anorexia, you may find it difficult to appreciate the compelling force of the illness, incorrectly believing that weight restriction, bingeing, and purging are self-imposed. If we see such self-destructive behaviours as a lifestyle or personal choice, it is only natural to blame the patient for any consequent health problems. The common personality traits of these patients, perfectionism, obsessive thoughts and actions relating to food, intense feelings of shame, people pleasing, and the need to have complete control over their therapy, pose additional challenges.

In your efforts to motivate patients and take advantage of their decision to seek help and be healthier take care not to allow encouragement to cross the line into authoritarianism and the assumption of a parental role. A patient's terror at gaining weight and their resistance to clinical interventions may engender significant frustration in the nurse struggling to build a therapeutic relationship and be empathic. Guard against any tendency to be coercive in your approach, and be aware that one of the primary goals of treatment, weight gain, is the very thing the patient fears. When patients appear to be resistant to change, it is helpful to acknowledge the constant struggle that so characterizes the treatment.

ASSESSMENT GUIDELINES

Anorexia Nervosa

Determine whether:
- The patient has a medical or psychiatric condition that warrants hospitalization (see Box 16.4)
- A thorough physical examination with appropriate blood work has been done
- Other medical conditions have been ruled out
- The patient is amenable to receiving or adherent to appropriate therapeutic modalities
- The family and patient need further teaching or information regarding the patient's treatment plan
- The patient and family want to participate in a support group and have been given a referral

Diagnosis

Imbalanced nutrition: less than body requirements is usually the most appropriate initial nursing diagnosis for individuals with anorexia (Herdman & Kamitsuru, 2014). This diagnosis generates further nursing diagnoses, for example, *Decreased cardiac output*, *Risk for injury* (electrolyte imbalance), and *Risk for imbalanced fluid volume* (which would take first priority when problems are addressed). Other nursing diagnoses include *Anxiety*, *Chronic low self-esteem*, *Disturbed body image*, *Deficient knowledge*, *Ineffective coping*, *Powerlessness*, and *Hopelessness*.

Outcomes Identification

To evaluate the effectiveness of treatment, outcome criteria are established. Relevant categories of the *Nursing Outcomes Classification (NOC)* (Moorhead et al., 2013) include *Weight gain behaviour*, *Weight maintenance behaviour*, *Anxiety self-control*, *Nutritional status: nutrient intake*, and *Self-esteem*. Refer to Table 16.2 for examples of short-term NOC indicators for the patient with anorexia nervosa.

Planning

Planning is affected by the acuity of the patient's situation. When a patient with anorexia is experiencing extreme electrolyte imbalance or weighs less than 85% of their ideal body weight, the plan is to provide immediate medical stabilization, most likely in an inpatient unit. A person's ideal body weight is based chiefly on height but is modified by factors such as gender, age, build, and degree of muscular development. With the initiation of therapeutic nutrition, malnourished patients may need treatment on a medical unit, owing to *refeeding syndrome*, a potentially catastrophic treatment complication involving a metabolic alteration in serum electrolytes, vitamin deficiencies, and sodium retention.

TABLE 16.2 NOC Outcomes Related to Anorexia Nervosa

Nursing Outcome and Definition	Short-Term Indicators
Nutritional status: nutrient intake: Nutrient intake to meet metabolic needs	Caloric intake
	Protein intake
	Fat intake
	Carbohydrate intake
Weight gain behaviour: Personal actions to gain weight following voluntary or involuntary significant weight loss	Selects a healthy target weight
	Commits to a healthy eating plan
	Monitors exercise for caloric requirements
	Sets achievable weight gain goals
Anxiety self-control: Personal action to eliminate or reduce feelings of apprehension, tension, or uneasiness from an unidentifiable source.	Monitors intensity of anxiety
	Plans coping strategies for stressful situations
	Uses effective coping strategies
Self-esteem: Personal judgement of self-worth	Verbalization of self-acceptance
	Description of self
	Acceptance of compliments from others
	Feelings about self-worth

Source: Data from Moorhead, S., Swanson, E., Johnson, M., & Maas, M. L. (Eds.). (2018). *Nursing Outcomes Classification (NOC): Measurement of health outcomes* (6th ed.). St. Louis: Elsevier.

Once a patient is medically stable, the plan addresses the psychological issues underlying the eating disorder, usually on an outpatient basis. The nature of the treatment is determined by the intensity of the symptoms, which may vary over time, and the experienced disruption in the patient's life.

Discharge planning (living arrangements, school, work, finances, follow-up care) is a critical component of treatment. Often family members also benefit from counselling.

Implementation
Acute Care
Typically, a patient with an eating disorder is admitted to the inpatient psychiatric facility when in a crisis state. The health care team's initial focus, then, depends on the results of a comprehensive assessment that addresses the physical, cognitive, psychological, and social components as well as general mental status baseline. Any acute psychiatric symptoms, such as suicidal ideation, are addressed immediately. The nurse is challenged to establish trust and monitor the patient's eating pattern. Norris and colleagues (2013) conducted a survey of intensive eating disorder programs specifically for adolescents across Canada, ultimately surveying 11 programs with a 90-item survey that addressed program characteristics and components, governance, staffing, referrals, assessments, therapeutic modalities in place, nutritional practices, and treatment protocols. They discovered a wide diversity of programming available but also the lack of a unified approach or protocols to intensive eating disorder treatment in youth.

Psychosocial Interventions
After addressing any acute symptoms, the patient with anorexia begins a weight-restoration program that allows for incremental weight gain. Based on the patient's height, a treatment goal is set at 90% of ideal body weight, the weight at which most women are able to menstruate.

As patients begin to eat again, they ideally participate in milieu therapy, in which the cognitive distortions (errors in thinking) that perpetuate the illness are consistently addressed by all members of the interprofessional team. Box 16.5 identifies some types of cognitive distortions characteristic of people with eating disorders. Focus should be on the eating behaviour and underlying feelings of anxiety, dysphoria, low self-esteem, and lack of control. When possible, the distortions in body image are avoided because attempts to change this perception are often misinterpreted, as shown in the following vignette.

> **VIGNETTE**
> Alicia, a 17-year-old cheerleader, did not come to treatment for weight loss until she fainted at a football game. She insisted that she only needed to "get more energy, not get fat." When the nurse pointed out that Alicia's ribs were clearly visible and that her backbone looked like a skeleton's, Alicia grinned and said, "Thank you."

Pharmacological Interventions
Research has not yet demonstrated that medications are effective as the first course of treatment of anorexia nervosa. Further studies are needed to determine if there is a medication that is effective to treat the core symptoms of the disorder. Despite the lack of rigorous scientific studies, the selective serotonin reuptake inhibitor (SSRI) fluoxetine (Prozac) has been found clinically useful in reducing obsessive-compulsive behaviour after the patient has reached a maintenance weight. Conventional antipsychotics such as chlorpromazine or haloperidol may be helpful for delusional or overactive patients. Atypical antipsychotic medications such as olanzapine (Zyprexa) are helpful in improving mood and decreasing obsessional behaviours and resistance to weight gain.

Health Teaching and Health Promotion
Self-care activities are an important part of the treatment plan. These activities include learning more constructive coping skills, improving social skills, and developing problem-solving and decision-making skills. These skills become the focus of therapy sessions. The following vignette illustrates the need for supportive education.

> **VIGNETTE**
> A nursing assessment of three young women and one young man in a nutrition group finds that all of the participants are very knowledgeable about the caloric value of common foods; as a group, they all avoid any "fatty" foods. The topic of fat-soluble vitamins and the consequences of vitamin deficiencies on the body introduced new information to all of the participants, and one of the young women started to cry, saying, "I had no idea I was doing that to my body." This show of emotion promoted a supportive interaction among the other group members as they shared their own stories of symptoms they could now identify as vitamin deficits.

Milieu Management: Reconceptualized as an Optimal Healing Environment
Milieu is a French word that means middle place or middle ground, which brings to mind a safe place, where every component of the person's environment is therapeutic in nature. Gunderson's (1978) identified five functions of the therapeutic milieu: containment, support, structure, involvement, and validation. Containment suggests that a milieu provides for the physical well-being of a patient, including food and shelter. Support highlights clinician efforts to improve a patient's well-being and self-esteem. Structure denotes that milieu activities are predictable. Involvement indicates that patients are an active part of their treatment, attending treatment team and therapy group meetings.

> **BOX 16.5 Cognitive Distortions**
>
> **Overgeneralization**
> A single event affects unrelated situations.
> - "He didn't ask me out. It must be because I'm fat."
>
> **All-or-Nothing Thinking**
> Reasoning is absolute and extreme, in mutually exclusive terms of black or white, good or bad.
> - "If I allow myself to gain weight, I'll blow up like a balloon."
>
> **Catastrophizing**
> The consequences of an event are magnified.
> - "If I gain weight, my weekend will be ruined."
>
> **Personalization**
> Events are overinterpreted as having personal significance.
> - "I know everybody is watching me eat."
>
> **Emotional Reasoning**
> Subjective emotions determine reality.
> - "When I'm thin, I feel powerful."
>
> **Source:** Adapted from Bowers, W. A. (2001). Basic principles for applying cognitive-behavioural therapy to anorexia nervosa. *Psychiatric Clinics of North America, 24,* 293–303. https://doi.org/10.1016/S0193-953X(05)70225-2

Validation emphasizes the individuality and value of each patient. Gunderson's (1978) concept of therapeutic milieu has been reconceptualized by Mahoney et al. (2009) to a systems approach. The systems approach extends beyond the physical characteristics and interpersonal atmosphere of an inpatient unit and addresses the interactions with broader systems such as health care delivery and information technology to create an optimal healing approach. An optimal health environment consists of people in relationships, their health-creating behaviors, and the surrounding physical environment (Jonas et al., 2014).

Milieu management of an eating-disorder unit is often organized to defeat troubling symptoms yet often reinforces themes of being in a battle in order to assist the patient in establishing more adaptive behavioural patterns, including normalization of eating. The highly structured milieu includes precise mealtimes, adherence to the selected menu, observations during and after meals, regularly scheduled weigh-ins, and participation in a combination of therapeutic modalities provided by an interprofessional team. Close monitoring of patients includes monitoring all trips to the bathroom after eating to prevent self-induced vomiting. Often patient privileges are linked to weight gain and treatment-plan adherence. These modalities are designed to normalize eating patterns and begin to address the medical, family, and social issues raised by the illness.

An optimal healing environment would include fostering healing and relationship building between patients and clinicians, clinicians and clinicians, and clinicians and community. The purpose is not to battle the problems or illness but rather to discover, heal, and transform. An optimal health environment recognizes the need for medical care; however, it moves beyond the inpatient unit including family in the treatment program and directly involved in the refeeding process. This type of therapy has the most evidence to support its use in children and adolescents with anorexia nervosa (Le Grange et al., 2016). Integrative healthcare is part of an optimal health environment by providing a platform for the integration of conventional, complementary, traditional, and alternative therapies through strong collaborative interdisciplinary teams and a practice of patient-centered care (Sakallaris et al., 2015). The interdisciplinary team would be trained to select the most appropriate intervention regardless of origin, providing onsite complementary and alternative practitioners available for ordering by the physician. A patient on an eating disorder unit would be supported to incorporate aromatherapy for sleep (Cheong et al., 2021), yoga for relaxation, or meditation for anxiety.

Advanced-Practice Interventions

Anorexia nervosa is a chronic illness. The 1-year relapse rate approaches 50%, and long-term studies show that up to 20% of patients continue to meet full criteria for anorexia nervosa after several years (Jagielska & Kacperska, 2017). Recovery is evaluated as a stage in the process rather than as a fixed event. Factors that influence the stage of recovery include percentage of ideal body weight that has been achieved, the extent to which self-worth is defined by shape and weight, and the amount of disruption existing in the patient's personal life.

The patient will require long-term treatment that might include periodic, brief hospital stays, admission to a partial hospitalization program, outpatient services, and pharmacological interventions.

Agras and Robinson (2008) reviewed the progress of treatment for eating disorders over the past 40 years. Table 16.3 outlines their findings.

Psychotherapy. The goals of psychotherapy treatment are weight restoration with normalization of eating habits and initiation of the treatment of psychological, interpersonal, and social issues that affect each individual patient. Assisting the patient with a daily meal plan, reviewing a journal of meals and dietary intake maintained by the patient, and providing for weekly weigh-ins (ideally two to three times a week) are essential if the patient is to reach a medically stable weight.

Families frequently report feeling powerless in the face of behaviour that is mystifying. For instance, patients are often unable to experience compliments as supportive and therefore are unable to internalize the support. They often seek attention from others but feel shamed when they receive it. Patients express that they want their families to care for and about them but are unable to recognize expressions of care. When others do respond with love and support, patients do not perceive this as positive. The following vignette demonstrates this phenomenon.

> **VIGNETTE**
>
> In a multi-family group on an inpatient unit Pearl (who last saw her daughter before she had gained 18 kg) is asked by the group leader how she regards her daughter, Lily. Pearl replies, "She looks healthy." Lily responds with an angry, sullen look. She ultimately verbalizes that she interprets comments about her "healthy" appearance as "You look fat." The group leader points out that it is interesting that Lily equates "healthy" with "fat." In the multi-family group there is a commonly expressed view that the illness "is not about weight" but that thinness confers a feeling of being special and that being at a normal weight (i.e., healthy) means this special status is lost.

Often family members and significant others seek ways to communicate clearly with the patient with anorexia but find that they are frequently misunderstood and that overtures of concern are misinterpreted. Consequently, families experience the tension of saying or doing the wrong thing and then feeling responsible if a setback occurs. Psychiatric mental health nurses have an important role in assisting families and significant others to develop strategies for improved communication and to search for ways to be comfortably supportive to the

TABLE 16.3 The State of Treatment for Eating Disorders, 2008

Disorder	Evidence-Informed Treatments Available (One or More Large-Scale Controlled Trials)	One or More Controlled Trials
Anorexia nervosa	None	Moderate number of controlled trials, although sample size and drop-out rates in adults present problems; family therapy for adolescents appears promising
Bulimia nervosa	Cognitive behavioural therapy (CBT); antidepressant medication (fluoxetine is approved for treatment in Canada); interpersonal therapy	Brief CBT-based therapies appear promising
Binge eating	CBT; antidepressant medication (topiramate) and stimulant medication (lisdexamfetamine dimesylate) reduce both binge eating and weight; interpersonal therapy	Antidepressants appear promising, with the added advantage of weight loss; brief CBT-based therapies appear promising

Source: Adapted from Agras, W. S., & Robinson, A. H. (2008). Forty years of progress in the treatment of the eating disorders. *Nordic Journal of Psychiatry, 62*(47), 19–24. https://doi.org/10.1080/08039480802315632

> **BOX 16.6 Coping With a Family Member Who Has an Eating Disorder**
>
> - Be patient. Eating disorders can be a long-term illness. Recovery takes time.
> - Encourage the person to seek professional help. If the family member is truly endangering their life, be insistent.
> - Seek outside help for yourself. Find a family or friend support group, a counsellor, or other professional who has experience in helping families.
> - Recognize that when addressing the problem with the person you suspect has an eating disorder (especially if it is for the first time), the reaction may be one of denial or perhaps even hostility.
> - Don't lay blame. This only reinforces the person's feelings of failure.
> - Try to ensure that you don't allow the person's problems to interfere with your routine functioning.
> - Let the person know that they are important to the family, but not more so than any other family member.
> - Do not dwell on food-related discussions. Encourage the person to get involved with non-food-related activities.
> - Avoid commenting on the person's weight or appearance—your comments may not be taken in the proper context.
> - People with eating disorders must feel control over their daily routine. This can be very frustrating for those around the individual, but the situation often only becomes worse when it is perceived that someone is trying to take that control away.
> - Be aware that low self-esteem is often a problem for those with eating disorders. Be careful not to make comparisons to other members of the family or to others within their peer group. Recognize the person for who they are.
> - Learn about eating disorders. Understanding is a key to coping.
>
> **Source:** Adapted from Woodside, D. B., & Shekter-Wolfson, L. (1988/2003). *Families and eating disorders. Know the facts.* Retrieved from http://www.nedic.ca/knowthefacts/documents/Familiesandeatingdisorders.pdf

> **BOX 16.7 Medical Complications of Bulimia Nervosa**
>
> - Sinus bradycardia
> - Orthostatic changes in pulse or blood pressure
> - Cardiac arrhythmias
> - Cardiac arrest from electrolyte disturbances or ipecac intoxication
> - Cardiac murmur, mitral valve prolapse
> - Electrolyte imbalances
> - Elevated serum bicarbonate levels (although can be low, indicating a metabolic acidosis)
> - Hypochloremia
> - Hypokalemia
> - Dehydration, which results in volume depletion, leading to stimulation of aldosterone production, which in turn stimulates further potassium excretion from kidneys; thus there can be both an indirect renal loss of potassium and a direct loss through self-induced vomiting
> - Severe attrition and erosion of teeth, producing irritating sensitivity and exposing the pulp of the teeth
> - Loss of dental arch
> - Diminished chewing ability
> - Parotid gland enlargement associated with elevated serum amylase levels
> - Esophageal tears caused by self-induced vomiting
> - Severe abdominal pain indicative of gastric dilation
> - Russell's sign (callus on knuckles from self-induced vomiting)
>
> **Source:** Data from Mitchell, J. E., & Wonderlich, S. A. (2014). Feeding and eating disorders. In R. E. Hales, S. C. Yudofsky, & L. W. Roberts (Eds.), *Textbook of psychiatry* (6th ed., pp. 557–587). Washington, DC: American Psychiatric Publishing.

patient. Box 16.6 lists strategies for families trying to cope with a family member who has an eating disorder.

Evaluation

The process of evaluation is built into the outcomes specified by *NOC*. Evaluation is ongoing, and short-term indicators are revised as necessary to achieve the treatment outcomes established. The indicators provide a daily guide for evaluating success and must be continually re-evaluated for their appropriateness. Case Study and Nursing Care Plan 16.1 presents a patient with anorexia nervosa.

BULIMIA NERVOSA

Bulimia first entered the *DSM* as a diagnosis in the third edition in 1980 but without purging or inappropriate compensatory behaviours as criteria. The diagnosis became bulimia nervosa with the addition of the preceding criteria in 1987. In the *DSM-IV-TR* it was further subcategorized as purging or non-purging type.

APPLICATION OF THE NURSING PROCESS

Assessment

General Assessment

Initially, patients with bulimia nervosa do not appear to be physically or emotionally ill. They are often at or slightly above or below ideal body weight. However, as the assessment continues and the nurse makes further observations, the physical and emotional problems of the patient become apparent. On inspection, the patient demonstrates enlargement of the parotid glands, with dental erosion and caries if the patient has been inducing vomiting. Box 16.7 identifies a number of medical complications that can occur and the laboratory findings that may result in individuals with bulimia nervosa. The disclosed history may reveal great difficulties with both impulsivity and compulsivity. Family relationships are frequently chaotic and reflect a lack of nurturing. Patients' lives reflect instability and troublesome interpersonal relationships as well. It is not uncommon for patients to have a history of impulsive stealing of items such as food, clothing, or jewellery.

> **VIGNETTE**
>
> During the initial assessment, the nurse wonders if Brittany is actually in need of hospitalization on the eating-disorders unit. The nurse is struck by how well the patient appears, seeming healthy, well dressed, and articulate. As Brittany continues to relate her history, she tells of restricting her food intake all day until early evening, when she buys her food and begins to binge as she is shopping. She arrives home and immediately induces vomiting. For the remainder of the evening and into the early morning hours, she "zones out" while watching television and binge eating. Periodically, she goes to the bathroom to vomit. She does this about 15 times during the evening. The nurse admitting Brittany to the unit reminds her of the goals of the hospitalization, including interrupting the binge–purge cycle and normalizing eating. The nurse further explains to Brittany that she has the support of the interdisciplinary treatment team that have been trained in optimal healing environments to assist her toward recovery.

Box 16.8 lists several thoughts and behaviours associated with bulimia nervosa, and Table 16.4 identifies possible signs and symptoms found on assessment and their causes.

BOX 16.8 Thoughts and Behaviours Associated With Bulimia Nervosa

- Binge eating behaviours
- Often self-induced vomiting (or laxative or diuretic use) after bingeing
- History of anorexia nervosa in one fourth to one third of individuals
- Depressive signs and symptoms
- Problems with:
  - Interpersonal relationships
  - Self-concept
  - Impulsive behaviours
- Increased levels of anxiety and compulsivity
- Possible chemical dependency
- Possible impulsive stealing

TABLE 16.4 Possible Signs and Symptoms of Bulimia Nervosa

Clinical Presentation	Cause
Normal to slightly low or slightly high weight	Excessive caloric intake with purging, excessive exercising
Dental caries, tooth erosion	Vomiting (hydrochloric acid reflux over enamel)
Parotid swelling	Increased serum amylase levels
Gastric dilation, rupture	Binge eating
Calluses, scars on hand (Russell's sign)	Self-induced vomiting
Peripheral edema	Rebound fluid, especially if diuretic used
Muscle weakening	Electrolyte imbalance
Abnormal laboratory values (electrolyte imbalance, hypokalemia, hyponatremia)	Purging: vomiting, laxative and/or diuretic use
Cardiovascular abnormalities (cardiomyopathy, electrocardiography [ECG] changes)	Electrolyte imbalance—*can lead to death*
Cardiac failure (cardiomyopathy)	Ipecac intoxication

Self-Assessment

In working with someone with bulimia be aware that the patient is sensitive to the perceptions of others regarding this illness and may feel significant shame and loss of control. In building a therapeutic alliance, try to empathize with the patient's feelings of low self-esteem, unworthiness, and dysphoria. If you believe that the patient is not being honest (e.g., active bingeing or purging goes unreported) or is being manipulative, acknowledge such obstacles and the frustration they provoke, and construct alternative ways to view the patient's thinking and behaviour. An accepting, non-judgemental approach, along with a comprehensive understanding of the subjective experience of the patient with bulimia, will help to build trust.

ASSESSMENT GUIDELINES
Bulimia Nervosa

1. Medical stabilization is the first priority. Problems resulting from purging are disruptions in electrolyte and fluid balance and cardiac function. Therefore a thorough physical examination is vital, including pertinent laboratory testing:
   - Electrolyte levels
   - Glucose level
   - Thyroid function tests
   - Complete blood count
   - Electrocardiography (ECG)
2. Psychiatric evaluation is advised because treatment of psychiatric comorbidity is important to outcome.

RESEARCH HIGHLIGHT
Screening Eating Disorders

Problem

People with eating disorders request services from primary care providers. The best way to assess the presence of an eating disorder in a primary care setting, however, is not known.

Purpose of Study

This study set out to compare the performance of two short eating-disorder screening tools (the SCOFF [sick, control, one stone, fat, food] Questionnaire and the Eating Disorder Screen for Primary Care [ESP]) in a primary care setting.

Methods

The 233 participants included primary-care-clinic patients and university students. The patients were approached in the clinic waiting room, and the university students were recruited using posters and announcements made in classes. Each participant completed both questionnaires.

Key Findings

It was determined that, for both the primary care patients and the university students, the ESP was a more useful tool than the SCOFF Questionnaire for helping clinicians determine the necessity of a more detailed assessment for a possible eating disorder. The ESP asked the following questions:
1. Are you satisfied with your eating patterns?
2. Do you ever eat in secret?
3. Does your weight affect the way you feel about yourself?
4. Have any members of your family suffered with an eating disorder?
5. Do you currently suffer with or have you ever suffered in the past with an eating disorder?

Implications for Nursing Practice

Using the five ESP questions can be an effective and quick method for screening people for eating disorders. If the patient identifies three or more abnormal responses, a more detailed assessment should be considered.

Source: Cotton, M-A., Ball, C., & Robinson, P. (2003). Four simple questions can help screen for eating disorders. *Journal of General Internal Medicine, 18*, 53–56. https://doi.org/10.1046/j.1525-1497.2003.20374.x

Diagnosis

The assessment of the patient with bulimia nervosa yields nursing diagnoses that result from the disordered eating and weight-control behaviours. Problems resulting from purging are a first priority because electrolyte and fluid balance and cardiac function are affected. Common nursing diagnoses include *Decreased cardiac output, Powerlessness, Chronic low self-esteem, Anxiety,* and *Ineffective coping* (substance use, impulsive responses to problems).

Outcomes Identification

Relevant *NOC* outcomes include *Vital signs, Electrolyte and acid/base balance, Weight maintenance behaviour, Self-esteem, Hope,* and *Coping*. Table 16.5 lists selected short-term indicators for patients with bulimia nervosa.

TABLE 16.5 NOC Outcomes Related to Bulimia Nervosa

Nursing Outcome and Definition	Short-Term Indicators
Vital signs: Extent to which temperature, pulse, respiration, and blood pressure are within normal range	Body temperature
	Apical heart rate
	Apical heart rhythm
	Respiratory rate
	Systolic blood pressure
Impulse self-control: Self-restraint of compulsive or impulsive behaviours	Identifies harmful impulsive behaviours
	Identifies feelings that lead to impulsive actions
	Identifies consequences of impulsive actions
	Controls impulses
Weight maintenance behaviour: Personal actions to maintain optimum body weight	Maintains recommended eating pattern
	Retains ingested foods
	Maintains fluid balance
	Plans for situations that affect food and fluid intake
	Expresses realistic body image
Hope: Optimism that is personally satisfying and life supporting	Expresses faith
	Expresses will to live
	Expresses optimism
	Sets goals

Source: Data from Moorhead, S., Swanson, E., Johnson, M., & Maas, M. L. (Eds.). (2018). *Nursing Outcomes Classification (NOC): Measurement of health outcomes* (6th ed.). St. Louis: Elsevier.

Planning

The criteria for inpatient admission of a patient with bulimia nervosa are included in Box 16.4. Like the patient with anorexia nervosa, the patient with bulimia nervosa may be treated for life-threatening complications such as gastric rupture (rare), electrolyte imbalance, and cardiac dysrhythmias. Planning will also include appropriate referrals for continuing outpatient treatment.

> **VIGNETTE**
>
> Kelsie weighs 85% of her ideal body weight. She has a history of diuretic abuse, and she becomes very edematous when she stops their use and enters treatment. The nurse informs Kelsie that the edema is related to the use of diuretics and thus is transient and will resolve after Kelsie begins to eat normally and discontinues the diuretics. Kelsie cannot tolerate the weight gain and the accompanying edema that occurs when she stops taking diuretics. She restarts the diuretics, perpetuating the cycle of fluid retention and the risk for kidney damage. The nurse empathizes with Kelsie's inability to tolerate the feelings of anxiety and dread she experiences because of her markedly swollen extremities.

Implementation

Acute Care

A patient who is medically compromised as a result of bulimia nervosa is referred to an inpatient eating-disorder unit for comprehensive treatment of the illness. The cognitive behavioural model of treatment is highly effective and frequently serves as the cornerstone of the therapeutic approach. Inpatient units designed to treat eating disorders are specially structured to interrupt the cycle of binge eating and purging and to normalize eating habits. Therapy is begun to examine the underlying conflicts and distorted perceptions of shape and weight that sustain the illness. The patient is also evaluated for treatment of comorbid disorders, such as major depression and substance use. In Canada the addictions and mental health systems have traditionally functioned as two separate systems, each with its own range of services and particular approaches to treatment and support; however, current best practice supports collaboration in concurrent disorder programs in Canada (refer to Chapter 18 for more information). In addition to specialty or general treatment, there are several centres and programs for those experiencing all types of eating disorders. The National Initiative for Eating Disorders (2020) provides information and education for immediate support and early intervention with a number of pan-Canadian resource links.

Pharmacological Interventions

Antidepressant medication together with cognitive behavioural psychotherapy has been shown to bring about improvement in bulimic symptoms. Limited research suggests that the SSRIs and tricyclic antidepressants help reduce binge eating and vomiting over short terms. Fluoxetine (Prozac) treatment may help prevent relapse. Bupropion (Wellbutrin) may be effective, but due to an increased risk for seizures, it is contraindicated in patients who purge.

Counselling

Compared with the patient with anorexia, the patient with bulimia nervosa often more readily establishes a therapeutic alliance with the nurse because the eating-disordered behaviours are seen as a problem. The therapeutic alliance allows the nurse, along with other members of the interprofessional team, to provide counselling that gives useful feedback regarding the patient's distorted beliefs.

Health Teaching and Health Promotion

Health teaching focuses on not only the eating disorder but also meal planning, use of relaxation techniques, maintenance of a healthy diet and exercise, coping skills, the physical and emotional effects of bingeing and purging, and the impact of cognitive distortions.

Once patients reach therapeutic goals, it is recommended that they seek long-term care to solidify those goals and address the attitudes, perceptions, and psychodynamic issues that maintain the eating disorder and attend the illness.

Advanced-Practice Interventions

Psychotherapy. Cognitive behavioural therapy is the most effective treatment for bulimia nervosa. Restructuring faulty perceptions and helping individuals to develop accepting attitudes toward themselves and their bodies is a primary focus of therapy. When patients do not engage in bulimic behaviours, issues of self-worth and interpersonal functioning become more prominent.

Box 16.9 presents relevant *Nursing Interventions Classification (NIC)* interventions for the management of eating disorders.

> **VIGNETTE**
>
> Nadia, a 23-year-old patient with a 6-year history of bulimia nervosa, struggles with issues of self-esteem. She expresses much guilt about "letting her father down" in the past by drinking alcohol excessively and binge eating and purging. She is determined that this time she is not going to fail at treatment. After her initial success in stopping the disordered behaviours, she says defiantly, "I'm doing this for me." Nadia usually experiences her behaviour as either pleasing or disappointing to others, but she begins to realize that her feeling of self-worth is very much dependent on how others see her and that she needs to develop a better sense of herself.

BOX 16.9 NIC Interventions for Eating-Disorders Management

Definition: Prevention and treatment of severe diet restriction and overexercising or bingeing and purging of food and fluids.

Activities:

- Develop a supportive relationship with patient.
- Collaborate with other members of health care team to develop treatment plan; involve patient and significant others as appropriate.
- Confer with team and patient to set a target weight if patient is not within a recommended weight range for age and body frame.
- Establish the amount of daily weight gain that is desired.
- Confer with dietitian to determine daily caloric intake necessary to attain or maintain target weight.
- Teach and reinforce concepts of good nutrition with patient (and significant others as appropriate).
- Encourage patient to discuss food preferences with dietitian.
- Monitor physiological parameters (vital signs, electrolyte levels) as needed.
- Weigh on a routine basis (e.g., at same time of day and after voiding).
- Monitor intake and output of fluids, as appropriate.
- Monitor daily caloric intake.
- Encourage patient self-monitoring of daily food intake and weight gain or maintenance as appropriate.
- Establish expectations for appropriate eating behaviours, intake of food and fluids, and amount of physical activity.
- Use behavioural contracting with patient to elicit desired weight gain or maintenance behaviours.
- Restrict food availability to scheduled, pre-served meals and snacks.
- Observe patient during and after meals and snacks to ensure that adequate intake is achieved and maintained.
- Accompany patient to bathroom during designated observation times following meals and snacks.
- Limit time spent in bathroom during periods when not under direct supervision.
- Monitor patient for behaviours related to eating, weight loss, and weight gain.
- Use behaviour modification techniques to promote behaviours that contribute to weight gain and limit weight-loss behaviours as appropriate.
- Provide reinforcement for weight gain and behaviours that promote weight gain.
- Provide support (e.g., relaxation therapy, desensitization exercises, opportunities to talk about feelings) as patient integrates new eating behaviours, changing body image, and lifestyle changes.
- Encourage patient use of daily logs to record feelings and circumstances surrounding urge to purge, vomit, or overexercise.
- Limit physical activity as needed to promote weight gain.
- Provide a supervised exercise program when appropriate.
- Allow opportunity to make limited choices about eating and exercise as weight gain progresses in desirable manner.
- Assist patient (and significant others as appropriate) to examine and resolve personal issues that may contribute to the eating disorder.
- Assist patient to develop a self-esteem that is compatible with a healthy body weight.
- Confer with the health care team on a routine basis about patient's progress.
- Initiate maintenance phase of treatment when patient has achieved target weight and has consistently shown desired eating behaviours for designated period of time.
- Monitor patient weight on a routine basis.
- Determine acceptable range of weight variation in relation to target range.
- Place responsibility for choices about eating and physical activity with patient as appropriate.
- Provide support and guidance as needed.
- Assist patient to evaluate the appropriateness and consequences of choices about eating and physical activity.
- Reinstitute weight-gain protocol if patient is unable to remain within target weight range.
- Institute a treatment program and follow-up care (medical, counselling) for home management.

Source: Adapter from Butcher, H. K., Bulechek, G. M., Dochterman, J. M., & Wagner, C. M. (Eds.). (2018). *Nursing Interventions Classification (NIC)* (7th ed.). St. Louis: Elsevier.

Evaluation

Evaluation of treatment effectiveness is ongoing and built into the *NOC* categories. Outcomes are revised as necessary to reach the desired outcomes. Case Study and Nursing Care Plan 16.2 presents a patient with bulimia nervosa.

BINGE EATING DISORDER

Binge eating disorder is characterized by recurring episodes of eating significantly more food than most in a relatively short period of time and without regular compensatory behaviors (such as purging). Binge eating disorder is accompanied by feelings of loss of control, anxiety, depression, and guilt. Overeating is frequently noted as a symptom of an affective disorder (e.g., atypical depression). Depression has been associated with binge eating disorder in a number of studies (Singleton et al., 2019). Social anxiety (Spettigue et al., 2020) and family history of anxiety (Blomquist & Grilo, 2015) also have strong associations with the disorder, and thus assessment practices are concerned with clearly determining the points for relevant intervention.

Because of its efficacy with bulimia, the use of SSRIs at or near the high end of the dosage range has been studied to treat binge eating disorder and seem to help in the short term; however, patients regained significant weight after discontinuance of medication. Other medications that are under investigation include the tricyclic antidepressants, antiepileptic medication, and appetite suppressants (McElroy, 2017).

Cognitive behavioural therapy and interpersonal therapy have been determined to be effective in eliminating binge eating; however, on average, these therapies do not produce clinically significant weight loss (Grilo, 2017). Dialectical behavioural therapy has been found to be effective in reducing binge eating for those patients seeking weight-loss services (Peckmezian & Paxton, 2020).

Binge eating is one of the most common forms of eating disorders documented in individuals who are being considered for bariatric surgery. Approximately 10 000 bariatric surgeries were performed in Canadian hospitals in 2017 (Obesity Canada-Obésité Canada, 2019). However, binge eating after bariatric surgery has been associated with poor weight outcomes (Freire et al., 2021). Pre-operative and post-operative cognitive behavioural therapy, dialectical behavioural therapy, and acceptance and commitment therapy all show promise in reducing binge eating, although their direct impact on longer-term weight loss is unknown (Freire et al., 2021). Many advanced-practice nurses are qualified to provide these therapies. Box 16.10 outlines the recommended pre-operative and post-operative standards of care for bariatric surgery.

BOX 16.10 Pre-operative and Post-operative Standards of Care for Bariatric Surgery

Pre-operative Period

Patients:
- Should have a full understanding of the post-operative dietary requirements, the necessary post-surgical supports, and the importance of stress-management strategies
- Should be screened for severe psychiatric comorbidities
- Must have a minimum 12-month period of recovery from any eating disorder, substance use, manic episode, psychosis, psychiatric hospitalization, suicide attempt, or trauma-related issue before having bariatric surgery
- Should receive counselling or education to assist with lifestyle changes

Post-operative Period

Patients:
- Will receive close follow-up and support from members of an interprofessional team (surgery, medicine, psychiatry or psychology, nutrition and exercise science) monthly for the first 6 months, then every 2 months for the remainder of the first year after surgery

---

CASE STUDY AND NURSING CARE PLAN 16.1
Anorexia Nervosa

Ella, a 20-year-old woman who uses the pronoun she/her, is brought to the inpatient eating-disorder unit of a local hospital by two older brothers, who are supporting her and walking closely, holding Ella up on either side. She is profoundly weak, holding her head up with her hands.

Assessment

Self-Assessment

Nurse Puneet is assigned to care for Ella. Although a young nurse, Puneet has spent the past 3 years working on the eating-disorders unit. When she first began, she had difficulty overidentifying with patients. Puneet has struggled with bulimia, but with treatment, she has done well. She seeks guidance from her nursing supervisor and the interprofessional team, which have helped her to maintain appropriate boundaries while creating a therapeutic alliance with patients.

Objective Data
- Height: 157 cm
- Weight: 26.3 kg—50% of ideal body weight
- Blood pressure: 74/50 mm Hg
- Pulse: 54 beats per minute
- Anemic—hemoglobin: 90 g/L (9 g/dL)
- Cachectic appearance, pale, with fine lanugo
- Sad facial expression
- Bruising on inside of each knee from sleeping on her side with knees touching

Subjective Data
- Denies being underweight: "I need treatment because I get fatigued so easily."
- "I check my legs every night. I'm so afraid of getting fat. I hate it if my legs touch each other."
- "I don't like to start anything until I know I can do it perfectly the first time. I wouldn't want anyone to see me make a mistake."
- Depressed mood

Diagnosis
1. *Imbalanced nutrition: less than body requirements* related to restriction of caloric intake secondary to extreme fear of weight gain
2. *Chronic low self-esteem* related to perception that others are always judging her

Outcomes Identification
Patient will reach 75% of ideal weight (41.7 kg) by discharge.

Planning
The initial plan is to address Ella's unstable physiological state.

Implementation
Ella's care plan is personalized as follows:

Short-Term Goal	Intervention	Rationale	Evaluation
1. Patient will gain a minimum of 1 kg and a maximum of 1.5 kg weekly through inpatient stay.	1a. Acknowledge the emotional and physical difficulty patient is experiencing. Use patient's extreme fatigue to engage cooperation in the treatment plan.	1a. A first priority is to establish a therapeutic alliance.	**Week 1** Patient increases caloric intake with liquid supplement only. Patient unable to eat solid food. Patient does not gain weight. Patient remains hypotensive, bradycardic, anemic (hemoglobin [Hgb] = 90 g/L [9 g/dL]).
	1b. Weigh patient daily for the first week, then three times a week. Patient should be weighed in bra and underwear only. There should be no oral intake, including a drink of water, before the early morning weigh-in.	1b. These measures ensure that weight is accurate.	**Week 2** Patient gains 1 kg drinking liquid supplement—minimal solid food. Patient remains hypotensive, bradycardic (Hgb = 100 g/L [10 g/dL]).

Continued

CASE STUDY AND NURSING CARE PLAN 16.1—cont'd
Anorexia Nervosa

Short-Term Goal	Intervention	Rationale	Evaluation
	1c. Do not negotiate weight with patient or reweigh. Patient may choose not to look at the scale or request that she not be told the weight.	1c. Patient may try to control and sabotage treatment.	**Week 3** Patient gains 0.5 kg drinking liquid supplement. Patient selects meal plan but is unable to eat most solid foods. Patient's blood pressure (BP) = 84/60 mm Hg; pulse = 68 beats per minute, regular; Hgb = 110 g/L (11 g/dL).
	1d. Measure vital signs three times a day (tid) until stable, then daily. Repeat electrocardiography (ECG) and laboratory tests until stable.	1d. As patient begins to increase in weight, cardiovascular status improves to within normal range, and monitoring is less frequent.	**Weeks 4–6** Patient gains an average of 1 kg/week. Patient samples more solid foods selected from meal plan. Patient's BP = 90/60 mm Hg; pulse = 68 beats per minute, regular; Hgb = 115 g/L (11.5 g/dL).
	1e. Provide a pleasant, calm atmosphere at mealtimes. Patient should be told the specific times and duration (usually a half-hour) of meals.	1e. Mealtimes become episodes of high anxiety, and knowledge of regulations decreases tension in the milieu, particularly when patient has given up so much control by entering treatment.	**Week 7** Patient weighs 32.2 kg (almost 60% of ideal body weight); calories are mostly from liquid supplement. Patient selects balanced meals, eating more varied solid food: turkey, carrots, lettuce, fruit. Patient's Hgb = 125 g/L (12.5 g/dL); normal range of BP and pulse are maintained. Patient continues to increase participation in social aspects of eating.
	1f. Administer liquid supplement as ordered.	1f. Patient may be unable to eat solid food at first.	
	1g. Observe patient during meals to prevent hiding or throwing away of food and for at least 1 hour after meals and snacks to prevent purging.	1g, h. The compelling force of the illness is such that behaviours related to hiding or discarding food are difficult to stop. A power struggle between staff and patient may emerge, in which patient appears to adhere but defies the rules (appearing to eat but throwing away food).	**Weeks 8–12** Patient gains an average of 1 kg/week and weighs 37.1 kg (approx. 68% of ideal body weight). Patient is eating more varied solid food, but most caloric intake is still from liquid supplement. Patient maintains normal vital signs and Hgb levels. Patient maintains social interaction during mealtimes and snacks.
	1h. Encourage patient to try to eat some solid food. Preparation of patient's meals should be guided by likes and dislikes list because patient is unable to make own selections to complete menu.		
	1i. Be empathic with patient's struggle to give up control of her eating and her weight as she is expected to make minimum weight gain on a regular basis. Permit patient to verbalize feelings at these times.	1i. Patient is expected to gain at least 0.25 kg on a specific schedule, usually three times a week (Monday, Wednesday, Friday).	**Weeks 13–16** Patient has reached medically stable weight at the end of 16th week—41.7 kg (approx. 75% of ideal body weight). Patient continues to eat more solid food with relatively less liquid supplement. Patient is not able to participate in planned exercise program until she reaches 85% of ideal body weight.
	1j. Monitor patient's weight gain. A weight gain of 1 kg/week to 1.5 kg/week is medically acceptable.	1j. Weight gain of more than 2.25 kg in 1 week may result in pulmonary edema.	
	1k. Provide teaching regarding healthy eating as the basis of a healthy lifestyle.	1k. Healthy aspects of eating (e.g., increased energy, rather than gaining weight) are reinforced.	
	1l. Use a cognitive behavioural approach to address patient's expressed fears regarding weight gain. Identify and examine dysfunctional thoughts; identify and examine values and beliefs that sustain these thoughts.	1l. Confronting irrational thoughts and beliefs is crucial to changing eating behaviours.	
	1m. As patient approaches her target weight, there should be encouragement to make her own choices for menu selection.	1m. Patient can assume more control of her meals, which is empowering for the patient with anorexia.	

CASE STUDY AND NURSING CARE PLAN 16.1—cont'd
Anorexia Nervosa

Short-Term Goal	Intervention	Rationale	Evaluation
	1n. Emphasize social nature of eating. Encourage conversation that does not have the theme of food during mealtimes.	1n. Eating as a social activity, shared with others and with participation in conversation, serves as both a distraction from obsessional pre-occupations and a pleasurable event.	
	1o. Focus on the patient's strengths, including her good work in normalizing her weight and eating habits.	1o. Patient who is beginning to normalize weight and eating behaviours has achieved a major accomplishment, of which she should be proud. Non-eating activities are explored as a source of gratification.	
	1p. Provide for a planned exercise program when patient reaches target weight.	1p. Patient experiences a strong drive to exercise; this measure accommodates this drive by planning a reasonable amount.	
	1q. Encourage patient to apply all the knowledge, skills, and gains made from the various individual, family, and group therapy sessions.	1q. Patient has been receiving intensive therapy and education, which have provided tools and techniques that are useful in maintaining healthy behaviours.	

Evaluation
By the end of the sixteenth week, Ella has achieved a stable weight of 41.7 kilograms. This weight is approaching congruency with Ella's height, frame, and age. Her vital signs and hemoglobin levels are consistently normal. She is participating in therapy and consistently communicating satisfaction with her body appearance.

CASE STUDY AND NURSING CARE PLAN 16.2
Bulimia Nervosa

Reena is a 30-year-old university graduate who reports that she is an aspiring actress working currently as a "temp" for an insurance agency. She is being admitted to a partial hospitalization program designed for patients with eating disorders. Reena has bulimia nervosa.

Assessment
Self-Assessment
Matthew, a seasoned nurse in the area of eating disorders, is assigned to care for Reena. Matthew enjoys working with patients with bulimia because he believes that he can help patients move toward health. When he first encounters Reena, he experiences an immediate negative response that surprises him. He speaks to his supervisor about these feelings and raises the question of whether he is the appropriate nurse to care for Reena. As he and the supervisor discuss his feelings, Matthew is able to recognize that Reena reminds him of a girlfriend he had many years earlier. The relationship ended badly. Matthew experiences an emotional release with this realization and believes that he will be able to separate his earlier negative experience from his work with Reena.

Objective Data
Height: 165 cm
Weight: 57.6 kg—95% of ideal body weight
Blood pressure: 120/80 mm Hg sitting; 90/60 mm Hg standing
Pulse: 70 beats per minute (sitting); 96 beats per minute (standing)
Potassium level of 2.7 mmol/L (normal range, 3.3–5.5 mmol/L)
ECG: abnormal—consistent with hypokalemia
Erosion of enamel, enlarged parotid glands, consistent with a history of binge eating and purging

Subjective Data
"I can't stand to be fat."
"I'm ashamed that I can't control my bingeing and vomiting—I know it's not good."

Diagnosis
1. *Risk for injury* related to low potassium and other physical changes secondary to binge eating and purging
2. *Powerlessness* related to inability to control bingeing and vomiting cycles

Continued

CASE STUDY AND NURSING CARE PLAN 16.2—cont'd
Bulimia Nervosa

Outcomes Identification

Reena will demonstrate an ability to regulate eating patterns, resulting in consistently normal electrolyte balance.

Planning

Reena is admitted to a partial hospitalization program designed for patients with eating disorders. She attends the program 3 or 4 days a week and participates in individual and group therapy. She will continue to work as a "temp" for an insurance agency.

Implementation

Reena's care plan is personalized as follows:

Short-Term Goal	Intervention	Rationale	Evaluation
1. Patient will identify signs and symptoms of low potassium level (K^+), and K^+ level will remain within normal limits throughout hospitalization.	1a. Educate patient regarding the ill effects of self-induced vomiting, low K^+ level, dental erosion. 1b. Educate patient about binge–purge cycle and its self-perpetuating nature. 1c. Teach patient that fasting sets one up to binge eat. 1d. Explore ideas about trigger foods. 1e. Challenge irrational thoughts and beliefs about "forbidden" foods. 1f. Teach patient to plan and eat regularly scheduled, balanced meals.	1a. Health teaching is crucial to treatment. The patient needs to be reminded of the benefits of normalization of eating behaviour. 1.b, c. The compulsive nature of the binge–purge cycle is maintained by the sequence of intake restriction, hunger, bingeing, purging accompanied by feelings of guilt, and then repetition of the cycle over and over. 1d. Patient needs to understand beliefs about trigger foods to challenge irrational thoughts. 1e. Challenge forces patient to examine own thinking and beliefs. 1f. This teaching helps to ensure success in maintaining abstinence from binge–purge activity.	**Week 1** Patient begins to select balanced meals. Patient demonstrates knowledge of untoward effects of vomiting and K^+ deficiency. Patient begins to demonstrate understanding of repetitive nature of binge–purge cycle. **Week 2** Patient begins to challenge irrational thoughts and beliefs. Patient continues to plan nutritionally balanced meals, including dinner at home. Patient begins to sample "forbidden foods" and discuss thoughts and attitudes about same. **Week 3** Patient discusses triggers to binge and resultant behaviour. Patient continues to challenge irrational thoughts and beliefs in individual and group sessions. Patient plans meals, including "forbidden foods." **Week 4** Patient reports no binge–purge behaviours at day program or outside. Patient demonstrates understanding of repetitive nature of binge–purge cycle. Patient continues to challenge irrational thoughts and beliefs.

Evaluation

At the end of 4 weeks, Reena reports no binge–purge cycles, and her potassium level remains consistently within normal limits. She is beginning to plan meals and challenge irrational thoughts and beliefs.

KEY POINTS TO REMEMBER

- A number of theoretical models help explain the origins of eating disorders.
- Neurobiological theories identify an association among eating disorders, depression, and neuroendocrine abnormalities.
- Psychological theories explore issues of control related to eating disorders.
- Genetic theories postulate the existence of vulnerabilities that may predispose people toward eating disorders.
- Sociocultural models look at our present societal ideal of being thin.
- Men with eating disorders share many of the characteristics of women with eating disorders.
- The suicide rate of patients with eating disorders is much higher than predicted rates in similar age groups.
- Anorexia nervosa is a potentially life-threatening eating disorder that includes severe underweight; low blood pressure, pulse, and temperature; dehydration; low serum potassium level; and dysrhythmias.
- Anorexia may be treated in an inpatient treatment setting in which milieu therapy, psychotherapy (cognitive), development of self-care skills, and psychobiological interventions can be implemented.

- Long-term treatment is provided on an outpatient basis and aims to help patients maintain healthy weight. It includes treatment modalities such as individual therapy, family therapy, group therapy, psychopharmacology, and nutrition counselling.
- Patients with bulimia nervosa are typically within the normal weight range, but some may be slightly below or above ideal body weight.
- Assessment of the patient with bulimia may show enlargement of the parotid glands and dental erosion and caries if the patient has induced vomiting.
- Acute care may be necessary when life-threatening complications such as gastric rupture (rare), electrolyte imbalance, and cardiac dysrhythmias are present.
- The goal of interventions is to interrupt the binge–purge cycle.
- Psychotherapy and self-care skill training are included in the treatment plan.
- Long-term treatment focuses on therapy aimed at addressing any coexisting depression, substance use, or personality disorders that are causing the patient distress and interfering with the quality of life. Self-worth and interpersonal functioning eventually become issues that are useful for the patient to target.
- People with binge eating disorder report a history of major depression significantly more often than people who do not binge eat.
- Effective treatment for obese patients with binge eating disorder integrates modification of the disordered eating, improvement of depressive symptoms, and achievement of an appropriate weight.

CRITICAL THINKING

1. Logan, a 19-year-old male model, has experienced a rapid decrease in weight over the past 4 months after his agent told him he would have to lose some weight or lose a coveted account. Logan is 188 cm tall and weighs 60 kg, down from his usual 80 kg. He is brought to the emergency department with a pulse of 40 beats per minute and severe arrhythmias. His laboratory workup reveals severe hypokalemia. He has become extremely depressed, saying, "I'm too fat! I don't want anything to eat—if I gain weight, my life will be ruined. There is nothing to live for if I can't model." Logan's parents are startled and confused, and his best friend is worried and feels powerless to help: "I tell Logan he needs to eat or he will die. I tell him he is a skeleton, but he refuses to listen to me. I don't know what to do."
   a. Which physical and psychiatric criteria suggest that Logan should be hospitalized immediately?
   b. What are five questions that could be asked to help determine if further assessment is needed regarding the possibility of an eating disorder?
   c. What are some of the questions you would eventually ask Logan when evaluating his biopsychosocial functioning?
   d. What are your feelings toward someone with anorexia? Can you make a distinction between your thoughts and feelings toward women with anorexia and toward men with anorexia?
   e. What are some things you could do for Logan's parents and friend in terms of offering them information, support, and referrals? Identify specific referrals.
   f. Explain the kinds of interventions or restrictions that may be used while Logan is hospitalized.
   g. How would you describe partial hospitalization programs when asked if Logan will have to be hospitalized for an extended period?
   h. What are some of Logan's cognitive distortions that would be a target for therapy?
   i. Identify at least five criteria that, if met, would indicate that Logan was improving.

2. You and Ambreen have been close friends since nursing school and are now working on the same surgical unit. Ambreen told you that in the past she had made several suicide attempts. Today, you come upon her bingeing off-unit, and she looks embarrassed and uncomfortable when she sees you. On several occasions, you notice that she spends time in the bathroom, and you hear sounds of retching. In response to your concern, she admits that she has been bingeing and purging for several years but that she is now getting out of control and feels profoundly depressed.
   a. Although Ambreen does not show any physical signs of bulimia nervosa, what would you look for when assessing an individual with bulimia?
   b. What kinds of emergencies could result from bingeing and purging?
   c. What would be the most useful type of psychotherapy for Ambreen initially, and what issues would need to be addressed?
   d. What kinds of new skills does a person with bulimia need to learn to lessen the compulsion to binge and purge?
   e. What would be some signs that Ambreen is recovering?

3. The high school principal shares with you that several students (male and female) have disclosed to faculty that they have an eating disorder. The principal is concerned about the health of all of the students in the school and asks you to hold a general information session.
   a. What type of health promotion material will be helpful?
   b. How could you deliver this information to the students?

CHAPTER REVIEW

1. Which female patient should the nurse recognize as having the highest risk to have or develop bulimia nervosa? The one who:
   a. Grew up in an underserved area
   b. Lives in a society influenced by Eastern cultural beliefs
   c. Is 20 years old
   d. Is Asian Canadian

2. The nurse is caring for a 16-year-old female patient with anorexia nervosa. What should the initial nursing intervention be upon the patient's admission to the unit?
   a. Build a therapeutic relationship.
   b. Increase the patient's caloric consumption.
   c. Involve the patient in group therapy to build a support group.
   d. Self-assess to decrease tendencies toward authoritarianism.

3. The nurse is caring for a patient with bulimia. Which nursing intervention is appropriate?
   a. Monitor patient on bathroom trips after eating.
   b. Allow patient extensive private time with family members.
   c. Provide meals whenever the patient requests them.
   d. Encourage patient to select foods that they like.

4. The nurse is admitting a patient who weighs 45 kg, is 167 cm tall, and is below ideal body weight. The patient's blood pressure is 130/80 mm Hg, pulse is 72 beats per minute, potassium is 2.5 mmol/L, and ECG is abnormal. Her teeth enamel is eroded, her hands are visibly shaking, and her parotid gland is enlarged. The patient states, "I am really worked up about coming to this unit." What is the priority nursing diagnosis?
   a. Powerlessness
   b. Risk for injury
   c. Imbalanced nutrition: Less than body requirements
   d. Anxiety

5. The nurse is planning care for a patient with an eating disorder. What outcomes are appropriate? **Select all that apply**.
   a. The patient will experience a decrease in depression.
   b. The patient will identify four methods to control anxiety.

c. The patient will collect different kinds of cookbooks.
d. The patient will identify two people to contact if suicidal thoughts occur.
6. What patient statement acknowledges the characteristic behavior associated with a diagnosis of pica?
a. "Nothing could make me drink milk."
b. "I'm ashamed of it, but I eat my hair."
c. "I haven't eaten a green vegetable since I was 3 years old."
d. "I regurgitate and rechew my food after almost every meal."

https://evolve.elsevier.com/Canada/Varcarolis/psychiatric/

REFERENCES

Agras, W. S., & Robinson, A. H. (2008). Forty years of progress in the treatment of the eating disorders. *Nordic Journal of Psychiatry, 62*(47), 19–24. https://doi.org/10.1080/08039480802315632

American Psychiatric Association. (APA). (2013). *DSM-5 table of contents.* Retrieved from https://www.psychiatry.org/dsm5

Anderson, L. E. A., Smith, A. P. L., & Crow, S. (2017). Suicidality, self-injurious behavior, and eating disorders. In L. K. Anderson, S. B. Murray, & W. H. Kaye (Eds.) *Clinical handbook of complex and atypical eating disorders* (p. 79). New York: Oxford University Press.

Bahji, A., Mazhar, M. N., Hudson, C. C., et al. (2019). Prevalence of substance use disorder comorbidity among individuals with eating disorders: A systematic review and meta-analysis. *Psychiatry Research, 273*, 58–66.

Blomquist, K. K., & Grilo, C. M. (2015). Family histories of anxiety in overweight men and women with binge eating disorder: A preliminary investigation. *Comprehensive Psychiatry, 62*, 161–169. https://doi.org/10.1016/j.comppsych.2015.07.007

Bruch, H. (1978). *The golden cage: The enigma of anorexia nervosa.* Cambridge: Harvard University Press.

Calzo, J. P., Blashill, A. J., Brown, T. A., et al. (2017). Eating disorders and disordered weight and shape control behaviors in sexual minority populations. *Current Psychiatry Reports, 19*(8), 49. https://doi.org/10.1007/s11920-017-0801-y

Canadian Senate. (2016). *Report of the Standing Senate Committee on Social Affairs, Science and Technology: Obesity in Canada: A whole-of-society approach for a healthier Canada.* Retrieved from https://sencanada.ca/content/sen/committee/421/SOCI/Reports/2016-02-25_Revised_report_Obesity_in_Canada_e.pdf

Cheong, M. J., Kim, S., Kim, J. S., et al. (2021). A systematic literature review and meta-analysis of the clinical effects of aroma inhalation therapy on sleep problems. *Medicine, 100*(9), e24652.

Cliffe, C., Shetty, H., Himmerich, H., et al. (2020). Suicide attempts requiring hospitalization in patients with eating disorders: A retrospective cohort study. *International Journal of Eating Disorders, 53*(5), 728–735.

Cucchi, A., Ryan, D., Konstantakopoulos, G., et al. (2016). Lifetime prevalence of non-suicidal self-injury in patients with eating disorders: A systematic review and meta-analysis. *Psychological Medicine, 46*(7), 1345. https://doi.org/10.1017/S0033291716000027

Dahlgren, C. L., Wisting, L., & Rø, Ø. (2017). Feeding and eating disorders in the DSM-5 era: A systematic review of prevalence rates in non-clinical male and female samples. *Journal of Eating Disorders, 5*(1), 1–10.

Doris, E., Shekriladze, I., Javakhishvili, N., et al. (2015). Is cultural change associated with eating disorders? A systematic review of the literature. *Eating and Weight Disorders: EWD, 20*(2), 149–160. https://doi.org/10.1007/s40519-015-0189-9

Erskine, H. E., Whiteford, H. A., & Pike, K. M. (2016). The global burden of eating disorders. *Current Opinion in Psychiatry, 29*(6), 346–353.

Francisco, R. (2018). Studies on body image, eating, and weight in models, dancers, and aesthetic athletes. In M. Cuzzolaro, & S. Fassino (Eds.), *Body image, eating, and weight* (pp. 401–411). Cham: Springer.

Freire, C. C., Zanella, M. T., Segal, A., et al. (2021). Associations between binge eating, depressive symptoms and anxiety and weight regain after Roux-en-Y gastric bypass surgery. *Eating and Weight Disorders-Studies on Anorexia, Bulimia and Obesity, 26*(1), 191–199.

Galmiche, M., Déchelotte, P., Lambert, G., et al. (2019). Prevalence of eating disorders over the 2000–2018 period: A systematic literature review. *The American Journal of Clinical Nutrition, 109*(5), 1402–1413.

Gárriz, M., Andrés-Perpiñá, S., Plana, M. T., et al. (2021). Personality disorder traits, obsessive ideation and perfectionism 20 years after adolescent-onset anorexia nervosa: A recovered study. *Eating and Weight Disorders-Studies on Anorexia, Bulimia and Obesity, 26*(2), 667–677.

Grilo, C. M. (2017). Psychological and behavioral treatments for binge-eating disorder. *The Journal of Clinical Psychiatry, 78*(1), 20–24.

Gunderson, J. G. (1978). Defining the therapeutic processes in psychiatric milieus. *Psychiatry, 41*(4), 327–335.

Harrington, B. C., Jimerson, M., Haxton, C., et al. (2015). Initial evaluation, diagnosis, and treatment of anorexia nervosa and bulimia nervosa. *American Family Physician, 91*(1), 46–52.

Haworth-Hoeppner, S. (2017). *Family, culture, and self in the development of eating disorders.* New York: Routledge.

Herdman, T. H., & Kamitsuru, S. (Eds.). (2014). *NANDA international nursing diagnoses: Definitions and classification* (pp. 2015–2017). Oxford: Wiley-Blackwell.

Jagielska, G., & Kacperska, I. (2017). Outcome, comorbidity and prognosis in anorexia nervosa. *Psychiatria Polska, 51*(2), 205–218.

Jonas, W. B., Chez, R. A., Smith, K., et al. (2014). Salutogenesis: The defining concept for a new healthcare system. *Global Advances in Health and Medicine, 3*(3), 82–91.

Kappou, K., Ntougia, M., Kourtesi, A., et al. (2021). Neuroimaging findings in adolescents and young adults with anorexia nervosa: A systematic review. *Children, 8*(2), 137.

Karrer, Y., Halioua, R., Mötteli, S., Iff, S., Seifritz, E., Jäger, M., & Claussen, M. C. (2020). Disordered eating and eating disorders in male elite athletes: A scoping review. *BMJ Open Sport & Exercise Medicine, 6*(1), e000801. https://doi.org/10.1136/bmjsem-2020-000801

Le Grange, D., Hughes, E. K., Court, A., et al. (2016). Randomized clinical triafvl of parent-focused treatment and family-based treatment for adolescent anorexia nervosa. *Journal of the American Academy of Child & Adolescent Psychiatry, 55*(8), 683–692.

Lindstedt, K., Kjellin, L., & Gustafsson, S. A. (2017). Adolescents with full or subthreshold anorexia nervosa in a naturalistic sample–Characteristics and treatment outcome. *Journal of Eating Disorders, 5*(1), 1–10.

Mahoney, J. S., Palyo, N., Napier, G., et al. (2009). The therapeutic milieu reconceptualized for the 21st century. *Archives of Psychiatric Nursing, 23*(6), 423–429.

Mayhew, A. J., Pigeyre, M., Couturier, J., et al. (2018). An evolutionary genetic perspective of eating disorders. *Neuroendocrinology, 106*(3), 292–306.

Melisse, B., de Beurs, E., & van Furth, E. F. (2020). Eating disorders in the Arab world: A literature review. *Journal of Eating Disorders, 8*(1), 1–19.

McElroy, S. L. (2017). Pharmacologic treatments for binge-eating disorder. *The Journal of Clinical Psychiatry, 78*(1), 14–19.

Moorhead, S., Johnson, M., Maas, M. L., et al. (2013). *Nursing Outcomes Classification (NOC)* (5th ed.). St. Louis: Mosby.

Morris, J., & Anderson, S. (2021). An update on eating disorders. *BJPsych Advances, 27*(1), 9–19. https://doi.org/10.1192/bja.2020.24

Nakai, Y., Nin, K., Noma, S. I., et al. (2018). Changing profile of eating disorders between 1963 and 2004 in a Japanese sample. *International Journal of Eating Disorders, 51*(8), 953–958.

National Initiative for Eating Disorders. (2020). *Resources*. Retrieved from https://nied.ca/resources/

Norris, M., Strike, M., Pinhas, L., et al. (2013). The Canadian eating disorder program survey: Exploring intensive treatment programs for youth with eating disorders. *Journal of the Canadian Academy of Child and Adolescent Psychiatry/Journal de l'Académie Canadienne de Psychiatrie de l'Enfant et de l'Adolescent, 22*(4), 310.

Obesity Canada-Obésité Canada. (2019). *Report card on access to obesity treatment for adults in Canada 2019*. Retrieved from https://obesitycanada.ca/wp-content/uploads/2019/04/OC-Report-Card-2019-Eng-F-web.pdf

Organisation for Economic Co-operation and Development (OECD). (2017). *OECD data: Obesity update*. Retrieved from https://www.oecd.org/els/health-systems/Obesity-Update-2017.pdf

Ostermann, T., Vogel, H., Boehm, K., et al. (2019). Effects of yoga on eating disorders—A systematic review. *Complementary Therapies in Medicine, 46*, 73–80. https://doi.org/10.1016/j.ctim.2019.07.021

Parker, L. L., & Harriger, J. A. (2020). Eating disorders and disordered eating behaviors in the LGBT population: A review of the literature. *Journal of Eating Disorders, 8*, 51. https://doi.org/10.1186/s40337-020-00327-y

Peckmezian, T., & Paxton, S. J. (2020). A systematic review of outcomes following residential treatment for eating disorders. *European Eating Disorders Review, 28*(3), 246–259.

Pisetsky, E. M., Haynos, A. F., Lavender, J. M., et al. (2017). Associations between emotion regulation difficulties, eating disorder symptoms, non-suicidal self-injury, and suicide attempts in a heterogeneous eating disorder sample. *Comprehensive Psychiatry, 73*, 143–150. https://doi.org/10.1016/j.comppsych.2016.11.012

Pop, L. M., Iorga, M., Jain, A., et al. (2020). Adverse childhood experiences in relationship with eating disorders. *Medical Surgical Journal, 124*(1), 123–133.

Rodgers, R. F., DuBois, R., Thiebaut, S., Jaussent, I., Maimoun, L., Seneque, M., Lefebvre, P., Renard, E., Courtet, P., & Guillaume, S. (2019). Structural differences in eating disorder psychopathology after history of childhood abuse: Insights from a Structural differences in eating disorder psychopathology after history of childhood abuse: Insights from a Bayesian network analysis. *Journal of Abnormal Psychology, 128*(8), 795–805. https://doi.org/10.1037/abn0000470

Romano, C. (2015). Current findings in pediatric non organic feeding disorders: The gastroenterologist point of view. *Italian Journal of Pediatrics, 41*(2), A61. https://doi.org/10.1186/1824-7288-41-S2-A61

Rosenvinge, J., & Petterson, G. (2015). Epidemiology of eating disorders part II: An update with a special reference to the DSM-5. *Advances in Eating Disorders, 3*(2), 198–220. https://doi.org/10.1080/21662630.2014.940549

Sakallaris, B. R., Macallister, L., Voss, M., et al. (2015). Optimal healing environments. *Global Advances in Health and Medicine, 4*(3), 40–45.

Samuels, K. L., Maine, M. M., & Tantillo, M. (2019). Disordered eating, eating disorders, and body image in midlife and older women. *Current Psychiatry Reports, 21*(8), 1–9.

Santomauro, D. F., Melen, S., Mitchison, D., et al. (2021). The hidden burden of eating disorders: An extension of estimates from the Global Burden of Disease Study 2019. *The Lancet Psychiatry, 8*(4), 320–328.

Singleton, C., Kenny, T. E., Hallett, D., et al. (2019). Depression partially mediates the association between binge eating disorder and health-related quality of life. *Frontiers in Psychology, 10*, 209.

Smith, A. J., Farstad, S. M., & Von Ranson, K. M. (2021). Self-reported eating disorder psychopathology prevalence in community-based female and male Albertans: Gender and age group comparisons. *International Journal of Eating Disorders, 54*(3), 438–444. https://doi.org/10.1002/eat.23434

Spettigue, W., Obeid, N., Santos, A., et al. (2020). Binge eating and social anxiety in treatment-seeking adolescents with eating disorders or severe obesity. *Eating and Weight Disorders-Studies on Anorexia, Bulimia and Obesity, 25*(3), 787–793.

Uchôa, F. N. M., Uchôa, N. M., Daniele, T. M. D. C., et al. (2019). Influence of the mass media and body dissatisfaction on the risk in adolescents of developing eating disorders. *International Journal of Environmental Research and Public Health, 16*(9), 1508.

Vrabel, J. K., & Zeigler-Hill, V. (2020). Conscious versus unconscious determinants of behavior. In V. Zeigler-Hill, & T. K. Shackelford (Eds.), *Encyclopedia of personality and individual differences* (pp. 855–858). Cham: Springer.

Wells, K. R., Jeacocke, N. A., Appaneal, R., et al. (2020). The Australian Institute of Sport (AIS) and National Eating Disorders Collaboration (NEDC) position statement on disordered eating in high performance sport. *British Journal of Sports Medicine, 54*(21), 1247–1258.

World Health Organization. (2018). *ICD-11 for mortality and morbidity statistics*. Retrieved from https://icd.who.int/browse11/l-m/en

Yilmaz, Z., Hardaway, J. A., & Bulik, C. M. (2015). Genetics and epigenetics of eating disorders. *Advances in Genomics and Genetics, 5*, 131.

Zipfel, S., Schmidt, U., & Giel, K. E. (2022). Comment: The hidden burden of eating disorders during the COVID-19 pandemic. *The Lancet, 9*(1), 9–11. https://doi.org/10.1016/S2215-0366(21)00435-1

17

Neurocognitive Disorders

Gabriel Barrington-Moss
Originating US chapter by Jane Stein-Parbury

 http://evolve.elsevier.com/Canada/Varcarolis/psychiatric/

OBJECTIVES

1. Compare and contrast the clinical picture of delirium with that of dementia and brain injury.
2. Discuss three critical needs of a person with delirium, stated in terms of nursing diagnoses.
3. Identify three outcomes for patients with delirium.
4. Summarize the essential nursing interventions for a patient with delirium.
5. Recognize the signs and symptoms occurring in the stages of Alzheimer's disease.
6. Give an example of the following symptoms assessed during the progression of Alzheimer's disease: (1) amnesia, (2) apraxia, (3) agnosia, and (4) aphasia.
7. Formulate three nursing diagnoses suitable for a patient with Alzheimer's disease, and define two outcomes for each.
8. Formulate a teaching plan for a caregiver of a patient with Alzheimer's disease, including interventions for communication, health maintenance, and a safe environment.
9. Compose a list of appropriate referrals in the community, including a support group, hotline for information, and respite services, for people with dementia and their caregivers.

KEY TERMS AND CONCEPTS

agnosia
Alzheimer's disease
aphasia
apraxia
catastrophic reactions
confabulation
delirium
dementia
major neurocognitive disorders
mild neurocognitive disorders
neurocognitive disorders
perseveration
pseudodementia
sundowning

The clarity and purpose of an individual's personal journey through life depend on the ability to reflect on its meaning. Cognition therefore is a fundamental human feature that distinguishes living from existing. This mental capacity has a distinctive, personalized impact on the individual's physical, psychological, social, and spiritual conduct of life. For example, the ability to remember the connections between related actions and how to initiate them depends on cognitive processing. Moreover, this cognitive processing has a direct relationship to activities of daily living.

Cognitive functioning involves a variety of domains. Attention and orientation are basic lower-level cognitive domains. Higher-level cognitive domains are more complex and include the ability to:
- Plan and problem-solve (executive functioning)
- Learn and retain information in long-term memory
- Use language
- Visually perceive the environment
- Interpret social cues (social cognition)

Although primarily an intellectual and perceptual process, cognition is closely integrated with an individual's emotional and spiritual values. **Neurocognitive disorders** result from changes in the brain and are marked by disturbances in orientation, memory, intellect, judgement, and affect. These disorders may be described as ranging from

 HOW A NURSE HELPED ME
What Happened to the Person I Married?

My husband and I have been married for more than 45 years. Over the past couple of years, he has become more irritable and difficult to live with. In the past, he was always very particular about his appearance and was very kind to everyone. Now, he rarely showers or bathes, almost never brushes his teeth, and wears his dirty clothes for several days. His kindness has been replaced by irritability and sarcasm. We have always had a physical relationship, but now he says sexually explicit comments that are rude and offensive. His comments are sometimes about children; he was never like that. He has also begun to masturbate in public.

I was very upset with these changes in behaviour. Our doctor said that he had a form of dementia that makes his impulses hard to control. Knowing this did not make it easier for me to cope, however. Fortunately, there was a mental health outreach nurse in our area. She came to see my husband and me. She helped me understand my husband's illness and provided me with information on dementia and the impulsive behaviours that are associated with different kinds of dementias. We also discussed how I could set boundaries for myself and understand that my husband's behaviours were not something I had caused. She informed me that my husband's behaviours would change as his dementia got worse. The nurse also helped me figure out what I was going to tell my daughters, who were upset that I did not want the grandchildren staying overnight anymore. We practised role-playing the discussion that I needed to have with my children. This helped build my confidence, knowing that I understood what was happening with my husband's dementia and that I was able to explain it to my kids.

minor to *major* in terms of the level of cognitive decline and subsequent impact on global impairment.

The three main neurocognitive classifications are delirium, **mild neurocognitive disorders**, and **major neurocognitive disorders**. The first syndrome, delirium, tends to be short-term and reversible. Mild neurocognitive disorders may or may not progress to being major. Major neurocognitive disorders are commonly referred to as dementia, which is progressive and irreversible. In both mild and major neurocognitive disorders there is a decline in cognitive functioning from a previous level, although they differ in how much they interfere with independence in everyday activities (American Psychiatric Association [APA], 2013).

The labyrinth of current knowledge about cognitive disorders requires compassionate understanding of the patient and family. Nursing interventions are focused on attending to the needs, desires, and choices of the individual with a cognitive disorder and their family. The goals of the interventions are to protect welfare, preserve functional status, and promote well-being for cognitively impaired patients regardless of the reason for the impairment.

This chapter addresses the broad categories of delirium and major neurocognitive disorders, by far the most common conditions nurses encounter. It also introduces psychiatric symptoms of people with brain injuries and compares them with those of people with delirium and major neurocognitive disorders. Table 17.1 offers some guidelines for distinguishing among delirium, major neurocognitive disorders, depression, and brain injury (these last two may have similar symptoms and may co-occur in older persons).

TABLE 17.1 Comparison of Delirium, Major Neurocognitive Disorders, Depression, and Brain Injury

	Delirium	Major Neurocognitive Disorders	Depression	Brain Injury
Onset	Sudden, over hours to days	Slowly, over months	May have been gradual, with exacerbation during crisis or stress	Usually sudden; symptoms increase as damage becomes more pervasive
Cause or contributing factors	Hypoglycemia, fever, dehydration, hypotension; infection, other conditions that disrupt body's homeostasis; adverse drug reaction; head injury; change in environment (e.g., hospitalization); pain; emotional stress	Alzheimer's disease, vascular disease, human immunodeficiency virus (HIV) infection, neurological disease, chronic alcoholism, head trauma	Lifelong history, losses, loneliness, crises, declining health, medical conditions	Traumatic injury (external physical force) or acquired injury (conditions other than degenerative, such as stroke, anoxia, hypoxia, tumour, toxin)
Cognition	Impaired memory, judgement, calculations, attention span; can fluctuate through the day	Impaired memory, judgement, calculations, attention span, abstract thinking; agnosia	Difficulty concentrating, forgetfulness, inattention	May have difficulty thinking and learning; poor judgement; easily distractible; disoriented, confused, or amnesic depending on injury
Level of consciousness	Altered	Not altered	Not altered	Variable alterations depending on injury
Activity level	Can be increased or reduced; restlessness, which may worsen in evening (sundowning); sleep–wake cycle may be reversed	Not altered; behaviours may worsen in evening (sundowning)	Usually decreased; lethargy, fatigue, lack of motivation; may sleep poorly and awaken in early morning	Depending on injury, may have sleep disturbances, swallowing or appetite changes, weakness or paralysis, balance or coordination difficulties
Emotional state	Rapid swings; can be fearful, anxious, suspicious, aggressive; may have hallucinations, delusions, or both	Flat; delusions	Extreme sadness, apathy, irritability, anxiety, paranoid ideation	Anxiety, depression, agitation, hyper-reactivity, disinhibition, impulsivity, labile mood depending on injury
Speech and language	Rapid, inappropriate, incoherent, rambling	Incoherent, slow (sometimes due to effort to find the right word), inappropriate, rambling, repetitious	Slow, flat, low	Depending on the injury, may experience difficulties with expressive speech, word finding, comprehension
Prognosis	Reversible with proper and timely treatment	Not reversible; progressive	Reversible with proper and timely treatment	Varies depending on the location and the extent of brain damaged

DELIRIUM

> **SAFETY TIP**
>
> Be aware: a patient with delirium's health status can change rapidly, as can their behaviour. Be attentive to early signs of confusion driven by frustration and agitation, those that could lead to an unintended act of aggression, from the patient towards a care provider. Stay aware, stay safe!

Clinical Picture

Delirium is an acute cognitive disturbance characterized as a syndrome composed of a constellation of symptoms rather than a disorder. An important distinguisher between delirium and dementia is the nature, correlating variables, and presentation of the symptomology. Dementia presents as a sudden shift in behavior, cognition, emotional regulation, and physiological stability. This shift is sudden, as is the patient's physiological decline should the causative agent(s) of the delirious state not be addressed. Delirium is not a disease of progressive neurological decline, unlike the nature of dementia. Although these two disorders may present with shared symptomology, the causative nature, illness trajectory, and treatment approaches vary significantly. Recognizing and understanding these differences is a critical opportunity for nurses to apply their knowledge of disease pathology and process.

The cardinal symptoms of delirium are an inability to direct, focus, sustain, and shift attention; an abrupt onset with clinical features that fluctuate with periods of lucidity; and disorganized thinking and poor executive functioning. Other characteristics include disorientation (often to time and place, but rarely to person), anxiety, agitation, poor memory, and delusional thinking. When hallucinations are present, they are usually visual. *Diagnostic and Statistical Manual of Mental Disorders, fifth edition (DSM-5)*: Diagnostic Criteria for Delirium identifies the diagnostic criteria for delirium.

Delirium, also referred to as acute confusional state, is a serious medical event, and timely intervention must be initiated if reversible, neurological damage is to be avoided (Kennedy et al., 2020). In hospitalized patients who develop delirium 35% to 40% will die within 1 year of developing delirium. Mortality and morbidity are markedly high with the development of this medical emergency (Goldberg et al., 2020). A recent comprehensive review of the literature suggests that one-third of patients who develop delirium go on to then develop post-traumatic stress disorder (PTSD). Delirium as a result of mechanical ventilation further increases the risk of the subsequent development of PTSD, and as such, attention of the early warning signs of shifting attention, concentration, and level of consciousness are essential in mitigating this risk (Grover et al., 2019).

Epidemiology

Delirium is a common complication of hospitalization, especially in older patients. The reported incidence of delirium in older patients is between 15% and 50%, in terms of the development of delirium during their hospital admission. It is also important to note that when delirium occurs in a younger patient, it is most often associated with drug use or an acute systemic medical decompensation (Kennedy et al., 2020). The high degree of variability in the reported incidence of delirium is most likely due to its under-recognition (see Research Highlight box).

Comorbidity and Etiology

Delirium is always secondary to another physiological condition and is often a transient disorder. If the underlying condition is corrected, complete recovery from delirium should also occur. Delirium can be an early indicator of a more worrisome underlying medical condition or disorder. As delirium may not present as it would in a younger person, with altered concentration and attention, it is important to take note of social withdrawal and depressive symptoms as early indicators of delirium in the older patient (Kennedy et al., 2020). The common acute causes of delirium are nervous system disease, systemic disease (such as cardiac failure) (Box 17.1), and intoxication or withdrawal from a chemical substance (Chapter 18).

The key to helping patients avoid the consequences of delirium is recognizing and investigating potential causes as soon as possible. Early recognition and diagnosis are challenging for clinicians because of the lack of knowledge about cognitive impairment and its clinical assessment and failure to interpret the signs and symptoms. The best evidence for the prevention and management of delirium in hospitalized patients is having clinical protocols for minimizing modifiable risk factors. Early detection of delirium may be improved by implementing the regular use of health care analytic tools that encourage a collaborative and interdisciplinary approach to documenting and analyzing early indicators of delirium (Hendrie et al., 2021).

APPLICATION OF THE NURSING PROCESS

Assessment

While symptoms of delirium must be managed, the goal of treatment is to determine the underlying cause and rectify it when possible. Clinicians who suspect delirium should conduct a thorough examination, including mental and neurological status examinations, as well as a physical examination. Blood tests and a urinalysis should also be done. If possible, additional information should be obtained from a person who knows the patient, such as a family member or friend. The patient's medication regimen should be reviewed carefully for drug interactions or toxicity profiles.

General Assessment

There are four cardinal features of delirium that clinicians focus on when using the Confusion Assessment Method (CAM):
1. Acute onset and fluctuating course
2. Inattention
3. Disorganized thinking
4. Disturbance of consciousness

 DSM-5

Diagnostic Criteria for Delirium

A. A disturbance in attention (i.e., reduced ability to direct, focus, sustain, and shift attention) and awareness (reduced orientation to the environment).

B. The disturbance develops over a short period of time (usually hours to a few days), represents a change from baseline attention and awareness, and tends to fluctuate in severity during the course of a day.

C. An additional disturbance in cognition (e.g., memory deficit, disorientation, language, visuospatial ability, or perception).

D. The disturbances in Criteria A and C are not better explained by another pre-existing, established, or evolving neurocognitive disorder and do not occur in the context of a severely reduced level of arousal such as coma.

E. There is evidence from the history, physical examination, or laboratory findings that the disturbance is a direct physiological consequence of another medical condition, substance intoxication, withdrawal (i.e., due to a drug of abuse or to a medication), or exposure to a toxin or is due to multiple etiologies.

Specify whether:

Substance Intoxication Delirium: This diagnosis should be made instead of substance intoxication when the symptoms in Criteria A and C predominate in the clinical picture and when they are sufficiently severe to warrant clinical attention.

Source: American Psychiatric Association. (2013). *Diagnostic and statistical manual of mental disorders* (5th ed.). Washington, DC: Author.

RESEARCH HIGHLIGHT

Recognition, Prevention, and Treatment of Delirium in Emergency Department: An Evidence-Based Narrative Review

Background
Delirium is classified as an acute disorder, primarily impacting attention, concentration, behavior, and cognition. This disorder is commonly under-diagnosed, presumed to be related to uncontrolled mental illness, and, if not accurately assessed and treated, may be fatal and/or cause permanent neurological damage. Delirium is frequently seen in the emergency department (ED), as the person presents with acute delirium-related symptoms that have gone unrecognized in their earlier presentation.

Objective of Study
The authors engaged in an evidence-based narrative review that focused on the key aspects of delirium screening, prevention, and treatment.

Methods
The authors searched PubMed and reference lists from relevant original research articles and systematic reviews using the terms "delirium," "encephalopathy," and "organic brain syndrome" for articles published in English from 1996 to June 2019.

Key Findings
The key research findings from this review include many delirium assessment tools with high sensitivity and specificity, including the delirium triage screen and brief Confusion Assessment Method, which are helpful in assessing delirium in the ED. To reduce the incidence of delirium in the geriatric population, modifying the ED environment to reduce precipitating factors is an essential focus. Orientation, hydration, and early mobilization have also been shown to be important strategies in preventing delirium in the ED.

Implications for Nursing Practice
Geriatric ED patients are at high risk for developing delirium and the outcomes for this population include high mortality rates; as such, a focused assessment of the patient's cognitive state and physiological symptoms is essential. Focused and timely screening, prevention, and intervention for those who are at risk of developing delirium or who present with delirium, particularly geriatric patients who can decompensate quickly, are the priority foci in moving forward.

Source: Lee, S., Gottlieb, M., Mulhausen, P., et al. (2020). Recognition, prevention, and treatment of delirium in emergency department: An evidence-based narrative review. *American Journal of Emergency Medicine, 38*(2), 349–357. https://doi.org/10.1016/j.ajem.2019.158454

BOX 17.1 Common Causes of Delirium

Postoperative States, Drug Intoxications, and Withdrawals
- Anticholinergics, benzodiazepines, alcohol, anxiolytics, opioids, and central nervous system stimulants (e.g., cocaine, crack cocaine)

Infections
- Systemic: pneumonia, typhoid fever, malaria, urinary tract infection, and septicemia
- Intracranial: meningitis and encephalitis

Metabolic Disorders
- Dehydration
- Hypoxia (pulmonary disease, heart disease, and anemia)
- Hypoglycemia
- Sodium, potassium, calcium, magnesium, and acid–base imbalances
- Hepatic encephalopathy or uremic encephalopathy
- Thiamine (vitamin B_1) deficiency (Wernicke's encephalopathy)
- Endocrine disorders (e.g., thyroid or parathyroid)
- Hypothermia or hyperthermia
- Diabetic acidosis

Drugs
- Digitalis, steroids, lithium, levodopa, anticholinergics, benzodiazepines, central nervous system depressants, tricyclic antidepressants
- Central anticholinergic syndrome due to use of multiple drugs with anticholinergic adverse effects

Neurological Diseases
- Seizures
- Head trauma
- Hypertensive encephalopathy

Tumour
- Primary cerebral

Psychosocial Stressors
- Relocation or other sudden changes
- Sensory deprivation or overload
- Sleep deprivation
- Immobilization
- Pain

Suspect the presence of delirium when a person's ability to focus, sustain, or shift attention becomes abruptly impaired and their awareness of the environment is reduced. Conversation is made more difficult because the person may be easily distracted by irrelevant stimuli. Questions must be repeated because the individual's attention wanders, and the person might easily get off track and need to be refocused. The person may also have difficulty with orientation, first to time, then to place, and last to person. For example, a man with delirium may think that the year is 1972, that the hospital is home, and that the nurse is his wife. Orientation to person is usually intact to the extent that the person is aware of their own identity.

A person with delirium may also appear withdrawn, agitated, or psychotic. Fluctuating levels of consciousness are unpredictable. Disorientation and confusion are usually markedly worse at night and during the early morning. In fact, some patients may be confused or delirious only at night and may remain lucid during the day. The phenomenon in which symptoms become more pronounced in the evening is called **sundowning** (also known as *sundown syndrome*). Sundowning often begins in the late afternoon as the evening approaches. This symptom-exacerbation pattern may occur in people who have either delirium or dementia. Sundowning can significantly impact an individual's quality of life. When impacted, the individual will often become paranoid, suspicious, and may even exhibit a break from reality, as they respond to unsubstantiated sensory stimuli. Some of the possible causes of sundowning include end-of-day fatigue that leads to decreased coping, altered sensory perception exacerbated by dim lighting and shadow casting, alteration in sleep–wake cycle, and decreased activity levels in the afternoon, leading to nighttime restlessness. (Alzheimer Society of Canada, 2021a).

As nurses, our frequent interaction with those in hospital places us in a prime position to prevent, detect, and treat the effects of delirium. Nursing assessment includes observation and evaluation of (1) cognitive and perceptual disturbances, (2) physical needs, and (3) moods and physical behaviours.

Cognitive and perceptual disturbances. Patients experiencing delirium may be difficult to engage in conversation because they are easily distracted, display marked attention deficits, and exhibit memory impairment. In mild delirium memory deficits are noted only on careful questioning. In more severe delirium memory problems usually take the form of obvious difficulty in processing and remembering recent events. For example, the person might ask when a son is coming to visit, even though the son left only an hour earlier.

Another helpful tool clinicians can use to determine the presence of a component of dementia is the Montreal Cognitive Assessment (MoCA). The MoCA assesses short-term memory, visuospatial abilities, executive functioning, attention, concentration, working memory, language, and orientation to time and place (Nasreddine et al., 2005). The MoCA can be completed by an experienced clinician in approximately 10 minutes. An important consideration when using MoCA, and other cognitive testing tools, is that these tools necessitate the individual's ability to accurately hear and respond to the questions asked. Many older patients may struggle with hearing loss and this can impact their MoCA score (Alzheimer Society of Canada, 2021a).

Perceptual disturbances are also common. *Perception* is the processing of information about one's internal and external environments. Various misinterpretations of reality may take the form of illusions. For example, a person may mistake folds in the bedclothes for white rats or the cord of a window blind for a snake. Alternatively, misinterpretations may take the form of hallucinations. For example, individuals experiencing delirium may become terrified when they "see" giant spiders crawling over the bedclothes or "feel" bugs crawling on or under their skin.

The individual with delirium generally is aware that something is very wrong. Statements like "My thoughts are all jumbled" may signal cognitive problems. When perceptual disturbances are present, the emotional response is often one of fear and anxiety, which may be manifested by psychomotor agitation.

Physical needs. A person with delirium becomes disoriented and may try to "go home." Alternatively, a person may think that they *are* home and jump out of a window in an attempt to get away from "invaders." Wandering, pulling out intravenous lines and Foley catheters, and falling out of bed are common dangers that require nursing vigilance.

An individual experiencing delirium has difficulty processing stimuli in the environment, and confusion magnifies the inability to recognize reality. The physical environment should be made as simple and clear as possible. Objects such as clocks and calendars can maximize orientation to time. Glasses, hearing aids, and adequate lighting without glare can maximize the person's ability to interpret more accurately what is going on in the environment. The nurse should interact with the patient whenever the patient is awake. Short periods of social interaction help to reduce anxiety and misperceptions (Canadian Institute for Health Information, 2010).

Self-care deficits, injury, hyperactivity, or hypoactivity may lead to skin breakdown and possible infection. Often this condition is compounded by poor nutrition, forced bed rest, and possible incontinence. These situations require nursing assessment and intervention.

Autonomic signs, such as tachycardia, sweating, flushed face, dilated pupils, and elevated blood pressure, are often present in delirium. These changes must be monitored and documented carefully and may require immediate medical attention, as they may be an indication that the underlying physiological condition is worsening.

Changes in the sleep–wake cycle should be assessed and documented. In some cases a complete reversal of the night–day, sleep–wake cycle can occur. The patient's level of consciousness may range from lethargy to stupor or from semi-coma to hypervigilance. In hypervigilance patients are extraordinarily alert, and their eyes constantly scan the room; they may have difficulty falling asleep or may be actively disoriented and agitated throughout the night.

You should always suspect medications as a potential cause of delirium. This is especially true when there is polypharmacy or the use of psychoactive agents. To recognize drug reactions or anticipate potential interactions before delirium actually occurs, it is important to assess all medications, both prescription and over the counter, and other substances (i.e., street drugs, alcohol, herbal or natural therapies) the patient is taking.

Moods and physical behaviours. The individual's moods and physical behaviours may change dramatically within a short period. A person with delirium may display motor restlessness (agitation), or they may be "quietly delirious" and appear calm and settled. When there is agitation, delirium is considered hyperactive; when there is no agitation, delirium is considered hypoactive. Moods may swing back and forth between fear, anger, anxiety, euphoria, depression, and apathy. A person may strike out from fear or anger or may cry, call for help, curse, moan, and tear off clothing one minute and become apathetic or laugh uncontrollably the next. In short, behaviour and emotions are erratic and fluctuating. The following vignette illustrates the fear and confusion a patient may experience during and after an episode of delirium.

> **VIGNETTE**
> Peter Wright, age 43, survived numerous life-threatening complications after open-heart surgery to replace his mitral valve. He spent 3 weeks in an ICU and then moved to a general medical unit.
> Peter became suspicious about his bed being moved. "Why are you taking me to another country?" He expressed concern that his organs would be removed and donated for transplantation. He began to yell for his wife. Peter knew that the very people who had saved his life were now out to get him.
> When he was sure nobody was looking, he climbed out of bed and attempted to leave the unit. The nurses responded by calling security personnel to escort him back to bed. Once he was safely in bed, the nurses applied mechanical restraints and sedated him.
> Peter's confusion disappeared the next day. While he realized how distorted his thinking had been during the episode, the anxiety and fear he experienced remained with him for months after discharge from the hospital.
> What are some more helpful interventions the nurses could have used? What could the nurses have done differently? What would you have done?

Self-Assessment

Because the behaviours exhibited by the patient with delirium can be directly attributed to temporary medical conditions, intense personal reactions in staff are less likely to arise. In fact, intense, conflicting emotions are less likely to occur in nurses working with a patient with delirium than in nurses working with a patient with dementia, which is discussed later in this chapter. Nonetheless, interacting with these patients can be frustrating for health care providers, especially given the fluctuating nature of the clinical picture.

ASSESSMENT GUIDELINES
Delirium

1. Assess for acute onset and fluctuating levels of consciousness, which are key in delirium.
2. Assess the person's ability to attend to the immediate environment, including responses to nursing care.
3. Establish the person's normal level of consciousness and cognition by interviewing family members or other caregivers.
4. Assess for past cognitive impairment, especially an existing dementia diagnosis, and other risk factors.
5. Identify disturbances in physiological status, especially infection, hypoxia, and pain.
6. Identify any physiological abnormalities documented in the patient's record.
7. Assess vital signs, level of consciousness, and neurological signs.
8. Assess potential for injury, especially in relation to potential for falls and wandering.
9. Maintain comfort measures, especially in relation to pain, cold, or positioning.
10. Monitor situational factors that worsen or improve symptoms.
11. Assess for availability of immediate medical interventions to help prevent irreversible brain damage.
12. Remain non-judgemental. Confer with other staff readily when questions arise.

Diagnosis

Safety needs play a substantial role in nursing care. Patients with delirium often perceive the environment in a distorted way, and objects are often misperceived (due to illusions or hallucinations). People and objects may be misinterpreted as threatening or harmful, and patients often act on these misinterpretations. For example, if feeling threatened or thinking that common medical equipment is harmful, the patient may pull off an oxygen mask, pull out an intravenous or nasogastric tube, or try to flee. In such a case the person demonstrates a *risk for injury* related to confusion as evidenced by sensory deficits or perceptual deficits.

Hallucinations, distractibility, illusions, disorientation, agitation, restlessness, and misperception are major aspects of the clinical picture. When some of these symptoms are present, *acute confusion* related to delirium is an appropriate nursing diagnosis.

If fever and dehydration are present, fluid and electrolyte balance will need to be managed. If the underlying cause of the patient's delirium results in fever, decreased skin turgor, decreased urinary output or fluid intake, and dry skin or mucous membranes, then the nursing diagnosis of *deficient fluid volume* is appropriate. Fluid volume deficit may be related to fever, electrolyte imbalance, reduced intake, or infection.

In cases of delirium restful sleep is not achieved, day or night; the patient may be less responsive during the day and may become disruptively wakeful during the night. *Insomnia* or *sleep deprivation* related to impaired cerebral oxygenation or disruption in consciousness is a likely diagnosis.

Engaging in communication with a delirious patient is difficult. An example of a nursing diagnosis addressing this problem is *impaired verbal communication* related to cerebral hypoxia or decreased cerebral blood flow as evidenced by confusion or clouding of consciousness.

Fear is one of the most common of all nursing diagnoses and may be related to illusions, delusions, or hallucinations, as evidenced by verbal and non-verbal expressions of fearfulness. Other nursing concerns include *self-care deficit, disturbed thought processes*, and *impaired social interaction*. Table 17.2 identifies nursing diagnoses for any confused patient with delirium or dementia.

Outcomes Identification

The overall outcome is that the delirious patient will return to the pre-morbid level of functioning. Table 17.3 includes outcomes for acute confusion from the *Nursing Outcomes Classification (NOC)* (Moorhead et al., 2018). However, for many of the diagnoses we would use for the person experiencing delirium, *NOC* is not specific enough. Although the person can demonstrate a wide variety of needs, *risk for injury* is always present. Appropriate outcomes are as follows:

- During periods of lucidity, the patient will be oriented to time, place, and person with the aid of nursing interventions, such as the provision of clocks, calendars, maps, and other types of orienting information.
- Patient will remain free from falls and injury while confused, with the aid of nursing safety measures while in the hospital.

Because the level of consciousness can change throughout the day, the patient needs to be checked frequently for orientation.

Planning

Planning nursing care for a patient who is experiencing delirium involves special attention to the safety and security of the environment. You should address the following questions:

- Does the person have the necessary visual and auditory aids?
- Are family members available to stay with the patient?
- Does the environment provide visual cues as to the time of day and season of the year?
- Has the person experienced continuity of care providers?

Implementation

The priorities of treatment are to keep the patient safe while attempting to identify the cause. If the underlying disorder is corrected, complete recovery is possible. If, however, the underlying disorder is not corrected and persists, irreversible neuronal damage can occur. Nursing concerns therefore centre on:

- Preventing physical harm due to confusion, aggression, or electrolyte and fluid imbalance
- Performing a comprehensive nursing assessment to aid in identifying the cause
- Assisting with proper health management to eradicate the underlying cause
- Using supportive measures to relieve distress

The *Nursing Interventions Classification (NIC)* (Bulechek et al., 2013) can be used as a guide to developing interventions for a person experiencing delirium (Box 17.2). Medical management of delirium involves treating the underlying organic causes. If the underlying cause of delirium is not treated, permanent brain damage may ensue. In addition, thoughtful use of antipsychotic or anti-anxiety agents may also aid in controlling behavioural symptoms.

A patient in acute delirium should never be left alone. Because most hospitals and health facilities are unable to provide one-to-one supervision of the patient, family members can be encouraged to stay with the patient.

Evaluation

Long-term outcome criteria for a person experiencing delirium include:

- Patient will remain safe.
- Patient will be oriented to time, place, and person by discharge.
- Underlying cause will be treated and ameliorated.

TABLE 17.2 Potential Nursing Diagnoses for the Confused Patient

Symptoms	Nursing Diagnoses
Wanders, has unsteady gait, acts out fear from hallucinations or illusions, forgets things (leaves stove on, doors open)	Risk for injury
Awake and disoriented during the night (*sundowning*), frightened at night	Disturbed sleep pattern Fear Acute confusion
Unable to take care of basic needs	Self-care deficit (bathing/hygiene, dressing, feeding, toileting) Ineffective coping Functional urinary incontinence Imbalanced nutrition: less than body requirements Risk for deficient fluid volume
Sees frightening things that are not there (*hallucinations*), mistakes everyday objects for something sinister and frightening (*illusions*), may become paranoid and think that others are doing things to confuse them (*delusions*)	Anxiety Disturbed sensory perception Impaired environmental interpretation syndrome Disturbed thought processes
Does not recognize familiar people or places, has difficulty with short- or long-term memory or both, is forgetful and confused	Impaired memory Impaired environmental interpretation syndrome Acute or chronic confusion
Has difficulty with communication, cannot find words, has difficulty recognizing objects or people, is incoherent	Impaired verbal communication Impaired social interaction
Devastated over losing place in life as known (during lucid moments), fearful and overwhelmed by what is happening to him or her	Spiritual distress Hopelessness Situational low self-esteem Grieving
Family and loved ones overburdened and overwhelmed, unable to care for patient's needs	Disabled family coping Interrupted family processes Impaired home maintenance Caregiver role strain

TABLE 17.3 NOC Outcomes Related to Acute Confusion

Acute confusion: Abrupt onset of reversible disturbance of consciousness, attention, cognition, and perception that develops over a short period of time.

Nursing Outcome and Definition	Intermediate Indicators	Short-Term Indicators
Cognitive orientation: Ability to identify person, place, and time accurately	Identifies correct day Identifies correct month Identifies correct year Identifies correct season Identifies current place Identifies significant current events	Identifies self Identifies significant other
Neurological status and level of consciousness: Arousal, orientation, and attention to the environment	Oriented cognitively Communicates appropriately for situation Attends to environmental stimuli	Opens eyes to external stimuli Obeys commands Makes motor responses to noxious stimuli

Source: Moorhead, S., Swanson, E., Johnson, M., & Maas, M. L., (Eds.). (2018). Nursing Outcomes Classification (NOC): Measurement of health outcomes (6th ed.). St. Louis: MO: Elsevier.

MILD AND MAJOR NEUROCOGNITIVE DISORDERS

Dementia is a broad term used to describe the progressive deterioration of cognitive functioning and global impairment of intellect. It is a term that does not refer to specific disease but rather to a collection of symptoms. The *DSM-5* (APA, 2013) incorporates dementia into the diagnostic categories of mild and major neurocognitive disorders. These disorders are characterized by cognitive impairments that signal a decline from previous functioning.

When mild, the impairments do not interfere with essential activities of daily living, although the person may need to make extra efforts. While such impairments may be progressive, a mild cognitive impairment does not necessarily mean that it will progress to a major neurocognitive disorder (Alzheimer's Association, 2021). *DSM-5:* Diagnostic

BOX 17.2 NIC Interventions for Delirium Management

Definition of *delirium management*: Provision of a safe and therapeutic environment for the patient who is experiencing an acute state of confusion.

Activities:
- Identify etiological factors causing delirium.
- Initiate therapies to reduce or eliminate factors causing delirium.
- Monitor neurological status on an ongoing basis.
- Provide unconditional positive regard.
- Verbally acknowledge patient's fears and feelings.
- Provide optimistic but realistic reassurance.
- Allow patient to maintain rituals that limit anxiety.
- Provide patient with information about what is happening and what can be expected to occur in the future.
- Avoid demands for abstract thinking if patient can think only in concrete terms.
- Limit need for decision making if frustrating or confusing to patient.
- Administer prn (as needed) medications for anxiety or agitation.
- Encourage visitation by significant others, as appropriate.
- Recognize and accept patient's perceptions or interpretation of reality (hallucinations or delusions).
- State your perception in a calm, reassuring, and non-argumentative manner.
- Respond to the theme or feeling tone, rather than the content, of the hallucination or delusion.
- When possible, remove stimuli that create misperception in a particular patient (e.g., pictures on the wall or television).
- Maintain a well-lit environment that reduces sharp contrasts and shadows.
- Assist with needs related to nutrition, elimination, hydration, and personal hygiene.
- Maintain a hazard-free environment.
- Place identification bracelet on patient.
- Provide appropriate level of supervision and surveillance to monitor patient and allow for therapeutic actions, as needed.
- Use physical restraints, as needed.
- Avoid frustrating patient by quizzing with orientation questions that cannot be answered.
- Reorient patient to person, place, and time, as needed.
- Provide a consistent physical environment and daily routine.
- Provide caregivers who are familiar to the patient.
- Use environmental cues (e.g., signs, pictures, clocks, calendars, colour coding of environment) to stimulate memory, reorient, and promote appropriate behaviour.
- Provide a low-stimulation environment for patients disoriented by overstimulation.
- Encourage use of aids that increase sensory input (e.g., glasses, hearing aids, dentures).
- Approach patient slowly and from the front.
- Address patient by name when initiating interaction.
- Reorient patient to health care provider with each contact.
- Communicate with simple, direct, descriptive statements.
- Prepare patient for upcoming changes in usual routine and environment before their occurrence.
- Provide new information slowly and in small doses, with frequent rest periods.
- Focus interpersonal interactions on what is familiar and meaningful to patient.

Source: Bulechek, G. M., Butcher, H. K., & Dochterman, J. M. (2013). *Nursing Interventions Classification (NIC)* (6th ed.). Toronto: Elsevier.

DSM-5
Diagnostic Criteria for Mild Neurocognitive Disorder

A. Evidence of modest cognitive decline from previous level of performance in one or more cognitive domains (complex attention, executive function, learning and memory, language, perceptual-motor, or social cognition) based on:
  1. Concern of the individual, a knowledgeable informant, or clinician that there has been a mild decline in cognitive function; and
  2. A modest impairment in cognitive performance, preferably documented by standardized neuropsychological testing or, in its absence, another quantified clinical assessment.

B. The cognitive deficits do not interfere with capacity for independence in everyday activities (i.e., complex instrumental activities of daily living such as paying bills or accommodation may be required).

C. The cognitive deficits do not occur exclusively in the context of delirium.

D. The cognitive deficits are not better explained by another mental disorder (e.g., major depressive disorder, schizophrenia).

Source: American Psychiatric Association. (2013). *Diagnostic and statistical manual of mental disorders* (5th ed.). Washington, DC: Author.

DSM-5
Diagnostic Criteria for Major Neurocognitive Disorder

A. Evidence of significant cognitive decline from previous level of performance in one or more cognitive domains (complex attention, executive function, learning and memory, language, perceptual-motor, or social cognition) based on:
  1. Concern of the individual, a knowledgeable informant, or clinician that there has been significant decline in cognitive function; and
  2. A substantial impairment in cognitive performance, preferably documented by standardized neuropsychological testing or, in its absence, another quantified clinical assessment.

B. The cognitive deficits interfere with independence in everyday activities (i.e., at a minimum, requiring assistance with complex instrumental activities of daily living such as paying bills or managing medications).

C. The cognitive deficits do not occur exclusively in the context of delirium.

D. The cognitive deficits are not better explained by another mental disorder (e.g., major depressive disorder, schizophrenia).

Source: American Psychiatric Association. (2013). *Diagnostic and statistical manual of mental disorders* (5th ed.). Washington, DC: Author.

Criteria for Mild Neurocognitive Disorder lists diagnostic criteria for mild neurocognitive disorders.

When progressive, these disorders become major neurocognitive disorders because they interfere with daily functioning and independence. While often characterized by memory deficits, neurocognitive disorders affect other areas of cognitive functioning, for example, problem solving (executive functioning) and complex attention. DSM-5: Diagnostic Criteria for Major Neurocognitive Disorder describes the diagnostic criteria for major neurocognitive disorders.

Mild and major neurocognitive disorder criteria are general. Specific disorders such as Alzheimer's disease (AD) are listed in Table 17.4.

While the underlying etiology varies in neurocognitive disorders, nursing care is based on their behavioural manifestations. Therefore approaches to care are not necessarily different for various etiologies. It is for this reason that the remainder of this chapter focuses on the most frequently occurring major neurocognitive disorder, AD.

TABLE 17.4 Types of Neurocognitive Disorders

Type of Dementia	Symptoms
Alzheimer's disease	*Early:* Difficulty with recent memory, impaired learning, apathy, and depression *Moderate to severe:* Visual/spatial and language deficits, psychotic features, agitation, and wandering *Late:* Gait disturbance; poor judgement; disorientation; confusion; incontinence; and difficulty speaking, swallowing, and walking
Frontotemporal dementia	Impaired social cognition, disinhibition, apathy, compulsive behaviour, poor comprehension, and language difficulties
Dementia with Lewy bodies	Fluctuating cognition, early changes in attention and executive function, sleep disturbance, visual hallucinations, muscle rigidity, and other Parkinsonian features
Vascular dementia	One or more documented cerebrovascular events. Impaired judgement; poor decision making, planning, and organizing (executive functions); and personality and mood changes
Traumatic brain injury	Trauma to the head with loss of consciousness, post-traumatic amnesia, disorientation and confusion, and/or neurological signs
Substance-medication-induced dementia	Symptoms of neurocognitive impairment persist beyond the usual duration of intoxication and acute withdrawal. Substances include alcohol, inhalants, sedative, hypnotic, or anti-anxiety agents
HIV infection	A documented infection with HIV. Impaired executive function, slowing of processing, problems with attention, difficulty learning new information, aphasia. Symptoms dependent on area of brain affected by HIV pathogenic processes
Prion	Insidious onset and rapid progression of impairment. Motor features such as myoclonus or ataxia. Memory and coordination behaviour changes, rapidly fatal
Parkinson's disease	Progression of Parkinson's disease results in dementia with symptoms similar to dementia with Lewy bodies or Alzheimer's disease; apathetic, depressed, or anxious mood; and sleep disorder
Huntington's disease	Abnormal involuntary movements, severe decline in thinking and reasoning, mood changes such as irritability and depression, due to genetic defect

Clinical Picture

Dementia is the general term used to describe a decline in cognitive functioning that interferes with daily living. **Alzheimer's disease**, the most common cause of dementia in older persons, is a progressive degenerative neurocognitive disorder marked by impaired memory and thinking skills. It accounts for 60% to 80% of all dementias (Alzheimer's Association, 2021). It is a devastating disease that not only affects the person who has it but also places an enormous burden on the families and caregivers of those affected. Nurses practising in any setting will care for patients with AD and must be prepared to respond.

It is important to distinguish between normal forgetfulness and the memory deficit of AD and other dementias. Severe memory loss is *not* a normal part of aging. Slight forgetfulness is a common phenomenon of the aging process (age-associated memory loss), but memory loss that interferes with one's activities of daily living is not. Table 17.5 outlines memory changes in normal aging and memory changes seen in dementia.

Many people who live to a very old age never experience significant memory loss or any other symptom of dementia. Most of us know of people in their eighties and nineties who lead active lives with their intellect intact. Pablo Picasso, Duke Ellington, Ansel Adams, and George Burns are just a few examples of people who were still active in their careers when they died, and all were older than 75 years of age (Picasso was 91; George Burns was 100). The slow, minor cognitive changes associated with aging should not impede social or occupational functioning.

Although dementia often begins with a worsening of ability to remember new information, it is marked by progressive deterioration in intellectual functioning, memory, and the ability to solve problems and learn new skills; a decline in the ability to perform activities of daily living; and a progressive deterioration of personality accompanied by impairment in judgement. A person's declining intellect often leads to emotional changes such as mood lability, depression, and aggressive acting out, as well as neurological changes that produce hallucinations and delusions.

There are several types of dementias, including dementia of the Alzheimer's type, vascular dementia, Lewy body disease, Pick's disease, alcohol-related dementias (including Korsakoff's syndrome),

TABLE 17.5 Memory Deficit: Normal Aging Versus Major Neurocognitive Disorder

Parameter	Normal Aging	Major Neurocognitive Disorder
Area of impairment	Difficulty in word finding, but no aphasia, dyspraxia, agnosia	Aphasia, dyspraxia, agnosia often found
Extent of impairment	Slowing	Minor to major deceleration
	Cautiousness	Variable cautiousness
	Reduced ability to solve new problems	Minor to major problem-solving impairment
	Mildly impaired memory	Minor to major intellectual impairment
	Mild decline in fluid intelligence	Minor to major decline in fluid intelligence
Rate of impairment	Slow change over many years	More rapid though still gradual changes

CONSIDERING CULTURE
Understanding Dementia Within Indigenous Peoples in Canada

Over 500 000 people are experiencing age-related dementia. This number is believed to double over the next 30 years, to over 1 125 184 people. In Indigenous populations in Canada, the incidence of dementia is upwards of 34% higher than in the general population.

From an epidemiological perspective, we see an earlier age of onset and higher prevalence in males within Indigenous populations. For many researchers and community members, dementia is being viewed as a new or emerging challenge for this population; however, the shift in trajectory towards a longer life expectancy and increased exposure of the aging population to dementia care assessment is arguably a large component of the aforementioned findings.

As many Indigenous peoples view dementia symptoms as a normal part of the aging process, and the care of their elders is managed in the community through cultural care models, the willingness to engage in a biomedical, institutionalization-centered approach has, understandably, not been widely accepted or viewed through a positive lens.

Therapeutic engagement on dementia care with Indigenous peoples will require the Indigenous ways of managing the care of their elderly be advocated for and actively integrated, and that Indigenous persons are seen as leading partners when creating a plan of care for the individual.

Source: Jacklin, K., & Walker, J. (2020). Cultural understandings of dementia in Indigenous peoples: A qualitative evidence synthesis. *Canadian Journal on Aging, 39*(2), 220–234. https://doi.org/10.1017/S071498081900028X

TABLE 17.6 Stages of Alzheimer's Disease

Stage	Hallmarks
Mild Alzheimer's disease (early stage)	The person and their loved ones notice memory lapses. The person may still be able to function independently but will experience: • Difficulties retrieving correct words or names, previously known • Trouble remembering names when introduced to new people • Greater difficulty performing tasks in social or work settings • Forgetting material that one has just read • Losing or misplacing a valuable object • Trouble with planning or organizing • Mild coordination challenges
Moderate Alzheimer's disease (middle stage)	The person confuses words, gets frustrated or angry, or acts in unexpected ways such as refusing to bathe. The person will often require assistance with many aids to daily living at this point. Symptoms become noticeable to others and the person may: • Forget events or own personal history • Become moody or withdrawn, especially in socially or mentally challenging situations • Be unable to recall their own address or telephone number or the high school or university from which they graduated • Become confused about where they are or what day it is • Need help choosing proper clothing for the season or the occasion • Have trouble controlling bladder and bowels • Change sleep patterns, such as sleeping during the day and becoming restless at night • Be at risk of wandering and becoming lost • Become suspicious and delusional or compulsive, for example, repetitive behaviour such as hand-wringing or tissue shredding
Severe Alzheimer's disease (late stage)	The person loses the ability to respond to their environment, to carry on a conversation, and, eventually, to control movement. The person may still say words or phrases, but communicating pain becomes difficult. Non-verbal communication strategies become critical at this stage. Personality changes may take place and individuals need extensive help with daily activities. The person may: • Require full-time, around-the-clock assistance with daily personal care • Lose awareness of recent experiences and of their surroundings • Require high levels of assistance with daily activities and personal care • Experience changes in physical abilities, including the ability to walk, sit, and, eventually, swallow • Have increasing difficulty communicating • Become vulnerable to infections, especially pneumonia

Source: Adapted from Alzheimer Society of Canada. (2021). *What to expect as a person's dementia progresses.* https://alzheimer.ca/en/help-support/im-caring-person-living-dementia/what-expect-persons-dementia-progresses

Creutzfeldt–Jakob disease, and the dementias associated with Parkinson's disease, Huntington's disease, acquired immunodeficiency syndrome (AIDS), and traumatic and acquired brain injury.

Progression of Alzheimer's Disease

AD is classified according to the stage of the degenerative process. Table 17.6 outlines the three stages. These stages can be used as a guide to understanding the progressive deterioration seen in those diagnosed with AD. The three stages are mild, moderate, and severe. The first stage roughly corresponds to the *DSM-5* criteria for mild neurocognitive disorders. The second and third stages relate to the *DSM-5* criteria for major neurocognitive disorders.

The loss of intellectual ability is insidious. The person with mild AD loses energy, drive, and initiative and has difficulty learning new things. Because personality and social behaviour remain intact, others tend to minimize and underestimate the loss of the individual's abilities. The individual may continue to work, but the extent of the dementia becomes evident in new or demanding situations. Depression may occur early in the disease but usually resolves over time.

More severe symptoms appear as AD progresses. The person experiences agnosia, which is the inability to identify familiar objects or people, even a spouse. Apraxia is a common symptom whereby a person needs repeated instructions and directions to perform the simplest tasks: "Here is the washcloth. Pick up the soap. Now, put water on the face cloth, and rub the face cloth with soap."

Often the individual cannot remember the location of the toilet or is unaware of the process of urinating and defecating, resulting in incontinence. It is usually at this point that total care is necessary. For the family, this burden can be emotionally, financially, and physically devastating. For the individual with AD, the world is very frightening and nothing makes sense. In response, agitation, paranoia, and delusions are common.

> **VIGNETTE**
>
> Mrs. White, 78 years old, a retired teacher, has always enjoyed an active life and good health other than an underactive thyroid, which has been successfully controlled. Remarkably, her only hospitalizations were for the births of her two children, now grown and married. She is a vibrant person who takes pride in her appearance and in her beautiful home. She is beginning to forget things that she previously has taken for granted but jokes about her failing memory as "senior moments."
>
> Recently, her daughter found Mrs. White quite distressed as she attempted to make her famous specialty, lasagna. The ingredients were strewn all over the kitchen, and Mrs. White was frantically searching for a recipe. Her daughter was surprised because neither of them had ever used a written recipe. Her daughter managed to help Mrs. White with step-by-step instructions in the construction of the lasagna. Her daughter was worried about her mother's failing memory, fearing that it was more than usual aging. She tried to broach the subject with her dad, a loving and loyal companion to Mrs. White. His reply was simply, "I don't know what you're talking about."
>
> The situation reached a crisis point when her daughter discovered that Mrs. White was no longer taking her thyroid medication. Since Mrs. White had taken medication for her thyroid for 30 years and could not remember to do so now, this signalled a progression in her condition.
>
> It was painful, but her husband, too, began to realize that Mrs. White was not functioning. Her once-clean house was in a state of disarray. She could no longer coordinate her clothing and usually wore the same outfit for a number of days. Often her clothes were dirty, and her makeup was applied in a disorganized manner.

> **VIGNETTE**
>
> Mrs. White would stare at both the paper and the television, attempting to understand but unable to retain any information. She was often restless during the day, going from one random activity to another, often rearranging her favourite knick-knacks in her curio cupboard. She would attempt to wash clothes but forget to put laundry detergent in the machine. She would empty half-filled drinking glasses into the gas range top. If these mistakes were pointed out, she would become angry, stating, "I have always done it this way."
>
> Eating became difficult, as she did not seem to recognize food on her plate, and she was unable to use a knife and fork to cut her food. Sometimes she would pick up a spoon and ask what it was. Her weight began to decrease.
>
> Although Mrs. White always slept well throughout her adult life, she began to wander at night, often waking her husband to ask questions. She would go to the kitchen and empty the cupboards. She would enter her wardrobe and rearrange her clothing, often leaving articles of clothing lying on the floor.
>
> When she set kitchen paper towels on fire on the gas range, her husband and family realized that she could no longer function safely at home. Her husband was unable to leave her alone even for short periods of time, as she would be become extremely distressed, almost to the point of panic. She and her husband moved into an assisted-living facility.

Epidemiology

- Globally, it is estimated that 50 million people have dementia (a figure greater than the entire population of Canada) and more than 60% of those people live in low- to middle-income-earning countries (WHO, 2020).
- More than 500 000 Canadians are currently living with dementia. Of these, 71 000 are under the age of 65.
- Among Canadians over the age of 65, 1 in 11 has dementia.
- Women comprise 72% of all Canadians living with the Alzheimer's subtype of neurocognitive disorder.
- The Alzheimer's subtype of neurocognitive disorder is experienced across race, culture, gender, and socioeconomic backgrounds.
- Although AD can occur at a younger age (early onset), most of those with the disease are 65 years of age or older (late onset).

Etiology

Although the cause of AD is unknown, most experts agree that, like other chronic and progressive conditions, it is a result of multiple factors: genetics, lifestyle, and environment. However, the greatest risk factor is advancing age. Protective factors appear to include healthy lifestyle, exercise, balanced diet, adequate sleep, neurological stimulation, and stress reduction (Alzheimer Society of Canada, 2021b).

Biological Factors

Neurobiological. In the brains of people with AD there are signs of neuronal degeneration that begins in the hippocampus, the part of the brain responsible for recent memory. The degeneration then spreads into the cerebral cortex, the part of the brain responsible for problem solving and higher-order cognitive functioning.

There are two processes that contribute to cell death. The first is the accumulation of the protein amyloid outside the neurons, which interferes with synapses. The second is an accumulation of the protein tau inside the neurons, which forms tangles that block the flow of nutrients. Interestingly we have seen vascular risk factors such as hypertension, diabetes, and smoking begin to demonstrate a marked increase in risk for the development of AD (Kinney et al., 2018).

Genetic. There is an increased risk for AD among those people with an immediate family member who has or had dementia. There are three known genetic mutations that guarantee that a person will develop AD, although these account for less than 1% of all cases. These mutations lead to the devastating early-onset form of AD, which occurs before the age of 65 and as young as 30 years (Alzheimer's Association, 2020).

Head injury and traumatic brain injury. Brain injury and trauma are associated with a greater risk for developing AD and other dementias. People who suffer repeated head trauma, such as boxers and football players, may be at greater risk. Traumatic brain injury (TBI) has been associated with an earlier onset of AD and an increase in neuropsychiatric symptoms such as disinhibition, depression, anxiety, and motor disturbances. Neuropsychiatric symptoms can often precede the confirmed diagnosis of AD and can be underreported by the individual impacted or their caregivers (Bray et al., 2021).

Cardiovascular disease. The health of the brain is closely linked to overall heart health, and there is evidence that people with cardiovascular disease are at greater risk for AD. Previous stroke has also been associated with the development of brain plaques that are believed to be responsible for some of the dysfunction caused by AD. Likewise, lifestyle factors associated with cardiovascular disease, such as inactivity, high cholesterol, diabetes, and obesity, are considered risk factors for AD (Alzheimer's Association, 2021).

Environmental Factors

There is some evidence that brain health is affected by modifiable factors, such as remaining mentally and socially active and consuming a healthy diet. Avoiding smoking and excess alcohol intake has also been found to reduce to risk of developing AD (Alzheimer's Association, 2021).

APPLICATION OF THE NURSING PROCESS

Assessment

General Assessment

AD is commonly characterized by progressive deterioration of cognitive functioning. Initial deterioration may be so subtle and insidious that others may not notice. In the early stages of the disease the affected person may be able to compensate for loss of memory, sometimes even hide it. This hiding is actually a form of denial, which is an unconscious protective defence against the terrifying reality of losing one's place in the world. Family members may also unconsciously deny that anything is wrong as a defence against the painful awareness that a loved one is deteriorating. As time goes on, symptoms become more obvious, and other defence mechanisms become evident, including (1) denial, (2) *confabulation* (the creation of stories or answers in place of actual memories, in an attempt to maintain self-esteem; it is not the same as lying because it is done unconsciously), (3) *perseveration* (the repetition of phrases or behaviour), and (4) avoidance of questions. The following exchange between a nurse and a patient who has remained in a hospital bed all weekend provides an example of confabulation:

Nurse: Good morning, Ms. Jones. How was your weekend?
Patient: Wonderful. I discussed politics with the prime minister, and he took me out to dinner.

or

Patient: I spent the weekend with my daughter and her family.

Symptoms observed in AD include:

- Amnesia or memory impairment. Initially, the person has difficulty remembering recent events. Gradually, deterioration progresses to include both recent and remote memory.
- *Aphasia* (loss of language ability), which progresses with the disease. Initially, the person has difficulty finding the correct word, then is reduced to a few words, and finally is reduced to babbling or mutism.
- *Apraxia*, which is the loss of purposeful movement in the absence of motor or sensory impairment. The person is unable to perform once-familiar and purposeful tasks. For example, in apraxia of gait, the person loses the ability to walk. In apraxia of dressing the person is unable to put clothes on properly (may put arms in trousers or put a jacket on upside down).
- *Agnosia*, which is the loss of the sensory ability to recognize objects. For example, the person may lose the ability to recognize familiar sounds (auditory agnosia), such as the ring of the telephone, a car horn, or the doorbell. Loss of this ability extends to the inability to recognize familiar objects (visual or tactile agnosia), such as a glass, magazine, pencil, or toothbrush. Eventually, people are unable to recognize loved ones or even parts of their own bodies.
- Disturbances in executive functioning (planning, organizing, abstract thinking). The degeneration of neurons in the brain results in the wasting away of the brain's working components. These cells contain memories, receive sights and sounds, cause hormones to secrete, produce emotions, and command muscles into motion.

A person with AD loses a personal history, a place in the world, and the ability to recognize the environment and, eventually, loved ones. AD robs family and friends, husbands and wives, and sons and daughters of valuable human relatedness and companionship, which results in a profound sense of grief. It robs society of productive and active participants. Because of these devastating effects, mental health care providers and social agencies, the medical and nursing professions, and researchers are challenged to look for possible causes and treatments.

Diagnostic Tests

A wide range of problems may be mistaken for dementia or AD. For example, in older adults depression and dementia may have similar symptoms. It is important that nurses and other health care providers be able to assess some of the important differences among depression, neurocognitive disorder, and delirium (see Table 17.1).

Other disorders that often mimic dementia include drug toxicity, metabolic disorders, infections, and nutritional deficiencies. A disorder that mimics dementia is sometimes referred to as a *pseudodementia*. Making a diagnosis of AD requires ruling out all other pathophysiological conditions through careful assessment, including medical and family history, as well as through physical and laboratory tests, many of which are identified in Box 17.3.

Brain imaging with computed tomography (CT), positron emission tomography (PET), and other developing scanning technologies have diagnostic capabilities because they reveal brain atrophy and rule out other conditions such as neoplasms. The use of mental status questionnaires, such as the Mini-Mental State Examination and various other tests to identify deterioration in mental status and brain damage, is an important part of the assessment.

In addition to performing a thorough physical and neurological examination, it is important to obtain a complete medical and psychiatric history, a description of recent symptoms, a review of medications used, and a nutritional evaluation. The observations and history provided by family members are invaluable to the assessment process.

As mentioned, depression in the older person is the disorder most frequently confused with dementia. Medical and nursing personnel should be cautioned, however, that dementia and depression or dementia and delirium can co-exist. In fact, studies indicate that many people diagnosed with Alzheimer's dementia also meet the *DSM-5* criteria for a depressive disorder.

Self-Assessment

Working with cognitively impaired people in any setting places a tremendous amount of responsibility on caregivers. The behavioural problems that people with dementia may display can cause stress for professionals and family caregivers alike.

Nurses working in facilities designed for people who are cognitively impaired (e.g., assisted-living, supported-living, long-term care, and extended care facilities) need special education and skills. Education must include information about the process of the disease and effective

---

BOX 17.3 Basic Medical Workup for Dementia

- Chest and skull radiographic studies
- Electroencephalography
- Electrocardiography
- Urinalysis
- Sequential multiple analyzer 12-test serum profile
- Thyroid function tests
- Folate level
- Venereal Disease Research Laboratory (VDRL) and human immunodeficiency virus (HIV) tests
- Serum creatinine assay
- Electrolyte assessment
- Vitamin B_{12} level
- Liver function tests
- Vision and hearing evaluation
- Neuroimaging (when diagnostic issues are not clear)

interventions, as well as knowledge regarding antipsychotic drugs. Support and educational opportunities should be readily available, not just to nurses but also to nursing aides, who are often directly responsible for administering basic care.

Because stress is common among those working with patients with cognitive impairments, staff need to be proactive in minimizing its effects through the use of the following strategies:

- Having a clear understanding of the disease so that expectations for the person are realistic
- Establishing realistic outcomes (perhaps as minor as *patient feeds self with spoon*) for the person and recognizing when they are achieved, remembering that even the smallest achievement can be a significant accomplishment for the impaired individual
- Maintaining good self-care and protecting ourselves from the negative effects of stress by obtaining adequate sleep and rest, eating a nutritious diet, exercising, engaging in relaxing activities, and addressing our own emotional and spiritual needs.

ASSESSMENT GUIDELINES
Neurocognitive Disorders

1. Evaluate the person's current level of cognitive and daily functioning.
2. Identify any threats to the person's safety and security and arrange for their reduction.
3. Evaluate the safety of the person's home environment (e.g., with regard to wandering, eating inedible objects, falling, engaging in provocative behaviours toward others).
4. Review the medications (including herbs and complementary agents) the person is currently taking.
5. Interview family to gain a complete picture of the person's background and personality.
6. Explore how well the family is prepared for and informed about the progress of dementia, depending on cause (if known).
7. Discuss with the family members how they are coping with the requirements of caregiving and what their main issues are at this time.
8. Review the resources available to the family. Ask family members to describe the help they receive from other family members, friends, and community resources. Determine if caregivers are aware of community support groups and resources.
9. Identify the needs of the family for teaching and guidance, for example, how to manage **catastrophic reactions** (over-reactions to a seemingly normal, non-threatening situation commonly experienced in AD), lability of mood, aggressive behaviours, and sundowning.

Diagnosis

One of the most important areas of concern identified by both staff and families is safety. Many people with AD wander and may be lost for hours or days. Wandering, along with behaviours such as rummaging, may be perceived as purposeful to the person with AD. Wandering may result from changes in the physical environment, fear caused by hallucinations or delusions, or lack of exercise.

Seizures are common in the later stages of this disease. Injuries from falls and accidents can occur during any stage as confusion and disorientation progress. The potential for burns exists if the person is a smoker or is unattended when using the stove. Prescription drugs can be taken incorrectly, or bottles of noxious fluids can be mistakenly ingested, resulting in a medical crisis. Therefore *risk for injury* is always present.

As the person's ability to recognize or name objects decreases, *impaired verbal communication* becomes a problem. As memory diminishes and disorientation increases, *impaired environmental interpretation syndrome*, *impaired memory*, and *confusion* occur.

Additional family issues may emerge. Perhaps some of the most crucial aspects of caregiving are support, education, and referrals for the family. The family loses an integral part of its unit, as well as the love, function, support, companionship, and warmth that this person once provided. *Caregiver role strain* is always present, and planning with the family and arranging community supports are vital parts of appropriate care. *Anticipatory grieving* is also an important phenomenon to assess and may be a significant target for intervention. Helping the family grieve can make the task ahead somewhat clearer and at times less painful. Review Table 17.2 for potential nursing diagnoses for confused patients.

Outcomes Identification

Families who have a member with dementia face an exhaustive list of issues that need to be addressed. Table 17.7 provides a checklist that may help nurses and families to identify areas for intervention. Self-care needs, impaired environmental interpretation, chronic confusion, ineffective individual coping, and caregiver role strain are just a few of the areas nurses and other health care providers will need to target (Box 17.4).

Planning

Planning care for a person with a major cognitive disorder is geared towards the person's immediate needs. Refer to Table 17.7 for help in identifying potential areas of care. Functional dementia scales can be used by nurses and families to plan strategies for addressing immediate needs and to track the progression of the dementia. The Cognitive Performance Scale, derived from the inter-RAI assessments, which reflect memory, decision-making skills, communication, and eating, can also be used as a tool to track the progression of dementia (Canadian Institute for Health Information, 2013).

Identifying a patient's level of functioning and assessing caregivers' needs help health care providers to focus on planning and identify appropriate community resources. Does the patient or family need the following?

- Transportation services
- Supervision and care when primary caregiver is out of the home
- Referrals to adult day programs
- Information on support groups within the community
- Meals on Wheels
- Information on respite and residential services
- Telephone numbers for helplines
- Home health aides
- Home care services
- Additional psychopharmaceuticals to manage distressing or harmful behaviours

Implementation

Caring for a person with dementia requires a great deal of patience, creativity, and maturity. The needs of such a person can be enormous for nursing staff and for families who care for their loved ones in the home. As the disease progresses, so do the needs of the person and the demands on the caregivers, staff, and family. The attitude of unconditional positive regard is the nurse's single most effective tool in caring for people with dementia. Positive regard induces patients to cooperate, reduces catastrophic outbreaks, and increases family members' satisfaction with the care provided. Box 17.5 lists *NIC* interventions related to the management of neurocognitive disorders.

A considerable number of individuals with dementia have secondary behavioural disturbances, including depression, hallucinations, delusions, agitation, insomnia, and wandering. Because these symptoms impair the person's ability to function, increase the need for

TABLE 17.7 Problems That May Affect People With Major Neurocognitive Disorders and Their Families

Problem	Examples	Problem	Examples
Memory impairment	Forgets appointments, visits, etc.	Uncontrolled behaviour	Restlessness during day or night
	Forgets to change clothes, wash, go to the toilet		Vulgar table or toilet habits
	Forgets to eat, take medications		Undressing
	Loses things		Sexual disinhibition
Disorientation	Time: mixes night and day, mixes days of appointments, wears summer clothes in winter, forgets age		Shoplifting
		Incontinence	Urine
			Faeces
	Place: loses way around house		Urination or defecation in the wrong place
	Person: has difficulty recognizing visitors, family, spouse	Emotional reactions	Catastrophic reactions
			Demands for attention
Need for physical help	Dressing		Depression
	Washing, bathing		Distress and anxiety
	Toileting		Frustration and anger
	Eating		Embarrassment and withdrawal
	Performing housework		Lack of emotional control
	Maintaining mobility	Other reactions	Suspiciousness
Risks in the home	Falls		Hoarding and hiding
	Fire from cigarettes, cooking, heating	Mistaken beliefs	Still at work
	Flooding		Parents or spouse still alive
	Admission of strangers to home		Hallucinations
	Wandering out	Decision making	Indecisive
Risks outside the home	Competence, judgement, and risks at work		Easily influenced
	Driving, road sense		Refuses help
	Getting lost		Makes unwise decisions
Apathy	Little conversation	Burden on family	Disruption of social life
	Lack of interest		Distress, guilt, rejection
	Poor self-care		Family discord
Poor communication	Aphasia		
Repetitiveness	Repetition of questions or stories		
	Repetition of actions		

supervision, and influence the need for institutionalization, the control of these symptoms is a priority in managing AD. Helping the individual achieve the highest possible level of independence and function is the foundation of care.

However, intervention with family members is also critical. The effects of losing a family member to dementia, that is, watching the deterioration of a person who has had an important role within the family unit and who is loved and is a vital part of their family's history, can be devastating. The following interventions are useful: counselling, health teaching, community supports, family support, and pharmacological interventions and integrative therapies.

Counselling and Communication Techniques

How one chooses to communicate with a person with dementia affects that person's ability to maintain self-esteem and their ability to participate in care. People with dementia often find it difficult to express themselves. Potential reasons for this difficulty are listed here.
- Cannot find the right words
- Invent new words to describe things
- Frequently lose their train of thought
- Rely on non-verbal gestures

Guidelines for Communication: People With Dementia provides special guidelines for nurses, family members, and other caregivers to use in communicating with a cognitively impaired person.

Health Teaching and Health Promotion

Educating families who have a cognitively impaired member is one of the most important health-teaching duties nurses encounter. Families who are caring for a member in the home need to know about strategies for communicating and for structuring self-care activities (see Patient and Family Teaching: Guidelines for Self-Care for Individuals With Cognitive Impairment).

Most important, families need to know where to get help. Help includes professional counselling and education regarding the process and progression of the disease. Families especially need to know about and be referred to community-based groups that can help shoulder this burden (e.g., adult support programs, senior citizen groups, organizations providing home visits and respite care, family support groups).

> ### BOX 17.4 *NOC* Outcomes Related to Neurocognitive Disorders[a]
>
> **Injury**
> - Person will remain safe in the hospital or at home.
> - With the aid of an identification bracelet and neighbourhood or hospital alert, the person will be returned within 1 hour of wandering.
> - With the aid of interventions, person will remain burn free.
> - With the aid of guidance and environmental manipulation, person will not hurt themself if a fall occurs.
> - Person will ingest only correct doses of prescribed medications and appropriate food and fluids.
>
> **Communication**
> - Person will communicate needs.
> - Person will state needs in alternative modes when they are aphasic (e.g., will signal correct word on hearing it or will refer to picture or label).
> - Person will wear prescribed glasses or hearing aid each day.
>
> **Agitation Level**
> - Person will have rest periods if pacing and restless.
> - Person will cooperate with caregiving activities.
> - Person will experience minimal frustrating experiences.
> - Person will express frustrations in an appropriate manner.
>
> **Caregiver Role Strain**
> - Family members will have the opportunity to express "unacceptable" feelings in a supportive environment.
> - Family members will have access to professional counselling.
> - Family members will name two organizations within their geographical area that can offer emotional support and help with legal and financial burdens.
> - Family members will participate in ill member's plan of care, with encouragement from staff.
> - Family members will state that they have outside help that allows them to take personal time for themselves each week or month.
>
> **Impaired Environmental Interpretation: Chronic Confusion**
> - Person will acknowledge the reality of an object or a sound that was misinterpreted (illusion), after it is pointed out.
> - Person will state that they feel safe after experiencing delusions or illusions.
> - Person will remain non-aggressive when experiencing paranoid ideation.
>
> **Self-Care Needs**
> - Person will participate in self-care at optimal level.
> - Person will be able to follow step-by-step instructions for dressing, bathing, and grooming.
> - Person will put on own clothes appropriately, with aid of fastening tape (Velcro) and nursing supervision.
> - Person's skin will remain intact and free from signs of pressure.
>
> [a]Partial list.
>
> **Source:** Moorhead, S., Swanson, E., Johnson, M., & Maas, M. L., (Eds.). (2018). *Nursing Outcomes Classification (NOC): Measurement of health outcomes* (6th ed.). St. Louis: MO: Elsevier.

A list with definitions of some of the types of services available in the person's community, as well as the names and telephone numbers of the providers of these services, should be given to the family.

Referral to community supports. The Alzheimer Society of Canada is a national umbrella agency that provides various forms of assistance to people with the disease and their families. The society offers educational resources on AD, and related dementias, guidelines for providing quality care, ethical guidelines to help people address sensitive issues, and information and referrals for support programs and services, some of which may help prevent total emotional and physical fatigue in caregivers. The society also advocates on behalf of persons and caregivers impacted by AD, in terms of research funding, expansion of supportive services provided to those with AD, and legislative developments such as Medical Assistance in Dying (MAiD). Of note, the society is currently advocating actively on behalf of those who desire to apply for MAiD, in advance of significant disease progression, as the act does not currently allow for an advance request. Those with AD are often unable to request MAiD, once they meet the current criteria, as set out by the Government of Canada, because of their reduced ability to make what is considered an informed decision at the time of the request (Alzheimer Society of Canada, 2021c). In partnership with the Royal Canadian Mounted Police the Alzheimer Society of Canada also has developed the Safely Home registry, a national registry, to help find lost Alzheimer's patients and assist them in returning home (Alzheimer Society of Canada, 2021). More information about this registry can be found on the Alzheimer Society of Canada's website: https://alzheimer.ca/en/help-support/programs-services/medicalert-safely-home#How_MedicAlert%C2%AE_Safely_Home%C2%AE_works. The support programs and services available from the Alzheimer Society vary from community to community; examples of services it provides are found in Table 17.8.

Although many families manage the care of their loved one until death, other families eventually find that they can no longer deal with the labile and aggressive behaviour, incontinence, wandering, unsafe habits, or disruptive nocturnal activity. Family members need to know where and how to place their loved one for care if such a move becomes necessary. Families need information, support, and legal and financial guidance at this time. When the nurse is unable to provide the relevant information, proper referrals by the social worker are needed. Information regarding advance directives, durable power of attorney, and guardianship should be included in the communication with the family. Patient and Family Teaching: Guidelines for Care at Home provides useful guidelines for families for structuring a safe environment and planning appropriate activities.

Pharmacological Interventions

There is currently no cure for AD. There are, however, four drugs approved by Health Canada that slow the progression of the illness. Although these medications are used widely and have been shown to have statistically significant effects when compared with placebos, they produce only a clinically marginal improvement in cognition and functioning. The benefits of these medications wane after 1 to 2 years, so patients should weigh the potential side effects against the potential benefits. Refer to Figure 17.1 for a brief summary of the neurobiology of Alzheimer's and the effects of medication on the brain (Buckley & Salpeter, 2015).

BOX 17.5 NIC Interventions for Neurocognitive Management

Definition of *neurocognitive management*: Provision of a modified environment for the patient who is experiencing a chronic confusional state.

Activities:
- Include family members in planning, providing, and evaluating care, to the extent desired by the patient and family.
- Identify usual patterns of behaviour for such activities as sleep, medication use, elimination, food intake, and self-care.
- Determine physical, social, and psychological history of patient, usual habits, and routines.
- Determine type and extent of cognitive deficit(s), using standardized assessment tool.
- Monitor cognitive functioning, using standardized assessment tool.
- Determine behavioural expectations appropriate for patient's cognitive status.
- Provide a low-stimulation environment (e.g., quiet, soothing music; non-vivid and simple decor with familiar patterns; performance expectations that do not exceed cognitive processing ability; dining in small groups).
- Provide adequate but non-glare lighting.
- Identify and remove potential dangers for patient in environment.
- Place identification bracelet on patient.
- Provide a consistent physical environment and daily routine.
- Prepare for interaction with eye contact and touch, as appropriate.
- Introduce self when initiating contact.
- Address patient distinctly by name when initiating interaction, and speak slowly.
- Give one simple direction at a time.
- Speak in a clear, low, warm, respectful tone of voice.
- Use distraction, rather than confrontation, to manage behaviour.
- Provide unconditional positive regard.
- Avoid touch and proximity if they cause stress or anxiety.
- Provide caregivers who are familiar to the patient (e.g., avoid frequent rotations of staff assignments).
- Avoid unfamiliar situations when possible (e.g., room changes and appointments without familiar people present).
- Provide rest periods to prevent fatigue and reduce stress.
- Monitor nutrition and weight.
- Provide space for safe pacing and wandering.
- Avoid frustrating patient by quizzing with orientation questions that cannot be answered.
- Provide cues, such as current events, seasons, location, and names, to assist orientation.
- Seat patient at a small table in groups of three to five for meals, as appropriate.
- Allow patient to eat alone if appropriate.
- Provide finger foods to maintain nutrition for patient who will not sit and eat.
- Provide patient with a general orientation to the season of the year by using appropriate cues (e.g., holiday decorations; seasonal decorations and activities; access to contained, outdoor area).
- Decrease noise levels by avoiding paging systems and call lights that ring or buzz.
- Select television or radio programs based on cognitive processing abilities and interests.
- Select one-to-one and group activities geared to patient's cognitive abilities and interests.
- Label familiar photos with names of the individuals in the photos.
- Select artwork for patient's rooms featuring landscapes, scenery, or other familiar images.
- Ask family members and friends to see patient one or two at a time, if needed, to reduce stimulation.
- Discuss with family members and friends how best to interact with patient.
- Assist family in understanding that it may be impossible for patient to learn new material.
- Limit number of choices patient has to make so as not to cause anxiety.
- Provide boundaries, such as red or yellow tape on the floor when low-stimulus units are not available.
- Place patient's name in large block letters in room and on clothing, as needed.
- Use symbols, rather than written signs, to assist patient in locating room, bathroom, or other area.
- Monitor carefully for physiological causes of increased confusion that may be acute and reversible.
- Remove or cover mirrors if patient is frightened or agitated by them.
- Discuss home safety issues and interventions.

Source: Bulechek, G. M., Butcher, H. K., Dochterman, J. M., et al. (2012). *Nursing Interventions Classification (NIC)* (6th ed.). St. Louis: Mosby.

GUIDELINES FOR COMMUNICATION
People With Dementia

Intervention	Rationale
Always identify yourself and call the person by name at each meeting.	The person's short-term memory is impaired—requires frequent orientation to time and environment.
Speak slowly.	The person needs time to process information.
Use short, simple words and phrases.	The person may not be able to understand complex statements or abstract ideas.
Maintain face-to-face contact.	Verbal and non-verbal clues are maximized.
Be near the person when talking, one or two arm-lengths away.	This distance can help the person focus on the speaker while maintaining personal space.
Focus on one piece of information at a time.	The person's attention span is poor, and he or she is easily distracted—bite-sized information helps the person focus. Too much data can be overwhelming and can increase anxiety.
Talk with the person about familiar and meaningful things.	Self-expression is promoted, and reality is reinforced.
Encourage reminiscing about happy times in life.	Remembering accomplishments and shared joys helps distract the person from deficit and gives meaning to existence.

Continued

GUIDELINES FOR COMMUNICATION—cont'd

Intervention	Rationale
When the person is delusional, acknowledge the person's feelings and reinforce reality. Do not argue or refute delusions.	Acknowledging feelings helps the person feel understood. Pointing out realities may help the person focus on realities. Arguing can enhance adherence to false beliefs.
If the person gets into an argument with another person, stop the argument and temporarily separate those involved. After a short while (5 minutes), explain to each person matter-of-factly why you had to intervene.	Escalation to physical acting out is prevented. The person's right to know is respected. Explaining in an adult manner helps maintain self-esteem.
When the person becomes verbally aggressive, acknowledge the person's feelings, and shift the topic to more familiar ground (e.g., "I know this is upsetting for you, because you always cared for others. Tell me about your children.")	Confusion and disorientation easily increase anxiety. Acknowledging feelings makes the person feel more understood and less alone. Topics the person has mastery over can remind them of areas of competent functioning and can increase self-esteem.
Have the person wear prescription glasses or hearing aid(s).	Environmental awareness, orientation, and comprehension are increased, which in turn increase awareness of personal needs and the presence of others.
Keep the person's room well lit.	Environmental clues are maximized.
Have clocks, calendars, and personal items (e.g., family pictures, meaningful books) in clear view of the person while they are in bed.	These objects assist in maintaining personal identity.
Reinforce the person's pictures, non-verbal gestures, Xs on calendars, and other methods used to anchor the person in reality.	When aphasia starts to hinder communication, alternative methods of communication need to be instituted.

Source: Butcher, H. K., Bulechek, G. M., Dochterman, J. M., & Wagner, C. M. (Eds.). (2019). *Nursing Interventions Classification (NIC)* (7th ed.). St. Louis: MO: Elsevier.

PATIENT AND FAMILY TEACHING
Guidelines for Self-Care for Individuals With Cognitive Impairment

Intervention	Rationale
Dressing and Bathing	
Always have the person perform all tasks within their present capacity.	Maintains the person's self-esteem and uses muscle groups Impedes staff burnout Minimizes further regression
Always have the person wear own clothes, even if in the hospital.	Helps maintain the person's identity and dignity
Use clothing with elastic, and substitute fastening tape (Velcro) for buttons and zippers.	Minimizes the person's confusion Eases independence of functioning
Label clothing items with the person's name and name of item.	Helps identify the person if they wander Gives the person additional clues when aphasia or agnosia occurs
Give step-by-step instructions whenever necessary (e.g., "Take this blouse. Put in one arm … now the other arm. Pull it together in front. Now …").	Uses the person's ability to focus on small pieces of information more easily Allows the person to perform at optimal level
Make sure that water in faucets is not too hot.	Ensures safety for person who is lacking judgement or is unaware of many safety hazards
If the person is resistant to performing self-care, come back later and ask again.	Respects that the person's moods may be labile—the person often complies after a short interval
Nutrition	
Monitor food and fluid intake.	Helps to prevent anorexia or refusal to eat because of confusion
Offer finger food that the person can take away from the dinner table.	Increases intake throughout the day—the person may eat only small amounts at meals
Weigh the person regularly (once a week).	Monitors fluid and nutritional status
During periods of hyperorality, watch that the person does not eat non-food items (e.g., ceramic fruit or food-shaped soaps).	Ensures safety of the person who puts everything into mouth or who is unable to differentiate inedible objects made in the shape and colour of food
Bowel and Bladder Function	
Begin bowel and bladder program early; start with bladder control.	Helps prevent incontinence by establishing same time of day for bowel movements and toileting—in early morning, after meals and snacks, and before bedtime

Intervention	Rationale
Evaluate use of disposable incontinence products.	Prevents embarrassment
Label bathroom door, as well as doors to other rooms.	Maximizes independent toileting by offering additional environmental clues
Sleep	
Because the person may awaken, be frightened, or cry out at night, keep area well lit.	Reinforces orientation Minimizes possible illusions
Maintain a calm atmosphere during the day.	Encourages a calming night's sleep
Order non-barbiturates (e.g., chloral hydrate) if necessary.	Avoids paradoxical reaction of agitation, often caused by barbiturates
If medications are indicated, consider neuroleptics with sedative properties, which may be the most helpful (e.g., haloperidol [Haldol]).	Helps clear thinking Sedates
Avoid the use of restraints.	Avoids inciting fear in the person, who may fight against restraints until exhausted to a dangerous degree

TABLE 17.8 Types of Services That May Be Available to People With Dementia

Type of Service	Services Provided
Family/caregiver	Caregivers have a right to: Easy access to services Respite care Full involvement in decision making Assessment of the needs of both the caregiver and the person with dementia Information and referral Case management: coordination of community resources and follow-up
Community services	Adult support programs: provide activities, socialization, and supervision in an outpatient setting Physician services Protective services: prevent, eliminate, or remedy effects of abuse or neglect Recreational services Transportation Mental health services Legal services
Home care	Meals on Wheels Home health aide services Homemaker services Respite services Occupational therapy Paid companion or sitter services Physiotherapy Skilled nursing care Personal care services: assistance in basic self-care activities Social work services Telephone reassurance: regular telephone calls to individuals who are isolated and homebound[a] Personal emergency response systems: telephone-based systems to alert others that a person who is alone is in need of emergency assistance[a]

[a]Vital for those living alone.

Cholinesterase inhibitors. Because a deficiency of acetylcholine has been linked to AD, medications aimed at preventing its breakdown have been developed. Drugs in this classification work by preventing an enzyme called acetylcholinesterase or, more simply, cholinesterase from breaking down acetylcholine in the brain. As a result, an increased concentration of acetylcholine leads to temporary improvement of some symptoms of AD.

The cholinesterase inhibitors produce small, but short-lived, improvements in cognitive functioning, including learning and memory function. There is minimal benefit after 2 years, and risk for side effects doubles in people over 85 years of age (Alzheimer Society of Canada, 2021b).

The most commonly prescribed cholinesterase inhibitor is donepezil (Aricept). Indications for donepezil include mild, moderate, and severe AD. It also appears to improve cognitive functions without the potentially serious liver toxicity attributed to tacrine. Some individuals may experience diarrhea and nausea while taking the drug. These side effects are dose related, so a decreased dose helps minimize them.

PATIENT AND FAMILY TEACHING
Guidelines for Care at Home

Intervention	Rationale
Safe Environment	
Gradually restrict use of the car.	Ensures safety as the person's judgement becomes impaired
Remove throw rugs and other objects in person's path.	Minimizes tripping and falling
Minimize sensory stimulation.	Decreases sensory overload, which can increase anxiety and confusion
If the person becomes verbally upset, listen briefly, give support, and then change the topic.	Aims to prevent escalation of anger
	Distracts person to more productive topics and activities
Label all rooms and drawers. Label often-used objects (e.g., hairbrushes, toothbrushes).	May keep the person from wandering into other people's rooms
	Increases environmental clues to familiar objects
Install safety bars in bathroom.	Prevents falls
Supervise the person when they smoke.	Minimizes danger of burns
If the person has history of seizures, keep padded tongue blades at beside. Educate family on how to deal with seizures.	Ensures safety—seizure activity is common in advanced Alzheimer's disease
Wandering	
If the person wanders during the night, put their mattress on the floor.	Prevents falls when the person is confused.
Have the person wear medical alert bracelet that cannot be removed (with name, address, and telephone number).	Ensures easy identification by police, neighbours, or hospital personnel
Provide police department with recent pictures.	
Alert local police and neighbours about wanderer.	May reduce time necessary to return the person to home or hospital
If the person is in hospital, have them wear brightly coloured vest with name, unit, and phone number printed on back.	Makes the person easily identifiable
Put complex locks on door.	Reduces opportunity to wander
Place locks at top of door.	Ensures safety—in moderate and late Alzheimer's-type dementia, ability to look up and reach upwards is lost
Encourage physical activity during the day.	May decrease wandering at night
Explore the feasibility of installing sensor devices.	Provides warning if the person wanders
Useful Activities	
Provide picture magazines and children's books when the person's reading ability diminishes.	Allows continuation of usual activities that the person can still enjoy
	Provides focus
Provide simple activities that allow exercise of large muscles.	Provides socialization (e.g., exercise groups, dance groups, walking groups)
	Increases circulation and maintains muscle tone
Encourage group activities that are familiar and simple to perform.	Increases socialization (e.g., activities such as group singing, dancing, reminiscing, working with clay and paint)
	Minimizes feelings of alienation

Rivastigmine (Exelon) is another cholinesterase inhibitor used in the mild to moderate stages of AD. The most common side effects are nausea, vomiting, loss of appetite, and weight loss. In most cases these side effects are temporary. Patients should always take rivastigmine with food to reduce gastrointestinal side effects. The Exelon transdermal patch is applied once a day and has no food requirement. It is useful for people who have trouble swallowing pills. Patients and families should be cautioned to always remove the old patch before applying the new one to prevent serious side effects.

Despite slight variations in the mode of action of the cholinesterase inhibitors, there is no evidence of any differences between them with regards to effectiveness. All of the cholinesterase inhibitors have the potential to cause nausea, diarrhea, and vomiting, depending on the dosage level. Bradycardia and syncope have been associated with this class of drugs. They should be used with caution when patients are taking non-steroidal anti-inflammatory drugs.

N-methyl-D-aspartate (NMDA) receptor antagonist. Memantine (Namenda) is typically added after trying the cholinesterase inhibitors. It regulates the activity of glutamate, a neurotransmitter that plays a role in information processing, storage, and retrieval. Memantine blocks NMDA receptors to protect against excessive neuronal stimulation by glutamate. It is approved for use in moderate to severe dementia but not mild dementia.

Refer to Chapter 11 for a more detailed discussion of psychotropic medications.

Medications for behavioural symptoms. Other medications are often useful in managing the behavioural symptoms of individuals with cognitive impairment, but these need to be used with extreme caution. The rule of thumb is "start low and go slow." Another is to use the smallest dose for the shortest duration possible and discontinue if the medications are not effective. In addition, because people with cognitive impairment are at high risk for developing delirium, always add medications with caution.

Neurobiology of Alzheimer's and the Effects of Medication on the Brain

Two essential neurotransmitters implicated in Alzheimer's disease are acetylcholine and glutamate.
Acetylcholine: is involved with learning, memory, and mood. As Alzheimer's disease progresses, the brain produces less and less acetylcholine. What little acetylcholine is left is rapidly destroyed by the enzyme acetylcholinesterase.
Cholinesterase: inhibitors keep the acetylcholinesterase enzyme from breaking down acetylcholine, thereby increasing both the level and the duration of action of the neurotransmitter acetylcholine.
Glutamate: is involved with cell signalling, learning, and memory. Glutamate binds to cells at the *N*-methyl-D-aspartate (NMDA) receptor and allows calcium to enter the cell. In Alzheimer's disease excess glutamate from damaged cells leads to chronic overexposure to calcium.
NMDA: antagonists help reduce excess calcium by blocking some NMDA receptors.

Brain Dysfunction

Amyloid plaques are sticky clumps found between nerve cells that may either cause or be the result of the disease. The clumps block communication at synapses that are normally protected by tau proteins and healthy microtubules. They may also activate immune system cells that trigger inflammation and devour disabled cells.

Neurofibrillary tangles are abnormal collections of protein threads inside nerve cells. They are composed mainly of a protein called tau. Tangles disrupt the transport of food molecules, cell parts, and other key elements. This disruption results in cell death.

Brain atrophy is the cerebral cortex shrivelling up, damaging areas involved in thinking, planning, and remembering. The hippocampus, an area of the cortex that is essential for memory, experiences severe shrinkage. Ventricles, the fluid-filled spaces within the brain, grow larger.

FDA-Approved Drugs for the Treatment of Alzheimer's Disease

Drug Name	Brand Name	Classification	Approved For
galantamine	Razadyne	Cholinesterase inhibitor	Mild to moderate
donepezil	Aricept	Cholinesterase inhibitor	All stages
rivastigmine	Exelon	Cholinesterase inhibitor	All stages
memantine	Namenda	Namenda, an NMDA antagonist, helps reduce excess calcium by blocking some NMDA receptors	Moderate to severe
donepezil and memantine	Namzaric	Cholinesterase inhibitor and NMDA receptor antagonist combination	Moderate to severe

Fig. 17.1 Neurobiology of Alzheimer's and the effects of medication on the brain.

Most people with cognitive impairment will experience behavioural symptoms that reduce their quality of life, are distressing to them and their caregivers, and may lead to placement in a residential care facility. Some of the troubling behaviours are psychotic symptoms (hallucinations, paranoia), severe mood swings (depression is common), wandering, anxiety, agitation, and verbal or physical aggression (combativeness). Not only are these behaviours distressing, but they may also lead to injuries from falls, infections, and incontinence.

Psychotropic medications may be prescribed. Drug classifications that are used off-label include antidepressants, antipsychotics, antianxiety agents, and anticonvulsants. Of these, antipsychotics have been used most often. These medications are associated with risk for mortality, mostly from cardiovascular and infectious causes. As a result, all antipsychotics, both first and second generation, are no longer approved for dementia-related psychosis (Burchum & Rosenthal, 2019).

With the legalization of cannabis on October 17, 2018, the question of using this substance as a form of treatment for Alzheimer's has come into question. Of clinical relevance to nurses is currently there is no verifiable evidence to suggests that the use of cannabis to prevent or treat AD has any benefit to the individual. The Alzheimer Society of Canada's position on the use of cannabis is that it is not recommended as a treatment option for AD, in part because to date, there has been no proven efficacy in the treatment of AD, in combination with cannabis use demonstrating a negative impact on memory and an increase in anxiety in some individuals with AD (Alzheimer Society of Canada, 2021d).

The future of drug therapy. Additional research is ongoing, with focuses on:
- The development of other cholinesterase inhibitors
- The use of cholesterol-lowering agents
- The use of anti-inflammatory agents as a preventive measure
- The use of neurotrophic agents with the potential to regenerate brain cells
- The use of diabetic treatments that might decrease blood vessel inflammation in the brain

Additional information about current clinical studies can be found on the Alzheimer Society of Canada website: http://www.alzheimer.ca.

Alternative Treatment for Alzheimer Disease

According to the Alzheimer Society of Canada (2021b), alternative or integrative therapies can be of some benefit to some individuals with AD. Some of the more common alternative therapies include aromatherapy, coconut oil, massage, medicinal cannabis, music therapy, natural health products, and pet therapy. These benefits largely centre on enhanced mood, sense of relaxation, and improved sleep. Little evidence exists in the research to substantiate these alternative treatments as a recommended treatment for AD, and at all times, the individual with AD should consult their primary care provider before supplementing their treatment plan with an alternative therapy, as there may be risk to the individual in doing so.

Evaluation

Outcome criteria for a person with cognitive impairments need to be measurable, within the capabilities of the individual, and evaluated frequently. As the person's condition continues to deteriorate, outcomes must be altered to reflect the person's diminished functioning. Frequent evaluation and reformulation of outcome criteria and short-term indicators also help reduce staff and family frustration and minimize the person with dementia's anxiety by ensuring that tasks are not more complicated than the person can accomplish.

The overall outcomes for treatment are to promote the person's optimal level of functioning and to delay further regression whenever possible. Working closely with family members and providing them with the names of available resources and support sources may help increase the quality of life for both the family and the patient with AD (Case Study and Nursing Care Plan 17.1).

CASE STUDY AND NURSING CARE PLAN 17.1
Cognitive Impairment

During the past 4 years, Mr. Ludwig has demonstrated rapidly progressive memory impairment, disorientation, and deterioration in his ability to function, related to Alzheimer's disease. He is a 67-year-old man who retired at age 62 to spend some of his remaining "youth" with his wife and to travel, garden, visit family, and finally get to do the things they always wanted to do. At age 63, he was diagnosed with Alzheimer's disease.

Mr. Ludwig has been taken care of at home by his wife and his daughter, Kelly. Kelly is divorced and has returned home with her two young daughters.

The family members find themselves close to physical and mental exhaustion. Mr. Ludwig is becoming increasingly incontinent as he cannot consistently find the bathroom. He wanders away from home, despite close supervision. The police and neighbours bring him back home an average of four times a week. Once, he was lost for 5 days after he had somehow boarded a bus for Vancouver, 1 000 kilometres from home. He was robbed and beaten before being found by the police and returned home.

He frequently wanders into his granddaughters' rooms at night while they are sleeping and tries to get into bed with them. Too young to understand that their grandfather is lonely and confused, they fear that he is going to hurt them. Four times in the past 2 weeks, he has fallen while getting out of bed at night, thinking he is in a sleeping bag, camping out in the mountains. After a conflicted and painful 2 months, the family places him in a care facility for people with Alzheimer's disease.

Mrs. Ludwig tells the admitting nurse, Mr. Behar, that her husband wanders almost all the time and that he has difficulty finding the right words for things (aphasia) and becomes frustrated and angry when that happens. Sometimes he does not seem to recognize the family (agnosia). Once, he thought that Kelly was a thief breaking into the house and attacked her with a broom handle. The telling of this story causes Kelly to break down into heavy sobs: "What's happened to my father? He was so kind and gentle. Oh, God ... I've lost my father."

Mrs. Ludwig tells Mr. Behar that her husband can sometimes participate in dressing himself; at other times, he needs total assistance. At this point, Mrs. Ludwig begins to cry uncontrollably, saying, "I can't bear to part with him, but I can't do it anymore. I feel as if I've betrayed him."

Mr. Behar then focuses his attention on Mrs. Ludwig and her experience. He states, "This is a difficult decision for you." Mr. Behar suggests that Mrs. Ludwig talk to other families who have a cognitively impaired member. "It might help you to know that you are not alone, and having contact with others to share your grief can be healing." One of the organizations he suggests is the Alzheimer Society of Canada, a well-known group that provides support and information to caregivers.

Assessment
Self-Assessment
Mr. Behar has worked on his particular unit for 4 years. It is a unit designed especially for cognitively impaired individuals, which makes nursing care of these patients easier than in a regular unit. He applied for this position shortly after his

CASE STUDY AND NURSING CARE PLAN 17.1—cont'd
Cognitive Impairment

own father died of complications secondary to Alzheimer's disease. Mr. Behar refers to the process of living and dying with this disease as horrifying; his goal is to help other people go through it with caring, dignity, and the highest level of functioning possible.

Caring for Mr. Ludwig and his family is becoming especially personal. Mr. Behar is struck by the similarity between this family's situation and his own. Mr. Ludwig is about the same age his father had been, looks similar to him, and has many of his mannerisms. Mrs. Ludwig and her daughter Kelly seem to be responding in much the same way his family did. He finds that he is having stronger than usual counter-transference feelings with this family and even became teary when Mrs. Ludwig did.

The evening after he met the Ludwigs, Mr. Behar went home utterly exhausted and continued to think about them and his own father. He shared these feelings with his wife, and the two of them spent some time talking about his father and all they had been through together, good and bad. In the end, Mr. Behar sat back, breathed a long, deep sigh of relief, and thanked his wife for being there for him. He told her that he supposed he will never really get over the death of his father, but he is getting better every day.

When Mr. Behar returned to work, he nearly walked right into Mr. Ludwig, who was standing at the doorway wearing two shirts, a pair of pyjama bottoms, and a baseball cap. "Are you the man who's taking me to pick up my car?" he asks. Mr. Behar smiles and says, "It looks like you have quite a day planned. Let's start with a cup of coffee," and redirects him to the day hall.

Objective Data
Patient:
- Wanders away from home about four times a week
- Was lost for 5 days and was robbed and beaten
- Is often incontinent when he cannot find the bathroom
- Has difficulty finding words
- Has difficulty identifying members of the family at times
- Has difficulty dressing himself at times
- Falls out of bed at night
- Has memory impairment
- Is disoriented much of the time
- Gets into bed with granddaughters at night when wandering
- Family is undergoing intense feelings of loss and guilt

Subjective Data
"I can't bear to part with him."
"I feel as if I've betrayed him."
"I've lost my father."

Diagnosis
1. *Risk for injury* related to confusion, as evidenced by wandering
   - Supporting Data
   - Wanders away from home about four times a week
   - Wanders despite supervision
   - Falls out of bed at night
   - Gets into other people's beds
   - Wanders at night
2. *Functional urinary incontinence* related to disturbed cognition, as evidenced by inability to find the toilet
   - Supporting Data
   - Incontinent when he cannot find the bathroom
3. *Self-care deficit* (self-dressing) related to impaired cognitive functioning, as evidenced by impaired ability to put on and take off clothing
   - Supporting Data
   - Sometimes he is able to dress with help of wife
   - At other times he is too confused to dress self at all
4. *Anticipatory grieving* related to loss and deterioration of family member
   - Supporting Data
   - "I can't bear to part with him."
   - "I feel as if I've betrayed him."
   - "I've lost my father."
   - Family undergoing intense feelings of loss and guilt

Outcomes Identification
Although Mr. Ludwig has many unmet needs that require nursing interventions, Mr. Behar decides to focus on the four initial nursing diagnoses. As other problems arise, they will be addressed.

Continued

CASE STUDY AND NURSING CARE PLAN 17.1—cont'd

Cognitive Impairment

Nursing Diagnosis	Long-Term Goals	Short-Term Goals
1. *Risk for injury* related to confusion, as evidenced by wandering	1. Resident will remain safe in nursing home.	1a. Throughout nursing home stay, resident will not fall out of bed. 1b. Throughout nursing home stay, resident will wander only in protected area. 1c. Resident will be returned within 2 hours if he succeeds in escaping from the unit.
2. *Functional urinary incontinence* related to disturbed cognition, as evidenced by inability to find the toilet	2. Resident will experience less incontinence (fewer episodes) by fourth week of hospitalization.	2a. By the end of 4 weeks, resident will participate in unit orientation to find toilet. 2b. By the end of 4 weeks, resident will find the toilet most of the time.
3. *Self-care deficit* (self-dressing) related to impaired cognitive functioning, as evidenced by impaired ability to put on and take off clothing	3. Resident will participate in dressing himself 80% of the time.	3a. By the end of 4 weeks, resident will follow step-by-step instructions for dressing most of the time. 3b. By the end of 4 weeks, resident will dress in own clothes with aid of fastening tape.
4. *Anticipatory grieving* related to loss and deterioration of family member	4. In 3 months' time all family members will state that they feel they have more support and are able to talk about their grieving.	4a. After 3 months, family members will state that they have opportunity to express "unacceptable" feelings in supportive environment. 4b. After 3 months, family members will state that they have found support from others who have a family member with Alzheimer's disease.

Planning
Mr. Behar plans care to ensure Mr. Ludwig's safety, provide for the maintenance of his hygiene needs and incontinence, and assist Mrs. Ludwig as she deals with her husband's deterioration.

Implementation
Using the concepts of *NIC*, Mr. Behar's plan of care (nursing diagnosis: *Risk for injury* related to confusion, as evidenced by wandering) was personalized as follows:

Short-Term Outcome	Intervention	Rationale	Evaluation
1. Throughout stay in nursing home, resident will not fall out of bed.	1a. Spend time with resident on admission.	1a. Time spent with resident lowers anxiety and provides orientation to time and place. Resident's confusion is increased by change.	**Goal Met** Mattress on floor prevents falls out of bed.
	1b. Label resident's room in big, colourful letters.	1b. Labels offer clues in new surroundings.	
	1c. Remove mattress from bed and place on floor.	1c. Placing the mattress on the floor prevents falls out of bed.	
	1d. Keep room well lit at all times.	1d. Lighting provides important environmental clues and helps lower possibility of illusions.	
	1e. Show resident clock and calendar in room.	1e. These items foster orientation to time.	
	1f. Keep window shade up.	1f. This visibility allows day–night variations.	
2. Throughout nursing home stay, resident will wander only in protected area.	2a. At night, take resident to large, protected, well-lit room.	2a. Resident is able to wander safely in protected environment.	**Goal Met** Resident continues to wander at night but, with supervision, keeps out of other residents' rooms most of the time. By 4th week, resident starts to nap on couch in large room after snacks during the night.
	2b. Alert physician to check resident for cardiac decompensation.	2b. Physical check addresses possible underlying cause of nocturnal wakefulness and wandering.	
	2c. Offer snacks when resident is up—milk, decaffeinated tea, sandwich.	2c. Snacks help replace fluid and caloric expenditure.	
	2d. Allow soft music on radio.	2d. Music helps induce relaxation.	
	2e. Spend short, frequent intervals with resident.	2e. Time with others decreases resident's feelings of isolation and increases orientation.	
	2f. Take resident to bathroom after snacks.	2f. Bathroom visits after eating help prevent incontinence.	
	2g. During day, offer activities that include use of large muscle groups.	2g. For some residents, using large muscle groups helps decrease wandering.	

CASE STUDY AND NURSING CARE PLAN 17.1—cont'd
Cognitive Impairment

Short-Term Outcome	Intervention	Rationale	Evaluation
3. Resident will be returned within 2 hours if he succeeds in escaping from the unit.	3a. Order MedicAlert bracelet for resident (with name, unit, hospital, and phone number).	3a. If resident gets out of hospital, he can be identified.	**Goal Met** By 4th week, resident wanders off unit only once; is found in lobby and returned by security guard within 45 minutes.
	3b. Place brightly coloured vest on resident with name, unit, and phone number taped on back.	3b. If resident wanders in hospital, he can be identified and returned.	
	3c. Check resident's whereabouts periodically during the day and especially at night.	3c. Regular checks help monitor resident's activities.	

Evaluation
Although Mr. Ludwig continues to display wandering behaviours, his wandering is contained to safe areas of the unit, except for one instance when he wanders to the lobby. However, then he is stopped by security and safely returned to the unit within 45 minutes. He has not fallen out of bed. Nursing interventions such as placing his mattress on the floor and ensuring adequate lighting increase his safety while at the same time acknowledging that he continues to exhibit wandering behaviours.

KEY POINTS TO REMEMBER

- *Neurocognitive disorder* is a term that refers to disorders resulting from changes in the brain and is marked by disturbances in orientation, memory, intellect, judgement, and affect.
- Delirium and neurocognitive disorders are most frequently seen by health care workers.
- Delirium is marked by acute onset, disturbance in consciousness, and symptoms of disorientation and confusion that fluctuate by the minute, hour, or time of day.
- Delirium is always secondary to an underlying condition; therefore it is transient and may last from hours to days once the underlying cause is treated. If the cause is not treated, permanent damage to neurons can result.
- Signs and symptoms change according to the three stages of Alzheimer's disease: mild, moderate, and severe.
- Behavioural manifestations of Alzheimer's disease include confabulation, perseveration, aphasia, apraxia, agnosia, hyperorality, and sundowning.
- No known cause or cure exists for Alzheimer's disease, although a number of drugs that increase the brain's supply of acetylcholine (a nerve-communication chemical) or regulate glutamate are helpful in slowing the progress of the disease.
- Specific nursing interventions for cognitively impaired individuals can increase communication, safety, and self-care and are described in the chapter. The need for family teaching and support is crucial.

CRITICAL THINKING

1. Mrs. Kendel is an 82-year-old woman who has Alzheimer's disease. She lives with her husband, who has been trying to care for her in their home. Mrs. Kendel is having trouble dressing. She has put her blouse on backwards and sometimes puts her bra on over her blouse. She often forgets where things are. She makes an effort to cook but has recently attempted to "put out" the electric burners of the stove with pitchers of water. Once in a while, she cannot find the bathroom in time, often mistaking a closet for it. At times, she cries because she is aware that she is losing her sense of place in the world. She and her husband have always been close, loving companions, and he wants to keep her at home for as long as possible.
   a. Assist Mr. Kendel by writing out a list of suggestions that he can try at home that might help with (a) communication, (b) activities of daily living, and (c) maintenance of a safe home environment.
   b. Identify at least three interventions that are appropriate to this situation for each of the problems Mrs. Kendel is having.
   c. Identify resources available for maintaining Mrs. Kendel in her home for as long as possible. Provide the name of a self-help group that you would urge Mr. Kendel to join.
2. Share with your class or clinical group the name and function of at least three community agencies in your area that could be an appropriate referral for a family with a member with dementia. (For one, you can contact the Alzheimer Society of Canada: http://www.alzheimer.ca)

CHAPTER REVIEW

1. A 73-year-old woman with pneumonia becomes agitated after being admitted to the intensive care unit through the emergency department. She continually tries to leave her bed despite being too weak to walk. Her vital signs are erratic, and her thinking seems disorganized. During her first 24 hours in the continuing care unit, the patient varies from somnolent to agitated and from laughing to angry. Her daughter reports that the patient "was never like this at home." What is the most likely explanation for the situation?
   a. Pneumonia has worsened the patient's early-stage dementia.
   b. The patient is experiencing delirium secondary to the pneumonia.
   c. The patient is sundowning due to the decreased stimulation of the critical care unit.
   d. The patient does not want to be in the hospital and is angry that staff will not let her leave.
2. Intervention(s) appropriate for a hospitalized patient experiencing delirium include which of the following? **Select all that apply.**
   a. Immediately placing the patient in restraints if she begins to hallucinate or act in an irrational or unsafe manner.
   b. Ensuring that a clock and a sign indicating the day and date are displayed where the patient can see them easily.

c. Being prepared for possible hostile responses to efforts to take vital signs or provide direct physical care.
d. Preventing sensory deprivation by placing the patient near the nurses' station and leaving the television and multiple lights turned on 24 hours per day.
e. Speaking with the patient frequently for short periods for reassurance, assisting the patient in remaining oriented, and ensuring the patient's safety.
f. Anticipating that the patient may try to leave if agitated and providing a secure environment with direct observation to prevent wandering.
g. Promoting normalized sleep patterns by encouraging the patient to remain awake during the day and facilitating rest at night.

3. Which statement about dementia is accurate?
   a. The majority of people over age 85 are affected by dementia.
   b. Disorientation is the dominant and most disruptive symptom of dementia.
   c. People with dementia tend to be distressed by it and complain about its symptoms.
   d. Hypertension, diminished activity levels, and head injury increase the risk for dementia.

4. Mrs. Smythe dies at the age of 82. In the 2 months following her death her husband, aged 84 and in good health, has begun to pay less attention to his hygiene and seems less aware of his surroundings. He complains of difficulty concentrating and sleeping and reports that he lacks energy. His family sometimes has to remind and encourage him to shower, take his medications, and eat, all of which he then does. Which response is most appropriate?
   a. Arrange for an appointment with a therapist for evaluation and treatment of suspected depression.
   b. Reorient Mr. Smythe by pointing out the day and date each time you interact with him.
   c. Meet with family and support persons to help them accept, anticipate, and prepare for the progression of his stage 2 dementia.
   d. Avoid touch and proximity, which are likely to be uncomfortable for Mr. Smythe and may provoke aggression when he is disoriented.

5. Which of the following interventions would be beneficial for those caring for a loved one with Alzheimer's disease? **Select all that apply.**
   a. Guide the family to restrict the patient's driving as soon as signs of forgetfulness are exhibited.
   b. Recommend switching to hospital-type gowns to facilitate bathing, dressing, and other physical care of the patient.
   c. Discourage wandering by installing complex locks or locks placed at the tops of doors, where the patient cannot readily reach them.
   d. For situations in which the patient becomes upset, teach loved ones to listen briefly, provide support, and then change the topic.
   e. Encourage caregivers to care for themselves, as well as the patient, via the use of support resources such as adult day care or respite care.
   f. If the patient is prone to wander away, encourage the family to notify the police and neighbours of the patient's condition, wandering behaviour, and description.

http://evolve.elsevier.com/Canada/Varcarolis/psychiatric/

REFERENCES

Alzheimer's Association. (2020). Alzheimer's disease facts and figures. *Alzheimer's & Dementia: The Journal of the Alzheimer's Association, 16*(3), 391–460. https://doi.org/10.1002/alz.12068

Alzheimer's Association. (2021). *Causes and risk factors for Alzheimer's disease.* https://www.alz.org/alzheimers-dementia/what-is-alzheimers/causes-and-risk-factors

Alzheimer Society of Canada. (2021a). *Restlessness or "sundowning."* https://alzheimer.ca/en/help-support/im-caring-person-living-dementia/understanding-symptoms/restlessness-or-sundowning

Alzheimer Society of Canada. (2021b). *Alternative treatments for dementia.* https://alzheimer.ca/en/about-dementia/how-can-i-treat-dementia/alternative-treatments-dementia

Alzheimer Society of Canada. (2021c). *Medical assistance in dying.* https://alzheimer.ca/en/help-support/im-caring-person-living-dementia/end-life-care/medical-assistance-dying

Alzheimer Society of Canada. (2021d). *Cannabis and the treatment of dementia.* https://alzheimer.ca/en/about-dementia/how-can-i-treat-dementia/cannabis-treatment-dementia

American Psychiatric Association (APA). (2013). *Diagnostic and statistical manual of mental disorders* (5th ed.). Washington, DC: Author.

Bray, M. J. C., Richey, L. N., Bryant, B. R., Krieg, A., Jahed, S., Tobolowsky, W., LoBue, C., & Peters, M. E. (2021). Traumatic brain injury alters neuropsychiatric symptomatology in all-cause dementia. *Alzheimer's & Dementia: The Journal of the Alzheimer's Association, 17*(4), 686–691.

Buckley, J. S., & Salpeter, S. R. (2015). A risk–benefit assessment of dementia medications: Systematic review of the evidence. *Drugs and Aging, 32*, 453–467.

Bulechek, G. M., Butcher, H. K., & Dochterman, J. M. (2013). *Nursing Interventions Classification (NIC)* (6th ed.). Toronto: Elsevier.

Burchum, J. R., & Rosenthal, L. D. (2019). *Lehne's pharmacology for nursing care* (10th ed.). Elsevier.

Canadian Institute for Health Information. (2010). *Caring for seniors with Alzheimer's disease and other forms of dementia: Describing outcome scales (RAI-HC).* Ottawa: Author.

Canadian Institute for Health Information. (2013). *Caring for seniors with Alzheimer's disease and other forms of dementia.* Ottawa: Author.

Goldberg, T. E., Chen, C., Wang, Y., Jung, E., Swanson, A., Ing, C., Garcia, P. S., Whittington, R. A., & Moitra, V. (2020). Association of delirium with long-term cognitive decline: A meta-analysis. *JAMA Neurology, 77*(11), 1–9. Advanced online publication. https://doi.org/10.1001/jamaneurol.2020.2273

Grover, S., Sahoo, S., Chakrabarti, S., & Avasthi, A. (2019). Post-traumatic stress disorder (PTSD) related symptoms following an experience of delirium. *Journal of Psychosomatic Research, 123,* 109725. https://doi.org/10.1016/j.jpsychores.2019.05.003

Hendrie, K., Chadha, G., Sridhar, M., Agarwal, S., Rangan, P., & Agarwal, N. (2021). Using smart EHR tools for early detection of delirium in hospitalized older adults. *The American Journal of Geriatric Psychiatry, 29*(4). https://doi.org/10.1016/j.jagp.2021.01.080

Kennedy, M., Helfand, B. K., Gou, R. Y., Gartaganis, S. L., Webb, M., Moccia, J. M., Bruursema, S. N., Dokic, B., McCulloch, B., Ring, H., Margolin, J. D., Zhang, E., Anderson, R., Babine,

R. L., Hshieh, T., Wong, A. H., Taylor, R. A., Davenport, K., Teresi, B., & Inouye, S. K. (2020). Delirium in older patients with Covid-19 presenting to the emergency department. *JAMA Network Open. 3*(11). https://doi.org/10.1001/jamanetworkopen.2020.29540

Kinney, J. W., Bemiller, S. M., Murtishaw, A. S., Leisgang, A. M., Salazar, A. M., & Lamb, B. T. (2018). Inflammation as a central mechanism in Alzheimer's disease. *Alzheimer's & Dementia: Translational Research & Clinical Interventions, 4,* 575–590. https://doi.org/10.1016/j.trci.2018.06.014

Moorhead, S., Swanson, E., Johnson, M., & Maas, M. L. (Eds.). (2018). *Nursing outcomes classification (NOC): Measurement of health outcomes* (6th ed.). St. Louis: MO: Elsevier.

Nasreddine, Z. S., Phillips, N. A., Bédirian, V., Charbonneau, S., Whitehead, V., Collin, I., Cummings, J. L., & Chertkow, H. (2005). The Montreal Cognitive Assessment, MoCA: A Brief Screening Tool For Mild Cognitive Impairment. *Journal of the American Geriatrics Society* (JAGS), *53*(4), 695–699. https://doi.org/10.1111/j.1532-5415.2005.53221.x

World Health Organization. (2020). *Key facts.* https://www.who.int/news-room/fact-sheets/detail/dementia

18

Psychoactive Substance Use and Treatment

Rick Csiernik

 https://evolve.elsevier.com/Canada/Varcarolis/psychiatric/

OBJECTIVES

1. Compare and contrast the terms substance *use, misuse, dependence*, and *addiction*.
2. Understand the significance of tolerance and withdrawal and their contribution to the process of physical dependency in creating an addiction.
3. Distinguish between addiction and a compulsive behaviour.
4. Understand the economic implications of substance use and misuse in Canada.
5. Reflect on the implications of Canada's legalization of cannabis.
6. Understand biological, psychological, and social perspectives on why substance misuse occurs.
7. Discuss four components of the assessment process, including assessment of readiness for change, to be used with a person who is experiencing substance misuse.
8. Describe the signs of alcohol withdrawal and options to respond to it.
9. Identify two short-term goals for a person who misuses alcohol in terms of (1) withdrawal, (2) active treatment, and (3) health maintenance.
10. Distinguish between the symptoms of opioid intoxication and those of opioid withdrawal.
11. Compare and contrast the signs and symptoms of intoxication, overdose, and withdrawal for cocaine and amphetamines.
12. Recognize signs of substance use or impaired practice in colleagues and the appropriate steps to take to assist.
13. Present and discuss the stages of the Transtheoretical Model of Change (TTM).
14. Explore the principles and practices of motivational interviewing as an evidence-informed intervention and an approach to communication for recovery.
15. Recognize the phenomenon of relapse as it affects people who use substances during different phases of treatment.
16. Evaluate four indications that a person is successfully recovering from substance use.
17. Identify the components of the addiction treatment continuum of care, including the various harm reduction options.
18. Identify different treatment approaches for patients with concurrent disorders.
19. Identify distinct treatment needs of Indigenous peoples.

KEY TERMS AND CONCEPTS

addiction	contemplation	opioid
alcohol poisoning	drug misuse	physical dependency
alcohol withdrawal	hallucinogens	pre-contemplation
alcohol withdrawal delirium	harm reduction	preparation
Alcoholics Anonymous	inhalants	psychological dependency
blood alcohol level	integrated use	relapse prevention
Cannabis sativa	integration	standard drink
collaboration	maintenance/adaption	tolerance
compulsive behaviour	motivational interviewing	Transtheoretical Model of Change
concurrent disorder	mutual aid	withdrawal
consultation	neurotransmitters	

Canada is a complex, diverse society whose citizens use a variety of psychoactive agents for various biological, psychological, and social purposes: to restore health, reduce pain and anxiety, increase energy, aid weight loss or gain, create a feeling of euphoria, take part in social customs and rituals, induce relaxation or sleep, and create community and intimacy. Most of us, both personally and professionally, have been affected by the use, and misuse, of psychoactive agents and the impact of addiction personally and on our communities. The impact of drugs and also of compulsive behaviours is vast, affecting us not only individually but also on a family level, in the workplace, in our interpersonal relationships, and as a society. This chapter begins by differentiating between an addiction and a compulsive behaviour and then explores the clinical trajectory and implications of psychoactive substances, as well as the screening for addiction and the assessment of and nursing care for those experiencing addiction, including nurses themselves.

❤ HOW A NURSE HELPED ME

Kari Cared Enough to Take Action

I was introduced to opioids years ago after an injury to my back in a work-related accident. All through my nursing education, I continued to use opioids to control the pain. Eventually, my need for more Dilaudid forced me to see doctors in different cities and towns. I didn't want my family or friends to know; but more importantly I didn't want my employer to know. When my own family doctor suggested going on Suboxone as an alternative to Dilaudid use for my pain, I willingly agreed. At first, the Suboxone seemed to be working, but my anxiety and fear about being found out caused nausea and vomiting. One day, I took an ampoule of dimenhydrinate 50 mg home from work. I was pleased with the effects; my anxiety abated (as did the nausea and vomiting). I started carrying two or three ampoules of dimenhyrindate 50 mg in my uniform pocket (just in case I needed it at work). Each shift, I would restock my supply, and even though it was only an antihistamine, I knew how wrong this was; still, the feeling of relief I got from the dimenhydrinate was profound.

One day, I mentioned this to the nurse at the opioid substitution clinic. I thought by telling her, maybe they would increase my dose or the clinic doctor would prescribe something better. The nurse, Kari, was kind and non-judgmental but was very worried about my mixing of these two central nervous systems depressants and my working under their influence. Kari asked how much I had used the day before, my plan for stopping, and solutions I had tried to diminish my anxiety at work. The next day, Kari invited me into her office at the clinic, where we discussed our nursing practice standards and her responsibility for reporting me to the professional nursing association. I think I was angry at first; the clinic is supposed to be confidential; my right to privacy and confidentiality was supposed to be first and foremost!

Then the next day, Kari asked what I had planned to do: was I going to report my using and pilfering of dimenhydrinate from my work, or did I want her to? I didn't realize until later how much relief I felt; no more avoiding. It was time to get more help. Thanks to Kari, I booked myself into an inpatient addiction treatment program with the help of my family doctor. I went to my union and my association and told them what was happening. The association suspended my license, as I knew they would, but because Kari cared enough about my patients—and me—to take action, the association accepted my plan of recovery. I can't begin to imagine my life had that one nurse not taken the initiative to put professional practice into my vision of recovery. My use affected not only myself and my family but my patients and my colleagues. I used to be ashamed and angry about my personal life at work, and my work life at home. Now my recovery is having a positive effect on all aspects of my life and the lives of my patients.

Source: Nova Scotia College of Nurses. (2020). *Problematic substance use: A guide for nurses.* https://cdn1.nscn.ca/sites/default/files/documents/resources/Problematic_Substance_Use.pdf

DISTINGUISHING BETWEEN AN ADDICTION AND A COMPULSIVE BEHAVIOUR

Psychoactive drugs are unique substances that alter the central nervous system (CNS), changing thought, mood, and behaviour. Chronic use leads to **psychological dependency**, which can range from a mild wish to a compelling emotional need for the periodic or continuous use of a drug. Psychological dependence occurs when a drug becomes so important to an individual's thoughts and actions that the person believes that they cannot manage without the substance. Psychoactive drugs also affect the peripheral nervous system (PNS), creating changes to core biological functioning. Chronic substance use, except with hallucinogens, produces **physical dependency**, which is a physiological state of cellular adaptation that arises when the CNS and PNS become habituated to a psychoactive agent such that the person physically needs the drug to function or to avoid the physical pain of withdrawal as described in the opening case study. The use of psychoactive drugs also is affected by the social environment. The classic example of this arose out of the Vietnam War. A visit by an American congressman to Vietnam in 1971 on a fact-finding mission led to urine-screening of all troops to detect the use of heroin prior to their redeployment to the United States. In one study 75% of soldiers, most of whom were drafted and by the age of 21 were combat veterans, tested positive. Upon returning to the United States, only one-third continued to use heroin, but of these individuals, less than 10% were classified as dependent. Once they were removed from a constant life-threatening situation, there was no longer a need to use the drug. Thus a comprehensive conceptualization of **addiction** must include three elements: biological, psychological, and social (Figure 18.1) (Csiernik, 2021).

> **SAFETY TIP**
>
> As addiction has a distinct and often powerful biological component, individuals who are in active, acute withdrawal may engage in drug seeking behaviour, so be cognizant if your workplace administers psychoactive agents and, if so, ensure that they are not readily accessible or visible during your intake or assessment.

In contrast, **compulsive behaviours** do not have the biological element but only the psychological and social elements. This is not to diminish the severity of these issues, for they can have substantive impacts on individuals, families, and society, but they simply do not have direct biological risk and thus require distinct treatment approaches, treatment systems, and policies. Examples of compulsive behaviours that are labelled by some as addictive behaviours, even in the academic literature, are exercising, gaming, gambling, Internet use, pornography viewing, shopping, smartphone use, studying, and work. However, with these compulsive behaviours, there are no biological risks of withdrawal or overdose as would occur with a psychoactive substance. As well, food and sex, which certainly have distinct biological components, have been labelled as addictions by some in the popular and academic literature. The question to ask yourself as you review the remainder of the chapter, given the context of what an addiction entails, is, should essential biological processes necessary for our continued survival as individuals, and as a species, be considered an addiction? If the primary addiction treatment protocol remains abstinence, then what are the implications if we label a person as being addicted to food or sex?

The Process of Addiction Development

The diagnosis of a substance-related disorder requires the knowledge of the class of drug used, patterns of use, the severity of symptoms (mild, moderate, or severe), and the development of tolerance and withdrawal. Figure 18.2 highlights the process of addiction from experimentation to addiction.

No Contact

Prior to a person coming into contact with a psychoactive agent, there is no use and thus no risk. In this stage the individual does not use any psychoactive substances. Just as someone can be predisposed to substance use due to biological (genetic), psychological, or social factors, one's personal disposition or social environment may dissuade the use of certain substances or behaviours. There are many protective factors for not using drugs, including culture, family, other positive social

Fig. 18.1 Holistic view of addiction.

supports, and faith, as well as fear of legal consequences and abiding by one's professional standard of practice.

Experimentation
Individuals begin to experiment with drugs for a range of biological, psychological, or social reasons, such as to feel the effects of different substances; to fit in with peers; to reduce the anxiety of intimacy; and to escape from issues of stress, violence, trauma, and oppression.

Integrated Use
Some people may use a substance to enhance an already pleasurable and ongoing experience and therefore consider their use to be a social habit, integrated into their lives and not creating any biological, psychological, or social issues. This can include a glass of wine with dinner or using cannabis before going to sleep. This *integrated use* of a substance in a socially and culturally accepted manner has few negative consequences.

Excessive Use
The *misuse* or excessive use of a substance results in problems for users and often for those associated with them. People who misuse drugs may experience lapses in memory; experience conflict in their personal, school, or vocational relationships because of impairment; or engage in acts they would not consider when not under the influence of a psychoactive substance. Treatment intervention becomes appropriate when a person has reached this degree of psychoactive drug consumption.

Addiction
At the stage of addiction, a person has reached the state where they are physically and psychologically dependent. The person has lost the ability to choose to use, and the drug becomes the central organizing principle of the person's life. With regular use of a psychoactive substance, a person develops *tolerance*. *Tolerance* is a physiological experience that occurs when a person's reaction to a substance decreases with repeated administrations of the same dose. At this point, if the person attempts to stop using the substance, they may experience symptoms of *withdrawal*, which entails cravings for the substance of misuse that are accompanied by decreased physical and emotional health. Withdrawal also produces physiological changes as the blood and tissue concentrations of a drug decrease after heavy and prolonged use of a substance.

Epidemiology
Health Canada's (2018) national survey reported that 78% of Canadians 15 and older consumed alcohol in the past year, with the average age of first drink being 16. In 2018 21% of adult drinkers exceeded the low-risk drinking guidelines of five or more standard drinks at least once. The rate of alcohol-impaired driving was 177 incidents per 100 000 people nationally, with alcohol accounting for 13.2% of all overdose deaths in Canada. Approximately 4.6 million Canadians (15%) smoked cigarettes in 2017, slightly more than what the 2015 national survey found but still a dramatic decrease from 1965 when nearly half of Canadians did so. Men (17%) were more likely to smoke tobacco than women (13%). Daily smokers averaged 13.7 cigarettes per day while 1% reported using chewing tobacco regularly. Interestingly, the same percentage of individuals who reported smoking also indicated they had used an e-cigarette, including 23% (460 000) of youth aged 15 to 19, and 29% (704 000) of young adults aged 20 to 24 (Health Canada, 2018).

Illicit drug use remains low among the general Canadian population, though the percentage has increased from 1% in the 1990s to approximately 3% in 2017. However, this number should not negate the seriousness of opioid misuse that continues to occur across the country. The number of fatal and non-fatal opioid-related toxicity events has risen dramatically over the past decade. Between January 2016 and September 2020, over 19 000 opioid-related deaths were recorded in Canada, with one in six being individuals under the age of 25. During that same time period, over 17 000 opioid poisonings lead to formal hospitalizations. Coronavirus disease 2019 (COVID-19) prevention measures were introduced to address the increasing opioid crisis in Canada in April 2020. Despite these initiatives, in the following 6 months there were over 3300 opioid deaths, an increase of 74% from

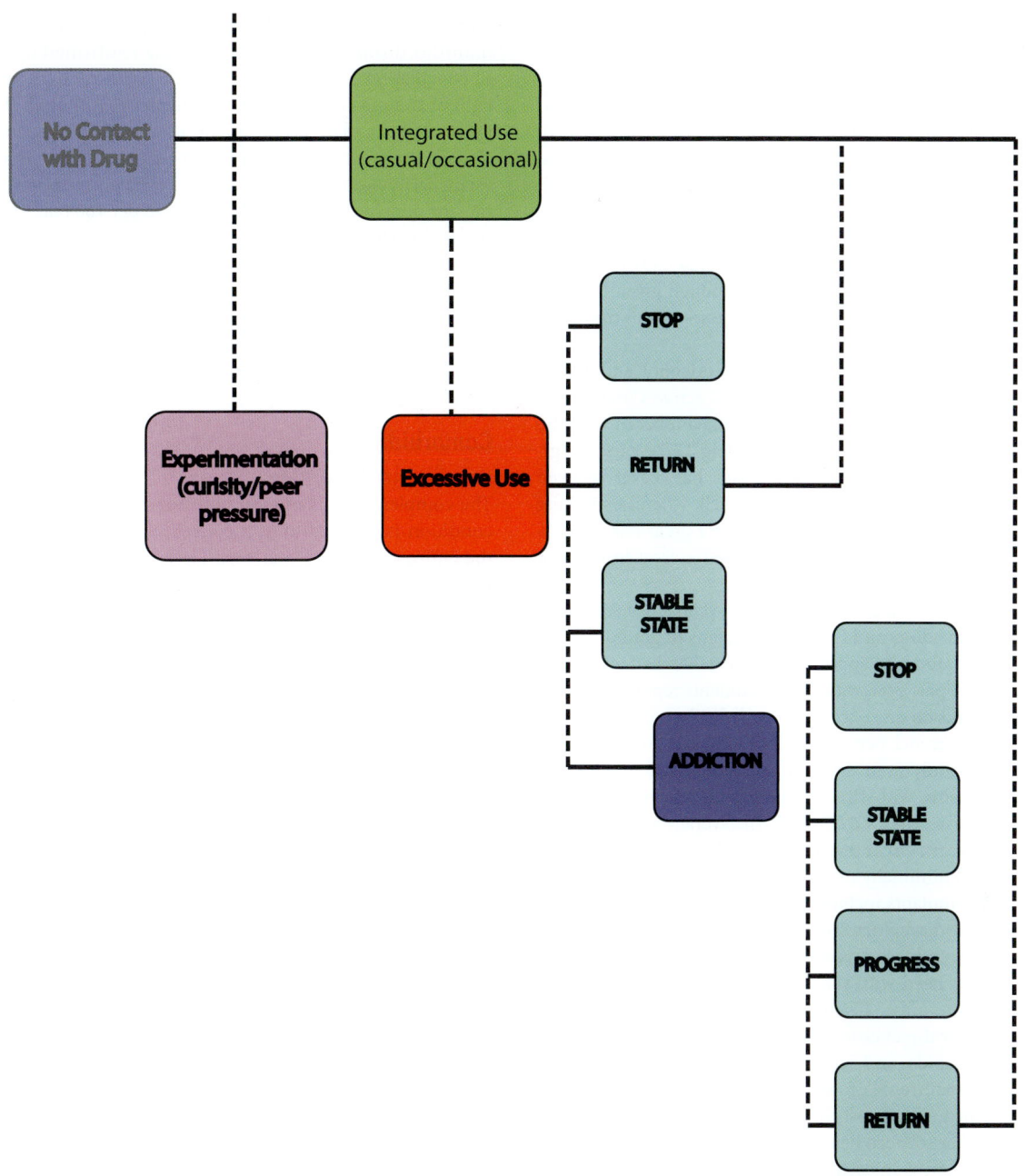

Fig. 18.2 Stages in the process of drug use. (**Source:** Csiernik, R., & Rowe, W. S. [2017]. *Responding to the oppression of addiction*. Toronto: Canadian Scholars Press.)

the previous 6 months. Of these, 96% were deemed unintentional. Leading causes for this surge in preventable deaths were the increasing toxicity of the drug supply; increased feelings of isolation, stress, and anxiety; and reduced access to treatment services (Health Canada, 2018; Special Advisory Committee on the Epidemic of Opioid Overdoses, 2019; Statistics Canada, 2021).

Although opioids have garnered most of the media attention in Canada, the largest increase in illicit drug use was a stimulant, cocaine, and whereas utilization increased 50% in 1 year, only 3% of Canadians who used this illegal psychoactive agent. Canadian men continue to report using more illegal drugs than women, with the majority of these users being under the age of 25. The overall pattern of illicit drug use has been consistent across time as less than 1% of Canadians reported the use of crystal methamphetamine or hallucinogens such as lysergic acid diethylamide (LSD) and methylenedioxymethamphetamine (MDMA [ecstasy]) in the 1990s, which is similar to the current study's findings (Statistics Canada, 2018).

About 6.5 million Canadians (22%) 15 years of age and older were estimated to have used a prescription psychoactive drug in 2017, with a greater proportion of women than men using these legal drugs. The most commonly prescribed psychoactive drugs were opioids, with 12% of the Canadian adult population reporting use of at least one such drug in 2017. In this study approximately 100 000 people (3%) stated that they had misused a prescribed opioid (Health Canada, 2018).

Regular recreational cannabis use more than doubled from 1985 (5.6%) to 2014 (15.0%) among Canadians aged 15 years and older, with use having steadily crept up since then. Lifetime use among Canadians is reported as 41.5% of the adult population. Cannabis use remains more prevalent among males (19%) than females (11%). Another substantive change has been the number of individuals using cannabis for medical purposes; 1.6 million Canadians (5%) in 2018 (Statistics Canada, 2018, 2019). Not surprisingly, with legalization, reported cannabis use has increased. In a 2020 Statistics Canada survey 27% of those surveyed reported using cannabis with provincial/territorial estimates ranging from 21% to 37%, a slight increase from the reported prevalence in 2019. More men (31%) than women (23%) reported using cannabis with those aged 20 to 24 (52%) were using cannabis the most, followed by 16- to 19-year-olds (44%). In 2020 COVID-19 had not had a substantive impact on cannabis use, though given the prolonged nature of the pandemic it is impossible to assess if this trend will continue (Statistics Canada, 2020).

The 2018–2019 Canadian Student Tobacco, Alcohol and Drugs Survey sampled 62 580 students in grades 7 to 12 across Canada. The study extrapolated that 19% of students had smoked tobacco with the average age for beginning experimentation being 13.7 years of age. Of those using e-cigarettes, 42% indicated they had never smoked an actual cigarette; they exclusively vaped. As well, whereas smoking cigarettes on a regular basis was perceived to be a great risk by 66% of students, only 14% reported that vaping posed a great health risk (Health Canada, 2019).

Alcohol remains the most commonly used psychoactive substance among both Canadian adults and Canadian students in grades 7 to 12. Forty-four percent of students, approximately 880 000, had used alcohol at least once in the past year, with 23% of students reporting having had five or more drinks on one occasion (the definition of at-risk alcohol use), with little difference between males (24%) and females (23%). The next most commonly used drug, not including caffeine, for this population was cannabis, with 18% of young people having used this drug at least once during the study period. The average age of first use of cannabis was 14.3 years. Other than energy drinks containing caffeine, other drugs were still minimally used by Canadian students: synthetic cannabinoids: 4%, stimulants including Ritalin 4%, hallucinogens 3%, opioids 3%, and benzodiazepines 2% (Health Canada, 2019).

A comprehensive study was completed in 2018 that examined the costs and harms associated with substance use in Canada. The study examined four specific areas: healthcare, lost productivity, criminal justice costs, and other direct costs associated with the use of alcohol, tobacco, cannabis, opioids, and other psychoactive agents. Lost productivity due to premature death and disability related to substance use accounted for the greatest costs in all Canadian provinces and territories, with alcohol or tobacco being responsible for the greatest proportion of costs and harms in each jurisdiction. However, this should not diminish concerns with illicit drug use for although between 2007 and 2014 healthcare costs associated with cocaine decreased 57% from $180 billion to $78 billion, costs associated with other CNS stimulants, specifically methamphetamine, increased 110% from $51 billion to $107 billion (Canadian Substance Use Costs and Harms Scientific Working Group [CSUCHSWG], 2018).

In 2017–2018 there were more than 155 000 hospital stays for harm caused by substance use, more than for all cardiovascular issues including heart attack and stroke. Median hospital stay is longer than 5 days, creating a total of 2 million days of hospital stays a year (Canadian Institute for Health Information, 2019). On average, 10 patients die in the hospital every day because of substance use. The vast majority (77%) from health complications were related to alcoholism. This is in part because many of those who die prematurely from substance use outside of hospital are using illicit drugs, highlighted by opioid poisonings.

The group most affected by psychoactive drug use is Canada's Indigenous peoples. Over a quarter-century ago, the Royal Commission on Aboriginal Peoples (1996) concluded that alcoholism was the factor creating the greatest problem for Indigenous individuals and communities throughout Canada, an issue reaffirmed by the Truth and Reconciliation Commission of Canada (2015), and discussed further in light of trauma-informed care in Chapter 8. Although there is a much greater age-standardized hospitalization rate for Indigenous Peoples of Canada for most mental health and behavioural conditions, the greatest disparity occurs with psychoactive substance–related disorders. The rate for non-Indigenous Canadians is 50 per 100 000, compared to 191 per 100 000 for Indigenous Peoples living outside of First Nations communities, and 348 per 100 000 for those living in First Nations communities (Carrière et al., 2018). Indigenous post-secondary students were more likely to report binge drinking alcohol and using cannabis and recreational drugs compared to non-Indigenous post-secondary students (Hop Wo et al., 2019).

Comorbidity

Psychiatric Comorbidity

The complex combination of both substance use and a mental health condition is referred to as a concurrent disorder. This incorporates the entire range of mental health issues from post-traumatic stress to mood disorders to psychosis, for example, an individual dependent upon alcohol with depression or misusing cannabis with schizophrenia. In the United States the terms dual diagnosis, dual disorder, or mentally ill chemical abuser may be used instead; however, in Canada the term dual diagnosis refers to an individual with a mental health disorder and a co-occurring developmental disability.

Of Canadians aged 15 to 64, over one-quarter of a million individuals (1.2%) experience a concurrent disorder. These individuals consistently have poorer psychological health and higher use of health services and are more likely to report partially met/unmet needs than those with only a substance use disorder or a mental health issue, even when demographic and socioeconomic factors and a number of chronic health conditions are considered. Relapse rates are greater among those individuals who also have mental health issues, and likewise there is a greater risk of mental health issues returning when psychoactive substances are used (Khan, 2017).

Medical Comorbidity

Alcohol is pharmacologically unique, giving it the ability to affect all organ systems, particularly the CNS, resulting in disorders such as Wernicke's encephalopathy and Korsakoff's syndrome when there is chronic use. Wernicke's (alcoholic) encephalopathy is an acute and reversible condition, whereas Korsakoff's syndrome is a chronic condition with a recovery rate of only about 20%. The pathophysiological connection between the two problems is a thiamine deficiency, which may be caused by poor nutrition associated with alcohol use or by the malabsorption of nutrients. Wernicke's encephalopathy is characterized by altered gait, vestibular dysfunction, confusion, and several ocular motility abnormalities (horizontal nystagmus, lateral orbital palsy, and gaze palsy). These eye-focused signs are bilateral but not necessarily symmetrical. Sluggish reaction to light and anisocoria (unequal pupil size) are also symptoms. Wernicke's encephalopathy may clear up within a few weeks or may progress into Korsakoff's syndrome, the more severe and chronic version of this problem. Wernicke's encephalopathy responds rapidly to large doses of intravenous thiamine two to three times daily for 1 to 2 weeks. Treatment of Korsakoff's syndrome is also thiamine for 3 to 12 months. Most patients with Korsakoff's syndrome never fully recover, although cognitive improvement may occur with thiamine and nutritional support. Chronic alcohol use also produces esophagitis, gastritis, pancreatitis, alcoholic hepatitis, and cirrhosis of the liver and is associated with tuberculosis, cancer, all types of accidents, suicide, and homicide.

Alcohol use during pregnancy can have negative consequences for the fetus and result in fetal alcohol spectrum disorder (FASD), which is a lifelong issue affecting cognitive ability. FASD is the umbrella term for several different diagnoses, which include fetal alcohol syndrome (FAS), partial FAS, alcohol-related neurodevelopmental disorder (ARND), and alcohol-related birth defects (ARBDs). Women who are planning a pregnancy or are already pregnant are strongly advised to abstain from drinking any alcohol. Consuming four or more drinks per occasion and regular heavy drinking place a fetus at the greatest risk for severe problems, although the risk of adverse birth outcomes, including low birth weight, miscarriage, and premature birth, increase with alcohol consumption of more than two standard drinks per week. Alcohol exposure during pregnancy is related to decreased placental weight and a smaller placenta-to-birthweight ratio. Alcohol exposure is also associated with an increased risk of placental hemorrhage. Consuming alcohol during pregnancy can cause brain damage to the developing infant, leading to a range of developmental, cognitive, and behavioural problems that can appear at any time during childhood. People with FASD often have difficulty in a broad range of areas, including coordination, emotional control, socialization, academic achievement, and maintaining employment. Children born with FAS have restricted growth, facial abnormalities, and learning and behavioural disorders that may be severe and lifelong. FAS can lead to issues with learning, memory, attention span, communication, vision, or hearing, as well as interpersonal relationship difficulties. Children diagnosed with FAS are easily overstimulated and slow to settle, have difficulties understanding personal boundaries, and have issues with information processing, abstract thinking, and executive function. Individuals with ARND have a range of intellectual disabilities and problems with behaviour and learning. They typically do poorly in school and have difficulties with math, memory, attention, and judgment and exhibit poor impulse control. Individuals with an ARBD might have a range of physical problems, typically with the heart, kidneys, or bones, and often have hearing issues as well (Brancato et al., 2018; Brown & Trickey, 2018; Carter et al., 2016; Jansson, 2018; Wang et al., 2019).

For people who use drugs, the route of drug administration influences the possible comorbid medical complications. Those who use intravenous drugs have a higher incidence of infections and associated problems from infection, including hepatitis and human immunodeficiency virus (HIV), cellulitis, and sclerosing of veins. Those who use intranasal substances may be prone to sinusitis and perforated nasal septum. Smoking substances increases the likelihood of respiratory problems and saliva or airborne infections if sharing pipes, cigarettes, or e-cigarettes. Table 18.1 lists physical complications associated with various classes of drugs and their routes of administration.

Etiology

Substance use disorders are characterized by use, misuse, and physical and psychological dependence and also by certain patterns of behaviour: (1) loss of control of substance consumption, (2) continued substance use despite associated problems, and (3) cravings and a tendency to lapse and relapse after efforts to change behaviour. The reason a person may experience a substance use disorder relates to the intersection of biological, psychological, and social factors.

Biological Factors

From 2000 into the 2020s, neurobiological studies of addiction have undergone tremendous development and have yielded enormous amounts of valuable information about neuronal response mechanisms and their adaptive changes through an array of techniques ranging from in vitro molecular methods to brain imaging procedures in conscious subjects actively performing a range of behavioural tasks.

TABLE 18.1 Physical Complications Related to Psychoactive Substances by Method of Administration

Sample Substance	Route	Physical Complications
Cannabis	Inhalation	Impaired lung structure
		Micronucleic white blood cells—increased risk for disease due to decreased resistance to infection
		Possible long-term effects on short-term memory
Nicotine	Inhalation	Cancer of the larynx and esophagus
		Cancer of the mouth
		Cardiovascular disease
		Emphysema
		Hypertension
Cocaine hydrochloride	Intranasal (mucous membrane)	Cardiovascular collapse
		Hyperpyrexia
		Perforation of nasal septum
		Respiratory paralysis
Heroin	Intravenous injection	Abscesses—osteomyelitis
		Bacterial endocarditis
		Cardiac arrest
		Dermatitis
		Hepatitis
		Human immunodeficiency virus (HIV)
		Pulmonary emboli
		Renal failure
		Respiratory arrest
		Seizures
		Septicemia
		Tetanus
Caffeine	Oral	Gastroesophageal reflux
		Increased intraocular pressure in unregulated glaucoma
		Increased plasma glucose and lipid levels
		Peptic ulcer
		Tachycardia

This research has demonstrated that brain structures do change over time due to exposure to psychoactive drugs until they reach a threshold, at which point the primary symptom of dependence occurs, making it difficult to stop excessive drug use without professional assistance. The brain continually attempts to keep the body at or return the body to a point of balance or homeostasis, and in doing so it will adapt to the prolonged or excessive presence of drugs by making changes in brain cells and neural pathways. When people administer a psychoactive drug, it activates the same reinforcement system in the brain that is normally activated by food, water, and sex, sometimes to a lesser extent but sometimes to a far greater degree. Biological theories have examined the role of the limbic system, particularly the amygdala, the part of the brain responsible for emotions such as fear and anxiety, as being crucial to this process, and the effect of reinforcement of dopamine receptors in the mesolimbic system that originate in the ventral tegmental area and terminate in the nucleus accumbens. All of these reinforcers share one physiological effect, that is, increased amounts of dopamine being released in the brain either directly or indirectly through other neurotransmitters being activated. During this process, prominent physical changes occur in areas of the brain that are critical to judgement, decision making, learning and memory, and behavioural control. Neurobiological research focuses on four primary areas:

- Drug actions on intracellular signaling systems that mediate cell responses
- Synaptic plasticity in the course of chronic drug exposure
- The role of dopaminergic and other components of the human reward system
- Genetic factors that will be examined as a distinct theoretical construct (Csiernik, 2021)

Regardless of which neurobiological theory you favour, scientists now know that psychoactive drugs affect specific neurotransmitters and areas of the brain. **Neurotransmitters** are chemical signaling molecules in the brain that are used to relay, amplify, and modulate signals between neurons and can be grouped into three categories:

- Monoamines, including acetylcholine, norepinephrine, dopamine, histamine, and serotonin
- Peptides and hormones, including endorphins, cortisone, and nitric oxide
- Amino acids, including gamma-aminobutyric acid (GABA) and glutamate (Volkow et al., 2017)

All of the approximately 100 identified neurotransmitters that carry chemical information between cells follow the same chemical transmission pathway. However, they can act in different ways on this pathway. First, a neurotransmitter is released from the sending neuron into the synaptic cleft from a storage vesicle located in the axon terminal. The neurotransmitter then diffuses (travels) across the synaptic cleft. On the receiving neuron, there are specialized receptor areas that are designed to receive one type of neurotransmitter and bind with it. As more and more binding occurs, an electrical signal begins to form in the receiving neuron, and when a sufficient amount of the neurotransmitter is bound, an internal electrical charge is generated and the message is sent forward, following the same pattern of transmission. Once the charge is generated, the neurotransmitter may be broken down by enzymes in the cleft and thus deactivated or actively transported back to its point of origin, the axon terminal of the sending neuron (Figure 18.3).

Fig. 18.3 Chemical transmission between cells. (**Source:** Sproule, B. [2004]. *Pharmacology and drug abuse* [2nd ed.]. Toronto: Centre for Addiction and Mental Health.)

The chemical structure of many psychoactive drugs is similar to that of neurotransmitters. The similarity in structure allows them to be recognized by neurons and to alter normal brain messaging. This leads to five distinct chemical processes that influence the CNS and change behaviour, which are termed pharmacodynamic interactions:

- Blocking the reuptake of a neurotransmitter back into the axon terminal, allowing more of the neurotransmitter to be available for binding, thus enhancing the message (cocaine)
- Pushing more neurotransmitters out of the storage vesicles into the synaptic cleft, increasing the opportunity for binding and thus enhancing the message (amphetamines)
- Enhancing the binding to the neurotransmitters to further enhance binding to the receptor site to enhance the message (diazepam)
- Blocking the enzyme from breaking down the drug in the synaptic cleft, allowing more neurotransmitters to bind to their receptors to enhance the message (monoamine oxidase inhibitors [MAOIs], which are antidepressants, such as phenelzine [Nardil] and tranylcypromine [Parnate])
- Mimicking neurotransmitters and binding directly to receptor sites, but not allowing a message to be transmitted (naloxone).

The main systems that seem to be involved in substance use are the endorphin, catecholamine (especially dopamine), serotonin, endocannabinoid, and GABA systems. Cocaine, amphetamines, and lesser stimulants increase levels of norepinephrine, serotonin, and dopamine. **Opioid** drugs act on endorphin receptors with a secondary effect on dopamine. Alcohol and other CNS depressants will act on GABA receptors and, as a result, increase the bioavailability of glutamate, norepinephrine, and dopamine. Hallucinogens act to varying degrees on serotonin, whereas cannabis acts on endocannabinoids (Csiernik, 2019).

Psychological Factors

Among the earliest investigations into why people became addicted to substances were learning theories that studied stimuli that give pleasure, relief, or excitement and how reliably and quickly these effects could be produced. Fundamental to this perspective is the belief that people will repeat any behaviour that brings them some kind of pleasure or reward and will discontinue any behaviour that brings them discomfort or punishment. If a drug brings pleasure or relief in a stressful situation, reduces anxiety or fear, or provides status or popularity in an insecure or lonely situation, its use will become a repeated behaviour. Tolerance is also an important process and is associated with habituation. Habituation is seen through reduced responses to a drug either because of prior exposure to the substance or because of the presentation of environmental stimuli that in the past have reliably predicted the presence of the drug. Under specific circumstances, people who are dependent on opioids have been observed to respond to the mere anticipation of drug effects, to an injection of saline or to an opioid injected while an antagonist is present, as if they had actually administered the drug. Extinction also plays a role and is the process whereby the link between the previously established behaviours of drug seeking and drug using is weakened until a point is reached when the behaviour no longer has any reinforcing benefit or purpose. This is what the treatment process attempts to accomplish in terminating an individual's misuse of a psychoactive agent.

Another prominent psychological theory is personality theory. Human personality traits have been grouped into five categories: extraversion, agreeableness, conscientiousness, emotional stability, and openness to experience. Of these five, it is the extraversion trait that has been most closely associated with excessive substance use, particularly the attribute of impulsivity. However, the idea of a person having an alcoholic personality had been extremely popular well before the development of the five personality dimensions and contributed to the rise in the popularity of personality tests for those with addiction issues in the mid-twentieth century. The literature generally sides with the view that personality does not predict illness, with research continuing in this area and attempting to determine if those with certain personality characteristics become drug misusers or if drug use creates a specific type of personality.

A third long-established psychological perspective on addiction is based in psychodynamic theory. This view arises from the early work of Freud, although Freud himself did not devote much attention to addiction in his extensive writings, despite his own drug dependency on tobacco and cocaine. From this perspective, there are three potential explanations for all maladaptive behaviour:
- Seeking sensuous satisfaction
- Conflicts among the components of the self
- Fixation in the infantile past

Freud stated that alcoholism may be due to the inability to successfully resolve issues among the three components of the self: the id or instinctual striving for at times pleasure and at other times pain relief, the superego or conscience, and the ego or coping component of the person. Failure of the ego to resolve issues between conscience and basic instincts can lead to maladaptive coping responses, including the use of psychoactive drugs.

A fourth perspective is attachment theory, which focuses on long-term emotional bonds. The core idea of attachment theory is that primary caregivers who are available and responsive to an infant's needs allow the child to develop a sense of security, which some label as love, enabling the child to explore their environment in a confident manner, knowing that they are protected. Children who are securely attached as infants tend to develop stronger self-esteem and are more sociable and self-reliant as they grow older. They generally become independent and have good school performance, which establishes a foundation for successful adulthood interactions. Individuals who are more securely attached in childhood tend to have good self-esteem, positive romantic relationships, and the ability to self-disclose to others. Attachment theory views addiction as an attempt to fill the empty space left by the lack of a secure attachment due to deprivation during childhood, including painful, rejecting, or shaming relationships. Excessive drug use, then, is seen as an individual's attempt to self-repair psychological deficits and fill an emptiness from childhood (Csiernik, 2021).

Sociocultural Factors

Culture is a set of thoughts shared by members of a social unit that include common understandings, patterns of beliefs, and expectations. Cultural guidelines are generally unwritten rules of conduct and direction for acceptable behaviours and actions that reflect the morals, norms, and values of a specific group. Cultural theory begins with this premise in attempting to describe and explain the process of drug use in relation to societal norms. Sociocultural factors express the social relationships, politics, and environments beyond individual psychological environments, and thus sociocultural theories attempt to explain differences in the incidence of substance use in various groups. Sociocultural theorists support the demystification of substance use and the study of drugs within an integrated life model. As early as 1943, Horton asserted that the primary function of alcohol in a culture was to reduce anxiety. Thus substance use would be more prevalent in societies in which anxiety abounds and few alternatives to drinking alcohol and using drugs as tension-releasers exist. These societies would also exhibit the highest rates of intoxication. Culture influences alcohol and other socially accepted psychoactive drug use in three distinct ways:
- By the degree to which they operate to bring about the acute need for adjustment of inner tensions such as guilt, suppression, aggression, conflict, and sexual tension in their members
- By the attitudes toward drinking that they produce in the members seen in information exchange, including advertising
- By the degree to which the culture provides substitute means of satisfaction beyond substance use in the form of positive alternative lifestyle options

Using alcohol as an example, four prominent cultural patterns of drug use can be observed:

1. Abstinent cultures in which the overall attitude toward drugs, including alcohol, is negative and all alcoholic beverages are forbidden. An example is Saudi Arabia.
2. Ambivalent cultures in which the attitude toward alcohol use is positive in social settings but negative in others. The African nation of Morocco is an example of this cultural pattern. Morocco is a democratic Islamic nation that has a parliament but where the hereditary king's decisions supersede those of parliament. Islam forbids the drinking of alcohol; however, it is widely available throughout the nation and is an important source of income in some areas.
3. Permissive cultures in which using alcoholic beverages is acceptable, although a negative attitude toward drunkenness remains. An example is Canada.
4. Ultra-permissive cultures in which the attitude is permissive toward both drinking and alcohol-related problems. This last model is most likely to be observed in a culture that is experiencing rapid social change, especially where there is a heavy economic interest in alcohol production and distribution. An example is Russia after the end of communism.

Cultures tend to have lower rates of drug use when the rules governing the use of substances are clear, uniform, and prohibitive and specific social sanctions are associated with use. Lower rates are also more prevalent when members of the culture are exposed to the drug at an early stage and observe adults using it in moderate amounts in settings that discourage the use of the drug as an intoxicant, such as at meals or during religious ceremonies. Sociocultural theories also examine the role of media in the development of drug use, misuse, and addiction. Marketing cues also influence the paths that individuals take both toward becoming addicted and moving away from maladaptive consumption and addiction, such as in labels on products or public service advertising about drinking alcohol while pregnant, as well as similar labels on smoking or vaping products warning about health risks of smoking.

APPLICATION OF THE NURSING PROCESS

Assessment

Assessment of Substance Use and Substance-Induced Disorders

Assessment of chemical impairment, substance use, misuse, dependence, tolerance, and withdrawal is becoming more complex because of the increase in polydrug misuse, co-occurring psychiatric disorders, and comorbid physical illnesses, including HIV and hepatitis C infections, dementia, and encephalopathy. Also, changes in the diagnostic criteria for substance use and substance-induced disorders lead to changes in practice. Depending on the context of the assessment, acute care, critical care unit, community clinic, or street engaged, different practice guidelines need to be considered. Regardless of the setting, the assessment of the safety of the patient and others is always the priority.

Sensitivity to cultural and contextual concerns of patients and families is also important in assessing, interpreting symptoms, making diagnoses, providing clinical care, and designing prevention strategies (see Chapter 8). Steps to follow in assessment include (1) level of acute intoxication, (2) history and past substance use, (3) medical history,

(4) psychiatric history, and (5) psychosocial assessment. General nursing assessment can be augmented with specific substance use assessment and addiction screening, family assessment, and assessment of readiness for change in preparation for interventions (Box 18.1).

Assessment of Acute Intoxication and Active and Historical Substance Use

Acute intoxication and history of substance use are critical aspects of assessment. Although acute intoxication may or may not be obvious, it is crucial for intoxication to be ascertained to ensure an accurate clinical picture and to prevent possible drug interactions or misdiagnoses. Intracranial hematomas, subdural hematomas, and other conditions can go unnoticed if symptoms of acute alcohol intoxication and withdrawal are not distinguished from the symptoms of a brain injury. Therefore neurological signs such as pupil size, equality, and reaction to light need to be assessed, especially in comatose patients suspected of having traumatic injuries. In addition, questions pertaining to alcohol misuse should be asked as part of the assessment of any trauma. **Blood alcohol level** (BAL), a measurement of the percentage of alcohol in the bloodstream, tested through urinalysis and breath screening devices, can be useful for acute assessment purposes.

Assessment strategies must include collection of data pertaining to both patterns of substance use and psychiatric impairment. Unexplained exacerbations of psychiatric disorders may be due to acute

---

BOX 18.1 Key Areas for Comprehensive Assessment

Patient's Goals
- Reasons for seeking care
- Immediate and long-term goals related to health care concerns, including both physical and mental health
- Perceived obstacles to and supports in achieving current goals
- Discussion of the impact of the patient's substance use goals on their other health care goals
- Patient's values and beliefs about the best outcome for themself
- Readiness and stage of change regarding substance use

Demographic and Socioeconomic Information
- Age
- Gender: sexual orientation, gender identity, gender expression
- Cultural and ethnic background
- Education, employment, income
- Housing
- Relationships
- Legal: past or current involvement with the justice system
- Circle-of-care supports: health care providers, family, and other social supports
- Cultural and diversity needs
- Spirituality

Substance Use History
- Substances used by patient
- Age of first use of each substance
- Pattern of use, including amount, frequency, duration of use, and historic use looking for issues of tolerance
- Route of substance use: intravenous (IV), intramuscular (IM), subcutaneous (SC), inhalation, via mucous membrane, oral, transdermal
- Withdrawal symptoms associated with substance use
- Tolerance to substances
- Substances of concern, as identified by the patient
- Access and use of harm reduction strategies, including safer drug use education and supplies, or supplies as required in each individual case, including but not limited to clean needles
- Triggers of substance use
- Adverse consequences related to use
- Increasing loss of control over use
- Periods of abstinence and factors that supported abstinence
- Past history of seeking help for substance use
- Paradoxical effects to substances

Physical Health History and Medical Conditions
- Diagnosed health conditions past and present
- Medication: past and current, including over-the-counter medications and alternative or complementary medications
- Interventions and procedures
- Experiences with interventions and services
- Chronic pain
- History of seizures
- Dental issues
- Sexually transmitted infections

Potential Infections Resulting From IV Drug Use
- Localized and systemic infections or abscesses
- Cellulitis
- Human immunodeficiency virus (HIV)
- Hepatitis B
- Hepatitis C
- Infective endocarditis
- Osteomyelitis

Mental Health History
- History of mental health problems
- Current mental health concerns
- Current and past interventions for mental health problems, both pharmacological and non-pharmacological
- Experiences with interventions and services for mental health problems
- Trauma: emotional, physical, psychological, and sexual
- History of self-harm
- Suicide attempts or thoughts of suicide
- Feelings of anxiety or depression
- Current ability to cope with emotions
- Resilience and hopefulness

Family History of Substance Use and Mental Health Concerns
- Information about relatives who have or have had issues due to substance use or a substance use disorder, and how they have managed, including use of different medications and therapies and current health status
- Information about relatives who have or have had mental health concerns, and how they have managed, including use of different medications and therapies and current health status

Resilience and Strengths
- Patient-identified personal strengths and sources of resilience
- Patient-identified needs and supports to enhance resilience and strengths

Source: American Psychiatric Associaction. (2018). *Practice guidelines for the pharmacological treatment of patients with alcohol use disorders.* Washington: APA.

substance use or to dependence. Substance use can go undetected in patients with depression, anxiety, mania, or suicidal ideation unless a thorough history is taken. Similarly, the understanding and treatment of people with substance use disorders are enhanced by inquiries about symptoms of depression and anxiety.

Once specific data are obtained, it is helpful to know whether the person is actively using the substance and the severity of symptoms from mild to severe as assessed by the symptoms present. In addition to an overall assessment interview, any number of more focused rudimentary screening tools may also be used. One of the earliest and still most commonly used measures for assessing alcohol misuse is the Michigan Alcoholism Screening Test (MAST). The MAST, validated for use with many populations, is a 25-point questionnaire designed to provide a rapid and effective screening for lifetime alcohol-related problems and alcoholism (Selzer, 1971; Teitelbaum & Mullen, 2000). Another popular tool is the CAGE questionnaire (Ewing, 1984). The four questions to be asked in the screening process are remembered by using the mnemonic CAGE:

1. Have you felt you ought to *C*ut down on your drinking, substance use, or behaviour?
2. Have people *A*nnoyed you by criticizing your drinking, substance use, or behaviour?
3. Have you felt *G*uilty about your drinking, substance use, or behaviour?
4. Have you had a drink (or used another substance or behaviour) first thing in the morning to steady your nerves or get yourself going for the day (an *E*ye-opener)?

Each question with an answer of yes scores 1 point, and the higher the score, the greater the problems with the substance or behaviour. A score of 2 or more is considered clinically significant. If the patient is not able to respond to questions or provide a description of current or historical substance use, the nurse should assess for observable indications of substance use, such as dilated or constricted pupils, abnormal vital signs, needle marks, tremors, or alcohol on the breath, and obtain information from family and friends.

ASSESSMENT GUIDELINES

Acute Chemical Impairment

1. Assess for a severe or major withdrawal syndrome.
2. Assess for a drug poisoning that warrants immediate medical attention.
3. Assess the patient for suicidal thoughts or other self-harming behaviours.
4. Evaluate the patient for any physical complications related to drug misuse.
5. Explore the patient's interest in doing something about their drug problem.
6. Assess the patient's and family's knowledge of community resources for addiction treatment.

Signs of Intoxication and Withdrawal

Each class of drugs has its own physiological signs and symptoms of intoxication, which are summarized in the tables for each substance class. Both intoxication and withdrawal may require observation and medical attention or nursing care and can constitute psychiatric emergencies.

Central nervous system depressants. CNS depressant drugs include alcohol, sedative hypnotics (benzodiazepines, Z-drugs, and barbiturates), and inhalants. Symptoms of intoxication, overdose, and withdrawal and possible treatments are presented in Table 18.2.

Withdrawal reactions from alcohol and other CNS depressants are the most problematic and are associated with severe morbidity and mortality, unlike withdrawal from other psychoactive agents (Csiernik, 2019). The syndrome for alcohol withdrawal is the same as that for the entire class of CNS depressant drugs; therefore alcohol is used in this discussion as the prototype as it will be the most commonly observed. Alcohol withdrawal, if uncomplicated, is typically complete within 5 to 7 days. Symptoms of withdrawal, however, continue for a longer period and are more severe for older than younger patients; as well, psychological craving can last for months and even years. Withdrawal may

TABLE 18.2 Central Nervous System Depressants

Drugs	Signs of Intoxication	Effects of Overdose	Possible Treatments for Overdose	Effects of Withdrawal	Possible Treatments for Withdrawal
Barbiturates Benzodiazepines Chloral hydrate Glutethimide Meprobamate Alcohol	*Physical:* Slurred speech Incoordination Unsteady gait Drowsiness Decreased blood pressure *Psychological–perceptual:* Disinhibition of sexual or aggressive drives Impaired judgement Impaired social or occupational function Impaired attention or memory Irritability	Cardiovascular or respiratory depression or arrest (mostly with barbiturates) Coma Shock Convulsions Death	Monitor vital signs every 15 minutes. Monitor for respiratory depression. Oxygen, intubation, or mechanical ventilation may be prescribed. If recent ingestion, induced vomiting, gastric lavage, or activated charcoal may be prescribed. Monitor ECG and lab values for shock. Intravenous (IV) fluids may be prescribed. Continue monitoring VS frequently for respiratory complications, cardiac arrest, and possible seizures.	*Cessation of prolonged or heavy use:* Nausea and vomiting Tachycardia Diaphoresis Anxiety or irritability Tremors in hands, fingers, eyelids Marked insomnia Grand mal seizures *After 5–15 years of heavy use:* Delirium	The physician may prescribe a carefully titrated drug in a similar classification so as to minimize symptoms of withdrawal. *Note:* Abrupt withdrawal can lead to death.

ECG, Electrocardiogram; *VS,* vital signs.
Source: Rowe, B., Lang, E. S., Brown, M. D., Houry, D., Newman, D. H., & Wyer, P. C. (2009). *Evidence-based emergency medicine* (Vol. 63). Oxford: Wiley-Blackwell.

be delayed, however, when another CNS depressant is the main drug of choice or when the patient is withdrawing from a combination of alcohol and other CNS depressants. Multiple drug and alcohol dependencies can result in simultaneous withdrawal syndromes that present a complicated clinical picture among polydrug users and may pose additional problems for safe withdrawal.

Several CNS depressants have become associated with facilitating sexual assaults. These include the benzodiazepine flunitrazepam (Rohypnol, or "roofies") and the solvent gamma-hydroxybutyric acid (GHB) and its congeners. These drugs are odourless, tasteless, and colourless; mix easily with alcoholic drinks; and can render a person unconscious in a matter of minutes due to the pharmacodynamic interaction of two CNS depressants. Perpetrators use these drugs in combination with alcohol because they rapidly produce disinhibition and relaxation of voluntary muscles; they also cause the victim to have lasting anterograde amnesia for events that occur (see also Chapter 25).

Alcohol poisoning. Alcohol poisoning is a state of toxicity that can result when an individual has consumed large amounts of alcohol either quickly or over time. It can produce death from aspiration of emesis or a shutdown of body systems due to severe CNS depression. Signs of alcohol poisoning include an inability to rouse the individual, severe dehydration, cool or clammy skin, respirations less than 10 per minute, cyanosis of the gums or under the fingernails, and emesis while semiconscious or unconscious (see also Table 18.2).

Alcohol withdrawal. The early signs of alcohol withdrawal, a physical reaction to the cessation or reduction of alcohol (ethanol) intake, can develop within a few hours of the last intake. Symptoms peak after 24 to 48 hours and then rapidly and dramatically disappear unless the withdrawal progresses to *alcohol withdrawal delirium*. The severity of withdrawal tends to be dose related, with heavier drinkers experiencing more severe symptoms. Withdrawal severity is also related to age, with those over 65 years of age typically experiencing more severe symptoms. During withdrawal, the patient may appear hyperalert, manifest jerky movements and irritability, startle easily, and experience subjective distress often described as "shaking inside." Grand mal seizures may appear 7 to 48 hours after cessation of alcohol intake, particularly in people with a history of seizures. Careful assessment, including this history and any other risk factors, followed by appropriate medical and nursing interventions, can prevent the more serious withdrawal reaction of delirium.

A competent, supportive manner on the part of the nurse can allay anxiety and provide a sense of security. Consistently and frequently orienting the patient to time and place may be necessary. Encouraging family or close friends, one at a time, to remain with the patient in quiet surroundings can also help to increase orientation and minimize confusion and anxiety.

During withdrawal, some patients may experience illusions, which can be both disorientating and terrifying. Illusions are misinterpretations, usually of a threatening nature, of objects in the environment due to excess activation of the CNS by the drug. For example, a person may think that spots on the wallpaper are blood-sucking ants. However, illusions can be clarified to reduce the patient's terror: "See, they are not ants; they are just part of the wallpaper pattern." Some patients withdrawing from alcohol may be argumentative, hostile, or demanding due to the difficult physical experiences but also because of deep-seated anxiety. The nurse can relieve some of these feelings by demonstrating a non-judgmental attitude, validating the experiences of the patient, maintaining a positive affect and encouragement for efforts at recovery. The Clinical Institute Withdrawal Assessment for Alcohol (CIWA-Ar) provides an efficient, objective means of assessing alcohol withdrawal to prevent under- or overtreating patients with benzodiazepines (Table 18.3).

Alcohol intoxication. Alcohol is the only drug for which exact objective measures of intoxication (BAL) currently exist. The relationship between BAL and behaviour in a non-tolerant individual is illustrated in Table 18.4. Assessing the patient's behaviour can assist the nurse in (1) ascertaining whether the person accurately reported recent drinking and (2) determining the level of intoxication and possible tolerance,

TABLE 18.3 Clinical Institute Withdrawal Assessment for Alcohol (CIWA-Ar)

Nausea/Vomiting	
Ask "Do you feel sick to your stomach? Have you vomited?"	
No nausea and no vomiting	0
Mild nausea and no vomiting	+1
(Severe symptoms)	+2
(More severe symptoms)	+3
Intermittent nausea with dry heaves	+4
(Severe symptoms)	+5
(More severe symptoms)	+6
Constant nausea, frequently dry heaves, and vomiting	+7
Tremor	
Arms extended and fingers spread apart.	
No tremor	0
Not visible, but can be felt fingertip to fingertip	+1
(Severe symptoms)	+2
(More severe symptoms)	+3
Moderate, with patient's arms extended	+4
(Severe symptoms)	+5
(More severe symptoms)	+6
Severe, even with arms not extended	+7
Paroxysmal Sweats	
No sweat visible	0
Barely perceptible sweating, palms moist	+1
(Severe symptoms)	+2
(More severe symptoms)	+3
Beads of sweat obvious on forehead	+4
(Severe symptoms)	+5
(More severe symptoms)	+6
Drenching sweats	+7
Anxiety	
Ask, "Do you feel nervous?"	
No anxiety, at ease	0
Mildly anxious	+1
(Severe symptoms)	+2
(More severe symptoms)	+3
Moderately anxious, or guarded, so anxiety is inferred	+4

TABLE 18.3 Clinical Institute Withdrawal Assessment for Alcohol (CIWA-Ar)—cont'd

(Severe symptoms)	+5	Continuous hallucinations	+7
(More severe symptoms)	+6	**Visual Disturbances**	
Equivalent to acute panic states as seen in severe delirium or acute schizophrenic reactions	+7	Ask "Does the light appear to be too bright? Is its color different? Does it hurt your eyes? Are you seeing anything that is disturbing to you? Are you seeing things you know are not there?"	
Agitation			
Normal activity	0	Not present	0
Somewhat more activity than normal activity	+1	Very mild sensitivity	+1
(Severe symptoms)	+2	Mild sensitivity	+2
(More severe symptoms)	+3	Moderate sensitivity	+3
Moderately fidgety and restless	+4	Moderately severe hallucinations	+4
(Severe symptoms)	+5	Severe hallucinations	+5
(More severe symptoms)	+6	Extremely severe hallucinations	+6
Paces back and forth during most of the interview, or constantly thrashes about	+7	Continuous hallucinations	+7
Tactile Disturbances		**Headache/Fullness in Head**	
Ask, "Have you any itching, pins and needles sensations, any burning, any numbness, or do you feel bugs crawling on or under your skin?"		Ask "Does your head feel different? Does it feel like there is a band around your head?" Do not rate for dizziness or lightheadedness. Otherwise, rate severity.	
None	0	Not present	0
Very mild itching, pins and needles, burning, or numbness	+1	Very mild	+1
Mild itching, pins and needles, burning, or numbness	+2	Mild	+2
Moderate itching, pins and needles, burning, or numbness	+3	Moderate	+3
Moderately severe hallucinations	+4	Moderately severe	+4
Severe hallucinations	+5	Severe	+5
Extremely severe hallucinations	+6	Very severe	+6
Continuous hallucinations	+7	Extremely severe	+7
Auditory Disturbances		**Orientation/Clouding of Sensorium**	
Ask, "Are you more aware of sounds around you? Are they harsh? Do they frighten you? Are you hearing anything that is disturbing to you? Are you hearing things you know are not there?"		Ask "What day is this? Where are you? Who am I?"	
		Oriented, can do serial additions	0
Not present	0	Can't do serial additions or is uncertain about date	+1
Very mild harshness or ability or frighten	+1	Disoriented for date by no more than 2 calendar days	+2
Mild harshness or ability or frighten	+2	Disoriented for date by more than 2 calendar days	+3
Moderate harshness or ability or frighten	+3	Disoriented to place or person	+4
Moderately severe hallucinations	+4	**Scoring**	
Severe hallucinations	+5	0–9	Absent or minimal withdrawal
Extremely severe hallucinations	+6	10–19	Mild to moderate withdrawal
		20+	Severe withdrawal

Sources: Reoux, J. P., & Miller, K. (2000). Routine hospital alcohol detoxification practice compared to symptom triggered management with an objective withdrawal scale (CIWA-Ar). *The American Journal on Addictions, 9*(2), 135–144; Sullivan, J. T., Sykora, K., Schneiderman, J., Naranjo, C. A., & Sellers, E. M. (1989). Assessment of alcohol withdrawal: The revised Clinical Institute Withdrawal Assessment for Alcohol scale (CIWA-Ar). *British Journal of Addiction, 84*(11), 1353–1357.

as patient behaviours may indicate greater or lesser levels of tolerance. As tolerance develops, a discrepancy is seen between the BAL and expected behaviour: a person with tolerance to alcohol may have a high BAL but minimal signs of impairment. Alternatively, a person who is highly sensitive to alcohol or compromised medically may have a low BAL but demonstrate a high level of intoxication.

Alcohol content varies from product to product; nevertheless, a drink is a drink is a drink, with 1.5 ounces of liquor (40% alcohol), a 12-ounce bottle of beer (5% alcohol), and a 5-ounce glass of table wine (12% alcohol) all containing the same amount of ethanol and being considered a standard drink. Thus all affect human physiology in a consistent manner as measured by blood alcohol content, although there are distinct differences between men and women (Table 18.5). Differences in effects from person to person produced by beverage alcohol do not generally result from the type of drink consumed but rather from the person's size, previous drinking experiences, and rate

TABLE 18.4 Relationship Between Blood Alcohol Level and Effects in a Non-tolerant Drinker

Blood Alcohol Level (%)	Blood Alcohol Accumulation (Number of Drinks)	Effects
0.05	1–2	Changes in mood and behaviour; impaired judgement
0.10	5–6	Clumsiness in voluntary motor activity
0.20	10–12	Depressed function of entire motor area of the brain, causing staggering and ataxia; emotional lability
0.30	15–18	Confusion, stupor
0.40	20–24	Coma
0.50	25–30	Death due to respiratory depression

TABLE 18.5 Blood Alcohol Content (BAC) (Milligrams of Alcohol/100 Millilitres of Blood)

Lean Body Weight		FEMALE — Number of Drinks									
Pounds	Kilos	1	2	3	4	5	6	7	8	9	10
100	45.4	50	101	152	203	253	304	355	406	456	507
125	56.7	40	80	120	162	202	244	282	324	364	404
150	68.1	34	68	101	135	169	203	237	271	304	338
175	79.4	29	58	87	117	146	175	204	233	262	292
200	90.8	26	50	76	101	126	152	177	203	227	253
225	102.1	22	45	68	91	113	136	159	182	204	227
250	113.4	20	41	61	82	101	122	142	162	182	202

Lean Body Weight		MALE — Number of Drinks									
Pounds	Kilos	1	2	3	4	5	6	7	8	9	10
100	45.4	43	87	130	174	217	261	304	348	391	435
125	56.7	34	69	103	139	173	209	242	278	312	346
150	68.1	29	58	87	116	145	174	203	232	261	290
175	79.4	25	50	75	100	125	150	175	200	225	250
200	90.8	22	43	65	87	108	130	152	174	195	217
225	102.1	19	39	58	78	97	117	136	156	175	195
250	113.4	17	35	52	70	87	105	122	139	156	173

Note: Blood alcohol content is described here as the amount of alcohol in mg per 100 mL of blood, though often reported in the conversion to a percent from grams.
Rate of elimination 15 mg per hour
Standard drink 1 beer (12 oz 5% alcohol) = 1 wine (5 oz 12% alcohol) = 1 shot (1.5 oz 40% alcohol)

Source: Csiernik, R. (2019). *The essential guide to psychoactive drugs in Canada.* Toronto: Canadian Scholars Press.

of consumption. A person's feelings and activities and the presence of other people also play a role in the way the alcohol affects behaviour.

Alcohol withdrawal delirium. Alcohol withdrawal delirium, also referred to as *delirium tremens (DTs)*, is a medical emergency that can result in death in 20% of untreated patients. It is an altered level of consciousness that presents with seizures following acute alcohol withdrawal. Death is usually due to cardiopathy, cirrhosis, or other comorbidities requiring mechanical ventilation (Foertsch et al., 2019). The state of delirium usually peaks 48 to 72 hours after cessation or reduction of intake, although it can peak later, and lasts 2 to 3 days. Features of alcohol withdrawal delirium include the following:

- Autonomic hyperactivity (tachycardia, diaphoresis, elevated blood pressure)
- Severe disturbance in sensorium (disorientation, clouding of consciousness)
- Perceptual disturbances (visual or tactile hallucinations)
- Fluctuating levels of consciousness (ranging from hyperexcitability to lethargy)

TABLE 18.6 Inhalants: Intoxication, Overdose, and Treatment

Drugs	Intoxication	Adverse Effects/Overdose	Treatment
Organic solvents (gases or liquids that vaporize at room temperature): Toluene, Gasoline, Lighter fluid, Paint thinner, Nail polish remover, Benzene, Acetone, Chloroform, Model airplane glue	Alcohol-like effects: euphoria, impaired judgement, slurred speech, flushing, central nervous system (CNS) depression. Visual hallucinations and disorientation	Chronic use is toxic to heart, liver, and kidneys. Toxicity may result in sudden death from anoxia, vagal stimulation, respiratory depression, and dysthymia.	Support affected systems; no antidotes
Volatile nitrites: Room deodorizers, Products sold for recreational use	Enhancement of sexual pleasure	Venodilation causes profound systolic blood pressure drop (dizziness, lightheadedness, palpitations, pulsate headache). Toxic dose may result in methemoglobinemia.	Toxicity may be treated with oxygen.
Anaesthetics: Gas—especially nitrous oxide (used in dental procedures and as a propellant for whipped cream), Liquid, Local	Giggling, laughter. Euphoria	Numbness, weakness, sensory loss, loss of balance. May cause physical dependence. Possible polyneuropathy and myelopathy when use is chronic.	Neuropathy may be treated with vitamin B_{12}.

Sources: Data from Burchum, J., & Rosenthal, L. (2019). *Lehne's pharmacology for nursing care* (10th ed.). Philadelphia: Saunders; Ruiz, P., & Strain, E. C. (2014). *The substance abuse handbook* (2nd ed.). Philadelphia: Lippincott Williams & Wilkins.

- Delusions
- Anxiety and agitated behaviours
- Fever (38°C to 39°C)
- Insomnia
- Anorexia

If these symptoms are observed, immediate medical attention, including ongoing assessment and supervised treatment, is warranted.

Inhalants. A distinct CNS depressant subgroup is **inhalants**, which include volatile gases, substances that exist in a gaseous form at body temperature, refrigerants, solvents, general anaesthetics, and propellants. Except for nitrous oxide, more commonly known as laughing gas, and related aliphatic nitrates, all inhalants are hydrocarbons. The misuse of these collective substances has been labelled volatile substance use. As this is typically one of the first drugs misused by adolescents, particularly Indigenous youth, it is a significant public health concern. In addition, long-term exposure to solvents in the workplace has also been linked to a range of health issues in older persons, particularly dementia. It is generally believed that solvents alter CNS functioning through one of three means: altering the structure of lipid membranes by impairing ion channels, altering enzymes that bind to the brain's membrane, or producing toxic metabolites (Csiernik, 2019; Hancock & McKim, 2018).

These substances not only have depressant effects but also can produce minor hallucinogenic effects on the CNS. As solvents are inhaled, entry into the brain is extremely quick and the onset of effects is virtually immediate, producing feelings of relaxation and warmth within 8 to 15 seconds and with effects generally lasting for several hours. This class of psychoactive drugs has a significant misuse liability. The initial mood-enhancement effect is typically characterized by lightheadedness, exhilaration, fantasy images, and excitation. Negative effects include nausea, increased salivation, sneezing and coughing, loss of coordination, depressed reflexes, and sensitivity to light, along with skin irritation and burns around the mouth and nose. In some users feelings of invincibility may lead to reckless, dangerous, violent, or erratic behaviour. Physical effects include pallor, thirst, weight loss, nosebleeds, bloodshot eyes, and sores on the nose and mouth. Chronic use creates a range of medical problems, including damage to the cardiovascular, pulmonary, renal, and hepatic systems as well as to cognitive functioning (Hancock, & McKim, 2018). Types of inhalants, signs of intoxication, and adverse effects are outlined in Table 18.6.

Opioids. Opioids are a distinct family of CNS depressants that includes codeine, fentanyl, heroin, meperidine, methadone, and oxycontin (Box 18.2). An opioid is a derivative or synthetic that affects the CNS and the PNS. Medically, it is used primarily as an analgesic (pain masker). Consistent use causes tolerance and severe, physically painful withdrawal symptoms. Table 18.7 lists signs and symptoms of intoxication, overdose, withdrawal, and possible treatments.

Distinct phases are experienced when injecting an opioid such as heroin. The initial rush that occurs almost immediately is frequently characterized in terms of feelings of sexual arousal and as being superior to sexual intimacy. This initial euphoric phase is characterized physiologically by facial flushing and a deepening of the voice. The second, more prolonged, phase entails a sense of extreme well-being as an intense endorphin reaction is occurring in the brain. This phase can extend for several hours. The third phase reflects the fact that opioids are CNS depressants and is characterized by a range of responses, from lethargy to virtual unconsciousness. The fourth phase occurs when the heroin is nearly fully metabolized and the person who has used the substance begins to seek additional heroin in order to avoid the painful withdrawal process.

TABLE 18.7 Opioids: Intoxication, Overdose, and Withdrawal

Drugs	Effects of Intoxication	Effects of Overdose	Possible Treatments for Overdose	Effects of Withdrawal	Possible Treatments for Withdrawal
Opium (Paregoric) Heroin Meperidine (Demerol) Morphine Codeine Methadone (Metadol) Hydromorphone (Dilaudid) Fentanyl (Fentora—sublingual) Fentanyl analogues	*Physical:* Constricted pupils Decreased respiration Drowsiness Decreased blood pressure Slurred speech Psychomotor retardation *Psychological–perceptual:* Initial euphoria followed by dysphoria and impairment of attention, judgement, and memory	Possible dilation of pupils due to anoxia Respiratory depression or arrest Coma Shock Convulsions Death	Opioid antagonist (e.g., naloxone [Narcan, Suboxone]) to quickly reverse CNS depression	Yawning Insomnia Irritability Rhinorrhea Panic Diaphoresis Cramps Nausea and vomiting Muscle aches ("bone pain") Chills Fever Lacrimation Diarrhea	Methadone tapering[a] Clonidine–naltrexone detoxification Suboxone substitution[a]

[a]Methadone tapering is managed very slowly and in careful consultation with the patient with regard to their readiness.
Sources: Taha, S. (2018). *Best practices across the continuum of care for treatment of opioid use disorder.* Ottawa: Canadian Centre on Substance Use and Addiction; Veilleux, J. C., Colvina, P. J., Andersona, J., et al. (2010). A review of opioid dependence treatment: Pharmacological and psychosocial interventions to treat opioid addiction. *Clinical Psychology Review, 30,* 155–166. https://doi.org/10.1016/j.cpr.2009.10.006

BOX 18.2 Canada's Fentanyl Public Health Crisis

Developed in 1959 for use as a general anesthetic, fentanyl is therapeutically used to provide physical and emotional relief from acute pain, principally for palliative-care patients or those with long-term chronic pain who experience breakthrough pain when using other less potent opioids. It has rapid onset and short duration of action; thus it is primarily administered transdermally in a hospital setting to make its use more convenient for those who are severely ill, with each patch designed to slowly release the potent substance over 72 hours.

In 2017 the illicit street use of the potent licit synthetic opioid fentanyl became a national public health crisis, with overdose deaths in Canada reaching new levels. A decade before, a less potent licit synthetic opioid oxycontin had likewise become a public health issue, which led to its use being prohibited but without the development of a concurrent treatment strategy for those who had become addicted. In fact, during this time, the Harper government appealed all the way to the Supreme Court of Canada in an attempt to shutter the nation's lone supervised injection site; after losing that appeal, the government introduced legislation creating additional barriers to opening any new facility anywhere in Canada.

Historically, whenever a psychoactive substance is prohibited, in its void an alternative arises (Csiernik, 2021). Unfortunately, in this case the prohibition of oxycontin, which was accompanied by its manufacturer, Purdue Pharma, paying a $600 million fine for product misbranding, led to an increase in heroin use. However, heroin is both expensive and illicit, whereas fentanyl, a synthetic drug that is 3 times as potent as uncut heroin and 100 times as potent as morphine, is both far cheaper to manufacture and can be legally produced in nations such as China. Across Canada, the cheaper fentanyl was being mixed with heroin, and at times cocaine, so that less of the expensive drug needed to be used and thus drug dealers could increase their profit margins. Combining the two drugs in street-level labs, however, often creates "hot spots" where more fentanyl is incorporated, into the mix and thus the risk of overdose is further increased. Along with fentanyl, another synthetic opioid, even more potent, carfentanil, began to be used for this purpose, again increasing the likelihood of each injection leading to an overdose.

As with alcohol, a protocol has been established to assist with opioid withdrawal. The Clinical Opiate Withdrawal Scale was developed for buprenorphine/naloxone induction, though it can also be used in a variety of clinical settings such as assessing acute opioid withdrawal during an opioid detoxification, methadone maintenance, or methadone treatment, as well as during the treatment of chronic pain (Table 18.8).

Central nervous system stimulants. This family of drugs includes cocaine hydrochloride as well as crack, amphetamines including crystal meth, caffeine, and nicotine. CNS stimulants are drugs that increase the activity of both the CNS and the PNS primarily through the direct activation of dopamine. Mood enhancement occurs because of these changes as well as increased activity of serotonin and norepinephrine. Upon initial ingestion, there is euphoria, followed by excitement and then agitation. Higher doses produce irritability, violent behaviour, spasms, convulsions, and, in infrequent and extreme cases, death. More common and frequent short-term effects include enhanced concentration, increased vigilance, increased blood pressure, increased strength, reduced fatigue, reduced appetite, and feelings of power. While all stimulants increase alertness, as a family, they exhibit considerable differences in the nature of their effects and in their relative potencies.

Table 18.9 outlines the physical and psychological effects of intoxication from amphetamines and other psychostimulants, possible life-threatening results of overdose, and emergency measures for both overdose and withdrawal. Upon the abrupt discontinuation of drug administration, abstinence symptoms observed include fatigue, severe mood depression, lethargy, and irritability; these are commonly referred to as the "crash," which can also include abdominal and muscle cramps, dehydration, and a general apathy. However, unlike with depressants, there is generally no risk for fatal withdrawal, although when someone who has ingested a stimulant experiences chest pain, has an

TABLE 18.8 Clinical Opiate Withdrawal Scale (COWS) for Opioid Withdrawal

Resting Pulse Rate (bpm)		**Nasal stuffiness or unusually moist eyes**		+1
Measure pulse rate after patient is sitting or lying down for 1 minute		Nose running or tearing		+2
≤80	0	Nose constantly running or tears streaming down cheeks		+4
81–100	+1	**GI Upset**		
101–120	+2	Over last 0.5 hours		
>120	+4	No GI symptoms		0
Sweating		Stomach cramps		+1
Sweating not accounted for by room temperature or patient activity over the last 0.5 hours		Nausea or loose stool		+2
		Vomiting or diarrhea		+3
No report of chills or flushing	0	Multiple episodes of vomiting or diarrhea		+5
Subjective report of chills or flushing	+1	**Tremor Observation of Outstretched Hands**		
Flushed or observable moistness on face	+2	No tremor		0
Beads of sweat on brow or face	+3	Tremor can be felt, but not observed		+1
Sweat streaming off face	+4	Slight tremor observable		+2
Restlessness Observation During Assessment		Gross tremor or muscle twitching		+4
Able to sit still	0	**Yawning Observation During Assessment**		
Reports difficulty sitting still, but is able to do so	+1	No yawning		0
Frequent shifting or extraneous movements of legs/arms	+3	Yawning once or twice during assessment		+1
Unable to sit still for more than a few seconds	+5	Yawning three or more times during assessment		+2
Pupil Size		Yawning several times per minute		+4
Pupils pinned or normal size for room light	0	**Anxiety or Irritability**		
Pupils possibly larger than normal for room light	+1	None		0
Pupils moderately dilated	+2	Patient reports increasing irritability or anxiousness		+1
Pupils so dilated that only the rim of the iris is visible	+5	Patient obviously irritable/anxious		+2
Bone or Joint Aches		Patient so irritable or anxious that participation in the assessment is difficult		+4
If patient was having pain previously, only the additional component attributed to opiate withdrawal is scored		**Gooseflesh Skin**		
		Skin is smooth		0
Not present	0	Piloerection of skin can be felt or hairs standing up on arms		+3
Mild diffuse discomfort	+1	Prominent piloerection		+5
Patient reports severe diffuse aching of joints/muscles	+2	**Score Interpretation**		
Patient is rubbing joints or muscles and is unable to sit still because of discomfort	+4	• <5: no active withdrawal • 5–12: mild withdrawal • 13–24: moderate withdrawal • 25–36: moderately severe withdrawal • >36: severe withdrawal		
Runny Nose or Tearing				
Not accounted for by cold symptoms or allergies				
Not present	0			

GI, Gastrointestinal.

Sources: Tompkins, D. A., Bigelow, G. E., Harrison, J. A., et al. (2009). Concurrent validation of the Clinical Opiate Withdrawal Scale (COWS) and single-item indices against the Clinical Institute Narcotic Assessment (CINA) opioid withdrawal instrument. *Drug and Alcohol Dependence, 105*(1), 154–159; Wesson, D. R., & Ling, W. (2003). The Clinical Opiate Withdrawal Scale (COWS). *Journal of Psychoactive Drugs, 35*(2), 253–259.

irregular pulse, or has a history of heart trouble, the person should immediately be taken to an emergency department.

Cocaine and crack. Cocaine is a naturally occurring stimulant extracted from the leaf of the coca bush, whereas crack is an alkalinized form of coca administered via inhalation. When smoked, crack alters the CNS in as little as 6 to 10 seconds, producing a short sense of euphoria, followed by a crash, and then a period of deep depression as the body works to return to homeostasis that reinforces the drug-using behaviour.

Cocaine works by blocking the reuptake of norepinephrine, dopamine, and serotonin, causing an imbalance of neurotransmitters that, when the drug is metabolized, results in physical withdrawal symptoms including depression, lethargy, anxiety, insomnia, sweating and chills, and a renewed craving for the drug (Cunningham et al., 2020). There are three distinct phases of withdrawal from cocaine:

1. The first phase, the *crash phase*, can last up to 4 days. Those who use cocaine report depression, anergia, and an acute onset of agitated depression. Craving for the drug peaks during this phase, as do anxiety and paranoia. Inpatient care to prevent access to further doses of the drug is helpful during the first and second phases of withdrawal.
2. During the second phase, the user feels a prolonged sense of dysphoria and anhedonia, a lack of motivation, and intense cravings

TABLE 18.9 Central Nervous System Stimulants: Intoxication, Overdose, and Withdrawal

Drugs	Effects of Intoxication	Effects of Overdose	Possible Treatments for Overdose	Effects of Withdrawal	Possible Treatments for Withdrawal
Cocaine, crack (short-acting) High obtained by (method) in (time frame): snorted, 2–3 minutes; injected, 15–30 seconds; smoked (for crack), 4–10 seconds Average high lasts 15–30 minutes for cocaine; 5–7 minutes for crack	Physical: Tachycardia Dilated pupils Elevated blood pressure Nausea and vomiting Insomnia Psychological–perceptual: Agitation and aggression Grandiosity Impaired judgement Impaired social and occupational functioning Euphoria	Respiratory distress Ataxia Hyperpyrexia Convulsions Coma Stroke Myocardial infarction Death	Antipsychotics, medical and nursing management for: Fever (ambient cooling) Convulsions (diazepam) Respiratory distress or cardiovascular shock (resuscitation and medical treatment to control hypertension, tachycardia, and respirations) Acidification of urine (ammonium chloride for amphetamine)	Fatigue Depression Agitation Apathy Anxiety Sleepiness Disorientation Lethargy Craving	Supportive measures Diazepam (Valium) or lorazepam (Ativan) may be prescribed for mild to moderate withdrawal symptoms
Amphetamines (long-acting) Dextroamphetamine Methamphetamine/crystal meth	Increased energy Severe effects: State resembling paranoid schizophrenia Paranoia with delusions Psychosis Visual, auditory, and tactile hallucinations Severe to panic levels of anxiety Potential for violence Note: Paranoia and ideas of reference may persist for months afterward	Same as above	Same as above	Same as above	Same as above

Source: Sofuoglu, M., Poling, J., Gonzalez, G., et al. (2006). Cocaine withdrawal symptoms predict medication response in cocaine users. *American Journal of Drug and Alcohol Abuse, 32*, 617–628. https://doi.org/10.1080/00952990600920680

for the drug. This phase can last up to 10 weeks. Lapse and relapse is most likely during the second phase of withdrawal.
3. The third phase is characterized by intermittent craving and can last indefinitely.

Amphetamines and methamphetamine. Amphetamines are chemically related to the naturally occurring catecholamine neurotransmitter and work by increasing synaptic levels of dopamine, serotonin (5-HT), and norepinephrine. They are used to raise energy levels and reduce both appetite and the need for sleep, as well as to provide feelings of clear-headedness and power. Norepinephrine is responsible for methamphetamine's alerting, anorectic, locomotor, and sympathomimetic effects; dopamine also stimulates locomotor effects but, in excess, can produce psychosis and perception disturbances; and changes to serotonin (5-HT) are responsible for the delusions and psychosis associated with the use of amphetamines. Methamphetamine's effects are similar to those of cocaine, but its onset is slower and the duration is longer (Table 18.10).

Bath salts (methylenedioxypyrovalerone and mephedrone). Pharmacologically, bath salts are most closely related to khat, a plant that grows and is used widely in the Horn of Africa region. Its psychoactive property is derived from the same source, cathinone, though the synthetic version is much more potent. Although cathinone was synthesized by pharmaceutical companies in the late twentieth century, its derivatives did not become broadly used within the drug trade until the beginning of the twenty-first century. It also shares some pharmacological similarity with MDMA (ecstasy) but with less hallucinogenic and more stimulant properties closer to the effects of methamphetamine. In a study of the rewarding and reinforcing effects of methylenedioxypyrovalerone (MDPV) rats showed self-administration patterns and escalation of drug intake nearly identical to those seen with methamphetamine (Colon-Perez et al., 2016).

This drug can be administered orally, across mucous membranes, or via inhalation or injection. The energizing and often agitating effects occur because of increased levels of dopamine, which also increase a user's heart rate and blood pressure. The surge in dopamine creates feelings of euphoria, increased physical activity, heightened sexual interest, a lack of hunger and thirst, muscle spasms, sleeplessness, and, when sleep does occur, disrupted dream cycles. Behavioural effects include erratic behaviour, teeth grinding, a lack of recall of how much of the substance has been consumed, panic attacks, anxiety, agitation, severe paranoia, hallucinations, psychosis, self-harm, and behaviour that can be aggressive, violent, and in extreme cases move beyond suicidal ideation to suicidal actions. Overdose is possible due to heart and blood vessel problems because of a lack of any type of regulation

TABLE 18.10 Cocaine–Methamphetamine Comparison

Action	Cocaine	Methamphetamine
Length of action		
20–30 minutes	X	
4–6 hours		X
Produces self-esteem	X	X
Increases alertness	X	X
Postpones sleep	X	X
Decreases appetite	X	X
Increases blood pressure	X	X
Produces seizures	X	X
Local anaesthetic	X	
Increases body temperature	X	X
Cardiac arrhythmias	X	X
Elicit paranoid psychosis	X	X
Depression during withdrawal	X	X
High dependency liability	X	X

Source: Csiernik, R. (2019). *The essential guide to psychoactive drugs in Canada*. Toronto: Canadian Scholars Press.

of this drug, leading to inconsistency of the psychoactive ingredient between brands. In 2012 the Government of Canada made it illegal to possess, traffic, import, or export MDPV unless authorized by regulation (Colon-Perez et al., 2016; Government of Canada, Department of Justice, 2019).

Caffeine. Caffeine is the most used psychoactive drug not only in Canada but across the world. It is found in coffee, tea, energy drinks, and soft drinks. Caffeine blocks the actions of adenosine, an inhibitory neurotransmitter, by binding to its receptor and preventing post-binding changes from taking place, which leads to increased firing of dopaminergic neurons, particularly in the nucleus accumbens. Due to its ability to constrict cerebral blood vessels, caffeine is used in combination with other drugs to combat migraine and other cerebrovascular headaches associated with high blood pressure. However, contrary to popular belief, caffeine is not effective in ameliorating headaches due to other causes, and in some instances it may even exacerbate pain. In other medical uses caffeine is employed to counteract certain symptoms, such as respiratory depression, associated with CNS depressant poisoning. It is also used:

- As a respiratory stimulant in babies who have had apnea episodes (periods when spontaneous breathing ceases)
- As an emergency bronchodilator in asthmatic children
- As a substitute for methylphenidate for children with attention-deficit/hyperactivity disorder
- As an antifungal agent in the treatment of skin disorders
- As an aid in fertility, because of its ability to enhance sperm mobility
- As a mild stimulant for an assortment of medical problems (Csiernik, 2019)

When taken in moderate amounts, caffeine can produce stimulant effects on the CNS similar to those of small doses of amphetamines. These can include mild mood elevation; feelings of enhanced energy; an increased alertness and reduced performance deficit due to boredom or fatigue; postponement of feelings of fatigue and the need for sleep; and a decrease in hand steadiness, suggesting impaired fine motor performance. Small doses of caffeine can also increase motor activity, alter sleep patterns (including delaying the onset of sleep), diminish sleep time, and reduce the depth of sleep (including altering rapid eye movement sleep patterns) while also increasing respiration, blood pressure, and metabolism. However, with the increasing use of dietary supplements, caffeine pills, and energy drinks containing far more caffeine than coffee, tea, or cola, there has been an increase in hospitalizations involving the drug and in overdoses leading to death (Eichner, 2014; Fagerstrom, 2018; Parsh, 2019).

Nicotine. Nicotine, in combination with its agent of delivery, tobacco, is the leading cause of premature death from any psychoactive agent in Canada and in the world. Nicotine has a pale-yellow colour and an oily consistency. It turns brown on contact with air, and doses of 60 mg can be fatal, while amounts as low as 4 mg can produce severe illness. Tobacco smoke comprises some 500 compounds, including tar, ammonia, acetaldehyde, acetone, benzene, toluene, benzo(a)pyrene, dimethylnitrosamine, methylethylnitrosamine, naphthalene, carbon monoxide, and carbon dioxide.

This drug is thought to affect the brain reward system by increasing dopamine concentrations through interaction with nicotine acetylcholine receptors. Since nicotine is a CNS stimulant, it increases heart rate, pulse rate, and blood pressure; depresses the spinal reflex; reduces muscle tone; decreases skin temperature; increases acid in the stomach; reduces urine formation; precipitates a loss of appetite; increases adrenaline production; and stimulates, then reduces, brain and nervous system activity. In non-smokers small doses, even less than one cigarette, may produce an unpleasant reaction that includes coughing, nausea, vomiting, dizziness, abdominal discomfort, weakness, and flushing (Csiernik, 2019).

Nicotine crosses the placenta, and women who smoke during pregnancy tend to have babies smaller in body weight, height, and head circumference and are more likely to give birth prematurely. Cigarette smoking during pregnancy also increases the risk of sudden infant death syndrome, whereas exposure to second-hand smoke during pregnancy increases the risk of infant stillbirth, congenital malformations, low birth weight, and respiratory illnesses. Newborns exposed *in utero* to nicotine are more irritable and have poorer attention than unexposed infants, and they exhibit increased muscle tension, increased tremors and startle responses, and deficient speech processing (Lee et al., 2018; Reece et al., 2018).

Cannabis. *Cannabis sativa* is a member of the hemp family of plants, with one major distinction: it contains delta-9-tetrahydrocannabinol (THC). This is the psychoactive ingredient found in the resin secreted from the flowering tops and leaves of the female cannabis plant. While this substance has historically been classified as part of the hallucinogen family of drugs, THC also produces depressant effects and is the only hallucinogen that produces physical dependency; thus it is a fully addicting agent. Cannabis is generally smoked, but it also can be ingested orally, typically in baked goods or other sweets such as chocolates or jelly candies. Desired effects include euphoria, detachment, and relaxation. Other effects include talkativeness, slowed perception of time, inappropriate hilarity, heightened sensitivity to external stimuli, and anxiety or paranoia. Long-term use of cannabis can result in lethargy, anhedonia, difficulty concentrating, amotivational syndrome, and memory impairment.

Medical cannabis is used in response to a broad range of issues, including fighting antibiotic-resistant infections, as an antiemetic, controlling chemotherapy-induced nausea, reduction of intraocular pressure in glaucoma, appetite stimulation in acquired immunodeficiency syndrome (AIDS) wasting syndrome, muscle spasms associated with spinal cord injury, and multiple sclerosis, and to decrease seizures caused by some forms of epilepsy. Cannabis can also help alleviate gastrointestinal

> ### RESEARCH HIGHLIGHT
> **Smoking Cessation Support via Mobile Texting**
>
> **Problem**
> Most of those killed prematurely due to tobacco use started smoking as teenagers, with smoking tobacco contributing to the death of one of every two of those who smoke past 35 years of age. Stopping smoking at an early age conveys greater health benefits.
>
> **Purpose of Study**
> For many people, mobile phone use has become a core component of their daily routine, allowing for text intervention to occur any place and at any time. The purpose of this study was to assess the effectiveness of a mobile phone–based smoking intervention.
>
> **Methods**
> Participants were recruited through various media, including websites, primary care facilities, and pharmacies. Inclusion criteria were that participants were age 16 or older, had a mobile phone, and were willing to attempt to stop smoking. In the next month 5800 participants were randomized into two groups based on age, sex, education, and nicotine dependency score. Individuals in the treatment group received motivational and behavioural text messages, whereas the control group received text messages related only to the importance of participation in the trial. At 6 months post-trial, salivary tests were used to confirm self-reported abstinence.
>
> **Key Findings**
> Text messages via mobile phones doubled smoking cessation rates in the treatment group, but these cessation rates were similar to those seen with other behavioural interventions, such as group, one-to-one, or telephone advice programs. Mobile phones simply provided a new channel for individualized programs to be delivered inexpensively and wherever the person is located.
>
> **Implications for Nursing Practice**
> The findings suggest that the use of mobile text messages should be considered as part of an adjunct to existing cessation programs, and particularly during times such as the global COVID-19 pandemic where face-to-face counselling and gatherings are restricted. The researchers also suggested that using mobile technology may be effective in changing other behavioural risk factors.
>
> **Source:** Free, C., Knight, R., Robertson, S., et al. (2011). Smoking cessation support delivered via mobile phone text messaging (txt2stop): A single-blind, randomised trial. *The Lancet, 378,* 49–55. https://doi.org/10.1016/S0140-6736(11)60701-0

disorders, symptoms of Tourette's syndrome, depression, anxiety, and post-traumatic stress disorder; can decrease chronic pain and the pain from fibromyalgia; and can aid insomnia (Csiernik, 2019). Canada was among the first nations to prohibit the use of cannabis and now has become one of the first to legalize its use. Bill C-45, The *Cannabis Act*, along with its companion legislation Bill C-46, *An Act to Amend the Criminal Code*, was passed by the House of Commons of Canada in late November 2017 with Royal Assent on June 21, 2018. The *Cannabis Act* created a formal legal framework for controlling the production, distribution, sale and possession of cannabis with three stated goals:

- to keep cannabis out of the hands of youth
- to eliminate the illegal market of cannabis sales
- to protect public health and safety by allowing adults access to legal cannabis with known and stated THC levels

Each individual of legal age is allowed to possess up to 30 g of dried cannabis or equivalent in non-dried form in public, to share up to 30 g of legal cannabis with other adults, and to buy dried or fresh cannabis and cannabis oil from a provincially licensed retailer. Individuals are also allowed to grow up to four cannabis plants per residence for personal use and to make their own homemade products using dried cannabis. While cannabis is now a legal product in Canada, there remains a range of penalties for cannabis offences ranging from warnings and fines for minor offences such as possession of small amounts over the limit, to a maximum sentence of 14 years for illegal cultivation and distribution and selling cannabis to a minor. As with alcohol, there are also specific penalties for cannabis-impaired driving. There are two prohibited levels for THC and it is a less serious offence to have between 2 and 5 ng of THC per mL of blood, while it is a more serious offence to have 5 ng of THC or more per mL of blood. The prohibited levels of alcohol and cannabis, when found in combination, is 50 mg or more of alcohol per 100 mL blood with 2.5 ng or more of THC per mL of blood. Having any detectable amount of LSD, psilocybin, ketamine, phencyclidine (PCP), cocaine, methamphetamine or 6-mam (a metabolite of heroin) in your system within 2 hours of driving is also prohibited (Government of Canada, Department of Justice, 2019).

Hallucinogens. Hallucinogens are distinct psychoactive agents in that they do not primarily produce euphoria but rather disrupt the CNS and PNS, producing a disconnect between the physical world and the user's perception of the physical world. Effects can include distortion in space and time, hallucinations, delusions, both paranoid and grandiose, and synesthesia, which is a blurring and intermingling of the senses, such as smelling a colour or tasting a feeling. Table 18.11 outlines the signs and symptoms of hallucinogen intoxication and overdose.

Hallucinogens, excluding cannabis, are divided into three groups. Indolealkylamines, such as LSD and psilocybin, have no secondary psychoactive effects. Phenylethylamines, such as mescaline and jimson weed, have structural similarities to amphetamines, producing secondary stimulant effects on the body. Dissociative anaesthetics, psychoactive drugs such as PCP and ketamine that are members of the arylcyclohexylamine family, possess depressant properties along with their hallucinatory effects.

A hallucinogen that has received extensive public attention is MDMA (3,4-methylenedioxymethamphetamine), referred to as ecstasy, molly, Adam, yaba, and XTC. Related hallucinogens with stimulant properties include MDA (methylenedioxyamphetamine), the "love drug," and MDE (3,4-methylenedioxyethamphetamine), whose slang name is "Eve." MDMA causes a significant release of the neurotransmitters serotonin, dopamine, and norepinephrine. The brain's saturation with these neurotransmitters causes those who use MDMA to exhibit major empathy toward others; reduces inhibitions; elicits introspection; and results in an outpouring of good feelings about others, the current environment, and the world. The release of serotonin also intensely sharpens the senses of those using the substance.

Those using MDMA may be hyperactive and have inexhaustible energy (dancing all night long), dilated pupils with impaired reaction to light, elevated temperature, elevated pulse, elevated blood pressure, diaphoresis, dystonia, and bruxism (grinding of the teeth). Other symptoms of stimulant use, such as tachycardia, mydriasis (dilation of the pupils), tremors, arrhythmias, parkinsonism, esophoria (eyes turning inward), serotonin syndrome, and severe hyponatremia, may also present with MDMA use. Those using MDMA must drink a large quantity of water during use to prevent dehydration and hyperthermia, which have contributed to occasional deaths. After the effects of MDMA wear off, the person using the substance commonly goes through a period of depression, referred to as "suicide Tuesdays." This affective state is

TABLE 18.11 Hallucinogens: Intoxication, Overdose, and Withdrawal

Drugs	Physical Effects of Intoxication	Psychological–Perceptual Effects of Intoxication	Effects of Overdose	Possible Treatments for Overdose
Lysergic acid diethylamide (LSD) Psilocybin (mushrooms) Mescaline (peyote)	Pupil dilation Tachycardia Diaphoresis Palpitations Tremors Incoordination Elevated temperature, pulse, respiration	Fear of going crazy Paranoid ideas Marked anxiety, depression Synesthesia (e.g., colours are heard, sounds are seen) Depersonalization Hallucinations, although sensorium is clear Grandiosity (e.g., thinking one can fly)	Psychosis Brain damage Death	Keep patient in room with low stimuli—minimal light, sound, activity. Have one person stay with patient. Provide reassurance. Speak slowly and clearly in quiet voice. Diazepam or chloral hydrate may be prescribed for extreme anxiety or tension.
Phencyclidine piperidine (PCP) Ketamine	Vertical or horizontal nystagmus Increased blood pressure, pulse, and temperature Ataxia Muscle rigidity Seizures Blank stare Chronic jerking Agitated, repetitive movements Belligerence, assaultiveness, impulsiveness Impaired judgement, impaired social and occupational functioning	*Severe effects*: Hallucinations, paranoia Bizarre behaviour (e.g., barking like a dog, grimacing, repetitive chanting speech) Regressive behaviour Violent bizarre behaviours Very labile behaviours	Psychosis Possible hypertensive crisis or cardiovascular accident Respiratory arrest Hyperthermia Seizures	*If alert:* Put in room with minimal stimuli. Do not attempt to talk down! Speak slowly, clearly, and in a quiet voice. *Monitor and be prepared to intervene for:* Hyperthermia High blood pressure Respiratory distress Hypertension

Source: Meehan, Y. J., Bryant, S. M., & Aks, S. E. (2010). Drugs of abuse: The highs and lows of altered mental states in the emergency department. *Emergency Medicine Clinics of North America, 28*, 663–682. https://doi.org/10.1016/j.emc.2010.03.012

caused by a depletion of serotonin, levels of which do not return to normal within the CNS for at least 3 to 4 days.

Two distinct pharmacological processes are most closely associated with this family of drugs. The first process is tachyphylaxis, the rapid reduction in the effect produced by the substance, regardless of how much of the drug is consumed. Essentially, this is total tolerance that occurs in a short period of time, such that there is no physical withdrawal to the drug. If a drug is taken for a consecutive number of days, after 3 or 4 days, no psychoactive effects of any type are perceived. The secondary effects of hallucinogens such as MDMA or ketamine can still be perceived even when the primary hallucinogenic effect is not. The second process is a flashback, or hallucinogen persisting perceptual disorder (HPPD). These are transitory recurrences of perceptual disturbance that can be caused by a person's earlier hallucinogenic drug use but occur after the fact, when the person is in a drug-free state. Flashbacks can be experienced as pleasant but most often entail recurrences of frightening images, visual distortions, time expansion, loss of ego boundaries, and intense emotions. However, HPPD is typically discussed more than it is actually experienced (Csiernik, 2019).

Helping Patients Change

Self-Assessment and Self-Awareness

To offer support and motivation toward recovery, a nurse must begin by examining their own attitudes, feelings, and beliefs about addiction and persons with addiction issues. Such reflection often means that nurses must examine their own substance use and the substance use of others in their lives, particularly their partners and family members, which is a potentially difficult task. A history of substance use in a nurse's own family can interfere with the helping relationship and contribute to counter-transference (see Chapter 9). The negative or positive experiences a nurse has had with family members or others with addiction issues can influence interpersonal interactions with patients and affect treatment outcomes. Therefore attending to personal feelings that arise when working with people experiencing addiction issues is vital, as are ongoing self-reflection and supervision that encourages reflection on the nurse's responses as well as the patients'. Nurses who do not attend to, and work through, expected negative feelings that arise while providing care are more likely to engage in power struggles with patients, resulting in an ineffective therapeutic process, and are more likely to suffer from vicarious trauma (Wheeler & Phillips, 2019).

Psychological Changes

Distinct psychological characteristics are associated with substance use, often arising from trauma or oppression, including hopelessness, low self-esteem, anxiety, and depression.

People who use substances often feel threatened on many levels in their interactions with nurses in formal hospital and treatment settings. First, they are concerned about being rejected because not all nurses are willing to care for people with addiction issues. In fact, many patients have reported experiences of rejection in past encounters with nursing personnel (Lewis & Jarvis, 2019; Menard-Kocik & Caine, 2019). Second, people who use substances may be anxious about giving up the substance they believe they need to survive; this relates to psychological dependency. Third, people with addiction issues often are concerned about failing at recovery, as addiction is a chronic, relapsing condition. In fact, relapse is one of the criteria for diagnosing an addiction. Most individuals with an addiction have tried to become abstinent at least once and often several times before experiencing relapse. As a result, many become discouraged about their chances of ever succeeding. Such feelings of discouragement and a high level of hopelessness can act as substantive barriers to recovery and contribute to the risk of suicide.

Concerns about failure or potential relapse on the path of recovery can threaten the person's sense of security and sense of self, increasing anxiety levels. To protect against these feelings, the person with an addiction may establish self-defensive responses, including defence mechanisms (refer to Chapter 4) such as projection or rationalization, or thought processes such as all-or-none thinking, selective attention, or conflict minimization and avoidance. Typically, the person is unable to give up these maladaptive coping styles until more positive and functional skills are learned.

The Transtheoretical Model of Change

Prochaska and DiClemente (1984) revolutionized thinking regarding addiction treatment with their integrative model of intentional change based on their work with tobacco smokers who stopped without any formal or self-help assistance. They took the idea of motivation and made it into an active counselling skill. Rather than being located exclusively within the patient, they expressed the idea that motivation was an interpersonal, interactional process within which the probability existed for behaviours to lead to positive outcomes. Prochaska and DiClemente identified six specific steps necessary for any type of radical change to occur, which represented a natural process of change that could be adapted by nurses to assist any patient in moving forward (Figure 18.4).

Pre-contemplation. In the first stage of the model it is recognized that an individual will be resistant to change and typically has no intention of altering behaviour in the near future; there is typically no or little recognition from the patient's perspective that any type of problem exists. This idea has historically been called denial. Critical to the entire premise of the Transtheoretical Model of Change (TTM) is the replacement of the long-standing idea that patients are in denial regarding their addiction with the concept of pre-contemplation.

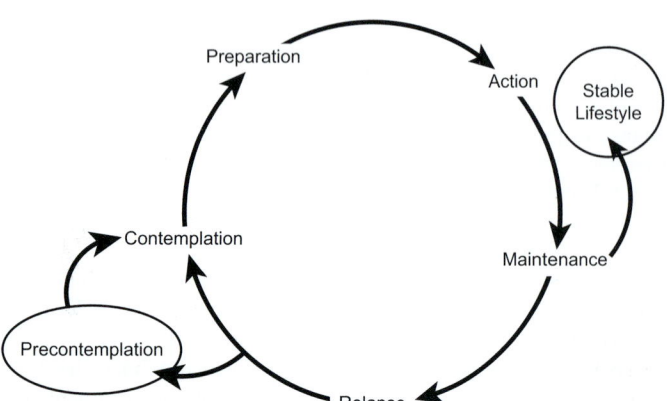

Fig. 18.4 Transtheoretical Model of Change. (**Source:** Association of Faculties of Medicine of Canada. (2016). *Primer on population health*. Retrieved from http://phprimer.afmc.ca/en/)

Prochaska and DiClemente (1984) reconceptualized the idea of denial to frame it so that patients are not viewed as willfully deceiving themselves and others and in the process destroying themselves or their families; instead, these individuals are considered to be truly unaware of the impact of their behaviour and the effect it has on those around them. People with substance use disorders are often ambivalent about changing their harmful behaviour regarding alcohol or other drug use. They may continue their drug use for a range of reasons, such as being attracted to a particular lifestyle, wanting to be included in a peer group, coping with life's daily stresses, or responding to trauma and oppression in their lives. When the destructive effect of these behaviours becomes obvious, they are then faced with the reality of giving up most of the people, places, and things they have come to enjoy and with which they may strongly identify. Without a clear picture of the future, these individuals are typically reluctant to engage in any type of change process. Thus considerable effort is required by the individual with a substance use disorder, their family members, friends, and helping professionals to become willing to make a commitment to change. Approaches to supporting the patient at this stage include:

- Validating the lack of readiness
- Encouraging re-evaluation of current behaviour
- Encouraging self-exploration rather than immediate action
- Explaining and personalizing the risk

Contemplation. In the second stage, contemplation, patients become aware that they are stuck in a situation and must decide whether they wish to change or remain where they are at. Nurses support patients in gaining an understanding of the consequences of their drug use but do not force the patient to make a commitment to change. The nurse helps to balance in the patient's mind the delicate equilibrium between the desire to change and the fear of changing and the associated unknown consequences. Nurses need to reflect this ambivalence to help patients be able to move forward to the next stage while recognizing and acknowledging the fear associated with change. Nurses also need to be open to the fact that some patients will drop out at this highly stressful stage, and thus a willingness to work with the patient in the future must be presented, again, once the person is ready and able to move forward. Supportive approaches include:

- Encouraging evaluation of the pros and cons of behaviour change
- Re-evaluating group image through group activities
- Identifying and promoting new, positive-outcome expectations

Preparation. The third stage, preparation, also known as the determination stage, involves some commitment from the patient that changing the drug-using behaviour is being considered along with the anticipation of what this future action may look like and what actions need to occur. However, the nurse needs to be aware that a significant level of ambivalence may still exist to the idea and process of actual change. During the preparation phase, probing, reviewing consequences, and self-evaluation are areas of work to perform with the patient, and a specific time frame is established for when the patient agrees to begin changing existing practices and actions, with a maximum target of 1 month. Supportive approaches at this phase include:

- Encouraging the evaluation of the pros and cons of behaviour change
- Identifying and promoting new positive-outcome expectations
- Encouraging realistic, practical, and small initial steps
- Offering referrals to and support of action-oriented programs such as smoking cessation

Action. The fourth stage is when the work and behavioural change begin, with a heavy emphasis on problem solving and problem-solving skills. However, action also entails changing awareness, emotions, self-image, and thinking. Support of positive decisions and positive reinforcement dominate this stage of moving forward by the patient. Emphasis is on the positive: what patients are doing rather than what they are not (i.e., not using drugs). Supportive approaches include:

- Helping the patient with restructuring cues and triggers and solidifying social support
- Enhancing self-efficacy for dealing with obstacles
- Helping to guard against feelings of loss and frustration, especially if a lapse occurs

Maintenance/adaption. The fifth stage, maintenance/adaption, focuses on supporting and consolidating the gains made during the action stage and on avoiding lapses or a more significant relapse. Social skills training underscores this stage of continued change. This is the skills practice phase of the TTM during which patients are less tempted to lapse and become increasingly confident that they can continue their changed behaviour. Approaches to use include:

- Planning for follow-up support
- Reinforcing internal rewards
- Discussing strategies for coping with triggers and relapse
- Generalizing positive behaviours into more situations

Evaluation/termination. The final stage of the TTM has the patient move past problem solving with a focus on relapse prevention and dealing with the reality of abstinence and sobriety. During this phase, patients assess their strengths and areas that may be problematic in the future as they develop a relapse prevention plan that can be undertaken on their own and begin once a lapse occurs. Supportive approaches that are particularly helpful to assist the patient and family include:

- Evaluating triggers for relapse
- Reassessing motivation and barriers to change
- Planning and rehearsing new and stronger coping strategies

Motivational Interviewing

Closely associated with the TTM, and integral to its success, is the idea of motivational interviewing (MI), initially conceptualized by William Miller (1983). MI is a brief, patient-centred, directive method for enhancing change in intrinsic motivation by exploring and resolving patient ambivalence using the ideas of empathy, attribution, cognitive dissonance, and self-efficacy. In MI motivation is conceptualized not as a personality trait but as an interpersonal process. The model de-emphasizes labelling, replacing confrontation with empathy, and places a much greater emphasis on individual responsibility and internal attribution for change. It has become a foundation practice approach in community-based addiction counselling approaches across Canada.

Cognitive dissonance is a core technique in the MI approach. It is created by contrasting the ongoing problem behaviour of a patient with salient awareness of the behaviour's negative consequences. Empathic processes, motivation, and objective assessment feedback are used to channel this dissonance toward a behaviour change, being cognizant of and avoiding the typical patient barriers of low self-esteem, low self-efficacy, and pre-contemplation. MI is a strength-based counselling style in which the nurse works with the patient rather than doing things for or to the patient. The focus is to look for natural motivating issues within a patient's life or the patient's system. The nurse needs to anticipate and respond to a patient's genuine hesitation and insecurity to engage in a fundamentally life-altering change in behaviour because simply giving patients advice to change is typically unrewarding and ineffective. MI is non-confrontational in nature and acknowledges the fact that creating conflict, rather than ambivalence, in the therapeutic relationship is counterproductive and is more likely to create patient resistance than patient change. MI seeks to increase a patient's awareness of their problematic behaviour along with unrecognized strengths and opportunities for change. Miller and Rollnick (2002) established eight steps for the MI process: establishing rapport, setting the agenda, assessing readiness to change, sharpening focus, identifying ambivalence, eliciting self-motivating statements, handling resistance, and shifting focus and transition (Box 18.3).

Communication Techniques for Assessment and Interventions

Accurate assessment and effective intervention planning and implementation for colleagues and patients depends on the development of a therapeutic relationship (see Chapter 9) and effective communication (see Chapter 10), which can be enhanced by incorporating MI and the TTM in a nurse's practice. The nurse's ability to develop a therapeutic relationship with a patient with addiction issues can help the patient feel safe enough to start looking at problems with some degree of openness and honesty. The following is a portion of an intake interview with a patient upon admission to a treatment program.

Dialogue	Therapeutic Tool or Comment
Nurse: "Elyse, I get the impression that life must have been very difficult for you lately." **Elyse:** (long pause) "I don't think you would understand."	Validating and empathizing
Nurse: "I guess sometimes it feels as if no one understands, but I would like to try." **Elyse:** "At times I feel I can't go on anymore … so many losses."	Reflecting and empathizing
Nurse: "Loss is difficult. Elyse, take a moment, take a breath, and then tell me about your losses." **Elyse:** "My brother's sudden death … We were so close. … I depended on him so much."	Encouraging the patient to share her painful feelings
Nurse: "It must have been difficult for you to lose him so suddenly." **Elyse:** (long pause) "No one knows …. Then Joseph, he left …." (Elyse starts to cry)	Empathizing
Nurse: (sitting in silence as Elyse cries, then asking for more information about the feelings expressed) "Tell me about this experience." **Elyse:** "I don't know …. I just wonder, why does everyone leave me? Oh, I hate them all …. I wish I had a Valium now."	Encouraging the expression of feelings while feelings are close to the surface. The use of silence is often difficult but is a key therapeutic tool
Nurse: "And what does the Valium do to help you?"	Beginning to explore the drug dependence in a gentle, non-threatening manner

The following example demonstrates the use of therapeutic leverage, making abstinence and sobriety worthwhile for those abusing the substance. It is presented as a dialogue between a nurse and a 17-year-old man whose parents are divorced and whose father emotionally abuses him when drinking. He was picked up three times during the preceding 7 months for possession of crystal.

BOX 18.3 The Motivational Interviewing (MI) Process

1. **Establish rapport.** Chapters 9 and 10 discuss establishing rapport with patients, but in the case of MI, rapport may be fostered by simply asking permission to discuss the patient's behaviour or concern. For example:
"Do you mind if we spend a few minutes talking about …?"
"How do you feel about the behaviour (or desired behaviour change)?"
2. **Set the agenda.** Working with the patient to create an agenda helps the nurse and patient to clarify the immediate concerns of interest for the patient and sets the boundaries of the helping relationship. For example:
"What do you know about …?"
"Are you interested in learning more about …?"
"Are you able to come back to the clinic to discuss your plans further?"
3. **Assess readiness to change.** Motivation is not static and can change rapidly from day to day. Patients enter treatment at different levels of motivation or readiness to change, and many are ambivalent about changing, as there are often aspects about the addiction that the patient is still benefiting from in some way. Assessing the patient's readiness to change prepares the nurse to tailor treatment to that stage. Such assessment can be made using a Readiness to Change Ruler, much like a pain scale. This scaling strategy conceptualizes readiness or motivation to change along a continuum and asks patients to use a ruler with a 10-point scale, where 1 equals "definitely not ready to change" and 10 equals "definitely ready to change."
4. **Sharpen the focus.** The nurse can work with the patient to draw a table of costs and benefits of substance use or addiction and also to identify specific facilitators of and barriers to change. For example:
"Over the past 2 months, you have been talking about stopping using crack, and it seems that just recently you have started to recognize that the fewer good things about using are outweighing the bad things. What is changing for you now that has you leaning toward stopping?"
5. **Identify ambivalence.** While identifying motivators is important, it is also important to address the fluctuation in motivation common in any behaviour change. Uncovering ambivalence and paradox can be achieved through statements that point out the contradictions in the patient's motivations for change. For example:
"You have been continuing to engage in drinking binges, and yet you say that you want to get your driver's licence back and regain the trust of your parents."
6. **Elicit self-motivating statements.** This approach encourages the patient to state their own cognitive recognition of the problem, affective expression of concern, a direct intention toward change, and a sense of optimism. A *cognitive recognition of the problem* may be heard in a statement such as "I guess this is more serious than I thought." While a patient may have heard others express concern many times, self-recognition is a more powerful drive for change. An *affective expression of concern* about the perceived problem, such as, "I'm really worried about what is happening to me," anchors the significance of the problem in the patient's own words. A *direct intention to change behaviour*—for example, "I've got to do something about this"—sets out a goal. Last, an expression of *optimism* about one's ability to change reinforces a sense of hope. A nurse may be able to elicit a statement of optimism by asking a patient what they can achieve in treatment. A patient may respond with "I know that if I try, I can really do it" or "I have maintained my sobriety for a long period of time before and know it is possible." The nurse can repeat these statements or have the patient write these statements down for future reference.
7. **Handle resistance.** There is a risk involved in recognizing the patient's resistance to change and inviting the patient to argue their case, but the nurse, nevertheless, should address resistance head-on and be ready to roll with the counterarguments. The patient may not be able to argue for ongoing change and motivation and may instead retreat to a previous phase of change. In that case the nurse must be accepting and work with the patient to handle the resistance and the shifting phase of change. Handling resistance requires the nurse to ask questions about readiness and desire for change. The following questions provide examples of addressing the resistance honestly in the interview and reviewing motivation:
"I know you have been coming to treatment for 2 months, but you are still drinking heavily. Maybe now is not the right time to change?"
"So it sounds as though you have a lot going on with trying to balance a career and family, and these priorities are competing with your treatment at this time."
8. **Shift focus and transition.** Through all phases of change, there will be times to illuminate a shift in focus or transition to a new phase of motivation. Making a declaration about such shifts allows the patient to hear your evaluation and to argue for whatever change is developing. One example of shifting focus for motivation is provided by the following long-term outpatient treatment scenario:
"Your goal to be able to regain visitation of your son, coupled with your girlfriend leaving you because you continued to use crack, makes it easy to understand why you are now committed to not using crack anymore."

Source: Adapted from Sobell, L. C., & Sobell, M. B. (2008). *Motivational interviewing strategies and techniques: Rationales and examples.* Retrieved from http://www.nova.edu/gsc/forms/mi_rationale_techniques.pdf

Dialogue	Therapeutic Tool or Comment
Nurse: "I understand you entered the treatment program yesterday afternoon following your court appearance."	Placing the event in time and sequence; validating the precipitating event
Kang: "Yeah—it was my dad's idea."	
Nurse: "Well, what do you think of the idea?"	Encouraging evaluation (actions first; thoughts; then feelings)
Kang: "I don't like it. I don't need this place. I'm not a junkie—I just use a little crystal when I'm with my friends … that's the only time. I can handle it."	
Nurse: "From what I've heard, your involvement with crystal has gotten you into trouble with the police and courts."	Pointing out realities
Kang: "Yeah, it has … but I still don't think I need this place."	
Nurse: "Are you saying that you don't think you need a treatment program?"	Validating the patient's perception
Kang: "Well, I don't know. I don't think so but things have gotten a little messed up."	
Nurse: "Messed up."	Restating
Kang: "Yeah."	
Nurse: "What is one thing that makes you feel messed up?"	Encouraging the patient to be specific rather than global while also focusing on affect
Kang: (silence) "I guess I feel like I don't belong anywhere."	
Nurse: "Tell me more about what that feels like."	Clarifying

Diagnosis

Formulation of appropriate nursing diagnoses depends on accurate assessment and screening. Whereas the criteria for medical diagnosis emphasize patterns of use and physical symptoms, nursing diagnoses identify how dependence on substances interferes with a person's ability to deal with the activities and demands of daily living. Nursing diagnoses for patients with psychoactive substance use disorders are many and varied because of the range of physical and psychological effects of drug misuse or dependence on people using these substances, as well as on their families. Concurrent disorders also need to be directly addressed. Potential nursing diagnoses for people with substance use disorders are listed in Table 18.12.

Outcomes Identification

Nursing Outcomes Classification (NOC) categories (Moorhead et al., 2018) for outcome criteria for patients with substance use disorders can be divided into withdrawal, initial and active treatment, and health maintenance. When the patient has a concurrent disorder, the nurse will also develop nursing outcomes for that mental health disorder. Specific *NOC* outcomes and examples of patient goals follow.

Withdrawal

Fluid balance: Patient's blood pressure will not be compromised.
Neurological status: Consciousness: Patient will have no seizure activity.
Distorted thought self-control: Patient will consistently describe the content of hallucinations.

Initial and Active Treatment

Risk control: Substance use: Patient will consistently demonstrate a commitment to substance use control strategies.
Risk control: Substance use: Patient will consistently acknowledge personal consequences associated with substance use.
Substance addiction consequences: Patient will demonstrate no difficulty supporting themselves financially.

Health Maintenance

Knowledge: Substance use control: Patient will describe actions to prevent and manage relapses in substance use.
Family coping: Family will consistently demonstrate care for the needs of all family members.

Planning

Planning care requires attention to the patient's social status, income, ethnic background, faith or religion, sex, sexual orientation, age, substance use history, and current condition. Planning must also address the patient's major psychological, social, and medical problems, as well as the substance-using behaviour. The involvement of appropriate family members is also essential whenever possible.

Unfortunately, a person's social status and social relations often deteriorate as a result of addiction. Job demotion or loss of employment, with resultant reduced or non-existent income, may occur. Meeting basic needs for food, shelter, and clothing is affected. Marriage and other close interpersonal relationships often deteriorate, and the patient is then left alone and isolated. A lack of interpersonal and social supports is a complicating factor in treatment planning for people experiencing addiction. Case Study and Nursing Care Plan 18.2 presents a discussion of a patient with concurrent alcohol dependence and depression.

Implementation

The aim of treatment is self-responsibility and motivation, not adherence to an imposed program. A major challenge is improving

TABLE 18.12 Potential Nursing Diagnoses Related to Psychoactive Substance Use

Signs and Symptoms	Nursing Diagnoses
Vomiting	Imbalanced nutrition: less than body requirements
Diarrhea	
Poor nutritional and fluid intake	Deficient fluid volume
Audiovisual hallucinations	Disturbed thought processes
Impaired judgement	Disturbed sensory perception
Memory deficits	
Cognitive impairments related to substance intoxication or withdrawal (e.g., deficits in problem solving, ability to attend to tasks, and grasp ideas)	
Changes in sleep–wake cycle (e.g., interference with stage 4 sleep, inability to sleep, long periods of sleeping related to effects of or withdrawal from substance)	Disturbed sleep pattern
Lack of self-care (hygiene, grooming, failure to care for basic health needs)	Ineffective health maintenance
	Self-care deficit
	Non-adherence to health care regimen
Feelings of hopelessness, inability to change	Hopelessness
	Spiritual distress
Feelings of worthlessness	Situational low self-esteem
Feeling that life has no meaning or future	Chronic low self-esteem
	Risk for self-directed violence
	Risk for suicide
Family crises and family pain	Interrupted family processes
Ineffective parenting	Impaired parenting
Emotional neglect of others	Risk for other-directed violence
Increased incidence of physical and sexual abuse of others	
Increased self-hate projected to others	
Excessive substance use affecting all areas of a person's life: loss of friends, poor job performance, increased illness rates, proneness to accidents and overdoses	Ineffective coping
	Impaired verbal communication
	Social isolation
	Risk for loneliness
	Anxiety
	Risk for suicide
Increased health problems related to substance used and route of use, as well as overdose	Activity intolerance
	Ineffective airway clearance
	Ineffective breathing pattern
	Impaired oral mucous membrane
	Risk for infection
	Decreased cardiac output
	Sexual dysfunction
Total preoccupation with (and majority of time consumed by) taking and withdrawing from drug	Delayed growth and development
	Ineffective coping
	Impaired social interaction
	Dysfunctional family processes

treatment effectiveness by matching subtypes of patients to specific types of treatment. Although those experiencing substance-related disorders may share some characteristics and dynamics, significant differences exist with regard to physiological, psychological, and sociocultural processes for all individuals. As with most complex issues and illnesses, the best solutions are the ones that can be readily implemented and sustained.

Proposing abstinence as a treatment goal is safest for those with more than one substance use disorder. Abstinence is strongly related to good work adjustment, positive health status, comfortable interpersonal relationships, and general social stability, though it may also often be too great a commitment for many patients with long-term drug use. Often the choice of treatment approach depends on the patient's needs, treatment goals, motivation, and personal circumstances, including family needs and financial resources. Outpatient programs work best for people with substance use disorders who are employed and have an active social support system or those opting for a harm reduction approach. Individuals who have little to no support and structure in their daily lives may do better in inpatient or longer-term residential programs focused exclusively upon abstinence goals.

Beyond personal concerns and choice of treatment, neuropsychological deficits have been associated with long-term alcohol misuse and may affect treatment choices or potential benefits. Such deficits have been found in abstract reasoning ability, ability to use feedback in learning new concepts, attention and concentration spans, cognitive flexibility, and subtle memory functions. These cognitive impairments undoubtedly have an impact on the process of treatment for alcohol or another substance use. At all levels of practice, the nurse can play an important role in the intervention process by recognizing the signs of substance use in both the patient and the family and by being familiar with the resources available to help with the problem.

Substance Use Interventions
Pharmacological Interventions

Alcohol. Antidipsotropics are drugs that were traditionally prescribed to create an adverse physical reaction when the individual consumed alcohol intended to deter further drinking. The two prominent drugs in this category are disulfiram (tetraethylthiuram disulphide) and citrated calcium carbimide. When an antidipsotropic interacts with alcohol, a person's face and neck become warm and flushed, and the individual can experience dizziness, a pounding heart, a throbbing head, and nausea, essentially an exaggerated hangover effect. The severity of the reaction varies; the more alcohol consumed, the more severe the reaction. If a person continues to consume alcohol, the person can experience escalating unpleasant and dangerous symptoms such as vomiting, tachycardia, hyperventilation, shortness of breath, hypotension, and in severe instances arrhythmias, unconsciousness, and even myocardial infarction, which explains, in part, why these drugs are no longer commonly used (Csiernik, 2019).

Acamprosate is a newer, less toxic pharmacological option for responding to alcohol dependency. Taken orally three times a day, the drug ameliorates the symptoms of alcohol withdrawal and aids in limiting reactions to drink-related cues. Acamprosate makes consuming alcohol less pleasurable, with a goal of stopping lapses from becoming relapses. Acamprosate also has far fewer side effects than antidipsotropics. It is thought to stabilize the chemical balance in the CNS that is disrupted by both alcohol and benzodiazepine withdrawal, though the exact mechanism of action remains uncertain. The American Psychiatric Association (2018) recommends the use of acamprosate with individuals who have moderate to severe alcohol-related issues who have a goal of reducing alcohol consumption or becoming abstinent. Antabuse is now only recommended when patients specifically request it as part of their treatment regimen, with both acamprosate and naltrexone (see next) having better outcomes with fewer risks.

Naltrexone is an opioid antagonist that had been demonstrated to have some success in decreasing cravings for alcohol. Antagonists are drugs that block the effects of other pharmacologically similar psychoactive agents by occupying the same receptor sites in the brain. Antagonists extinguish the behavioural aspects of drug use for when they are administered ahead of the psychoactive agent, the individual obtains no positive reinforcement from the psychoactive drug. However, as with antidipsotropics, the effectiveness of this method of intervention rests solely with the dependent person's willingness to take the drug. As well, there is always a risk of overdose when using these drugs as dependent persons attempt to overcome the antagonistic effect by increasing the amount of psychoactive drug they consume.

When using naltrexone, which is marketed under the name ReVia, the pleasurable effects some people experience when they drink are diminished or do not occur. As well, there is no experience of nausea such as with the use of antidipsotropics. However, unlike its interaction with heroin, fentanyl, and other opioids, naltrexone does not prevent one from becoming impaired or intoxicated with the use of alcohol, as alcohol does not attach itself to only one type of receptor site in the brain as do opioids. When naltrexone is present in the brain, alcohol cannot stimulate the release of dopamine. The use of ReVia has been demonstrated to reduce the frequency and intensity of drinking, to reduce the risk of relapse to heavy drinking, and to increase the percentage of days abstinent. However, this drug does not discriminate and when it is being used, it decreases the release of dopamine regardless of the activity (Froehlich et al., 2019).

Baclofen is an orally administered muscle relaxant primarily used to prevent muscle spasms resulting from neurological conditions. It was also found to aid alcohol-dependent persons in maintaining abstinence and is well tolerated, even in cases of lapse. Effectiveness in producing abstinence appears to be dose dependent; an American study of 30 mg a day did not produce significant abstinence, whereas a German study administering three doses of 90 mg, up to 270 mg/day did. However, even in the German study, one-quarter of participants dropped out due to lapses and only half of the participants maintained abstinence throughout the entire study. Individuals taking Baclofen are found to have greater rates of abstinence compared to those not receiving any type of pharmacological assistance, though it does not consistently decrease episodes of heavy drinking, craving, anxiety, or depression (Rose & Jones, 2018).

Topiramate is a non-benzodiazepine anticonvulsant medication. Preliminary clinical trials have demonstrated that its use decreases alcohol's reinforcement of the CNS, leading to a decrease in alcohol consumption (Johnson et al., 2007). Topiramate appears to antagonize alcohol-rewarding effects by inhibiting dopamine release while also enhancing the inhibitory function of GABA, which in turn antagonizes glutamate receptors, further inhibiting dopamine release. Side effects of topiramate include an increased likelihood of cognitive dysfunction and numbness, tingling, dizziness, taste abnormalities, and decreased appetite or weight loss compared to those in a control group. However, the major limitation of topiramate is that tolerance seemingly builds rapidly to its effects (American Psychiatric Association, 2018).

Opioids. Drug dependence that involves heroin and other opioid drugs is a chronic, relapsing condition with a generally unfavourable prognosis. The outstanding characteristic elements include an overpowering drive to continue to administer the drug and to obtain it by any means for pleasure or to avoid the extreme discomfort of withdrawal. The basic premise for opioid substitution therapy is that appropriate drug substitutes suppress withdrawal symptoms, reducing the use of illicit and higher-risk opioids. The two primary substances employed in opioid substitution therapy are methadone and Suboxone, both of which are themselves opioids. These alternative opioids, both of which are administered orally, do not produce the same euphoria as other opioids and are safer as they are given in standardized doses with no impurities and do not have to be taken as frequently. The use of methadone and Suboxone eliminates withdrawal though the drugs need to be taken every day because if a person misses a dose, the individual will experience the same physically painful withdrawal effects as from any other opioid.

Methadone is currently the most widely used pharmacotherapeutic medication for maintenance treatment, with a history dating back to the Vietnam War era (Dole & Nyswander, 1965). The World Health Organization considers it an essential medication for global health as it effectively reduces illicit drug use, treats opioid use disorder, and retains individuals in treatment, even if they do remain physically dependent upon this opioid. Among methadone's pharmacological strengths is that, unlike morphine, it is highly effective when administered orally and it is metabolized and excreted slowly, making it therapeutically effective for up to 24 hours. However, tolerance and withdrawal do occur in methadone users, though their development is much slower than with other opioids. Without other forms of intervention, chronic users eventually become both psychologically and physically dependent on methadone. Methadone's side effects include weight gain due to lowered metabolism, dental issues due to decreased salivation, constipation, numbness in extremities, sedation, and, for some, hallucinations when initially prescribed the drug. Long-term use will also create sexual dysfunction due to decreased testosterone levels in males, as occurs with chronic use of any opioid (Csiernik, 2019).

The major alternative to methadone is Suboxone, which is comprised of the partial μ-opioid receptor agonist buprenorphine in combination with the opioid antagonist naloxone in a 4:1 ratio. Buprenorphine, derived from thebaine, is a partial opioid agonist, producing less sedation than methadone, which is a full opioid agonist. The effects of buprenorphine peak 1 to 4 hours after the initial dose with adverse effects are similar to other opioids: nausea, vomiting, and constipation. Naloxone is a true antagonist with a chemical structure similar to oxymorphone. However, it produces neither pain relief nor any type of psychoactive effects. When taken orally, it produces no discernable effects; however, if naloxone is crushed, dissolved, or injected, it produces severe opioid withdrawal effects almost immediately. As a result, naloxone has several therapeutic uses not only in combination with buprenorphine in Suboxone but also as a means of reversing the opioid-induced respiratory depression, sedation, and hypotension that is commonly observed in cases of opioid overdose. Naloxone can begin working in as little as 30 seconds after administration though it has a far shorter half-life than the vast majority of opioids: 30 to 90 minutes (Kerensky & Walley, 2017; McDonald et al., 2017). A recent study in the United Kingdom found that Suboxone users suffered fewer poisonings and had a lower risk of mortality than did methadone users, though on average, the period of usage was shorter for Suboxone than for methadone (Hickman et al., 2018).

Nicotine. Nicotine replacement therapy has become a prominent pharmacological treatment approach for those wishing to stop smoking tobacco products with several administration options (Table 18.13). In each of these approaches one form of nicotine is simply being replaced by another, though all the other harmful side effects of smoking are eliminated, except with electronic cigarettes (e-cigarettes), where it is reduced. E-cigarettes have the look and feel of cigarettes but do not burn tobacco. Instead, e-cigarettes use a battery and an electronic device to produce a warm vapour from a cartridge containing nicotine, often propylene glycol, and some flavouring additive. Cartridges can be refilled with different flavours and nicotine concentrations. E-cigarettes still contain some carcinogens (including nitrosamines), toxic chemicals (such as diethylene glycol), and tobacco-specific components that are harmful to humans. E-cigarettes deliver nicotine to the blood more rapidly than nicotine inhalers but less rapidly than cigarettes. As a result, the effect of the e-cigarette on nicotine craving is similar to that of the nicotine inhaler but less than that of cigarettes. This has led researchers to conclude that e-cigarette use leads to decreased tobacco consumption among existing smokers (McKeganey et al., 2019). The issues of course have not been this reduction, which is a positive harm reduction approach, but rather the number of new vapers this method of nicotine administration has created, primarily adolescents and young adults.

E-cigarettes are a safer nicotine delivery mechanism but still not a totally safe option. Individuals who have moved to vaping rather than smoking are still consuming nicotine, with a variety of health issues associated with this administration option, from minor mouth and throat irritation to airway obstruction, increased cardiovascular risks, and lung damage (Ghosh et al., 2019). While carcinogens remain in the product, the overall health effects are less than smoking a cigarette, though here again, as with cigarettes and cigars, vapour in the air contains harmful irritants, though it is not yet known if these are as problematic as second-hand smoke. For individuals addicted to tobacco, completely substituting e-cigarettes for combustible tobacco cigarettes reduces their users' exposure to thousands of toxicants and carcinogens present in traditional tobacco cigarettes (Koval et al., 2018). E-cigarettes can be an aid in both reducing and totally stopping the use of tobacco products (Manzoli et al., 2017) with the potential to decrease tobacco-related deaths (Levy et al., 2018). Preliminary studies have indicated that the use of e-cigarettes is more effective in promoting smoking cessation than the other nicotine-replacement options summarized in Table 18.13 (Hajek et al., 2019). However, this benefit has been undermined by the direct targeting of the product to non-smokers, primarily adolescents, creating a group of new nicotine users who otherwise may never have used this drug.

Benzodiazepines (sedative-hypnotics). Benzodiazepines with long half-lives (clonazepam) are used to assist persons to withdraw from dependencies on benzodiazepines with short half-lives (Xanax). A typical five-step intervention model incorporating benzodiazepine drug substitution with ongoing counselling would consist of the following:

1. For 2 weeks, patients monitor and record their daily drug consumption.
2. Eight one-on-one therapy sessions follow at a rate of one per week.
3. Gradual reduction of drug use begins by switching to drugs with longer half-lives.

TABLE 18.13 Nicotine Replacement Therapy Options

Nicotine Replacement Therapy Option	Dose	Side Effects
Gum	2 or 4 mg	Mouth soreness
	4 mg for those smoking >25 cigarettes daily	
	1 piece every 1–2 hours as needed for 12 weeks	Jaw ache
	Maximum: 24 pieces per day	Indigestion
Lozenges	2 or 4 mg	Nausea
	9 lozenges/day for 6–12 weeks then taper	Heartburn
	Maximum 20 lozengers/day	Coughing
		Oral cavity irritation
Nasal spray	0.5 mg dose to each nostril 1–2 doses/hour	Nasal irritation
	Increase until symptom relief	Nasal congestion
	8–40 doses/day for 3–6 months	Altered sense of smell
Sublingual tablets	2 mg for a minimum of 12 weeks then taper	Oral cavity irritation
Transdermal patch	7, 14, and 21 mg options	Local skin irritation
	Typically begin at 21 mg and wean down	Insomnia

Source: Sachdev, R., Garg, D., & Singh, G. (2018). Nicotine replacement therapy—Effective tool in smoking cessation: A short review. *Dental Science, 7*(7), 47–48.

4. Ongoing supportive care and reassurance continues until the cessation of any drug use.
5. A 1-year follow-up period commences, using a support group model (Ashton, 2013).

Stimulants. No medications have yet been proven effective in pharmacologically treating addiction to either cocaine or methamphetamine. Ritalin has been used in an attempt to improve brain function among those addicted to cocaine, while both D-amphetamine and methylphenidate are being used to treat heavy amphetamine users, with some limited success. When given disulfiram for the treatment of their alcoholism, individuals who misused both cocaine and alcohol also reduced their cocaine use from 2.5 days per week to less than once per week. As well, modafinil, a mild stimulant used to treat chronic fatigue, has been found to have some value in treating those physically dependent on crack. While several clinical trials have found those using modafinil to be far more likely to become abstinent, the vast majority (over three quarters in the experimental group) did lapse or relapse during the study period (Chan et al., 2019; Singh et al., 2016).

Implementation at Primary, Secondary, and Tertiary Levels of Prevention

Primary prevention. Prevention models in health care are classified as primary, secondary, or tertiary. In terms of substance use and addiction prevention primary approaches are those efforts focused on reducing the demand for a substance as well as stopping the occurrence of alcohol or drug use or misuse. Examples include implementing healthy public policy, offering health education related to addiction, taxing and health-related warning labelling of licit products such as cigarettes and alcohol, and promoting educational campaigns such as addiction and mental health in the workplace.

Secondary prevention. Secondary prevention seeks to limit further health deterioration and social harm from the use of, misuse of, dependence on, and addiction to psychoactive substances. Examples include programs of early recognition, awareness campaigns, relapse prevention, community support approaches, and strategies for safe prescribing guidelines. The most prominent and most controversial among secondary prevention approaches is harm reduction.

Harm reduction. Harm reduction refers to a range of programs, policies, and interventions designed to reduce or minimize the adverse consequences associated with drug use, such as overdose, infections, and spread of communicable diseases. Officially one of the four pillars of Canada's drug plan, the approach involves any strategy or behaviour that an individual uses to reduce the potential harm that may exist for them. Harm reduction is more than just a programming approach, it is also a philosophy, and seven prominent values that shape harm reduction programming are highlighted here:

1. All humans have intrinsic value.
2. All humans have the right to comprehensive, non-judgmental medical and social services.
3. Licit and illicit drugs are neither good nor bad.
4. Psychoactive drug users are sufficiently competent to make choices regarding their use of drugs.
5. Outcomes are in the hands of the substance user.
6. Options are to be provided in a non-judgmental, non-coercive manner (Denis-Lalonde et al., 2019).

Needle exchange programs. Needle exchange programs allow injection drug users (IDUs) to trade used syringes for new, sterile syringes and related injection equipment, although in recent years many of these fixed and mobile outreach programs have also begun to offer crack pipes and straws for cocaine use. Needle exchange is a harm reduction strategy that arose as a direct result of the blood-borne infections of HIV, hepatitis C virus, and hepatitis B virus that were an unintended outcome of injection drug use. However, this is not only a form of intervention for IDUs but also part of a broader public health model, as funding for these initiatives occurs so as to limit the transfer of these diseases into the general populace.

Opioid substitution therapy: methadone treatment and methadone maintenance/Suboxone treatment and Suboxone maintenance. Both methadone/Suboxone maintenance (MM/SM) and methadone/Suboxone treatment (MT/ST) consist of an individual administering a sufficient dose of the alternative opioid on a daily basis to eliminate opioid withdrawal symptoms. The basic premise of opioid substitution therapy is that methadone or Suboxone administered daily by mouth is effective in the suppression of withdrawal symptoms and in the reduction of the use of illicit opioids. MM/SM involves determining a correct dose for each individual and providing regular health care and treatment for other addiction issues, while MT/ST programs also entail the provision of counselling and support, mental health services, health promotion, and disease prevention and education, along with advocacy and links to community-based supports and services such as housing.

Heroin-assisted treatment (HAT). Some individuals do not respond well to methadone or Suboxone, as it may not ease the physical or psychological pain of withdrawal, it may not negate the craving, or an individual may have a negative reaction to the synthetic nature of the drug. Historically, these individuals either endured a cold turkey withdrawal or more typically went back to using street opioids. By returning to use, they again put themselves at risk for life-threatening health issues, including drug overdose, blood-borne viral infections, and endocarditis, as well as the violence that accompanies illicit drug transactions. One controversial alternative is heroin-assisted treatment (HAT). Under a HAT protocol, street opioid users are prescribed pharmaceutical quality heroin, which is injected in safe, clean specialized medical clinics. Service users typically attend up to two to three times per day to self-inject their dose of heroin. Average heroin dosage ranges from 400 and 600 mg/day, with supervised consumption administered on average at around 150 to 300 mg/dose. Clinical staff can also supplement this further with a small 20- to 60-mg oral methadone dose as needed. Methadone administration is prevalent as a means to prevent withdrawal between the administrations of heroin which has a far shorter half-life. The heroin-assisted programs are usually supported by access to psychological support in the form of counseling and group work, as well as general social welfare support from social services (Hill, 2016).

The overall value of HAT remains inconclusive, in part due to a lack of multiple outcomes studies. Existing research suggests that the majority of dependent users seeking treatment can use either methadone or Suboxone and these options should be offered first. However, HAT can be considered as a secondary option for those who fail to make significant progress with the standard options. Research completed on HAT programs found that program participants demonstrated improved:

- Use of structured drug treatment programs
- Physical and psychological health outcomes
- Social integration including improved capacity for work, better living conditions, and debt management
- Pro-social behaviours highlighted by a significant reduction in offending-related activity (Hill, 2016).

Supervised consumption sites (SCS). Supervised consumption sites (SCSs) began as supervised (or safe) injection sites (SISs) in Canada. These clinics were designed to provide IDUs with clean needles and sterilized works to inject their drugs in a safer manner. SISs that have evolved to SCSs provide individuals with a healthier environment in which to inject, inhale, intranasally, or orally consume drugs while also providing related health and social services, all in one location. While the first Canadian site opened in Lethbridge, Alberta, in 2017, Switzerland, Germany, and the Netherlands adopted the concept of safe injection rooms during the 1970s, again as a general public health initiative. However, since then, the strategy demonstrated a decrease in new HIV and HCV infections and reduced the number of overdose-related deaths while providing access to primary and emergency health care for a traditionally oppressed population. After the opening of a new site, once the public backlash has subsided, there is generally a decrease in public nuisance issues related to drug use, including public injecting, discarded syringes, and injection-related litter (Rowe & Rapp, 2017).

SCSs offer a safe place where drug-dependent individuals can administer drugs under the supervision of trained multi-disciplinary health and social services staff who can provide education regarding safer use practices, as well as respond appropriately in the event of an overdose. Each SCS varies in the way it operates. However, in general, individuals bring pre-obtained drugs to the site, are provided with sterile equipment to use, and consume their drugs with nurses and other trained staff nearby. Typically, needles, syringes, candles, sterile water, paper towels, cotton balls, cookers/spoons, ties, alcohol swabs, filters, ascorbic acid, and bandages are available in the injection-specific areas. SCSs allow substance users to have their privacy while also offering the comfort of knowing that trained medical staff are available to respond in case of an emergency. SCSs do not allow the sharing of drugs or equipment and prohibit assisted injection. SCSs lead to a reduction in syringe sharing among users, which also reduces the spread of diseases and infections. SCSs attempt to protect and promote the health of drug users by employing a non-judgmental, person-centered approach rooted in a harm-reduction philosophy (Rowe & Rapp, 2017).

As with other forms of harm reduction, SCSs benefit a hard-to-reach population by offering services with minimal barriers to access and avoidance of interactions with the criminal justice system. Contact with these hard-to-reach persons can lead to important social and health referrals and treatment opportunities, which ultimately result in positive social and community opportunities. The introduction of SCSs has contributed to individual improvements in health, social functioning, and stabilization, along with a decreased number of overdoses and pre-mature deaths (Kennedy et al., 2019). The Registered Nursing Association of Ontario has now prepared a set of best practice guidelines to assist in the development of this important community-based service (https://rnao.ca/sites/rnao-ca/files/bpg/Implementing_supervised_injection_services.pdf).

Controlled drinking. Controlled drinking is an adapted behavioural technique used with persons experiencing low levels of alcohol misuse. Assessment of the patient's level of alcohol dependence is necessary to determine if a goal of controlled drinking is feasible. This approach proposes that training in drinking skills is required to teach alcohol misusers to drink in a non-abusive manner as an alternative to abstinence as part of a more broad-based treatment program. The first step in controlled drinking is determining whether a person is using alcohol excessively or is alcohol dependent. This is accomplished by imposing a 2- to 3-week period of abstinence. If the person can go without drinking, they are moved into the next phase. Those who cannot abstain during this baseline period generally do not qualify for a controlled drinking treatment program. In the program itself patients are provided with a set of goals and rules to help them control their alcohol intake. A common drinking goal of a set number of standard drinks per week is established, with numerous limitations. For a young, healthy male approximately 6 feet tall and weighing 180 pounds, the following regimen might be applied:

- No more than two standard drinks per day (one for women)
- No more than one drink per hour
- Sip drinks and avoid carbonated beverages
- Drink only on a full stomach
- Two days per week must be set aside on which no alcohol is consumed
- Limit weekly intake to 14 standard drinks per week (7 for women).

Low-risk, or reduced, drinking is achievable for some individuals as they undergo treatment for alcohol dependence. Individuals with lower dependence severity, less baseline drinking, fewer negative mood symptoms and fewer heavy drinkers in their social networks have a higher probability of achieving low-risk drinking during treatment. Reduced drinking may be a viable alternative for those who do not have alcohol-related physical damage and who have not experienced any serious personal, financial, legal, or employment problems as a result of their alcohol misuse. However, controlled drinking training is not an alternative for those who are physically and psychologically dependent on alcohol or on any other psychoactive substance (Witkiewitz et al., 2017).

Managed alcohol programs (MAPs). The primary purpose of managed alcohol programs (MAPs) is to offer continuing health and housing services for individuals who have a history of homelessness and alcohol misuse along with chronic health issues and are in many cases deemed to be near the end of their lives. The aim is to provide humane treatment and reduce harm to the patients by eliminating the need to binge drink and to drink non-beverage alcohol products. Nursing, medical, and rehabilitation care are provided along with a regular, limited amount of alcohol. MAPs' goal is to provide their residents with permanent rather than transient housing, and in this way it falls into the Housing First philosophy. Some MAPs offer private rooms, though the standard is shared accommodation, with all programs being staffed 24 hours per day. Care plans are individualized and typically include a recreational component. The overall goal is to improve the quality of life of patients while allowing them to live in a respectful, supportive environment. General strategies for relapse prevention are cognitive and behavioural: recognizing and learning how to avoid or cope with threats to recovery, changing lifestyle, learning how to participate in activities without drugs, and securing help from other people or from social support services. In Canada MAPs are almost exclusively used by men.

Relapse prevention and aftercare. Long-term recovery is not a straight line but is preceded by periods of flux and discontinuity before change is stabilized. These periods can last longer than the length of time the individual was actually in treatment initially. This reality has placed increasing importance and emphasis upon follow-up, aftercare, or, as it has become more prominently known, relapse prevention. Relapse, which is a return to previous drug use patterns, poses a fundamental barrier to the treatment of addiction. It is distinct from lapse, which is a singular or short-term use of drugs that is viewed as a learning opportunity around a specific event or trigger (Kougiali et al., 2017).

Depending on the definition one uses for recovery, statistics indicate that upwards of 90% of individuals have the potential to relapse. Historically, relapse had been attributed to factors such as cravings or withdrawal symptoms arising due to the disease of addiction. However, relapse is a complicated, multi-faceted process rather than a discrete event and is now generally considered not a failure but rather a setback. Thus aftercare needs to be a continuation of work initiated during the initial treatment regimen, with a focus on resettling and reintegrating individuals back into society. The goal is to provide continuous encouragement, support, and additional services as needed following a patient's completion of a treatment plan. Preventing relapse or minimizing its extent is a necessity for successful, long-term change (Csiernik, 2021).

The contemporary approach to relapse prevention also rejects the idea of a person being either successfully abstinent or failing and being a drug misuser. Rather, the transition is viewed as a process where lapses are not end points but learning opportunities. If a lapse becomes a relapse, it is still only a temporary setback, which is not unique to the individual but a common part of the process toward the end goal of abstinence. It is simply another learning opportunity, which, when resolved, becomes part of the person's behavioural repertoire. The primary goals of treatment are functional analysis, determining triggers and consequences of use, and skill building.

Relapse prevention as an intervention is a tertiary strategy, intended to reduce the likelihood and severity of relapse following the cessation or reduction of problematic substance use. Cognitive-behavioural principles guide contemporary evidence-informed relapse prevention models (Figure 18.5). Marlatt and Witkiewtiz's (2005) model views relapse as a complex, circular process in which various factors interact, creating the opportunity for the person to return to regular drug use. Thus the key becomes to assist patients

Fig. 18.5 Marlatt & Witkiewtiz's cognitive-behavioral model of relapse. (**Source:** Marlatt, G., & Witkiewtiz, K. [2005]. Cognitive-behavioral model of relapse.)

in recognizing and quickly addressing high-risk situations in their lives. There are two sets of variables that need to be considered. The first are called tonic factors and are constants in a person's life while the second group, phasic, are transient influences in a person's life. Tonic processes include personality, genetic and familial risk factors, drug sensitivity, metabolism, neurotransmitter levels, and the effects produced by physical withdrawal. Tonic processes also include cognitive factors that show relative stability over time, such as drug-related outcome expectancies, a person's degree of self-efficacy, and personal beliefs about one's ability to remain abstinent. Tonic processes provide a baseline of risk, but it is typically phasic responses that produce the relapse event. Phasic processes can be both cognitive and affective, including urges/cravings often triggered by an event or mood, both negative (distress) or positive (eustress). A minimally acceptable aftercare program would involve a monthly contact for 1 year, with the provision that the patient can contact the relapse prevention worker whenever needed. Box 18.4 outlines relapse prevention strategies that are of value in a nursing environment. Alcoholics Anonymous (AA) and related 12-step groups are a self-help format that also serves as an ongoing relapse prevention support system. While AA is the most prominent and well-known form of mutual aid, it is not the best fit for all, especially women with trauma histories. As such, it is valuable to familiarize yourself with a range of options such as Women for Sobriety (WFS), SMART Recovery, the Secular Organization for Sobriety (SOS), Rational Recovery (RR), Moderation Management (MM), and Refuge Recovery.

BOX 18.4 Relapse Prevention Strategies

Basics

It is important to keep the program simple at first. Remember that many patients who use substances have mild to moderate cognitive problems while actively using substances. Providing prompts and assistance for the patient's recall may be beneficial. For example:

- Reviewing instructions from health team members
- Encouraging use of a notebook to write down important information, appointments, schedules, and telephone numbers

Skills

Patients may take advantage of cognitive behavioural therapy to increase their coping skills. The patient can identify which important life skills are needed by inquiring about the following:

- Which situations are challenging and stress-producing?
- What situations command new skills or abilities?
- What abilities and skills are currently strong?

Enhancement of Personal Insight

Counselling can help a patient gain insight and control over a variety of psychological concerns. For example:

- What triggers the use or addiction?
- What constitutes a healthy, supportive relationship?
- How can self-esteem, self-worth, and coping be strengthened?
- What does the addiction offer that would be difficult to give up? What would be the loss without the use or addiction? What could replace the loss?

Relapse Prevention Groups

Support membership in a relapse prevention group. These groups help patients work on:

- Rehearsing stressful situations using a variety of techniques
- Finding ways to deal with current problems or ones that are likely to arise without the drugs, alcohol, or behavioural addiction
- Providing role models to support change

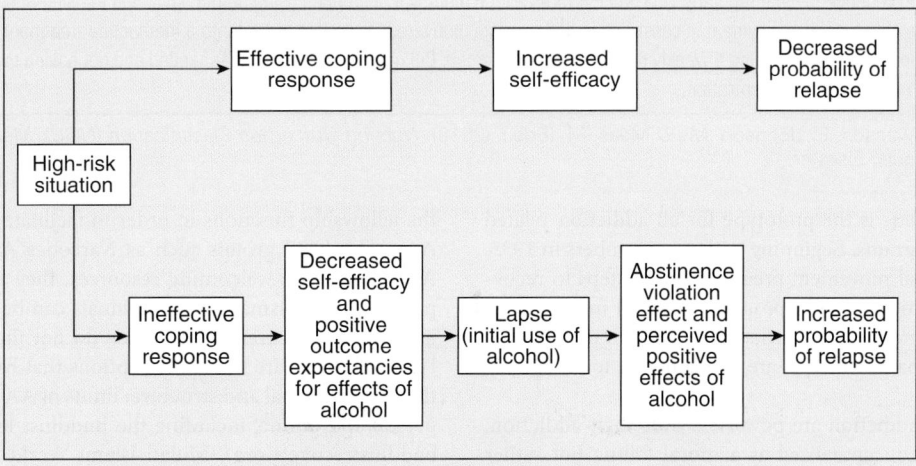

Source: Adapted from Zerbe, K. J. (1999). *Women's mental health in primary care* (pp. 94–95). Philadelphia: Saunders.

CASE STUDY AND NURSING CARE PLAN 18.1

Bill, a 20-year-old single man, was brought to the emergency department after having been found unconscious in his room at home. He was accompanied by his mother, with whom he shares a small apartment. When his mother was not able to rouse him, she dialed 911 for an ambulance. A syringe and some white powder were found next to Bill.

On admission, Bill had laboured breathing, and his pupils were constricted. Vital signs were taken; his blood pressure was 60/40 mm Hg, and his pulse was 132 beats per minute. Bill's situation was determined to be life threatening. Although extremely distressed, Bill's mother was able to report to the staff that Bill had a substance use problem and had been injecting heroin for 6 months before recently entering a methadone maintenance program 1 year ago. It was decided at this point to administer an opioid antagonist, and naloxone was given intramuscularly. Bill's breathing improved, and he was able to respond to verbal stimuli. Bill's mother later told staff that Bill had not been attending his methadone maintenance program for the past week. At the staff's urging, she called the program, and an outreach worker, Sylvain, arranged to talk to her and Bill at the hospital. Bill made an appointment to follow up with Sylvain at the methadone clinic on the following Monday. Sylvain recognized that Bill's future would ultimately depend on Bill's own actions but that he could offer some motivation and guide Bill's insight.

On Monday, Sylvain spoke with Bill about his situation, what changes he wanted for himself, his drug use, some of the factors that led him to lapse, and what Bill thought he might need in order to get back into recovery. Bill stated, "I know I can do it if I can concentrate on health and life. If I lose that concentration, it just is old habit to use again. I can see how I slipped off track." Their interaction included the following exchange:

Dialogue	Therapeutic Tool or Comment
Sylvain: "I was in the emergency department Friday afternoon when you were brought in by ambulance."	Placing the event in time and sequence, validating the precipitating event
Bill: "Were you? I guess a lot of people thought it was over for me."	
Sylvain: "It certainly looked quite serious."	Emphasizing the reality—prevents minimizing the situation
Bill: "Yeah. I should never have left the program. I was doing better, and I just didn't think I needed the methadone every day anymore."	
Sylvain: "You said you were doing well."	Reflecting
Bill: "Yeah. I had a job, and I was beginning to save some money. Wow! I can't believe I blew this whole thing."	
Sylvain: "I don't know that you really did, it was just one slip and you already seem motivated to keep trying. Your counsellor in the program phoned your doctor this morning to find out how you were doing."	Pointing out reality
Bill: "Do you think they'll take me back?"	
Sylvain: "Why don't we talk some more, and after we finish, I'll speak with the other staff about your situation. If you would like to get back into the program, you can call your counsellor, and we'll support your decision. There is a big difference between a lapse and a relapse and the fact you are talking to me shows you are still committed to changing."	Gathering information Supporting decision making

Sylvain and Bill agreed to continue to meet regularly, and while it took several months, Bill stopped using heroin; switched to using Suboxone, as he found the side effects less harsh; and was able to find employment in construction. Bill appears motivated, as he has moved into a methadone treatment program that uses motivational interviewing and is now regularly attending a weekly relapse prevention group. Bill reports that being clear headed and not having to always think about getting and using the drug is worth the time and concentration.

Source: Moorhead, S., Swanson, E., Johnson, M., & Maas, M. (Eds.). (2018). *Nursing Outcomes Classification (NOC): Measurement of health outcomes* (6th ed.). St. Louis: Elsevier.

Alcoholics Anonymous is the prototype for all addiction-related **mutual aid** self-help programs. Beginning with two members in 1935, it has grown into a global movement premised on 12 steps to recovery (Box 18.5). These programs offer properly matched individuals a behavioural, cognitive, and dynamic structure to assist in maintaining their abstinence. Three basic concepts are fundamental to all 12-step programs:

1. Individuals with an addiction are powerless over their addiction, which is no longer conceptualized as a moral failing but rather as a disease, and their lives are unmanageable because of their addiction.
2. Although individuals with an addiction are not responsible for their disease, they are responsible for their recovery.
3. Individuals can no longer blame people, places, and things for their addiction; they must face their problems and their feelings and do so in conjunction with a Higher Power.

Before referring any patient to any mutual aid group, a nurse should attend an open meeting to learn what occurs there and how the fellowship functions in order to facilitate a proper referral. While AA and related groups such as Narcotics Anonymous and Cocaine Anonymous are welcoming resources, they are not a good fit for all patients, and mismatched individuals can be discouraged from seeking professional treatment if they do not find AA of value to them. However, there are now other options that have arisen in response to the organizational and structural limits of AA that are available both in person and online, including the Buddhist Recovery Network (www.buddhistrecovery.org), Millati Islami World Services (www.millatiislami.org), MM (www.moderation.org), RR (www.rational.org), SOS (www.sossobriety.org), SMART Recovery (www.smartrecovery.org), and WFS (www.womenforsobriety.org).

Self-help groups for the patient and family or friends. Counselling and support should be encouraged for all family and friends of a person experiencing problems with alcohol, other substance use, or addictions. Al-Anon (https://al-anon.org) and Alateen (https://al-anon.org/for-members/group-resources/alateen/) are self-help groups that offer support and guidance for adults and teenagers,

> **BOX 18.5 The 12 Steps of Alcoholics Anonymous**
>
> 1. We admitted we were powerless over alcohol—that our lives had become unmanageable.
> 2. Came to believe that a Power greater than ourselves could restore us to sanity.
> 3. Made a decision to turn our will and our lives over to the care of God as we understood Him.
> 4. Made a searching and fearless moral inventory of ourselves.
> 5. Admitted to God, to ourselves, and to another human being the exact nature of our wrongs.
> 6. Were entirely ready to have God remove all these defects of character.
> 7. Humbly asked Him to remove our shortcomings.
> 8. Made a list of all persons we had harmed and became willing to make amends to them all.
> 9. Made direct amends to such people wherever possible, except when to do so would injure them or others.
> 10. Continued to take personal inventory and when we were wrong, promptly admitted it.
> 11. Sought through prayer and meditation to improve our conscious contact with God as we understood Him, praying only for knowledge of His will for us and the power to carry that out.
> 12. Having had a spiritual awakening as a result of these steps, we tried to carry this message to alcoholics and to practise these principles in all our affairs.

respectively. Self-help groups assist family members and friends in dealing with many common issues. Their work is based on a combination of educational and operational principles centred on the acceptance of the disease model of addiction, including pragmatic methods for avoiding enabling behaviours. However, they are not a replacement for, but rather an adjunct to, family counselling, especially in situations where the patient is not ready yet to commit to changing but where the family needs support.

Tertiary prevention. Tertiary prevention is concerned with limiting and reducing complications and dysfunction related to the experience of addiction. Effective care, treatment, and rehabilitation programs and services are characteristic of tertiary prevention approaches. Specialized addiction detoxification programs, recovery programs, and concurrent disorder programs are examples of tertiary-level services.

Assessment and referral. Once an individual has been identified as having a substance use issue, the depth and breadth of the situation needs to be determined. Assessment and referral agencies provide services that use specific instruments and processes to determine the major issues as well as the strengths and supports of the person with a substance issue. These agencies develop individualized plans for assistance, which may entail referral to other organizations for more intensive or residential treatment. A standardized assessment procedure can take anywhere from 2 to 3 hours to complete, typically including a history of the use of alcohol and other drugs, including the age of onset, duration, patterns, consequences of use, use of alcohol and drugs by family members, and types of and responses to previous treatment initiatives. It is also recommended that assessments determine a patient's physical health, environmental supports (including partner and family), accommodation, employment (if employed), school status (if attending school), leisure activities, legal problems, sexual orientation, gender identification, and any history of sexual or other physical abuse or trauma. It is also essential to initially assess the level and intensity of withdrawal management and stabilization services required. This systematic process must also identify the patient's strengths and take into consideration what the patient actually wants.

Withdrawal management services: daytox and detox. Withdrawal management or detoxification services are often a first step in the treatment process. This entails total abstinence from not only the drug of misuse but also often all other drugs, including, in some facilities, tobacco. The detoxification process should be of sufficient length to allow all of the psychoactive drugs to be eliminated by the body. A patient's safety is the first priority of all withdrawal management staff, though once an individual becomes more stable, staff also typically offer social and environmental support during the stay, including referrals to mutual aid groups. Daytox programs provide support and programming during the day, while detox programs have a residential component that lasts 3 to 7 days depending upon the province and the drug.

Community-based (outpatient) treatment. This is treatment provided on a non-residential basis, usually in regularly scheduled sessions of 1 to 2 hours per week but sometimes two times per week. Treatment may entail individual and/or group sessions to explore all aspects of the person's substance use and related problems. Sessions offer information and strategies to assist each individual in their recovery process. This is the least intense and intrusive treatment intervention option, primarily offered by non-medical, community-based counselling agencies. Appropriate matches for this service include patients who:

- Are free of any significant medical problem
- Are self-motivated
- Have a support system in place, including family, friends, or work
- Live within easy access to the facility
- Have not yet had their personal or work life extensively affected by their substance use

Day treatment. This is a more intensive, structured non-residential treatment, typically provided 5 days per week or alternatively 4 or 5 evenings per week for 3 to 4 hours per session. Treatment involves group activities ranging from formal group treatment sessions to education groups to recreational activities. As patients are at home on weekends, evenings, and days, the home environment must be stable, with support from family and friends. This treatment option allows the social aspect of addiction to be acknowledged and addressed early in the treatment process. Day treatment is appropriate for individuals who are able to maintain social competence despite their dependency.

Concurrent disorder programs. Another specialized form of community-based counselling entails work done by agencies whose patients have both an addiction and a mental health issue. Services offered by institutional and community-based psychologists, psychiatrists, social workers, and nurses have long been a part of the extended continuum of care, but traditionally these helping professionals dealt with either the mental health issue or the addiction issue alone, rarely the two together. Concurrent disorder programs move beyond working only with the addiction issue and provide counselling that also addresses issues such as anxiety, depression, loneliness, suicidal ideation and attempts, paranoia, and violent behaviours. Whether these behaviours are primary or secondary to the use of psychoactive agents is no longer an issue; rather, the mental health problems are categorized as coexisting with the drug misuse and vice versa, and thus intervention focuses on both. The Reis Typology (Box 18.6) is used to determine the best service for a patient with a concurrent disorder (Sinha et al., 2019).

Short-term residential treatment. These programs run for 18 to 28 days, can be sex specific or co-ed, and offer a wide variety of services, including medical evaluation, assessment of the extent of the drug dependency, detoxification in some facilities, individual and group counselling, drug education, spiritual guidance, family involvement, vocational guidance, and even employer involvement. The centres provide a safe, relatively stress-free environment in which the person can recover from

> **BOX 18.6 Reis Typology**
>
> | MI High Severity, SUD High Severity | MI Low Severity, SUD High Severity |
> |---|---|
> | Serious and persistent mental illness with substance dependence | Psychiatrically complicated substance dependence |
> | Service: Integrated care | Service: Collaboration |
> | **MI High Severity, SUD Low Severity** | **MI Low Severity, SUD Low Severity** |
> | Serious and persistent mental illness with substance use | Mild psychopathology with substance use |
> | Service: **Collaboration** | Service: **Consultation** |

MI, Mental illness; *SUD*, substance use disorder.

the physical and emotional effects of prolonged substance use. Planning for rehabilitation upon return to the natural environment is also typically part of the process. Education on the effects of drugs varies between programs but usually includes the short- and long-term effects of drug use physiologically, socially, spiritually, and psychologically. Often, attendance at a 12-step group is either recommended or mandated. The same requirement of commitment and attendance may also be part of other programs that are not premised on the philosophy of AA. In Canada residential treatment programs can be both government sponsored or private agencies, with costs for the latter being up to and over $20 000.

Recovery homes. For many struggling with ongoing issues in their recovery, the ability to avoid a relapse is often jeopardized by untenable housing or unsupportive living environments. Recovery residences, also called social model recovery or sober living houses, are designed to provide safe and supportive housing to help individuals initiate and sustain recovery primarily through peer-to-peer interactions guided by staff who themselves have recovery histories. They are sex-specific, residential programs in which the goal is to provide a safe, supportive, therapeutic program of addiction education and life skills counselling. They provide an array of services to individuals with addiction problems within a structured environment either before or after the person has attended a withdrawal management program or has received more intensive treatment through the auspices of a short-term residential program. One issue that is highlighted among recovery homes, but pertains to all addiction residential programming, is that there are currently more facilities and more beds for men than for women.

Alternative living environment. For many people with a substance use problem, the environment they live in is counterproductive to their successful treatment and recovery. These people may have unstable home lives or no support from family and friends who themselves may also be regular substance users. Others come into treatment having no real home at all, having no role models for healthy living, or needing to relearn or learn socialization skills. Alternative living environments or therapeutic communities provide a protective living environment for people whose substance use is not an isolated problem but a major disruption of their entire life. These programs help in setting limits and defining behaviour while satisfying daily needs and desires in a quasi-home setting. Relationships that develop provide a basis on which the members can build the learning or relearning of living with others. Real-life issues of daily existence take precedence at these facilities, the premise being that people best learn about how to sustain and manage the stresses of daily living and relationships while experiencing actual everyday life (rather than an isolated bubble, no matter how safe that may seem). Many alternative living settings are affiliated with a religious order, the most prominent being the Salvation Army.

Addiction supportive housing (ASH). Addiction supportive housing (ASH) programs are another component of the treatment continuum that recognizes the importance of safe and sustainable housing in the recovery process. This resource is part of the Housing First initiative and, while still limited, it provides longer support in a therapeutic environment than do short-term residential programs or recovery homes. The goal is to encourage program participants to develop long-term skills that are necessary to maintain one's own residence but without necessarily demanding abstinence in order to be housed. By providing housing supports, ideally in conjunction with but not contingent on addiction treatment, service providers can increase the probability that someone who is marginally housed or homeless will follow through with addiction treatment.

Onen'tó:kon Healing Lodge: an Indigenous treatment approach. The Onen'tó:kon Healing Lodge situated in the Mohawk community of Kanehsatake is one of a network of specialized Indigenous treatment programs in Canada. The 6-week residential program takes a cultural perspective on treatment, including talking and healing circles. Not only is the chemical dependency addressed, but the specific issues that the individual identifies, such as anger; resentment; grief; physical, emotional, and sexual abuse; and low self-esteem, are addressed as well. Talking circles are a variant of group therapy where a person speaks about the issues that are causing pain. The other members of the circle provide individual feedback and confront behaviours that are not helpful in the individual's recovery program. However, healing circles are conducted without confrontation unless an individual behaves in a manner that is disruptive.

Individuals may choose to smudge prior to joining the circle. The act of smudging has a deeply spiritual significance for most Indigenous peoples. The smoke from sage is used to cleanse oneself of evil spirits, and the smoke from sweet grass is used to invite positive influences to help the individual engage in the event in a more positive, integrated, spiritual way that respects the Creator, ancestors, and other participants. People use smudging to find calmness from negative feelings by using the medicines of sweet grass, sage, and cedar. Sweet grass braids and sage are available for people who smudge as a way of communicating with the Creator. Sweat lodges are also available for people who want to do a sweat during the week that they complete treatment. A sweat takes place in an enclosure with hot rocks where people can pray to their higher power. The sweat is used as a healing circle, a peaceful and calm place. It is a safe place to let go of issues.

During the 5th week of a person's treatment program at Onen'tó:kon, an "affirmation circle" takes place in one of the talking circles. Each individual is placed in the centre of the circle, and the other circle members whisper words of affirmation in their ear, such as, "I am so happy that you were born," "I love you," "You are so special," "You are precious to me," and "I am so proud of you." This activity has a profound effect on the patient because for some it may be the first time someone has said those positive words to them. The treatment program is geared toward helping people rid themselves of negative thinking and negative "self-talk."

At the conclusion of the 6-week residential treatment program, there is a graduation ceremony at which individuals obtain certificates of achievement. This is a very important occasion when the participants' loved ones and friends are invited to help in celebrating each person's accomplishment. The graduates usually feel great pride in having completed the treatment program, as for some it is the first time they have completed something that they have started. During the ceremony, graduates participate through drumming, through singing, and in a greeting circle. The leader starts the greeting with the graduates and continues on to the guests and staff members. The circle gives each individual an opportunity to say the words that need saying, face to face, because those in the circle may not cross paths again (Brownbill & Etienne, 2017).

CHAPTER 18 Psychoactive Substance Use and Treatment

CASE STUDY AND NURSING CARE PLAN 18.2
Alcohol Dependence With Depression

Mr. Jiratatprasot, age 49 years, and his wife arrive at the emergency department one evening, fearful that he has had a stroke. His right hand is limp, he is unable to hyperextend his right wrist, and sensation to the fingertips in the hand is impaired.

Mr. Jiratatprasot looks much older than his stated age; in fact, he looks about 65. History taking is difficult. Mr. Jiratatprasot and his wife's English is limited and he answers only what is asked of him, volunteering no additional information. He states that he took a nap that afternoon, and when he awakened, he noticed the problems with his right arm.

Shilo, the admitting nurse, begins the assessment. Mr. Jiratatprasot reveals that he has been unemployed for 4 years because the company he worked for went bankrupt. He has been unable to find a new job but has a job interview in 10 days. His wife is now working full time as a personal support worker, so the family finances are stable but far less than they were used to when he was employed. They have two grown children who no longer live at home. As he relates this information, his lips momentarily start to tremble and his eyes fill with tears.

Mr. Jiratatprasot does not acknowledge any significant medical illness except for high blood pressure, just diagnosed last year. His father has a history of depression, and his mother has a substance use issue but has been abstinent for many years. However, as they both still live in Thailand, Mr. Jiratatprasot does not have regular contact with them. Shilo shares with him the fact that depression and alcohol dependency run in families. She asks Mr. Jiratatprasot (1) whether he knows this and (2) whether it concerns him with regard to his own drinking. He says that he knows and that he does not want to think about it.

Shilo speaks separately with Mrs. Jiratatprasot and asks if there is anything she would like to add. Mrs. Jiratatprasot's shoulders slump; she sighs and says, "Earlier this week I spend 1 day talking to counsellor at treatment centre to see if they can help my husband but I did not understand everything they told me on the phone. My husband says he does not have a problem and drinking is what he and his friends have done all their lives when not working." Mrs. Jiratatprasot recounts a 6-year history of steadily increasing alcohol use. She says that she could not admit to herself until now that her husband was an excessive drinker.

She describes her feelings, which are like an emotional roller coaster—she feels happy when he is not drinking but sad when he loses control. Mrs. Jiratatprasot is afraid to go to work some days, especially on night shifts due to fear of what her husband might do while she is gone. She says she is terrified that one day he will get into a car wreck and kill himself, because he often drives when intoxicated. He tells her not to worry, because the life insurance policy is paid up and she will be taken care of.

Meanwhile, the physician in the emergency department has concluded his initial examination of Mr. Jiratatprasot. The diagnosis is radial nerve palsy. Mr. Jiratatprasot most likely passed out while lying on his arm. Because he was intoxicated, he did not feel the signals that his nerves sent out to warn him to move (numbness, tingling). He was in this position for so long that the resultant cutoff of circulation was sufficient to cause some temporary nerve damage.

Mr. Jiratatprasot's blood alcohol level (BAL) is 0.15%—nearly twice the legal limit (0.08%) for intoxication. Even though he has a high BAL, Mr. Jiratatprasot is alert and oriented, not slurring his speech or giving any other outward signs of intoxication. The difference between Mr. Jiratatprasot's BAL and his behaviour indicates the development of tolerance, a symptom of physical dependence.

Assessment
Self-Awareness

Shilo has developed capacity and skills in working with people who misuse alcohol. She grew up in a home in which alcohol transformed her father from a caring and responsible parent to one who was physically and verbally abusive to his wife and children. He eventually lost his job and left home. Shilo was determined to be everything her father was not and firmly resolved never to drink or use drugs.

As a new nurse, Shilo became extremely frustrated and angry with patients like Mr. Jiratatprasot and found herself being overly protective of the patient's family. At the end of a particular day on which she had to work with yet another intoxicated patient, she felt drained, depressed, and despondent. It became such a problem that she knew she needed to either leave her job or deal with the dynamics underlying her responses. She began to attend the support group Al-Anon. There, she was able to talk about her feelings with others who had similar backgrounds. Shilo was also provided with tools for dealing with her own feelings, gaining a greater understanding of the pathology and trauma behind alcohol misuse.

As Shilo approaches her work with the Jiratatprasot family, she does so with new confidence. She feels empathy and understanding for Mrs. Jiratatprasot, but she is able to maintain emotional boundaries and does not feel drained by their interactions. While she still feels a little frustration with Mr. Jiratatprasot, she recognizes these feelings and focuses on him as a person with a serious disorder.

Shilo organizes her data into objective and subjective components.

Objective Data	Subjective Data
Driving when intoxicated	Pre-contemplative with regards to alcohol problem
Covert references to death	Pre-contemplative with regards to depression
Nerve damage from passing out while lying on arm	
Increased alcohol use since becoming unemployed	
Ability to find employment impaired by alcohol use	
Disruption in marital relationship because of alcohol use	
Inability to see effects of his drinking	
Family history of alcoholism and depression	
BAL twice the legal limit of intoxication; has developed tolerance	

Diagnosis

From the data, the nurse formulates the following nursing diagnoses:
1. *Risk for suicide* related to depressed mood

CASE STUDY AND NURSING CARE PLAN 18.2—cont'd
Alcohol Dependence With Depression

Supporting Data
- Dangerous behaviour: driving when drinking
- Full payment of life insurance policy

2. *Ineffective coping* related to alcohol use

Supporting Data
- Increased alcohol use during stressful period of unemployment
- Impairment in capacity to obtain employment caused by alcohol use
- Disruption in marital relationship because of alcohol use
- Inability to see effect of his drinking on his life functioning

Outcomes Identification
1. The patient will refrain from attempting suicide.
2. The patient will report increase in psychological comfort.

Planning

The initial plan is to allow Mr. Jiratatprasot to remain in the emergency department until his BAL drops to 0.0% in order to discuss his goals. Once he is no longer impaired, the nurse will establish realistic outcomes with him. The risk is that his tolerance has become so substantive he can only function when there is some degree of alcohol in his system. Thus Mr. Jiratatprasot's withdrawal needs to be carefully monitored and managed as per the CIWA-Ar protocol.

Implementation

Mr. Jiratatprasot's plan of care is personalized as follows:

1. **Nursing diagnosis:** *Risk for suicide*
   Outcome: Patient will consistently demonstrate suicide self-restraint.

Short-Term Goal	Intervention	Rationale	Evaluation
1. Patient will seek treatment for depression from a community mental health care provider.	1a. Determine presence and degree of suicidal risk. 1b. Refer patient to mental health care provider for evaluation and treatment.	1a. Risk for suicide is increased in substance-using patients. 1b. Addressing both substance use and mental health treatment needs improves outcomes.	**Goal Met** After 3 weeks, patient attends appointment at Canadian Mental Health Association and has started taking an antidepressant.

2. **Nursing diagnosis:** *Ineffective coping*
   Outcome: Patient will demonstrate mild to no change in health status and social functioning due to substance addiction.

Short-Term Goal	Intervention	Rationale	Evaluation
1. Patient will consistently acknowledge personal consequences associated with alcohol misuse.	1a. Identify with patient those factors (genetics, stress, unemployment) that contribute to chemical dependence. 1b. Assist patient in identifying negative effects of chemical dependency.	1a. Emphasis on alcoholism having biological (genetics), psychological (stress), and social (unemployment) aspects lowers guilt and increases self-esteem. 1b. Identifying negative effects helps patient move from pre-contemplative to preparation and early action stages (TTM).	**Goal Met** Patient understands how his alcohol use is effecting his ability to find employment.
2. Patient will commit to alcohol use control strategies.	2a. Determine history of alcohol use. 2b. Patient attends community addiction treatment program to complete assessment.	2a. Determining history identifies high-risk situations. 2b. Alcohol dependence requires outpatient counselling in conjunction with mutual aid involvement.	**Goal Met** After 3 weeks, patient states that he has arranged for an assessment and has been to one AA meeting and one Rational Recovery meeting and is still deciding which best fits his way of thinking about alcohol but that he will continue to attend both until he decides. His wife has joined the family support group offered at the assessment centre

Evaluation

See individual outcomes and evaluation in the care plan.

Source: Moorhead, S., Swanson, E., Johnson, M. & Maas, M. (Eds.). (2018). *Nursing Outcomes Classification (NOC): Measurement of health outcomes* (6th ed.). St. Louis: Elsevier.

Nurses and addiction in the workplace. The issue of nurses developing an addiction is not as taboo a topic as in the past, helped in part by the dramatization of this issue in media such as Nurse Jackie (2009 to 2015). However, fear of disciplinary action up to and including job loss still prevents nurses in the real world from either seeking help for themselves or from reporting a colleague or friend. Supporting the treatment and recovery of a fellow nurse experiencing an addiction can be challenging, but the situation is not uncommon, nor is being supportive impossible. The choices for action are varied, and the only choice that is clearly wrong is doing nothing. Without intervention or treatment, the problems associated with addiction escalate, including systemic and institutionalized problems such as over-work, workplace bullying, and the potential for not only self-harm but also patient harm increases (Ross et al., 2019; Strobbe & Crowley, 2017).

A nurse experiencing an addiction may often volunteer to work additional shifts to be nearer to the supply of the substance of use. The nurse may leave the unit frequently or spend excessive time in the bathroom. When the nurse with an addiction is on duty, more patients may complain that their pain is unrelieved by their opioid analgesic or that they are unable to sleep, despite receiving sedative medications. Increases in inaccurate drug counts and reports of vial breakage may occur.

The Canadian Nurses Association's (2017) code of ethics requires nurses to recognize when their own personal problems might interfere with their effectiveness and to take appropriate action. The code of ethics also requires nurses to recognize signs of substance use or impaired practice in colleagues and to report such behaviour to the nurse manager. Intervention is the responsibility of the nurse manager and other nursing administrators. However, clear documentation by co-workers (specific dates, times, events, consequences) is crucial. The nurse manager's major concerns are with job performance and patient safety. Once the nurse manager has been informed, the legal and ethical responsibilities for in-house reporting have been met. If the nurse experiencing an addiction remains in the situation and no action is taken by the nurse manager, co-workers must take the information to the next level in the management structure or look to the provincial or territorial regulatory body for consultation and guidance. These measures can prevent harm to patients under the care of the nurse who is using substances and can save a colleague's professional career or even life.

Reporting a colleague who has a problem with substance use or addiction is not easy, even though it is a professional responsibility. In efforts to avoid conflict or difficult emotions, nurse colleagues may deny or rationalize the problem, thus allowing the nurse who is using substances to continue to put themselves at risk. The nurse is also at risk for endangering the lives of those in their care. In light of the duty of professional responsibility nurses can ask themselves the difficult questions: if they have ever co-signed controlled substance "wastes" that were not actually witnessed, if they have ever corrected the narcotic count to account for a discrepancy, or if they have ever excused or rationalized behaviour that might be related to substance use. While not an exhaustive list, Box 18.7 can be used to assess whether there is a specific drug diversion or a potential misuse of drugs for personal gain in the workplace by a nurse colleague.

Fortunately, most large employers have Employee Assistance Programs, confidential counselling initiatives that are available at no cost, as a viable option through which to seek help for a developing substance-use issue before or after it becomes a performance and health issue. Though criticized for flawed and AA-dominated approaches, formal treatment programs for professionals experiencing addictions have been developed in most Canadian provinces (Ross et al., 2019). Some provincial and territorial professional nursing associations support nurses who are experiencing substance use or addiction and may withhold any disciplinary action if treatment is sought. The aims of supportive policy and specific treatment programs for nurses are to protect patients and to keep the nurse in active practice (perhaps with limitations) or return the nurse to practice after suspension and professional help. More severe consequences, for example, restricting or withholding the ability of the nurse to provide direct patient care, are put into place for nurses who show signs of ongoing impairment.

> **BOX 18.7 Signs of Workplace Diversion of Drugs**
>
> - Repeated attendance issues with a pattern (sick after days off); calling in sick a lot
> - Volunteering for overtime
> - Moving to a position where there is less visibility or supervision
> - Arriving late for work, leaving early
> - Long breaks or lunch hours; sometimes without telling colleagues
> - Frequent or unexplained disappearances from the unit
> - Excessive number of incidents/mistakes
> - Failing to have narcotic wastage observed/co-signed; or performing narcotic counts alone
> - Tampering of packages or vials
> - Waiting until alone to open narcotic cupboard and/or draw up medication
> - Using fictional patient names on narcotic records
> - Frequent revisions/discrepancies on narcotic records
> - Inconsistencies between narcotic records and patients' medication administration records (MARs)
> - Frequent reports of lost or wasted medications
> - Asking to be assigned to patients receiving large amounts of pain medication
>
> **Source:** British Columbia College of Nursing Professionals. (2020). *Signs and symptoms of possible substance abuse.* Retrieved from https://www.bccnm.ca/RN/learning/dutytoreport/drug_diversion/Pages/signs_symptoms.aspx

Evaluation

Favourable treatment outcome is judged by increased use of harm reduction strategies, fewer lapses and relapses, increased lengths of time of abstinence (if not following a harm reduction approach), acceptable occupational functioning, improved family relationships, and ultimately the ability to sustain healthy relationships and behaviour. Although continuous monitoring and evaluation increase the chances for prolonged success, it must be stated that no single approach has been found to be universally successful in the treatment of those misusing psychoactive substances. Research is conclusive, however, that intervention is superior to no treatment.

Given that addiction is a biopsychosocial phenomenon, an integrated approach of several types of helping modalities will be more successful than recourse to any one alone. Two things are certain: that the treatment used must be tailored to meet the specific needs of each individual and that no patient should be forced into a particular type of rehabilitation merely because of the nurse's convenience or prejudicial choice. Critical factors to always consider are:

- The patient choosing to enter treatment with an expectation of being helped to change their behaviour, thus having a motivation to change
- The credibility of the technique being used to both the nurse and the patient
- Consistent application of an empirically proven technique
- The ability to create optimism for a successful outcome
- The ability to create a foundation so that change may occur
- The nurse's discretion, flexibility, and emotional support
- The ability of the nurse to create a supportive environment
- The choice of harm reduction or abstinence

Thus regardless of the approach used by the nurse, it should always be consistently applied and patient centred such that the focus is on the individual in relation to their needs and wants, both perceived and actual. Evidence from decades of research has slowly begun to indicate that the actual intervention used, while important, is far less vital than the process (Hubble et al., 2010; Smedslund et al., 2011). The process includes the nurse–patient relationship, patient expectations, the model used, and extratherapeutic variables (other factors) such as the patient's attributes, the patient's social system and social environment, and the treatment environment (Figure 18.6). The personal attributes of the nurse, the nurse's background, understanding, and patience all play significant roles in the success of the treatment, as the better the reported nurse–patient relationship at all stages of treatment is, the better the outcome for the patient and the patient system. As well, rather than the types of treatment, what tends to matter to a greater degree is the nurse's capacity to structure the treatment so that, regardless of the method or model used, the patient feels heard and supported and that a sense of hope is instilled in the helping relationship (Chamodraka et al., 2017; Parkin & Swift, 2017). The patient's expectations, beliefs, and desires determines a great deal of what can occur and contributes a great deal to the final outcome of treatment. Research indicates that what motivates people to change is positive thoughts, not negative ones. The more one focuses on problems, the more stuck people feel. It is hope that causes people to change, not the pain of addiction or the losses it brings them.

KEY POINTS TO REMEMBER

- Substance use and dependence occur on a continuum, and addiction develops over a period of time and is distinct from compulsive behaviours.
- The cause of substance use disorders is a combination of biological, psychological, and social/environmental factors.
- Assessment of patients with substance use disorders needs to be comprehensive, aimed at identifying common medical and psychiatric comorbidities but also considering the social context of the patient.
- Patients with concurrent disorders have more severe symptoms, experience more crises, require longer treatment for successful outcomes, and need to be properly assessed and integrated into both treatment systems as per their individual needs.
- Substance use disorders affect the patient's entire family system.
- Assessment of readiness for change is an essential part of the assessment process and can support appropriate treatment strategies.
- Lapse and relapse are expected stages of change from addiction, and treatment needs to include a significant focus on teaching relapse prevention.
- Motivational interviewing, a form of intervention, can lead to appropriate treatment strategies and improved outcomes.
- There is an extensive addiction continuum of care that a nurse should become familiar with, including both professional and mutual aid resources.
- Nurses need to be aware of their own feelings about substance use so that they can provide empathy and motivate change for patients.
- Nurses should be vigilant for signs of impairment and addiction in colleagues to ensure patient safety and referral to treatment for the nurse experiencing an addiction.

CRITICAL THINKING

1. The addiction field is a very ambiguous one, filled with myth, belief, half-truths, and ignorance. What are your core beliefs, perception, and knowledge about what addiction is? How has your definition of addiction changed after reading this chapter?

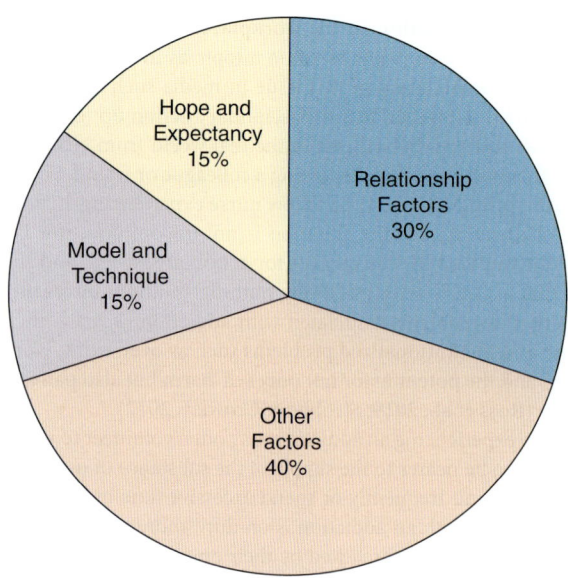

Fig. 18.6 Contributing factors to positive addiction treatment outcome. (**Source**: Adapted from Hubble, M., Duncan, B., Miller, S., & Wampold, B. [2010]. Introduction. In B. Duncan, S. Miller, B. Wampold, & M. Hubble (Eds.), *The heart and soul of change: Delivering what works in therapy* [2nd ed., pp. 23–46]. Washington, DC: American Psychological Association.)

2. Write a paragraph describing reactions you might have to a drug-dependent patient to whom you are assigned.
   a. Would your response be different depending on the substance (alcohol vs. heroin or cannabis vs. cocaine)? Give reasons for your answers.
   b. Would your response be different if the substance-dependent person were a professional colleague? How?
3. Aline is a 15-year-old girl who has started using heroin.
   a. When Aline asks you why she needs to take more and more to get "high," how would you explain to her the concept of tolerance?
   b. If she had recently used heroin, what would you find on assessment of physical and psychological–perceptual signs and symptoms?
   c. If she were brought to the emergency department for overdosing on heroin, what would be the emergency care? What might be effective long-term care?
4. Roberto is a 45-year-old mechanic. He has a 20-year history of heavy drinking, and he says he wants to quit.
   a. Role-play with a classmate an initial assessment. Identify the kinds of information you would need to have in order to plan holistic care.
   b. Roberto decided to stop drinking abruptly. He is now in the emergency department with delirium tremens. What are the dangers for him? What are the appropriate medical interventions?
   c. What are some possible treatment alternatives for Roberto when he is safely detoxified? How would you explain to him the usefulness and function of Alcoholics Anonymous? What are some additional treatment options that might be useful to Robert? What are available as referrals for him in your community?
5. Given the legalization of cannabis and the normalization of alcohol in Canada, how would you discuss the pros and cons of drug use with a teenager who has begun to experiment with substances?

CHAPTER REVIEW

1. Addiction is best explained as
   a. Occurring with games of chance such as roulette or poker
   b. A chronic brain disease
   c. A biopsychosocial phenomenon
   d. The domain of neurobiologists
2. The nurse is caring for a patient with an addictive disorder who is currently drug free. The patient is experiencing repeated occurrences of vivid, frightening images and thoughts. Which term would the nurse use to document this finding?
   a. Tolerance
   b. Flashbacks
   c. Withdrawal
   d. Physical dependency
3. The condition most concerning for the nurse who is caring for a patient who misuses alcohol would be
   a. Cirrhosis of the liver
   b. Suicidal potential
   c. Wernicke's encephalopathy
   d. Korsakoffs syndrome
4. Which patient response to the question, "Have you ever drunk more alcohol or used more drugs than you meant to?" should immediately cause the nurse to assess further?
   a. "No, I have never used drugs or alcohol."
   b. "I have drunk alcohol before but have never let myself get drunk."
   c. "I figured you'd ask me about that."
   d. "Yes, I did that once and will never do it again."
5. Which patient behaviours should the nurse suspect as being related to alcohol withdrawal?
   a. Hyperalert state, jerky movements, easily startled
   b. Tachycardia, diaphoresis, elevated blood pressure
   c. Peripheral vascular collapse, electrolyte imbalance
   d. Paranoid delusions, fever, fluctuating levels of consciousness
6. A patient at your community mental health centre smokes up to half a pack of cigarettes daily but has tried, with limited success, to cut back over the past 2 weeks. Today he asked the pharmacist about the various products that could aid his attempts to quit smoking in time for him to manage a long overseas flight next month and travel with friends who are allergic to smoke. What phase of change is this patient demonstrating?
   a. Pre-contemplation
   b. Contemplation
   c. Preparation
   d. Action

REFERENCES

American Psychiatric Association. (2018). *Practice guidelines for the pharmacological treatment of patients with alcohol use disorders*. Washington: APA.

Ashton, H. (2013). *Benzodiazepines: How they work and how to withdraw*. The Ashton Manual Supplement. Retrieved from www.benzo.org.uk/ashsupp11.htm

Brancato, A., Castelli, V., Cavallaro, A., Lavanco, G., Plescia, F., & Cannizzaro, C. (2018). Pre-conceptional and peri-gestational maternal binge alcohol drinking produces inheritance of mood disturbances and alcohol vulnerability in the adolescent offspring. *Frontiers in Psychiatry, 9*, 150.

Brown, R., & Trickey, H. (2018). *Devising and communicating public health alcohol guidance for expectant and new mothers: A scoping report*. London: Alcohol Research UK.

Brownbill, K., & Etienne, M. (2017). Understanding the ultimate oppression: Alcohol and drug addiction in Native land. In R. Csiernik, & W. Rowe (Eds.), *Responding to the oppression of addiction* (3rd ed.). Toronto: Canadian Scholars Press.

Canadian Institute for Health Information. (2019). *Hospital morbidity database and Ontario mental health reporting system, 2017–2018*. Ottawa: Canadian Institute for Health Information.

Canadian Nurses Association. (2017). *Code of ethics for registered nurses*. Ottawa: Author.

Canadian Substance Use Costs and Harms Scientific Working Group. (2018). *Canadian substance use costs and harms in provinces and territories (2007–2014)*. Ottawa: Canadian Institute for Substance Use Research, University of Victoria and the Canadian Centre on Substance Use and Addiction.

Carrière, G., Bougie, B., & Kohen, D. (2018). *Acute care hospitalizations for mental and behavioural disorders among First Nations people*. Ottawa: Statistics Canada.

Carter, R., Wainwright, H., Molteno, C., Georgieff, M., Dodge, N., Warton, F., Meintjes, E., Jacobson, J., & Jacobson, S. (2016). Alcohol, methamphetamine, and marijuana exposure have distinct effects on the human placenta. *Alcoholism: Clinical and Experimental Research, 40*(4), 753–764.

Chamodraka, M., Fitzpatrick, M., & Janzen, J. (2017). Hope as empowerment model: A client-based perspective on the process of hope development. *The Journal of Positive Psychology, 12*(3), 232–245.

Chan, B., Freeman, M., Kondo, K., Ayers, C., Montgomery, J., Paynter, R., & Kansagara, D. (2019). Pharmacotherapy for methamphetamine/amphetamine use disorder—A systematic review and meta-analysis. *Addiction, 114*(12), 2122–2136.

Colon-Perez, L., Tran, K., Thompson, K., Pace, M., Blum, K., Goldberger, B., Gold, M., Bruijnzeel, A., Setlow, B., & Febo, M. (2016). The psychoactive designer drug and bath salt constituent MDPV causes widespread disruption of brain functional connectivity. *Neuropsychopharmacology, 41*(9), 2352–2365.

Csiernik, R. (2019). *The essential guide to psychoactive drugs in Canada*. Toronto: Canadian Scholars Press.

Csiernik, R. (2021). *Substance use and misuse: Everything matters* (3rd ed.). Toronto: Canadian Scholars Press.

Cunningham, K., Howell, L., & Anastasio, N. (2020). *Serotonin neurobiology in cocaine use disorder*. In Handbook of behavioral neuroscience (Vol. 31, pp. 745–802). Oxford: Elsevier.

Denis-Lalonde, D., Lind, C., & Estefan, A. (2019). Beyond the buzzword: A concept analysis of harm reduction. *Research and Theory for Nursing Practice, 33*(4), 310–323.

Dole, V., & Nyswander, M. (1965). A medical treatment for diacetylmorphine (heroin) addiction. *Journal of the American Medical Association, 193*(8), 646–650.

Eichner, E. R. (2014). Fatal caffeine overdose and other risks from dietary supplements. *Current Sports Medicine Reports, 13*(6), 353–354.

Ewing, J. A. (1984). Detecting alcoholism: The CAGE questionnaire. *Journal of the American Medical Association, 252*, 1905–1907.

Fagerstrom, K. (2018). A comparison of dependence across different types of nicotine containing products and coffee. *International Journal of Environmental Research and Public Health, 15*(8), 1609.

Foertsch, M., Winter, J., Rhoades, A., Martin, L., Droege, C., & Ernst, N. (2019). Recognition, assessment, and pharmacotherapeutic treatment of alcohol withdrawal syndrome in the intensive care unit. *Critical Care Nursing Quarterly, 42*(1), 12–29.

Froehlich, J., Nicholson, E., & Dilley, J. (2019). Dual therapy for alcohol use disorders: Combining Naltrexone with other medications. In *Neuroscience of alcohol* (pp. 653–660). Cambridge: Academic Press.

Ghosh, A., Coakley, R., Ghio, A., Muhlebach, M., Esther Jr., C., Alexis, N., & Tarran, R. (2019). Chronic e-cigarette use increases neutrophil elastase and matrix metalloprotease levels in the lungs. *American Journal of Respiratory and Critical Care Medicine, 200*(11), 1392–1401. https://doi.org/10.1164/rccm.201903-0615OC

Government of Canada, Department of Justice. (2019). *Cannabis legalization and regulation*. Retrieved from https://www.justice.gc.ca/eng/cj-jp/cannabis/

Hajek, P., Phillips-Waller, A., Przulj, D., Pesola, F., Myers Smith, K., Bisal, N., Li, J., Parrott, S., Sasieni, P., Dawkins, L., Ross, L., Goniewica, M., Wu, Q., & McRobbie, H. (2019). A randomized trial of e-cigarettes versus nicotine-replacement therapy. *New England Journal of Medicine, 380*(7), 629–637.

Hancock, S., & McKim, W. (2018). *Drugs and behaviour: An introduction to behavioral pharmacology* (8th ed.). New York: Pearson.

Health Canada. (2018). *Canadian Tobacco, Alcohol and Drugs Survey (CTADS): Summary of results for 2017*. Ottawa: Health Canada.

Health Canada. (2019). *The Canadian student tobacco, alcohol and drugs survey 2018-2019*. Ottawa: Health Canada.

Hickman, M., Steer, C., Tilling, K., Lim, A., Marsden, J., Millar, T., Strang, J., Tefler, M., Vicerman, P., & Macleod, J. (2018). The impact of buprenorphine and methadone on mortality: A primary care cohort study in the United Kingdom. *Addiction, 113*(8), 1461–1476.

Hill, D. (2016). *Heroin-assisted treatment*. In S. Boslaugh (Ed.), *The SAGE encyclopedia of pharmacology and society* (Vol. 4, pp. 694–696). Thousand Oaks: SAGE Publications Ltd.

Hop Wo, N., Anderson, K., Wylie, L., & MacDougall, A. (2019). The prevalence of distress, depression, anxiety, and substance use issues among Indigenous post-secondary students in Canada. *Transcultural Psychiatry, 57*(2), 263–274. https://doi.org/10.1177/1363461519861824

Hubble, M., Duncan, B., Miller, S., & Wampold, B. (2010). Introduction. In B. Duncan, S. Miller, B. Wampold, & M. Hubble (Eds.), *The heart and soul of change: Delivering what works in therapy* (2nd ed., pp. 23–46). Washington, DC: American Psychological Association.

Jansson, L. (2018). Maternal alcohol use during lactation and child development. *Pediatrics, 142*(2), e20181377.

Johnson, B., Rosenthal, N., Capece, J., Wiegand, F., Mao, L., Bevers, K., McKay, A., Ait-Daoud, N., Anton, R., Ciraulo, D., Kranzler, H., Mann, K., O'Malley, S., & Swift, R. (2007). Topiramate for treating alcohol dependence: A randomized controlled trial. *Journal of the American Medical Association, 298*(14), 1641–1651.

Kennedy, M., Hayashi, K., Milloy, M., Wood, E., & Kerr, T. (2019). Supervised injection facility use and all-cause mortality among people who inject drugs in Vancouver, Canada: A cohort study. *PLoS Med, 16*(11), e1002964. https://journals.plos.org/plosmedicine/article?id=10.1371/journal.pmed.1002964

Kerensky, T., & Walley, A. (2017). Opioid overdose prevention and naloxone rescue kits: What we know and what we don't know. *Addiction Science and Clinical Practice, 12*(4), 1–7. https://doi.org/10.1186/s13722-016-0068-3

Khan, S. (2017). *Concurrent mental and substance use disorders in Canada*. Ottawa: Statistics Canada.

Kougiali, Z., Fasulo, A., Needs, A., & Van Laar, D. (2017). Planting the seeds of change: Directionality in the narrative construction of recovery from addiction. *Psychology & Health, 32*(6), 639–664.

Koval, R., Willett, J., & Briggs, J. (2018). Potential benefits and risks of high-nicotine e-cigarettes. *Journal of the American Medical Association, 320*(14), 1429–1430.

Lee, S., Sirieix, C., Nattie, E., & Li, A. (2018). Pre- and early postnatal nicotine exposure exacerbates autoresuscitation failure in serotonin-deficient rat neonates. *The Journal of Physiology, 596*(23), 5977–5991.

Levy, D., Borland, R., Lindblom, E., Goniewicz, M., Meza, R., Holford, T., Zhe, Y., Lua, Y., O'Connor, R., Niaura, R., & Abrams, D. (2018). Potential deaths averted in USA by replacing cigarettes with e-cigarettes. *Tobacco Control, 27*(1), 18–25.

Lewis, L., & Jarvis, L. (2019). Undergraduate nursing students' experiences and attitudes towards working with patients with opioid use disorder in the clinical setting: A qualitative content analysis. *Nurse Education Today, 73*(1), 17–22.

Manzoli, L., Flacco, M., Ferrante, M., La Vecchia, C., Siliquini, R., Ricciardi, W., Marzuillo, C., Villari, P., & Fiore, M. (2017). Cohort study of electronic cigarette use: Effectiveness and safety at 24 months. *Tobacco Control, 26*(3), 284–292.

Marlatt, G., & Witkiewitz, K. (2005). Relapse prevention for alcohol and drug problems. *Relapse Prevention: Maintenance Strategies in the Treatment of Addictive Behaviors, 2*, 1–44.

McDonald, R., Campbell, N., & Strang, J. (2017). Twenty years of take-home naloxone for the prevention of overdose deaths from heroin and other opioids: Conception and maturation. *Drug and Alcohol Dependence, 178*(1), 176–187.

McKeganey, N., Russell, C., & Haseen, F. (2019). Vaping and the number of cigarettes not now smoked: An additional means of assessing the public health impact of e-cigarettes. *Journal of Pulmonary and Respiratory Medicine, 3*, 104. https://doi.org/10.29011/PROA-104.100004

Menard-Kocik, J., & Caine, V. (2019). Obstetrical nurses' perspectives of pregnant women who use illicit substances and their provision of care: A thematic analysis. *Canadian Journal of Nursing Research, 53*(1), 47–55. https://doi.org/10.1177/0844562119870419

Miller, W. R. (1983). Motivational interviewing with problem drinkers. *Behavioural Psychotherapy, 11*, 147–172.

Miller, W. R., & Rollnick, S. (2002). *Motivational interviewing: Preparing people for change* (2nd ed.). New York: Guilford Press.

Moorhead, S., Johnson, M., Maas, M. L., & Swanson, E. (2018). *Nursing Outcomes Classification (NOC)-E-Book: Measurement of health outcomes*. Elsevier Health Sciences.

Parkin, S., & Swift, J. (2017). Utilizing patient hope and outcome expectations to facilitate treatment gains. *Medical Research Archives, 5*(6). Retrieved from https://journals.ke-i.org/mra/article/view/1337

Parsh, B. (2019). How to recognize caffeine overdose. *Nursing, 49*(4), 52–55.

Prochaska, J. O., & DiClemente, C. C. (1984). *The transtheoretical approach: Towards a systematic eclectic framework*. Homewood: Dow Jones Irwin.

Reece, S., Morgan, C., Parascandola, M., & Siddiqi, K. (2018). Second-hand smoke exposure during pregnancy: A cross-sectional analysis of data from Demographic and Health Survey from 30 low-income and middle-income countries. *Tobacco Control, 28*(4), 420–426.

Rose, A., & Jones, A. (2018). Baclofen: Its effectiveness in reducing harmful drinking, craving, and negative mood. A meta-analysis. *Addiction, 113*(8), 1396–1406.

Ross, C., Jakubec, S. L., Berry, N., & Smye, V. (2019). The business of managing nurses' substance use problems. *Nursing Inquiry, 27*(1). Retrieved from https://onlinelibrary.wiley.com/doi/full/10.1111/nin.12324

Rowe, W., & Rapp, L (2017). Supervised injection sites: Harm reduction and health promotion. In R. Csiernik, & W. Rowe

(Eds.), *Responding to the oppression of addiction: Canadian social work perspectives* (3rd ed., pp. 48–59). Toronto: Canadian Scholars' Press.

Royal Commission on Aboriginal Peoples. (1996). *Report of the Royal Commission on Aboriginal Peoples.* Ottawa: Indian and Northern Affairs Canada.

Sachdev, R., Garg, D., & Singh, G. (2018). Nicotine replacement therapy—Effective tool in smoking cessation: A short review. *Dental Science, 7*(7), 47–48.

Selzer, M. L. (1971). The Michigan Alcoholism Screening Test (MAST): The quest for a new diagnostic instrument. *American Journal of Psychiatry, 127,* 1653–1658.

Singh, M., Keer, D., Klimas, J., Wood, E., & Werb, D. (2016). Topiramate for cocaine dependence: A systematic review and meta-analysis of randomized controlled trials. *Addiction, 111*(8), 1337–1346.

Sinha, P., Garg, A., Khanna, P., & Khanna, A. (2019). Management of chronic mental illnesses and substance use disorders. In Information Resources Management Association (Ed.), *Substance abuse and addiction: Breakthroughs in research and practice* (pp. 1–23). IGI Global.

Smedslund, G., Berg, R., Hammerstrøm, K., Steiro, A., Leiknes, K. A., Dahl, H. M., & Karlsen, K. (2011). Motivational interviewing for substance abuse. *The Cochrane Database of Systematic Reviews*(5), CD008063. https://doi.org/10.1002/14651858.CD008063.pub2

Special Advisory Committee on the Epidemic of Opioid Overdoses. (2019). *National report: Opioid-related harms in Canada.* Ottawa: Public Health Agency of Canada. Retrieved from https://health-infobase.canada.ca/substance-related-harms/opioids

Statistics Canada. (2018). *Police-reported crime statistics in Canada, 2018.* Retrieved from https://www150.statcan.gc.ca/n1/pub/85-002-x/2019001/article/00013-eng.htm

Statistics Canada. (2019). *Prevalence of cannabis consumption in Canada.* Table 36-10-597-01. Retrieved from https://www150.statcan.gc.ca/t1/tbl1/en/tv.action?pid=3610059701

Statistics Canada. (2020). *Canadian cannabis survey 2020.* Retrieved from https://www.canada.ca/en/health-canada/services/drugs-medication/cannabis/research-data/canadian-cannabis-survey-2020-summary.html#f5

Statistics Canada. (2021). *Opioid- and stimulant-related harms in Canada.* Retrieved from https://health-infobase.canada.ca/substance-related-harms/opioids-stimulants/

Strobbe, S., & Crowley, M. (2017). Substance use among nurses and nursing students: A joint position statement of the Emergency Nurses Association and the International Nurses Society on Addictions. *Journal of Addictions Nursing, 28*(2), 104–106.

Teitelbaum, L., & Mullen, B. (2000). Validity of the MAST in psychiatric settings: A META-analytic integration. *Journal of Studies on Alcohol, 61*(2), 254–261.

Truth and Reconciliation Commission of Canada. (2015). *Truth and Reconciliation Commission of Canada.* House of Commons.

Volkow, N., Wise, R., & Baler, R. (2017). The dopamine motive system: Implications for drug and food addiction. *Nature Reviews Neuroscience, 18,* 741–752.

Wang, R., Shen, Y. L., Hausknecht, K. A., Chang, L., Haj-Dahmane, S., Vezina, P., & Shen, R. Y. (2019). Prenatal ethanol exposure increases risk of psychostimulant addiction. *Behavioural Brain Research, 356,* 51–61.

Witkiewitz, K., Hallgren, K. A., Kranzler, H. R., Mann, K. F., Hasin, D. S., Falk, D. E., Litten, R. Z., O'Malley, S. S., & Anton, R. F. (2017). Clinical validation of reduced alcohol consumption after treatment for alcohol dependence using the World Health Organization risk drinking levels. *Alcoholism, Clinical and Experimental Research, 41*(1), 179–186. https://doi.org/10.1111/acer.13272

Wheeler, K., & Phillips, K. E. (2019). The development of trauma and resilience competencies for nursing education. *Journal of the American Psychiatric Nurses Association, 27*(4), 322–333. https://doi.org/10.1177/1078390319878779

19

Personality Disorders

Cheryl L. Pollard
Originating US chapter by Margaret Jordan Halter, Christine A. Tackett

 http://evolve.elsevier.com/Canada/Varcarolis/psychiatric/

OBJECTIVES

1. Analyze the interaction of biological determinants and psychosocial stress factors in the etiology of personality disorders.
2. Identify and distinguish among the three clusters of personality disorders.
3. Identify 10 personality disorders.
4. Describe the emotional and clinical needs of nurses and other staff when working with patients who meet criteria for personality disorders.
5. Formulate a nursing diagnosis for each of the personality disorders.
6. Discuss two nursing outcomes for patients with borderline personality disorder.
7. Plan basic nursing care interventions for a patient with impulsive, aggressive, or manipulative behaviours.
8. Identify the role of the advanced-practice nurse when working with patients with personality disorders.

KEY TERMS AND CONCEPTS

anger control assistance
callousness
dialectical behaviour therapy
diathesis–stress model
emotional dysregulation
emotional lability
impulse-control training
impulsivity
limit setting
persona
personality
personality disorders
personality trait
personality type
splitting
temperament

Often, we meet someone and think, "That's quite a strange person" or "What an unusual character." When we make evaluations such as these about other people, we are reacting to their personalities. *Personality* comes from the Latin word **persona**, which means "mask" and may refer to the person as other people see them. What is a personality? **Personality** is an individual's characteristic patterns of relatively permanent thoughts, feelings, and behaviours that define the quality of experiences and relationships. In mental health nursing there are two key underlying concepts related to an individual's personality. They are personality trait and personality type. A **personality trait** is a stable characteristic of a person, such as neuroticism, extraversion, openness to experience, agreeableness, and conscientiousness. These can be compared to personality states, which are temporary behaviours and feelings. A **personality type** is a way to describe a cluster of traits. For example, a person with an authoritarian personality has traits that relate to maintaining orderliness, command, and power. In contrast, a person's character involves defining an individual's integrity.

A personality is considered unhealthy when interpersonal and social relationships and functioning are consistently maladaptive, complicated, or dysphoric. We know that personality can be protective for a person in times of difficulty but may also be a liability if one's personality results in ongoing relationship problems or leads to emotional distress on a regular basis.

Until quite recently, we believed that personalities were fairly fixed entities. More contemporary views challenge this notion. Rather than unchanging patterns of behaviours and thoughts, the rate of personality's change slows over time but does not cease (Newton-Howes et al., 2015). If personality traits evolve continually across the lifespan, we have an opportunity to develop and support more adaptive functioning and social relationships.

 HOW A NURSE HELPED ME
My Reality Check

I was 22 and going through a bitter divorce. I was very angry and felt hopeless. Becoming more depressed, I had thoughts about harming myself and my husband (soon to be ex-husband). I was drinking to help numb my anger. One night, I was drunk and cut my wrists. As I lay bleeding in the bathtub, I phoned my parents to say goodbye. They phoned the ambulance, and I was taken to the hospital and admitted to the "psych" unit. My parents had often told me that I did not make good decisions for myself. I chose the wrong kind of man and the wrong kinds of friends, drank too much, and spent too much. Behind my back, my friends would say that I had a "personality problem." I didn't expect to hear the nurses tell me I had a personality problem, too. I hated being in hospital, but my family felt it was the best thing for me, as they were at their wits' end with me (well, that's what they told me).

I felt I was fairly bright and thought that I would be able to beat the system. I didn't feel I needed any help, and I certainly didn't need to be in hospital. Manipulation was the key: I knew how to sweet-talk to get my way—well, it worked with my family! I went with the routine; I played by the rules, and, yes, I was able to justify my behaviour to the doctor, social worker, and most of the nurses. I behaved the way I did because I had been abandoned. The divorce was my husband's fault, not mine. My parents didn't understand the emotional turmoil I was going through. I had no support. My nurse applied what I felt were strict rules: if I wanted anything, I had to go through her; I couldn't ask the other nurses. This gave me only more reason to try to manipulate my nurse and play the "sweet card." This game, as I referred to it, went on for weeks, but I finally realized she was always one step ahead of me.

My nurse would sit down and talk to me about how I showed patterns of being overly dramatic and displayed erratic behaviour. She gave me some examples of her claim, something I found hard to take, and I became quietly resistive to her "talks." But now, looking back many years later, I see that her description seems fairly close to how I acted. It took me a long time, with two more admissions to hospital (because of self-harming), to understand some of my behaviours. There were other discussions, or as my nurse called them, "therapy," about my manipulative behaviours. I blamed my parents, my friends, and my ex-husband for my behaviour, and I still do to an extent. But I have learned to control my blaming and emotional behaviours to a degree.

I never said thank you to that particular nurse, who gave me a "reality check," as I didn't think the sessions were in my best interest at the time. But I now realize that the nurse was helping me take control of my life and provided me with various coping skills that I have since applied in my interactions with others. I still have good and bad days, but I know that this particular nurse helped guide me to be stronger and more controlled. I'm now a person who takes responsibility for her behaviours, something I didn't realize she was teaching me through those "therapy" sessions.

CLINICAL PICTURE

Individuals with **personality disorders** display significant challenges in self-identity or self-concept, they have problems with empathy and have difficulty establishing healthy, stable relationships. Individuals with personality disorders believe that the problems originate outside of themselves. They believe that if others behaved differently toward them or treated them differently, then all their problems would be solved. In the treatment of personality disorders, a key factor to success is that the person with the personality disorder recognizes and takes responsibility for the contributions they make to their relational and social difficulties. Treating personality disorders is difficult and complex, as people with these disorders have difficulty recognizing or owning the fact that their difficulties are problems of their personality. People with personality disorders experience intrapsychic pain. At times this pain may be so severe and their coping skills so limited that death may seem like a way of communicating their pain or may be viewed as a way to escape their difficulties. People with personality disorders may injure themselves. The life expectancy of a person living with a personality disorder is approximately 9 to 13 years shorter than people without a personality disorder (Potvin et al., 2019).

Judgements about an individual's personality functioning must take into account the person's ethnic, cultural, and social background. Patients who differ from the majority culture or the culture of the clinician may be at risk for overdiagnosis of a personality disorder. Therefore it is important to obtain additional information from others who are knowledgeable about the particular cultural or ethnic norms before determining the presence of a personality disorder.

> ⚡ **SAFETY TIP**
>
> Thinking about personality as being made up of self-identity and self-concept is an important consideration when interacting with a person with a personality disorder. How they form opinions, and what actions they take, are influenced by how they see themselves in relation to the world. This impacts how the therapeutic relationship can be established and used. It is essential that the healthcare team establish parameters to help staff deal with "splitting" behaviours.

According to the American Psychiatric Association (APA, 2013), there are 10 personality disorders. These 10 disorders are grouped into three clusters of similar behaviour patterns and personality traits. These clusters are:

Cluster A: Individuals with these disorders share characteristics of eccentric behaviours, such as social isolation and detachment. They may also display perception distortions, unusual levels of suspiciousness, magical thinking, and cognitive impairment.
- Paranoid personality disorder
- Schizoid personality disorder
- Schizotypal personality disorder

Cluster B: People living with cluster B personality disorders show patterns of responding to life demands with dramatic, emotional, or erratic behaviour. Problems with impulse control, emotion processing and regulation, and interpersonal difficulties characterize this cluster of disorders. Insight into these issues is generally limited. To get their needs met, individuals with cluster B personality disorders may resort to behaviours that are considered desperate or entitled, including acting out, committing anti-social acts, or manipulating people and circumstances.
- Borderline personality disorder (BPD)
- Narcissistic personality disorder
- Histrionic personality disorder
- Anti-social personality disorder

Cluster C: An individual with these types of personality disorders will demonstrate a consistent patterns of anxious and fearful behaviours, rigid patterns of social shyness, hypersensitivity, need for orderliness, and relationship dependency.
- Avoidant personality disorder
- Dependent personality disorder
- Obsessive-compulsive personality disorder

In this chapter we begin with an overview of personality disorders, including epidemiology, comorbidity, and risk factors. Afterward, the personality disorders are presented along with prevalence, characteristic pathological responses, nursing care guidelines, and medical treatments. A vignette is provided to illustrate each of these disorders. After reviewing these disorders, application of the nursing process is described.

EPIDEMIOLOGY

Many patients receiving inpatient or outpatient psychiatric care have co-occurring mental illnesses. Personality disorders are often accompanied by experiences of depression and anxiety. The lifetime prevalence of personality disorders is between 4% and 15% (Potvin et al., 2019). While narcissistic and schizotypal personality disorders (STPDs) are relatively rare, borderline, avoidant, and obsessive-compulsive personality disorders have been established by meta-analyses (which pull together the best and most relevant research) to be common among both community and clinical populations (Keefe et al., 2020).

Culture has an influence on the rate of diagnosing personality disorders. For example, personality disorders are more often diagnosed in high-income countries when compared to low to moderate-income countries (Winsper et al., 2019). Differences may reflect the view of personality and behaviour as deviant rather than normal in a particular culture and within certain study methods; or, it may reflect better diagnosing practices or a system that has more resources to assist people with personality disorders. Further studies are needed to better understand the influence of ethnicity and race on the development and experience of personality disorders.

COMORBIDITY

Personality disorders frequently co-occur with disorders of mood and eating, anxiety, and substance use. Personality disorders often amplify emotional dysregulation, a term that describes poorly modulated mood characterized by mood swings. Individuals with emotion regulation problems have ongoing difficulty managing painful emotions in ways that are healthy and effective.

The aging process has some effect on the prevalence of personality disorders. The dramatic, emotional, or erratic cluster B disorders may mute with age as individuals become less impulsive. This dampening may be due to a general tuning down of neurotransmitters (Rosowsky et al., 2013). Other disorders such as obsessive-compulsive personality disorder or paranoid personality disorder may worsen with age, perhaps due to anxiety regarding declining sensory and cognitive capacity.

Personality traits are amplified during the experience of a crisis and any illness; therefore it is pre-mature and not in the best interest of the individual for a personality disorder to be diagnosed during the active phase of another illness, especially a psychiatric episode or major stressful life event such as grief and loss or trauma.

ETIOLOGY

Personality disorders are the result of complex biological and psychosocial phenomena that are influenced by multi-faceted variables involving genetic, neurobiological, neurochemical, and environmental factors.

Biological Factors

Genetics

Several possible hypotheses attempt to account for the personality differences among people in the same family (Henry et al., 2018). The relationship among genes and personality traits is a complex one. For example, a child's temperament can elicit different responses from family members. Individual children may perceive family experiences in unique ways and therefore respond differently from other family members. Children are also affected by forces outside the family that influence personality development. It may be that personality is influenced even by the intrauterine environment, although there are fewer data to support this hypothesis.

Neurobiology and Neurochemistry

Biological influences on personality expression are a promising area of research in understanding these disorders. Influences on the development of personality disorders probably incorporate a complex interaction of genetics, neurobiology, and neurochemistry. The chemical neurotransmitter theory proposes that certain neurotransmitters, including neurohormones, may regulate and influence temperament (Render & Jansen, 2019). Research in brain imaging has also revealed some differences in the size and function of specific structures of the brain in people with some personality disorders.

Psychological Factors

Several psychological theories may help to explain the development of personality disorders. Learning theory emphasizes that children develop maladaptive responses based on modelling of or reinforcement by important people in the child's life. Cognitive theories emphasize the role of beliefs and assumptions in creating emotional and behavioural responses that influence one's experiences within the family environment.

Psychoanalytic theory focuses on the use of primitive defence mechanisms by individuals with personality disorders. Defence mechanisms such as repression, suppression, regression, undoing, and splitting have been identified as dominant (Kernberg, 1985). The role of psychoanalytic theory, while historically relevant and interesting, is not confirmable through evidence-informed research methods.

Environmental Factors

Behavioural genetics research has shown that about half of the variance accounting for personality traits emerges from the environment (Render & Jansen, 2019). These findings suggest that while the family environment is influential on development, there are other environmental factors besides upbringing that shape an individual's personality. One need only think about the individual differences among siblings raised together to illustrate this point.

Childhood neglect and trauma have been established as risk factors for personality disorders (Henry et al., 2018). This association has been linked to possible neurotransmitter changes in response to early life stress and emotional reactivity (Haliczer et al., 2020).

System Factors

Diathesis–Stress Model

The diathesis–stress model is a general theory that explains psychopathology using a systems approach. This theory helps us understand how personality disorders emerge from the multi-faceted factors of biology and environment (Kender, 2020). *Diathesis* refers to genetic and biological vulnerabilities and includes personality traits and temperament. Temperament is our tendency to respond to challenges in predictable ways. Examples of descriptors of temperament may be *laid back*, referring to a calm temperament, or *uptight*, referring to an anxious temperament. These characteristics remain stable throughout a person's life. In this model *stress* refers to immediate influences on personality such as the physical, social, psychological, and emotional environment. *Stress* also includes what happened in the past, such as growing up in one's family with exposure to unique experiences and patterns of interaction. The diathesis–stress model proposes that, under conditions of stress, some people have maladaptive personality development, resulting in the emergence of a personality disorder (Kender, 2020).

There is a two-way directionality among stressors and diatheses. Genetic and biological traits are believed to influence the way an individual responds to the environment while, at the same time, the environment is thought to influence the expression of inherited traits. Many studies have suggested a strong correlation between trauma, neglect, and other dysfunctional family or social patterns of interaction and the development of personality disorders among individuals with particular personality traits and temperament.

The following is a summary of factors that are theorized to influence the development of each disorder (Skodol et al., 2014):

- STPD is a schizophrenia spectrum disorder and is genetically linked, meaning that there is a higher incidence of schizophrenia-related disorders in family members of people with STPD.
- Anti-social personality disorder is genetically linked, and twin studies indicate a predisposition to this disorder. This predisposition is set into motion by a childhood environment of inconsistent parenting, significant abuse, and extreme neglect.
- BPD has traditionally been thought to develop as a result of early abandonment, which results in an unstable view of self and others. This abandonment is made more intense by a biological predisposition, and twin studies identify a heritability of 69%.

- Narcissistic personality disorder may be the result of childhood neglect and criticism. The child does not learn that other people can be a source of comfort and support. As an adult, the individual hides feelings of emptiness with an exterior of invulnerability and self-sufficiency. Little is known about inborn traits or heritability for this disorder.
- Avoidant personality disorder has been linked with parental and peer rejection and criticism. A biological predisposition to anxiety and physiological arousal in social situations has also been suggested. Genetically, this disorder may be part of a continuum of disorders related to social phobia (social anxiety disorder; see Chapter 12).
- Obsessive-compulsive personality disorder may be related to excessive parental criticism, control, and shame. The child responds to this negativity by trying to control their environment through perfectionism and orderliness. Heritable traits such as compulsivity, oppositionality, lack of emotional expressiveness, and perfectionism have all been implicated in this disorder.

CLUSTER A PERSONALITY DISORDERS

Paranoid Personality Disorder

Paranoid personality disorder is characterized by a long-standing distrust and suspiciousness of others based on the belief, which is unsupported by evidence, that others want to exploit, harm, or deceive the person. These individuals are hypervigilant, anticipate hostility, and may provoke hostile responses by initiating a counterattack.

The prevalence of paranoid personality disorder has been estimated at about 2% to 4% (APA, 2013). Slightly more men than women are diagnosed with this disorder. Relatives of patients with schizophrenia are more frequently affected by this disorder. A diagnosis of paranoid personality disorder often precedes a schizophrenia diagnosis.

Symptoms may be apparent in childhood or adolescence. Parents may notice that their child does not have friends and experiences social anxiety. Young people with this disorder are frequently teased due to their odd behaviour.

As adults, relationships are difficult due to jealousy, controlling behaviours, and unwillingness to forgive. Projection is the dominant defence mechanism whereby people attribute their own unacknowledged feelings to others. For example, they may accuse their partner of being hypercritical when they themselves are attentively fault finding.

Guidelines for Nursing Care
- Considering the degree of mistrust, promises, appointments, and schedules should be strictly adhered to.
- Being too nice or friendly may be met with suspicion. Instead, give clear and straightforward explanations of tests and procedures beforehand.
- Use simple language and project a neutral but kind affect.
- Limit setting is essential when threatening behaviours are present.

Treatment

Individuals with paranoid personality disorder tend to reject treatment. If they somehow end up in a psychiatric treatment setting, they may appear puzzled and obviously suspicious about why this is happening. Paranoid people are difficult to interview because they are reluctant to share information about themselves for fear that the information will be used against them.

Psychotherapy is the first line of treatment for paranoid personality disorder (Boland & Verduin, 2021). Individual therapy focuses on the development of a professional and trusting relationship. Due to their fears, patients may behave in a threatening manner. Therapists should respond by setting limits and dealing with delusional accusations in a realistic manner without humiliating the patients.

Group therapy is threatening to people with paranoid personality disorder. However, the group setting may be useful in improving social skills. Role-playing and group feedback can help reduce suspiciousness. For example, if the patient says, "I think the therapist is singling me out," other groups members may provide a reality check or describe similar feelings in the past.

An anti-anxiety medication such as diazepam (Valium) may be used to reduce anxiety and agitation (Boland & Verduin, 2021). More severe agitation and delusions may be treated with antipsychotic medication such as haloperidol in small doses for brief periods of time to manage the mildly delusional thinking or severe agitation. The first-generation antipsychotic medication pimozide may be useful in reducing paranoid ideation.

> **Vignette**
> Ms. Alonzo is a 54-year-old unemployed female who comes to a mental health clinic complaining of depression and pain. She believes that her health maintenance organization has circulated her medical record to all health care providers to prevent her from being treated. She refuses to give any social history and is reluctant to share her telephone number. When the nurse indicates that the psychiatrist does not prescribe pain medications, she smiles bitterly and says, "So they already got to you."

Schizoid Personality Disorder

People with schizoid personality disorder exhibit a lifelong pattern of social withdrawal. They are somewhat expressionless and operate with a restricted range of emotional expression. Others tend to view them as odd or eccentric due to their discomfort with social interaction.

The prevalence rate may be nearly 5% of the population (APA, 2013). Males are more often affected. Symptoms of schizoid personality disorder appear in childhood and adolescence. These young people tend to be loners, do poorly in school, and are the objects of ridicule by their peers for their odd behaviour. There is increased prevalence of the disorder in families with a history of schizophrenia or STPD. Abnormalities in the dopaminergic systems may underlie this problem.

Relationships are particularly affected due to the prominent feature of emotional detachment. People with this disorder do not seek out or enjoy close relationships. Neither approval nor rejection from others seems to have much effect. Friendships, dating, and sexual experiences are rare. If trust is established, the person may divulge numerous imaginary friends and fantasies.

Employment may be jeopardized if interpersonal interaction is necessary. Individuals with this disorder may be able to function well in a solitary occupation such as being a security guard on the night shift. They often endorse feelings of being an observer rather than a participant in life. The patient may describe feelings of depersonalization or detachment from oneself and the world.

Guidelines for Nursing Care
- Nurses should avoid being too "nice" or "friendly."
- Do not try to increase socialization.
- Patients may be open to discussing topics such as coping and anxiety.
- Conduct a thorough assessment to identify symptoms the patient is reluctant to discuss.
- Protect against ridicule from group members due to patient's distinctive interests or ideas.

Treatment

Patients with schizoid personality disorder tend to be introspective (Boland & Verduin, 2021). This trait may make them good, if distant, candidates for psychotherapy. As trust develops, these patients may describe a full fantasy life and fears, particularly of dependence. Psychotherapy can help improve sensitivity to others' social cues. Group therapy may also be helpful, even though the patient may frequently be silent. Group therapy provides experience in practising interactions with and receiving feedback from others. Group members may become quite important to the person with schizoid personality disorder and may be the only form of socialization they have.

Antidepressants such as bupropion (Wellbutrin) may help increase pleasure in life. Second-generation antipsychotics, such as risperidone or olanzapine (Zyprexa), are used to improve emotional expressiveness.

> **Vignette**
> Mr. Gray, a 30-year-old single male, is a graduate student in mathematics at a large university. He lives alone and has never been married. He works as an assistant in a math classroom in which the professor teaches the course remotely via television. Mr. Gray wears thick glasses, and his clothing is inconspicuous. He rarely smiles and seldom looks directly at the students, even when answering questions. He does get somewhat animated when he writes lengthy solutions to math problems on the blackboard. He is content with his low-paying job and has never been in psychiatric treatment.

Schizotypal Personality Disorder

People with STPD do not blend in with the crowd. Their symptoms are strikingly strange and unusual. Magical thinking, odd beliefs, strange speech patterns, and inappropriate affect are hallmarks of this disorder.

Estimates of the prevalence of STPD vary from 0.6% to 4.6% (APA, 2013). It is more common in men than women. Like the other cluster A personality disorders, symptoms are evident in young people. People who have first-degree relatives with schizophrenia are at more risk for this disorder. Abnormalities in brain structure, physiology, chemistry, and functioning are similar to schizophrenia. For example, both disorders share reduced cortical volume.

The *Diagnostic and Statistical Manual of Mental Disorders*, fifth edition *(DSM-5)* (APA, 2013), identifies this problem as both a personality disorder and the first of the schizophrenia spectrum disorders. The ICD-10 (World Health Organization, 2016), used throughout the world, classifies schizotypal disorder along with schizophrenia and no longer lists schizotypal disorder as a personality disorder. Chapter 15 discusses the schizophrenia spectrum disorders in greater detail.

Like schizoid personality disorder, individuals with STPD have severe social and interpersonal deficits. They experience extreme anxiety in social situations. Contributions to conversations tend to ramble, with lengthy, unclear, overly detailed, and abstract content. An additional feature of this disorder is paranoia. Individuals with STPD are overly suspicious and anxious. They tend to misinterpret the motivations of others as being out to get them and blame others for their social isolation. Odd beliefs (e.g., being overly superstitious) or magical thinking (e.g., "He caught a cold because I wished he would") are also common.

Psychotic symptoms seen in people with schizophrenia, such as hallucinations and delusions, may also exist with STPD, but to a lesser degree and only briefly. A major difference between this disorder and schizophrenia is that people with STPD can be made aware of their suspiciousness, magical thinking, and odd beliefs. Schizophrenia is characterized by far stronger delusions.

Guidelines for Nursing Care

- Respect the patient's need for social isolation.
- Nurses should be aware of the patient's suspiciousness and employ appropriate interventions.
- Perform careful assessment as needed to uncover any other medical or psychological symptoms that may need intervention (e.g., suicidal thoughts).
- Be aware that strange beliefs and activities, such as strange religious practices or peculiar thoughts, may be part of the patient's life.

Treatment

The principles of psychotherapy used are similar to those for schizoid personality disorder (Boland & Verduin, 2021). However, clinicians should be aware that these patients may also be actively involved in groups such as cults and unusual religious groups and engage in occult activities.

While there is no specific medication for STPD, associated conditions may be treated. People with STPD seem to benefit from medications that help to control their symptoms. For example, antipsychotic medications for such symptoms as ideas of reference or illusions. Co-morbid symptoms related to depression and anxiety may be treated with antidepressants and anti-anxiety medications.

> **Vignette**
> Raymond is a 55-year-old single male who lives with his mother. He is the youngest of seven children raised in a farming community. Three of his siblings are deaf, and Raymond also has some hearing loss. Raymond started therapy with Wei, an advanced-practice registered nurse in psychiatric mental health, after he suffered a career-ending injury, from which he is completely disabled. Wei and Raymond have been working together for several years on quality-of-life issues and depression. Raymond is frequently distressed by his unwavering belief that everyone in his hometown greets him with sexual gestures and believes that he is gay. This belief extends to truck drivers who come through the town; he believes that they talk about his sexuality on their CB radios. These beliefs create great distress and anxiety for him. He occasionally yells at people or gestures back. Wei has been helping Raymond to understand how his perceptions may be faulty and how his hearing loss may contribute to his perceptual difficulties and anxiety. Raymond and Wei have invited his mother into the discussion so she can support him at home.

CLUSTER B PERSONALITY DISORDERS

Borderline Personality Disorder

BPD is the most well known and dramatic of the personality disorders. BPD prevalence may be as high as 5.9% in the general population and be about 20% among people receiving inpatient psychiatric care (APA, 2013). The major features of this disorder are patterns of marked instability in emotion regulation, unstable interpersonal relationships, identity or self-image distortions, and unstable mood. These symptoms result in severe functional impairments, a high mortality rate (approximately 30%), and extensive use of health care services (Public Health Agency of Canada, 2015). People with BPD seek out treatment for depression, anxiety, suicidal and self-harming behaviours, and other impulsive behaviours including substance use. Although hospitalization may decrease self-destructive risk for patients with BPD, it is not regarded as an effective long-term solution. With effective treatment, people with BPD can experience high rates of remission and low rates of relapse (Keefe et al., 2020).

BPD is around five times more common in first-degree biological relatives with the same disorder compared with the general population (APA, 2013). This disorder is highly associated with genetic factors such as hypersensitivity, impulsivity, and emotional dysregulation.

There is evidence of serotonergic dysfunction that accompanies the borderline trait of impulsivity. It may also contribute to the depression and aggression that commonly accompany this disorder. The serotonin transporter gene *5-HTT* may have shorter alleles, which have been associated with lower levels of serotonin and increased impulsive aggression.

Structural and functional magnetic resonance imaging have revealed abnormalities in the pre-frontal cortex and limbic regions. The frontal region is implicated in regulatory control processes, and the limbic region is essential for emotional processing (Schulze et al., 2019). Limbic hyper-reactivity and diminished control by the frontal brain may explain poor emotion processing, impulsivity, and interpersonal disturbances.

See the Neurobiology of Borderline Personality Disorder feature for more information about the neurobiology of BPD.

Neurobiology of Borderline Personality Disorder

Borderline personality disorder (BPD) is a serious and disabling brain disorder marked by impulsivity and emotional dysregulation.

Serotonin: Altered functioning of serotonin in the brain has been linked to depression, aggression, and difficulty in controlling destructive urges. The serotonin transporter gene *5-HTT* is thought to have shorter alleles in BPD, which have been associated with lower levels of serotonin and increased impulsive aggression.

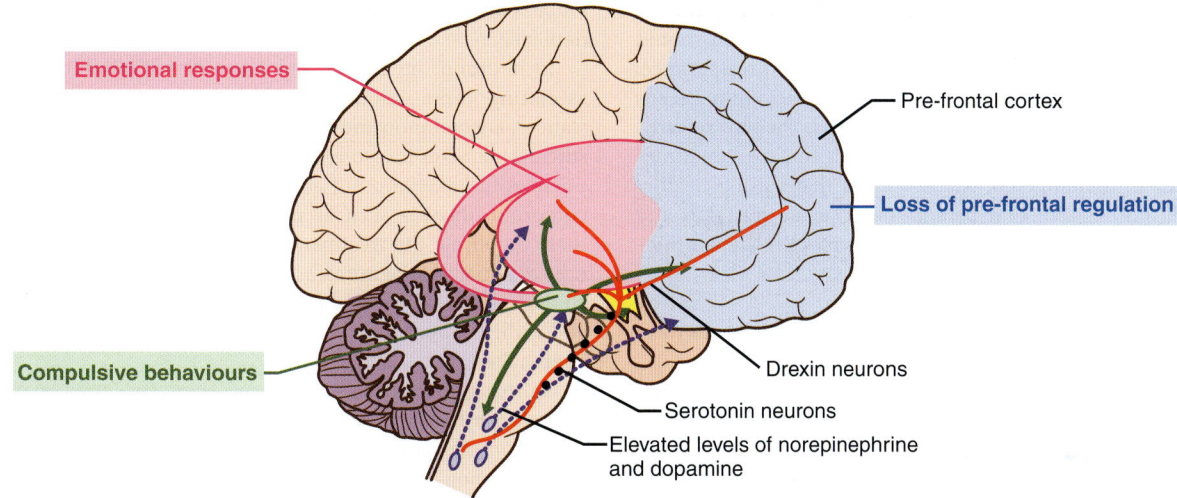

Emotional dysregulation: Emotional responses that are poorly modulated (e.g., angry outbursts, rage, marked fluctuation of mood, self-harm) and that can shift within seconds, minutes, or hours

Brain imaging (functional magnetic resonance imaging) findings
Pre-frontal cortex: In times of stress this part of the brain helps us regulate emotions and refrain from inappropriate actions. The pre-frontal cortex helps with reality testing and guides attention and thought. In people with BPD this part of the brain does not respond. Instead, there is an extreme perception and intensity of negative emotions.

Limbic system/amygdala: In BPD parts of the emotional centre of the brain are overstimulated and take longer to return to normal. Also, **certain neurotransmitters** that act as constraints in normal circumstances may underfunction in BPD, leaving a person in a prolonged fight-or-flight response.

Medications/therapy to help individuals regulate their emotions

Method	What's Involved	What It Does
Medications	Selective serotonin reuptake inhibitors, anticonvulsants, second-generation antipsychotics, lithium	Helps brain switch from sympathetic nervous system (arousal) to parasympathetic nervous system (relaxation mode)
Dialectical behavioural therapy (DBT)	Mindfulness, deep breathing, relaxation techniques	Helps dampen angry, impulsive, labile behaviour

Sources: Dialectical Living. (n.d.). *Emotion dysregulation.* http://www.dialecticalliving.ca/emotion-regulation-disorder-bpd/; Ruocco, A. C., Amirthavasagam, S., Choi-Kain, L. W., et al. (2013). Neural correlates of negative emotionality in borderline personality disorder: An activation-likelihood-estimation meta-analysis. *Biological Psychiatry, 73*(2), 153–160; and Nauert, R. (2015). Brain scans clarify borderline personality disorder. *Psych Central.* https://psychcentral.com/news/2017/09/04/brain-scans-clarify-borderline-personality-disorder#1.

Margaret Mahler (1895–1985), a Hungarian-born child psychologist who worked with emotionally disturbed children, developed a framework that is useful in considering BPD. Mahler and colleagues (1975) believed that psychological problems are a result of the disruption of the normal separation-individuation of the child from the mother.

According to Mahler, an infant progresses from complete self-absorption with an inability to separate themself from the mother to a physically and psychologically differentiated toddler. Mahler emphasized the role of the significant other (traditionally the mother) in providing a secure emotional base of support that promotes enough confidence for the child to separate. This support is achieved through a balance of holding (emotionally and physically) a child enough for the child to feel safe, while at the same time fostering and encouraging independence and natural exploration.

Problems may arise in this separation-individuation process. If a toddler leaves their mother on the park bench and wanders off to the sandbox, ideally two things should happen. First, the child should be encouraged to go off into the world with smiles and reassurance: "Go on, honey, it's safe to go away a little." Second, the mother needs to be reliably present when the toddler returns, thereby rewarding their efforts. Clearly, parents are not perfect and are sometimes distracted and short tempered. Mahler notes that raising healthy children does not require that parents never make mistakes and that "good enough parenting" will promote successful separation-individuation.

Stages of this process are as follows:

- **Stage 1 (birth–1 month): Normal autism.** The infant spends most of their time sleeping.
- **Stage 2 (1–5 months): Symbiosis.** The infant perceives the mother-infant as a single fused entity. Infants gradually distinguish the inner world from the outer world.
- **Stage 3 (5–10 months): Differentiation.** The infant recognizes distinctness from the mother. Progressive neurological development and increased alertness draw the infant's attention away from self to the outer world.
- **Stage 4 (11–18 months): Practising.** The ability to walk and explore greatly expands the toddler's sense of separateness.
- **Stage 5 (18–24 months): Rapprochement.** Toddlers move away from their mothers and come back for emotional refuelling. Periods of helplessness and dependence alternate with the need for independence.
- **Stage 6 (2–5 years): Object constancy.** When children comprehend that objects (in this case, the object is the mother) are permanent even when they are not in their presence, the individuation process is complete.

Children who later develop BPD may have had this process disrupted. The rapprochement stage is particularly crucial and coincides with the "terrible twos," which are characterized by darting away and clinging and whining. Some experts suggest that this phase is not a desirable time for extended separation between parent and child.

Consider the previous ideal example of the child who wants to play in the sandbox. If the child wanders off to the sandbox and returns to a caregiver who is emotionally unavailable, perhaps hurt by the attempt at independence, the child feels unsafe to explore. Alternately, if the caregiver has personal issues related to dependency and abandonment, they may be threatened by the child's attempts at independence and respond with clinging and halting exploration. The child cannot safely move on to the next stage of development. A fear of abandonment from others, along with a sense of anger, carries over into adulthood.

Pathological Personality Traits Seen in People With BPD

One of the pathological personality traits seen in people with BPD is negative affect. This affect is characterized by emotional lability, that is, moods that alternate rapidly from one emotional extreme to another. Other characteristics of a negative affect include responding to situations with emotions that are out of proportion to the circumstances, pathological fear of separation, and intense sensitivity to perceived personal rejection. Other disruptive traits common in people with BPD are impulsivity and antagonism. Impulsivity is manifested in acting quickly in response to emotions without considering the consequences. This impulsivity results in damaged relationships and even suicide attempts.

BPD is also characterized by feelings of antagonism, manifested in hostility, anger, and irritability in relationships. Physical violence toward intimate partners and non-intimate partners alike may occur. Rarely, a homicide of family members or others occurs. Violence is also manifested in destructive behaviours such as property damage.

In addition, ineffective and harmful self-soothing habits, such as cutting, promiscuous sexual behaviour, and numbing with substances, are common and may result in unintentional death. Chronic suicidal ideation is also a common feature of this disorder and influences the likelihood of accidental death. There are high rates of comorbid illnesses such as mood, anxiety, or substance disorders that complicate the treatment and prognosis of BPD. A number of non-psychiatric diagnoses are also associated with BPD. They include diabetes, high blood pressure, chronic back pain, fibromyalgia, and arthritis, and must be considered when determining treatment approaches.

Splitting, the primary defence or coping style used by people with BPD, is the inability to incorporate positive and negative aspects of oneself or others into a whole image. This kind of dichotomous thinking and coping behaviour is believed to be partly a result of the person's failed experiences with adult personality integration and is likely influenced by exposure to earlier psychological, sexual, or physical trauma. For example, the individual may tend to idealize another person (e.g., friend, lover, health care provider) at the start of a new relationship, hoping that this person will meet all of their needs. However, at the first disappointment or frustration, the individual quickly shifts to devaluation, despising the other person.

Guidelines for Nursing Care

- A therapeutic relationship is essential with patients who have BPD because most of them have experienced failed relationships, including therapeutic alliances.
- The therapeutic relationship often follows an initial hesitancy on the part of the patient, then an upward curve of idealization by the patient toward the caregiver. This idealization is invariably followed by a devaluation of the staff member when the patient is disappointed by unmet, frequently impossible, expectations.
- Conduct a thorough assessment of current or past physical, sexual, or emotional abuse and level of current risk for harm from self or others.
- Clinical supervision and additional education are helpful and supportive to health care providers.
- Awareness and monitoring of one's own stress responses to patient behaviours facilitate more effective and therapeutic intervention, regardless of the therapeutic approach being used.
- Evaluating treatment effectiveness in this patient population is difficult. Nurses may never know the real results of their interventions.

Treatment

People with BPD are usually admitted to psychiatric treatment programs because of symptoms with comorbid disorders or dangerous behaviour. Emotions such as anxiety, rage, and depression and behaviours such as withdrawal, paranoia, and manipulation are among the most frequent that health care workers must address. When patients blame and attack others, the nurse needs to understand the context of their complaints. These attacks originate from the feeling of being threatened. The more intense the complaints are, the greater the patients' fear of potential harm or loss is. Be aware of manipulative behaviours such as flattery, seductiveness, and instilling guilt. Case Study and Nursing Care Plan 19.1 presents a patient with BPD.

Realistic outcomes are established for individuals with BPD based on the perspective that personality change occurs with one behavioural solution and one learned skill at a time. This can be expected to take a lot of time and repetition. In the acute care setting the focus is on the presenting problem, which may be depression or severe anxiety. Health care providers do not expect resolution of chronic behaviour problems during the hospital stay, but rather expect to be met with appropriate therapeutic feedback and incremental steps toward recovery in an outpatient setting.

People with BPD are impulsive and may be suicidal, self-mutilating, aggressive, manipulative, and even psychotic during periods of stress. Provide clear and consistent boundaries and limits. Use straightforward communication. When behavioural problems emerge, calmly review the therapeutic goals.

There are no approved medications for treating BPD. When medications are used, their purposes are to maintain patients' cognitive function, relieve symptoms, and improve quality of life. People with BPD often respond to antidepressants such as selective serotonin reuptake inhibitors (SSRIs), anti-convulsants, and lithium for mood and emotional dysregulation symptoms. Naltrexone, an opioid receptor antagonist, has been found to reduce self-injurious behaviours. Second-generation antipsychotics may control anger and brief psychosis.

When individuals with BPD are admitted to the hospital, partially hospitalized, or in day treatment settings, team management is a significant part of treatment. The primary goal is management of the patient's affect in a group context. Community meetings, coping skills groups, and socializing groups are all helpful for these patients. They have the opportunity to interact with peers and staff to discuss goals and learn problem-solving skills. Dealing with emotional issues that arise in the milieu requires a calm, united approach by the staff to maintain safety and enhance self-control.

Common problems resulting from staff splitting can be minimized if the unit leaders hold weekly staff meetings in which staff members are allowed to express their feelings about conflicts with patients and each other. This process is often acted out in the treatment milieu and can interrupt the delivery of care. For example, a female patient may briefly idealize her male nurse on the inpatient unit, telling staff and patients alike that she is "the luckiest person because she has the best nurse in the hospital." The rest of the team understands that this comment is an exaggeration. After days of her constant dramatic praise for the nurse and subtle insults to the rest of the staff, some members of the team may start to feel inadequate and resentful of the nurse. They begin to make critical remarks about minor events to prove that the nurse is not perfect. A similar scenario can occur if the person constantly complains about one staff member; some colleagues are then torn between defending and criticizing the targeted staff member. Consistency and a team approach help to ensure the productive use of therapeutic time and structure for the patient. Patient-centred approaches allow the patient to be part of the treatment planning.

Evaluating treatment effectiveness in this patient population is difficult. Freedom from harm to self and others is a tangible and satisfying positive evaluation. Nurses may never know the real results of their intervention, particularly in acute care settings. Even in long-term outpatient treatment, patients with BPD experience too many disruptions to relationships to remain long enough for successful treatment. As noted earlier, however, some motivated patients may be able to learn to change their behaviour, especially if positive experiences are repeated.

> **Vignette**
> Shaina is a 38-year-old married woman with one young son. She works full time as a dietitian in a primary care network. Shaina was diagnosed with fibromyalgia 2 years ago and is in treatment at a pain clinic. Most days, she comes home from work fatigued and goes to bed, leaving her son to play by himself after school or with friends until her husband gets home from work. Shaina also has struggled with an eating disorder since she was a teenager. When she feels guilty for ignoring her son's needs, she binges and then purges to relieve her negative emotions. Shaina recognizes that this behaviour helps only temporarily and adds to her fatigue, but she still feels helpless to stop it. When her son asks her to play with him or take him to an activity, she becomes angry with him and then feels angry at herself. Shaina has been referred by the palliative care nurse at the pain clinic to a dialectical behaviour therapy group (discussed later in this chapter) to learn skills to deal with her chronic pain and discover alternative self-soothing strategies for her bingeing and purging behaviours.

Anti-social Personality Disorder

Anti-social personality disorder is a pattern of disregard for, and violation of, the rights of others. People with this disorder may be more commonly referred to as sociopaths. This diagnosis is reserved for adults, but symptoms are evident by the mid-teens. Symptoms tend to peak during the late teenage years and into the mid-twenties. By around 40 years of age, the symptoms may abate and improve even without treatment. The prevalence of anti-social personality disorder is between 0.2% and 3.3% (APA, 2013). While the disorder is much more common in men (3% vs. 1%), women may be underdiagnosed due to the traditional close association of this disorder with males.

Anti-social personality disorder is genetically linked, and twin studies indicate a predisposition to this disorder. Kendler and colleagues (2012) note that there are two main dimensions of genetic risk. One is the trait of aggressive disregard, which refers to violent tendencies without concern for others; the other is the trait of disinhibition, which is a lack of concern for consequences. It is likely that the genetic predisposition for characteristics of anti-social personality disorder such as a lack of empathy may be set into motion by childhood maltreatment. Inconsistent parenting and discipline, significant abuse, and extreme neglect are associated with this disorder. Children reflect parental attitudes and behaviours in the absence of more prosocial influences. Virtually all individuals who eventually develop this disorder have a history of impulse control and conduct problems as children and adolescents.

The main pathological traits that characterize anti-social personality disorder are antagonistic behaviours such as being deceitful and manipulative for personal gain or being hostile if needs are blocked. The disorder is also characterized by disinhibited behaviours such as high level of risk taking, disregard for responsibility, and impulsivity. Criminal misconduct and substance use are common in this population.

People with this disorder are mostly concerned with gaining personal power or pleasure, and in relationships they focus on their own

CONSIDERING CULTURE
Gender Bias in Diagnosing Personality Disorders

There may be a culture-bound gender bias in the diagnosing of personality disorders. BPD is an example of such a bias: well-respected diagnostic manuals report a 3:1 gender ratio of females to males for BPD (Sansone & Sansone, 2011). However, Grant and colleagues (2008), in a well-executed epidemiological survey, found BPD to be equally prevalent in men and women. Thus a subtle clinician bias has increased the predominance of BPD diagnosis in women. This bias may have developed because women with BPD undertake more self-harming behaviours, which result in their admission to treatment, whereas men with BPD have more substance use and anti-social features, which result in their incarceration. This difference may lead staff working in a psychiatric treatment facility to think that there are more females with BPD. Also, the emotional aspects of BPD may present differently in women and men (Verona et al., 2012), and, as a result, it is important for health care providers to think of this disorder more broadly than as primarily a women's issue. More recently Barker et al. (2018) have identified that women with a diagnosis of personality disorder upon discharge contributed to increased recidivism when compared to men.

Sources: Grant, B., Chou, S., Goldstein, R., et al. (2008). Prevalence, correlates, disability, and comorbidity of DSM-IV borderline personality disorder: Results from the wave 2 national epidemiologic survey on alcohol and related conditions. *Journal of Clinical Psychiatry, 69*(4), 533–545. Retrieved from https://www.ncbi.nlm.nih.gov/pubmed/18426259; Sansone, R., & Sansone, L. (2011). Gender patterns in borderline personality disorder. *Innovations in Clinical Neuroscience, 8*(5), 16–20. Retrieved from https://www.ncbi.nlm.nih.gov/pmc/articles/PMC3115767/; Verona, E., Sprague, J., & Javdani, S. (2012). Gender and factor-level interactions in psychopathy: Implications for self-directed violence risk and borderline personality disorder symptoms. *Personality Disorders, 3*(3), 247–262. https://doi.org/10.1037/a0025945; and Barker, L. C., Gruneir, A., Fung, K., et al. (2018). Predicting psychiatric readmission: Sex-specific models to predict 30-day readmission following acute psychiatric hospitalization. *Social Psychiatry & Psychiatric Epidemiology, 53*(2), 139–149. https://doi.org/10.1007/s00127-017-

gratification to an extreme. They have little to no capacity for intimacy and will exploit others if it benefits them in relationships. One of the most disturbing qualities associated with anti-social personality disorder is a profound lack of empathy, also known as callousness. This **callousness** results in a lack of concern about the feelings of others, the absence of remorse or guilt except when facing punishment, and a disregard for meeting school, family, and other obligations.

These individuals tend to exhibit a shallow, unexpressive, and superficial affect. They may also be adept at portraying themselves as concerned and caring if these attributes help them to manipulate and exploit others. A person with anti-social personality disorder may be able to act witty and charming and be good at flattery and manipulating the emotions of others.

Guidelines for Nursing Care
- Nurses should be aware and monitor their responses to patient behaviours to facilitate effective and therapeutic responses.
- Conduct a thorough assessment of current life stressors, history of violent thoughts and behaviours (including suicidal ideation), and substance use.
- Be aware that distrust, hostility, and a profound inability to connect with others will impair the usual process of developing a therapeutic relationship.
- Evaluating treatment effectiveness in this patient population is difficult. Nurses may never know the real results of their interventions.

Treatment

In the context of anti-social personality disorder the role of the nurse will be to provide consistency, support, boundaries, and limits. Providing realistic choices (e.g., selection of a particular group activity) may enhance adherence to treatment. People with anti-social personality disorder may be involuntarily admitted to psychiatric units for evaluation. With their freedom limited, they tend to be angry, manipulative, aggressive, and impulsive. Try to prevent or reduce untoward effects of manipulation (flattery, seductiveness, instilling of guilt). Set clear and realistic boundaries and consequences and ensure that all staff follow these limits. Carefully document behaviours and signs of manipulation. Be aware that anti-social patients can manipulate with feelings of guilt when they are not getting what they want.

The safety of patients and staff is a prime consideration in working with individuals in this population. To promote safety, the entire treatment team should follow a solid treatment plan that emphasizes realistic limits on specific behaviour, consistency in responses, and consequences for actions. Careful documentation of behaviours will aid in providing effective interventions and in promoting teamwork.

Therapeutic communication techniques are valuable tools for working with individuals with anti-social personality disorder. Simply being heard can defuse an emotionally charged situation. For example, the nurse can listen to a patient's emotional complaints about the staff and the hospital without correcting errors, simply noting that the patient truly feels hurt. Showing empathy may also decrease aggressive outbursts if the patient feels that staff members are trying to understand feelings of frustration.

There are no approved medications for treating anti-social personality disorder. Medications are used to treat concurrent comorbid disorders. The advanced-practice psychiatric mental health registered nurse may care for individuals with this type of personality disorder in a variety of inpatient and community settings. Research shows that individuals with this disorder do benefit from therapies to address other mental health conditions. These individuals often require intense and long-term treatment.

> **Vignette**
> Manwell is a 27-year-old divorced cab driver who is referred to the hospital by the court for a mental health evaluation after an assault charge. He told the arresting officer that he has bipolar disorder. He has a history of substance use and multiple arrests for disorderly conduct or assault. During his intake interview, he is polite and even flirtatious with the female nurse. He insists that he is not responsible for his behaviour because he is manic. The only symptom he describes is irritability. He points out that he cannot tolerate any psychotropic medications because of the adverse effects. He also notes that he has dropped out of three clinics after several visits because "the staff don't understand me."

Histrionic Personality Disorder

People with histrionic personality disorder are excitable and dramatic yet are often high functioning. They may be referred to in terms of being a "drama queen" or "drama major." Classic characteristics of this population include extraversion, flamboyancy, and colourful personalities. Despite this bold exterior, those with histrionic personality disorder tend to have limited ability to develop meaningful relationships.

Histrionic personality disorder occurs at a rate of nearly 2% in community samples (APA, 2013). In clinical settings it tends to be diagnosed more frequently in women than in men. Symptoms begin by early adulthood. Inborn character traits such as emotional expressiveness and egocentricity have also been identified as predisposing an individual to this disorder.

This disorder is characterized by emotional attention-seeking behaviours, including self-centredness, low frustration tolerance, and excessive emotionality. The person with histrionic personality disorder is often impulsive and may act flirtatiously or provocatively. Relationships do not last because the partner often feels smothered or reacts to the insensitivity of the histrionic person. The individual with histrionic personality disorder does not have insight into a personal role in breaking up relationships.

In general, individuals with this disorder do not think they need psychiatric help. They may go into treatment for associated problems such as depression, which may be precipitated by losses such as the end of a relationship.

Guidelines for Nursing Care

- Nursing care should reflect an understanding that seductive behaviour is a response to distress.
- Keep communication and interactions professional.
- Patients may exaggerate symptoms and difficulty in functioning.
- Encourage and model the use of concrete and descriptive rather than vague and impressionistic language.
- Assist patients to clarify feelings because they often have difficulty identifying them.
- Teach and role model assertiveness.
- Assess for suicidal ideation. What was intended as a suicide gesture may inadvertently result in death.

Treatment

Individuals with histrionic personality disorder may be out of touch with their feelings (Boland & Verduin, 2021). Psychotherapy may promote clarification of inner feelings and appropriate expression. Group therapy may be useful in this population, although distracting symptoms may be disruptive to group functioning.

There are no specific pharmacological treatments available for people with histrionic personality disorder. Medications such as antidepressants can be used for depressive symptoms. Anti-anxiety medications may be helpful in treating anxiety. Antipsychotics may be used if the patient exhibits derealization or illusions.

> **Vignette**
> Ms. Lombard is a 35-year-old twice-divorced female admitted to an inpatient unit after an overdose of asthma medications and antibiotics. She took all of her pills after her primary care provider refused to order a sleeping pill for her. On the first night, she is withdrawn and tearful in her room. By the next morning, she is neatly groomed, even wearing makeup, and is socializing with everyone. She denies thoughts of self-harm. Over the next 2 days, Ms. Lombard monopolizes the community meetings by talking about how unappreciated she is by her family. She seeks special attention from a male evening-shift registered nurse, asking if he can stay late after his shift to sit with her. When he refuses, she demands to be placed back on one-to-one precautions because she feels suicidal again.

Narcissistic Personality Disorder

Narcissistic personality disorder is characterized by feelings of entitlement, an exaggerated belief in one's own importance, and a lack of empathy. In reality, people with this disorder suffer from a weak self-esteem and hypersensitivity to criticism. Narcissistic personality disorder is associated with less impairment in individual functioning and quality of life than the other personality-based disorders.

The prevalence of narcissistic personality disorder ranges from 0% to about 6% in community samples (APA, 2013). It tends to be more common in males than in females. Age of onset is difficult to determine due to the narcissistic traits that are typically found in adolescents. There may be a familial tendency for this disorder, as parents with narcissism may attribute an unrealistic sense of talent, importance, and beauty to their children. These attributions put the children at higher risk for the disorder.

People with narcissistic personality disorder come across as arrogant and as having an inflated view of their self-importance. The individual with this disorder has a need for constant admiration along with a lack of empathy for others, a factor that strains most relationships over time. They are very sensitive to rejection and criticism and can be disparaging to others. A sense of personal entitlement paired with a lack of social empathy may result in the exploitation of other people.

Underneath the surface of arrogance, people with narcissistic personality disorder feel intense shame and have a fear of abandonment. In keeping with these descriptions the main pathological personality trait of narcissism is antagonism, represented by grandiosity and attention-seeking behaviours. Those with narcissistic personality disorder tend to tolerate rejection poorly. As a result, narcissistic individuals may seek help for depression or may seek to be validated by therapists and loved ones for their emotional pain of not being appreciated by others for their efforts or special qualities.

Guidelines for Nursing Care

- Nurses should remain neutral and recognize the source of narcissistic behaviour, shame and fear of abandonment.
- Use the therapeutic nurse–patient relationship as an opportunity to practise engaging in meaningful interaction.
- Avoid engaging in power struggles or becoming defensive in response to the patient's disparaging remarks.
- Role model empathy.

Treatment

Because patients need to confront their problem to make progress, treating people specifically for this disorder is difficult (Boland & Verduin, 2021). Because individuals are not likely to seek help for their own problems, they are more likely to be involved in couples or family therapy than in individual treatment. In these family-oriented approaches narcissistic individuals are likely to deflect suggestions that they contribute to family problems and will instead blame others.

If a person with narcissistic personality disorder somehow seeks treatment, individual cognitive behavioural therapy is helpful in deconstructing faulty thinking. Group therapy can also assist the person in sharing with others, seeing their own qualities in others, and learning empathy.

There are no approved medications for treating narcissistic personality disorder. Medications are used to treat concurrent comorbid disorders.

> **Vignette**
> Dr. Abigail McLaughlin is a 40-year-old female attending psychiatrist at a university outpatient centre. She is twice divorced and has no children. Her grooming and makeup are impeccable, and she likes to chat about her expensive shopping habits. She is quite intelligent and is the only doctor on the staff trained in psychoanalysis. In clinical team meetings she often discusses this fact, repeatedly telling others that psychoanalysis is the best treatment for mental illness. She frequently makes derogatory remarks to psychiatric residents if they suggest alternative treatment approaches for new cases. She is usually late to staff meetings, and when she is not speaking, she yawns and shifts noisily in her seat. She has a reputation for exhibiting angry outbursts at therapists in the hallway over minor mistakes, such as a scheduling error for a patient. She underwent 7 years of psychoanalysis but does not consider it to have been therapy, it "was for training purposes only."

CLUSTER C PERSONALITY DISORDERS

Avoidant Personality Disorder

The main pathological personality traits associated with avoidant personality disorder are low self-esteem related to functioning in social situations, feelings of inferiority compared with peers, and a reluctance to engage in unfamiliar activities involving new people. Some individuals with avoidant personality disorder can function in a protective environment. However, if their support system fails, they can suffer from depression, anxiety, and anger. They are especially sensitive to and preoccupied with rejection, humiliation, and failure. They often avoid new interpersonal relationships or activities due to their fears of criticism or disapproval (APA, 2013).

Avoidant personality disorder occurs in approximately 2.4% of the population (APA, 2013). It is found equally among men and women. Early symptoms of the disorder are often evident in infants and children. These symptoms include shyness and avoidance that, unlike common shyness, increases during adolescence and early adulthood.

Guidelines for Nursing Care

- Nurses should use a friendly, accepting, reassuring approach and remember that being pushed into social situations can cause extreme and severe anxiety for these patients.
- Convey an attitude of acceptance toward patient fears.
- Provide the patient with exercises to enhance new social skills, but use these with caution because any failure can increase feelings of poor self-worth.
- Assertiveness training can assist the person to learn to express needs.

Treatment

Individual and group therapy is useful in processing anxiety-provoking symptoms and in planning methods to approach and handle anxiety-provoking situations (Boland & Verduin, 2021). Psychotherapy focuses on trust and assertiveness training.

Anti-anxiety medications can be helpful. Beta-adrenergic receptor antagonists (e.g., atenolol) help reduce autonomic nervous system hyperactivity. Antidepressant medications, such as SSRIs like citalopram (Celexa) and serotonin–norepinephrine reuptake inhibitors (SNRIs) like venlafaxine (Effexor), may reduce social anxiety. Serotonergic medications may help individuals with avoidant personalities feel less sensitive to rejection. Chapter 11 describes the use of psychotropic medication in more detail.

> **Vignette**
> Annemarie is a 35-year-old single female who works as a receptionist for a computer repair company. As a child, she had few friends and never participated in extracurricular activities. Annemarie lives alone in her own apartment and has never had an intimate adult relationship. On the job, she rarely talks to coworkers and prefers to work alone. If she has any questions, she asks the supervisor and carefully follows directions. Although she has 7 years of experience and a good work record, she refuses the offer of a promotion because it would require her to interact with customers.

Dependent Personality Disorder

Dependent personality disorder is characterized by a pattern of submissive and clinging behaviour related to an overwhelming need to be cared for. This need results in intense fears of separation.

Dependent personality disorder is fairly rare, with an estimated prevalence rate of about 0.5% (APA, 2013). Dependent personality disorder may be the result of chronic physical illness or punishment for independent behaviour in childhood. The inherited trait of submissiveness may also be a factor.

People with dependent personality disorder have a high need to be taken care of. This need can lead to patterns of submissiveness with fears of separation and abandonment by others. Because they lack confidence in their own ability or judgement, those with dependent personality disorder may manipulate others to assume responsibility for such activities as finances or child rearing. This may create problems by leaving them more vulnerable to exploitation by others because of their passive and submissive nature. Feelings of insecurity about their self-agency and lack of self-confidence may interfere with attempts to become more independent. They may experience intense anxiety when left alone for even brief periods of time (APA, 2013).

Guidelines for Nursing Care

- Nurses can help the patient identify and address current stressors.
- Be aware that strong counter-transference may develop because of the patient's demands for extra time and crisis states.
- The therapeutic nurse–patient relationship can provide a testing ground for increased assertiveness through role modelling and teaching of assertive skills.

Treatment

Psychotherapy is the treatment of choice for dependent personality disorder (Boland & Verduin, 2021). Cognitive behavioural therapy can help patients develop more healthy and accurate thinking by examining and challenging automatic thoughts that result in fearful behaviour. This process can help in developing new perspectives and attitudes about the need for other people.

There are no specific medications indicated for this disorder, but symptoms of depression and anxiety may be treated with the appropriate antidepressant and anti-anxiety medications. Panic attacks can be helped with the tricyclic antidepressant imipramine.

> **Vignette**
> Bawaajige is a 32-year-old, married former engineer, and she is mother to two young children, ages 3 years and 11 months. Bawaajige's depression and anxiety have been more severe since she stopped working. She feels inadequate and overwhelmed by her responsibilities, so her mother moved in with the young family at Bawaajige's request. Her therapist, an advanced-practice psychiatric mental health registered nurse, recommended that she receive brief treatment for depression and anxiety at the partial hospitalization program. Bawaajige quickly bonded with the advanced-practice nurse, who is an older woman. She frequently asks her for reassurance that she is doing the right thing by coming to treatment and seeks her out frequently for extra individual sessions. Gradually, as the result of individual and group therapy, Bawaajige begins to realize that excessive dependence on her mother contributes to long-standing feelings of ineffectiveness, helplessness, and invalidation of her own parenting skills.

Obsessive-Compulsive Personality Disorder

Obsessive-compulsive personality disorder is characterized by limited emotional expression, stubbornness, perseverance, and indecisiveness. Pre-occupation with orderliness, perfectionism, and control are the hallmarks of this disorder.

Obsessive-compulsive personality disorder is one of the most prevalent personality disorders. The prevalence rate ranges from 2.1% to 7.9% (APA, 2013). It is more common in men than in women. Oldest siblings tend to be affected more often than subsequent siblings. Risk factors for this disorder include a background of harsh discipline and having a first-degree relative with this disorder. Obsessive-compulsive personality disorder has been associated with increased relapse rates of depression and an increase in suicidal risks in people with co-occurring depression.

The main pathological personality traits are rigidity and inflexible standards of self and others. People with obsessive-compulsive personality disorder rehearse over and over how they will respond in social situations. They persist in goal seeking long after it is necessary, even if it is self-defeating or relationship defeating. The pre-occupation often results in losing the major point of the activity. Projects are often incomplete due to overly strict standards.

There is a difference between obsessive-compulsive disorder and obsessive-compulsive personality disorder. Obsessive-compulsive disorder is characterized by obsessive thoughts and by repetition or adherence to rituals. Those with obsessive-compulsive disorder are aware that these thoughts and actions are unreasonable. Obsessive-compulsive personality disorder is characterized more by an unhealthy focus on perfectionism. Those with obsessive-compulsive personality disorder think that their actions are right and feel comfortable with such self-imposed systems of rules.

People with obsessive-compulsive personality disorder often do feel genuine affection for friends and family, yet leisure activities and friendship are dropped in favour of excessive devotion to work and productivity.

Guidelines for Nursing Care

- Nurses should guard against power struggles with these patients, as their need for control is very high.
- Patients with this disorder have difficulty dealing with unexpected changes.
- Provide structure, yet allow patients extra time to complete habitual behaviour.
- Assist patients to identify ineffective coping and to develop effective coping techniques.

Treatment

Typically, patients seek help for obsessive-compulsive personality disorder, as they are aware of their own suffering. They may also seek treatment for anxiety or depression. The treatment course is often long and complicated. Both group therapy and behavioural therapy can be helpful, so that the person can learn new coping skills for their anxiety and see direct benefits for change from feedback within the group.

Clomipramine (Anafranil) may help reduce the obsessions, anxiety, and depression associated with this disorder. Other serotonergic medications such as fluoxetine (Prozac) may also be effective.

Vignette

Robert is a 45-year-old, single, male postal worker in a small town. He lives alone and has never married. He is well groomed and wears a clean, neatly ironed uniform every day. He carefully follows all policies and procedures and is quite resistant whenever there is an update or change. He frequently challenges the supervisor about policy details and has been referred to the regional personnel office countless times for resolution of these conflicts. In staff meetings he gives excessive circumstantial details and writes extra material on the back of any required report form. When dealing with the public, he sometimes gets into arguments with customers about postal rules or the schedule. Other staff members do not consider him to be a team player because he seldom volunteers to help others. Even if he is asked to help someone, he is quick to criticize his peer's performance. Although he has worked in the same office for 10 years, he has never advanced beyond the front-line position. He is fairly content with his work and has never been in psychiatric treatment.

APPLICATION OF THE NURSING PROCESS

Assessment

Assessment Tools

The preferred method for determining a diagnosis of personality disorder is the semistructured interview obtained by clinicians. These types of interviews have standard questions and a standard format for asking the questions. These interviews go beyond asking the patient to self-report symptoms because individuals with personality disorders often lack insight into their behaviours and motivations and therefore have difficulty accurately describing themselves. One way to elicit more objective information is to ask the person if family members and colleagues perceive them in a certain way. For example, "You said that you don't think you're emotionally distant. How would your wife describe you?" Cultural norms and expectations also need to be considered when evaluating the presence of a personality disorder. Personality disorders are often assessed through identifying pathology within one or more personality dimensions. The five main dimensions of personalities are (1) extraversion versus introversion, (2) antagonism versus adherence, (3) constraint versus impulsivity, (4) emotional dysregulation versus emotional stability, and (5) unconventionality versus closedness to experience. See Table 19.1.

Open-ended or subjective interviews, which do not have standard questions or a standard question format, are more likely to result in biased and culturally based decisions about diagnosis and treatment delivery. Self-report inventories, such as the well-known Minnesota Multi-phasic Personality Inventory, are useful because they have built-in validity and reliability scales for the clinician to refer to when interpreting test results. Other more focused questionnaires and rating scales can be used to assess several symptoms. These include:

- Feelings of emptiness
- An inclination to engage in risky behaviours such as reckless driving, unsafe sex, substance use, binge eating, gambling, or overspending
- Intense feelings of abandonment that result in paranoia or feeling spaced out
- Idealization of others and becoming close quickly
- A tendency toward anger, sarcasm, and bitterness
- Self-mutilation and self-harm
- Suicidal behaviours, gestures, or threats
- Sudden shifts in self-evaluation that result in changing goals, values, and career focus
- Extreme mood shifts that occur in a matter of hours or days
- Intense, unstable romantic relationships
- Feelings of insecurity
- Rigidity
- Perfectionism

Patient History

Taking a full medical history can help determine if the problem is a psychiatric one, a non-psychiatric medical one, or both. Non-psychiatric illness should never be ruled out as the cause for problem behaviour until the data support this conclusion. Important issues in assessing for personality disorders include a history of suicidal or aggressive ideation or actions, current use of medications and illegal substances, ability to handle money, and legal history.

Significant topics about which further details must be obtained include current or past physical, sexual, or emotional abuse and level of current risk for harm from self or others. At times, immediate interventions may be needed to ensure the safety of the person or others. Information regarding prior use of any medication, including non-prescription substances, is important.

TABLE 19.1 Five Dimensions of Personality

Personality Dimensions	Attitudes and Behaviours
Extraversion versus introversion	Activity, aloofness, assertiveness, detachment, entitlement, excitement seeking, exhibitionism, exploratory excitability, extravagance, gregariousness, histrionic sexualization, intimacy problems, optimism, positive emotionality, restricted expression, schizoid orientation, shyness, sociability, social avoidance, social closeness, social potency, stimulus seeking, warmth, well-being
Antagonism versus adherence	Adherence, aggression, agreeableness, alienation, altruism, attachment, callousness, compassion, conduct problems, dependency, diffidence, empathy, entitlement, helpfulness, insecure attachment, interpersonal disesteem, manipulativeness, mistrust, modesty, narcissism, passive oppositionality, psychopathy, pure-heartedness, rejection, sentimentality, social acceptance, social closeness, straightforwardness, submissiveness, suspiciousness, tender-mindedness, trust
Constraint versus impulsivity	Achievement striving, childishness, competence, compulsivity, conscientiousness, deliberation, disorderliness, dutifulness, eagerness of effort, harm avoidance, impulsivity, irresponsibility, obsessionality, order, perfectionism, propriety, resourcefulness, responsibility, risk taking, self-discipline, traditionalism, workaholism
Emotional dysregulation versus emotional stability	Affective lability, alienation, angry hostility, anticipatory worry, anxiousness, dependency, depressiveness, dysphoria, emotional dysregulation, fear of uncertainty, hostility, hypochondriasis, identity problems, inferiority, introspection, irritability, negative affect, pessimism, self-acceptance, self-consciousness, self-harm, sensitivity, stress reaction, unhappiness, vulnerability, worthlessness
Unconventionality versus closedness to experience	Absorption, dissociation, eccentric perceptions, eccentricity, openness to experience, perceptual cognitive distortion, rigidity, spiritual acceptance, thought disorder, transpersonal identification

Source: Adapted from Simms, L., Goldberg, L., Roberts, J., et al. (2011). Computerized adaptive assessment of personality disorder: Introducing the CAT-PD project. *Journal of Personality Assessment, 93*(4), 380–389. https://doi.org/10.1080/00223891.2011.577475. Reprinted by permission of the publisher (Taylor & Francis Ltd., https://www.tandf.co.uk/journals).

Self-Assessment

Because enduring patterns of interpersonal difficulties are central to the problems faced by people diagnosed with personality disorders, it is understandable that their relationship problems with their caregivers surface in the treatment milieu. Anticipating that people with personality disorders will likely have a disrupted, intense interpersonal experience with caregivers is helpful to the caregivers as they monitor their own personal stress responses. It is important to keep in mind that these dysfunctional behaviours may really represent the person's best efforts to cope because they lack the necessary skills to be effective in their lives.

Finding an approach that works with people in the setting in which they are treated is important. Therapies such as dialectical behaviour therapy (DBT) and mindfulness-based therapies offer staff evidence-informed interventions, clinical structure, and formalized support for identifying best practices.

Diagnosis

When people with personality disorders are admitted to hospital, it is usually because of symptoms of comorbid disorders, dangerous behaviour, or court-ordered treatment. BPD and anti-social personality disorder both present a challenge for health care providers because the behaviours central to these disorders often cause disruption in psychiatric and medical-surgical settings. Emotions such as anxiety, rage, and depression and behaviours such as withdrawal, paranoia, and manipulation are among the most frequent concerns that health care workers must address. Table 19.2 lists common potential nursing diagnoses related to personality disorders.

Outcomes Identification

Realistic outcomes are established for individuals with personality disorders based on the perspective that personality change occurs with one behavioural solution and one learned skill at a time. This change can be expected to take much time and repetition. In the acute care setting the focus is on the presenting problem, which may be depression or severe anxiety. During the hospital stay, the chronic behaviour problems of individuals with personality disorders are not expected to be resolved but rather to be met with appropriate therapeutic feedback.

Pertinent categories of nursing outcomes based on the *Nursing Outcomes Classification (NOC)* include aggression self-control, impulse self-control, social interaction skills, personal resiliency, fear level, abusive behaviour self-restraint, and self-mutilation restraint (Moorhead et al., 2018). Table 19.3 gives examples of other potential nursing outcomes for manipulative, aggressive, and impulsive behaviours.

Planning

It is often difficult to create a therapeutic relationship with individuals who have personality disorders because most of them have experienced failed relationships, including therapeutic alliances. Individuals with BPD or anti-social personality disorder will distrust relationships and demonstrate hostility toward others, thus making the establishment of a therapeutic relationship difficult. People with personality disorders require a sense of control over what is happening to them. Giving them realistic choices (e.g., selection of a particular group activity) may enhance adherence to treatment. It is also important to plan individual patient treatment within the context of their family. Patients, families, and health care providers can access further information on personality disorders from the Internet; two reliable Canadian sites are the Canadian Mental Health Association (https://www.cmha.ca) and HeretoHelp (https://www.heretohelp.bc.ca). Refer to Table 19.4 for guidelines for nursing care for the major clusters of personality disorders. Case Study and Nursing Care Plan 19.1 presents a person with BPD.

Implementation

People with BPD are impulsive (e.g., suicidal, self-mutilating), aggressive, manipulative, and even psychotic during periods of stress. Individuals with anti-social personality disorder are often involuntarily admitted and are manipulative, aggressive, and impulsive. Refer to Boxes 19.1 to 19.3 for interventions to address these behaviours, based on the *Nursing Interventions Classification (NIC)* (Butcher et al., 2019).

RESEARCH HIGHLIGHT
How Do Psychiatric Nurses Respond to Patients With Borderline Personality Disorder?

Problem
People diagnosed with borderline personality disorder (BPD) have problems relating to people in their everyday lives. There is anecdotal evidence that they are also unpopular among mental health nurses.

Purpose of Study
To determine whether mental health nurses respond to people with BPD in problematic ways.

Methods
A systematic integrated literature review of quantitative and qualitative studies was conducted. Forty articles through April 2015 were included. Papers were gathered describing primary research focused on psychiatric nurses' attitudes, behaviour, experience, and knowledge regarding adults with BPD.

Key Findings
- Psychiatric nurses find patients with this diagnosis very challenging to work with.
- Psychiatric nurses report poorer attitudes than other health care providers toward this population.
- Psychiatric nurses hold poorer attitudes toward patients with BPD than other diagnostic groups.
- Nurses who use a coherent therapeutic framework to guide their practice experience improvement in caregiving.

Implications for Nursing Practice
Mental health nurses have all heard a dismissive, "Oh, she's just a borderline" in response to certain patients. We need a fresh approach to this problem. The authors conclude that developing nurses to lead in the design, implementation, and teaching of coherent therapeutic frameworks will improve the therapeutic relationship.

Source: Dickens, G. L., & Lamont, E. (2016). Mental health nurses' attitudes, behaviour, experience and knowledge regarding adults with a diagnosis of borderline personality disorder: Systematic, integrative literature review. *Journal of Clinical Nursing, 25*(13–14), 1848–1875. https://doi.org/10.1111/jocn.13202

TABLE 19.2 Potential Nursing Diagnoses for Personality Disorders

Signs and Symptoms	Nursing Diagnoses
Crisis, high levels of anxiety	Ineffective coping
	Anxiety
	Self-mutilation
Anger and aggression; child, older adult, or spouse abuse	Risk for other-directed violence
	Ineffective coping
	Impaired parenting
	Disabled family coping
Withdrawal	Social isolation
Paranoia	Fear
	Disturbed sensory perception
	Disturbed thought processes
	Defensive coping
Depression	Hopelessness
	Risk for suicide
	Self-mutilation
	Chronic low self-esteem
	Spiritual distress
Difficulty in relationships, manipulation	Ineffective coping
	Impaired social interaction
	Defensive coping
	Interrupted family processes
	Risk for loneliness
Failure to keep medical appointments, late arrival for appointments, failure to follow prescribed medical procedure or medication regimen	Ineffective therapeutic regimen management
	Non-adherence

ASSESSMENT GUIDELINES
Personality Disorders

1. Assess for suicidal or homicidal thoughts. If such thoughts are present, the person needs immediate attention.
2. Determine whether the person has a medical disorder or another psychiatric disorder that may be responsible for the symptoms (especially a substance use disorder).
3. View the assessment about personality functioning from within the person's ethnic, cultural, and social background.
4. Ascertain whether the person experienced a recent important loss. Personality disorders are often exacerbated after the loss of significant supporting people or in a disruptive social situation.
5. Evaluate for a change in personality, in middle adulthood or later, that signals the need for a thorough medical workup or assessment for an unrecognized substance use disorder.

Safety and Teamwork

When individuals with personality disorders are receiving treatment from a team of health professionals, milieu management is a significant part of treatment. Most individuals with personality disorders are admitted to hospital because of a risk to themselves or others. Patient and staff safety is a priority.

When patients are actively involved in developing their treatment plans (e.g., being included in daily staff rounds to set goals and evaluate progress), they typically take more responsibility for themselves and the success of implementing the plan. Having limits and being confronted about negative behaviour are better accepted by the person if staff members first employ empathic mirroring (i.e., reflecting back to the person an understanding of the person's distress without a value judgement). For example, the nurse can listen to a person's emotional complaints about the staff and hospital without correcting any errors but simply noting that the person truly feels hurt. Showing empathy may also decrease aggressive outbursts if the person feels that staff members are trying to understand feelings of frustration. Table 19.5 depicts a therapeutic nurse–patient interaction after an anti-social patient initiates a fight with a peer on an inpatient unit.

A final approach that is useful for people with BPD relates to the response to superficial self-destructive behaviours. Acting in accordance with unit policies, the nurse remains neutral and dresses the cutting wound in a matter-of-fact manner. Then the person is instructed to

TABLE 19.3 NOC Outcomes for Manipulative, Aggressive, and Impulsive Behaviours

Nursing Outcome and Definition	Intermediate Indicators	Short-Term Indicators
Social interaction skills: Personal behaviours that promote effective relationships	Uses conflict-resolution methods	Exhibits receptiveness Exhibits sensitivity to others Cooperates with others Uses assertive behaviours as appropriate Uses confrontation as appropriate
Personal resiliency: Positive adaptation and function of an individual following significant adversity or crisis	Uses effective coping strategies	Expresses emotion Seeks emotional support Uses strategies to promote safety Takes responsibility for own actions Uses strategies to avoid violent situations Identifies available community resources Obtains needed support Self-initiates goal-directed behaviour Expresses belief in ability to perform action Expresses that performance will lead to desired outcome
Aggression self-control: Self-restraint of assaultive, combative, or destructive behaviours toward others	Communicates needs appropriately	Identifies when frustrated Identifies when angry Identifies responsibility to maintain control Identifies alternatives to aggression Identifies alternatives to verbal outbursts Vents negative feelings appropriately Refrains from striking or harming others
Impulse self-control: Self-restraint of compulsive or impulsive behaviours	Controls impulses	Identifies harmful impulsive behaviours Identifies feelings that lead to impulsive actions Identifies consequences of impulsive actions to self or others Avoids high-risk environments and situations Seeks help when experiencing impulses

Source: Moorhead, S., Swanson, E., Johnson, M., & Maas, M. L. (Eds.). (2018). *Nursing Outcomes Classification (NOC): Measurement of health outcomes* (6th ed.). St. Louis: Elsevier.

write down the sequence of events leading up to the injury, as well as the consequences, before staff will discuss the event. This cognitive exercise encourages the person to think independently about their own behaviour instead of merely ventilating feelings. It facilitates the discussion with staff about alternative actions.

Pharmacological Interventions

There is no direct pharmacological treatment for personality disorders. However, people with personality disorders may be helped by a broad array of psychotropic medications, all geared toward maintaining cognitive function and relieving symptoms. Depending on the chief complaint, antidepressant, anxiolytic, or antipsychotic medication may be ordered for symptom relief and improved quality of life (Burchum & Rosenthal, 2018), but the treatment efficacy of these medications remains questionable, as they do not specifically treat the underlying personality disorder. Ripoll (2013) investigated trends in medication efficacy for the following personality disorders:

- People with STPD seem to benefit from low-dose atypical antipsychotic medications for their psychotic-like symptoms and day-to-day functioning.
- People with anti-social personality disorder respond to mood-stabilizing medications like lithium to help with aggression and impulsivity.
- People with BPD often respond to anti-convulsant mood-stabilizing medications, low-dose antipsychotic medications, and omega-3 supplementation for mood and emotion dysregulation symptoms. Naltrexone hydrochloride, an opioid receptor antagonist, has been found to reduce self-injuring behaviours.
- People with avoidant personality disorder seem to respond positively to medications similar to those used for anxiety disorders, such as SSRIs like citalopram (Celexa) and SNRIs such as duloxetine (Cymbalta).

Pharmacological evidence is lacking for the treatment of people with narcissistic and obsessive-compulsive personality disorders.

Case Management

Many people with personality disorders function at a high level, but a significant number need assistance to maintain their independence. Case management is helpful for individuals with personality disorders who are persistently and severely impaired. Many have had multiple hospitalizations, have been unable to maintain work or personal relationships, and are relatively alone in their attempts to care for themselves. In the acute care setting case management focuses on three goals: to gather pertinent history from current or previous providers; to support reintegration with family or loved ones as appropriate; and

TABLE 19.4 Nursing and Therapy Guidelines for Personality Disorder by Cluster

Personality Disorder	Characteristics	Nursing Guidelines	Suggested Therapies
Cluster A • Paranoid personality disorder • Schizoid personality disorder • Schizotypal personality disorder	Manifestation of ideas of reference Cognitive and perceptual distortions Social ineptness Anxiety Odd and eccentric behaviours	1. Respect patient's need for social isolation. 2. Be aware of patient's suspiciousness, and employ appropriate interventions. 3. Perform careful diagnostic assessment as needed to uncover any other medical or psychological symptoms that may need intervention (e.g., suicidal thoughts).	Supportive psychotherapy Cognitive and behavioural measures Group therapy to try to improve social skills Low-dose antipsychotics and anti-depressants

Cluster B
• Borderline personality disorder
• Narcissistic personality disorder
• Histrionic personality disorder
• Anti-social personality disorder
	Ability to seem normal
	Manipulative
	Exploitive of others
	Disparaging
	Impulsive (suicide, self-mutilation)
	Splitting (adoring then devaluing people)
	Grandiose
	Filled with rage
	Very sensitive to rejection, criticism
	Inability to experience empathy
		1. Try to prevent or reduce untoward effects of manipulation (flattery, seductiveness, instilling of guilt):
		  a. Set clear and realistic limits on specific behaviour.
		  b. Ensure that limits are adhered to by all staff.
		  c. Carefully document signs of manipulation or aggression.
		  d. Document behaviours (give times, dates, circumstances).
		  e. Provide clear boundaries and consequences.
		2. Be aware that patients can instill guilt when they are not getting what they want. Guard against being manipulated through feelings of guilt.
		3. Use clear and straightforward communication.
		4. When behavioural problems emerge, calmly review the therapeutic goals and boundaries of treatment.
		5. Avoid rejecting or rescuing.
		6. Assess for suicidal and self-mutilating behaviours, especially during times of stress.
		7. Remain neutral; avoid engaging in power struggles or becoming defensive in response to the patient's disparaging remarks.
		8. Convey unassuming self-confidence.
			Individual psychotherapy
			Dialectical behaviour therapy
			Group therapy
			Pharmacotherapy for anxiety, depression
			Careful use of addictive medications (e.g., benzodiazepines)
			Anti-convulsants may help impulsive behaviour
			Antipsychotics to control anger and brief psychosis

Cluster C • Avoidant personality disorder • Dependent personality disorder • Obsessive-compulsive personality disorder	Excessively anxious in social situations Hypersensitive to negative evaluation Desiring of social interaction Perfectionistic Has need for control Inflexible, rigid Pre-occupied with details Highly critical of self and others	1. Being pushed into social situations can cause extreme and severe anxiety. 2. Guard against power struggles with patient. Need for control is very high. 3. A friendly, accepting, reassuring approach is the best way to treat patients. 4. The most common defence mechanisms are intellectualization, rationalization, reaction formation, isolation, and undoing.	Supportive or insightful psychotherapy Group therapy Assertiveness training Anti-depressants Anti-anxiety medications Beta-adrenergic receptor antagonists help reduce autonomic nervous system hyperactivity

BOX 19.1 *NIC* Interventions for Manipulative Behaviour Limit Setting

Definition of limit setting: Establishing the parameters of desirable and acceptable personal behaviour

Activities[a]

- Discuss concerns about behaviour with person.
- Identify (with input when appropriate) undesirable personal behaviour.
- Discuss with person, when appropriate, what desirable behaviour is in a given situation or setting.
- Establish consequences (with person's input when appropriate) for occurrence or non-occurrence of desired behaviours.
- Communicate established behavioural expectations and consequences to person in language that is easily understood and non-punitive.
- Refrain from arguing or bargaining with person about established behavioural expectations and consequences.
- Monitor person for occurrence or non-occurrence of desired behaviour.
- Modify behavioural expectations and consequences, as needed, to accommodate reasonable changes in person's situation.

[a]Partial list.
NIC, Nursing Interventions Classification.
Source: Butcher, H. K., Bulechek, G. M., Dochterman, J. M., et al. (2019). *Nursing Interventions Classification (NIC)* (7th ed.). Toronto: Elsevier.

BOX 19.2 *NIC* Interventions for Aggressive Behaviour Anger Control Assistance

Definition of anger control assistance: Facilitation of the expression of anger in an adaptive, non-violent manner

Activities[a]

- Determine appropriate behavioural expectations for expression of anger, given person's level of cognitive and physical functioning.
- Limit access to frustrating situations until person is able to express anger in an adaptive manner.
- Encourage person to seek assistance from nursing staff during periods of increasing tension.
- Monitor potential for inappropriate aggression, and intervene before its expression.
- Prevent physical harm if anger is directed at self or others (e.g., restraint and removal of potential weapons).
- Provide physical outlets for expression of anger or tension (e.g., punching bag, sports, clay, journal writing).
- Provide reassurance to person that nursing staff will intervene to prevent person from losing control.
- Assist person in identifying source of anger.
- Identify function that anger, frustration, and rage serve for person.
- Identify consequences of inappropriate expression of anger.

[a]Partial list.
NIC, Nursing Interventions Classification.
Source: Butcher, H. K., Bulechek, G. M., Dochterman, J. M., et al. (2019). *Nursing Interventions Classification (NIC)* (7th ed.). Toronto: Elsevier.

BOX 19.3 *NIC* Interventions for Impulsive Behaviour Impulse-Control Training

Definition of impulse-control training: Assisting the person to mediate impulsive behaviour through application of problem-solving strategies to social and interpersonal situations

Activities[a]

- Assist person to identify the problem or situation that requires thoughtful action.
- Assist person to identify possible courses of action and their costs and benefits.
- Teach person to cue themself to "stop and think" before acting impulsively.
- Assist person to evaluate the outcome of the chosen course of action.
- Provide positive reinforcement (e.g., praise and rewards) for successful outcomes.
- Encourage person to self-reward for successful outcomes.
- Provide opportunities for person to practise problem solving (role-playing) within the therapeutic environment.
- Encourage person to practise problem solving in social and interpersonal situations outside the therapeutic environment, followed by evaluation of outcome.

[a]Partial list.
NIC, Nursing Interventions Classification.
Source: Butcher, H. K., Bulechek, G. M., Dochterman, J. M., et al. (2019). *Nursing Interventions Classification (NIC)* (7th ed.). Toronto: Elsevier.

Advanced-Practice Interventions

The mental health nurse treats individuals with personality disorders in a variety of inpatient and community settings. Research shows that treatment can be effective for many people with personality disorders, especially when a comorbid major mental illness is targeted. See Table 19.4 for a summary of nursing and therapy guidelines for personality disorders.

Advanced-practice nurses are likely to interact with staff members regarding the treatment of individuals with personality disorders as part of their practice and clinical supervision responsibilities. They can assist staff members in a therapeutic alliance. For example, they mentor and teach additional techniques that staff members can use to develop rapport and trust with patients diagnosed with STPD when these patients are experiencing heightened anxiety from being hospitalized. Nurses should understand that the patient's ability to interpret subtle, affective cues is limited and that straightforward communication is necessary (Potvin et al., 2019).

Psychotherapy. Advanced-practice nurses are highly involved in and are often the clinical leaders in providing individual and group psychotherapy using dialectical behaviour therapy. DBT is an evidence-informed therapy developed by Dr. Marsha Linehan to treat chronically suicidal people with BPD (Linehan, 1993). DBT is based on a biosocial theory that views the self-harming behaviour as a behaviour used to cope with or eliminate distress brought on by a negatively perceived environmental event, self-generated behaviours, and individual temperaments. There are three primary reasons why individuals use this means of coping: (1) low stress tolerance, (2) deficiencies in emotional regulation, and (3) self-harm is regarded as a reasonable means of problem solving. For example, if an individual is facing an intolerable and inescapable life problem, it would be only reasonable to think about suicide.

to ensure appropriate referrals to outpatient care, including substance disorder treatment, if needed. In the long-term outpatient setting case-management objectives include reducing hospitalization by providing resources for crisis services and enhancing the social support system.

TABLE 19.5 Dialogue With a Person With Manipulative, Aggressive, and Impulsive Traits

Dialogue	Therapeutic Tool/Comment
Nurse: "Borys, I would like to talk with you about what happened this morning." **Borys:** "Okay, shoot."	Be clear as to purpose of interview.
Nurse: "Tell me what started the incident." **Borys:** "Well, as I told you before, I always had to fight to get what I wanted in life. My father and mother abandoned me emotionally when I was a child."	Use open-ended statements. Maintain a non-judgemental attitude.
Nurse: "Yes, but tell me about this morning." **Borys:** "Okay. I disliked Richard from the first. He has it in for me, I just know it. He doesn't get along with anyone here. Just 2 days ago, he almost had a fight."	Redirect person to present problem or situation.
Nurse: "Borys, what do you mean, Richard has it in for you?" **Borys:** "When I'm talking to one of the nurses, he stares and makes comments under his breath."	Explore situation.
Nurse: "What does he say?" **Borys:** "How I'm 'in' with the nurses. I'm just trying to do what's expected of me here."	Encourage description.
Nurse: "You mean that Richard is envious of your relationship with the nurses?" **Borys:** "Right. He really doesn't want to be here. He doesn't care about all that therapeutic junk."	Validate person's meaning.
Nurse: "You seem to know a lot about how Richard thinks. I wonder how that is." **Borys:** "He reminds me of someone I knew when I was young. His name was Joe. We called him 'Bones.'"	Assist the person to recognize that they are assuming to know what others are thinking and that the interpretations may not be based in reality.
Nurse: "Tell me more about Bones." **Borys:** "We called him Bones because he was skinny. He was into drugs and never ate. He was also called Bones because he was selfish. He never shared anything. He never even had a girl that I knew about."	Explore situation further.
Nurse: "So Richard reminds you of someone who is selfish and lonely?" **Borys:** "That's right. I've had three marriages and girlfriends on the side. No one can take them away from me." (angrily) "Just let them try!"	Make interpretation of information. Note increasing anxiety.
Nurse: "What makes you so angry now?" **Borys:** "Richard! I know he wants to be like me, but he can't. I'll hurt him if he makes any more comments about me."	Identify feelings and explore threat or anxiety.
Nurse: "Borys, you will not hurt anyone here on the unit." **Borys:** "I'm sorry, I didn't mean that."	Set limits on, and expectations of, person's behaviour.
Nurse: "It's important that we examine your part in the incident this morning and ways to cope without threats or violence."	Focus on person's responsibility and suggest alternative methods of coping with situation.
Borys: "Listen, I know I've gotten into trouble because I can't control my temper, but that's because I won't get any respect until I can show them I don't fear them."	Person exhibits rationalization.
Nurse: "Who do you mean by 'them'?" **Borys:** "People like Richard."	Clarify pronoun.
Nurse: "You've told me that fighting was a way of survival as a child, but as an adult there are other ways of handling situations that make you angry."	Show understanding and suggest other means of coping.
Borys: "You're right. I've thought about this. Do you think it would help if you gave me some meds to control my anger?"	Person exhibits superficial and concrete thinking—possible manipulation.
Nurse: "I wasn't thinking of medications but of a plan for being aware of your anger and talking it out instead of fighting it out."	Clarify meaning toward behaviour change. Start to explore alternatives person can use when angry instead of fighting.
Borys: "I told you before, I have to fight. If I can't fight, I cut myself."	
Nurse: "Have you thought about the consequences of your fighting or cutting?"	Identify results of impulsive behaviour.
Borys: "I feel bad afterward. Sometimes I wish it hadn't happened."	Person continues to explore.

DBT combines cognitive and behavioural techniques with mindfulness, which emphasizes being aware of thoughts and actively shaping them. Interventions that are common to DBT and other behaviour therapies include cognitive restructuring, therapist reciprocal vulnerability, skills training, and reinforcement. Unique DBT interventions include the use of emotional regulation and opposite action skills, dialectics, distress tolerance skills, higher degree of therapist self-disclosure, validation as an explicit therapist skill set, and microanalytic chain analysis.

DBT encourages balance and synthesis of acceptance and change. Traditional behavioural treatment modalities focused on change in thoughts, feelings, and behaviours. There was no acknowledgement of why these occur. Patients felt invalidated and criticized and often would drop out of treatment. DBT therapists simultaneously acknowledge the pain and angst of the patient and strategize with the patient on ways of changing, thus there is acceptance and change. The primary philosophical underpinning of dialectical therapies is that in order to understand human suffering, one must understand the system as a whole. The system changes constantly, and each change influences other parts of the system. Patients are treated as a whole person; all aspects of their lives are interrelated and influence their behaviour and those around them.

The goals of DBT are to increase the person's ability to manage distress and improve interpersonal effectiveness. Treatment focuses on behaviour targets, beginning with identification of and interventions for suicidal behaviours and then progressing to a focus on interrupting destructive behaviours (Figure 19.1). Finally, DBT addresses quality-of-life behaviours across a hierarchy of care (Figure 19.2). Optimally, DBT is delivered as a skills training group program combined with individual therapy with a DBT-trained therapist who may be a nurse, social worker, or psychologist.

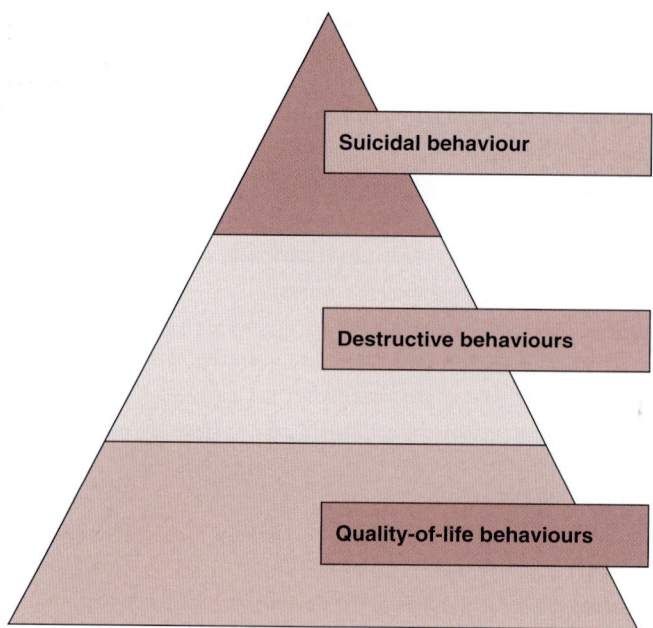

Fig. 19.1 Dialectical behaviour therapy treatment targets.

Fig. 19.2 Dialectical behaviour therapy treatment hierarchy. *QOL, Quality of life.*

Evaluation

Each therapeutic experience offers an opportunity for the person to observe themself interacting with caregivers who consistently try to teach positive coping skills. Effectiveness can be measured by how successfully the nurse is able to be genuine with the person, maintain a helpful posture, offer substanti-al instruction, and still maintain their own self care. Specific short-term outcomes may be accomplished, and overall, the person can be given the message of hope that quality of life can always be improved.

CASE STUDY AND NURSING CARE PLAN 19.1
Borderline Personality Disorder

Ada is a 24-year-old single administrative assistant who lives alone. She has been seen in the emergency department several times for superficial suicide attempts. She is admitted because she has cut her wrists, ankles, and vagina with glass and has lost a lot of blood. This event is precipitated by her graduation from business college.

Upon admission, she is sweet, serene, and grateful to all the nurses, calling them "angels of mercy." Within a week, she is angry at half of the nurses and demands a new primary nurse, saying that the one she has (to whom she had grown attached) hates her. She has a history of heavy drinking and has managed to sneak alcohol onto the unit. She has been found in bed with a young man. She continually breaks unit rules and then pleads to have this behaviour forgiven and forgotten. When angry, she threatens to cut herself again. When asked why she cut herself, Ada states, "I was tired." She appears restless and tense and frequently asks for anti-anxiety medication. When asked what she is anxious about, she says, "Uh … I don't know … I feel so empty inside." Ada frequently paces up and down the halls, looking both angry and bored. Her admitting diagnoses include substance use disorder and borderline personality disorder.

Assessment
Self-Assessment
Annie is a recent nurse graduate and Ada's primary nurse. Ada's therapist impresses upon Annie the difficulty that health care workers have in dealing effectively with people with BPD. These patients constantly act out their feelings in self-destructive and maladaptive ways. They usually are not aware of their feelings or what triggered their actions. Most difficult for many health care workers is dealing with the intense feelings and reactions that individuals with BPD can provoke in others. Annie sets up meetings twice a week with Ada's therapist to discuss the quality of the therapeutic relationship with Ada. At the next meeting, common goals and intervention strategies are discussed. This type of staff meeting, sometimes referred to as *supervision*, is a way to facilitate self-reflection for Annie and to help her work more effectively with Ada.

CASE STUDY AND NURSING CARE PLAN 19.1—cont'd
Borderline Personality Disorder

Objective Data

- Makes frequent, superficial suicide attempts
- Requests anti-anxiety medication frequently
- Paces up and down the hall much of the day
- Threatens self-mutilation when anxious
- Brings alcohol onto the unit
- Is found in bed with man

Subjective Data

- Initially was attached to her primary nurse; now says her primary nurse "hates" her, and she demands another nurse
- Appears restless and tense
- Complains of feeling empty inside
- Looks angry and bored much of the time

Diagnosis
Annie formulates two initial nursing diagnoses that have the highest priority during this time:
1. *Ineffective coping* related to inadequate psychological resources, as evidenced by self-destructive behaviours

Supporting Data
- After stating that her nurse hates her, Ada sneaks alcohol onto the unit, is found in bed with a man, and demands a new primary nurse.
Self-mutilation related to borderline personality disorder, as evidenced by suicidal gestures and poor impulse control

Supporting Data
- Is admitted following self-mutilation
- Threatens self-mutilation when anxious
- Threatens self-mutilation on unit

Outcomes Identification
1. Person will consistently demonstrate the use of effective coping strategies.
2. Person will refrain from injuring self.

Planning
The initial plan is to maintain personal safety and to encourage verbalization of feelings and impulses instead of action.

Implementation
Annie's plan of care is personalized as follows:
Nursing diagnosis: *Ineffective coping*
Outcome: Ada will consistently demonstrate the use of effective coping strategies.

Short-Term Goal	Intervention	Rationale	Evaluation
Ada will consistently demonstrate a decrease in stress as evidenced by talking about feelings with staff every day and an absence of acting-out behaviours.	1. Encourage verbalization of feelings, perceptions, and fears.	1. Discussing and understanding the dynamics of frustration help reduce the frustration by helping the person take positive action.	**Goal Met** Ada was able to experience problems and deal with them appropriately. Acting out was minimal or absent. *Example:* Ada had an appointment for a job interview. She wanted to stay in bed and avoid the interview, but instead she talked with the nurse about her fear of "growing up" and was able to get up and go to the interview.
	2. Support the use of appropriate defence mechanisms.	2. Discussing and understanding the meaning of defences help reduce the potential for acting out.	

Continued

CASE STUDY AND NURSING CARE PLAN 19.1—cont'd
Borderline Personality Disorder

Nursing diagnosis: *Self-mutilation*
Outcome: Ada will refrain from injuring herself.

Short-Term Goal	Intervention	Rationale	Evaluation
Ada will consistently demonstrate that she will seek help when feeling the urge to injure herself, as evidenced by the absence of self-injurious behaviours and talking to staff about her troubling feelings on a daily basis.	1. Assist the person to identify situations and feelings that may prompt self-harm.	1. Observing, describing, and analyzing thoughts and feelings reduce the potential for acting them out destructively.	**Goal Met** Ada was able to experience troubling thoughts and feelings without self-mutilation. She stated, "I was mad at my therapist today and decided to cut my arms after the session. Instead, I told her I was angry, and together we figured out why."
	2. Instruct the person in coping strategies.	2. Alternative behaviours are offered that can be more satisfying and growth promoting.	
	3. Provide ongoing surveillance of the person and environment.	3. Times of increased anxiety, frustration, or anger without external controls could increase the probability of the person using self-mutilating behaviours.	

Evaluation
See individual outcomes and evaluation in the care plan.

KEY POINTS TO REMEMBER

- All personality disorders share characteristics of inflexibility and difficulties in interpersonal relationships that impair social or occupational functioning.
- Personality disorders are most likely caused by a combination of biological and psychosocial factors.
- People with personality disorders often enter psychiatric treatment because of distress from a comorbid major mental illness.
- Nurses may experience intense emotional reactions to individuals with personality disorders and need to make use of clinical supervision to maintain objectivity.
- Despite the relatively fixed patterns of maladaptive behaviour, some individuals with personality disorders are able to change their behaviours over time as a result of treatment.

CRITICAL THINKING

1. Vasily is undergoing surgery for a broken leg. He is suspicious of the staff and believes that the intravenous (IV) he is receiving for hydration and pre-anaesthesia will be used for harmful purposes. He keeps his eyes closed and refuses to answer or look at his family, who describe him as guarded and odd. He has schizotypal personality disorder.
   a. Explain how being friendly and outgoing may be threatening to Vasily.
   b. Explain how being matter-of-fact and neutral and sticking to the facts would be effective with Vasily.
   c. What could be done to give Vasily some control over his situation as a hospitalized person?
   d. How could you best handle Vasily's suspiciousness, so that both you and he would feel most comfortable?
2. Cherie is brought to the emergency department by her brother after slashing her wrist with a razor. She has previously been in the emergency department for drug overdose and has a history of addictions. Cherie can be sarcastic, belittling, and aggressive to those who try to care for her. She has a history of difficulty with interpersonal relationships at her job. When the psychiatric triage nurse comes in to see her, Cherie is initially adoring and compliant, telling him, "You are the best nurse I've ever had, and I truly want to change." However, when he refuses to support her request for diazepam (Valium) and meperidine (Demerol) for "pain," she yells at him: "You are a stupid excuse for a nurse! I want to see the doctor immediately!" Cherie has borderline personality disorder (BPD).
   a. What defence mechanisms is Cherie using?
   b. How could the nurse handle this situation and Cherie's sarcasm and hostility, while setting limits and demonstrating concern?
   c. How do family members of a person with BPD typically describe their experiences?

CHAPTER REVIEW

1. A person complains that most staff do not like her or care what happens to her, but says that you are special and she can tell that you are a caring person. She talks with you about being unsure of what she wants to do with her life and her "mixed-up feelings" about relationships. When you tell her that you will be on vacation next week, she becomes very angry. Two hours later, she is found using

a curling iron to burn her underarms and explains that it "makes the numbness stop." Given this presentation, you would deduce that this person most likely has which personality disorder?
   a. Obsessive-compulsive
   b. Borderline
   c. Anti-social
   d. Schizotypal
2. Which statement about people with personality disorders is most accurate?
   a. Unlike those with mood or psychotic disorders, they are at very low risk for suicide.
   b. They tend not to perceive themselves as having a problem but instead believe that their problems are caused by how others behave toward them.
   c. They are believed to be purely psychological disorders, that is, disorders arising from psychological rather than neurological or other physiological abnormalities.
   d. Their symptoms are not as disabling as most other mental health disorders; therefore their care tends to be less challenging and less complicated for staff.
3. A person shows the nurse multiple fresh, serious (but non–life-threatening) self-inflicted cuts on her forearm. Which response would be most therapeutic?
   a. Convey empathy and explore issues that led to the self-injury as you administer first aid to the wounds.
   b. Care for the wounds; then search the person for sharp objects, and place the person on one-to-one observation or in seclusion for her own safety.
   c. Recognizing that the self-injury is, at its heart, a maladaptive attempt to obtain attention, extinguish the behaviour by minimizing the attention paid to it.
   d. Maintain a neutral demeanour while dressing the wounds, and then assign the person to write a list of circumstances that led to the injury before discussing it further.
4. A patient is flirting with a peer and is overheard asking him to intercede with staff so that she will be given privileges to leave the inpatient mental health unit. Later, she offers a back rub to a nurse if that nurse will give her the prn sedation (sedation as needed) early, although it has been ordered for 1000 hours. Which response to such behaviours would be most therapeutic?
   a. Inform the patient that she is being manipulative.
   b. Advise the other nurses that this patient is being manipulative and that they should ignore her when she behaves this way.
   c. Bargain with the patient to determine a reasonable compromise regarding how much of such behaviour is acceptable before the patient crosses the line.
   d. Ignore the behaviour for the time being so that the patient will find it unrewarding and in turn seek other, hopefully more adaptive, ways to meet her needs.
5. A person becomes frustrated and angry when trying to get his MP3 player and headset to function properly and angrily throws it across the room, nearly hitting a peer with it. Which intervention would be the most therapeutic?
   a. Place the person in seclusion for 1 hour to allow him to de-escalate and think about his behaviour.
   b. Point out that the behaviour is unacceptable.
   c. Offer to help him learn about the operation of the MP3 player.
   d. Explore with the person his feelings as he works out how to operate his MP3 player.

https://evolve.elsevier.com/Canada/Varcarolis/psychiatric/

REFERENCES

American Psychiatric Association (APA). (2013). *Diagnostic and statistical manual of mental disorders* (5th ed.). Arlington: American Psychiatric Publishing.

Barker, L. C., Gruneir, A., Fung, K., et al. (2018). Predicting psychiatric readmission: Sex-specific models to predict 30-day readmission following acute psychiatric hospitalization. *Social Psychiatry & Psychiatric Epidemiology, 53*(2), 139–149. https://doi.org/10.1007/s00127-017-1450-5

Boland, R., & Verduin, M. L. (2021). *Kaplan and Sadock's synopsis of psychiatry* (12th ed.). Philadelphia: Wolters Kluwer.

Burchum, J., & Rosenthal, L. (2018). *Lehne's pharmacology for nursing care* (10th ed.). Philadelphia: Saunders.

Butcher, H. K., Bulechek, G. M., Dochterman, J. M., et al. (2019). *Nursing Interventions Classification (NIC)* (7th ed.). Toronto: Elsevier.

Haliczer, L. A., Dixon-Gordon, K. L., Law, K. C., et al. (2020). Emotion regulation difficulties and borderline personality disorder: The moderating role of race. *Personality Disorders: Theory, Research, and Treatment, 11*(4), 280–289. https://doi.org/1037/per0000355

Henry, J., Dionne, G., Viding, E., et al. (2018). A longitudinal twin study of callous-unemotional traits during childhood. *Journal of Abnormal Psychology, 127*(4), 374–384. https://doi.org/1037/abn0000349.supp

Keefe, J. R., McMain, S. F., McCarthy, K. S., et al. (2020). A meta-analysis of psychodynamic treatments for borderline and cluster C personality disorders. *Personality Disorders: Theory, Research, and Treatment, 11*(3), 157–169. https://doi.org/10.1037/per0000382.supp

Kender, K. S. (2020). A prehistory of the diathesis-stress model: Predisposing and exciting causes of insanity in the 19th century. *American Journal of Psychiatry, 177*(7), 576–588. https://doi.org/10.1176/appi.ajp.2020.19111213

Kendler, K. S., Aggen, S. H., & Patrick, C. J. (2012). A multivariate twin study of the DSM-IV criteria for anti-social personality disorder. *Biological Psychiatry, 71*(3), 247–253.

Kernberg, O. (1985). *Internal world and external reality*. London: Aronson.

Linehan, M. M. (1993). *Cognitive behavioral treatment of borderline personality disorder*. New York: Guilford.

Mahler, M. S., Pine, F., & Bergman, A. (1975). *The psychological birth of the human infant*. New York: Basic Books.

Moorhead, S., Johnson, M., Maas, M., et al. (2018). *Nursing outcomes classification (NOC)* (6th ed.). St. Louis: Mosby.

Newton-Howes, G., Horwood, J., & Mulder, R. (2015). Personality characteristics in childhood and outcomes in adulthood: Findings from a 30 year longitudinal study. *Australian & New Zealand Journal of Psychiatry, 49*(4), 377–386. https://doi.org/10.1177/0004867415569796

Potvin, O., Vallée, C., & Larivière, N. (2019). Experience of occupations among people living with a personality disorder. *Occupational Therapy International, 2019*, 9030897. https://doi.org/10.1155/2019/9030897

Public Health Agency of Canada. (2015). *Report from the Canadian chronic disease surveillance system: Mental illness in Canada, 2015*. https://www.canada.ca/en/public-health/services/publications/diseases-conditions/report-canadian-chronic-disease-surveillance-system-mental-illness-canada-2015.html

Render, A., & Jansen, P. (2019). Dopamine and sense of agency: Determinants in personality and substance use. *PLoS ONE, 14*(3), e0214069. https://doi.org/10.1371/journal.pone.0214069.

Ripoll, L. H. (2013). Psychopharmacologic treatment of borderline personality disorder. *Dialogues in Clinical Neuroscience, 15*(2), 213–224. https://doi.org/10.31887/DCNS.2013.15.2/lripoll

Rosowsky, I., Abrams, R. C., & Zwieg, R. A. (2013). *Personality disorders in older adults*. New York: Routledge.

Schulze, L., Grove, M., Tamm, S., et al. (2019). Effects of transcranial direct current stimulation on the cognitive control of negative stimuli in borderline personality disorder. *Scientific Reports, 9*(1), 1. https://doi.org/10.1038/s41598-018-37315-x.

Skodol, A. E., Bender, D. S., Gunderson, J. G., & Oldham, J. M. (2014). Personality disorders. In R. E. Hales, S. C. Yudofsky, & L. W. Roberts (Eds.), *The American Psychiatric Publishing textbook of psychiatry* (pp. 851–894). American Psychiatric Publishing, Inc.

Winsper, C., Bilgin, A., Thompson, A., et al. (2019). The prevalence of personality disorders in the community: A global systematic review and meta-analysis. *The British Journal of Psychiatry, 216*(2), 1–10. https://doi.org/10.1192/bjp.2019.166.

World Health Organization. (2016). *International classification of diseases and related health problems, 10th revision—Clinical modification*. https://www.cdc.gov/nchs/icd/icd10cm.htm.

20

Sleep–Wake Disorders

Gabriel Barrington-Moss
Originating US chapter by Margaret Jordan Halter

https://evolve.elsevier.com/Canada/Varcarolis/psychiatric/

OBJECTIVES

1. Discuss the impact of inadequate sleep on health and well-being.
2. Describe the social and economic impact of sleep disturbance and chronic sleep deprivation.
3. Identify the risks to personal and community safety imposed by sleep disturbance and chronic sleep deprivation.
4. Describe normal sleep physiology, and explain the variations in normal sleep.
5. Differentiate between insomnia and hypersomnia, and identify at least two examples of each.
6. Identify the predisposing, precipitating, and perpetuating factors for patients with insomnia.
7. Identify and describe the use of two assessment tools in the evaluation of patients experiencing sleep disturbance.
8. Develop a teaching plan for a patient with insomnia, incorporating principles of sleep restriction, stimulus control, and cognitive behavioural therapy.
9. Formulate three nursing diagnoses for people experiencing a sleep disturbance.
10. Develop a nursing care plan for the person experiencing sleep disturbance incorporating basic sleep hygiene principles.

KEY TERMS AND CONCEPTS

- confusional arousal disorders
- dyssomnias
- excessive sleepiness
- hypersomnia disorders
- insomnia disorders
- melatonin
- polysomnography
- sleep architecture
- sleep continuity
- sleep deprivation
- sleep efficiency
- sleep fragmentation
- sleep hygiene
- sleep latency
- sleep restriction
- stimulus control

Sleep disturbances vary in severity, duration, quality, or timing, all of which can have adverse health consequences. These disturbances are broadly referred to as dyssomnias. Understandably, energy level and cognitive focus can be impaired as a result of dyssomnias, but mood can also be affected. Disturbed sleep certainly worsens the distress and impairment caused by mental illnesses and is also a potential warning sign for additional mental or physical conditions. For instance, disturbed sleep may be a sign of medical or neurological problems such as Parkinson's disease, heart failure, or osteoarthritis, among other conditions, and can also contribute to the development or exacerbation of symptoms related to post-traumatic stress disorder (Miller et al., 2020).

Sleep and sleep–wake disorders are receiving increased attention in medical, nursing, research, and social science literature. The Canadian Sleep Society was established in 1986 to facilitate research, training, dissemination of health information, and other activities with respect to the basic understanding of sleep and sleep–wake disorders. Over the past 30 years, there has been an exponential growth in our scientific understanding of these disorders. However, despite the investment in sleep-related research and tremendous growth in our understanding of sleep physiology and pathology, application of the findings has been slow.

In this chapter we briefly review the components of normal sleep, sleep regulation, and functions of sleep and give an overview of the

 HOW A NURSE HELPED ME
Worrying the Night Away

Kelly, a 30-year-old woman, was referred to the mental health nurse by her family physician for an assessment of her insomnia. Kelly reported a 3-month history of insomnia that had resulted in a progressively harder time falling asleep. Kelly reported that she would toss and turn for 2 to 3 hours before falling asleep. Due to her children's schedules, she was usually up early, so was becoming more fatigued and irritable because of her lack of sleep. Kelly was adamant with her physician that she did not want to take sleeping pills.

The mental health nurse visited Kelly at her home and conducted a complete mental status examination, including formal depression or anxiety inventories and psychosocial, sleep history, and sleep hygiene surveys. Kelly reported no other signs of mental health problems and no acute stressors other than the ongoing challenges of parenting two young children ages 2 and 3. She reported difficulty winding down in the evening and felt that, at bedtime, she was constantly thinking of things she should be getting done. During the winter, she had decreased her exercise and was drinking four or five cups of coffee a day due to her fatigue. The mental health nurse spent the first session with Kelly educating her about sleep hygiene and some cognitive strategies for decreasing worrying at bedtime. Kelly felt she could try decreasing her caffeine intake to two to three cups of coffee before 1600 hours and wanted to try getting out for a walk each day for 20 minutes. She agreed to try a worry list each day at 1500 hours rather than at bedtime.

> The second session, a week later, focused on Kelly's new bedtime routine practices, which included a warm shower and a book rather than TV and cleaning. She reported surprise at how the "worry time" strategies seemed to be working. At the final follow-up visit 1 month later, Kelly was reporting improved sleep and energy levels.

most common sleep disturbances encountered in the clinical environment, with a focus on their relationship to psychiatric illness. Pediatric sleep disorders and treatments are discussed in brief. Finally, in this chapter we discuss the nurse's role in the assessment and management of a patient with a sleep disturbance.

SLEEP

In a fast-paced society people subject themselves to schedules that disrupt normal sleep physiology, so sleep is often forfeited. The National Sleep Foundation (2016) recommends that the average adult get 7 to 9 hours of sleep each night, yet epidemiological surveys suggest that mean sleep duration among Canadian adults has decreased during the past century, with one in three adults in Canada reporting ongoing difficulties getting enough sleep (see Figure 20.1) (Government of Canada, 2019). Sleep has become an expendable commodity. People frequently cut back on sleep to meet other social and professional demands, with compensated work time and travel time being the most potent determinants of total sleep time (Centre for Sleep and Human Performance, 2021).

CONSEQUENCES OF SLEEP LOSS

The major consequence of acute or chronic sleep curtailment is **excessive sleepiness** (ES). ES is a subjective report of difficulty staying awake that is serious enough to affect social and vocational functioning and increase the risk for accident or injury. The terms *excessive sleepiness*, *excessive daytime sleepiness*, *hypersomnia*, and *hypersomnolence* are often used interchangeably. While hypersomnia is considered a disease classification, ES is a symptom of a sleep disorder or other disease but not itself a disease per se. While self-imposed sleep restriction is a common cause of ES, disruption of the normal sleep cycle (as seen in those who do shift work and people who use electronic devices late into the night), underlying sleep–wake disorders, medications, alcohol, and many medical and psychiatric disorders are important causes of ES (Gandhi et al., 2020).

We need only look to our own experiences with acute or total sleep loss to recognize its consequences. After a poor night's sleep, we feel tired, lethargic, and irritable. The effects of chronic sleep deprivation may be less obvious but may have a greater overall impact on health and well-being. The discrepancy between hours of sleep obtained and hours of sleep required for optimal functioning creates a state of **sleep deprivation**, which has widespread implications for health, safety, and quality of life. Poor general health, frequent physical distress, frequent mental distress, limitations in activities of daily living, depressive symptoms, anxiety, pain, and poor memory, learning, and motor function are all consequences of sleep deprivation (Medic et al., 2017). Specifically, chronic sleep deprivation has been linked to diabetes, obesity, and heart disease, which often relate to endocrine and breathing problems that affect sleep. For instance, the breathing-related sleep disorder sleep apnea is believed to cause and worsen medical disorders because the hypoxia, caused by the obstructive sleep apnea, activates and dysregulates the central nervous system, which is responsible for cardiovascular and endocrine hemostasis (Parajuli et al., 2019).

Sleep loss also diminishes safety, resulting in the loss of lives and property. Some of the most devastating environmental and human tragedies of our time can be linked to human error due to sleep loss and fatigue. The grounding of the *Exxon Valdez*, the nuclear meltdown at Chernobyl, and the explosion of the Union Carbide chemical plant in India are prime examples (Upender, 2017). The Canadian Council of Motor Transport Administrators reports that fatigue is the key factor in 21% of vehicle collisions, as problematic as impaired driving and distracted driving (CanadaDrives, 2022). In fact, sleep deprivation can produce psychomotor impairments equivalent to those induced by alcohol consumption at or above the legal limit for drivers. The sleep–wake cycles of all people, otherwise known as circadian rhythm, regulate cycles of wakefulness and sleep readiness throughout the day. The periods of the day that a person is most at risk for the consequences of reduced alertness are 0200 to 0400 hours and 1400 to 1600 hours. As such the Government of Canada (2017), has noted the use of jurisdictional signage, such as "Drowsy Driving Causes Crashes" or "Drowsy Drivers Next Exit 5 Kilometres," as being a valuable reminder for drivers to be aware of the implications of driving while fatigued.

Interestingly, the COVID-19 pandemic has highlighted the intrinsic relationship between quality sleep and mental health regulation. With the global pandemic impacting the macro and micro levels of functioning within individuals worldwide, we in Canada have seen a sharp increase in sleep-related disorders that have been connected to increased personal anxiety, increased alcohol intake and television exposure and decreased social support and physical activity (Kutana & Lau, 2021). Being aware of the importance of establishing a personalized plan for healthy sleep hygiene has become even more evident in the lived-experience of disrupted sleep and its collateral implications.

Formal training in sleep or sleep–wake disorders within nursing education is limited, and the number of trained clinicians and scientists is insufficient. Awareness among prospective nurses regarding the prevalence and burden of sleep disruption and the problem of inadequate sleep is lacking, and as such nursing students often rely on their own experience with sleep hygiene and sleep disorder management, rather than deferring to evidenced-based knowledge (Gellerstedt et al., 2019). Sleep is considered a basic human need and essential for holistic health and wellness. Nursing students, who are benefitted with the time to uniquely assess sleep quality in a patient, are positioned to identify altered sleep–wake cycles, their precipitating factors, and the impacts that altered sleep can have on patient challenges such as wound healing (Gellerstedt et al., 2019). See the Research Highlight for a clearer understanding of the current integration of sleep education in nursing education.

NORMAL SLEEP CYCLE

Sleep is a dynamic neurological process that involves complex interaction between the central nervous system and the environment. Behaviourally, sleep is associated with low or absent motor activity, a reduced response to environmental stimuli, and closed eyes. Neurophysiologically, sleep is categorized according to specific brainwave patterns, eye movements, and general muscle tone. Sleep is measured electrophysiologically through an electroencephalogram (EEG) and consists of two distinct physiological states: non–rapid eye movement (NREM) sleep and rapid eye movement (REM) sleep.

NREM sleep is divided into four stages characterized by progressive or deeper sleep. Stage N1, in healthy adults, begins with a brief transition between wakefulness and sleep. The time it takes to go to sleep is referred to as **sleep latency**. During stage N1 sleep, body temperature declines and muscles relax. Slow, rolling eye movements are common. People lose awareness of their environment but are generally

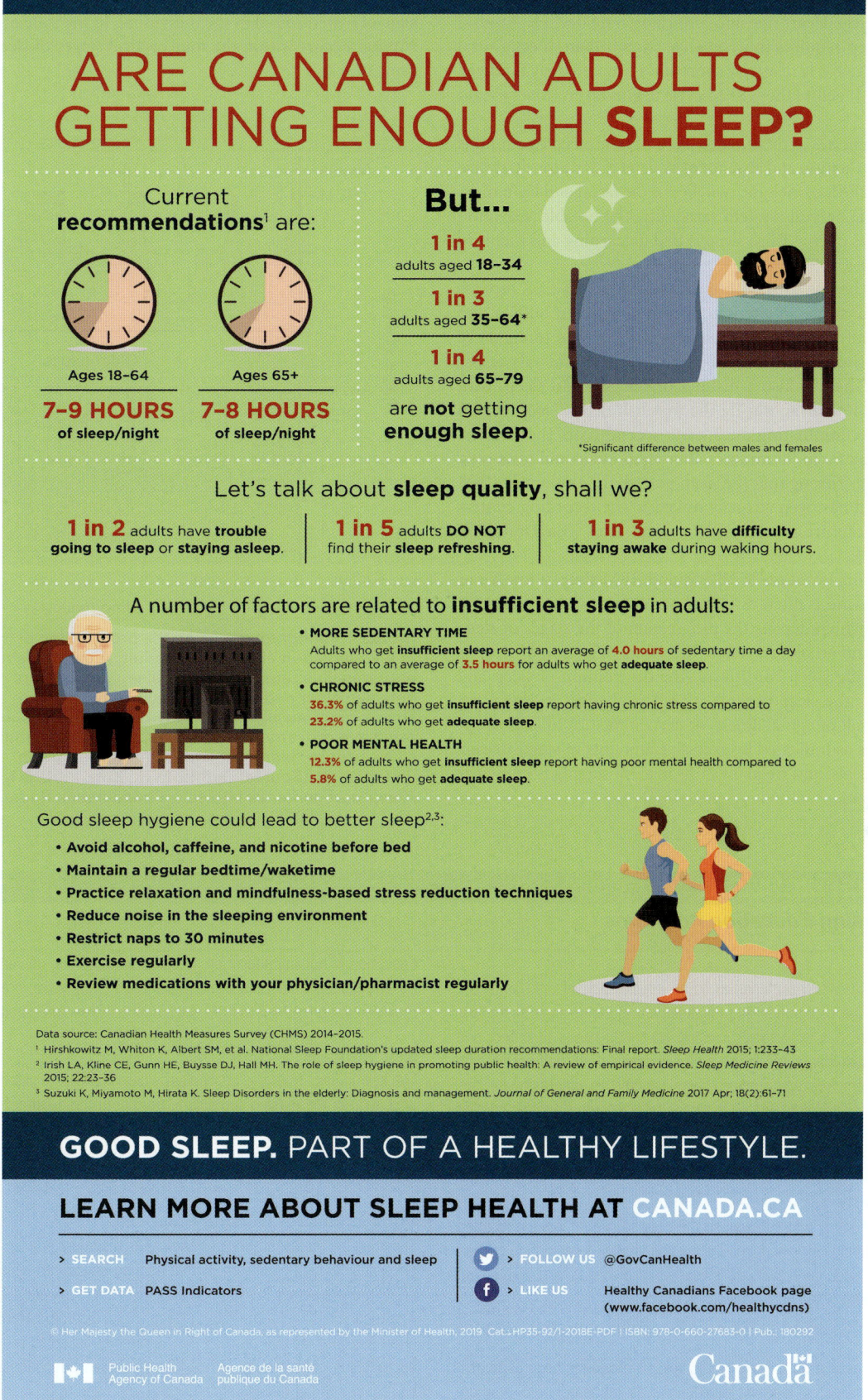

Fig. 20.1 Are Canadian adults getting enough sleep? **Source:** Government of Canada. (2019). *Are Canadians Getting enough sleep?* Retrieved from https://www.canada.ca/en/public-health/services/publications/healthy-living/canadian-adults-getting-enough-sleep-infographic.html

easily aroused. Stage N2 sleep occupies the largest amount of the total 90-minute sleep cycle. Heart rate and respiratory rate decline. Arousal from stage N2 sleep requires more intense stimuli than does arousal from stage N1. Stage N3 is relatively short and is immediately followed by a period of REM, before the NREM cycle begins again (MacDonald & Cote, 2021).

REM sleep comprises approximately 25% of total sleep time and is characterized by reduction and absence of skeletal muscle tone (muscle atonia), bursts of REM, myoclonic twitches of the facial and limb muscles, and autonomic nervous system variability. The notable activation of the hippocampus during REM sleep is tied to learning and memory (MacDonald & Cote, 2021).

Sleep normally begins with NREM sleep. Continuous EEG recordings of sleep demonstrate an alternating cycling between NREM and REM sleep. Typically, four to six cycles (potentially one to eight) of NREM and REM sleep occur over 90- to 120-minute intervals across the sleep period. There is also a distinct organization to sleep, with NREM sleep predominating during the first half of the sleep period and REM sleep predominating during the second half. The shortest REM period occurs 60 to 90 minutes after sleep onset and lasts only for several minutes. Throughout the sleep period, the amount of REM sleep increases and has been strongly linked to the recording centers of the brain that capture memory and dream states (MacDonald & Cote, 2021).

The structural organization of NREM and REM sleep is known as *sleep architecture* and is often displayed graphically as a hypnogram, as in Figure 20.2, which depicts the progression of the stages of sleep in a young adult and an older person. The visual depiction of sleep is helpful in identifying *sleep continuity* (the distribution of sleep and wakefulness across the sleep period) as well as changes in sleep that may occur as a result of aging, illness, or certain medications. Disruption of sleep stages as indicated by excessive amounts of stage 1 sleep, multiple brief arousals, and frequent shifts in sleep staging is known as *sleep fragmentation*.

Sleep can often be disrupted or fragmented as a by-product of a state of hyperarousal in the individual. In the state of hyperarousal disruption occurs within the four cyclical stages of sleep (Sleep Foundation, 2021).

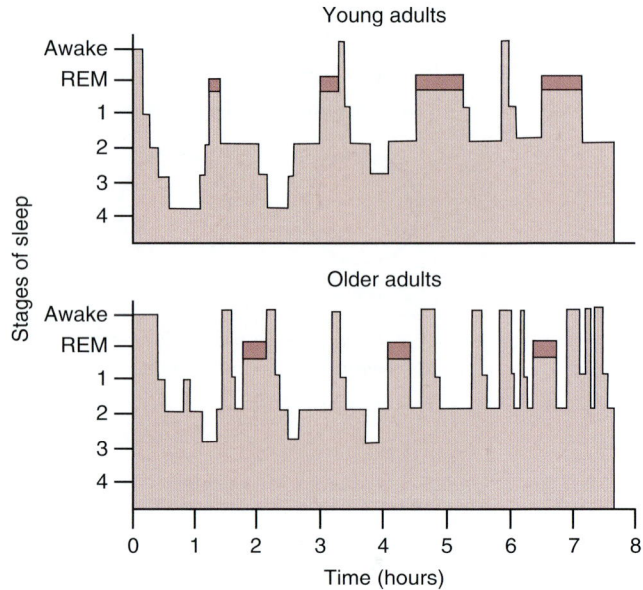

Fig. 20.2 Hypnogram depicting the progression of the stages of sleep in a young adult and an older adult. A comparison of the two hypnograms illustrates the typical sleep architecture differences found between older and young adults. The hypnogram for the older adult shows more awakenings (shown as the spikes in the graph), less rapid eye movement (REM) sleep (purple rectangles), and delayed sleep latency (length of line on far left of graph) than those of the young adult. (**Source:** Duthie, E. H., Katz, P. R., & Malone, M. (2007). *Practice of geriatrics* (4th ed.). Philadelphia: Saunders.)

RESEARCH HIGHLIGHT
Sleep in Nursing Education Programs

Problem
Nursing students are well positioned to be an integral part of the healthcare team, in terms of the recognition and management of sleep–wake disorders. In order to optimize this opportunity, nursing education needs to reflect and support the nursing students' requirements for engaging with their patients on sleep–wake disorders, from an evidenced-based perspective. Identifying the current level of nursing curriculum related to sleep–wake disorders and the nursing student's perceived preparedness to engage with patients on this topic is an essential undertaking if we are to elevate this opportunity.

Purpose of Study
The purpose of the study was to examine the current level of sleep education provided within nursing curriculum and the nursing student's perception of their preparedness to adequately evaluate sleep–wake disorders and implement meaning interventions when advantageous to the patient.

Methods
This study method was a descriptive study, using a mixed-methods approach. Information on anticipated learning outcomes was gathered from program and course syllabi, to determine the level and intentional integration of sleep education in nursing education, at three participating universities. Twenty-one nursing students from the same three universities were interviewed regarding their perception related to their sleep education and preparedness to practice.

Key Findings
The key findings from this study clearly demonstrated a significant lack of sleep education in the nursing curriculum, from both the quantitative and qualitative findings. In many programs, sleep education was entirely absent. Nursing students reported feeling significantly under prepared to engage with patients on sleep–wake disorders.

Implications for Nursing Practice
Elevating the representation of sleep–wake disorders as a significant mental and physiological health concern, within nursing education, will be essential if we are to prepare nurses to fulsomely engage in the recognition, assessment of, and treatment planning for those with sleep–wake disorders. Recognizing that sleep is an essential human process that is directly linked to patient health status, approaching engagement with evidenced-based educational preparation, will be required of our nursing students and will need to be made possible through nursing curricular change.

Source: Gellerstedt, L., Medin, J., Kumlin, M., et al. (2019). Sleep as a topic in nursing education programs? A mixed method study of syllabuses and nursing students' perceptions. *Nurse Education Today, 79*, 168–174. https://doi.org/10.1016/j.nedt.2019.05.030

REGULATION OF SLEEP

Although the regulation of sleep and wakefulness is not completely understood, it is believed to be a complex interaction between two processes: one that promotes sleep, known as the *homeostatic process* or *sleep drive*, and one that promotes wakefulness, known as the *circadian process* or *circadian drive*. The homeostatic process is dependent on the number of hours a person is awake. The longer the period of wakefulness, the stronger the sleep drive. During sleep, the sleep drive gradually dissipates.

Circadian drives are near-24-hour cycles of behaviour and physiology generated and influenced by endogenous and exogenous factors. The exogenous factors are various clues from the environment known as *zeitgebers* (time-givers) that help set our internal clock to a 24-hour cycle. The strongest external cue for wakefulness is light, whereas darkness is a cue for sleep. Other environmental cues include the timing of social events, such as meals, work, or exercise (Czeisler & Buxton, 2017). The endogenous component, known as the *master biological clock*, is located in the suprachiasmatic nucleus (SCN) of the hypothalamus. This clock regulates not only sleep but also a host of other biological and physiological functions within the body. Information about the lighting conditions of the external environment is relayed to the SCN from the retina via the retinohypothalamic tract. The SCN also receives information from the thalamus and the midbrain. These two pathways transmit photic (light-related) and non-photic information to the circadian clock through an expansive network. They also exert control over endocrine regulation, body temperature, sleep–wake cycles, metabolism, autonomic regulation, psychomotor and cognitive performance, attention, memory, and emotion (Czeisler & Buxton, 2017).

In addition to the circadian and homeostatic processes, several neurotransmitter systems are responsible for sleep and wakefulness. Wakefulness is established by wake-promoting neurons (WPN). WPN include noradrenergic neurons, serotonergic neurons, histaminergic neurons, and orexin/hypocretin-producing neurons (Oh et al., 2019). Sleep-promoting neurons (SPN) include melanin-concentrating hormone (MCH) producing neurons, gamma aminobutyric acid (GABA) energic neurons (Oh et al., 2019). The current dominant theory is that SPN and WPN compete for central inhibition and through this competition trip the switch for the corresponding sleep–wake cycle to begin (Oh et al., 2019). Any medication that crosses the blood–brain barrier may affect sleep and wakefulness through the modulation of these neurotransmitters. Many of the medications used in psychiatry manipulate these neurotransmitter systems. For example, amphetamines, which promote wakefulness, increase the release of dopamine and norepinephrine. Caffeine (methylxanthine), which promotes alertness, functions by blocking adenosine. Prescribers of medications must be aware of the effects of medication on neurotransmitters that are involved in sleep and wakefulness.

FUNCTIONS OF SLEEP

Despite remarkable advances in the understanding of sleep–wake disorders and the biological and physiological process of sleep, very little is known about the true function of sleep. Most of the information on the function of sleep, to date, demonstrates that sleep is responsible for energy conservation, restoration of performance, immune and neural pruning, and the solidification and translation of learning and memory (Song & Tagliazucchi, 2020). In brief, the essence of these theories suggest general adaptation and regulation processes. Sleep serves to restore what the body loses while awake, giving the body a chance to rejuvenate and repair itself. Energy conservation is one of the main functions of sleep and allows for synaptic downscaling and improved signal-to-noise-ratio in the brain, which in the absence of environmental stimuli and reduced energy demands, creates stronger connections in memory consolidation (Song & Tagliazucchi, 2020).

SLEEP REQUIREMENTS

Sleep architecture and efficiency may change over time, but there is little change in the amount of sleep required once we reach adulthood. Sleep requirement varies considerably from individual to individual and to some degree is probably genetically mediated. Most adults require 7 to 8 hours, and adolescents require 8 to 10 hours of sleep for optimal functioning (Arora et al., 2020). The amount of sleep required is determined by the amount after which a person feels fully awake and able to sustain normal levels of performance during the period of wakefulness. Considerable variability also exists in children's sleep duration requirements, infants aged 0 to 3 months require 14 to 17 hours, 4 to 11 months require 12 to 15 hours, children aged 1 to 2 years require 11 to 14 hours, 3 to 5 years require 10 to 13 hours, and 6 to 13 years require 9 to 11 hours' sleep over a 24-hour period (Furlong, 2019).

CONSIDERING CULTURE

Intersection Between Immigration and Gender in the Context of Troubled Sleep: Some Evidence from Canada

When examining the relative health and wellness of new immigrants, it is commonly seen that the immigrant individual will present to Canada with a higher level of measured health than a Canadian-born citizen. This is believed to be related to the nature of self-selection in the immigration process. Those able and privileged to apply and organize the necessary process to successfully immigrate often come from a background of privilege in their home countries. Canada also requires an extensive health screening process as well as an in-depth analysis of the individual's financial capital that they will bring with them to Canada. These factors position the newly landed immigrant in a position of enhanced health, when compared to a Canadian-born citizen.

Interestingly this initial health advantage appears to disappear after 5 to 10 years of their arrival to Canada. This marked decline in health status is believed to be correlated to the challenges experienced by new immigrants related to securing optimal employment, language and cultural barriers, barriers to accessing appropriate and timely healthcare, and racial discrimination. The stressors experienced by the immigrants, have been linked to the adoption of unhealthy lifestyle habits, such as smoking, high-fat/low-nutrient diets, and a sedentary lifestyle.

When we look at sleep specifically, what we see in the literature is that new immigrants do not have enhanced sleep upon arrival to Canada, and this facet of their overall health and wellness is not in alignment with their elevated health status in other domains. Even more specifically, we see that female-identified immigrants report an even lower measure of restful sleep than their male-identified counterparts.

When explored further, female immigrants described a high level of stress, related to social isolation, language barriers, reduced independence, and decreased health literacy as challenges that contributed to poor sleep duration and quality.

As nurses, we have the opportunity to assess for and identify supportive measures to reduce the barriers to restful sleep and reduced healthcare access, as experienced by new immigrants, regardless of their gender. We can capitalize on the ability to recognize the barriers experienced by our immigrants and advocate for culturally appropriate health education, social support groups and public health measures to specifically address the needs of this marginalized population.

Source: Kyeremeh, E., Sano, Y., Antabe, R., et al. (2021). Exploring the intersection between immigration and gender in the context of troubled sleep: Some evidence from Canada. *Journal of Immigrant & Minority Health, 23*(2), 257–264. https://doi.org/10.1007/s10903-020-00975-x

Many people have a misconception regarding sleep need and tend to allow circumstances to dictate the amount of sleep obtained. The most accurate way to determine one's sleep requirement is to establish a routine bedtime and allow oneself to sleep undisturbed without an alarm for several days. The average of several nights' undisturbed sleep is a good estimate of total sleep requirement, as the amount of sleep required to feel rested and minimize day-time fatigue will be based upon individual metabolic, cognitive, and functional demands of daily living (Furlong, 2019).

SLEEP PATTERNS

Sleep architecture changes over the lifespan. The percentage of each stage of sleep, as well as the overall sleep efficiency, or ratio of sleep duration to time spent in bed, varies according to age. For example, infants sleep 16 to 18 hours a day, enter sleep through REM (not NREM) sleep, and spend up to 50% of sleep time in REM sleep. By age 3, the percentage of REM sleep decreases to 20% to 25% and stays relatively constant throughout the lifecourse. The amount of slow wave sleep is maximal in young children and declines with age to almost none, particularly in men. This deficit results in a tendency for middle-of-the-night awakenings and reduced sleep efficiency with age (Bliwise & Scullin, 2017).

SLEEP–WAKE DISORDERS

The causation of sleep–wake disorders is multi-factorial, with distinct and often overlapping biological (neurological or neurochemical), psychological, and social origins. Distinct aspects of causation affect specific disorders, and since different causes call for different treatment approaches, the assessment phase of the nursing process must be emphasized.

Sleep testing is often indicated for people complaining of sleep disturbance or ES that impairs social and vocational functioning. Four common diagnostic procedures are used in the evaluation of sleep–wake disorders: polysomnography, the multiple sleep latency test (MSLT), the maintenance of wakefulness test (MWT), and actigraphy.

The polysomnogram (PSG) is the most common sleep test. It is used to diagnose and evaluate people with sleep disorders related to breathing, nocturnal seizure disorders, and various parasomnias, or unusual sleep patterns that interrupt functioning.

A PSG is a non-invasive, pain-free procedure that usually requires spending a night or two in a sleep facility for what are commonly referred to as sleep studies (National Sleep Foundation, 2020). During a PSG, a technologist records multiple biological functions during sleep, such as brainwave activity, eye movement, muscle tone, heart rhythm, and breathing, via electrodes and monitors placed on the head, chest, and legs.

After a full night's sleep is recorded, the data are tabulated and presented to a physician for interpretation. Depending on the interpretation and needs, patients may be even given therapy during the course of the study, which could include medication, oxygen, or a device for continuous positive airway pressure (CPAP) therapy. If CPAP is ineffective for obstructive sleep apnea (OSA), alternative breathing devices such as adaptive servo-ventilation (ASV) or bilevel positive airway pressure (BPAP) have demonstrated proven efficacy for some individuals (National Sleep Foundation, 2020).

An MSLT assesses daytime sleepiness by capturing and averaging how long it takes for an individual to fall asleep during four to five nap opportunities provided, and whether they enter into the state of REM sleep during the nap (National Sleep Foundation, 2020). The MSLT is routinely performed for patients suspected of having narcolepsy. An MWT evaluates a person's ability to remain awake in a situation conducive to sleep and is used to document adequate alertness in individuals with careers for which sleepiness would pose a risk to public safety (Sadeghniiat-Haghighi et al., 2020).

As an adjunct to clinical interviews, sleep diaries and, even alongside the overnight sleep studies mentioned here, actigraph devices are also used to measure sleep and track alterations, in particular for those with insomnia or circadian rhythm disorders. These watch-like devices are worn on the wrist and record movements that can be used to estimate sleep parameters with specialized algorithms in computer software programs. The watch-like device is often worn for several weeks, to get an accurate picture of activity during periods of wakefulness and sleep (Stanford Health Care, 2021).

> **SAFETY TIP**
>
> When providing care for a patient with compromised sleep, consider the impact this may have on the patients' ability to perform ADLs safety, communicate their needs effectively, heal and recover from surgery, etc. The assessment and the promotion of adequate sleep is an important and focal nursing intervention that can significantly improve clinical outcomes in the client. Promote Sleep, Stay Safe.

CLINICAL PICTURE

In the *Diagnostic and Statistical Manual of Mental Disorders*, fifth edition (*DSM-5*) sleep–wake disorders are classified into three major categories: insomnia, hypersomnia, and confusional arousal disorders, with a variety of subtypes for each (Reynolds et al., 2010). Additional clusters of sleep–wake disorders include those related to breathing and circadian rhythm. Diagnostic criteria for all include disturbed sleep causing marked distress and impaired daytime functioning. As mentioned at the start of this chapter, sleep–wake disorders may be experienced independently or as co-occurring disorders and require clinical attention so as to achieve optimal outcomes for sleep, mental health, and physical health. The most common insomnia, hypersomnia, and confusional arousal disorders, as well as breathing and sensory and movement disorders affecting sleep, are described in more detail in this chapter, with particular attention to diagnostic criteria, care, and interventions for insomnia disorders.

Insomnia Disorders

Insomnia disorders are those sleep disturbances not directly attributable to another medical, psychiatric, or substance use disorder. Individuals who experience insomnia complain that they have difficulty with sleep initiation, sleep maintenance, early awakening, or non-refreshing, non-restorative sleep. People experiencing insomnia disorders will also have altered daytime functioning associated with the sleep disturbance, such as impaired social or vocational functioning, decreased concentration or memory impairment, somatic complaints, or mood disturbance. A disorder is not manifested by a few nights of poor sleep. To be classified as a disorder, symptoms must be present for 3 or more nights a week for more than 3 months, with an impairment in functioning.

Insomnia is best understood as a state of constant hyperarousal, that disrupts the individual's ability to fall asleep and remain asleep (Sleep Foundation, 2021). Current exploration in the research has brought forward the concept of "sleep reactivity," which is a particular vulnerability of some individuals to have their sleep quality and duration negatively impact by acute or chronic stress (Sleep Foundation, 2021). In addition to a thorough medical, psychiatric, and substance use history, it is helpful to use Spielman's 3P model of insomnia to comprehensively assess the causes of insomnia, suggest appropriate interventions, and provide rationales for treatment (Sadock et al., 2017). This model suggests that three factors contribute to the insomnia complaint: predisposing, precipitating, and perpetuating factors.

Predisposing factors are individual factors that create a vulnerability to insomnia. These may include a prior history of poor-quality sleep, a history of depression and anxiety, or a state of hyperarousal. People at risk for insomnia may describe themselves as light sleepers and "night owls." Pediatric insomnia has other precipitating factors that include neurological and other disorders. For example, parents of children with attention-deficit/hyperactivity disorder (ADHD) reported that 70% of their children experienced disruptive sleep patterns in the form of, difficulty falling asleep, day-time sleepiness, delayed-onset sleep, and obstructive breathing sleep challenges (Martin et al., 2021).

Precipitating factors are external events that trigger insomnia. Personal and vocational difficulties, medical and psychiatric disorders (often comorbidly experienced with mood disorders, anxiety, post-traumatic stress disorder, cognitive disorders, and others), grief, and changes in role or identity (as seen with retirement) are examples. *Perpetuating factors* are sleep practices and attributes that maintain disordered sleep, such as dysfunctional beliefs about self and ability to sleep, fatigue, presleep arousal, and worry about the consequences of insomnia (Ellis et al., 2021).

Successful treatment of insomnia involves an integration of the basic principles of sleep hygiene (conditions and practices that promote continuous and effective sleep) (Box 20.1), behavioural therapies, and, in some instances, the use of hypnotic medication. Treatment is always targeted to the particular subtype, so, in some cases, lifestyle and breathing interventions are indicated (for instance, with sleep apnea disorders). Sedative and hypnotic medication is always used with caution, particularly when the patient has breathing-related insomnia, when addiction may be a concern, or when physical health or illness compromise breathing or central nervous system functioning. Both sedative or anxiolytic medications and over-the-counter sleeping aids have adverse effects; over-the-counter products also demonstrate limited effectiveness. Melatonin, a naturally occurring hormone, is a popular over-the-counter nutraceutical, but few data support its use in the management of insomnia (see Integrative Therapy: Melatonin for Insomnia).

Hypersomnia Disorders

Hypersomnia

Hypersomnia disorders are defined as ES that occurs three or more times per week for 3 or more months despite a main sleep lasting 7 hours or longer. The disorder is evidenced by either prolonged nighttime sleep episodes or daytime sleep episodes that occur almost daily and cause significant distress and social and vocational impairment. Key diagnostic features of hypersomnia disorders are a report of continuous yet not refreshing nor restorative sleep and difficulty waking up, either in the morning or at the end of a nap. Some individuals with these disorders can sleep up to 20 hours a day. Diagnosis is determined by clinical evaluation and a PSG and MSLT. Treatment is through lifestyle modification and stimulant medication.

BOX 20.1 Sleep Hygiene

- Maintain a regular sleep–wake schedule.
- Develop a pre-sleep routine that signals the end of the day.
- Reserve the bedroom for sleep and a place for intimacy.
- Create an environment that is conducive to sleep (taking into consideration light, temperature, and clothing).
- Avoid clock watching.
- Limit caffeinated beverages to one or two a day and none in the evening.
- Avoid heavy meals before bedtime.
- Use alcohol cautiously, and avoid use for several hours before bed.
- Avoid daytime napping.
- Exercise daily but not right before bed.
- Restrict use of light-emitting devices.

Source: Epstein, L. (2007). *The Harvard Medical School guide to a good night's sleep.* New York: McGraw-Hill.

Narcolepsy

The classic tetrad of narcolepsy includes episodes of irresistible attacks of refreshing sleep, cataplexy (muscle weakness), sleep paralysis (waking in a state of temporary paralysis), and hypnagogic hallucinations (dreaming while awake). While everyone with narcolepsy reports impairing degrees of ES, not everyone experiences cataplexy, sleep paralysis, and hypnagogic hallucinations, making diagnosis sometimes difficult. Diagnosis focuses on narcolepsy with or without cataplexy, so all points of assessment are important. When cataplexy is present, narcolepsy is almost always caused by an immune-mediated destruction of orexin (also referred to as hypocretin) neuropeptides located in the lateral hypothalamus. This condition is not considered a hypersomnia but rather its own category of disorder, and the cataplexy is then typically managed with sodium oxybate (Xyrem) and antidepressant medications.

Narcolepsy is also distinguished from other hypersomnia disorders in that patients generally feel refreshed upon waking. Associated symptoms include disturbed nighttime sleep with multiple middle-of-the-night awakenings and automatic behaviours characterized by memory lapses. Diagnosis is determined by clinical evaluation and a PSG and MSLT. Treatment is through lifestyle modifications and stimulant medication.

Confusional Arousal Disorders

Confusional arousal disorders are recurrent episodes of incomplete awakening from sleep with or without terror or movement, usually occurring during the first third of the major sleep episode and contributing to impaired nighttime and daytime safety or functioning. Varying subtypes exist and include sleepwalking, sleep terrors, nightmare disorder, sleep paralysis, and rapid eye movement behaviour disorder (RBD).

Sleepwalking

Also referred to as *somnambulism*, sleepwalking consists of a sequence of complex behaviours that begin in the first third of the night during deep NREM sleep (stages 3 and 4) and usually progress, without full consciousness or later memory, to leaving bed and walking about (activities may include dressing, going to the bathroom, screaming, and even driving). Because of the possibility of accident or injury, somnambulism in adults should be evaluated by a sleep specialist. A PSG is sometimes indicated to rule out the possibility of an underlying disorder of sleep fragmentation. Treatment consists of instructing the person and family regarding safety measures such as installing alarms or locks on windows and doors and gating stairways. Attention to sleep hygiene, limiting alcohol prior to bed, obtaining adequate amounts of sleep, and stress reduction help to prevent episodes.

Sleep Terrors

Sleep terrors are recurrent episodes of abrupt awakening from sleep, usually occurring during the first third of the major sleep episode and beginning with a panicky scream. There is intense fear and signs of autonomic arousal, such as mydriasis, tachycardia, rapid breathing, and sweating, during each episode.

Nightmare Disorder

Characterized by long, frightening dreams from which people awaken scared, nightmares almost always occur during REM sleep, usually after a long REM period late in the night. For some people, nightmare disorder is a lifetime condition; for others, nightmares occur only at times of stress and illness. Diagnosis is determined by clinical evaluation. Recurring nightmares can occur with post-traumatic stress disorder, so a thorough psychiatric exam and psychosocial history is necessary. Treatment is dependent on the frequency and severity of the symptoms, as well as the underlying cause. Treatment can include cognitive behavioural strategies, pharmacotherapy, or both. Many people do well with lifestyle modification measures, attention to sleep hygiene, and stress reduction.

Sleep Paralysis

Sleep paralysis is the sensation of paralysis at sleep onset or upon waking. The patient describes a complete awareness of their surroundings but is unable to move. For many people, sleep paralysis causes extreme anxiety and even panic. For a number of people, sleep paralysis events are rare or isolated and do not require any long-term treatment. Reassurance that the sensation is harmless and temporary is helpful. For those individuals with more frequent or severe episodes, further evaluation and treatment by a sleep specialist are warranted. Because sleep paralysis can be seen in people with narcolepsy, screening for narcolepsy is also indicated.

Rapid Eye Movement Behaviour Disorder

RBD is characterized by the absence of muscle atonia during sleep. People with this disorder display elaborate motor activity associated with dream mentation. These people are actually acting out their dreams. RBD is most frequently seen in older-adult men but can be the heralding symptom of neurological pathology such as Parkinson's disease. Serotonergic medications (such as selective serotonin reuptake inhibitors [SSRIs] or selective serotonin–norepinephrine reuptake inhibitors [SNRIs]) can induce or exacerbate episodes. Diagnosis is determined by clinical evaluation and a PSG with video recording. Treatment focuses on patient and sleep partner safety. Placing the mattress on the floor is sometimes necessary to prevent injury as a result of falling out of bed. The use of intermediate-acting benzodiazepines can be helpful, especially in cases of severe disruption to the sleep partner and concerns about safety.

Kleine–Levin Syndrome

Kleine–Levin syndrome is characterized by recurrent episodes of excessive sleep (more than 11 hours per day). These episodes of hypersomnia occur at least once a year and are between 2 days and 4 weeks in duration. When awake, during at least one of these episodes, cognition is abnormal, with a feeling of disorientation, unreality, or confusion. During episodes, patients may experience abnormal behaviour such as megaphagia or hypersexuality. Between episodes, the patient experiences normal alertness, cognitive functioning, and behaviours.

Sleep–Wake Disorders Related to Breathing
Obstructive Sleep Apnea–Hypopnea Syndrome

The most common disorder of breathing and sleeping is obstructive sleep apnea–hypopnea syndrome, which is characterized by repeated episodes of upper airway collapse and obstruction that result in sleep fragmentation. Essentially, patients with obstructive sleep apnea–hypopnea syndrome are not able to sleep and breathe at the same time. Typical symptoms include loud, disruptive snoring; witnessed apnea episodes; and excessive daytime sleepiness. Obesity is an important risk factor for OSA. Diagnosis is determined by clinical evaluation and a PSG. Treatment is with CPAP therapy.

Primary Central Sleep Apnea

Another form of sleep disorder related to breathing, primary central sleep apnea, is characterized by experiences of at least one of the following: excessive daytime sleepiness, frequent arousals and awakenings during sleep or insomnia complaints, or awakening short of breath. The PSG will show five or more central apneas per hour of sleep.

Primary Alveolar Hypoventilation

In the case of primary alveolar hypoventilation PSG monitoring demonstrates episodes of shallow breathing longer than 10 seconds in duration associated with arterial oxygen desaturation and frequent arousals from sleep associated with the breathing disturbances or bradytachycardia. Patients often report excessive daytime sleepiness, frequent arousals and awakenings during sleep, or insomnia complaints.

Circadian Rhythm Sleep Disorder

Circadian rhythm sleep disorder is characterized by a persistent or recurrent pattern-of-sleep disruption. It results from an altered function of the circadian timing system or from a mismatch between the individual's natural circadian sleep–wake cycle and external demands regarding the timing and duration of sleep, for example, as occurs with shift work or jet lag. Diagnosis is determined by clinical evaluation, sleep diaries, and actigraphy. Current treatment plans include addressing lifestyle factors that may be mitigated to reduce the negative impacts of this form of sleep disorder. Researchers are closely looking at the timing to administration of sleep aid medication, and how this impacts the resetting or offsetting of the circadian rhythm cycles (Garbarino et al., 2020).

Restless Legs Syndrome (Willis-Ekbom Disease)

Restless legs syndrome (RLS) is a sensory and movement disorder characterized by an uncomfortable sensation in the legs (occasionally affecting the arms and trunk) accompanied by an urge to move. Symptoms begin or worsen during periods of inactivity and are relieved or reduced by physical activity such as walking, stretching, or flexing. Symptoms are worse in the evening and at bedtime and can have a significant impact on the individual's ability to fall asleep and stay asleep. Diagnosis is determined by clinical evaluation. Many people with RLS also have periodic limb movements during sleep that are observed during a PSG and are at increased risk for depression and anxiety. Those individuals diagnosed with chronic medical conditions including cardiovascular disease, hypertension, multiple sclerosis, Parkinson's disease, spinal cord disease, and neuropathy have a marked increased risk of developing RLS (Massey & Robertson, 2020). Treatment is through lifestyle modification and dopamine agonist therapy, such as pramipexole (Mirapex) and ropinirole (generic), as well as addressing low serum ferratin which can be a causative agent, increasing the individuals activity level and managing their identified comorbidities (Massey & Robertson, 2020).

> **VIGNETTE**
>
> Nahla is a 32-year-old woman who was referred by her primary care provider for a psychiatric evaluation for complaints of anxiety and restlessness. She reported feeling fine during the day, but in the evening, she felt nervous and anxious. The symptoms always started at the same time. As soon as she would settle down for the evening to watch some television, she would begin to have a restless sensation in her legs that would make her jump up and pace back and forth. She described the sensation as having "soda pop fizzing through my veins." Sometimes she would go out for a walk at night even if it was very late in order to "calm down." These episodes began to occur almost nightly, and, as a result, she was having difficulty getting a good night's sleep. She began to dread the approach of nightfall. A full clinical evaluation suggested the diagnosis of RLS, and a course of the dopamine agonist pramipexole was initiated in the evening, resulting in dramatic improvement in her symptoms and total resolution of her sleep complaint.

EPIDEMIOLOGY

Sleep–wake problems are highly prevalent and occur across all age groups, cultures, and genders. It is estimated that 6% to 48% of Canadians experience some form of insomnia, and the range reported is dependent on the impact and presence of daytime symptoms, diagnosed insomnia, and general dissatisfaction with their sleep (Statistics Canada, 2018). Further, 23% of Canadian adults have been diagnosed with sleep apnea or are at high risk for experiencing OSA (Respiratory Therapy Society of Ontario, 2020). In Canada long wait times to be definitively diagnosed with OSA, and be effectively treated and provided with the necessary at home CPAP device, results in a marked increased risk for OSA individuals to be involved in motor vehicle collisions, are 50% more likely to be involved in work-related injuries, and are at a notably higher risk of stroke and death (Respiratory Therapy Society of Ontario, 2020).

COMORBIDITY

Multiple studies suggest that sleeping less than 7 hours per night, or being a short sleeper, may have a significant impact on an individual's income level, symptoms of depression, body mass index, propensity to substance use, anemia, hyperlipidemia, and musculoskeletal injuries (Chen et al., 2020). Short sleep duration has been associated with obesity, cardiovascular disease and hypertension, and impaired glucose tolerance and diabetes (Barone & Menna-Barreto, 2011). Many sleep–wake disorders increase the risk for the development of certain medical conditions. For example, obstructive sleep apnea has been associated with systemic hypertension, vascular disease, cognitive deficiencies, and metabolic syndromes (Respiratory Therapy Society of Ontario, 2020). In a study focusing on nursing night shift nurses were shown to be significantly impacted by sleep-related problems due to the disruption in their circadian rhythm and the reduced day time sleep available to them. These disruptions were linked to decreased cognitive functioning and in turn, increased workplace accidents (Alfonsi et al., 2021). Individuals with neurological disease, such as Alzheimer's and Parkinson's disease, frequently experience sleep disturbance that worsens with the progression of the illness. Sleep disturbance is a major factor contributing to placement of people with dementia in a long-term care facility.

Most psychiatric disorders are associated with sleep disturbance. Insomnia is the most frequent complaint, but reports of hypersomnia are also common. About 85% of people with a major mood disorder will report some type of a sleep disturbance over the course of the illness. In addition, there is evidence to demonstrate that sleep disruption itself may be a precipitating factor in triggering mood and other psychiatric disorders and increases the risk for relapse, making the identification and management of sleep disturbance in people with affective disorders critical (Herrick & Sateia, 2016; Kaplan et al., 2012; Staner, 2010). In a Canadian study researchers found that people with mood disorders who experience a sleep disturbance or fragmented sleep have a marked increase in risk for suicidal ideation over their life time, and when their psychiatric symptoms are well managed, they often go on to struggle with sleep problems (Bertrand et al., 2020). Sleep disturbance is common in people with alcoholism, and insomnia occurs in 36% to 72% of patients in early recovery and persists for months or even years. Sleep disturbance increases the risk for relapse to alcohol abuse. Targeting sleep disturbance during recovery may support continued abstinence, as the risk for the misuse of sleep aids during recovery, when sleep disturbances can arise, and the subsequent dependence on those sleep aids, can create a vicious circle in the recovery–relapse cycle (Reid-Varley et al., 2020).

Sleep–Wake Disorders and Mental Illness

People with sleep–wake disorders tend to focus on their sleep problems and may ignore the symptoms of other mental health or physical health disorders. It is not unusual for patients to present to a sleep–wake disorders centre for a sleep evaluation and later be diagnosed with an additional sleep–wake disorder, a psychiatric disorder, or both. For example, a person may be assessed for a breathing-related sleep–wake disorder and also diagnosed with insomnia, or may be diagnosed with comorbid RLS and insomnia. People with major depressive disorder frequently experience insomnia that involves relatively normal sleep onset followed by repeated awakenings during the second half of the night and early-morning waking. They usually then are in a difficult mood in the morning. Many patients point to the sleep disruption as the cause of the mood disturbance and report that if they could just get a good night's sleep, the mood symptoms would improve.

Difficulty with sleep latency is common with all anxiety disorders, and it is not unusual for people with a previously undiagnosed anxiety disorder to present for treatment of an insomnia complaint of lifelong duration. Management of the underlying anxiety diagnosis in conjunction with the insomnia complaint results in the best clinical outcome. Finally, people with schizophrenia have prolonged sleep latencies, sleep fragmentation, and multiple middle-of-the-night awakenings. In people with schizophrenia sleep disruptions have been positively correlated with an increase in positive and negative symptoms, and notably increase the risk for psychosis (Meyer et al., 2020). Thirty-six to 44% of people with schizophrenia experience difficulty initiating and maintaining sleep, resulting in daytime napping and exacerbation of symptomology (Meyer et al., 2020).

> **VIGNETTE**
>
> Margret had been living with treatment-resistant schizophrenia for many years. Despite multiple medication trials, she had poor control of her symptoms and was frequently hospitalized. Last year she was started on clozapine (Clozaril); within a few months, she had a dramatic reduction in her command hallucinations and total resolution of paranoid delusions. Her family was thrilled. She was finally working and living in a group home. Over the past few months, however, the group home staff noticed a change in Margret's sleep patterns. She frequently wakes during the night and, in the morning, complains of a headache and a sore throat. When she returns home from work in the afternoon, it is not unusual for her to take a nap for 60 minutes or longer. In addition, the group home staff members express concern that she has gained more than 18 kilograms in the past year and feel that she is out of shape. They have been trying to get her motivated to exercise, but she complains of feeling too tired. While Margret was home on a family visit, her mother noted loud snoring and discussed this detail with the psychiatrist. A PSG was performed and demonstrated a severe degree of obstructive sleep apnea, most likely related to her recent weight gain. Continuous positive airway pressure (CPAP) therapy was initiated, and she was able to return to her baseline level of functioning.

Hypersomnia is seen in many patients with mental conditions, including mood disorders. Many people report excessive daytime sleepiness in the beginning stages of a mild depressive disorder. A similar complaint is characteristic of the depressed phase of bipolar I disorder. Uncomplicated grief may temporarily be associated with hypersomnia. Personality disorders, dissociative disorders, somatoform disorders, and dissociative fugue are all associated with hypersomnia. Treatment is directed at both the sleep–wake disorder and the psychiatric disorder (Reynolds et al., 2010).

Sleep and General Health

Many medical conditions are also associated with insomnia. For instance, people with conditions accompanied by pain and discomfort, such as arthritis and cardiovascular and pulmonary disease, frequently complain of insomnia. Insomnia is also associated with neoplasms, vascular lesions, infections, and degenerative and traumatic conditions. Chronic fatigue syndrome and hypothyroidism have been associated with hypersomnia. The relationship between chronic medical disorders and sleep disturbance highlights the importance of screening people with medical disorders for sleep complaints. Treatment is directed at both the sleep–wake disorder and the underlying medical condition (Sadock et al., 2017).

> **VIGNETTE**
> Robbie Carson is a student nurse assigned to Mrs. Ventresca in a long-term care (LTC) residence. Robbie is in their psychiatric nursing rotation, part of which is spent in LTC taking care of people with dementia. When Robbie receives the report in the morning, they learn that Mrs. Ventresca has been experiencing significant sleep disturbance. She seems to have difficulty falling asleep and frequently wakes up groaning during the night. Robbie notes that Mrs. Ventresca is very confused, as well as agitated. She grimaces whenever she moves. Robbie believes that Mrs. Ventresca is in pain. They check her history to find that she has had arthritis for many years. They then check her medication profile and discovers that Mrs. Ventresca is not on any pain medication for her arthritis. They speak to the charge nurse, who calls the physician. Immediately, the physician orders acetaminophen at bedtime for Mrs. Ventresca. Over the next few days, not only is there a dramatic improvement in Mrs. Ventresca's sleep, but her confusion abates, and the agitation disappears.

A substance-induced sleep disorder can result from the use or recent discontinuance of a substance or medication. While it is obvious that many prescriptions and over-the-counter medications may affect sleep, there is less appreciation for the effects of commonly used substances on sleep. Alcohol, nicotine, and caffeine all have an impact on sleep quantity and quality. Alcohol, despite its great soporific effects, decreases deep sleep (stages 3 and 4) and REM sleep and is responsible for middle-of-the-night awakenings with difficulty returning to sleep. Nicotine is a central nervous system stimulant, increasing heart rate, blood pressure, and respiratory rate. As nicotine levels decline through the night, people wake in response to mild withdrawal symptoms. Caffeine blocks the neurotransmitter adenosine, promoting wakefulness. It also increases anxiety, headaches, gastrointestinal problems, sleep difficulties, weight concerns and depressed mood related to perceived dependency. In an attempt to reduce or cease the use of caffeine, individuals will experience withdrawal symptoms, including flu-like symptoms, irritably, increased anxiety, day-time sleepiness, and headaches (Rodda et al., 2020).

APPLICATION OF THE NURSING PROCESS

Regardless of the clinical environment or the presenting complaint, every patient can benefit from a sleep evaluation. Assessment of the person's sleep allows the nurse to identify short- and long-term health risks associated with sleep–wake disorders and sleep deprivation, provide health teaching and counselling regarding sleep needs, and improve clinical outcomes in those experiencing a sleep disturbance.

Assessment

General Assessment

Sleep patterns. People frequently do not report sleep difficulties or discuss their sleep-related concerns with health care providers. They tend to minimize or adapt to the consequences of sleep disturbance. Furthermore, there is a lack of knowledge about the impact that sleep disturbance and sleep deprivation have on overall functioning and health. Many people do not complain of sleep disturbance directly but, rather, complain of associated symptoms such as fatigue, decreased concentration, mood disturbance, or physical ailments.

In assessing the patient with a sleep complaint, you must recognize the 24-hour nature of the sleep disturbance. Sleep disturbance is not confined to the 7 or 8 hours devoted to sleep. Sleep diaries (Figure 20.3) are helpful in identifying sleep patterns and behaviours that may be contributing to the sleep complaint. Assigning the person the homework of completing a sleep diary for 2 weeks will help guide the assessment and direct the plan of care. The following questions and comments provide direction for the assessment:

- When did you begin having trouble with sleep? Have you had trouble with sleep in the past?
- Describe your pre-bedtime routine. What are the activities you customarily engage in before sleep?
- Describe your sleeping environment. Are there things in your sleep environment that are hampering your sleep (such as noise, light, temperature, overall comfort)?
- Do you use your bedroom for things other than sleep or sexual activity (such as working, eating, or watching television)?
- What time do you go to bed? How long does it take to fall asleep?
- Once asleep, are you disturbed by middle-of-the-night awakening? If so, what wakes you up? Are you able to return to sleep?
- If you are unable to sleep, what do you do?
- What time do you wake up? What time do you get out of bed?
- How much time do you actually think you sleep?
- Do you sleep longer on weekends or days off?
- Do you nap? If so, for how long? Do you feel refreshed after napping?
- Can you identify any stress or problem that may have initially contributed to your sleep difficulties? Is there any particular issue or problem troubling you now?
- How have you dealt with that stress or problem?
- Tell me about your daily habits. I am interested in your diet, exercise, and medications you take. I am interested in whether or not you smoke or drink caffeinated or alcoholic beverages.
- Can you describe for me the thoughts you experience when you are lying in bed unable to get to sleep?
- What changes, if any, have you made to improve your sleep? What were the results?

Identifying sleep–wake disorders. It is helpful to think about sleep–wake disorders according to the predominant symptoms of insomnia, hypersomnia, and arousal disorders. Box 20.2 provides pertinent screening questions for each diagnosis. An affirmative answer to any of these questions demands further investigation and evaluation.

Functioning and safety. As previously described, sleep disturbance can result in increased risk for accident and injury and impose serious limitations on quality of life. Several screening tools are available to assist the clinician in evaluating sleep quality and the safety risk associated with ES. The Pittsburgh Sleep Quality Index is a subjective measure of sleep quality. A global sum of five or greater indicates poor quality and patterns of sleep (Buysse et al., 1989). The Epworth Sleepiness Scale is a validated psychometric tool used to measure subject reports of sleepiness and has been validated by objective measures using the MSLT. Scores of less than 10 are considered normal, 10 to 15 is moderately sleepy, and greater than 15 is excessively sleepy. In addition to these screening tools, the following questions provide direction for further assessment:

- Have you had an accident or injury as a result of sleepiness?
- Are you sleepy when you drive a car? What do you do if you are sleepy while driving?

Two-week sleep diary

INSTRUCTIONS:
1. Write the date, day of the week, and type of day: Work, School, Day off, or Vacation.
2. Put the letter "C" in the box when you have coffee, cola, or tea. Put "M" when you take any medicine. Put "A" when you drink alcohol. Put "E" when you exercise.
3. Put a line (|) to show when you go to bed. Shade in the box that shows when you think you fell asleep.
4. Shade in all the boxes that show when you are asleep at night or when you take a nap during the day.
5. Leave boxes unshaded to show when you wake up at night and when you are awake during the day.

SAMPLE ENTRY BELOW: On a Monday when I worked, I jogged on my lunch break at 1 PM, had a glass of wine with dinner at 6 PM, fell asleep watching TV from 7 to 8 PM, went to bed at 10:30 PM, fell asleep around midnight, woke up and couldn't get back to sleep at about 4 AM, went back to sleep from 5 to 7 AM, and had coffee and medicine at 7:00 AM.

Fig. 20.3 Two-week sleep diary. (**Source:** Adapted from American Academy of Sleep Medicine. (n.d.). *Two week sleep diary.* Retrieved from http://yoursleep.aasmnet.org/pdf/sleepdiary.pdf)

> **BOX 20.2 Primary Symptoms of Sleep–Wake Disorders Screening Questions**
>
> **Insomnia**
> - Do you have difficulty falling asleep, difficulty staying asleep, or early-morning awakenings?
> - Do you feel not refreshed and not restored in the morning?
> - Have you noticed any problems with your energy, mood, concentration, or work quality as a result of your sleep problem?
> - Is your desired sleep schedule in conflict with your social and vocational goals? What is your preferred sleep schedule? *(also for circadian rhythm disturbance.)*
>
> **Hypersomnia**
> - Have you ever been told that you snore or that it looks as though you stop breathing in your sleep? *(Obstructive sleep apnea)*
> - Do you have an unpleasant or uncomfortable sensation in your legs (or arms) that prevents you from sleeping or wakes you up from sleep and makes you want to move? *(restless legs syndrome)*
> - Do you have episodes of sleepiness you cannot control? *(narcolepsy)*
> - Do you ever feel unrested even after an extended sleep period? *(hypersomnia)*
>
> **Confusional Arousal Disorders**
> - Have you ever been told that you have done anything unusual in your sleep, such as walking *(somnambulism)* or talking *(somniloquy)*?
> - Have you ever been told that you act out your dreams? *(REM sleep behaviour disorder)*
> - Have you ever had an unusual experience associated with sleep, such as the inability to move upon awakening or falling asleep? *(sleep paralysis)*
>
> *REM*, Rapid eye movement.

- What kind of work do you do? Do you operate heavy equipment or machinery? How many hours a week do you work? How long is your commute?
- How does your sleep disturbance affect your work performance?
- Do you avoid social obligations as a result of your sleep problems?
- Do you feel as though your sleep disturbance is affecting your physical health? How so?

Sleep Studies

Alongside screening questionnaires and tools such as sleep diaries, and in cases where more complex medical diagnostics are necessary, a patient may participate in diagnostic sleep studies, often using PSG or actigraphy (National Sleep Foundation, 2020), described earlier.

Self-Assessment

Nurses are especially vulnerable to the effects of sleep deprivation and sleep disruption. Rotating shifts and night work result in circadian rhythm disruption that can cause problems with insomnia and ES. Long shifts and overtime hours may lead to a decrease in total available sleep time, and on average, a night-shift worker sleeps for nearly 1.5 to 2 hours less over a 24-hour period than a daytime worker. This lack of sleep accumulates over the course of several working nights and cannot be entirely recovered during the worker's days off. Consequently, this lack of sleep can eventually accumulate over the years and may contribute to the development of certain health problems (Canadian Sleep Society, n.d.; Government of Alberta, 2022). Inadequate sleep time and sleep quality have been shown to impair performance and judgement, both of which may affect personal safety and quality of care. In addition, nurses who work rotating or night shifts may pose an increased risk for accident or injury to self and the community, as night-shift work increases driver drowsiness, degrading driving performance and increasing the risk of near-crash drive events (Alfonsi et al., 2021).

Nurses need to be able to track their own sleep patterns, recognize the effects of chronic partial sleep deprivation on their performance and functioning, and take measures to ensure that they are well rested and able to provide safe and competent care. Self-evaluation for a possible sleep disorder and for the ability to cope with the rigours of shift work is warranted. Consultation with a sleep professional is indicated if there is significant disruption to sleep, physical and mental health, job performance, job satisfaction, and social functioning.

Paying attention to issues of sleep hygiene, obtaining 7 to 8 hours of sleep within a 24-hour period, limiting overtime hours, and limiting shift work to 8 hours are general recommendations for nurses and others working extended, night, and evening shifts, all of which can alter sleep quality and duration. Going to bed as soon as possible after a night shift will ensure a longer and a deeper sleep. It is advised to plan a fixed duration (e.g., from 0900 till 1100 hours) that will always be dedicated to sleep, both during working days and days off. This strategy of a regular sleeping period helps stabilize the biological clock and allows a worker to sleep better after a night shift without causing major disruptions during the days off. Avoiding exposure to morning light (i.e., by wearing sunglasses) between finishing work and during bedtime enables less stimulation of the biological clock and improved sleep. Increasing exposure to light in the evening and during the first half of the working night is also beneficial, as is sleeping in the darkest possible environment (Canadian Sleep Society, n.d.).

Sleeping the evening before a night shift is another strategy that supports adaptation to the altered sleep pattern, and could be appropriate as workers age and natural changes in sleep patterns occur, and for anyone starting their first night shift after some time. This strategy can reduce fatigue and stress during the night shift and allows workers to benefit from greater exposure to daylight, especially in winter. It is a strategy that facilitates moving onto a daytime schedule. For this strategy to be effective, the workers must be exposed to morning light; however, during the summer, sunglasses must be worn in the evening. Once again, sleeping in the darkest possible room is necessary (Canadian Sleep Society, n.d.).

Diagnosis

There are four specific nursing diagnoses for sleep disturbance (Herdman & Kamitsuru, 2014):
1. *Sleep deprivation*—prolonged periods of time without sleep (sustained natural, periodic suspension of relative consciousness)
2. *Insomnia*—a disruption in amount and quality of sleep that impairs functioning
3. *Readiness for enhanced sleep*—a pattern of natural, periodic suspension of consciousness that provides adequate rest, sustains a desired lifestyle, and can be strengthened
4. *Disturbed sleep pattern*—Time-limited interruptions of sleep amount and quality due to external factor

Outcomes Identification

The *Nursing Outcomes Classification (NOC)* (Moorhead et al., 2013) identifies several appropriate outcomes for the person experiencing sleep disruption, including *Sleep, Rest, Risk control*, and *Personal well-being*. Table 20.1 provides selected intermediate and short-term indicators for these categories.

Planning

The majority of people with sleep–wake disorders are treated in the community. The exceptions are cases in which the person has a primary psychiatric disorder or a medical condition that requires

TABLE 20.1 NOC Outcomes for Sleep Disturbances

Nursing Outcome and Definition	Intermediate Indicators	Short-Term Indicators
Sleep: Natural periodic suspension of consciousness during which the body is restored	Sleeps through the night consistently with improvements to sleep pattern and sleep quality	Hours of sleep improve to enable restorative state Sleep routine established Appropriate and functional wakefulness resumes
Rest: Quantity and pattern of diminished activity for mental and physical rejuvenation	Physically rested Emotionally rested Mentally rested Energy restored after rest	Amount of rest sufficient Rest pattern supports functioning Rest quality supports functioning Rested appearance
Risk control: Personal actions to prevent, eliminate, or reduce modifiable health risks	Acknowledges risk factors Modifies lifestyle to reduce risk factors	Develops effective risk-control strategies Commits to risk-control strategies
Personal well-being: Extent of positive perception of one's health status and life circumstances	Spiritual life is satisfactory Physical health is satisfactory Cognitive functioning is improved	Performance of activities of daily living Performance of usual roles

NOC, Nursing Outcomes Classification.
Source: Data from Moorhead, S., Johnson, M., Maas, M., et al. (2013). *Nursing Outcomes Classification (NOC)* (5th ed.). St. Louis: Mosby.

hospitalization. Because long-standing sleep problems are associated with a host of occupational, social, interpersonal, psychiatric, and medical conditions, the treatment is multi-faceted and frequently requires a team approach under the leadership of a sleep disorder specialist. The role of the nurse is generally to conduct a full assessment, provide support to the patient and family while the appropriate interventions are determined, and teach the patient and family strategies that may improve sleep.

Implementation

Counselling

The nurse's counselling role begins with the assessment of the sleep disorder. The nurse's questions and responses to the patient and family provide support and reassurance that the sleep problems are treatable. For many people, the distress caused by chronic sleep difficulties sets up a conditioned barrier of hopelessness. Through the nurse's counselling approach, this hopelessness is identified and countered with encouragement, positive suggestions, and the belief that the person will be able to manage sleep difficulties.

Health Teaching and Health Promotion

The nurse's role in health teaching cannot be overemphasized. Most individuals do not think about their sleep. This means that they also do not recognize the importance of a sleep routine or consider factors that influence good sleep. Many patients with sleep problems that can affect their mental health or with mental illnesses that affect sleep can learn sleep-promoting practices that they can put into place, for instance, adding a routine or taking away a sleep-impairing routine (such as use of light-emitting devices before bed). In addition, there are many myths regarding what constitutes "good sleep" and what factors contribute to sleep quality (see Box 20.1). Education about sleep testing, sleep–wake disorders, and sleep hygiene can be done verbally or with the use of educational materials such as those available through the Canadian Sleep Society or Canadian Lung Association. The nurse may also be involved in teaching relaxation techniques, such as meditation, guided imagery, progressive muscle relaxation, or controlled breathing exercises. Use of these techniques has been linked to sustained benefits for patients with primary insomnia (Sadock et al., 2017).

Pharmacological Interventions

Many people use medication to address their sleep problems. Nurses frequently provide education about the benefits of a particular medication, the adverse effects, and the fact that medications are usually prescribed for no more than 2 weeks because tolerance and withdrawal may result (Sadock et al., 2017). In many settings the nurse also monitors the effectiveness of the medication.

The Drug Treatment box provides information about hypnotics approved by Health Canada for treatment of insomnia.

Generally, however, long-term use of hypnotic medication is discouraged because non-pharmacological treatments have shown efficacy in reducing insomnia. Many antidepressants and atypical antipsychotics are also used off-label (i.e., without specific approval from Health Canada) in the treatment of sleep–wake disorders because of their sedative properties.

Cognitive Behavioural Therapy for Insomnia

Cognitive behavioural therapy for insomnia (CBT-I), that has been demonstrated to be the preferred treatment for insomnia, includes educational, behavioural, and cognitive components; it targets factors that perpetuate insomnia over time (O'Brien & Boland, 2020). The counsellor's first objectives are to provide education regarding sleep and sleep needs and help the person to set realistic expectations regarding sleep. Patients should be asked what they believe constitutes healthy sleep, and counsellors should then clarify any misconceptions. Eliciting information about the total number of hours spent sleeping typically has little value. Many people are stuck on a set number of sleep hours rather than on the quality of sleep obtained. Focusing on the number of hours slept rather than the quality of sleep and daytime functioning increases the insomnia experience.

The next approach involves modifying poor sleep habits and establishing a regular sleep–wake schedule. Keeping a sleep diary (see Figure 20.2) for a period of 2 weeks is helpful in establishing overall sleep patterns and determining overall sleep efficiency ([total sleep time ÷ total time in bed] × 100). After reviewing sleep diaries, patients are sometimes surprised to discover that their sleep problems are not as bad as previously believed. **Sleep restriction**, or limiting the total sleep time, creates a temporary, mild state of sleep deprivation and strengthens the sleep homeostatic drive. This technique decreases sleep latency and improves sleep continuity and quality. If, for example, a person's

INTEGRATIVE THERAPY

Melatonin for Insomnia

Many people with insomnia turn to over-the-counter solutions. Melatonin is a hormone secreted by the pineal gland in response to information it receives from the suprachiasmatic nucleus regarding light and dark. It is available as a synthetic product at most health food stores and pharmacies. Normally, as night approaches, melatonin is secreted and blood levels rise, producing a sensation of sleepiness. Melatonin levels stay elevated throughout the night but begin to decline in the early morning hours and are essentially undetectable during the day. It would stand to reason, then, that melatonin supplementation would be a safe and effective complementary therapy. Many patients reach for melatonin supplements in some situations to help align the body's circadian rhythms with the outside environment.

Unfortunately, research into the role of melatonin in the management of insomnia has been disappointing, with most data pointing to little to no benefit at all. It does seem, however, that melatonin may be effective in the management of circadian rhythm disorders such as jet lag, shift-work disorder, and advances and delays in the sleep cycle.

Although there have been no documented reports of toxicity or overdose of synthetic melatonin, it is important to tell patients that (1) there is no identified effective dosage range and (2) because melatonin is available over the counter and unregulated by Health Canada, there is no standardization of nutraceutical ingredients. Reported adverse effects include nausea, headache, and orthostatic blood pressure changes. Potential contraindications to melatonin use have included excessive sedation with ingestion, pregnancy or breastfeeding, seizure disorders, and warfarin therapy. More recently, the question of the potential effects of melatonin on glucose tolerance has emerged in the literature.

There is evidence available indicating that melatonin can be effective in the treatment of chronic insomnia in children and, on the whole, is well tolerated. However, there are limited evidence-based guidelines about the dosage and timing of intake for children, which makes the practice concerning. Very little systematic research has been done into the possible impact of melatonin intake on puberty and the endocrine system. Therefore treatment with melatonin in children with ADHD and chronic insomnia is advised to be reserved for only those children with sleep disorders that have a severe impact on daily functioning.

MEDICATION TREATMENT OF PATIENTS WITH INSOMNIA

Generic (Brand) Name	Onset of Action (Minutes)	Duration of Action	Health Canada–Approved for Insomnia	Habit Forming
Benzodiazepine Receptor Agonists				
Oxazepam (Serax, generics)	30–60	Long	Yes	Yes, all medications in this class are Schedule IV
Temazepam (Restoril)	45–60	Intermediate	Yes	
Triazolam	15–30	Short	Yes	
Zolpidem (Sublinox, generics)	60	Intermediate	Yes	
Zopiclone (Imovane)	60	Intermediate	Yes	
Antidepressant				
Trazodone (Oleptro)	60–120	Long	No	No
Antihistamines				
Diphenhydramine (Benedryl, Nytol)	60–180	Long	Yes	Tolerance to hypnotic effects develops in 1–2 weeks

Source: Adapted from Government of British Columbia. (2020). *Medications for insomnia.* Retrieved from https://www2.gov.bc.ca/assets/gov/health/practitioner-pro/provincial-academic-detailing-service/pad_insomnia_handout.pdf

sleep diary indicates that they are in bed for 8 hours but sleeping only 6 hours, sleep is restricted to 6 hours, and the bedtime and wake time are adjusted accordingly. The sleep time should not be reduced below 5 hours, regardless of sleep efficiency, and patients should be cautioned about the dangers of driving while undergoing a trial of sleep restriction. Once sleep efficiency is improved, total sleep time is gradually increased by 10- to 20-minute increments.

CBT-I also involves using **stimulus control**. CBT-I trained practitioners educate patients about the value of establishing a healthy connection between sleep and their bedroom environment. Specifically, the patient is guided in suggestions such as, if they are unable to fall asleep within 10 to 15 minutes that they should get out of bed and leave the bedroom, and engage in an activity that would normally fatigue them and prepare them for sleep. The patient can then return to bed when they feel fatigued (Erten Uyumaz et al., 2021).

Other objectives of CBT-I are aimed at identifying and correcting maladaptive attitudes and beliefs about sleep that perpetuate insomnia. For example, people frequently amplify the consequences of their insomnia and attribute most daytime experiences to their sleep complaint. They may rationalize maladaptive coping behaviours such as excessive time in bed to "catch up" on lost sleep and may exhibit unrealistic expectations about sleep. The practitioner offers alternative interpretations regarding the sleep complaint to assist the person in thinking about the insomnia in a different way, empowering the patient to be in control of their own sleep, and break the vicious cycle that can occur when anxiety about insomnia triggers insomnia and insomnia exacerbates the severity of the anxiety (Erten Uyumaz et al., 2021). Because CBT-I approaches are not immediately effective and may take several weeks of practice before improvement is seen, success is dependent on both a high degree of motivation in the patient and a commitment on the part of the practitioner.

Other non-pharmacological interventions for insomnia include regular exercise, music therapy, cupping, and acupuncture. Cupping in particular has been found to increase neural circulation and decrease the neural inflammation, while improving sleep and deceasing symptoms of depression, when compared to pharmacological sleep aids (Feng et al., 2019).

> **VIGNETTE**
> Josette Harris is a 52-year-old woman who complains of difficulty falling asleep and staying asleep every night. It is not unusual for Josette to take several hours to fall asleep, and once she does fall asleep, she is able to sleep for only 2 to 3 hours at a time. She tosses and turns and lies in bed "hoping to fall asleep." She estimates that she is sleeping only about 4 or 5 hours a night. Josette reports that this has been going on for at least a year but that it seems to have been getting progressively worse over the past several months. Because she sleeps poorly at night, she has been staying in bed until 0900 or 1000 in the morning and has been late for work several times during the past 3 months. She feels tired during her waking hours and has difficulty focusing on the task at hand in her accounting job. To improve her work performance, she has been drinking five or six cups of coffee during the day. Even though she feels tired, she is unable to nap. Family members complain that she is irritable and short tempered with them. Interestingly, she reports that she was able to sleep fairly well while on vacation last month. Josette completes a sleep diary for a 2-week period and undergoes a complete assessment. There seems to be no underlying medical or psychiatric disorder associated with her sleep complaint. She is diagnosed with an insomnia disorder and begins a cognitive behavioural therapy program.

Advanced-Practice Interventions

Although psychotherapy offers little value in the treatment of primary insomnia, there is a component of primary insomnia that involves a conditioned response. The initial episode of insomnia is frequently associated with a stressful event or crisis that produces anxiety. This anxiety becomes associated with worry about not being able to get to sleep and leads to preoccupation with getting enough sleep. The more the person tries to sleep, the more elusive sleep becomes, and the greater the person's anxiety. The advanced-practice nurse may be closely involved in the use of cognitive behavioural therapy to manage insomnia.

Evaluation

Evaluation is based on whether the person experiences improved sleep quality as evidenced by decreased sleep latency, fewer nighttime awakenings, and a shorter time to get back to sleep after waking. This evaluation is accomplished through an individual's report and maintenance of a sleep diary. Just as important as objective changes in the person's sleep pattern is the person's perception of improvement. Objectively, the improvement may be quite modest, but the person may perceive that they are no longer controlled by sleep (or the lack of it) but are exerting control over sleep through lifestyle changes and a better sleep routine.

KEY POINTS TO REMEMBER

- Sleep disturbance has major implications for overall health, quality of life, and personal and community safety.
- Research into the physiology of normal sleep, as well as sleep–wake disorders, is expanding.
- Most people with a mood disorder will report sleep disturbance; recognition and treatment of sleep disturbance in people with psychiatric disorders improves clinical outcomes.
- Regardless of the clinical environment or the presenting complaint, all patients can benefit from an evaluation of their sleep needs.
- It is helpful to categorize sleep disturbance according to the three major symptom categories of insomnia, hypersomnia, and confusional arousal disorders.
- Primary insomnia can be effectively treated with non-pharmacological interventions such as CBT-I, sleep restriction, stimulus control, and attention to issues of sleep hygiene. Long-term pharmacological management is generally not indicated.

CRITICAL THINKING

1. Jabar is a 46-year-old man who complains of waking frequently at night. Consequently, he is tired all day and knows that he has not been functioning as well as he should. Whenever he can manage it, he goes out to his car at lunchtime to take a 60-minute nap because he has fallen asleep at his desk in the past and been given a disciplinary warning. He is drinking two to three cups of coffee in the afternoon so that he does not feel sleepy while driving home.
   a. What questions would you ask to determine whether Jabar might have a sleep disorder?
   b. What recommendations will you make for him to improve his sleep hygiene?
   c. What instructions and education should you give Jabar regarding personal and community safety?
2. Your patient, Vivian, has been using temazepam (Restoril) for several years to treat insomnia. She has been reading that long-term use of hypnotics is not healthy or productive and wants to quit taking them. However, she is focused on needing 9 hours of sleep each night and is extremely worried about what will happen when she quits the temazepam.
   a. What instructions would you provide to Vivian regarding stimulus control, sleep restriction, and cognitive restructuring of her sleep complaint?
   b. Identify alternative pharmacological therapies.
3. Mrs. Levine is a 72-year-old woman with a history of major depression. She takes fluoxetine (Prozac) 10 mg every day and has experienced significant relief from depression. While listing her medications, she tells you she is using a variety of over-the-counter sleep aids because she has been having some difficulty sleeping recently. These over-the-counter products include diphenhydramine, melatonin, valerian, and something that her neighbour gave her to try.
   a. In light of the person's age and history of depression, what are your concerns?
   b. What further assessment is required?
   c. What specific question would you need to ask concerning her use of Prozac?
   d. What instructions and education will you provide?
4. Suzie Au, a 47-year-old business executive and single mother of two teenage sons, has presented to the urban mental health centre complaining that she is "hanging on by my fingernails," that taking care of her business and her boys is taking all of her energy, and that she has suffered from constant insomnia for several years but that it has worsened over the past few months. Her lack of sleep has forced her to give up her social life, including gym workouts. She feels stressed and worries that her ability to cope will soon disappear unless she can improve the quality of her sleep. She has begun to drink four or five cups of coffee per day to keep awake and tries to catch a nap whenever possible.
   a. What strategy or tool would enable Suzie to provide an accurate self-appraisal of the characteristics of her sleep?
   b. What further assessments would you need to do?
   c. What immediate instructions and education will you offer Suzie in regard to her current coping strategies?
   d. What short-term goals would be appropriate for Suzie?

CHAPTER REVIEW

1. A person states that he needs only 5 to 6 hours of sleep per night to feel rested. How should the nurse interpret this statement?
   a. The person is not sleeping enough.
   b. The person is sleeping too much.
   c. The person is sleeping according to his own body's needs.
   d. The person is not getting enough REM sleep.
2. The nurse is planning care for a person with primary insomnia. What is an appropriate outcome?
   a. The person will sleep 12 hours nightly.
   b. The person will go to bed and wake up at consistent times daily.
   c. The person will take one nap daily to restore energy.
   d. The person will drink a cup of warm tea before bedtime.
3. The nurse is providing teaching for a person who has been taking a hypnotic medication to sleep. What statement by the nurse is appropriate?
   a. "You can use this medication for as long as you would like."
   b. "It would be better to take an over-the-counter medication instead."
   c. "Melatonin has been shown to be just as effective as hypnotic medications."
   d. "Be certain to follow up with your doctor regularly while you take this medication."
4. Because of the likelihood of underestimated or inaccurate self-assessment of sleep, what tool would be most appropriate for the nurse to use in obtaining an assessment from a patient suspected of having a sleep–wake disorder?
   a. A mini-mental state examination
   b. An anxiety inventory
   c. A sleep diary
   d. A family history assessment
5. Which behaviour would alert the nurse to a circadian rhythm sleep disorder?
   a. Excessive sleepiness for at least 1 month, accompanied by prolonged sleep episodes
   b. Multiple episodes of brief daytime sleeping followed by disturbed nighttime sleep
   c. Persistent patterns of sleep disruption after travelling for business
   d. Repeated episodes of upper airway collapse and obstruction that results in sleep fragmentation

https://evolve.elsevier.com/Canada/Varcarolis/psychiatric/

REFERENCES

Alfonsi, V., Scarpelli, S., Gorgoni, M., et al. (2021). Sleep-related problems in night shift nurses: Towards an individualized interventional practice. *Frontiers in Human Neuroscience, 15,* 644570.

Arora, A., Pell, D., van Sluijs, E. M. F., et al. (2020). How do associations between sleep duration and metabolic health differ with age in the UK general population?. *PLoS ONE, 15*(11), 1–16. https://doi.org/10.1371/journal.pone.0242852

Barone, M. T., & Menna-Barreto, L. (2011). Diabetes and sleep: A complex cause-and-effect relationship. *Diabetes Research and Clinical Practice, 91,* 129–137. https://doi.org/10.1016/j.diabres.2010.07.011

Bertrand, L., Bourguignon, C., Beaulieu, S., et al. (2020). Suicidal ideation and insomnia in bipolar disorders: Idéation suicidaire et insomnie dans les troubles bipolaires. *Canadian Journal of Psychiatry, 65*(11), 802–810. https://doi.org/10.1177/0706743720952226

Bliwise, D., & Scullin, M. K. (2017). Normal aging. In M. Kryger, T. Roth, & W. Dement (Eds.), *Principles and practice of sleep medicine* (6th ed.) (pp. 25–38). Philadelphia: Elsevier.

Buysse, D. J., Reynolds, C. F., III, Monk, T. H., et al. (1989). The Pittsburgh Sleep Quality Index: A new instrument for psychiatric practice and research. *Psychiatry Research, 28,* 193–213. https://doi.org/10.1016/0165-1781(89)90047-4

CanadaDrives. (2022). *Drowsy driving: The dangers and laws in Canada.* Retrieved from https://www.canadadrives.ca/blog/driving-tips/drowsy-driving

Canadian Sleep Society. (n.d.). *Strategies for night shift workers.* Retrieved from https://css-scs.ca/product/brochure-strategies-night-shift-workers/

Centre for Sleep and Human Performance. (2021). *Spotlight on insomnia.* Retrieved from https://centreforsleep.com/about/news/spotlight-on-insomnia.html

Chen, X., Wang, S.-B., Li, X.-L., et al. (2020). Relationship between sleep duration and sociodemographic characteristics, mental health and chronic diseases in individuals aged from 18 to 85 years old in Guangdong province in China: A population-based cross-sectional study. *BMC Psychiatry, 20*(1), 1–10. https://doi.org/10.1186/s12888-020-02866-9

Czeisler, C., & Buxton, O. M. (2017). The human circadian timing system and sleep–wake regulation. In M. Kryger, T. Roth, & W. Dement (Eds.), *Principles and practice of sleep medicine* (6th ed.) (pp. 362–376). Philadelphia: Saunders.

Ellis, J. G., Perlis, M. L., Espie, C. A., et al. (2021). The natural history of insomnia: Predisposing, precipitating, coping and perpetuating factors over the early developmental course of insomnia. *Sleep, 44*(9), zsab095. https://doi.org/10.1093/sleep/zsab095

Erten Uyumaz, B., Feijs, L., & Hu, J. (2021). A review of digital cognitive behavioral therapy for insomnia (CBT-I Apps): Are they designed for engagement?. *International Journal of Environmental Research and Public Health, 18*(6), 2929. https://doi.org/10.3390/ijerph18062929

Feng, F., Yu, S., Wang, Z., et al. (2019). Non-pharmacological and pharmacological interventions relieve insomnia symptoms by modulating a shared network: A controlled longitudinal study. *NeuroImage: Clinical, 22,* 101745. https://doi.org/10.1016/j.nicl.2019.101745

Furlong, S. (2019). Child sleep: A systemic exploration of the knowledge and experience of educational psychologists, parents and primary school staff. *Published DEdPsy Thesis, Cardiff University.* Retrieved from https://orca.cardiff.ac.uk/124060/14/ThesisFurlongDEdPsy.pdf

Gandhi, K. D., Mansukhani, M. P., Silber, M. H., et al. (2020). Excessive daytime sleepiness: A clinical review. *Mayo Clinic Proceedings, 96*(5), P1288–P1301. https://doi.org/10.1016/j.mayocp.2020.08.033

Garbarino, S., Lanteri, P., Prada, V., et al. (2020). Circadian rhythms, sleep, and aging. *Journal of Psychophysiology, 35*(3), 129–138. https://doi.org/10.1027/0269-8803/a000267

Gellerstedt, L., Medin, J., Kumlin, M., et al. (2019). Sleep as a topic in nursing education programs? A mixed method study of syllabuses and nursing students' perceptions. *Nurse Education Today, 79,* 168–174. https://doi.org/10.1016/j.nedt.2019.05.030

Government of Alberta. (2022). *Fatigue management program and training.* Retrieved from https://www.alberta.ca/fatigue-management-program-and-training.aspx

Government of Canada. (2017). *Road safety in Canada.* Retrieved from https://www.tc.gc.ca/eng/motorvehiclesafety/tp-tp15145-1201.htm

Government of Canada. (2019). *Are Canadians getting enough sleep?* Retrieved from https://www.canada.ca/en/public-health/services/publications/healthy-living/canadian-adults-getting-enough-sleep-infographic.html

Herdman, T. H., & Kamitsuru, S. (Eds.). (2014). *NANDA International Nursing Diagnoses: Definitions and classification, 2015–2017.* Oxford: Wiley-Blackwell.

Herrick, D. D., & Sateia, M. J. (2016). Insomnia and depression: A reciprocal relationship. *Psychiatric Annals, 46*(3), 164. https://doi.org/10.3928/00485713-20160121-01

Kaplan, K. A., Talbot, L. S., Gruber, J., et al. (2012). Evaluating sleep in bipolar disorder: Comparison between actigraphy, polysomnography, and sleep diary. *Bipolar Disorders, 14*(8), 870–879. https://doi.org/10.1111/bdi.12021

Kutana, S., & Lau, P. H. (2021). The impact of the 2019 coronavirus disease (COVID-19) pandemic on sleep health. *Canadian Psychology, 62*(1), 12–19. https://doi.org/10.1037/cap0000256

MacDonald, K. J., & Cote, K. A. (2021). Contributions of post-learning REM and NREM sleep to memory retrieval. *Sleep Medicine Reviews, 59,* 101453. https://doi.org/10.1016/j.smrv.2021.101453

Martin, C. A., Papadopoulos, N., Rinehart, N., et al. (2021). Associations between child sleep problems and maternal mental health in children with ADHD. *Behavioral Sleep Medicine, 19*(1), 12–25. https://doi.org/10.1080/15402002.2019.1696346

Massey, T. H., & Robertson, N. P. (2020). Restless legs syndrome: Causes and consequences. *Journal of Neurology, 267*(2), 575–577. https://doi.org/10.1007/s00415-019-09682-6

Medic, G., Wille, M., & Hemels, M. E. (2017). Short- and long-term health consequences of sleep disruption. *Nature and Science of Sleep, 9,* 151–161. https://doi.org/10.2147/NSS.S134864

Meyer, N., Faulkner, S. M., McCutcheon, R. A., et al. (2020). Sleep and circadian rhythm disturbance in remitted schizophrenia and bipolar disorder: A systematic review and meta-analysis. *Schizophrenia Bulletin, 46*(5), 1126–1143. https://doi.org/10.1093/schbul/sbaa024

Miller, K. E., Brownlow, J. A., & Gehrman, P. R. (2020). Sleep in PTSD: Treatment approaches and outcomes. *Current Opinion in Psychology, 34,* 12–17. https://doi.org/10.1016/j.copsyc.2019.08.017

Moorhead, S., Johnson, M., Maas, M. L., et al. (2013). *Nursing Outcomes Classification (NOC)* (5th ed.). St. Louis: Mosby.

National Sleep Foundation. (2016). *How much sleep do we really need?* Retrieved from https://sleepfoundation.org/how-sleep-works/how-much-sleep-do-we-really-need

National Sleep Foundation. (2020). *Obstructive sleep apnea.* Retrieved from https://www.thensf.org/do-i-have-obstructive-sleep-apnea/

O'Brien, E. M., & Boland, E. M. (2020). CBT-I is an efficacious, first-line treatment for insomnia: Where we need to go from here. A commentary on the application of Tolin's criteria to cognitive behavioral therapy for insomnia. *Clinical Psychology: Science and Practice, 27*(4), e12370. https://doi.org/10.1111/cpsp.12370

Oh, J., Petersen, C., Walsh, C. M., et al. (2019). The role of co-neurotransmitters in sleep and wake regulation. *Molecular Psychiatry, 24*(9), 1284–1295. https://doi.org/10.1038/s41380-018-0291-2

Parajuli, S., Tiwari, R., Clark, D. F., et al. (2019). Sleep disorders: Serious threats among kidney transplant recipients. *Transplantation Reviews, 33*(1), 9–16. https://doi.org/10.1016/j.trre.2018.09.002

Reynolds, C. F., 3rd, Redline, S., & DSM-V Sleep-Wake Disorders Workgroup and Advisors (2010). The DSM-V sleep-wake disorders nosology: An update and an invitation to the sleep community. *Journal of Clinical Sleep Medicine, 6*(1), 9–10.

Reid-Varley, W.-B., Martinez, C. P., & Khurshid, K. A. (2020). Sleep disorders and disrupted sleep in addiction, withdrawal and abstinence with focus on alcohol and opioids. *Journal of the Neurological Sciences, 411,* 116713. https://doi.org/10.1016/j.jns.2020.116713

Respiratory Therapy Society of Ontario. (2020). *Obstructive sleep apnea: Are Canadians underdiagnosed and undertreated?* Retrieved from https://www.rtso.ca/obstructive-sleep-apnea-are-canadians-underdiagnosed-and-undertreated/

Rodda, S., Booth, N., McKean, J., et al. (2020). Mechanisms for the reduction of caffeine consumption: What, how and why. *Drug and Alcohol Dependence, 212,* 108024. https://doi.org/10.1016/j.drugalcdep.2020.108024

Sadeghniiat-Haghighi, K., Eftekhari, S., Mirzaaghaee, F., et al. (2020). Adaptation of a clinical practice guideline for Maintenance of Wakefulness Test (MWT). *Occupational Medicine, 12*(1), 87–97.

Sadock, B. J., Sadock, V. A., & Ruiz, P. (2017). *Concise textbook of clinical psychiatry* (4th ed.). Philadelphia: Lippincott Williams & Wilkins.

Sleep Foundation. (2021). *What causes insomnia?* Retrieved from https://www.sleepfoundation.org/insomnia/what-causes-insomnia

Song, C., & Tagliazucchi, E. (2020). Linking the nature and functions of sleep: Insights from multimodal imaging of the sleeping brain. *Current Opinion in Physiology, 15,* 29–36. https://doi.org/10.1016/j.cophys.2019.11.012

Staner, L. (2010). Comorbidity of insomnia and depression. *Sleep Medicine Reviews, 14*(1), 35–46. https://doi.org/10.1016/j.smrv.2009.09.003

Stanford Health Care. (2021). *Actigraphy.* Retrieved from https://stanfordhealthcare.org/medical-tests/s/sleep-disorder-tests/procedures/actigraphy.html

Statistics Canada. (2018). *Prevalence of insomnia for Canadians aged 6 to 79.* Retrieved from https://www150.statcan.gc.ca/n1/pub/82-003-x/2018012/article/00002-eng.htm

Upender, R. P. (2017). Sleep medicine, public policy, public health. In M. Kryger, T. Roth, & W. Dement (Eds.), *Principles and practice of sleep medicine* (6th ed.) (pp. 638–645). Philadelphia: Elsevier.

UNIT 5

Trauma Interventions

21. Crisis and Disaster

22. Suicide and Non-Suicidal Self-Injury

23. Anger, Aggression, and Violence

24. Interpersonal Violence: Child, Older Persons, and Intimate Partner Abuse

25. Sexual Assault

Crisis and Disaster

Meaghan Thumath

 https://evolve.elsevier.com/Canada/Varcarolis/psychiatric/

OBJECTIVES

1. Differentiate among the three types of crises.
2. Delineate six aspects of crisis relevant for nurses involved in crisis intervention.
3. Understand areas of assessment and approaches to assessment during crisis.
4. Discuss four common problems in the nurse–patient relationship encountered by beginning nurses when starting crisis intervention. Discuss resolutions to these problems.
5. Compare and contrast the differences among primary, secondary, and tertiary intervention, including appropriate intervention strategies.
6. Identify modalities of crisis intervention.
7. List at least five resources in the community that could be used as referrals for a patient in crisis.

KEY TERMS AND CONCEPTS

adventitious crisis
coping
coping methods
crisis
crisis intervention
critical incident stress debriefing
disaster risk reduction
disasters
emergency response
maturational crisis
mental health emergency
mental health first aid
pandemic
phases of crisis
primary care
public health emergency
secondary care
situational crisis
tertiary care
trauma

On March 11, 2020, the World Health Organization declared the novel coronavirus (COVID-19) outbreak a global pandemic and at time of writing, COVID-19 has been responsible for over 2.1 million reported deaths worldwide. Canada has simultaneously been facing a national overdose crisis with devastating impacts on communities and families, with over 21 000 lives lost to overdose between 2016 and 2020. On June 30, 2021, a fire destroyed the entire village of Lytton in British Columbia during a record-breaking heat wave that resulted in thousands of premature deaths across the Pacific Northwest. A train derailment in Lac-Mégantic, Quebec, left 47 people dead on July 6, 2013. Floods in Calgary and High River, Alberta, in June 2013, and in central Canada, in May 2017, left hundreds homeless and without their livelihoods.

What do these situations have in common? Each scenario could be the precipitant of a crisis, leaving individuals, families, or whole communities struggling to cope with the impact of the event. Prior to the global pandemic, more than 12.4 million Canadians aged 15 years and older reported having personally experienced a major emergency or disaster within their community in their lifetime (Statistics Canada, 2016).

Everyone experiences crises, which are not in themselves a mental illness but rather are representative of a struggle for equilibrium and adaptation. Crisis and disaster experiences do, however, create vulnerable populations and conditions that require mental health services (Kolski & Jongsma, 2014). Further, crises and disasters highlight vulnerabilities and risks for mental illness and disproportionately affect those who are marginalized (Raphael, 2015). Among those who are affected by war or other conflicts in the past 10 years, 22% will experience depression, schizophrenia, post-traumatic stress disorder (PTSD), or bipolar disorder (World Health Organization, 2019). A **crisis** is an acute state of psychological imbalance resulting in poor coping with evidence of distress and functional impairment. The primary cause of a crisis is an intensely felt threat or a stressful event (Registered Nurses' Association of Ontario, 2017). Two necessary conditions for a crisis identified by Yaeger and Roberts (2015) are (1) the individual's perception of the event as the cause of considerable upset, disruption, or both; and (2) the individual's inability to resolve the disruption by previously used coping mechanisms (p. 6).

Crisis both threatens personality organization and presents an opportunity for personal growth and development. Successful crisis resolution results from the development of adaptive coping methods, reflects ego development, and suggests the employment of physiological, psychological, and social resources. Crisis, or rather *coping* with crisis, is an essential component of individual growth and development. **Coping** can be defined as "finding ways to accomplish goals despite obstacles and challenges" (Goldner et al., 2016, p. 233). **Coping methods** are the thinking, behavioural, and emotional processes individuals use to support functioning in the face of stressors (Registered Nurses' Association of Ontario, 2002/2006; Algorani & Gupta, 2021).

Crises are typically defined as acute and time limited, usually lasting 4 to 6 weeks. They are associated with events that precipitate overwhelming emotions of increased tension, helplessness, and disorganization. As shown in Figure 21.1, resolution from the state of crisis depends on three factors:

1. The realistic perception of the event: People vary in the way they absorb, process, and use information from the environment (Aguilera, 1998).
2. Adequate situational supports: Situational supports include nurses, other health care providers, and community members who use *crisis intervention* to assist those in crisis. Crisis intervention is a process focused on resolution of the immediate problem through personal, social, and environmental resources. The goals of early intervention are (Registered Nurses' Association of Ontario, 2002/2006, p. 15):
   - Stabilization of the situation
   - Rapid resolution of the crisis experience
   - Prevention of further deterioration or trauma
   - Achievement of (at least) precrisis level of functioning
   - Promotion of effective problem solving and realistic understanding of the experience
   - Facilitation of a sense of self-reliance and belief in one's ability to return to independence and apply new coping skills to future challenges

Emergencies, violence, and conflict continue to affect millions around the globe, presenting a myriad of challenges that require innovative solutions to mitigate their impact. In recent years the management of hazardous emergencies has shifted away from reactive responses and towards more preventative approaches such as disaster risk reduction (DRR), aimed at reducing the risk of new and existing disasters and strengthening capacity and resilience from the individual to the global level (Inter-Agency Standing Committee, 2021).

In general, interventions are responsive to the situation, timing, environment, and resources available. Modalities may include mental health first aid (MHFA), including early identification and comfort measures; telephone support; home visits or mobile response interventions; reflection and goal setting to promote coping; or even emergency psychiatric services and hospitalization (Goldner et al., 2016; Mental Health Commission of Canada, 2017).

3. Adequate coping mechanisms: Coping skills are acquired through a variety of sources, such as cultural responses, modelling behaviours of others, and life opportunities that broaden experience and promote new adaptive coping responses (Aguilera, 1998). Many factors compromise a person's ability to cope with a crisis event, for example, the number of other stressful life events the person is currently coping with, the presence of other unresolved losses, the presence of coexisting psychiatric or medical problems, the presence of excessive fatigue or pain, and the quality and quantity of a person's usual coping skills.

THE DEVELOPMENT OF CRISIS THEORY

An early crisis theorist, Erich Lindemann, studied the grief reactions of relatives of victims who died in the 1942 fire at Boston's Coconut Grove nightclub. His research formed the foundation of crisis theory and intervention. Lindemann (1944) concluded that while acute grief is a normal reaction to a distressing situation, preventive interventions could eliminate or decrease the serious psychological consequences of the anxiety associated with crisis. He believed that the same interventions helpful in bereavement would prove helpful in crises.

In the 1960s Gerald Caplan advanced crisis theory and intervention strategies. Since then, clinicians and theorists have further extended our understanding of crisis and interventions. The significant impact of crisis on individual and population health has been well articulated. MHFA training, early intervention, and support crisis intervention are all priorities for strategic action in Canada's evolving national mental health framework for action (Mental Health Commission of Canada, 2017). Donna Aguilera and Janice Mesnick provided a classic framework for nurses related to crisis assessment and intervention, and Aguilera continues to set a standard in the practice of crisis assessment and intervention, including examination of the individual's reactions, education, coping, and problem solving. Albert R. Roberts's seven-stage model of crisis intervention (Figure 21.2) provides another useful model for addressing the suffering experienced in acute situational crises, as well as in acute stress disorder.

In an effort to establish consensus on mass disaster intervention principles, Hobfoll and colleagues (2007) identified five essential, empirically supported elements of mass trauma interventions that promote (1) a sense of safety, (2) calming, (3) a sense of self-efficacy and collective efficacy, (4) connectedness, and (5) hope.

The effects of a mass disaster such as the 2020 mass shooting that killed 22 people and resulted in the death of the shooter, wounded three others, and set fire to homes in 16 locations across Nova Scotia represent the need for crisis assessment and intervention at the community level. Regardless of the type of crisis and whether traumatized individuals are victims, families, rescue workers, or witnesses, those with access to crisis assessment and intervention are more likely to feel

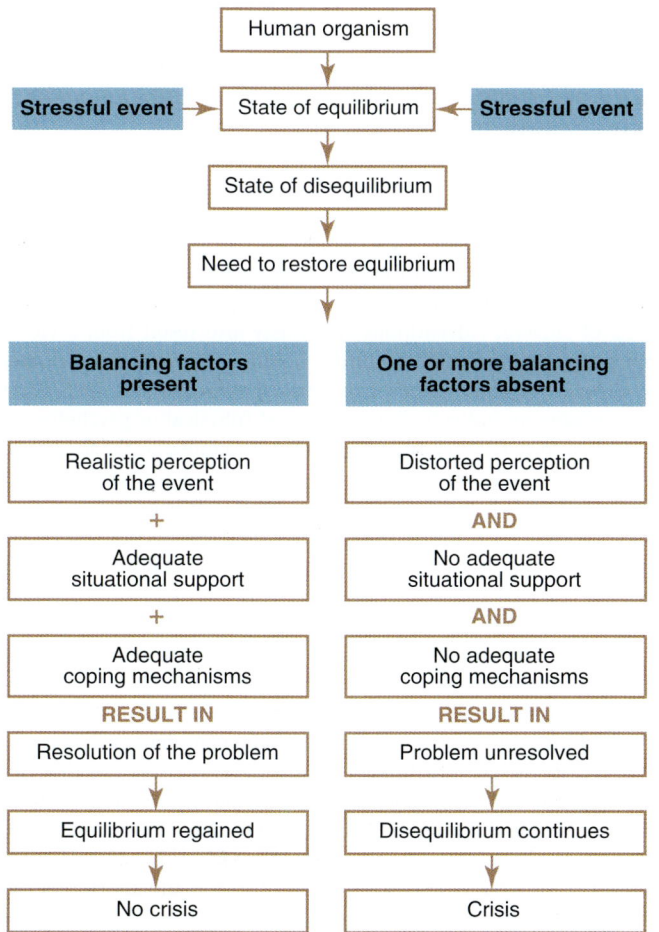

Fig. 21.1 Paradigm: the effect of balancing factors in a stressful event. (**Source:** Aguilera, D. C. [1998]. *Crisis intervention: Theory and methodology* (8th ed.). St. Louis: Mosby.)

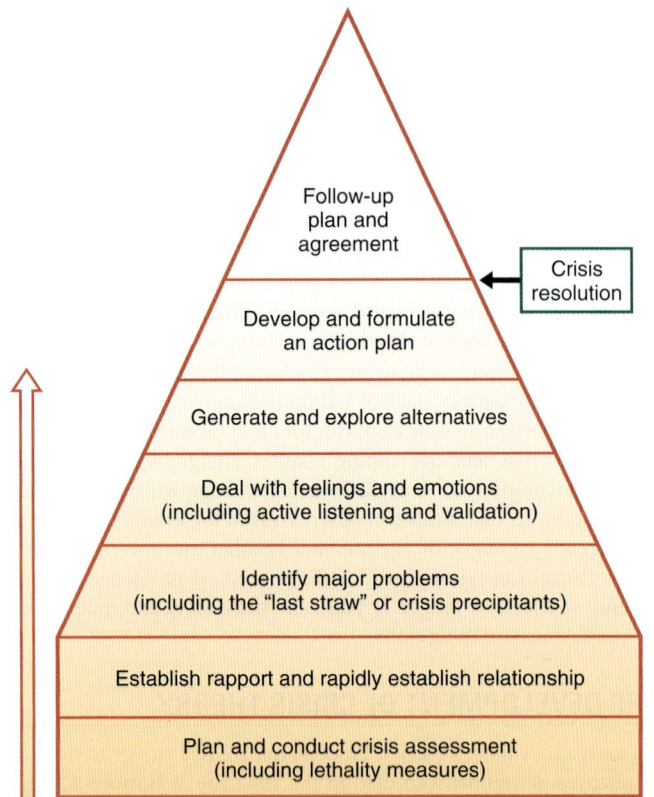

Fig. 21.2 Roberts' Seven-Stage Model of Crisis Intervention. (**Source:** Roberts, A. R., & Ottens, A. J. [2005]. The Seven-Stage Crisis Intervention Model: A road map to goal attainment, problem solving, and crisis resolution. *Brief Treatment and Crisis Intervention, 5,* 329–339.)

safe, supported, and able to make sense of their response to the disaster, as compared to those without such access (Hobfoll et al., 2007; Raphael, 2015).

Components of crisis assessment and intervention are derived from established crisis theory and evidence base. An understanding of three areas of crisis theory enables application of the nursing process: (1) types of crisis, (2) phases of crisis, and (3) aspects of crisis that have relevance for nurses.

Types of Crisis

There are three basic types of crisis situation: (1) developmental or maturational crises; (2) situational crises; and (3) disasters or adventitious crises. Marginalized people already affected by stigma such as those living in poverty or those with pre-existing mental health or substance use challenges are especially vulnerable to crisis (Registered Nurses' Association of Ontario, 2017).

Maturational Crisis

A process of maturation occurs across the life cycle. Erik Erikson conceptualized the process by identifying eight stages of ego growth and development (see Table 4.2). Each stage represents a time during which physical, cognitive, instinctual, and sexual changes prompt an internal conflict or crisis, which results in either psychosocial growth or regression. Therefore each developmental stage represents a maturational crisis (i.e., a critical period of increased vulnerability and heightened potential, a turning point).

When a person arrives at a new stage, formerly used coping styles are no longer effective, and new coping mechanisms have yet to be developed. Thus for a time, the person is without effective defenses. This deficit often leads to increased tension and anxiety, which may manifest as variations in the person's normal behaviour. Examples of events that can precipitate a maturational crisis include leaving home during late adolescence, marriage, the birth of a child, retirement, and the death of a parent. Successful resolution of these maturational tasks leads to the development of basic human qualities.

Erikson (1959) believed that the way these crises are resolved at one stage affects the ability to pass through subsequent stages, because each crisis provides the starting point for movement toward the next stage. If a person lacks support systems and adequate role models, successful resolution may be difficult or may not occur. Unresolved problems in the past and inadequate coping mechanisms then adversely affect what is learned in each developmental stage. Experiencing severe difficulty during a maturational crisis may disrupt progression through the maturational stages and warrant professional intervention. For example, the stage of life or retirement from worklife may initiate a maturational crisis for some people.

Situational Crisis

A situational crisis arises from events that are extraordinary, external rather than internal, and unanticipated (Owens & Parsons, 2018). Examples of precipitating events to a situational crisis are job loss or change, the death of a loved one, an unplanned pregnancy, financial troubles, relationship breakup, and severe physical or mental illness. Whether these events precipitate a crisis depends on factors such as the degree of support available from caring friends, family members, and others; general emotional and physical status; and the ability to understand and cope with the meaning of the stressful event. As in all crises, the stressful event involves loss or change that threatens a person's self-concept, self-esteem, and sense of security.

Adventitious Crisis

An adventitious crisis results from events not part of everyday life, such as a natural disaster (e.g., flood, fire, earthquake) or a national disaster (e.g., acts of terrorism, war, riots, airplane crashes). Disasters are those events that threaten (physically or psychologically) the well-being of citizens. Adventitious crises may also result from a violent crime (e.g., sexual assault or murder, bombing in public areas, domestic violence, or child abuse). Experiencing or witnessing such events that threaten an individual's very survival (physical or psychological) is referred to as trauma. An important development in the field of adventitious crisis theory has been the recognition of just how differently people respond to and are affected by disaster. It is known that traumatizing events may overwhelm an individual's usual coping skills and be of such intensity that lasting psychological harm occurs, including the potential for PTSD (Goldner et al., 2016). For more information on PTSD and interventions, see Chapter 12. PTSD is among several post-trauma disorders that also include acute stress disorder, dissociative disorder, and depression.

While certain people may be more vulnerable to crisis than others, the need for intervention for all people who experience crisis cannot be overemphasized. Situational and adventitious crises can challenge the basic assumptions that underlie individuals' world views. Vulnerability to a stressful event and challenges to one's ability to cope depend on the newness, intensity, and duration of the stressful event (Yaeger & Roberts, 2015). At times, the newness and shock that render a person vulnerable to a stressful event can result in numbness that protects the individual from being overwhelmed by the magnitude of the crisis or disaster. The response of numbness from a crisis may be adaptive in the short term; however, if sustained over a longer duration, it may ultimately interrupt daily functioning. In such cases coping can become exhausted, and further intervention may be required to re-establish balance (Yaeger & Roberts, 2015). Vulnerability also depends on the number of crises experienced simultaneously. Consider a 51-year-old patient who may be going through a midlife transition (maturational) when their partner dies suddenly of cancer (situational).

Phases of Crisis

Caplan (1964) first identified four distinct **phases of crisis**:

Phase 1

A person confronted by a conflict or problem that threatens the self-concept responds with increased feelings of anxiety. The increase in anxiety stimulates the use of problem-solving techniques and defense mechanisms to solve the problem and lower anxiety.

Phase 2

If usual defensive responses fail and the threat persists, anxiety continues to rise and produces feelings of extreme discomfort. Individual functioning becomes disorganized. Trial-and-error solutions, in an effort to restore a normal balance, begin.

Phase 3

If the trial-and-error attempts fail, anxiety can escalate to the severe or panic level, and the person may mobilize automatic relief behaviours, such as withdrawal and flight. Some form of resolution (e.g., compromising needs or redefining the situation to reach an acceptable solution) may be made in this stage.

Phase 4

If the problem remains unresolved and new coping skills are ineffective, an individual may transition to a **mental health emergency**, a state of overwhelming anxiety that can lead to serious personality disorganization, depression, confusion, and behavioural disturbances. In a mental health emergency there are urgent issues of safety, potentially because of risk for self-care limitations (e.g., lack of nutrition, exposure to physical risks), self-harm behaviour (e.g., substance use, risk for suicide), or violence against others (Goldner et al., 2016).

APPLICATION OF THE NURSING PROCESS

Because people typically experience increased stress and anxiety in medical, surgical, and psychiatric hospital settings, as well as in community settings, nurses are often positioned to implement MHFA and crisis intervention. Crisis theory defines aspects of crisis that are basic to crisis intervention and relevant to the nursing process (Box 21.1).

Assessment

General Assessment

As shown in Figure 21.1, a person's equilibrium may be adversely affected by one or more of the following: (1) an unrealistic perception of the precipitating event, (2) inadequate situational supports, and (3) inadequate coping mechanisms (Aguilera, 1998). It is crucial for nurses to assess these factors during a crisis. Data gained from the assessment guide the nurse and the patient in planning realistic and meaningful goals and interventions.

BOX 21.1 Foundation for Crisis Intervention

- A crisis is self-limiting and usually resolves within 4 to 6 weeks.
- At the resolution of a crisis, the patient will emerge at one of three different functional levels:
  - A higher level of functioning
  - The same level of functioning
  - A lower level of functioning
- The goal of crisis intervention is to return the patient to at least the precrisis level of functioning.
- The level of crisis resolution depends on the patient's actions and others' interventions.
- During a crisis, people are often more receptive than usual to outside intervention. With intervention, the patient can learn new approaches to the problem.
- The patient in a crisis situation is assumed to be mentally healthy and to have previously functioned well but is currently in a state of disequilibrium.
- Crisis intervention deals only with the patient's present problem and resolution of the immediate crisis (i.e., the here and now).
- The nurse must take an active, even directive role in intervention, which is in contrast to conventional therapeutic intervention that stresses a more non-directive role.
- Early intervention increases the potential for a good prognosis.
- The patient is encouraged to set realistic, focused goals and interventions with the nurse.

 SAFETY TIP

Suicide Nursing Assessment

Promote a sense of safety by assessing the patient's potential for suicide or homicide. If the patient is suicidal, homicidal, or unable to take care of personal needs, hospitalization should be considered (Aguilera, 1998). Sample questions to ask include:

- Do you feel you can keep yourself safe?
- Have you thought of killing yourself or someone else? If yes, have you thought of how you would do this?

After establishing that the patient poses no danger to self or others, the nurse assesses three main areas: (1) the patient's perception of the precipitating event, (2) the patient's situational supports, and (3) the patient's personal coping skills.

VIGNETTE

A 25-year-old woman named Caitlin is brought to the emergency department by police after being violently attacked by her husband. Caitlin is seen by the emergency physician and then interviewed by the emergency department's psychiatric mental health nurse. The nurse calmly introduces herself and tells Caitlin she would like to spend some time with her. The nurse says, "It looks as if things are pretty overwhelming. Is that how you're feeling?" The nurse makes the observation that Caitlin may be at risk if she returns home. Caitlin sits slumped in a chair, her hands in her lap, head hanging down, and tears in her eyes.

1. Assess the patient's perception of the precipitating event. The nurse's task is now to assess the individual or family and the problem. The more clearly the problem can be defined, the more likely effective

solutions will be identified. Sample questions that may facilitate assessment include:
- Can I get you anything (tea, snack, warm blanket)?
- Has anything particularly upsetting happened to you within the past few days or weeks?
- What was happening in your life before you started to feel this way?
- What leads you to seek help now?
- How does this situation affect your life?

> **VIGNETTE**
> **Nurse:** "Caitlin, tell me what has happened."
> **Caitlin:** "I can't go home. ... No one cares. No one believes me. I can't go through it again."
> **Nurse:** "Tell me what you can't go through again."
> (Caitlin cries, shaking with sobs. The nurse sits quietly for awhile and then speaks.)
> **Nurse:** "Tell me what is so troublesome. Let's look at it together."
> After a while, Caitlin tells the nurse that her husband, Dan, has been beating her regularly, particularly after drinking. The beatings have progressively become more violent, and Caitlin states, "I'm afraid he'll kill me."

2. Assess the patient's situational supports. Next, the nurse determines resources available to the patient. The following are sample questions:
   - Who do you live with?
   - Who do you talk to when you feel overwhelmed?
   - Who can you trust?
   - Who is available to help you?
   - Do you belong to a spiritual community?
   - Where do you go to school or to other community-based activities?
   - During difficult times in the past, who did you want most to help you?
   - Who is the most helpful?

> **VIGNETTE**
> **Nurse:** "Caitlin, who can you go to? Do you have any other family?"
> **Caitlin:** "No. My family is in another province. Dan and I are pretty much alone."
> **Nurse:** "Do you have anyone you can talk to?"
> **Caitlin:** "I really don't have any friends. Dan's jealousy makes it difficult for me to have friends. He doesn't like anyone who I would want as a friend."
> **Nurse:** "What about coworkers?"
> **Caitlin:** "My coworkers are nice, but I can't tell them things like this. They wouldn't believe me anyway."
> The nurse learns that Caitlin feels successful at her job and that work is a refuge from her troubles. Getting good job reviews also has another reward: it is the only time Dan says anything nice about her.

3. Assess the patient's personal coping skills. Finally, the nurse evaluates the patient's anxiety level and identifies their established coping patterns. Common coping mechanisms may be overeating, drinking, smoking, withdrawing, seeking out someone to talk to, yelling, fighting, or engaging in other physical activity (Behrman & Reid, 2002; Raja et al., 2015). It is important to remember that coping strategies vary widely, and that the specific coping strategy, particularly in the early phase of crisis assessment and intervention, is not as critical as whether it enables the person to cope (Minnesota Department of Health, 2019). In this way coping is assessed and addressed through harm reduction and trauma-informed approaches (Kimberg & Wheeler, 2019). Sample questions to ask include:
- What do you usually do to feel better?
- Did you try it this time? If so, what was different?
- What do you think might happen now?
- What helped you through difficult times in the past?
- What role does your culture play in handling situations like this? (See Considering Culture: How Acknowledging Culture Supports Crisis Resolution.)

CONSIDERING CULTURE
How Acknowledging Culture Supports Crisis Resolution

Consider your patient, who has lost his job with the closure of the local paper mill and presents in crisis at a rural health centre. Consider also your Indigenous patient at the clinic on a reserve who has experienced the stillbirth of her third child and the new-immigrant woman you are assessing in the psychiatric emergency department of a large urban hospital who has attempted suicide following a relationship breakdown. While rapid resolution of the crisis is the goal, there are many reasons a nurse should consider culture during such a crisis intervention. Culture can influence one's interpretation of and the meaning attributed to a disaster or crisis event. Culture can also influence an individual's personal coping or a community's reaction to an event. Despite the significance of culture on the assessment and intervention process, the immediacy of crisis intervention nursing often results in cultural factors and issues of cultural identity being overlooked in favour of efficient assessment and interventions. Ignoring the important role of culture, however, may get in the way of effective and efficient crisis resolution. The impact of the recent COVID-19 pandemic has reflected the structural inequalities that exist within Canada and is a critical example of how health crises are often fueled by systemic racism and thus require anti-racist, anti-oppressive, and culturally competent strategies to support racialized and marginalized communities.

Acknowledging the patient's personal history and context, as well as the distinct history, context, and cultures of the patient and nurse (i.e., occupation, income, age, gender, nationality, physical abilities, language, ethnic heritage, sexual orientation, education), allows for more rapid development of the trust and rapport necessary to communicate both verbally and non-verbally for assessment and intervention. Addressing context and culture in this way assists the nurse to convey acceptance and trust to assist with the immediate problems.

After the symptoms of crisis are stabilized and controlled, knowledge of the patient's culture can assist in identifying important resources available for follow-up care, such as family, religious community, or cultural heritage agencies, which can provide continuing support after the symptoms are controlled. In short, culture is crucial to the three balancing factors to a crisis: perception of the event, coping, and support. A nurse's capacity to acknowledge the patient's context, history, and culture will enhance crisis intervention and trauma-informed approaches and will support resolution and good patient outcomes. See also Chapter 8.

Sources: British Columbia Provincial Mental Health and Substance Use Planning Council. (2013). *Trauma-informed practice guide.* Retrieved from http://bccewh.bc.ca/wp-content/uploads/2012/05/2013_TIP-Guide.pdf; and Muskett, C. (2014). Trauma-informed care in inpatient mental health settings: A review of the literature. *International Journal of Mental Health Nursing, 23*(1), 51–59. https://doi.org/10.1111/inm.12012

> **VIGNETTE**
> **Nurse:** "What do you think would help your situation?"
> **Caitlin:** "I don't want to be in an abusive marriage. I just don't know where to turn."
> The nurse asks Caitlin for permission to work with her to find a solution and advises that she is concerned for Caitlin's safety and well-being.

Self-Assessment

Nurses' self-awareness when dealing with a patient in crisis is crucial. It is important for them to recognize their own anxiety level and negative feelings to prevent patients from closing off their expression of painful feelings.

There may be times when nurses feel they cannot deal effectively with a patient's situation. When this happens, the nurse could ask a colleague if they are available to work with the individual rather than limit the required assessment and intervention. Asking for support and supervision will help the nurse separate their own needs from the patient's and identify ways to address uncomfortable or painful personal issues to care more effectively for patients in crisis.

Essential aspects of the therapeutic relationship include clear verbal and non-verbal communication skills, assertiveness, responsiveness to patient needs, strong problem-solving abilities, attention to diversity and power relations, and genuine empathy for the lived experience of the patient. As examined in Chapters 9 and 10, the therapeutic relationship and communication demands are even more pronounced in crisis situations, in which rapid decisions and more extreme emotions are expected. It is crucial that the nurse engages in ongoing self-reflection and self-awareness and that expert supervision be available as an integral part of crisis intervention nursing.

Even experienced nurses can become overwhelmed when witnessing severe suffering, catastrophic loss of human life (e.g., pandemics, acts of war, plane crashes, workplace shootings), or mass destruction of people's homes and belongings (e.g., floods, fires, earthquakes). Mental health care providers may experience psychological distress from working with traumatized populations, a phenomenon called *secondary traumatic stress* or *vicarious traumatization* (Rauvola et al., 2019). Particular risk factors for secondary traumatic stress of mental health workers working with victims of trauma include a larger volume of patients in a caseload with trauma counselling needs, personal trauma or abuse history, perceived quality of work support and supervision, and social support outside of the clinical setting (Rauvola et al., 2019). Supervision and critical incident stress debriefing (CISD) are strategies that support nurses' ability to cope with overwhelming violent and disastrous situations (Registered Nurses' Association of Ontario, 2017).

ASSESSMENT GUIDELINES
Crisis

1. Identify whether the patient's response to the crisis warrants psychiatric treatment or hospitalization to minimize decompensation (e.g., suicidal or violent behaviour, psychotic thinking).
2. Identify whether the patient is able to identify the precipitating event.
3. Assess the patient's understanding of their present situational supports.
4. Identify the patient's usual coping styles, determining coping mechanisms suited to the present situation.
5. Determine any cultural beliefs or spiritual practices that should be responded to in assessing and intervening in this patient's crisis.
6. Assess whether this situation is one in which the patient needs primary (education, environmental manipulation, or new coping skills), secondary (crisis intervention), or tertiary (rehabilitation) interventions.

Diagnosis

When a person is in crisis, the nursing diagnosis of *Ineffective coping* is often useful (Herdman & Kamitsuru, 2014). This diagnosis is not to suggest that people in crisis are inadequate or do not have coping abilities, but because anxiety may escalate to moderate or severe levels in times of crisis, the ability to solve problems may be impaired. *Ineffective coping* may be experienced as an inability to meet basic needs, an inability to meet role expectations, an alteration in social participation, the use of inappropriate defence mechanisms, or the impairment of usual patterns of communication. The "related to" component of the diagnosis will vary according to the individual patient. Table 21.1 to follow, identifies potential nursing diagnoses for people in crisis and provides signs and symptoms that might be present to support the diagnosis.

In the preceding vignettes the assessment of Caitlin's perception of the precipitating event, situational supports, and personal coping skills provides the nurse with enough data to formulate two diagnoses and set goals and plan interventions with Caitlin.

> **VIGNETTE**
> Caitlin's nurse formulates the following nursing diagnoses:
> - *Anxiety (moderate or severe)* related to mental and physical abuse, as evidenced by ineffectual problem solving and feelings of impending doom
> - *Compromised family coping* related to the constant threat of violence

Outcomes Identification

Relevant outcomes of the *Nursing Outcomes Classification (NOC)* (Moorhead et al., 2018) for a person experiencing a crisis include *Coping*, *Decision making*, *Role performance*, and *Stress level*. The planning of realistic outcomes is done with the patient and family so as to determine outcomes congruent with the patient's cultural and personal values. Without the patient's involvement, the outcome criteria (i.e., goals at the end of 4 to 8 weeks) may be irrelevant or unacceptable solutions to that patient's crisis. Table 21.2 lists selected *NOC* outcomes with intermediate and short-term indicators for a patient in crisis.

MHFA is the help provided to a person developing a mental health problem or experiencing a mental health crisis. We know that physical first aid is administered to an injured person before medical treatment can be obtained; likewise, MHFA is given until appropriate treatment is found or until the crisis is resolved, and it is often life-saving. Many laypeople in communities are receiving this training that, like physical first aid, is found to support early intervention and disease prevention by preserving life when there is a danger or threat to life, to promote recovery and good mental health, and to provide comfort to those experiencing mental health problems. Psychological first aid (Shah et al., 2020) is another crisis response approach, one that is more specifically focused on unique crisis mental health responses to disasters (World Health Organization, 2019).

The MHFA approach and the training of people in MHFA represent a growing area of health promotion in Canada (Mental Health Commission of Canada, 2017). Overall, this approach aims to provide skills and knowledge to help people manage developing mental health problems in themselves, family members, friends, or coworkers. It does not attempt to train amateur therapists but, rather, teaches people to (1) recognize the signs and symptoms of mental health problems, (2) provide initial help, and (3) guide a person toward appropriate professional help. In 2016 the Mental Health Commission of Canada launched an

TABLE 21.1 Potential Nursing Diagnoses for Crisis Intervention

Signs and Symptoms	Nursing Diagnosis
Inability to meet basic needs, decreased use of social support, inadequate problem solving, inability to attend to information, isolation	Ineffective coping
	Risk for compromised resilience
Denial, exaggerated startle response, flashbacks, horror, hypervigilance, intrusive thoughts and dreams, panic attacks, feeling numb, substance use, confusion, incoherence	Post-trauma syndrome
	Rape-trauma syndrome
	Anxiety (moderate, severe, panic)
	Acute confusion
	Sleep deprivation
Minimizes symptoms, delays seeking care, displays inappropriate affect, makes dismissive comments when speaking of distressing events	Ineffective denial
Overwhelmed, depressed, nothing in life worthwhile, self-hatred, feelings of being ineffectual, sees limited alternatives, feels strange, perceives a lack of control	Risk for suicide
	Chronic low self-esteem
	Disturbed personal identity
	Hopelessness
	Powerlessness
Has difficulty with interpersonal relationships, isolated, has few or no social supports	Social isolation
	Impaired social interaction
Changes in family relationships and functioning, difficulty performing family caregiver role	Interrupted family processes
	Caregiver role strain

MHFA course adapted specifically for First Nations contexts (see the Research Highlight box).

RESEARCH HIGHLIGHT

Indigenous Mental Health First Aid: Community-Specific Adaptations to Mental Health First Aid in Canada

Problem

Indigenous peoples in Canada are disproportionately affected by mental health outcomes as a result of the psychological distress caused by colonialization in Canada. Previous mental health trainings developed for the general population have resulted in negative impacts on suicide prevention when used in Indigenous communities. There is a need for safe and culturally-relevant approaches to promoting mental health literacy in Indigenous contexts.

Purpose of Study

Mental health first aid First Nations (MHFAFN) training was adapted from the Mental Health First Aid Basic training program with the intention of creating a version that is relevant for Indigenous contexts and can be further adapted to the local context. A feasibility study of the MHFAFN course was conducted to assess the acceptability of the cultural adaptation, as well as its impacts on participants.

Methods

Ten MHFAFN courses were offered across four provinces in Canada in locations such as First Nations communities, urban centres, and rural communities. Of the 10 groups, 7 consisted solely of Indigenous participants. A survey of 91 participants was administered before and after the delivery of the course, and interviews with 89 participants were conducted in the latter half of the course. The survey discussed demographics, as well as knowledge, stigma, and self-efficacy related to mental health. Participants were also asked to provide feedback on the training experience and its impacts.

Key Findings

Participants' abilities to recognize signs and symptoms, social determinants of health, as well as identify available community support resources all increased following MHFAFN training. Overall, participants were satisfied with the integration of Indigenous culture and knowledge into the MHFA Basic course however, some felt that the cultural content in the course was underdeveloped.

Implications for Nursing Practice

The conclusion from the study was that MHFAFN training is an effective strategy for community-wide prevention in Indigenous communities by framing mental health in a colonial context and identifying local resources that can help participants respond to mental health crises in their communities. Nurses play an important role in teaching, training, and health promotion to support MHFA training.

Source: Crooks, C.V., Lapp, A., Auger, M., et al. (2018). A feasibility trial of mental health first aid First Nations: Acceptability, cultural adaptation, and preliminary outcomes. *American Journal Community Psychology, 61*(3–4), 459–471.

VIGNETTE

The nurse consults a social worker about Caitlin, and the three meet together. Caitlin decides she does not want to return to her home. Caitlin and the nurse then establish goals and plan interventions. The goals are as follows:
- With the support of the staff, Caitlin will find a safe environment.
- With the support of the staff, Caitlin will have at least two outside supports available within 24 hours.
- Caitlin will receive continued evaluation and support until the immediate crisis is over (6 to 8 weeks).

TABLE 21.2 NOC Outcomes for Patient in Crisis

Nursing Outcome and Definition	Intermediate Indicators	Short-Term Indicators
Coping: Personal actions to manage stressors that tax an individual's resources	Modifies lifestyle as needed Uses effective coping strategies Reports decrease in physical symptoms of stress Reports decrease in negative feelings	Identifies effective coping patterns Identifies ineffective coping patterns Reports decrease in stress Uses personal support system Verbalizes need for assistance
Decision making: Ability to make judgements and choose between two or more alternatives	Chooses among alternatives	Identifies relevant information Identifies alternatives Weighs alternatives
Role performance: Congruence of an individual's role behaviour with role expectations	Able to meet role expectations	Performs family role behaviours Describes role changes with illness or disability Describes role changes with older-person dependents, new family member, or family member who is leaving home Performs family, parental, intimate, community, work, or friendship role behaviours
Stress level: Severity of manifested physical or mental tension resulting from factors that alter an existing equilibrium	Able to modulate stress level	Reduction in elevated blood pressure Reduction in increased radial pulse rate Reduction in symptoms of upset stomach Reduced level of restlessness Improved sleep Reduction in interruption of thought process Reduced forgetfulness Infrequent cognitive mistakes Improved ability to concentrate on tasks Decrease in emotional outbursts

NOC, Nursing Outcomes Classification.
Source: Based on Moorhead, S., Johnson, M., Maas, M., et al. (2013). *Nursing Outcomes Classification (NOC)* (5th ed.). St. Louis: Mosby.

Planning

Nurses are called on to plan and intervene in a variety of crisis intervention modalities, such as disaster nursing, mobile crisis units, group work, training, health education and crisis prevention, victim outreach programs, and crisis lines or telephone outreach. The nurse may be involved in planning interventions for individuals (e.g., cases of physical abuse), groups (e.g., students after a classmate's suicide or shooting), or communities (e.g., disaster nursing after fires, shootings, or airplane crashes). Data from the answers to the following questions guide the nurse in determining immediate actions (Aguilera, 1998):

- How much has this crisis affected the patient's life? Can the patient still go to work? Attend school? Care for family members?
- How is the state of disequilibrium affecting significant people in the patient's life (e.g., partner, children, other family members, colleagues, employer)?

Implementation

Crisis intervention is a function of the basic-level nurse and has two initial goals:

1. Patient safety. External controls may be applied for protection of the patient in crisis if the patient is suicidal or homicidal.
2. Anxiety reduction. Anxiety-reduction techniques are used so that inner resources can be mobilized.

During the initial interview, the patient in crisis first needs to gain a feeling of safety. Solutions to the crisis may be offered so that the patient is aware of various options. Feelings of support and hope will temporarily diminish anxiety. The nurse needs to play an active role by indicating that help is available, conveyed by the competent use of crisis intervention skills and genuine interest and support. The availability of help is not conveyed by the use of false reassurances and platitudes, such as "Everything will be all right." Crisis intervention requires a creative and flexible approach through the use of traditional and non-traditional therapeutic methods. The nurse may act as educator, advisor, and role model, always keeping in mind that it is the patient who solves the problem, not the nurse. At times, highly directive interventions will be required to assist in problem solving, ensure safety, prioritize actions, and provide new information. Alongside this active and directive role, the following are important assumptions when working with a patient in crisis:

- The patient is in charge of their own life.
- The patient is able to make decisions.
- The crisis counselling relationship is one between partners.

The nurse helps the patient refocus to gain new perspectives on the situation, drawing on supportive interventions. In this way the nurse validates the patient experience and supports the patient during the process of finding constructive ways to solve or cope with the problem. It is important for nurses to be mindful of the fact that coping will look different for all patients and how difficult it is for the patient to change behaviours. Table 21.3 offers guidelines for nursing interventions and corresponding rationales. A broader collaborative crisis response is highlighted in Box 21.2.

BOX 21.2 Effective Emergency Response

World Health Organization (WHO), endorsed interagency mental health and psychosocial support guidelines for an effective response to emergencies recommend services at a number of levels, from basic services to clinical care. Clinical care for mental health should be provided by or under the supervision of mental health specialists including psychiatric nurses, psychologists, or psychiatrists.

Community self-help and social support should be strengthened, for example, by creating or re-establishing community groups in which members solve problems collaboratively and engage in activities such as emergency relief or learning new skills, while ensuring the involvement of people who are vulnerable and marginalized, including people with mental health challenges.

Psychological first aid offers first-line emotional and practical support to people experiencing acute distress due to a recent event and should be made available by field workers, including health staff, teachers, or trained volunteers.

Basic clinical mental health care covering priority conditions (e.g., depression, psychotic disorders, epilepsy, alcohol and substance use) should be provided at health-care facilities by trained and supervised general health staff.

Psychological interventions (e.g., problem-solving interventions, group interpersonal therapy, interventions based on the principles of cognitive-behavioural therapy) for people impaired by prolonged distress should be offered by specialists or by trained and supervised community workers in the health and social sector.

Links and referral mechanisms need to be established between mental health specialists, general health care providers, community-based support, and other services (e.g., schools, social services, and emergency relief services such as those providing food, water, and housing/shelter).

Source: World Health Organization. (2020). *Mental health in emergencies.* Retrieved from https://www.who.int/news-room/fact-sheets/detail/mental-health-in-emergencies.

VIGNETTE

After talking with the nurse and the social worker, Caitlin seems open to going to a safe house for women experiencing abuse. She also agrees to talk to a counsellor at a mental health centre. The nurse sets up an appointment at which she, Caitlin, and the counsellor will meet. The nurse will continue to see Caitlin twice a week.

Counselling

Primary care. Psychotherapeutic crisis interventions are directed toward three levels of care: (1) primary, (2) secondary, and (3) tertiary. Primary care promotes mental health and reduces mental illness to decrease the incidence of crisis. On this level, the nurse can:

1. Work with a patient to recognize potential problems by evaluating the patient's experience of stressful life events
2. Support the patient to develop specific coping skills, such as decision-making, problem-solving, assertiveness skills, meditation, and relaxation skills
3. Assist the patient in evaluating the timing or reduction of life changes to decrease the negative effects of stress as much as possible

The third intervention may involve working with a patient or client, such as a government or a health services department, to plan environmental changes, make important interpersonal decisions, and rethink changes in occupational roles. The Public Health Agency of Canada plays an important role in mass disaster planning and prevention, for instance, with COVID-19 pandemic planning and G8 meetings on disaster planning in Kananaskis and Toronto, and has recorded many lessons learned for future disaster planning (Public Health Agency of Canada, 2020).

Secondary care. Secondary care includes intervention during an acute crisis to prevent prolonged anxiety from diminishing personal effectiveness and personality organization. The nurse's primary focus is to ensure the safety of the patient. After safety issues are dealt with, the nurse works with the patient to assess the patient's problem, support systems, and coping styles. Desired goals are explored, and interventions are planned. This level of care lessens the time a patient is mentally disabled during a crisis. Secondary care occurs in hospital units, emergency departments, clinics, and mental health centres, usually

TABLE 21.3 Guidelines for Crisis Intervention

Intervention	Rationale
Assess for suicidal or homicidal thoughts or plans.	Safety is always the first consideration.
Take initial steps to make patient feel safe and less anxious.	A person who feels safe and less anxious is able to more effectively problem-solve solutions with the nurse.
Listen carefully (e.g., make eye contact, give frequent feedback to verify and convey understanding, summarize what patient says).	A person who believes someone is really listening is more likely to believe that someone cares about their situation and that help may be available. This belief offers hope.
Crisis intervention calls for directive and creative approaches. Initially, the nurse may make phone calls to arrange babysitters, schedule a visiting nurse, find shelter, or contact a social worker.	A person who is confused, frightened, or overwhelmed may be temporarily unable to perform usual tasks.
Identify needed social supports (with patient's input) and mobilize the priority.	A person's need for shelter, help with care for children or older-person dependents, medical workup, emergency medical attention, hospitalization, food, safe housing, and self-help groups is determined.
Identify needed coping skills (e.g., problem solving, relaxation, assertiveness, job training, newborn care, self-esteem building).	Increasing coping skills and learning new ones can help with current crisis and help minimize future crises.
Involve patient in identifying realistic, acceptable interventions.	The person's involvement in planning increases their sense of control, self-esteem, and adherence to the plan.
Plan regular follow-up (e.g., phone calls, clinic visits, home visits) to assess patient's progress.	Plan is evaluated to see what works and what does not.

during daytime hours. Psychological first aid programs are another approach to secondary care, aimed at helping survivors of disasters gain skills to manage distress and cope with post-disaster stress and adversity (Vernberg et al., 2008; World Health Organization, 2013; Substance Abuse and Mental Health Services Administration, 2015).

Tertiary care Tertiary care provides support for those who have experienced a severe crisis and are now recovering from a disabling mental state. Social and community facilities that offer tertiary intervention include rehabilitation centres, sheltered workshops, hospitals, and outpatient clinics. Primary goals are to facilitate optimal levels of functioning and prevent further emotional disruptions. People with severe and persistent mental problems are often extremely susceptible to crisis, and community facilities can provide a structured environment. Box 21.3 lists *Nursing Interventions Classification (NIC)* (Bulechek et al., 2018) interventions for responding to a crisis.

Critical incident stress debriefing. A CISD is a group-level crisis intervention carried out very soon after a traumatic event. Individuals involved in or witnessing the event (e.g., those in a school, workplace, or emergency responder group) are brought together in a safe and confidential environment to talk about what happened, discuss feelings and behavioural responses, and obtain health education about the crisis process for early intervention purposes. Generally, the discussion is guided by a professional or trained peer. There is evidence promoting CISD as an important strategy to prevent PTSD, one that should be implemented as part of a broad approach to crisis intervention that includes formal assessment and referrals for individual and family counselling and a range of other supports (Goldner et al., 2016).

 HOW A NURSE HELPED ME

Helping the Team Debrief From Not One Event but Accumulated Tragedies

As a member of our local critical incident stress management (CISM) committee representing our provincial parks managers, I was most intrigued by a recent debriefing. The participants included community members, ambulance staff, emergency physicians, nurses, and many of my coworkers with provincial and national parks who witnessed and supported the victims of a tragic incident last September. In that incident two teenagers were fatally injured in a mountaineering accident witnessed by park guides and other young people. Ginette, the community mental health nurse who is the leader of our CISM committee, facilitated the team process. It was intriguing because this process has changed my work with my parks colleagues, and changed me.

Even though I knew about crisis response and the need for debriefing, I had started to wear a figurative shield as a manager. These incidents occurred all too often and became things we just didn't talk about in our office. Sure, we talked about safety and strategy for prevention and education for mountaineers, but we never talked about the baggage we were carrying from these events. But it didn't stop these events, especially this event, from making me angry and sad. Truly, if I heard "they died doing what they loved" one more time, I was going to explode!

You see, during a crisis, our adrenaline pumps to help us provide the best response we can deliver, but then having to deliver horrible news to a family that their children have been severely injured and that they must get to the hospital, and must be prepared for the worst, is most certainly not an easy task for any of us. I had to do that twice on that day last September. The adrenaline only gets you so far!

But, in the debriefing last September, Ginette, guided us to think about many questions, even unanswerable ones. How exactly could we remain mentally healthy? How can we go on without the answers? Ginette was so calm, and just by raising these questions, she made me realize I had those questions all the time, but I just kept putting the baggage of our crisis work further back into the closet of my mind. I know now that we need to talk it out. We have to express feelings, or at least listen to the experiences of others. I needed to start listening, in a regular and real way, with my coworkers. The questions about what happened on scene in the park, and what happened in the hospital, must be discussed. Knowing the answers to the assumptions we naturally make may allow us to connect the dots to make more sense of an incident. I believe now that those questions are answered, or at least acknowledged, and we can start to move through the grieving period ourselves. I believe that the other incidents that have been stuffed into the baggage have also been let out. Ginette has been a great role model. I have learned new ways to respond better to the next incidents that will inevitably happen in our park … and to respond better to the whole team. I know I am a better manager because of how Ginette helped me. I have managed my anger by talking about even the unanswerable questions, instead of putting all my questions and feelings back in the baggage!

VIGNETTE

The nurse performs secondary crisis intervention and meets with Caitlin twice weekly for 4 weeks. At first, Caitlin is motivated to work with the social worker and the nurse to find another permanent place to live. The nurse suggests Caitlin see a counsellor in the outpatient clinic after the crisis is over so that she can talk about some of her pain. Caitlin becomes ambivalent and is already thinking she will return to her husband.

Evaluation

Guided by nursing best practice guidelines, the nurse might consider asking the following in the evaluation of interventions (Registered Nurses' Association of Ontario, 2002/2006, p. 28):

- Was the patient able to carry out the crisis plan, and what was the outcome?
- Does the patient have the supports and resources needed to work toward meeting their goals?
- Does the patient require additional or alternative links to community resources and supports?

NOC includes a built-in measurement for each outcome and for the indicators that support the outcome. Each indicator is measured on a five-point Likert scale, which helps the nurse evaluate the effectiveness of the crisis intervention. This evaluation is usually performed 4 to 8 weeks after the initial interview, although it can be done earlier (e.g., by the end of the visit, the anxiety level has decreased from 1 = severe to 3 = moderate). If the intervention has been successful, the patient's level of anxiety and ability to function should be at precrisis levels. A patient may wish to follow up on additional areas of concern and get referrals to other agencies for more long-term work. Crisis intervention frequently serves to prepare a patient for further treatment.

VIGNETTE

Caitlin returns to her husband 5 weeks after being assaulted. She is struggling to live alone and has convinced herself that he has changed his behaviour.

Caitlin continues to see the nurse, as planned; however, Caitlin is aloof and distant. After 6 weeks, Caitlin and the nurse decide that the crisis is over. The nurse evaluates Caitlin as being in a moderate amount of emotional pain, but Caitlin feels she is doing well. The nurse's assessment indicates that Caitlin has other serious issues (e.g., low self-esteem, childhood abuse), and the nurse strongly suggests that she could benefit from further counselling. The decision, however, belongs to Caitlin, who says she is satisfied with the way things are. Together they make a safety plan for Caitlin to return to the domestic violence shelter should the abuse resume and the nurse recommends additional mental health resources for her husband.

BOX 21.3 Crisis Intervention

Definition of crisis intervention: Use of short-term counselling and other interventions to help the patient cope with a crisis and resume precrisis state of functioning modalities. Interventions may include:

- Crisis lines—telephone support provided by trained volunteers (for first aid and support) or professionals (for assessment, triage, and referral)
- Mobile crisis outreach—outreach crisis response services often provided by collaborative teams, including police or other first responders
- Urgent or walk-in crisis care—services through which people can present their crisis needs to professionals for assessment, intervention, and referral
- Psychiatric emergency care—services such as emergency mental health care in hospital triage; assessment; crisis counselling; emergency medical treatment, often for brief-stay admissions

Activities

- Provide an atmosphere of support.
- Avoid giving false reassurances.
- Provide a safe haven.
- Determine whether the patient presents a safety risk to self or others.
- Initiate necessary precautions to safeguard the patient or others at risk for physical harm.
- Encourage expression of feelings in a non-destructive manner.
- Assist in identification of the precipitants and dynamics of the crisis.
- Encourage patient to focus on one implication at a time.
- Assist in identification of personal strengths and abilities that can be used in resolving the crisis.
- Assist in identification of past and present coping skills and their effectiveness.
- Assist in development of new coping and problem-solving skills, as needed.
- Assist in identification of available support systems.
- Link the patient and family with community resources, as needed.
- Provide guidance about how to develop and maintain support systems.
- Introduce the patient to people (or groups) who have successfully undergone the same experience.
- Assist in identification of alternative courses of action to resolve the crisis.
- Assist in evaluation of the possible consequences of the various courses of action.
- Assist the patient to decide on a particular course of action.
- Assist in formulating a time frame for implementation of the chosen course of action.
- Evaluate with the patient whether the crisis has been resolved by the chosen course of action.
- Plan with the patient how adaptive coping skills can be used to deal with crises in the future.

Sources: Adapted from British Columbia Ministry of Health. (2002). *Best practices in mental health: Crisis response and emergency services.* Retrieved from http://www.health.gov.bc.ca/library/publications/year/2000/MHABestPractices/bp_crisis_response.pdf; and Bulechek, G. M., Butcher, H. K., Dochterman, J. M., et al. (2013). *Nursing Interventions Classification (NIC)* (6th ed.). St. Louis: Mosby.

RESEARCH HIGHLIGHT

Crisis-Service Needs for Urban and Rural Areas—One Size Does Not Fit All

Problem
Law enforcement officers are often faced with difficult decisions about how to best respond to individuals experiencing a psychiatric crisis. The crisis intervention team (CIT) program fosters collaborative ties between law enforcement, the mental health treatment system, consumers, and consumer advocates. The CIT model was originally developed as an urban model for police officers responding to calls about persons experiencing a mental illness crisis. Little is known of the practical challenges of adapting this model in rural settings.

Purpose of Study
This study attempts to better understand the unique challenges of implementing the CIT model in a rural community and undertakes an exploration of the barriers and challenges that community stakeholders in rural areas may face in implementing CIT programs.

Methods
A qualitative analysis of data gathered through observations and focus groups of service providers.

Key Findings
The study revealed that there were both external and internal barriers to developing CIT programs in their respective communities. Some of these barriers were a consequence of working in small communities and working within small police departments. Participants actively overcame these barriers through the realization that CIT programs were needed in their community, through collaborative efforts across disciplines, and through the involvement of mental health advocacy groups.

Implications for Nursing Practice
These results indicate that CIT programs can be successfully implemented in rural communities.

Source: Skubby, D., Bonfine, N., Novisky, M., et al. (2013). Crisis intervention team (CIT) programs in rural communities: A focus group study. *Community Mental Health Journal, 49*(6), 756–764. https://doi.org/10.1007/s10597-012-9517-y

CASE STUDY AND NURSING CARE PLAN 21.1

Crisis

Gurpreet Sidhu, the psychiatric clinical nurse specialist, is called to the neurological unit. She is told that Alexzy, a 43-year-old man with Guillain-Barré syndrome, is demonstrating challenging behaviours, and the staff has requested a consult. The disease has caused severe muscle weakness to the point that Alexzy is essentially paralyzed; however, he is able to breathe on his own.

The nurse manager says that Alexzy is hostile and sexually abusive, and his abusive language, demeaning attitude, and angry outbursts are having an adverse effect on the unit as a whole. The staff nurses state that they feel ineffective and angry and have tried to be patient and understanding; however, Alexzy's difficult behaviours have persisted. The situation has affected the morale of the staff and, the nurses believe, the quality of their care.

Alexzy, a new Canadian from Eastern Europe, was employed as a taxicab driver. Six months before his hospital admission, he had given up drinking after years of episodic alcohol abuse. His fiancée visits him every day. He needs a great deal of assistance with every aspect of his activities of daily living: he has to be turned and repositioned every 2 hours and is fed through a gastrostomy tube.

CASE STUDY AND NURSING CARE PLAN 21.1—cont'd
Crisis

Assessment
Gurpreet gathers data from Alexzy, the nursing staff, and Alexzy's fiancée.

Perception of the Precipitating Event
During the initial interview, Alexzy speaks to Gurpreet angrily, using profanity and making lewd sexual suggestions. He also expresses anger about needing a nurse to "scratch my head and help me blow my nose." He cannot figure out how his illness suddenly developed. He says the doctors told him that it was too early to know for sure if he would recover completely but that the prognosis was good.

Support System
Gurpreet speaks with Alexzy's fiancée. Alexzy's relationships with his fiancée, within his Eastern European cultural group, and with his taxi company co-workers are strong. Neither Alexzy nor his fiancée has much knowledge of supportive agencies.

Personal Coping Skills
Alexzy comes from a strongly male-dominated subculture, in which the man is expected to be a strong leader. His independence and power to affect the direction of his life are central to his perception of being acceptable as a man.

Alexzy feels powerless, out of control, and enraged. He is handling his anxiety by displacing these feelings onto the environment, namely, the staff and his fiancée. This redirection of anger temporarily lowers his anxiety and distracts him from painful feelings. When he intimidates others, he feels temporarily in control and experiences an illusion of power. He uses displacement to relieve his painful levels of anxiety.

Alexzy's unconscious use of displacement is maladaptive and does not resolve the issues causing his distress. His anxiety continues to escalate. Furthermore, his behaviour leads others to avoid him, further increasing his sense of isolation and helplessness.

Self-Assessment
Gurpreet meets with the staff twice. The staff members discuss feelings of helplessness and lack of control stemming from their feelings of rejection by Alexzy. They talk of their anger about Alexzy's demeaning behaviour and frustration about the situation. Gurpreet points out to the staff that Alexzy's feelings of helplessness, lack of control, and anger at his situation are the same feelings the staff are experiencing. His displacement of his feelings of helplessness and frustration by intimidating the staff gives Alexzy a brief feeling of control. It also distracts him from his own feelings of helplessness.

The nurses become more understanding of the motivation for the behaviour Alexzy employs to cope with moderate to severe levels of anxiety. The staff begins to focus more on the patient and less on personal reactions and decides on two approaches to try as a group. First, they will not take Alexzy's behaviour personally. Second, Alexzy's displaced feelings will be refocused back to him.

On the basis of her assessment, Gurpreet identifies three main problem areas of importance and formulates the nursing diagnoses.

Diagnosis
1. *Ineffective coping* related to inadequate coping methods, as evidenced by inappropriate use of defence mechanisms (displacement).

Supporting Data
- Anger directed toward staff and fiancée
- Profanity and crude sexual remarks aimed at staff
- Isolation related to staff withdrawal
- Continued escalation of anxiety

2. *Powerlessness* related to lack of control over his health care environment, as evidenced by frustration over inability to perform previously uncomplicated tasks

Supporting Data
- Anger over nurses having to "scratch my head and help me blow my nose"
- Minimal awareness of available supports in larger community
- *Ineffective coping* related to exhaustion of staff's supportive capacity toward patient, as evidenced by staff withdrawal and limited personal communication with patient

Supporting Data
- Staff feels ineffective.
- Morale of staff is poor.
- Nurses believe that the quality of their care has been adversely affected.

Outcomes Identification
Gurpreet speaks to Alexzy and tells him she would like to spend 15 minutes with him every morning to talk about his concerns. She suggests that he might be able to handle his feelings in alternative ways and notes that they can also explore community resources. Alexzy gruffly agrees, saying, "You can visit me if it will make you feel better." They make arrangements to meet each morning at 0730 hours.

Continued

CASE STUDY AND NURSING CARE PLAN 21.1—cont'd
Crisis

The following outcomes are set:

Nursing Diagnosis

1. *Ineffective coping* related to inadequate coping methods, as evidenced by inappropriate use of defence mechanisms (displacement).
2. *Powerlessness* related to lack of control over health care environment, as evidenced by frustration over inability to perform previously uncomplicated tasks
3. *Ineffective coping* related to exhaustion of staff's supportive capacity toward patient, as evidenced by staff withdrawal and limited personal communication with patient

Short-Term Goal

1. Alexzy will be able to name and discuss at least two feelings about his illness and lack of mobility by the end of the week.
2. Alexzy will be able to name two community organizations that can offer him information and support by the end of 2 weeks.
3. Staff and nurse consultant will discuss reactions and alternative nursing responses to Alexzy's behaviour twice within the next 7 days.

Planning

Gurpreet creates a nursing care plan and shares it with the staff.
Nursing diagnosis: *Ineffective coping* related to inadequate coping methods, as evidenced by inappropriate use of defence mechanisms (displacement).
Outcome: By discharge, Alexzy will state that he feels more comfortable discussing difficult feelings.

Short-Term Goal	Intervention	Rationale	Evaluation
1. By the end of the week, Alexzy will be able to name and discuss at least two feelings about his illness and lack of mobility.	1a. Nurse will meet with patient daily for 15 minutes at 0730 hours.	1a. Night is usually the most frightening for patient; in early morning, feelings are closer to surface.	**Goal Met** Within 7 days, Alexzy speaks to nurse more openly about feelings.
	1b. When patient lashes out, nurse will remain calm.	1b. Patient perceives that nurse is in control of her feelings. This belief can reassure patient and increase patient's sense of security.	
	1c. Nurse will consistently redirect and refocus anger from environment back to patient (e.g., "It must be difficult to be in this situation").	1c. Refocusing feelings offers patient opportunity to cope effectively with his anxiety and decreases need to act out.	
	1d. Nurse will come on time each day and stay for allotted time.	1d. Consistency sets stage for trust and reinforces that patient's anger will not drive nurse away.	

Nursing diagnosis: *Powerlessness* related to lack of control over health care environment, as evidenced by frustration over inability to perform previously uncomplicated tasks.
Outcome: By discharge, Alexzy will contact at least one community support source.

Short-Term Goal	Intervention	Rationale	Evaluation
2. By the end of 2 weeks, Alexzy will name and discuss at least two community organizations that can offer information and support.	2a. Nurse will spend time with patient and fiancée. Role and use of specific agencies will be discussed.	2a. Both patient and fiancée will have opportunity to ask questions of nurse.	**Goal Met** By the end of 10 days, Alexzy and his fiancée can name two community resources they are interested in. At the end of 6 weeks, Alexzy has contacted the Guillain-Barré Society.
	2b. Nurse will introduce one agency at a time.	2b. Gradual introduction allows time for information to sink in and minimizes feeling of being pressured or overwhelmed.	
	2c. Nurse will not push patient to contact any of the agencies.	2c. Patient is able to make own decisions once he has appropriate information.	

CASE STUDY AND NURSING CARE PLAN 21.1—cont'd
Crisis

Implementation

Gurpreet goes into Alexzy's room at 0730 hours the following morning and sits by his bedside. At first, Alexzy's comments are hostile.

Dialogue	Therapeutic Tool or Comment
Nurse: "Alexzy, I'm here as we discussed. I'll be spending 15 minutes with you every morning. We could use this time to talk about some of your concerns."	Nurse offers herself as a resource, gives information, and clarifies her role and patient expectations. Night is Alexzy's most difficult time. In the early morning, he will be the most vulnerable and open for therapeutic intervention and support.
Alexzy: "Listen, sweetheart, my only concern is how to get a little sexual relief, get it?"	
Nurse: "Being hospitalized and partially paralyzed can be overwhelming for anyone. Perhaps you wish you could find some relief from your situation."	Nurse focuses on the process "need for relief," not the sexual content, and encourages discussion of feelings. Sexual issues often challenge new nurses, and discussing their feelings and appropriate interventions with an experienced professional is important for their growth and the quality of the care they give.
Alexzy: "What do you know, Ms. Know-it-all? I can't even scratch my nose without getting one of those fools to do it for me … and half the time those bitches aren't even around."	
Nurse: "It must be difficult to have to ask people to do everything for you."	Nurse restates what the patient says in terms of his feelings and continues to refocus away from the environment back to the patient.
Alexzy: "Yeah. … The other night a fly kept landing on my face. I had to shout for 5 minutes before one of those bitches came in, just to take the fly out of the room."	
Nurse: "Having to rely on others for everything can be a terrifying experience for anyone. It sounds extremely frustrating for you."	Nurse acknowledges that frustration and anger would be a natural response for anyone in this situation. This response encourages the patient to talk about these feelings instead of acting them out.
Alexzy: "Yeah. … It's a bitch … like a living hell."	

Gurpreet continues to spend time with Alexzy. He gradually talks more about his feelings and shows less hostility toward the staff. As he begins to feel more in control, he becomes less defensive about others caring for him. After 2 weeks, Gurpreet decreases her visits to twice a week. Alexzy is beginning to experience gross motor movements but is not walking yet. He still displaces much of his frustration and lack of control onto the environment, but he is better able to acknowledge the reality of his situation. He can also identify and briefly talk about his feelings.

Dialogue	Therapeutic Tool or Comment
Nurse: "What's happening? Your face looks tense this morning, Alexzy."	Nurse observes the patient's clenched fists, rigid posture, and tense facial expression.
Alexzy: "I had to wait 10 minutes for a bedpan last night."	
Nurse: "And you're angry about that."	Nurse verbalizes the implied.
Alexzy: "Well, there were only two nurses on duty for 30 people, and the nursing assistant was on his break. … You can't expect them to be everywhere, but still …"	
Nurse: "It may be hard to accept that people can't be there all the time for you."	Nurse validates the difficulty of accepting situations one does not like when one is powerless to make changes.
Alexzy: "Well … that's the way it is in this place."	

Evaluation

After 6 weeks, Alexzy is able to get around with assistance, and his ability to perform his activities of daily living is increasing. Although Alexzy still feels angry and overwhelmed at times, he is able to identify more of his feelings and acts them out less often, and he is able to talk to his fiancée about his feelings and lashes out at her less often. He is looking forward to going home, and his boss is holding his old job for him.

Alexzy makes arrangements for a meeting with the Guillain-Barré Foundation of Canada, and he is thinking about Alcoholics Anonymous but believes that he can handle this problem himself.

Staff members feel more comfortable and competent in their relationships with Alexzy. The goals have been met. Alexzy and Gurpreet agree that the crisis is over and terminate their visits. Alexzy is given the number of the crisis line and encouraged to call if he has questions or feels the need to talk.

Moorhead, S., Swanson, E., Johnson, M., & Maas, M., (Eds.). (2018). *Nursing Outcomes Classification (NOC): Measurement of health outcomes* (6th ed.). St. Louis: Elsevier.

KEY POINTS TO REMEMBER

- A crisis is not a pathological state but a struggle for emotional balance.
- Crises offer opportunities for emotional growth but can also lead to personality disorganization.
- There are three types of crisis: maturational, situational, and adventitious.
- Crises are usually resolved within 4 to 6 weeks.
- Assessment involves reviewing the balancing factors of the patient's perception of the problem, usual coping mechanisms, and situational supports.
- Social support and intervention can promote successful resolution.
- Resolution of a crisis takes three forms: a patient emerges at a higher level, at the precrisis level, or at a lower level of functioning.
- Crisis therapists take an active and directive approach with the patient in crisis.
- The patient is an active participant in setting goals and planning possible solutions.
- Crisis intervention is usually aimed at the mentally healthy patient who generally is functioning well but is temporarily overwhelmed and unable to function.
- The steps in crisis intervention are consistent with the steps of the nursing process.
- Specific qualities in the nurse that can facilitate effective intervention are a caring attitude, flexibility in planning care, an ability to listen, and an active, directive approach.
- The basic goals of crisis intervention are to reduce the individual's anxiety level and to support the effort to return the patient to their precrisis level of functioning.
- Crisis intervention therapy is short term, from 1 to 6 weeks, and focuses on the present problem only.
- Modalities of crisis intervention depend on the situation and services available at the time and locale (e.g., MHFA, which may be provided by professionals or community members; crisis lines; mobile response teams; urgent care clinics; in-hospital emergency psychiatric care, including medical and other interventions).
- The goals of mental health first aid are much like those of physical first aid: to assist in early intervention, health promotion, protection from harm, and application of comfort until other measures are obtained.
- A critical incident stress debriefing is a group approach that helps groups of people who have been exposed to a crisis situation.

CRITICAL THINKING

1. List the three important areas of crisis assessment once safety concerns have been identified. Give examples of two questions in each area that need to be answered before planning can take place.
2. Carley, a 21-year-old nursing student, tells her clinical instructor that her father (age 50 years) has just lost his job. Her father has been drinking heavily for years, and Carley is having difficulty coping. Because of her father's alcoholism and the increased stress in her family, Carley wants to leave school. Her mother has multiple sclerosis and thinks that Carley should quit school to take care of her.
    a. How many different types of crises are going on in this family? Discuss each crisis from the viewpoint of each individual family member.
    b. If you were providing crisis counselling for this family, what areas would you assess? What kinds of questions would you ask to evaluate each member's individual needs and the needs of the family as a unit (perception of events, social supports, coping styles)?
    c. Formulate some tentative goals you might set in conjunction with the family.
    d. Identify specific referral agencies in your area that would be helpful if members of this family were willing to expand their use of outside resources and stabilize the situation.
    e. How would you set up follow-up visits for this family? Would you see the family members together, alone, or in combination during the crisis period (4 to 6 weeks)? How would you decide whether follow-up counselling was indicated?
3. Why is it important for nurses to promote mental health first aid (MHFA) training in rural or resource-poor communities?
4. What are some of the unique characteristics of rural versus urban settings and the distinct facilitators and barriers each setting poses for crisis workers and services?

CHAPTER REVIEW

1. Jack had a psychotic episode when he was 15 years old. He did not respond well to treatments available at the time and continued to have a significant number of residual symptoms. At the age of 42, he began taking olanzapine (Zyprexa), which significantly reduced his remaining symptoms, allowing him to leave his group home and live independently for the first time. However, once his mental health became more stable and he was living in his own apartment, he was unsure of what to do with his time, how to go about getting a job, and how to meet his sexual and companionship needs appropriately. What type of crisis situation is represented by this case?
    a. Maturational crisis
    b. Situational crisis
    c. Adventitious crisis
    d. Phase 4 crisis
2. Rashid witnessed a car suddenly careen out of control and onto the sidewalk where he and his best friend were walking. Rashid's friend pushed him out of the way at the last second but was struck and killed instantly. Rashid was treated for minor injuries and released but was referred for mental health evaluation because he was very distraught over the death of his friend. Which response should be used first during your assessment of Rashid?
    a. "Tell me about what happened that day."
    b. "What would you like to accomplish during your treatment?"
    c. "Do you think you are coping well with this very tragic event?"
    d. "Tell me what has been going through your mind since the accident."
3. Rashid confides that he feels so guilty that his friend died while pushing him to safety that he has found himself having overwhelming impulses to kill himself by crashing his car, which he almost did yesterday. Which intervention would be most therapeutic?
    a. Admit Rashid to an inpatient mental health unit to ensure his safety until his condition can improve.
    b. Work with Rashid's family to ensure that he does not have access to a car, and set up emergency counselling sessions.
    c. Persuade Rashid to agree to remain safe pending counselling, as admitting him would only further traumatize him.
    d. Consult with a psychiatrist or prescribing physician so that Rashid can be started immediately on antianxiety and antidepressant medications.
4. Justine Lee, a mother of two teenagers and a nurse with 15 years of experience in the crisis centre, fails to show up for work several days in a row not long after providing crisis intervention to area

high school students following a shooting at their school. Coworkers complain that she is not taking her share of crisis calls. As Justine's manager, you attempt to address the issue, but she responds irritably and denies that anything is wrong. Justine most likely:
   a. Is becoming burned out on crisis work
   b. Is experiencing vicarious traumatization
   c. Has developed a hidden substance use problem
   d. Has lost her objectivity, owing to having children of her own
5. Suzanne experiences a crisis after witnessing the brutal assault of her friend during a robbery in their office tower parkade. Which outcome is the most appropriate for Suzanne?
   a. Suzanne reports greater satisfaction with her life within 2 months.
   b. Suzanne attends all treatment sessions specified in her treatment plan.
   c. Within 3 weeks, Suzanne reports that she no longer feels distressed.
   d. Suzanne returns to her precrisis level of functioning within 2 weeks.

REFERENCES

Aguilera, D. C. (1998). *Crisis intervention: Theory and methodology* (8th ed.). St. Louis: Mosby.

Algorani, E. B., & Gupta, V. (2021). Coping mechanisms. In *StatPearls*. StatPearls Publishing. Retrieved from https://www.ncbi.nlm.nih.gov/books/NBK559031/

Behrman, G., & Reid, W. J. (2002). Post-trauma intervention: Basic tasks. *Brief Treatment and Crisis Intervention, 2*, 39–48. https://doi.org/10.1093/brief-treatment/2.1.39

Bulechek, G. M., Butcher, H. K., Dochterman, J. M., et al. (2018). *Nursing Interventions Classification (NIC)* (7th ed.). St. Louis: Mosby.

Caplan, G. (1964). *Symptoms of preventive psychiatry*. New York: Basic Books.

Erikson, E. H. (1959). *Identity and the life cycle*. New York: International Universities Press.

Goldner, E. M., Palma, J., Jenkins, E., et al. (2016). *A concise introduction to mental health in Canada* (2nd ed.). Toronto: Canadian Scholars Press.

Herdman, T. H., & Kamitsuru, S. (2014). *NANDA International Nursing Diagnoses: Definitions and Classification, 2015–2017*. Oxford: Wiley-Blackwell.

Hobfoll, S., Watson, P., Bell, C., et al. (2007). Five essential elements of immediate and mid-term mass trauma intervention: Empirical evidence. *Psychiatry, 70*(4), 283–315.

Inter-Agency Standing Committee. (2021). *Technical note on linking disaster risk reduction (DRR) and mental health and psychosocial support (MHPSS)*. Retrieved from https://interagencystandingcommittee.org/system/files/2021-03/Technical%20Note%20Linking%20Disaster%20Risk%20Reduction%20(DRR)%20and%20Mental%20Health%20and%20Psychosocial%20Support%20(MHPSS)-%20Practical%20Tools,%20Approaches%20and%20Case%20Studies.pdf

Kimberg, L., & Wheeler, M. (2019). Trauma and trauma informed care. In M. R. Gerber (Ed.), *Trauma-informed healthcare approaches* (pp. 25–58). Cham: Springer.

Kolski, T. D., & Jongsma, A. E. (2014). *The crisis counseling and traumatic events treatment planner, with DSM-5 updates* (2nd ed.). Hoboken: Wiley.

Lindemann, E. (1944). Symptomatology and management of acute grief. *American Journal of Psychiatry, 101*(9), 141–148.

Mental Health Commission of Canada. (2017). *Advancing the mental health strategy for Canada: A framework for action*. Ottawa: Author. Retrieved from https://www.mentalhealthcommission.ca/wp-content/uploads/drupal/2016-08/advancing_the_mental_health_strategy_for_canada_a_framework_for_action.pdf

Minnesota Department of Health. (2019). *Public health interventions: Applications for public health nursing practice* (2nd ed.). St. Paul: Author.

Moorhead, S., Johnson, M., Maas, M. L., et al. (2018). *Nursing Outcomes Classification (NOC): Measurement of health outcomes* (6th ed.). St. Louis: Mosby.

Owens, E. W., & Parsons, R. D. (2018). *Crisis and trauma counseling*: West Chester University of Pennsylvania: Cognella, Inc. Retrieved from https://cognella-titles-sneakpreviews.s3-us-west-2.amazonaws.com/81845-1A-URT/81845-1A_SP.pdf

Public Health Agency of Canada. (2020). Lessons learned from the Public Health Agency of Canada's COVID-19 response (phase one). Retrieved from https://ourcommons.azureedge.net/data/Motion2020-10-26/2021-01-20-SPDP-8550-432-1-01/HESA_PHAC-ASPC_0000186_E.pdf

Raja, S., Hasnain, M., Hoersch, M., et al. (2015). Trauma informed care in medicine: Current knowledge and future research directions. *Family & Community Health, 38*(3), 216–226.

Raphael, B. (2015). Disaster, hope, help, reality. *Epidemiology and Psychiatric Sciences, 24*(6), 500–503. https://doi.org/10.1017/S204579601500075X

Rauvola, R. S., Vega, D. M., & Lavigne, K. N. (2019). Compassion fatigue, secondary traumatic stress, and vicarious traumatization: A qualitative review and research agenda. *Occupational Health Science, 3*, 297–336.

Registered Nurses' Association of Ontario. (2002/2006). *Crisis intervention*. Toronto: Author (Revised 2006 Supplement).

Registered Nurses' Association of Ontario. (2017). *Crisis intervention for adults using a trauma-informed approach: Initial four weeks of management* (3rd ed.). Toronto: Author.

Shah, K., Bedi, S., Onyeaka, H., et al. (2020). The role of psychological first aid to support public mental health in the COVID-19 pandemic. *Cureus, 12*(6), e8821. https://doi.org/10.7759/cureus.8821

Statistics Canada. (2016). *Canadians' experiences with emergencies and disasters, 2014*. https://www.statcan.gc.ca/pub/85-002-x/2016001/article/14469-eng.htm

Substance Abuse and Mental Health Services Administration. (2015). *Disaster Technical Assistance Center supplemental research bulletin: Disaster behavioral health interventions inventory*. Rockville: Author.

Vernberg, E. M., Steinberg, A. M., Jacobs, A. K., Brymer, M. J., Watson, P. J., Osofsky, J. D., Layne, C. M., Pynoos, R. S., & Ruzek, J. I. (2008). Innovations in disaster mental health: Psychological first aid. *Professional Psychology: Research and Practice, 39*(4), 381–388. https://doi.org/10.1037/a0012663

World Health Organization, War Trauma Foundation and World Vision International. (2013). *Psychological first aid: Facilitator's manual for orienting field workers*. Retrieved from https://www.who.int/publications/i/item/psychological-first-aid

World Health Organization. (2019). *Mental health in emergencies*. Retrieved from https://www.who.int/news-room/fact-sheets/detail/mental-health-in-emergencies

Yaeger, K. R., & Roberts, A. R. (2015). *Crisis intervention handbook: Assessment, treatment, and research* (4th ed.). New York: Oxford.

22

Suicide and Non-Suicidal Self-Injury

Sherri Melrose, Sharon Moore
With contributions by Sonya L. Jakubec

 https://evolve.elsevier.com/Canada/Varcarolis/psychiatric/

OBJECTIVES

1. Describe the profile of suicide in Canada, noting psychosocial and cultural factors that affect risk.
2. Identify three common precipitating events.
3. Describe risk factors and warning signs for suicide, including coexisting psychiatric disorders and trauma.
4. Name the most frequent coexisting psychiatric disorders.
5. Use the SAD PERSONS and IS PATH WARM scales to assess suicide risk.
6. Describe three expected reactions a nurse may have when beginning work with suicidal patients.
7. Give examples of primary, secondary, and tertiary (postvention) interventions.
8. Describe basic-level interventions that take place in the hospital or community.
9. Identify key elements of suicide precautions and environmental safety factors in the hospital.
10. Distinguish suicide from non-suicidal self-injury.
11. Identify appropriate interventions for non-suicidal self-injury in the clinical setting.

KEY TERMS AND CONCEPTS

cluster suicide
death by suicide
lethality
Medical assistance in dying
non-suicidal self-injury
postvention
primary intervention
SAD PERSONS scale
IS PATH WARM scale
secondary intervention
suicidal behaviour
suicidal ideation
suicide
survivors of suicide
tertiary intervention

Sadly, it is the rare individual who has yet to encounter, directly or indirectly, the significant public health problem that is suicide. More than 70 000 people die by suicide every year, one in every 100 deaths (World Health Organization [WHO], 2021b). In Canada approximately 11 people die by suicide each day (Public Health Agency of Canada, 2019). Although the overall suicide mortality rate in Canada is lower than it was a few decades ago, the decline has not continued in recent years (Liu et al., 2021). The impact of the novel Coronavirus disease 2019 (COVID-19) pandemic has the potential to significantly increase suicide rates, including suicidal ideation, attempts, and deaths, while immediate indicators show stability or decline during the initial years of the pandemic. (Government of Canada, 2020; Mental Health Commission of Canada [MHCC], 2020a). Nursing students and practising nurses at all levels encounter individuals suffering from the pain and hopelessness that all too frequently culminate in some type of suicidal behaviour. These individuals can be identified in inpatient settings, in outpatient treatment settings, and in the community. Studies have shown that 80% of people who die by suicide had contact with a primary care practitioner in the year prior to their death (Harmer et al., 2021; Stene-Larsen & Reneflot, 2019). This highlights the important role clinicians have in identifying risks and preventing these suicides. All too often, however, the focus of concern is concentrated on individuals who are at immediate risk (Hogan & Grumet, 2016). It is critical for nursing and primary health care providers to be advocates for this devastating problem and to mobilize the community to reduce factors that may contribute to suicide. Nurses at the primary, secondary, and tertiary levels of intervention can play a crucial role in the care of these patients, their families, and the **survivors of suicide** (family and friends of a person who has died by suicide). This chapter presents the facts about suicide and discusses approaches for the assessment and care of suicidal patients and their loved ones.

This chapter uses definitions that represent current thinking in reference to suicide and suicidal behaviours. The terms **suicide** or **death by suicide** are used to describe the act of taking one's own life. The term **suicidal behaviour** is used to describe potentially self-injurious actions with a non-fatal outcome for which there is evidence that a person intended to die by suicide (Turecki & Brent, 2016). Examples of suicidal behaviours include self-harm, suicidal ideation, desire to hasten death, risky behaviour, and suicide threats. Suicidal behaviour may or may not result in injury. **Non-suicidal self-injury** (NSSI) is discussed in brief at the end of the chapter and is characterized by self-harming behaviour with no intent to die.

Several terms used in association with suicide add to the stigma and alienation experienced both by people with suicidal ideation (referred to as self-stigma) and by survivors of suicide (Boyd et al., 2014). Terms such as *committed suicide*, *failed suicide*, and *successful suicide* are avoided. Words like *commit* and *attempt* evoke connotations of criminality, which are inappropriate and potentially stigmatizing to suicidal individuals and those touched by suicide. Certainly, the notions of failure and success in this regard are equally disrespectful and distort what could never be considered a success. Some suicide prevention activists use the term *completed suicide*; however, professionalized jargon is rarely helpful in this context, and the term *complete* expresses a connotation of incompleteness for those who non-fatally attempt suicide. For those surviving, there is nothing that feels "complete" amid the many unanswered questions and loss of hopes and dreams for and with their loved one. For these reasons, the neutral and factual expression "died by suicide" is preferred (Centre for Addiction and Mental Health, 2022; MHCC, 2020c). Changing the language that we use to describe suicide and suicidal behaviours is a first step in addressing the ways in which nurses can sensitively and empathically begin working with individuals who are suicidal.

EPIDEMIOLOGY

According to Statistics Canada (2020a), 4000 deaths by suicide were recorded in 2016. One-third of deaths by suicide are among people 45 to 59 years; suicide is the second leading cause of death among youth and young adults (15–34 years); and suicide rates are approximately three times higher among men compared with women (Public Health Agency of Canada, 2019). These numbers are thought to be understated, with the actual number of suicide deaths much higher. On their own, these numbers represent a considerable loss. Four thousand people is the equivalent of losing a small town from our national map every year. It is like twelve 747 jets crashing and killing everyone on board every year. It is more than double the annual number of traffic fatalities and nearly 10 times the annual number of homicides. These are unnecessary, preventable losses; the loss of life of the person who dies plus the grief of all the people touched by that person.

In Canada suicide is the ninth leading cause of death. For every 1 suicide death, there are 5 self-inflicted injury hospitalizations, 25 to 30 suicide attempts, and 7 to 10 people profoundly affected by suicide loss. Suicide and mental illness are deeply connected, and 90% of the 4000 individuals who die by suicide each year were living with a mental health problem or illness (Centre for Addiction and Mental Health, 2020; Government of Canada, 2016).

It is also important to consider that suicide reporting can be complex. Death by suicide can be challenging to determine as it may not be clear whether the person had the intent to die, and suicide death data take more than 2 years to become finalized (Olson, 2021). The number of suicides may actually be double or triple the reported statistics due to under-reporting in general (Rocket, 2010). Purposefully aiming a car at a bridge abutment and crashing may look like an accident. But, in fact, many reported accidents, homicides, and deaths ruled as "undetermined" are actually suicides.

Studies of suicide in the Canadian Armed Forces between 1995 and 2019 have demonstrated that suicide rates did not significantly increase over time, after age standardization. Suicide rates among the Armed Forces were also not statistically higher than those in the general Canadian population. History of deployment continued to be a possible risk factor for suicide in the Armed Forces, and deployment-related trauma and resulting mental health disorders are likely related to these associations (National Defence and the Canadian Armed Forces, 2021). Studies have indicated that Canadian veterans can, however, experience a higher prevalence of lifetime suicidal ideation, depression, anxiety, and post-traumatic stress disorders (PTSDs) than those who were not in the military (Hall et al., 2020). The *Life After Service Studies*, a joint research venture of Veterans Affairs Canada, the Department of National Defence/Canadian Forces, and Statistics Canada, continues to examine Canadian veterans' mental health issues as they transition to civilian life (Veterans Affairs, 2016).

Indigenous Peoples Statistics

First Nations, Inuit, and Métis peoples in Canada, collectively called Indigenous peoples (First Nations Health Authority, 2022), are especially vulnerable to death by suicide. Indigenous peoples experience poorer mental health outcomes, including anxiety, depression, and suicide, compared with non-Indigenous peoples in Canada (Graham et al., 2021). Differences in mental health outcomes exist among First Nations, Inuit, and Métis peoples (Statistics Canada, 2020b). For example, suicide rates were three times higher among First Nations; nine times higher among Inuit; and two times higher among Métis than those of non-Indigenous Canadians (Statistics Canada, 2020b). Suicide rates were highest among 15- to 24-year-old Inuit males and females and First Nations males (Kumar & Tjepkema, 2019). First Nations people living on tracts of land set aside by the Crown under the *Indian Act* have twice the suicide rate of those living elsewhere (Kumar & Tjepkema, 2019).

Poor mental health outcomes in Indigenous peoples have been linked to trauma associated with intergenerational effects of residential schools, forced relocation of communities, removal of children from families, childhood and adulthood maltreatment, discrimination, loss of culture and language, and mental health service gaps (Graham et al., 2021; Statistics Canada, 2019). Forced attendance at residential schools led to losses of culture, traditional values, and family stability, making it difficult for parents and Elders to pass along vital cultural knowledge and resilience to children who were taken away (Centre for Suicide Prevention, 2021). Intergenerational trauma, where the effects of trauma are passed on from one generation to the next, affects people's ability to cope and find healing. Maladaptive ways of coping with trauma that can lead to increased suicide risk include alcohol and substance use, isolation from support systems, and self-harm (Centre for suicide Prevention, 2021).

Since the COVID-19 pandemic, 6 in 10 Indigenous people reported that their mental health worsened (Arriagada et al., 2020b). In part, socioeconomic vulnerabilities impacted this worsening. Pre-pandemic, about one-quarter of Indigenous people in urban areas lived in poverty; about one-third lived in food-insecure households; and many reported being unable to cover an unexpected expense of $500 (Arriagada et al., 2020a). Post-pandemic, economic vulnerabilities, including the widespread job loss experienced throughout the pandemic, will continue to have far-reaching effects.

Indigenous people are disproportionately represented in toxic drug deaths. As the toxicity of street drugs increased, and more people used drugs in isolation due to public health measures to reduce exposure to COVID-19, British Columbia saw a 119% increase in toxic drug deaths from 2019 to 2020 (First Nations Health Authority, 2021). Indigenous people make up 3.3% of British Columbia's population yet accounted for almost 15% of the toxic drug deaths in 2020 (First Nations Health Authority, 2021).

The longstanding need to address the mental health and well-being of Canada's Indigenous peoples is a priority. The Truth and Reconciliation Commission of Canada Call to Action #19 called upon the federal government to "close the gap in health outcomes between Aboriginal and non-Aboriginal communities," including mental health, suicide, and addiction (Truth and Reconciliation Commission of Canada, 2015, pp. 2–3). A critical need to fund and support services in areas including trauma, addictions, and mental health treatment was further highlighted in the National Inquiry into Missing and Murdered Indigenous Women and Girls (2019).

Indigenous Services Canada (Government of Canada, 2022) mental wellness services are guided by two key documents that were developed by Indigenous partners. The First Nations Mental Wellness Continuum Framework (Health Canada, 2015) is a national framework that identifies ways to enhance coordination among various systems and supports culturally safe delivery of services. The National Inuit Suicide Prevention Strategy (Inuit Tapiriit Kanatami, 2016) promotes a shared understanding of the context and underlying risk factors for suicide in Inuit communities and guides policy at the regional and national levels on evidence-based approaches to suicide prevention. Although the demand for mental health interventions, particularly those related to suicide prevention, continues to grow, activities that respect and honour Indigenous Ways of Knowing have been introduced into Western healthcare systems. These activities include ceremony, being on the land, the Medicine Wheel, engaging in traditional food gathering, culturally grounded indoor and outdoor activities, group activities with other Indigenous people, and being connected with an Elder for conversation and guidance (Graham et al., 2021). Importantly, the activities share the common perspective that supporting wellness and promoting life is as important as suicide prevention. See Chapter 8 for further discussion on cultural influences on mental health and suicide.

Risk Factors

Suicide is not a psychiatric disorder per se; rather, self-harm is the manifestation of inner pain, hopelessness, and helplessness suffered by people experiencing suicidal ideation, also known as suicidal thoughts. These thoughts can range from a fleeting idea about one's own death (or about not being here) that does not include the act of taking one's own life to a detailed plan, possibly including disturbing preoccupations with self-annihilation fueled by delusions, which result in the final act of death by suicide (Harmer et al., 2021).

There is not one single risk factor that precipitates suicide. People with multiple risk factors and few protective factors, such as positive social support and coping skills, are at the highest risk for suicide. Prior suicide attempts and a history of deliberate self-harm and/or suicidal ideation are recognized as the strongest known risk factors for suicide (Centre for Addiction and Mental Health, 2020).

Mental illness, including co-occurring substance use disorder, is one of the most common risk factors for suicide. It is estimated that 90% of people who die by suicide are experiencing depression, another mental health illness, or a substance use disorder, all of which are potentially treatable (Centre for Addiction and Mental Health, 2020; Government of Canada, 2016). About 15% of patients who have major depression or bipolar disorder (during the depressed phase) will die by suicide (Brendel et al., 2016). Trauma, loss of relationships, financial difficulty, loss of housing, legal issues, physical health problems, a recent or impending life crisis, and impulsivity are contributing factors in this population.

Suicide risk is 50 times higher among people with schizophrenia than among the general population, especially during the first few years of the illness, and suicide is the leading cause of early death among those with the illness. The more risk factors that are present, the higher is the risk for suicide. All too frequently, death by suicide is associated with recent institutional release and a lack of medication adherence (Schmutte et al., 2021).

Keep in mind that suicide is not necessarily synonymous with a mental health disorder. Research has shown that numerous medical illnesses are associated with increased odds of suicide and that suicidal death extends through all demographic groups and includes virtually all psychiatric and medical diagnoses (Harmer et al., 2021). The act of purposeful self-destruction represented by taking one's own life is usually accompanied by intensely conflicted feelings of pain, hopelessness, guilt, and self-loathing, coupled with the belief that there are no solutions and that things will not improve. Self-harming actions have been associated with the feeling that there is no one to turn to for support (Muehlenkamp et al., 2013). People who survive serious suicide attempts often report that it is these feelings that fuelled the sense of isolation and despair. They describe an all-consuming psychic pain that shuts out thoughts of the loved ones and heartache they will leave behind. To understand this phenomenon, imagine the pain of your hand on a hot stove burner. At that moment, you are unlikely to think of anything but putting an immediate end to the pain. Emotional pain can render the individual void of thought and without even enough motivation to leave a suicide note. Antoon Leenaars, a Canadian psychologist and researcher who has studied suicide notes extensively, has stated that only between 12% and 37% of people who died by suicide left suicide notes (Canadian Association for Suicide Prevention [CASP], 2009).

Besides psychiatric disorders, other risk factors associated with the psychic pain that can trigger suicidal behaviour include trauma, victimization by bullying, incarceration, and non-heterosexuality. A trauma-informed perspective asks, "*What happened to you?*" instead of "*What's wrong with you?*" (Crisis Prevention Institute, 2020). Exposure to maltreatment; violence; physical, emotional, or sexual abuse; and other traumas, particularly in childhood, are associated with increased odds for suicidality in both young adults (Angelekis et al., 2020) and adults (Angelekis et al., 2019).

The term *bullycide* was coined by Marr and Field (2000) to refer to suicidal behaviour in response to bullying. A strong relationship exists between bullying and self-harm, for both those who have been victimized by bullying and those who bully others. Among adolescents engaging in self-harm, those who have been bullied are at six times higher risk for self-harm than those who have not been bullied, and those who bully are at three times higher risk for self-harm than those who do not bully (Myklestad & Straiton, 2021). Girls are at significantly greater risk than boys, and depression, anxiety, parental conflict, and school behavioral problems account for some of the association between experiences with bullying and self-harm (Myklestad & Straiton, 2021).

Suicide Among Older Persons

To be old, sad, and feel like life has no meaning can be reflected in the term triple jeopardy. Such is the experience of some older persons. Individuals over the age of 65 have a high rate of suicide, particularly men (Heisel et al., 2020). As the population ages, it is predicted that the number of people over the age of 65 will increase significantly and concomitantly, the number of older persons who die by suicide will increase (Canadian Coalition for Seniors Mental Health [CCSMH], 2021; Stats Canada, 2020c). In 2014 Canadians over the age of 65 (approximately 6 million) represented 15% of Canada's population. By 2030, it is estimated that this age group will represent almost 25% of the population (over 9.5 million) (Government of Canada, 2021).

While it is recognized that youth suicide is a major problem, few recognize the extent of the problem of suicide among older persons. Men over the age of 65 have rates of death by suicide at 20 per 100 000 and men over the age of 90 have rates of 338 per 100 000 people (MHCC, 2020b). For every three older persons who attempt suicide, one dies, as compared with youth suicide, where for every 200 attempts, one dies (Centre for Suicide Prevention, 2019). The reason that older men die more frequently is that they use more lethal means (suffocation, firearms). Suffocation has risen to the number one cause of death by suicide in Canada, surpassing firearms (Lie et al., 2021). It is clear that as men age, their risk of suicide increases dramatically into the eighth and ninth decades of life. The fastest-growing age group in Canada currently is the 85 and older age group. Clearly, suicide among older persons is a major public health concern and unnecessary cause of death that requires concerted efforts to address.

Risk Factors

There are risk factors specific to older persons that contribute to them being more at risk for suicidal thoughts and behaviours (Beghi et al., 2021; Flett & Heisel, 2020; Heuser & Howe, 2019; Lui et al., 2021).

- Experiences of loss such as loss of health, independence, friends, and loved ones
- Experiencing a life crisis
- Isolation and loss of social connections. Often, they live alone.
- Major life transitions and changes such as retirement, moving to a care facility, loss of financial capacity they once knew
- Chronic pain and illness
- Feeling of being a burden to family and others
- Substance use
- Depression

Usually, it is not just one risk factor that propels an older person toward suicide but rather an accumulation of losses or factors that become overwhelming.

Warning Signs

- Loss of a sense of meaning and purpose for living
- Feelings of hopelessness
- Loss of independence
- Death of a spouse or loved one
- Isolation
- Increased use of substances
- Expressing feelings of worthlessness and/or being a burden
- Comments like "everyone will be better off without me"
- Valuable possessions lose their meaning (may be given away or gotten rid of)

Interventions

- Focused interventions are needed to address this problem. While some intervention strategies may be the same as those for younger individuals, there are some that nurses can specifically target towards older persons through conversations with the older person (and sometimes their significant other or family).
- Have caring conversations with older persons. Speak with them and reflect a caring and non-judgmental attitude. Convey that they matter. Encourage their participation in meaningful activities (artistic, physical activities). Participation can often help to reduce depression.
- Connect them with resources. If they have lost a spouse, a grief support group may help. If a man has recently retired, a Meaning-Centred Men's Group may be available (which focuses on men recently retired or facing retirement). Other groups, such as Alzheimer's Support, Cancer Support, Parkinson's Support, all provide focused information and support for specific causes.
- Remove access to lethal means. Arrange to have firearms removed or secured in a location that does not make them easily accessible. The more difficult it is to access means for suicide, the more likely it is that a suicide attempt can be averted long enough to get help.
- Refer to a family physician for the treatment of depression (many suicidal older persons suffer from depression).
- COVID-19 has seen a burgeoning of online activities, courses, and resources, many of which are very accessible for disabled, youth, and older persons. Having conversations about their interests and desires can open up avenues to connect them with relevant online programs and activities.
- Limit use (and access) to substances that may impair judgement.
- Look for ways to foster hope regardless of ones' life circumstances.
- If you suspect that an older person is thinking of suicide, ask them directly. Be firm in your commitment to seek help for them. Suicides can be prevented.

RESEARCH HIGHLIGHT
Understanding Self-Harm and Suicidal Behaviour

Problem

Men account for almost 75% of suicides that occur in North America every year (Center for Disease Control and Prevention [CDC], 2017). Older men have the highest suicide rates in the world (Heisel et al., 2020; WHO, 2014). Given the rapidly aging population, suicide prevention efforts are needed that target this vulnerable group of men. Many men frequently have difficulty sharing personal difficulties and mental health needs. Retirement is a life transition that many men look forward to, yet it can create challenges where one's sense of identity has been found in their work and now is gone. Some men have not had interests or relationships outside of work and creating these after retirement can be daunting. For those men, retirement can become a time of depression and feeling worthless. "Interventions are needed that overcome the reluctance of some men to seek care, that are consistent with their values and goals, and are informed by an understanding of suicide risk and resiliency processes" (Heisel et al., 2020, p. 77). A non-traditional approach was developed by Dr. Marnin Heisel and the Meaning-Centred Men's Group (MCMG) Project Team to encourage men who were reluctant to pursue psychological interventions and support (Heisel et al., 2020).

Purpose of the Study

To assess the efficacy of an MCMG intervention, a 12-session, existentially oriented group based in the community was offered as a psychological group intervention that was targeted toward enhancing psychological resiliency and preventing suicide ideation among men facing retirement.

Methods

We recruited 30 men aged 55 and older with an average age of 63 (10 men were assigned to each of 3 groups) from community-based settings. Each group participated in the 12-session course offered through a community centre. Participants completed four assessments over the course of the group (eligibility, pre-, mid-, and post-group) focused on factors related to suicide ideation, psychological risk, and resiliency.

Key Findings

Promising results demonstrated that the men showed increases in meaning in life, life and retirement satisfaction, psychological well-being, and general health. They also showed decreases in loneliness, depression, and suicide ideation.

Implications for Nursing Practice

By recognizing that older men are at increased risk for suicide and often do not share their feelings of sadness or psychological distress, nurses can maintain an awareness of these vulnerabilities and recognize the important role that psychological resiliency can have in mitigating feelings of depression and suicide. Further, they can foster engagement in and access to meaningful activities and groups for men as a way of helping them connect with others who have like interests.

Source: Heisel, M. J., Moore, S. L., Flett, G. L., et al. (2020). Meaning-Centered Men's Groups: Initial findings of an intervention to enhance resiliency and reduce suicide risk in men facing retirement. *Clinical Gerontologist, 43*(1), 76–94. https://doi.org/10.1080/07317115.2019.1666443

Deaths by suicide among people in prison have long been shown to occur at higher rates than among general populations of similar ages (Zhong et al., 2021). There are 10 suicide deaths each year in federal penitentiaries, a rate 7 times higher than in the general population (Office of the Correctional Investigator Canada, 2014).

Researchers have established that suicidal behaviour is significantly higher in non-heterosexual populations. Members of diverse communities who are lesbian, gay, bisexual, transgender, queer, intersex, Two-Spirit, or those who identify with another non-binary gender or minority sexual identity (LGBTQ2) are vulnerable to self-harm. Of the 1 million LGBTQ2 people in Canada, 32% view their mental health as poor; 41% have been diagnosed with a mood or anxiety disorder; and 40% have seriously contemplated suicide in their lifetimes (Statistics Canada, 2021). Although most mortality data do not include sexual orientation, non-heterosexual youth are believed to experience suicidal ideation and engage in suicidal behaviour to a greater extent than heterosexual adolescents and young adults. The stigma and discrimination associated with their sexual orientation elevate risk and lower protective factors among this group.

Refer to Box 22.1 for a description of significant psychosocial risk and protective factors for suicide and to Box 22.2 for warning signs.

ETIOLOGY

Biological Factors

Researchers continue to study biological factors in order to better understand and screen for suicidal behaviour, although none of the biological markers identified to date are sensitive or precise enough for use in the clinical setting. People who died by suicide were found to have three specific DNA markers, suggesting that genetic variations may be associated with a broad range of suicidal thoughts and behaviours (Strawbridge et al., 2019). Evidence suggests a potentially causal association between suicidal behaviour and the serotonin neurotransmission system (Carballo et al., 2008). Further, hypothalamus–pituitary–adrenal (HPA) axis abnormalities, mainly characterized by hyperactivity of the HPA axis, may exert an important modulatory influence on suicide risk (Berardelli et al., 2020).

Studies indicate a combined effect of genetic and epigenetic (external gene-altering) factors. Guintivano and colleagues (2014) found that the *SKA2* gene expression was lower in individuals with suicidal ideation. This lowered gene expression along with anxiety and stress could account for about 80% of suicidal behaviours and the progression from suicidal ideation to suicide attempt. These findings are consistent with the diathesis–stress model or the dual-risk hypothesis.

Another consideration is the involvement of protein kinase A (PKA), a crucial enzyme in the adenylyl cyclase signal transduction pathway, which regulates gene transcription, cell survival, and plasticity. When stress affects PKA's synaptic and structural plasticity, an association with suicide has been identified (Dwivedi & Pandey, 2011).

Psychosocial Factors

Sigmund Freud originally theorized that suicide resulted from unacceptable aggression toward another person that is turned inward. Karl Menninger added to Freud's thought by describing three parts of suicidal hostility: the wish to kill, the wish to be killed, and the wish to die (Boland et al., 2022). Aaron Beck identified a central emotional factor underlying suicide intent: hopelessness. Certain cognitive styles that contribute to higher risk are rigid all-or-nothing thinking, inability to see different options, and perfectionism (Hewitt et al., 2014). Maladaptive perfectionist thinking, in which anything less than perfect is unacceptable, can leave individuals vulnerable to depression and suicide (Kiamanesh et al., 2015).

BOX 22.1 Suicide Risk Factors and Protective Factors

Risk Factors
- Suicidal ideation with intent
- Lethal suicide plan
- History of previous suicide attempt
- Co-occurring psychiatric illness
- Co-occurring medical illness
- History of maltreatment (violence; physical, emotional, or sexual abuse; and other traumas, particularly in childhood)
- Experiences being bullied or bullying
- Family history of suicide
- Lack of social support
- Unemployment
- Recent stressful life event (e.g., death, other loss, legal conflict, relationship breakup, conflict)
- Hopelessness
- Helplessness
- Panic attacks
- Feeling of shame or humiliation
- Impulsivity
- Aggressiveness
- Loss of cognitive function (e.g., loss of impulse control)
- Access to firearms and other highly lethal means
- Substance use (without formal disorder)
- Impending incarceration
- Low frustration tolerance
- Sexual orientation and gender identity issues
- Social isolation
- Key demographic risk (widowed, divorced, single, white, elderly, adolescent, young adult, Indigenous, LGBTQ2 [lesbian, gay, bisexual, transgender, queer, intersex, and Two-Spirited])

Protective Factors

Note that, although patients who exhibit protective factors may attempt and die by suicide, multiple protective factors generally contribute to patient resiliency in the face of stress and adversity. Protective factors may be considered in each of the domains of the individual, family, work, and community. Important protective factors may include:
- children in the home, except among those with postpartum psychosis
- responsibility to others
- pregnancy
- personal, social, cultural, and religious beliefs that discourage suicide and support self-preservation
- life satisfaction
- reality testing ability
- positive coping skills
- positive social support
- positive therapeutic relationship
- attachment to therapy, social, or family support
- hope for future
- self-efficacy
- supportive living arrangements
- fear of act of suicide
- fear of social disapproval

Sources: The Canadian Patient Safety Institute and the Mental Health Commission of Canada. (2021). *Suicide risk assessment toolkit: A resource for healthcare workers and organizations.* Retrieved from https://www.patientsafetyinstitute.ca/en/toolsResources/SuicideRisk/Documents/MHCC-CPSI%20-%20Suicide%20Risk%20Assessment%20Toolkit%20EN.pdf

BOX 22.2 Warning Signs

The American Association of Suicidology (AAS) uses the mnemonic **IS PATH WARM** to assist people in recognizing and identifying the warning signs of suicide.

Suicide Warning Signs

I	Ideation
S	Substance use
P	Purposelessness
A	Anxiety or agitation
T	Trapped
H	Hopelessness or helplessness
W	Withdrawal
A	Anger
R	Recklessness
M	Mood changes

The presence of any warning sign may signify that someone is thinking about suicide. The presence of more than one warning sign indicates a higher risk for suicide. The presence of one or more warning signs should signal the need to begin a dialogue into a person's circumstances and a follow-up with a more in-depth suicide risk assessment.

Source: American Association of Suicidology. (2020). *Know the warning signs*. Retrieved from https://suicidology.org/resources/warning-signs/suicide-warning-signs

Recent theories of suicide have focused on the lethal combination of suicidal fantasies accompanied by loss (e.g., of love, self-esteem, job, freedom due to imminent incarceration), rage or guilt, or identification with a suicide victim (**cluster suicide**). A cluster suicide, sometimes referred to as a copycat suicide, follows a highly publicized suicide of a public figure, an idol, or a peer in the community. Adolescents are at especially high risk for cluster suicide, owing to their immature prefrontal cortex, the portion of the brain that controls the executive functions involving judgement, frustration tolerance, and impulse control.

Current events also exert a psychosocial impact on the etiology of suicide. For example, in addition to the high infectivity and fatality rates people experienced throughout the COVID-19 pandemic, a "dual pandemic" of suicide-risk pandemic emerged as a global health threat. Pandemics lead to several risk factors for suicidality like isolation, loneliness, economic fallout, domestic abuse, stigma, and fear (Banerjee et al., 2021; Canadian Institute for Health Information, 2021). In 2020 and 2021, as many as 70% of Canadian children and adolescents experienced deterioration in their mental health, including increased depression, anxiety, irritability, attention, hyperactivity, and obsessions/compulsions (Cost et al., 2021). Distress, anxiety and depression, and PTSD, particularly among health care workers, occurred (Dubey et al., 2020). Catastrophic events, such as a pandemic, in combination with violence, alcohol use disorders, substance use, and feelings of loss, are important factors that can increase people's risk of deciding to take their own lives (Pan American Health Organization, 2020).

Athletes, at both elite and amateur levels, can feel constant pressure to perform. Loss of status in their sport, steroid use, or an injury such as post-concussion syndrome can leave them susceptible to suicidal fantasies. Persistent pain has been found to increase depression in retired professional athletes (Riley, 2016). The International Society of Sport Psychology identified that mental health is a core component of a culture of excellence in sport. The society emphasized that: "Winning 'at any cost' is incompatible with a modern responsible sport system that values the human behind the performer" (Henriksen et al., 2020, p. 554).

Societal Considerations

Medical Assistance in Dying (MAiD)

No discussion about current societal attitudes and trends would be complete without an examination of the way in which suicide is viewed in a general context. In Canada voluntary death for psychiatric conditions is legal. In 2016 the Parliament of Canada passed Bill C-14, a law permitting medical euthanasia and physician-assisted suicide, together known as **medical assistance in dying** (MAiD) (Komrad, 2021). A key eligibility criterion of this law was that a person's natural death is predicted to be reasonably foreseeable. When Bill C-14 was first passed, mental illnesses were not considered eligible conditions because they were not seen as strongly predictable. However, in 2019 the constitutionality of restricting MAiD requests was challenged, and a new federal bill was introduced to extend euthanasia eligibility, without limiting it to the end of life (Komrad, 2021). Yet, like Bill C-14, this new initiative, Bill C-7 (2021), excluded psychiatric disorders.

Later, in 2021 Parliament passed revised legislation that removed the requirement for a person's natural death to be reasonably foreseeable in order to be eligible for MAiD (Department of Justice Canada, 2021). Although euthanasia for those whose psychological or physical suffering is deemed intolerable and untreatable is permitted, an amendment excludes individuals suffering solely from mental illness for a period of 24 months, and expert review of protocols, guidance, and safeguards for MAiD for people suffering from mental illness continues (Department of Justice Canada, 2021).

Discussions related to the ethical and moral dilemmas of MAiD remain ongoing. Those in favor argue that people with psychiatric illnesses should not be discriminated against and should have the same options to access MAiD that are available to other Canadians (Komrad, 2021). Proponents maintain that data from jurisdictions where MAiD is available do not show an increase in suicide rates; that people are presumed to have the capacity to make medical decisions unless proven otherwise; and that suffering in severe mental illness can be equal to that of the most severe physical conditions (Dembo et al., 2018).

On the other hand, those opposed assert that allowing non-terminal, disabled individuals access to MAiD implies that their lives may be not worth living and that MAiD is a cost-saving alternative to suffering when adequate solutions are not available or affordable (Komrad, 2021). The practice is viewed as one that provides suicide to people rather than preventing suicide, which is incompatible with a commitment to healing (Komrad, 2021). The Canadian Mental Health Association (2021) emphasized how cases of severe and persistent mental illness that are initially resistant to treatment can show significant recovery over time. "Mental illness is very often episodic. Death, on the other hand, is not reversible" (Canadian Mental Health Association, 2021, para. 3). Despite a lack of consensus, most health professions agree that decisions related to accessing MAiD must be made on a person-by-person basis.

APPLICATION OF THE NURSING PROCESS

The process of suicide risk assessment is comprehensive and requires identifying specific risk factors, taking a psychosocial and medical history, and interacting with the patient during the interview. The nurse usually completes this assessment in conjunction with other clinicians since the comparison of data from two interviewers is often a significant element of the evaluation.

Not all patients who show suicidal ideation or who engage in suicidal behaviour truly want to die. Suicidal behaviour can include a variety of behaviours, including self-harm either with or without clear intent to cause bodily harm or death. Any previous suicidal behaviour is a risk factor for suicide; about half of all people who die by suicide have a history of some form of suicidal behaviour. Especially prevalent in the adolescent and young adult populations, self-harm (usually in the form of cutting) is most often done with the intent to handle inner pain and vulnerability (Stänicke, 2021). They do not engage in this behaviour as a means of seeking attention and will often go to great lengths to conceal the evidence. Self-harm often carries a lethal risk for death or permanent injury. It is important for nurses to try to understand what is behind the behaviour, as it is often a sign that the individual is trying to communicate their pain and despair.

Non-acute suicidal or self-destructive thoughts and feelings can be treated in the outpatient setting. Alternative services available to suicidal patients include crisis intervention, community mental health services, assertive community treatment, addiction treatment, social services, and legal assistance. Suicide risk assessment is a complex process that involves learning about a person, recognizing their needs and stressors, and working with them (and their family) to mobilize their strengths and supports. The purpose of suicide risk assessment is not to predict suicide. It is rather to assess and reduce the risk of suicide by identifying warning signs, risk and protective factors, the individual's medical and mental health history, their acute condition, access to lethal means, and available support networks (Canadian Patient Safety Institute & Mental Health Commission of Canada, 2021).

Assessment

The *Suicide Risk Assessment Guide: A Resource for Health Care Organizations* (Perlman et al., 2011) is a seminal guide that has been helping health care organizations understand and standardize the practice of high-quality suicide risk assessment for over 2 decades. The guide emphasizes the importance of thorough documentation in assessing suicide. The Suicide Risk Assessment Toolkit (Box 22.3) provides a sample of recommended documentation, summarizing eight important points to include in nursing assessments.

Organizations should also develop standard protocols for the location of documentation regarding suicide risk within the patient's record so that documentation is consistently located and therefore easily identified by others within the organization or by those involved in the care of the person.

Verbal and Non-verbal Clues

Almost all people considering suicide send out clues, especially to people they think of as supportive. Nurses and other health care workers often fit into this category. There may be overt or covert verbal clues and non-verbal signals. Examples include:
- Overt statements
  - "I can't take it anymore."
  - "Life isn't worth living anymore."
  - "I wish I were dead."
  - "Everyone would be better off if I died."
- Covert statements
  - "It's okay now. Soon everything will be fine."
  - "Things will never work out."
  - "I won't be a problem much longer."
  - "Nothing feels good to me anymore and probably never will."
  - "How can I give my body to medical science?"

Most often, it is a relief for people contemplating suicide to finally talk to someone about their despair and loneliness. Asking about suicidal thoughts does not "give a person ideas" and is, in fact, a professional responsibility similar to asking about chest pain in cardiac conditions. Talking openly leads to a decrease in isolation and can increase problem-solving alternatives for living. People who contemplate suicide, those who act on their suicidal thoughts, and even those

---

BOX 22.3 Sample of Recommended Documentation

1. The overall level of suicide risk
   The level of risk should be clearly documented, along with information to support this assertion, which can include:
   - The types of assessment tools used to inform risk assessment
   - Details from clinical interviews and from communication with others (e.g., the person's family and friends, other professionals), including:
     - The circumstances and timing of the event
     - Method chosen for suicide
     - Degree of intent
     - Availability of resources to carry out plan
     - Description of actions taken by the health care provider or family members
     - Consequences of previous suicidal ideation or self-harming behaviours (e.g., Were there any permanent injuries?)
2. Prior history of suicide attempt(s) and self-harming behaviour
   - The prior care or intervention plan that was in place
   - The length of time since previous suicide attempt(s) or self-harming behaviour(s)
   - The rationale for not being admitted to a more intensive environment or discharged to a less restrictive environment, and what safety plans were put into place
   - Details about family concerns and how these were addressed
3. Details about all potentiating risk factors, warning signs, and protective factors
4. The degree of suicide intent
   The degree of intent may include, for example, what the person thought or hoped would happen.
5. The person's feeling and reaction following suicidal behaviour
   Record, for example, whether the person feels a sense of relief or regret for being alive.
6. Evidence of an escalation in potential lethality of self-harm or suicidal behaviours
   Document whether the person has begun to consider, plan, or use increasingly lethal means (e.g., from cutting to hanging, seeking a gun).
7. Similarity of person's current circumstances to those surrounding previous suicide attempt(s) or self-harming behaviour(s)
8. History of self-harm or suicidal behaviour(s) among family or friends or significant loss of family or friends
   This history should include anniversary dates of these events as risk may be elevated at such times.

Source: The Canadian Patient Safety Institute and the Mental Health Commission of Canada. (2021). *Suicide risk assessment toolkit: A resource for healthcare workers and organizations*. Retrieved from https://www.patientsafetyinstitute.ca/en/toolsResources/SuicideRisk/Documents/MHCC-CPSI%20-%20Suicide%20Risk%20Assessment%20Toolkit%20EN.pdf

---

who regret the "failure" of their actions are often extremely receptive to talking about their suicide crisis. Specific questions to ask about suicidal ideation include:
- Have you ever felt that life was not worth living?
- Have you been thinking about death recently?
- Have you been feeling so bad that you have thought about taking your own life?
- Did you ever think about suicide?
- Have you ever tried to end your life?
- Do you have a plan for what you would do to end your own life?
- If so, what is your plan?
- Are the means to carry out your plan available to you?
- What stops you from following through with your plan?

Lethality of Suicide Plan

The evaluation of a suicide plan is extremely important in determining the degree of suicidal risk. The following elements must be considered when evaluating **lethality** (the degree of suicidal risk):

1. Presence of risk factors for suicide
2. Degree of suicidal ideation
3. Intent to carry out suicide plan
4. Means and availability of resources to carry out the selected method of suicide
5. Presence of protective factors
6. Degree of hope for improvement of psychological state

People who have definite plans for the time, place, and means are at high risk.

People experiencing psychotic episodes are at high risk, regardless of the specificity of details, because their impulse control and judgement are grossly impaired. A person suffering psychosis is particularly vulnerable when depressed or having command hallucinations. Regardless of whether the nurse considers a patient high or low risk, *all* threats of suicide should be taken seriously, and a suicide risk assessment should be completed.

Assessment Tools

Many tools have been developed to aid a health care worker in assessing suicidal potential. Patterson and colleagues (1983) devised an assessment aid with the acronym *SAD PERSONS* to evaluate 10 major risk factors for suicide (Table 22.1). The **SAD PERSONS scale** is a simple and practical guide for triaging potentially suicidal patients, particularly in an emergency department environment. Ten categories are described in the assessment tool, and the person being evaluated is assigned one point for each applicable characteristic. The total point score for the individual correlates with an action scale that assists health care workers in determining whether hospital admission is advisable. If a patient scores in the 3- to 4-point range, a psychiatric or mental health care provider must conduct a full mental status examination and interview.

TABLE 22.1 SAD PERSONS Scale

S	Sex	1 if male
A	Age	1 if <19 or >45 years
D	Depression	1 if present
P	Previous attempt	1 if present
E	Ethanol use	1 if present
R	Rational thinking loss	1 if psychotic for any reason
S	Social supports lacking	1 if lacking, especially recent loss
O	Organized plan	1 if plan with lethal method
N	No spouse	1 if divorced, widowed, separated, or single male
S	Sickness	1 if severe or chronic

Guidelines for Actions

Points	Clinical Action
0–2	Send home with follow-up
3–4	Closely follow up; consider hospitalization
5–6	Strongly consider hospitalization
7–10	Hospitalize or commit

Source: From Patterson, W. M., Dohn, H. H., Bird, J., et al. (1983). Evaluation of suicidal patients: The SAD PERSONS scale. *Psychosomatics, 24*(4), 343–345, 348–349.

The SAD PERSONS tool has its shortcomings. It does not address whether the patient is taking either illicit or prescribed drugs that may have a significant impact on them, and it is also dated (from 1983).

Prescription medications such as antidepressants should be evaluated for their contribution to suicide risk. No antidepressants are approved for use in anyone under 18 in Canada; however, health professionals often prescribe medicines for off-label use, meaning that they are not specifically approved but that may still be safe and effective (MyHealth.Alberta.ca, 2020). Health Canada and the US Food and Drug Administration (FDA) issued advisories to patients, families, and health professionals to closely monitor for warning signs of suicidal behaviour in children and adults younger than 25 who take antidepressants. This is especially important at the beginning of treatment or when doses are changed (MyHealth.Alberta.ca, 2020). Health Canada monitors the safety of these and other psychiatric medications and posts ongoing alerts on its website.

Medication-/substance-induced mental health disorders refer to depressive, anxiety, psychotic, or manic symptoms that occur as a physiological consequence of medications or the abuse of substances. Specified as "substance-induced" these mood disorders may occur during active use, intoxication, or withdrawal (Revadigar et al., 2021). Some patients taking psychiatric medications develop extreme restlessness and agitation (akathisia) that can make life intolerable and thereby increase the risk for suicide. Health care practitioners need to be aware that several medications can induce a manic state (e.g., antidepressants, interferon [IFN], corticosteroids, digoxin, and antiepileptic drugs) and ensure that responses to medications are carefully monitored and that screening for suicide potential is completed (Revadigar et al., 2021). The impulsivity associated with mania, and the regret that may be felt because of acts committed during a manic state, may also increase suicidal risk factors.

Self-Assessment

All health care providers who work with suicidal people need to collaborate with other clinicians. Fear, grief, anger, puzzlement, and condemnation of suicidal feelings or intent are common. If these intense emotional responses are not acknowledged, counter-transference may limit effective intervention. Understanding the suicidal patient, as well as acknowledging, understanding, and accepting the emotions that arise from working with and caring for these patients, is essential.

> **ASSESSMENT GUIDELINES**
> **Suicide**
>
> 1. Assess risk factors, including history of suicide (in family, friends), degree of hopelessness and helplessness, and lethality of plan.
> 2. If there is a history of a suicide attempt, assess intent, lethality, and injury.
> 3. Determine whether the patient's age, medical condition, psychiatric diagnosis, history of trauma, or current medications put the patient at higher risk.
> 4. Further assessment is necessary if the patient suddenly goes from sad or depressed to happy and peaceful. Often a decision to take one's own life gives a feeling of relief and calm.
> 5. If the patient is to be managed on an outpatient basis, also assess protective factors, social supports, and helpfulness of significant others.

Implementation

Nursing interventions for suicide take place at three different levels: primary, secondary, and tertiary. Because improving *overall* community mental health can reduce the incidence of suicide more effectively than extensive efforts directed at identifying imminently suicidal individuals, more attention focused on primary interventions that involve community-wide participation can improve outcomes at the community level (CASP, 2021a).

Primary Intervention

Primary intervention includes activities that provide support, information, and education to prevent suicide (Box 22.4). As you have seen by now, suicide is a grave concern. Its impact on individuals, families, and communities is huge. The pain and loss left in the wake of suicide is overwhelming. The World Health Organization (WHO) in June 2021 published a document, *Live Life*, and an accompanying video that addresses suicide prevention around the world. This document and video are well worth taking a look at, as you hear the stories of individuals who have lived this experience. The WHO suggests that governments and communities can contribute to suicide prevention by implementing *Live Life*—the WHO approach for starting suicide prevention with the goal of countries further developing it and using it as a basis for developing a national suicide prevention strategy (WHO, 2021a). Canada is one of the few industrialized countries that does not have a national strategy for suicide prevention. While the Canadian Association for Suicide Prevention (CASP, 2009) has developed a national Blueprint for Suicide Prevention, to date, the government has not.

Live Life is centred around the core pillars of:
- Situational analysis
- Multi-sectoral collaboration
- Awareness raising and advocacy
- Capacity building
- Financing
- Surveillance, monitoring, and evaluation

Live Life identifies the following key effective interventions for suicide prevention.
- Limit access to the means of suicide
- Interact with the media for responsible reporting of suicide
- Foster socioemotional life skills in adolescents
- Early identify, assess, manage, and follow up anyone who is affected by suicidal behaviours

Primary intervention can be practised in a wide variety of community settings, such as schools, homes, churches, hospitals, and work settings. Elementary school children are screened using evidence-informed tools that focus on both risk factors and warning signs. Several high schools are adopting suicide prevention curricula that

---

BOX 22.4 Goals of the National Strategy for Suicide Prevention

In 2009 the Canadian Association for Suicide Prevention (2009) released the second edition of the *Blueprint for a National Suicide Prevention Strategy* (the first edition having been released in 2004). This seminal document has been used across Canada as well as the United States, UK, Australia, New Zealand, and other European and Asian countries. It provides the foundation for the ongoing development of a National Suicide Prevention Strategy (Canadian Association for Suicide Prevention, n.d.). The Blueprint was developed out of the belief that many suicidal behaviours are potentially preventable and that it is the collective responsibility of Canadians to work together toward prevention, intervention, and postvention.

Six principles guided the development of the national strategy (Canadian Association for Suicide Prevention, 2009, p. 9):

1. Suicide prevention is everyone's responsibility.
2. Canadians respect our multi-cultural and diverse society and accept responsibility to support the dignity of human life.
3. Suicide is an interaction of biological, psychological, social, and spiritual factors and can be influenced by societal attitudes and conditions.
4. Strategies must be humane, kindly, effective, caring and should be:
   a. Evidence or experience based
   b. Active and informed
   c. Respectful of community- and culture-based knowledge
   d. Inclusive of research, surveillance, evaluation, accountability, and reporting
   e. Reflective of evolving knowledge and practices
5. Many suicides are preventable by knowledgeable, caring, compassionate, and committed communities.
6. We must have the courage to confront the stigma of suicide and the patience to address mental health literacy on both a national and local level.

Awareness and Understanding Goals
1. Promote awareness in every part of Canada that suicide and suicide-related behaviour is our problem and is preventable.
2. Develop broad-based support for suicide prevention, intervention, and postvention.
3. Develop and implement a strategy to reduce stigma, to be associated with all suicide prevention, intervention, and bereavement activities.
4. Increase media knowledge regarding suicide.

Prevention, Intervention, and Postvention Goals
1. Develop, implement, and sustain community-based suicide prevention, intervention, and postvention programs, respecting diversity and culture at local, regional, and provincial or territorial levels.
2. Reduce the availability and lethality of suicide methods.
3. Increase training for the recognition of risk factors, warning signs and at-risk behaviours and for the provision of effective intervention and postvention, targeting key gatekeepers, volunteers, and professionals.
4. Develop and promote effective clinical and professional practice (effective strategies, standards of care) to support patients, families, and communities.
5. Improve access and integration with strong linkages between the continuum-of-care components/services/families.
6. Prioritize intervention and service delivery for high-risk groups while respecting local, regional, and provincial or territorial uniqueness.
7. Increase crisis intervention and support.
8. Increase services and support to those bereaved by suicide or who have attempted suicide.
9. Increase the number of primary prevention activities.

Knowledge Development and Transfer
1. Improve and expand surveillance systems.
2. Promote and support the development of effective evaluation tools.
3. Promote and develop suicide-related research.
4. Increase opportunities for reporting.

Funding and Support
1. Increase funding and support for all activities connected with the *CASP Blueprint for a Canadian National Suicide Prevention Strategy* (2nd edition).
2. Ensure access to appropriate and adequate health, wellness, and recovery services for all Canadians in keeping with the *Canada Health Act*.

Source: Canadian Association for Suicide Prevention. (2009). *The CASP national suicide prevention strategy* (2nd ed., pp. 10–16). Winnipeg: Author. Retrieved from https://suicideprevention.ca/wp-content/uploads/2021/10/CASP-Blueprint-for-Cdn-National-Suicide-Prevention-Strategy_Final_2009pdf-1.pdf involve elements of education, peer support, and referral and discussions about risk factors and warning signs (Asarnow et al., 2018; Brann et al., 2021).

Secondary Intervention

Secondary intervention is the treatment of the actual suicidal crisis. It is practised in clinics, hospitals, and jails and on telephone hotlines. Involving the entire community, especially in primary and secondary interventions, is essential to reducing suicides. The foundation of any intervention for suicide or suicidal behaviours is establishing a therapeutic relationship. Understanding and appreciating patients' unique situations and treating individuals with respect and openness are essential. Nurses who remain informed, empathic, and non-judgmental are well positioned to initiate interventions at both the individual and the community levels. Often secondary interventions are the determinants of life or death, and nurses with good crisis intervention skills are in a position to use, role-model, and teach these skills to others.

In their review of suicide prevention initiatives Dabkowski and Porter (2021) noted several types of programs that show promise. One study suggested that programming should be targeted at long-term behavioural change in practitioners, recommending a need for improvements in organizational capacity. Strengthening the capacity of mental health professionals for crisis interventions was a strong recommendation.

Tertiary Intervention

Tertiary intervention (or **postvention**) refers to interventions with the family and friends of a person who has died by suicide. Postvention aims to both reduce the traumatic aftereffects and explore effective means of addressing survivor problems using primary and secondary interventions. Nurses understand grief or loss well and are in a position to refer, consult, and collaborate in the best interests of those left behind, a vital service since the suicide rate increases for those left behind (Jordan, 2017). Survivors of suicide are in immediate need of supportive avenues for coping with such complicated grief. (See section on Postvention.)

Milieu Management

Suicide precautions. In accordance with unit policies and procedures the patient is observed continuously by nursing staff. Refer to Table 22.2 for a general description of suicide precautions. This intense attention from the nurse provides for safety and allows for the constant reassessment of risk. Monitoring flow sheets for suicide precautions are more clinically useful if they include a description of affect as well as behaviour. For example, instead of noting, "Patient watching television," the nurse can describe the patient's affect at each observation interval (e.g., hostile, fearful, calm). Flow sheets should also indicate clear accountability for staff starting and ending their periods of observation. In addition to observing the patient, the nurse is responsible for monitoring the environment for safety hazards. Review Box 22.5 for guidelines on how to minimize physical risks in the milieu.

Studies show that acute care of suicidal patients is usually effective. Suicide risk is highest in the first few days of admission and during times of staff rotation, particularly rotation of psychiatric

---

BOX 22.5 Environmental Guidelines for Minimizing Suicidal Behaviour on the Psychiatric Unit

- Conduct frequent environmental tours of all areas of the unit, including patient bathrooms and other private spaces.
- Provide plastic eating utensils.
- Do not assign patient to a private room, and ensure that the door remains open at all times.
- Jump-proof and hang-proof the bathrooms by installing break-away shower rods and recessed shower nozzles.
- Keep electrical cords to a minimal length.
- Install unbreakable glass in windows. Install tamper-proof screens or partitions too small to pass through. Keep all windows locked.
- Lock all utility rooms, kitchens, adjacent stairwells, and offices. All non-clinical staff (e.g., housekeepers, maintenance workers) should receive instructions to keep doors locked.
- Take all potentially harmful gifts (e.g., flowers in glass vases) from visitors before allowing them to see patients.
- Go through personal belongings with patient present, and remove all potentially harmful objects (e.g., belts, shoelaces, metal nail files, tweezers, matches, razors, perfume, shampoo).
- Ensure that visitors do not bring in or leave potentially harmful objects in patient's room (e.g., matches, nail files).
- Search patient for harmful objects (e.g., drugs, weapons, sharp objects, cords) on return from pass.

TABLE 22.2 Suicide Precautions With Constant One-to-One Observation

Staff Assessment	Possible Patient Symptoms	Nursing Responsibilities
Patient with suicidal ideation or delusions of self-mutilation who, according to assessment by unit staff, presents clinical symptoms that suggest a clear intent to follow through with the plan or delusion	• Patient is currently verbalizing a clear intent to harm self. • Patient shows no insight into existing problems. • Patient has poor impulse control. • Patient has already attempted suicide in the recent past by a particularly lethal method (e.g., hanging, gun, carbon monoxide poisoning).	1. Conduct one-to-one nursing observation and interaction 24 hours a day (never let patient out of staff's sight). 2. Maintain arm's length observation at all times. 3. Chart patient's whereabouts and record mood, verbatim statements, and behaviour every 15–30 minutes per protocol. 4. Ensure that meal trays contain no glass or metal silverware. 5. When patient is sleeping, patient's hands should always be in view, not under the bedcovers. 6. Carefully observe patient swallow each dose of medication. 7. Respectfully maintain observation even when patient is in the bathroom. 8. The nurse and physician should explain to the patient what they will be doing and why; both document this explanation in the chart.

residents. Assessment of suicidal risk must be an ongoing process; assessment should be performed particularly before a change in level of observation or upon sudden improvement or worsening of symptoms.

Counselling

Counselling skills, including interviewing, crisis care, and problem-solving techniques, are used in both inpatient and outpatient settings. The key element is establishing a working alliance to encourage the patient to engage in more realistic problem solving. Helpful staff characteristics include warmth, sensitivity, interest, and consistency. Once patients leave the hospital, the nurse may see them in the clinic, in a partial hospital program, or in home care.

Talking openly and honestly about suicide and the feelings a patient is having is an important part of the process of ongoing assessment and intervention. Encouraging patients to consult with their physician, community mental health worker, or emergency department if they are experiencing suicidal ideation can be a first step in helping to link them with appropriate resources. While the use of "no-suicide contracts" has been a past practice in mental health work, these contracts are now discouraged, as there is limited evidence to support their value.

Health Teaching and Health Promotion

The nurse teaches the patient about psychiatric diagnoses, medications and complementary therapies, and age-related crises. Teaching regarding community resources, coping skills, stress management, and communication skills is also important. When possible, the family or significant others are included to strengthen the patient's support system. A focus on personal strengths and positive thoughts and emotions (e.g., hope) is essential.

The Mental Health Commission of Canada (MHCC) offers a short online course (free) on *Suicide: Facing the Difficult Topic Together—Empowering Nurses, Instilling Hope in Clients* (https://www.mdbriefcase.com/course/suicide-facing-the-difficult-topic-together-empowering-nurses-instilling-hope-in-clients/) (Mental Health Commission of Canada, n.d.). MHCC also offers numerous resources on Roots of Hope and toolkits focused on Suicide Prevention and Suicide Risk Assessment (https://mentalhealthcommission.ca).

Case Management

Case management is an important aspect of nursing care for the suicidal patient. The patient's perception of being alone without supports often blinds the person to the real support figures who are present. Reconnecting the patient with family and friends is a major focus, whether in the hospital or the community. Aftercare referral may be given and may include information on the following resources: substance treatment centres, crisis hotlines, support groups for patients or families, online resources and activities, and recreational activities to enhance socialization and self-esteem. Encouraging the patient to get re-acquainted with a previous spiritual support system can also be beneficial.

Pharmacological Interventions

A significant nursing intervention to assist the suicidal patient in regaining self-control is the careful administration of medication. All medications given to high-risk patients are monitored carefully, although lethal overdose is nearly impossible with selective serotonin reuptake inhibitors (SSRIs), unlike with the risky tricyclic antidepressants and monoamine oxidase inhibitors. Mouth checks may be used to be sure patients are not saving (hoarding) medications in the hospital; in the community provision of a limited day supply or family supervision is required.

Antidepressants should be ordered for patients who have depressive or anxiety disorders, with an emphasis on administering an adequate dosage and providing appropriate clinical evaluation when using SSRIs. Close monitoring must occur during the 2- to 3-week post-initiation period, when energy increases can lead to acting on suicidal ideation, and during times of dosage adjustment. Astute nursing care involves careful patient (and family, if appropriate) teaching about the identified benefits and risks of antidepressant therapy.

There is clear evidence that long-term lithium treatment for bipolar disorder and major depression significantly reduces suicide and suicide attempts. Some studies have shown a reduced suicide rate among patients with schizophrenia receiving clozapine. Thus far no clinical studies have examined the effect of antianxiety treatment on suicide risk.

An alternative somatic treatment for acute suicidal risk is electroconvulsive therapy (ECT). Evidence suggests that ECT decreases acute suicidal ideation. Refer to Chapter 13 for further discussion of ECT.

Postvention for Survivors of Suicide

A discussion of suicidal patients is incomplete without noting the issues surrounding a death by suicide. Surviving family and friends can experience overwhelming guilt and shame, compounded by the difficulty of discussing the frequently taboo subject of suicide (Overvad & Wagoner, 2020; van der Burgt et al., 2020). The usual social supports of neighbours and church are sometimes lacking for these mourners. Walking the path of grief left in the wake of a death by suicide is one of the most difficult paths families and loved ones may ever have to walk.

The CASP (2021b) offers a message to those who are bereaved by suicide that reflects the caring and sensitivity that is needed in working with survivors.

> *If you are very new to the tragedy of suicide loss, despair may be your companion. We hope you find some time to rest your burden and share it with those of us who need no explanation. You are not alone. The fact that someone died by suicide does not diminish our love for them, their value, the contribution they made to our families and communities and our right and need to celebrate and honour their lives and accomplishments. It is how a person lived not how they died that defines someone.*
>
> *Survivors are the most courageous people we know. Be well, be peaceful, be hopeful.*

Common reactions to a death by suicide are grief, shock and numbness, deep and profound sadness, anger, blame, fear, depression, guilt, shame, and denial. Further, survivors will have questions of why this happened and what they might have done. They may experience changes in relationships and feel alone and abandoned as others struggle to know how to respond to them. They may question their own spiritual beliefs and struggle to find meaning in life as a result of their grief. They may even contemplate thoughts of suicide (SPEAK, n.d.).

The COVID-19 world has witnessed an increased risk for suicide and complicated grief for survivors of suicide. This is often complicated further by the development of PTSD (Pinto et al., 2020). Regardless of the type of suicide, survivors are deeply grieving and need support on practical, emotional, and spiritual levels. A caring, sensitive nurse can make an important contribution to help these people as they walk their own grief paths. Several provinces across Canada have developed or adapted the Alberta Health Services booklet on *Hope and Healing: A Practical Guide for Survivors* (Alberta Health Services, 2018). These guides contain practical information for survivors and can be found online. Check online in your own province to see if there are additional resources that you can access and offer.

Staff members who have cared for a suicide victim may also be traumatized by suicide. Staff may experience symptoms of PTSD, with guilt, shock, anger, shame, and decreased self-esteem. A suicide has the potential to bring up painful memories for staff who have been personally affected by suicide. Group support is essential as the treatment team conducts a thorough psychological postmortem assessment. The event is carefully reviewed to identify the potential overlooked clues, faulty judgements, or changes that are needed in employer protocols.

Evaluation

Evaluation of a suicidal patient is ongoing. The nurse must be constantly alert to changes in the suicidal person's mood, thinking, and behaviour. The nurse also looks for indications that the patient is communicating thoughts and feelings more readily and that the patient's social network is widening. For example: it is a positive sign if the person is able to talk about their feelings and engage in problem solving with the nurse? Is the patient increasing their social activities and expanding their interests? The nurse must remember that suicidal behaviour is the result of interpersonal turmoil. If an episode of major depression is the main admitting diagnosis and a serious suicidal gesture resulted from this depression, both problems are initially assessed and treated. When the patient is no longer at acute risk of suicide, treating the depression becomes the main focus of care. Essentially, the nurse evaluates each short-term goal and establishes new ones as the patient progresses towards the long-term goal of resolving suicidal ideation.

Once stabilized, the patient may qualify for transfer to an intensive outpatient treatment program, which involves continuing treatment after discharge, or a partial hospitalization program, which allows patients to go home in the evenings to practise new coping skills. Community-based support groups are also available and are both effective and free of charge. Nurses need to be knowledgeable about, and proactive in, referring patients to these support groups.

NON-SUICIDAL SELF-INJURY

A problem closely related to suicidal behaviour is NSSI. NSSI is also commonly known as self-injurious behaviour, self-mutilation, parasuicide, deliberate self-harm, self-abuse, and self-inflicted violence (Klonsky et al., 2011). While ambiguity regarding the definition and conceptualization of NSSI exists, two points of consensus are that the injuries are intentional/deliberate and suicidal intent is absent (Lengel et al., 2021). Explanations of the extent of injury are vague and it remains unclear whether an actual wound is necessary (Lengel et al., 2021).

NSSIs are deliberate and direct attempts to inflict shallow yet painful injuries to the surface of the body without intending to end one's life. The behaviour most commonly consists of cutting, burning, scraping, or scratching skin; biting, hitting skin or hair picking; head banging; and interfering with wound healing. Often the self-injurers report multiple methods of self-injury.

For these behaviours to be considered significant, they typically last at least a year and happen repeatedly. The majority of self-injurers do not seek professional help. Even when they are not engaged in the behaviours, those who self-harm tend to be preoccupied with self-injury. Self-injurious actions are most often done with the intent to self-punish, to alleviate psychic pain, or to pierce the psychic numbness these individuals describe, in what is referred to as "antidissociation" (Doyle et al., 2017, p. 134). The majority of patients use this behavior with the aim of calming down, relaxing, and gaining control over their emotional difficulties (Babič et al., 2020).

Epidemiology

The lifetime prevalence of NSSI is difficult to accurately determine due to attempts to conceal the behaviour. However, some have estimated that between 13% and 17% of adolescents engage in NSSI (Tang et al., 2021). An upsurge of self-injurious behavior in youth is expected as a result of the COVID-19 pandemic (Fegert et al., 2020). It is a global problem, peaking between 20 and 29 years of age and declining thereafter.

Comorbidity

NSSI often occurs with other mental health disorders, including depression, anxiety, eating disorders, and substance use disorders. In the past researchers thought there was a direct relationship between borderline personality disorder and NSSI. However, Bracken-Minor and McDevitt-Murphy's (2014) research concluded that the emotional regulation and distress tolerance found in individuals with NSSI was distinctly different from characteristics found in borderline personality disorder.

Risk Factors

Biological Factors

Studies related to the physiological mechanism of action in NSSI are inconclusive; however, researchers continue to investigate the neurobiological mechanisms behind the disorder. Several neurochemical pathways in the brain play a role in the development of these behaviours. Although studies are inconclusive, the neurotransmitter group of monoamines including serotonin, dopamine, and norepinephrine may play a role in the mediation of self-injury, and research is ongoing. As practitioners continue to search for an effective treatment, clinical research will seek to find the neurobiological basis of NSSI.

Psychosocial. Psychosocial risk factors for NSSIs include both intrapersonal and interpersonal influences. Intrapersonal factors include neuroticism, self-esteem, alexithymia (an inability to recognize one's own emotions), impulsivity, depression, and subjective well-being. Interpersonal factors include family function, actual social support, virtual social support, and dissatisfaction with academic performance (Tang et al., 2021). In addition, high neuroticism (experiencing the world as distressing, threatening, and unsafe) and low self-esteem have been associated with people who engage in NSSI.

Societal. NSSIs such as cutting may be a social phenomenon that is rampant in society. Individuals often learn about the behaviour from a peer who is engaging in NSSI and begin using the behaviours themselves in an attempt to alleviate personal discomfort. In fact, when an individual who engages in NSSI is admitted to an inpatient unit, others on the unit have been known to engage in the behaviour as well.

Clinical Picture

NSSI is not an official disorder in the *Diagnostic and Statistical Manual of Mental Disorders (DSM-5)*. It is still under review to determine whether it will become a recognized disorder by the American Psychiatric Association (Zetterqvist et al., 2020). However, the behaviours associated with the disorder are often seen in both inpatient and outpatient settings. This self-harm differs from suicide attempt in terms of motivation, familial transmission (found only in suicidal behaviour), age of onset (younger in NSSI), psychopathology, and functional impairment (greater in suicide attempt) (Turecki & Brent, 2016).

Assessment

A history from the patient regarding the self-injurious behaviour includes types of self-injury, triggers for the behaviour, and frequency of the behaviour (Tofthagen et al., 2014). In addition, ask the patient what has worked effectively in stopping the behaviours in the past. Appropriate physical assessment to determine the condition of wounds, if present, allows you to plan appropriate interventions.

Self-Assessment

Nurses caring for patients who engage in self-injury report that they are emotionally affected by caring for these patients. Emotions experienced include feeling defeated by relapses, discouragement, and powerlessness (Tofthagen et al., 2014). Successful treatment is linked to the quality of the relationships healthcare providers establish with NSSI patients, who are often hesitant to disclose their behaviours and confide in others. It is important for nurses to reflect critically on their own views toward self-harm and explore any negative emotions they feel when delivering care (Babič et al., 2020). In addition, nurses need to be aware that transference may occur through the projection of the patient's emotions onto the nurse. Establishing appropriate professional boundaries with the patient is important for self-care, as is collaboration with other clinicians.

Diagnosis

The nursing diagnoses with the highest priorities are *Self-mutilation* and *Risk for self-mutilation*. Patients may be experiencing feelings of anxiety, tension, and self-reproach. Consider any nursing diagnosis that is appropriate for underlying comorbid psychiatric disorders as appropriate (see the chapters in Unit 4 for further information).

Outcomes Criteria

The relevant *Nursing Outcomes Classification (NOC)* is *Mutilation self-restraint*, which is defined as "personal actions to refrain from intentional self-inflected injury" (Moorhead et al., 2013, p. 1406). Measurements for this outcome include:

- Refrains from gathering means for self-injury
- Obtains assistance as needed
- Refrains from injuring self
- Uses available support groups
- Uses medication as prescribed
- Uses effective coping strategies

Planning

The plan of care for individuals who engage in self-injury includes the demonstration of a caring attitude toward the patient, bearing hope for recovery, observing for signs of self-harm, evaluating the need for medication, and providing appropriate interventions for patients' wounds and injuries. Engage patients in their recovery plan, which encompasses a six-step approach to recovery: (1) limiting setting for safety, (2) developing self-esteem, (3) discovery of the motive for self-injury and the role it served for the patient, (4) learning that self-injury can be self-controlled, (5) replacing the self-injury with coping skills, and (6) entering a maintenance phase (Gonzales & Bergstrom, 2013).

Interventions

Basic nursing interventions include establishing a positive trusting relationship, caring for the patient's wounds and injuries, and teaching coping skills to replace the self-injurious behaviours. Specific therapies that are used include cognitive behavioural therapy, dialectical behaviour therapy, and problem-solving therapy, which may take place in individual or group therapy. There are no specific medical treatments for self-harm or self-injury. Treating underlying psychiatric disorders using psychopharmacology is an additional role of the advanced-practice nurse.

Evaluation

Similar to suicidal behaviour, the evaluation of patients with NSSI behaviours is ongoing. The development of a therapeutic alliance with the patient allows for the patient to trust the care provider. The nurse must continue to evaluate whether the patient is communicating their thoughts and feelings accurately and whether the patient's perception is that their engagement in the behaviours is declining while they turn to appropriate coping skills.

KEY POINTS TO REMEMBER

- Suicide is a significant public health problem in Canada.
- Suicide is everyone's business.
- Specific biological, psychosocial, and cultural factors are known to increase the risk for suicide.
- Most suicidal patients can be helped by treatment of a co-existing psychiatric disorder.
- Certain medical conditions, psychiatric diagnoses, and traumatic events are associated with increased risk for suicide.
- Suicidal ideation must be taken seriously, even if the person has a history of multiple attempts.
- The nurse can have a real impact on suicide prevention through primary, secondary, and tertiary interventions.
- Nursing care of the suicidal patient is challenging but rewarding: patients' desperate feelings evoke intense reactions in staff, but most people with suicidal ideation respond to treatment and do not die by suicide.
- If a patient dies by suicide, family, friends, and health care workers are traumatized and need support, possibly including referrals for mental health intervention.

CRITICAL THINKING

1. Locate and review the suicide protocol at your hospital unit or community centre. Are there any steps you anticipate having difficulty carrying out? Discuss these difficulties with your peers or clinical group.
2. Knowing that nurses can suffer post-suicide stress and that they need support when those in their care are involved in suicidal behaviour, do you believe that help is available for nurses? What sort of support do you feel would be most helpful to you in this situation? How would you respond to another staff member who expresses guilt over the death by suicide of a patient on your unit?
3. Identify three common and expected emotional reactions that a nurse might have when initially working with people who are suicidal.
    a. How do you think you might react?
    b. What actions could you take to deal with the event and obtain support?
4. In addition to psychiatric mental health nursing practice areas, are there other practice areas in which nursing assessments for self-harm would strengthen patient care? How does knowing the reason for a patient self-harming make a difference in planning care?

CHAPTER REVIEW

1. Which assessment statements would be appropriate for a patient who may be suicidal? **Select all that apply**.
    a. Do you ever think about suicide?
    b. Are you thinking of hurting yourself?
    c. Do you sometimes wish you were dead?
    d. Has it ever seemed like life is not worth living?

e. Does it seem as though others might be better off if you were dead?
   f. If you were to take your own life, how would you do it?
   g. Are the means to take your own life available?
   h. What stops you from carrying out your plan?
2. Jon, 15 years old, asks the community health nurse what the greatest health risk for his age group is. How should the nurse respond?
   a. Suicide
   b. Substance use
   c. Eating disorders
   d. Unintentional injuries
3. Ms. Rallyea, 58 years old, is admitted with severe clinical depression and started on antidepressant medications. Her mood has remained low and she has not initiated conversation. On her 15th day of hospitalization, she informs the nurse that she is feeling great and energetic. What should the nurse do?
   a. Notify the social worker of the improvement to schedule a discharge planning conference.
   b. Invite Ms. Rallyea to talk and ask her if she is thinking of hurting herself.
   c. Report to the team that the antidepressant medication is effective.
   d. Chart the mood change and share the observation at the team meeting the next day.
4. A nurse has great difficulty distancing herself from the care of a patient when she leaves work. What should the nurse do?
   a. Recognize that she is too compassionate.
   b. Request that the patient be assigned to another nurse.
   c. Share her concern with the patient.
   d. Confide in a colleague she trusts.

REFERENCES

Alberta Health Services. (2018). *Hope and healing: A guide for people who have lost someone to suicide.* Calgary: Alberta Health Services. Hope and Healing: A Guide for People Who Have Lost Someone to Suicide. Retrieved from https://www.albertahealthservices.ca/assets/healthinfo/ip/hi-ip-pipt-chc-hope-and-healing-brochure.pdf

Angelekis, I., Austin, J., & Gooding, P. (2020). Association of childhood maltreatment with suicide behaviors among young people: A systematic review and meta-analysis. *JAMA Network Open, 3*(8), e2012563. https://doi.org/10.1001/jamanetworkopen.2020.12563

Angelekis, I., Gillespie, E. L., & Panagioti, M. (2019). Childhood maltreatment and adult suicidality: A comprehensive systematic review with meta-analysis. *Psychological Medicine, 49*(7), 1057–1078. https://doi.org/10.1017/S0033291718003823

Arriagada, P., Hahmann, T., & O'Donnell, V. (2020a). *Indigenous people in urban areas: Vulnerabilities to the socioeconomic impacts of COVID-19. StatCan COVID 19: Data to insights for a better Canada.* Statistics Canada. Catalogue no. 45280001. Retrieved from https://www150.statcan.gc.ca/n1/pub/45-28-0001/2020001/article/00023-eng.htm

Arriagada, P., Hahmann, T., & O'Donnell, V. (2020b). *Indigenous people and mental health during the COVID-19 pandemic. StatCan COVID 19: Data to insights for a better Canada.* Statistics Canada. Catalogue no. 45280001. Retrieved from https://www150.statcan.gc.ca/n1/pub/45-28-0001/2020001/article/00035-eng.htm

Asarnow, J. R., Fogelson, D., Fitzpatrick, O., et al. (2018). Child and adolescent suicide and self-harm: Treatment and prevention. *Psychiatric Times, 35*(12). 9+. Retrieved from https://link.gale.com/apps/doc/A574175731/EAIM?u=atha49011&sid=bookmark-EAIM&xid=c1cb39b7

Babič, M., Bregar, B., & Radobuljac, M. (2020). The attitudes and feelings of mental health nurses towards adolescents and young adults with nonsuicidal self-injuring behaviors. *Child and Adolescent Psychiatry and Mental Health, 14*(37). https://doi.org/10.1186/s13034-020-00343-5

Banerjee, D., Kosagisharaf, J. R., & Sathyanarayana Rao, T. S. (2021). The dual pandemic' of suicide and COVID-19: A biopsychosocial narrative of risks and prevention. *Psychiatry Research, 295*, Article 113577. https://doi.org/10.1016/j.psychres.2020.113577

Beghi, M., Butera, E., Giuseppe, C., et al. (2021). Suicidal behaviour in older age: A systematic review of risk factors associated to suicide attempts and completed suicides. *Neuroscience & Biobehavioral Reviews, 127*, 193–211.

Berardelli, I., Serafini, G., Cortese, N., et al. (2020). The involvement of hypothalamus–pituitary–adrenal (HPA) axis in suicide risk. *Brain Sciences, 10*(9), 653. https://doi.org/10.3390/brainsci10090653

Bill C-7. (2021, February 24). *An Act to amend the Criminal Code (medical assistance in dying).* Feb 24: House of Commons of Canada. First reading, first session, forty-third Parliament. Retrieved from https://parl.ca/DocumentViewer/en/43-1/bill/C-7/first-reading

Boland, R., Verduin, M. L., & Ruiz, P. (2022). *Kaplan and Sadock's concise textbook of clinical psychiatry* (5th ed.). Philadelphia: Lippincott Williams & Wilkins.

Boyd, J. E., Adler, E. P., Otilingam, P. G., et al. (2014). Internalized Stigma of Mental Illness (ISMI) Scale: A multinational review. *Comprehensive Psychiatry, 55*, 221–231.

Bracken-Minor, K., & McDevitt-Murphy, M. (2014). Differences in features of non-suicidal self-injury according to borderline personality disorder screening status. *Archives of Suicide Research, 18*, 88–103.

Brann, K. L., Baker, D., Smith-Millman, M. K., et al. (2021). A meta-analysis of suicide prevention programs for school-aged youth. *Children and Youth Services Review, 121*, 105826. https://doi.org/10.1016/j.childyouth.2020.105826

Brendel, R. W., Breezing, A., Lagomasino, I. T., et al. (2016). The suicidal patient. In T. A. Stern, J. R. Rosenbaum, & M. Fava et al. (Eds.), *Massachusetts General Hospital comprehensive clinical psychiatry* (2nd ed., pp. 589–598). St. Louis: Mosby.

Canadian Association for Suicide Prevention. (2009). *The CASP national suicide prevention strategy* (2nd ed.). Winnipeg: Author. Retrieved from https://suicideprevention.ca/wp-content/uploads/2021/08/CASP-Blueprint-for-Cdn-National-Suicide-Prevention-Strategy_Final_2009pdf-1.pdf

Canadian Association for Suicide Prevention (CASP). (2021a). *Advocacy: CASP strongly believes Canada needs a national suicide prevention strategy.* Retrieved from https://suicideprevention.ca/media/articles/life-promotion/casp-strongly-believes-canada-needs-a-national-suicide-prevention-strategy/

Canadian Association for Suicide Prevention (CASP). (2021b). *Survivors of suicide loss.* Retrieved from https://thelifelinecanada.ca/suicide-prevention-resources/survivors-of-suicide-loss/

Canadian Coalition for Seniors Mental Health (CCSMH). (2021). *Canadian guidelines for the assessment, prevention and treatment of depression among older adults (2021 Guideline Update).* Toronto: CCSMH.

Canadian Institute for Health Information. (2021). *Unintended consequences of COVID-19: Impact on self-harm behaviour.* Ottawa: Author.

Canadian Mental Health Association. (2021). *Statement on Medical Assistance in Dying (MAID)*. Retrieved from https://cmha.ca/news/statement-on-medical-assistance-in-dying-maid

Canadian Patient Safety Institute & Mental Health Commission of Canada. (2021). *Suicide risk assessment toolkit: A resource for healthcare workers and organizations*. Retrieved from https://www.patientsafetyinstitute.ca/en/toolsResources/SuicideRisk/Documents/MHCC-CPSI%20-%20Suicide%20Risk%20Assessment%20Toolkit%20EN.pdf

Carballo, J. J., Akamnonu, C. P., & Oquendo, M. A. (2008). Neurobiology of suicidal behavior: An integration of biological and clinical findings. *Archives of Suicide Research, 12*, 93–110. https://doi.org/10.1080/1381110701857004

Centre for Addiction and Mental Health. (2022). *Words matter*. Retrieved from https://www.camh.ca/en/today-campaign/help-and-resources/words-matter

Centre for Addiction and Mental Health. (2020). *Suicide prevention: A review and policy recommendations*. Retrieved from https://www.camh.ca/-/media/files/pdfs-public-policy-submissions/suicide-prevention-review-and-policy-recommendations-pdf

Centre for Suicide Prevention. (2019). *Older adults and suicide*. Retrieved from https://www.suicideinfo.ca/wp-content/uploads/2019/05/Older-Adults-Fact-Sheet_Web.pdf

Centre for Suicide Prevention. (2021). *Indigenous people, trauma and suicide prevention*. Retrieved from https://www.suicideinfo.ca/resource/trauma-and-suicide-in-indigenous-people/

Cost, K. T., Crosbie, J., Anagnostou, E., et al. (2021). Mostly worse, occasionally better: Impact of COVID-19 pandemic on the mental health of Canadian children and adolescents. *European Child Adolescent Psychiatry*. https://doi.org/10.1007/s00787-021-01744-3

Crisis Prevention Institute. (2020). *Trauma-informed care resources guide*. Milwaukee: Author. Retrieved from https://www.texomacc.org/wp-content/uploads/2020/10/pdf_ticrg_-1.pdf

Dabkowski, E., & Porter, J. E. (2021). An exploration into suicide prevention initiatives for mental health nurses: A systematic literature review. *International Journal of Mental Health Nursing, 30*, 610–623. https://doi.org/10.1111/inm.12872

Dembo, J., Schuklenk, U., & Reggler, J. (2018). "For their own good": A response to popular arguments against permitting medical assistance in dying (MAID) where mental illness is the sole underlying condition. *The Canadian Journal of Psychiatry, 63*(7), 451–456. https://doi.org/10.1177/0706743718766055

Department of Justice Canada (2021). *New medical assistance in dying legislation becomes law*. Retrieved from https://www.canada.ca/en/department-justice/news/2021/03/new-medical-assistance-in-dying-legislation-becomes-law.html

Doyle, L., Sheridan, A., & Treacy, M. P. (2017). Motivations for adolescent self-harm and the implications for mental health nurses. *Journal of Psychiatric and Mental Health Nursing, 24*(2–3), 134–142. https://doi.org/10.1111/jpm.12360

Dubey, S., Biswas, P., Ghosh, R., et al. (2020). Psychosocial impact of COVID-19. *Diabetes & Metabolic Syndrome, 14*(5), 779–788. https://doi.org/10.1016/j.dsx.2020.05.035

Dwivedi, Y., & Pandey, G. (2011). Elucidating biological risk factors in suicide: Role of protein kinase A. *Progress in Neuro-Psychopharmacology & Biological Psychiatry, 35*, 831–841. https://doi.org/10.1016/j.pnpbp.2010.08.025

Fegert, J. M., Vitiello, B., Plener, P. L., et al. (2020). Challenges and burden of the coronavirus 2019 (COVID-19) pandemic for child and adolescent mental health: A narrative review to highlight clinical and research needs in the acute phase and the long return to normality. *Child and Adolescent Psychiatry and Mental Health, 14*, 20. https://doi.org/10.1186/s13034-020-00329-3

First Nations Health Authority. (2021). *First Nations toxic drug deaths doubled during the pandemic in 2020*. Retrieved from https://www.fnha.ca/about/news-and-events/news/first-nations-toxic-drug-deaths-doubled-during-the-pandemic-in-2020

First Nations Health Authority. (2022). *Mental health and substance use*. Retrieved from https://www.fnha.ca/what-we-do/mental-wellness-and-substance-use

Flett, G. L., & Heisel, M. J. (2020). Aging and feeling valued versus expendable during the covid-19 pandemic and beyond: A review and commentary of why mattering is fundamental to the health and well-being of older adults. *International Journal of Mental Health and Addiction, 19*, 2443–2469. https://doi.org/10.1007/s11469-020-00339-4

Gonzales, A., & Bergstrom, L. (2013). Adolescent non-suicidal self-injury (NSSI) interventions. *Journal of Child and Adolescent Psychiatric Nursing, 26*, 124–130. https://doi.org/10.1111/jcap.12035

Government of Canada. (2016). *Working together to prevent suicide in Canada: The 2016 progress report on the federal framework for suicide prevention*. Retrieved from http://www.healthycanadians.gc.ca/publications/healthy-living-vie-saine/framework-suicide-progress-report-2016-rapport-d-etape-cadre-suicide/alt/64-03-15-1430-suicideprev-progressreport-eng.pdf

Government of Canada. (2020). *Working together to prevent suicide in Canada: The 2020 progress report on the federal framework for suicide prevention*. Retrieved from https://www.canada.ca/content/dam/hc-sc/documents/services/publications/healthy-living/64-03-18-2232-ProgressReport-SuicidePrevention_EN-06-eng.pdf

Government of Canada. (2021). *Action for seniors report*. Ottawa: Author.

Government of Canada. (2022). *Indigenous Services Canada*. Retrieved from https://www.canada.ca/en/indigenous-services-canada.html

Graham, S., Stelkia, K., Wieman, C., et al. (2021). Mental health interventions for First Nations, Inuit, and Métis peoples in Canada: A systematic review. *The International Indigenous Policy Journal, 12*(2). https://doi.org/10.18584/iipj.2021.12.2.10820

Guintivano, J., Brown, T., Newcomer, A., et al. (2014). Identification and replication of a combined epigenetic and genetic biomarker predicting suicide and suicidal behaviors. *American Journal of Psychiatry, 171*(12), 1287–1296.

Hall, A. L., Sweet, J., Tweel, M., et al. (2020). Comparing negative health indicators in male and female veterans with the Canadian general population. *BMJ Military Health, 168*, 82–87. https://doi.org/10.1136/bmjmilitary-2020-001526

Harmer, B., Lee, S., Duong, T., & Saadabadi, A. (2021). Suicidal ideation. In *StatPearls*. StatPearls: Publishing. Retrieved from https://pubmed.ncbi.nlm.nih.gov/33351435/

Health Canada. (2015). *First Nations mental wellness continuum framework* (Cat.: H34-278/1-2014E-PDF). Retrieved from https://thunderbirdpf.org/wp-content/uploads/2015/01/24-14-1273-FN-Mental-Wellness-Framework-EN05_low.pdf

Heisel, M. J., Moore, S. L., Flett, G. L., et al. (2020). Meaning-Centered Men's Groups: Initial findings of an intervention to enhance resiliency and reduce suicide risk in men facing retirement. *Clinical Gerontologist, 43*(1), 76–94. https://doi.org/10.1080/07317115.2019.1666443

Henriksen, K., Schinke, R., Moesch, K., et al. (2020). Consensus statement on improving the mental health of high performance athletes. *International Journal of Sport and Exercise Psychology, 18*(5), 553–560. https://doi.org/10.1080/1612197X.2019.1570473

Heuser, C., & Howe, J. (2019). The relation between social isolation and increasing suicide rates in the elderly. *Quality in Ageing and Older Adults, 20*(1), 2–9. https://doi.org/10.1108/QAOA-06-2018-0026

Hewitt, P. L., Caelian, C. F., Chen, C., et al. (2014). Perfectionism, stress, daily hassles, hopelessness, and suicide potential in depressed psychiatric adolescents. *Journal of Psychopathology and Behavioral Assessment, 36*(4), 663–674. https://doi.org/10.1007/s10862-014-9427-0

Hogan, M., & Grumet, J. G. (2016). Suicide prevention: An emerging priority for health care. *Health Affairs, 35*(6), 1084–1090.

Indigenous Services Canada. (n.d.). Government of Canada. https://www.canada.ca/en/indigenous-services-canada.html

Inuit Tapiriit Kanatami. (2016). *National Inuit suicide prevention strategy*. Retrieved from https://www.itk.ca/national-inuit-suicide-prevention-strategy/

Jordan, J. R. (2017). Postvention is prevention—The case for suicide prevention. *Death Studies, 41*(10), 614–621. https://doi.org/10.1080/07481187.2017.1335544

Kiamanesh, P., Dieserud, G., & Haavind, H. (2015). From a cracking façade to a total escape: Maladaptive perfectionism and suicide. *Death Studies, 39*(5), 316–322. https://doi.org/10.1080/07481187.2014.946625

Klonsky, E. D., Muehlenkamp, J. J., Lewis, S. P., et al. (2011). *Nonsuicidal self-injury*. Toronto: Hogrefe Publishing.

Komrad, M. (2021). First, do no harm: New Canadian law allows for assisted suicide for patients with psychiatric disorders. *Psychiatric Times, 38*(6). Retrieved from https://www.psychiatrictimes.com/view/canada-law-provide-not-prevent-suicide, https://www.psychiatrictimes.com/view/first-do-no-harm

Kumar, M. B., & Tjepkema, M. (2019). *Suicide among First Nations people, Métis and Inuit (2011–2016): Findings from the 2011 Canadian Census Health and Environment Cohort (CanCHEC)*. Statistics Canada. Retrieved from https://www150.statcan.gc.ca/n1/pub/99-011-x/99-011-x2019001-eng.htm

Lengel, G. J., Ammerman, B. A., & Washburn, J. J. (2021). Clarifying the definition of nonsuicidal self-injury: Clinician and researcher perspectives. Crisis. *The Journal of Crisis Intervention and Suicide Prevention*. Advance online publication. https://doi.org/10.1027/0227-5910/a000764

Liu, L., Capaldi, C. A., Orpana, H. M., et al. (2021). Changes over time in means of suicide in Canada: An analysis of mortality data from 1981 to 2018. *Canadian Medical Association Journal, 193*(10), E331–E338. https://doi.org/10.1503/cmaj.202378

Marr, N., & Field, T. (2000). *BullycideDeath at playtime*. Didcot: Success Unlimited.

Mental Health Commission of Canada. (2020a). *COVID-19 and suicide: Potential implications and opportunities to influence trends in Canada*. Ottawa: Author.

Mental Health Commission of Canada (MHCC). (2020b). *Older adults and suicide fact sheet*. Ottawa: MHCC.

Mental Health Commission of Canada (MHCC). (2020c). *Language matters*. Retrieved from https://www.mentalhealthcommission.ca/wp-content/uploads/drupal/2020-08/language_matters_cheat_sheet_eng.pdf

Mental Health Commission of Canada. (n.d.). *Suicide: Facing the difficult topic together—Empowering nurses, instilling hope in clients*. https://www.mdbriefcase.com/course/suicide-facing-the-difficult-topic-together-empowering-nurses-instilling-hope-in-clients/

Moorhead, S., Johnson, M., Maas, M. L., et al. (2013). *Nursing Outcomes Classification (NOC)* (5th ed.). St Louis: Mosby.

Muehlenkamp, J., Brausch, A., Quigley, K., et al. (2013). Interpersonal features and functions of nonsuicidal self-injury. *Suicide and Life-Threat Behavior, 43*(1), 67–80. https://doi.org/10.1111/j.1943-278X.2012.00128.x

MyHealth.Alberta.ca. (2020). *Health Canada and FDA Advisories for antidepressants*. Retrieved from https://myhealth.alberta.ca/health/pages/conditions.aspx?hwid=zu1129&lang=en-ca

Myklestad, I., & Straiton, M. (2021). The relationship between self-harm and bullying behaviour: Results from a population based study of adolescents. *BMC Public Health, 21*, 524. https://doi.org/10.1186/s12889-021-10555-9

National Defence and the Canadian Armed Forces. (2021). *2020 Report on suicide mortality in the Canadian Armed Forces (1995 to 2019)*. Retrieved from https://www.canada.ca/en/department-national-defence/corporate/reports-publications/health/2020-report-on-suicide-mortality-in-the-caf-1995-to-2019.html

National Inquiry into Missing and Murdered Indigenous Women and Girls. (2019). *Reclaiming power and place: The final report of the National Inquiry into Missing and Murdered Indigenous Women and Girls*. Retrieved from https://www.mmiwg-ffada.ca/final-report/

Office of the Correctional Investigator Canada. (2014). *A three-year review of federal inmate suicides (2011–2014)*. Retrieved from http://www.oci-bec.gc.ca/cnt/rpt/pdf/oth-aut/oth-aut20140910-eng.pdf

Olson, R. (2021). *The accuracy and reliability of suicide statistics: Why it matters*. Centre for Suicide Prevention, Canadian Mental Health Association. Retrieved from https://www.suicideinfo.ca/resource/accuracy-suicide-statistics/

Overvad, A. T., & Wagoner, B. (2020). Grief after suicide: A study of taboo and metaphor. *Culture & Psychology, 26*(3), 369–383. https://doi.org/10.1177/1354067X19861047

Pan American Health Organization. (2020). *COVID-19 exacerbates suicide risk factors*. Retrieved from https://www.paho.org/en/news/10-9-2020-covid-19-pandemic-exacerbates-suicide-risk-factors

Patterson, W. M., Dohn, H. H., Bird, J., et al. (1983). Evaluation of suicidal patients: The SAD PERSONS scale. *Psychosomatics, 24*(4), 343–345. 348–349.

Perlman, C. M., Neufeld, E., Martin, L., et al. (2011). *Suicide risk assessment guide: A resource for Canadian health care organizations*. Toronto: Ontario Hospital Association and Canadian Patient Safety Institute. Retrieved from http://www.oha.com/KnowledgeCentre/Documents/Final%20-%20Suicide%20Risk%20Assessment%20Guidebook.pdf

Pinto, S., Soares, J., Silva, A., et al. (2020). COVID-19 suicide survivors—A hidden grieving population. *Frontiers in Psychiatry, 11*, 626807. https://doi.org/10.3389/fpsyt.2020.626807

Public Health Agency of Canada. (2019). *Suicide in Canada: Key statistics*. Retrieved from https://www.canada.ca/en/public-health/services/publications/healthy-living/suicide-canada-key-statistics-infographic.html

Riley, E. T. (2016). Chronic traumatic encephalopathy and professional athletes: Suicides are contagious. *World Neurosurgery, 94*, 576–577. https://doi.org/10.1016/j.wneu.2016.04.055

Rocket, I. (2010). Counting suicides and making suicide count as a public health problem. *Journal of Crisis Intervention and Suicide Prevention, 31*, 227–230. https://doi.org/10.1027/0227-5910/a000071

Schmutte, T., Costa, M. P., & Davidson, L (2021). Comparisons between suicide in persons with serious mental illness, other mental disorders, or no known mental illness: Results from 37 U.S. states, 2003–2017. *Schizophrenia Research, 228,* 74–82. https://doi.org/10.1016/j.schres.2020.11.058

SPEAK (Suicide Prevention Education Awareness Knowledge). (2021). *After suicide: A practical and personal guide for survivors.* Manitoba: SPEAK.

Stänicke, L. (2021). The punished self, the unknown self, and the harmed self—Toward a more nuanced understanding of self-harm among adolescent girls. *Frontiers in Psychology, 12,* 967. https://doi.org/10.3389/fpsyg.2021.543303

Statistics Canada. (2019). *Suicide prevention in Indigenous communities.* Retrieved from https://www.sac-isc.gc.ca/eng/1576089685593/1576089741803

Statistics Canada. (2020a). *Leading causes of death, total population, by age group.* Table 13-10-0394-01. https://doi.org/10.25318/1310039401-eng

Statistics Canada. (2020b). *Health indicators, by Aboriginal identity, age-standardized rates, four-year period estimates.* https://doi.org/10.25318/1310045801-eng

Statistics Canada (2021). *A statistical portrait of Canada's diverse LGBTQ2+ communities.* Retrieved from https://www150.statcan.gc.ca/n1/daily-quotidien/210615/dq210615a-eng.htm

Stene-Larsen, K., & Reneflot, A. (2019). Contact with primary and mental health care prior to suicide: A systematic review of the literature from 2000 to 2017. *Scandinavian Journal of Public Health, 47*(1), 9–17. https://doi.org/10.1177/1403494817746274

Strawbridge, R., Ward, J., Ferguson, A., et al. (2019). Identification of novel genome-wide associations for suicidality in UK Biobank, genetic correlation with psychiatric disorders and polygenic association with completed suicide. *EBioMedicine, 41,* 517–525. https://doi.org/10.1016/j.ebiom.2019.02.005

Tang, W., Lin, M., You, J., et al. (2021). Prevalence and psychosocial risk factors of nonsuicidal self-injury among adolescents during the COVID-19 outbreak. *Current Psychology.* https://doi.org/10.1007/s12144-021-01931-0

Tofthagen, R., Talseth, A., & Fagerström, L. (2014). Mental health nurses' experiences of caring for patients suffering from self-harm. *Nursing Research and Practice, 2014,* 1–10. https://doi.org/10.1155/2014/905741

Truth and Reconciliation Commission of Canada. (2015). *Truth and Reconciliation Commission of Canada: Calls to action.* Retrieved from https://ehprnh2mwo3.exactdn.com/wp-content/uploads/2021/01/Calls_to_Action_English2.pdf

Turecki, G., & Brent, D. A. (2016). Suicide and suicidal behaviour. *The Lancet, 387*(10024), 1227–1239. https://doi.org/10.1016/S0140-6736(15)00234-2

van der Burgt, M. C. A., Beekman, A. T. F., Hoogendoorn, A. W., et al. (2020). The impact of a suicide prevention awareness campaign on stigma, taboo and attitudes towards professional help-seeking. *Journal of Affective Disorders, 279*(15), 730–736. https://doi.org/10.1016/j.jad.2020.11.024

Veterans Affairs. (2016). *2013 Life After Service Studies (LASS).* Retrieved from https://publications.gc.ca/site/eng/9.839366/publication.html

World Health Organization (WHO). (2021a). *Live life: An implementation guide for suicide prevention in countries.* Geneva: Author.

World Health Organization. (2021b). *Suicide worldwide in 2019. Global health estimates.* Retrieved from https://www.who.int/publications/i/item/9789240026643

Zetterqvist., M., Perini, I., Mayo, L., et al. (2020). Nonsuicidal self-injury disorder in adolescents: Clinical utility of the diagnosis using the Clinical Assessment of Nonsuicidal Self-Injury Disorder Index. *Frontiers in Psychiatry, 11,* 8. https://doi.org/10.3389/fpsyt.2020.00008

Zhong, S., Senior, M., Yu, R., et al. (2021). Risk factors for suicide in prisons: A systematic review and meta-analysis. *The Lancet Public Health, 6*(3), e164–e174. https://doi.org/10.1016/S2468-2667(20)30233-4

23

Anger, Aggression, and Violence

Melodie B. Hull

https://evolve.elsevier.com/Canada/Varcarolis/psychiatric/

OBJECTIVES

1. Compare and contrast three theories that explore the determinants for anger, aggression, and violence.
2. Differentiate between aggression and violence.
3. Explain the state of rage.
4. Identify precipitators to anger, aggression, or violence.
5. Differentiate between violence in the workplace and workplace violence.
6. Identify strategies for de-escalation.
7. Describe two criteria for the use of seclusion or restraint.

KEY TERMS AND CONCEPTS

aggression
anger
bullying
de-escalation
de-escalation techniques
emotional intelligence
locus of control
rage
violence
violence in the workplace
workplace violence

Anger is an emotion. Rage is a violent state of overwhelming anger. Aggression is behaviour and violence is extreme aggression. All people experience the emotion of anger and can be moved, under certain circumstances, to behave aggressively and engage in acts of violence. These acts can protect and save. Understanding the emotion of anger, its etiology, and its psychological and behavioural manifestations is key to accurate assessment, intervention, and treatment.

Anger is a normal, natural emotion that occurs on a continuum, from mild to severe: appropriate to inappropriate depending on the situation. It can be suppressed over periods of time or controlled in its release (emotional regulation). It does not always lead to violence. It can be triggered by someone else's anger, illness, pain, or fear. Personal appraisals of self-worth and self-efficacy also factor into the anger response. Anger is sometimes a coping response to embarrassment, jealousy, or fear of rejection or replacement. Anger is not always expressed loudly or by facial expression. Sometimes in the heat of anger a person will suddenly become silent, actively listening and watching, processing it all. A sudden eruption of anger, even aggression, may follow.

Anger can be functional when it prompts individuals to remove obstacles and barriers to achieving their goals but is also seen as an enhancer of creativity in, for example, problem solving, conflict resolution, and restructuring environments. In other words, anger can be a healthy way to draw attention to a matter of concern, elicit problem-solving, and collaboration. However, its expression comes with responsibility (Box 23.1). Proactive anger is present in social movements: petition-gathering, marches, media campaigns, and more. Anger that is used to oppress, embarrass, avoid, or achieve power over another is maladaptive and inappropriate but often used by people to cope. Anger can also be linked to resentment.

Suppressed anger is a learned, protective response to fear, abuse, or oppression. Historical trauma often leads to suppressed anger. This arises from decades of political and societal oppression. It is not uncommon for those who have experienced this, such as those who have come out of severely repressive regimes or that experienced by Indigenous peoples of this land, Canada.

Rage is an uncontrollable, violent state of anger and is quite uncommon. Once the person has begun expressing rage, they cannot think clearly or logically, and psychosocial or cognitive behavioural interventions are not possible. Rage must dissipate on its own. An example is road rage, a dangerous aggressive response to extreme anger. Rage begins with a trigger that is usually spontaneous. Contributing factors may include age, gender, self-centredness, attention deficits, antisocial personality, and more at the time the incident occurs. Implications for Nursing: protective strategies are necessary both for the raging person and for those around them.

Aggression is an intentional behaviour. The intent is to harm another person who does not want to be harmed. It does not include physical violence. Aggression is not the same as aggressive thought (anger leading to imagining acts of violence or revenge, for example). Under certain stressful or fearful conditions, negative emotions can initiate aggressive thought, but action does not always follow. Aggression is often used interchangeably with the term violence. This is not accurate. The use of the term aggression is common in everyday speech but not necessarily used in the true clinical, psychosocial sense of the word (Allen et al., 2017). Here are two examples. A person can aggressively seek employment. No harm is intended to anyone. Aggressive treatment of a disease does not indicate intent to actually harm a patient. Aggression is not an emotion but it is a descriptor often used for one. Rarely does someone say, "I feel aggressive" but instead say "I am aggressive." Instrumental aggression is that which is planned to achieve a goal of harm. Wanting what another person has and threatening and intimidating to get it is an example. Instrumental aggression is sometimes necessary for self-protection or that of others, such as shouting to get someone to stop a dangerous action. Emotional aggression is that which lacks any degree of planning and is generally more impulsive.

465

> **BOX 23.1 Expressing Anger**
>
> To avoid bottling up anger and losing control of it at some point, it is healthy to express it. However, this comes with a very important responsibility not to harm or burden others with one's own anger. Self-awareness and responsibility are necessary. Freedom from the feeling of anger is not about venting it *on* others or burdening or harming another but about voicing feelings and opening up for discussion with them. Teaching anger control assistance strategies or using cognitive behavioural therapeutic techniques for anger management can help.

Reactive aggression may be the result of a sudden insult or danger to self. If this type of aggression is hostile in nature, it is violence. Like all types of aggression, its origin is based in our emotional brain. The responses formed when experiencing reactive aggression are typically spontaneous and seek to regain equilibrium or retaliation.

Relational aggression occurs when one party intends to harm the other in the relationship by socially isolating them, belittling, demeaning, manipulating, controlling, and socially isolating them (Coyne et al., 2017) (see Chapter 24). The outcome can be verbal abuse. Under section 264.1(1) of the *Criminal Code of Canada* (2020a), uttering threats is considered a crime.

Workplace harassment is aggressive and often takes the form of discrimination. The intent is to ridicule and insult, to offend and intimidate. It is targeted. Verbal and non-verbal messages are used to convey this. Workers might find themselves being harassed by gender, ethnicity, minority status, age, ability, dress, and so forth (Hango & Moyser, 2018). Workplace harassment (discriminatory behaviour) can lead to bullying (power over behaviour) and physical violence, but it does not always do so.

Bullying is intentional and repetitive: it is aggression and it is ongoing. It is predatory. Power and power imbalance are key factors. The bully exerts power over someone else, the victim. Bullying is predatory and often dispute related in nature. Bullies are not seeking resolution. Attempts to facilitate this can be challenging. The action can put the victim at even higher risk for retaliation. It is very important to distinguish bullying from interpersonal conflict. Sometimes accusations are made of bullying when in actuality that is not the case. Using accurate terminology is important when interventions are warranted. Bullying and interpersonal conflict are not the same, nor is their management. The latter is situational and does not intend harm, and the parties are usually of equal power and wish to find resolution or a third party can step in to find it.

Cyberbullying is a behavioural subset of bullying. Like generic bullying, it is predatory aggression. It occurs through social media sites, computers, and cell phones. The intent is to cause psychological and social harm. Cyberbullying becomes physical violence when the bully intends a violent outcome, such as spurring the victim to self-harm or suicide. Cyberbullying can take the form of *revenge porn*. This is when intimate photos of a target are shared online without permission and accompanied by hostile and explicit commentary by a perpetrator. This is an aggressive act. The photos may be real or digitally altered; the intent is to demean, take revenge, punish, and cause severe psychological harm. Revenge porn becomes physical violence when the intent is to encourage or direct the target to physically self-harm.

Violence is a behaviour intended primarily, but not solely, to do physical harm to someone or something. Violence is aggression in its extreme form. An act can be planned or spontaneous. Violence can be used to dominate; to exert power and control over others; and to exact revenge. It can be used for correction or discipline by a parent, as in spanking a child. Note that this is not illegal in Canada (Barnett, 2016). An act of excessive spanking is. The *Criminal Code of Canada* (2020b) includes violence under its definition of *assault*: physical or verbal. Here, violence includes psychological and emotional abuse, damage to property, suicide, and self-harm. States of high arousal, hyperexcitability, psychosis, and confusion are all possible antecedents to acts of violence, although some violence is clearly planned. Violence is almost always an objectionable act. Exceptions include the work of armed forces and police officers. In a best-case scenario violence can be used to defend. Used instrumentally, it can protect self and others. Physical restraints used in healthcare or policing are examples. At its worst, violence can be used in self-service to cause the maiming or death of another.

Violence can be enacted by people identified with or without illness (Penney et al., 2016). Non–illness-based motivators might include the use of violence to counter violence, achieve need gratification, mete out punishment, find emotional or sexual gratification, or retaliate or take revenge. Lack of access to any of the social determinants of health (SDOH) can play a factor, as can age, gender, culture, religion, and response to being in an irate, hostile group or crowd. Exposure to violence and victimization, particularly in youth, can contribute to violent behaviour in adulthood (Caruso, 2017; Pabian & Vandebosch, 2016).

Workplace violence may take many forms. In healthcare workplace violence refers to overt acts of aggression and violence by patients directed at hurting staff or others. It also includes staff-to-staff actions including belittling, lashing out, or social exclusion. Although not limited to these situations, Geoffrion et al. (2017) identify that Canadian bus drivers, police, and healthcare workers' responses go beyond the physical ramifications and can lead to physical and mental health issues. Lateral workplace violence refers to psychologically violent acts that occur worker to worker. It is not uncommon in health care and in fact has been well studied in this field. Cultural relativism may be a contributing factor to why nursing seems so affected (Faletta, 2017). Traditions and beliefs held by nurses about new nurses and vice versa, age cohorts, and hierarchies in nursing and the environment are also thought to contribute to this phenomenon (Edmonson & Zelonka, 2019) (Box 23.2).

Workplace violence may also be perpetrated by a patient's family member(s) or their visitors. This type of violence can also occur patient to patient. In nursing workplace violence occurs more often in long-term/dementia care, in acute inpatient psychiatric units, and in emergency departments in hospitals than other places of care (Casey, 2019; Thomas, 2016). Several contributing factors have been associated with the increased incidence of violence in these settings.

In-group workplace violence also occurs. Dissatisfaction with an organization's practices and policies, workplace constraints, poor communication or collaboration among the team, and incivility can all contribute to workplace stress and violence. While interpersonal conflict

> **BOX 23.2 Lateral Violence**
>
> *Lateral violence* is a form of psychological violence within a group itself. It includes acts of incivility, bullying, harassment, scapegoating, withholding information, gossiping, and refusing to help, to name a few. It can be overt or covert and the intention is to cause harm to someone. It happens in a toxic or oppressive work environment where there are real or perceived power imbalances, devaluation of workers' contributions, and a sense that one's integrity is challenged. When means of coping and adapting fail, moral distress can occur. At this juncture, psychological violence against others is potentiated. With no relief in sight, physical violence in the workplace may ensue. Lateral violence is also known as horizontal violence.

may arise as a normal response to stresses that interfere with getting along, this does not mean that workplace violence such as harassment or bullying will necessarily occur (Baillien et al., 2017).

Some workplace violence is caused by the defense mechanisms of suppression and projection. When individuals feel powerless, voiceless, disrespected, undervalued, or unable to implement change, they turn on others close at hand: others that are more vulnerable. This is not so different from the causes of violence in general.

Approximately 61% of Canadian nurses were victims of assault, abuse, or harassment in 2015 alone (Reichert, 2017; Zwelling, 2017). In a 2019 poll taken by the Canadian Union of Public Employees and the Ontario Council of Hospital Unions 89% of personal support workers experienced violence and 62% experienced it weekly (Casey, 2019). Research by Brophy et al. (2017) found that close to 90% of Canadian long-term care providers in long-term care facilities have been victims of violence. Incidents of violence within health care settings can lead to occupational stress disorder or post-traumatic stress disorder in first responders, health care workers, and military personnel (Standing Committee on Public Safety and National Security, 2016). Implications for Nursing: employers, unions, and policymakers have moved to a zero-tolerance position on all types of workplace violence. While this applies in healthcare settings, it is not always possible to prevent it. The Canadian Nurses Association (CNA) and Canadian Federation of Nurses Unions' (CFNU's) (2015) joint position on zero tolerance for violence in the workplace remains in place.

Box 23.3 identifies milieu characteristics in the hospital or institutional setting that are conducive to violence.

Physical violence ranges from physically pushing or hitting to rape or murder and all things in between. It can include the destruction of property, injury, and death of animals.

Relational violence is also known as intimate partner violence or interpersonal violence. This includes a myriad of physical and psychological harms to the victim, including the potential for murder (see Chapter 24).

Collective violence is social, political, or economic. Violence is enacted by groups of people onto others. Examples are gang violence, dictatorships, and those like human traffickers, who prey on the disadvantaged and poor seeking work. It can include mob violence.

Implications for Nursing: incidents of anger, aggression, and violence are associated with the perpetrator experiencing an emotional reaction. These reactions occur in all areas of the healthcare system (O'Rourke et al., 2018; Schablon et al., 2018; Perelman School of Medicine, 2016). A long-held stigmatizing belief among health care workers and the general public is that it is more dangerous to work in psychiatry that any other specialty area. Thomas (2016) has identified that the incidents of violent acts are similar in the emergency room, long-term care, general medicine, and psychiatry. To deal effectively with this and maintain the wellness of self and others, nurses need skills in managing violence pre-, during-, and post-incident. But first, they need knowledge. Understanding the contributing factors to workplace violence and the policies and practices are essential for protection of self and others.

EPIDEMIOLOGY

The World Health Organization's (2002) definition of violence identifies the likelihood that individuals, groups, or communities will be injured, killed, deprived, or suffer abnormal human or social development. The effects of violence in society today pose a major health concern. Victims and witnesses may experience anxiety, depression, suicide, or post-traumatic stress disorder and increased risk for medical issues such as cardiovascular disease (Rivara et al., 2019). Other outcomes for victims can include substance use and physical and cognitive disabilities.

Comorbidity

Anger, aggression, and violence are natural phenomena. They can stand alone or coexist with multiple psychiatric and non-psychiatric disorders. Anger is a key diagnostic criterion in intermittent explosive disorder, oppositional defiant disorder, disruptive mood dysregulation disorder, borderline personality disorder, and bipolar disorder (refer to Chapter 27). Substance use, anxiety disorders, neurocognitive disorders, and personality disorders can be also factors in the expression of anger, aggression, and violence (Caruso, 2017; Volicer et al., 2017; Dutra et al., 2016) (Refer to Chapters 12, 17–19, 23–25.) Neurodevelopmental disorders, medical conditions, brain injury, medications, and pain are non-psychiatric conditions from which the healthcare practitioner needs to consider the patient's experience of anger, aggression, and violence when making a diagnosis and developing a treatment plan. For those people with mental health disorders, additional assessment related to the content of hallucinations and delusions is needed. The risk of violence is enhanced when psychosis is accompanied by delusions of a persecutory nature (Ullrich et al., 2018). Patients with acute, severe mental illnesses who concurrently use substances are also at a greater risk for being a victim of violence than the general public (see Chapter 18). Disorders that include mood dysregulation hold the potential for impulsive, maladaptive expressions of anger, aggression, and violence (Cassiello-Robbins & Barlow, 2016) (see the Vignette about Solange).

BOX 23.3 Milieu Characteristics that Contribute to Violence in the Hospital or Institutional Setting

- Overcrowding
- Provocative or controlling staff
- Unclear rules and boundaries
- Language or other communication barriers
- Cultural barriers
- Higher patient acuity
- Staff inexperience
- Long periods of waiting/queuing to get attention
- Restricted movement—locked unit
- Poor or limited food choices

VIGNETTE

Solange has been admitted as an involuntary patient to the psychiatric unit of a general hospital. She is a 41-year-old woman with a diagnosis of bipolar disorder and a history of eight hospital admissions to acute care psychiatry over the past 20 years. She is presently in an acute manic state, which includes affect dysregulation and demanding behaviours. She exhibits hyperactivity, racing thoughts, poor judgement, distractibility, pressured speech, and sleep deprivation. She has very low frustration tolerance and reacts spontaneously and impulsively to stressors. Being admitted against her wishes frustrates and angers her. Solange feels trapped. Her aggression is both reactive and a result of her mental state. She is able to voice her feelings of being overwhelmed and out of control, but she is quite incapable of dealing with these feelings. She refuses to take her mood-stabilizing medications or any prn medications. She attempts to intimidate the staff with verbal aggression and threats, including stepping into their personal space. She blames everyone for her situation, an external locus of control stance. Implications for Nursing: require setting clear and consistent limits to decrease the chaos she is experiencing. Offering of a low-stimulus environment (such as a quiet room) can increase a sense of personal control. The use of prn medication is indicated to help her settle. Choices of oral or injectable medication give some personal power back as well. Ultimately, restraint or seclusion might be appropriate should Solange escalate to the point of being a threat to self or others on the unit and unable to exhibit self-control of her behaviours. At that point, a decision about injectable medication, prn may be made for her.

ETIOLOGY

Biological Factors

Biologically, anger, aggression, and violence are associated with the corticolimbic areas of the brain. A biological predisposition to respond to life events with irritability, low frustration tolerance, and anger may be a function of neurological development or neurochemical changes due to brain tumours or brain injury.

Neurological

Any neurological condition affecting areas of the brain that are involved with impulse control and emotion regulation can result in increased violence, severe behavioural disorders, and low levels of frustration tolerance.

Temporal lobe dysfunction, violence, and aggression are correlated. Within the temporal lobes lies the amygdala, responsible for the regulation and perception of emotions. The lobes share some memory function with the limbic system. Memory of previous insult or assault is important in the cognitive appraisal of a threat and can play a determining role in the expression of anger. When there is damage to the frontal lobes of the brain, particularly a lesion in the frontal ventromedial area, the potential for aggression and violence is not uncommon (Brodie et al., 2016). Prefrontal cortex damage is also implicated in aggressive behaviour as this structure is needed for judgement, reasoning, emotional and body reaction, and impulse control.

Mild brain injury such as a concussion is extremely common. Dailey et al. (2018) found the integrity of the white matter in the area of the corpus callosum post-injury significantly to be correlated with greater aggression, particularly in the chronic phase of recovery.

Traumatic brain injury can lead to anger, aggression, and violence in the acute, recovery, and rehabilitation stages. This is dependent on the amount of damage, the severity, and, most importantly, the centres of the brain involved, particularly the prefrontal and temporal cortices. Injuries in these areas also affected attitudes about aggression and violence (Cristofori et al., 2016).

Epilepsy is a neurological disorder. For years, aggression and violence were thought to be symptoms. Understanding the true cause of the behaviour is essential to providing the most appropriate treatment. Aggression and violence are only factors for a minority of these patients. Violent outbursts occurring in the post-ictal phase of recovery are related to the adverse effects of certain antiepileptic medications, not the disease itself (Wahab et al., 2019; Brodie et al., 2016). The concurrent use of the beta-blocker pindolol can significantly decrease these episodes (Wahab et al., 2019; Brodie et al., 2016).

Neurochemical

The neurotransmitters serotonin, dopamine, gamma-aminobutyric acid (GABA), glutamate, and acetylcholine all have an impact on anger and aggression (Fanning & Coccaro, 2016; Klasen et al., 2019). Neurotransmitters stimulated in the alarm stage of the general adaptation syndrome can also trigger outbursts, particularly when the body is flooded with adrenalin and in the fight/flight mode (see Chapter 5). Dopamine too, has been linked to aggressive outbursts. There is some indication that this may be based on whether a reward–avoidance process is present during the dopamine transmission. Chester et al. (2016) found that individuals with low dopamine systems were more likely to seek external rewards through activities such as thrill-seeking, substance use, and acts of risk and violence.

The hormones adrenalin and testosterone play significant roles in the arousal of anger and subsequent excitability that can lead to aggression or violence (see Chapter 5). Fluctuating hormonal changes during pregnancy and menopause are examples. Steroid hormones can influence the ability to cope with or express anger, particularly in pubescent, adolescent, and young adult males who experience surges in testosterone. Research reveals that higher levels of testosterone combined with low levels of cortisol in males are positively associated with impulsivity and aggression (Geniole et al., 2019). Thyroid dysfunction can also contribute to anger, aggression, and violence.

Neurodevelopmental

Mental health disorders, cognitive disabilities, and conduct disorders should be assessed when anger, aggression, and violence are factors in caring for children and adolescents (see Chapter 27). There are implications for individuals diagnosed with fetal alcohol spectrum disorder or neonatal abstinence syndrome (see Chapter 18). This history can be helpful in adult assessment and treatment as well.

Psychological Factors

No one factor can be identified as the source of anger, aggression, or violence. All are at least to some extent, unique to the individual. Emotional intelligence, personality, and personal power are factors. Behavioural, cognitive, cognitive behavioural, and social learning theories offer insights into how anger, aggression, and violence manifest themselves.

Emotional intelligence perception is how we become aware of something. We perceive, then we interpret. The perception of emotions is called emotional intelligence and it plays a crucial role in the psychology of anger. Over time and with experience, a person develops a sense of how others are expressing emotions and learns to interpret these and respond accordingly. They also learn to imitate the emotions of others. Recognition accuracy is important to form appropriate responses. Misinterpretation of the emotions of others such as perceiving anger, insult, or rejection can arouse fear and an angry or aggressive response. Emotional intelligence and emotional regulation are issues present in cyberbullying, particularly among youth. Beck (1976) theorized that a perceived assault on areas of personal domain (e.g., values, moral code, self-esteem) can lead to anger (see Chapter 5). Implications for Nursing: research shows that the development of emotional intelligence and teaching emotional regulation with young people can mitigate issues later in life (Martínez-Monteagudo et al., 2019). At any age, counselling, individual or group psychotherapy, and psychoeducational programs are beneficial.

RESEARCH HIGHLIGHT

How Psychology Might Alleviate Violence in Queues: Perceived Future Wait and Perceived Load Moderate Violence Against Service Providers

Problem
Long queues in emergency departments (EDs); patient's perceptions of how busy the ED is and what the staff's workload is; and how long they perceive they must still wait can potentiate violence toward healthcare service providers.

Purpose of Study
Understanding the effect of long queues and wait times on the potential development of violence by waiting patients could lead to a decrease in incidents. Findings could also provide insight into and opportunities for intervention in the management of ED. Results could be extrapolated elsewhere in care where wait times and queues are an issue.

Methods
Two-hundred and twenty-six visitors to the ED in one large hospital were surveyed for their subjective, psychological perspective. These data were compared to the hospital's objective, operational data that identified the number of visitors, how busy the ED was, number of staff on duty, etc. Crowding in the ED and the waiting room and long wait times were considered.

Key Findings
Increased crowding in the ED area, longer queues, more skepticism about the actual workload of the ED staff, and the visitor's negative perception of what was occurring were factors contributing to incidents of violence and the more times security had to intervene. Visitors were amenable to the wait when they could see how busy the ED was, when staff articulated their workload more clearly, and when patients perceived the wait would not be much longer. Operationally, improvements could be made in how the ED sets up and responds to queues and wait times.

Implications for Nursing Practice
Understanding the wants and needs of a patient for attention from a nurse must not be forgotten, regardless of how busy the unit or facility is. A focus on people first rather than on task matters, even when busy. This should include waiting areas. A moment of person-to-person sharing, caring, and empathy could help alleviate the risk for violence.

Source: Efrat-Treister, D., Cheshin A., Harari D., et al. (2019). How psychology might alleviate violence in queues: Perceived future wait and perceived load moderate violence against service providers. *PLoS ONE, 14*(6), e0218184. https://doi.org/10.1371/journal.pone.0218184

Personality Theory

In general, personality is organized around a person's characteristic traits, way of thinking, feeling, and doing (see Chapter 19). Personality traits combine to create personality type. *Trait aggression* is typical of persons with psychopathy, narcissism, and others lacking empathy (Bushman, 2020).

The theory of **locus of control** (LOC) was first introduced by Rotter (1966) and has proven significant in the field of mental health. Today, it is conceptualized as empowerment: personal power. LOC and self-efficacy are related. We all wish to exert and maintain control over our lives. Loss of same can lead to mental health problems and sometimes, critical incidences. An internal LOC exists when one has a sense of control over the external world. A person who believes that they have a strong, positive internal LOC believes that any rewards and successes that occur are the result of self-efficacy. Happiness and satisfaction are based on a positive internal LOC (Shubina, 2018, Chapter 5). Internal LOC works conjointly with problem-solving abilities and is more likely to produce better coping and successful outcomes (Boysan & Kiral, 2016). A person with an external LOC is more likely to feel powerless and blame others for what occurs. This person sees themself as a victim of life or, at least, of the situation. When our personal power is threatened, we can experience psychological strain, even briefly, and that may precipitate an incident of anger, aggression, and violence. Consider that medication non-adherence, for example, may sometimes be an act of passive aggressiveness (Nafaradi et al., 2017). Or consider the adult patient on a psychiatric unit who is held under the *Mental Health Act* and wants to leave or have various freedoms restored for those patients who are restrained and secluded. Loss of freedom and loss of personal power and control decreases a person's aversion to risk, self-harm, or harming others. Implications for Nursing: interventions often reflect LOC theory as we strive to empower patients to manage their own care. This is also seen in non-violent crisis intervention; trying to allow as much personal control over a situation as deemed appropriate and safe (see Vignettes).

Behavioural Theories

Twentieth-century psychologists like B.F Skinner, I. Pavlov, and J. Watson studied how behaviour is connected to the mind by a stimulus-reward/avoidance response (see Chapter 5). Behaviourist theory explains how rewards for acting with aggression and violence can have perceived rewards of power, need gratification, and improved social status no matter how fleeting these may be. Behaviourism is still one of the relevant theories used when exploring crime. Its tenets are also applicable to bullying, social anxiety disorder, eating disorders, and more (Richie et al., 2017; Waller & Reykos, 2019). Implications for Nursing: behavioural approaches can be found when working with those with brain injury, cognitive deficits, intellectual disability, and some autism spectrum disorders when anger, aggression, and violence are issues. These can include variations of behaviour modification and step programming. Aspects of behaviourism form part of cognitive behavioural treatment modalities (see Chapter 4).

Cognitive and Cognitive Behavioural Theories

Albert Ellis's (1973) seminal works discussed irrational thinking (see Chapter 4). In this theory self is paramount and there is personal confusion about why others do not respond in ways one thinks they should. For example, a person who believes that they should be loved and accepted by absolutely everyone at all times is demonstrating irrational or faulty thinking. The irrationality here is the abiding belief in should and must. As a result, anger, hostile aggression, and violence are not uncommon behaviours, nor are suicide or self-harm. Acting out is a maladaptive attempt to deal with a perceived sense of rejection, devaluing, or disrespect and to deal with their inability to feel satisfied, loved, and accepted. Ellis (1990) believed that long-term suppression of anger may decrease the ability to deal effectively with new anger-provoking stimuli. Implications for Nursing: cognitive therapy examines the extremisms, faulty thinking, and personal belief systems and attempts to restore rational thinking. Cognitive behaviorism focuses on how thinking and behaving are intertwined and how reasoning and action may be faulty or based in false beliefs. Cutting edge theorists Beck, Emery, and Greenberg (2005) expanded Beck's original theory by looking at dysfunctional anger. They found it was rooted in our predispositions, beliefs, memories, learning, and interpretations of self and others in relation to self. For example, self-appraisal of efficacy leads to confidence. This contributes to how we deal with all situations, including perceived threats. For example, a person predisposed to speaking their mind, seeking immediate need gratification, and having learned it is indeed possible to get this through anger and acting out exhibits dysfunctional anger to achieve goals. Sometimes it is successful and oft times it is not. Still, the behaviour is not extinguished, and this maladaptive anger/aggression response can continue for years until a crisis or desire to change occurs. Implications for Nursing: cognitive behaviour therapy includes not just working also restoring rational thinking but also developing and practicing positive changes in behaviour as well.

Social Learning Theories

Social learning theory considers imitation, modelling, influence, associations, and rewards on behaviours. Bandura's (1973) original social learning theory asserted that children learned aggression by imitating others and that people repeated behaviour that was rewarded. In other words, children exposed to violence often grow up to be aggressive and violent because that behaviour was originally imitated and subsequently rewarded. Using this reasoning, children who are disciplined or punished with disproportionate force and those exposed to violence on television, in music lyrics, images, and video games learn that violence is an option for resolving conflict and that those violent acts have no real negative consequences. Even so, benefits for angry, aggressive, and violent actions are often intermittent and short lived and, in that regard, are not satisfying or adaptive overall. Other variations of social learning theory have been applied to understanding gang violence and interpersonal violence, assessing the effects of violence in the media (Delhove & Greitemeyer, 2021). Implications for Nursing: psychoeducational programs that focus on building empathy, cooperation, and respect are beneficial. Access to positive role-modelling in relationships, groups, and teams is therapeutic.

Sociocultural Factors

Social factors influencing responses of anger, aggression, or violence can also be external. The SDOH including parenting, poverty, education, health, and food affect one's sense of safety and security. When basic needs are not met, that is, when the determinants are not met, fear, anger, resentment, a sense of injustice, etc., can all lead to aggressive and violent actions. Other important demographics include a history of violence, male gender, age 14 to 24 years, substance use, inadequate support system, and a history of prison time. A history of limited coping skills increases risk for using violence. Implications for Nursing: comprehensive social history-taking for the present and past are important. Engaging members of the interdisciplinary team for in-patient and/or community care are essential for a well-balanced approach to reaching the SDOH. Co-occurring counselling or group therapies for anger management may be indicated.

Although all people experience the emotion of anger, it is not expressed in the same way across cultures. Biologically and psychologically based anger responses are inextricably entwined with folkways (group habits that are common to a society or culture) that mediate the actual expression of anger. In a multi-cultural context this difference in expression of anger provides a challenge to both nurses and patients. Language difficulties and culturally based acceptance of how anger is and can be expressed can easily confound a person's abilities to experience and deal successfully with an anger-producing situation. In Western cultures the functionality of anger is acknowledged and accepted. The expression of anger is a way to protect rights, personal freedoms, and self-esteem. Anger is seen as a means to find clarity. In other cultures the expression of anger would be seen as inappropriate and disrespectful. Implications for Nursing: achieving a degree of cultural awareness and cultural knowledge is the first step to providing culturally sensitive and appropriate care even within the Western context of healthcare.

> ### CONSIDERING CULTURE
>
> **Historical Trauma and Lateral Violence**
> Historical trauma is a lived experience of the Inuit, First Nations, and Métis peoples in Canada. It stems from systemic, cultural, and spiritual oppression. For Indigenous people, lateral violence (internalized colonialism) refers to how suppression of the effects of colonialism, oppression, inter-generational trauma, and racism has found release in acts against each other: acts of in-group violence. Incidents can transpire between individuals, within a group, or be endemic in communities. It can exist between the various Indigenous peoples as well. This type of lateral violence is not connected to any one immediate triggering situation but rather to multiple factors over a very long period. These include voicelessness and powerlessness of individuals and populations.

Sources: Monchalin, R., Smylie, J., & Nowgesic, E. (2020). "I guess I shouldn't come back here": Racism and discrimination as a barrier to accessing health and social services for urban Métis women in Toronto, Canada. *Journal of Racial and Ethnic Health Disparities, 7*, 251–261. https://doi.org/10.1007/s40615-019-00653-1; Holmes, C., & Hunt, S. (2017). *Indigenous communities and family violence: Changing the conversation*. National Collaborating Centre for Aboriginal Health. Retrieved from https://www.ccnsa-nccah.ca/docs/emerging/RPT-FamilyViolence-Holmes-Hunt-EN.pdf; Native Women's Association of Canada (NWAC). (n.d.). *Aboriginal lateral violence, what is it?* [Fact sheet]. Retrieved from https://www.nwac.ca/wp-content/uploads/2015/05/2011-Aboriginal-Lateral-Violence.pdf

APPLICATION OF THE NURSING PROCESS

Assessment

When the nursing assessment identifies the potential for anger, aggression, or violence, a more comprehensive risk assessment is warranted.

General Assessment

A person's history of violent behaviour is the most important indicator of risk for future incidents.

Initial and ongoing assessment of the patient can reveal problems before they escalate to anger and aggression. These can include increased demandingness, irritability, frowning, redness of the face, pacing, twisting of the hands, or clenching and unclenching of the fists. The rate and volume of speech may be increased or may be slowed, pointed, and quiet. Any change in behaviour from what is typical for that patient must be noticed. The Risk Assessment Guide highlights various predictors and risk assessment criteria for aggression or violence. Assessment of the environmental stimuli that precede a patient's agitation should be included. Once the assessment is complete, a nursing care plan (NCP) is developed.

General assessment should also include history. For some, traumatic histories can impede a patient's ability to self-soothe, resulting in negative coping responses and creating a vulnerability to coercive interventions by staff.

Trauma-informed care refers to care focused on the patient's past experiences of violence or trauma and the role it currently plays in their lives. When a history of trauma is present, it is important for the nursing team to be aware of this and to avoid any situations that may retraumatize the patient. Consider the following examples:
- A woman who was raped may be re-traumatized by being catheterized for a medical procedure years later. She lashes out in blind anger.
- An Indigenous person who was starved and beaten in a residential school as a small child may be re-traumatized by the lights and sounds in the environment when hospitalized, especially at night,

or may be triggered when meals are late or reflective of the types of food from that earlier traumatic time. He withdraws and is noncommunicative, staring and glaring, or abruptly throws his meal tray.
- A Canadian veteran who was wounded and confined as a prisoner by the enemy years ago may be re-traumatized if confined to a hospital bed in traction. They may be verbally aggressive and even lash out physically in response to the situation.

Self-Assessment

Nurses may have their own histories of anger, aggression, and violence, and these experiences can influence their ability to intervene safely and effectively in a similar incident. It is essential to be aware of personal dynamics that may trigger non-therapeutic emotions and reactions with specific patients. Nurses should use self-reflection to identify any personal triggers such as certain words, tone of voice, or non-verbal communication. Finally, the nurse must assess situational factors (e.g., personal fatigue, insufficient staff on duty) that may decrease one's normal ability to manage complex patient problems such as acting out. Self-assessment promotes calm responses to patient anger and potential aggression. These responses are further supported by the creation of an environment that encourages staff to express feelings with each other, use humour, and develop a professional support system.

RISK ASSESSMENT GUIDE
Aggression or Violence

Initial Risk Assessment	Assaultive Stage—Risk Assessment
History of aggressive behaviours Feelings of … • Frustration, fear, anxiety, embarrassment, shame, or rejection • Irritability, hypersensitivity to perceived criticism, or attempts by others to control Voicing … • Lack of control over life or situation • Defiance • Need for support of anger from others Behaviours indicative of … • Hyperactivity, impulsivity, or withdrawal • Confusion or delusions • Intoxication or other impairment • Sullenness or pacing Thinking…. • Rumination • Decreasing concentration	History of limited coping skills increases risk for using violence Voicing … • Verbal abuse (profanity, argumentativeness, threats) • Loud voice; change of pitch; or very soft • Negative or hostile response in the context of limit setting by the nurse Thinking (cognition or decision making) … • Narrowed field of perception; judgement • Diminishing ability to recognize the anger • Diminishing ability or desire to diffuse own anger • Inability to differentiate between assertiveness and aggressive expressions of anger • Plan, wish, or intent to harm and capacity or means to do so • Possession of a weapon or object that may be used as a weapon (fork, knife, rock) Behaviours … • Hyperactivity most important predictor of imminent violence (pacing, restlessness) • Increasing anxiety and tension (clenched jaw or fist, rigid posture, fixed or tense facial expression, mumbling to self, shortness of breath, sweating, and rapid pulse) • Intense or avoidant eye contact • Assault (hitting, punching, striking, throwing, intimidating, or threatening) • Voice, forcing others to strain to hear

Nursing Diagnosis

A nursing diagnosis may identify maladaptive coping with anger, frustration, or any other emotion/situation that might trigger inappropriate behaviour by the at-risk patient. Or it might target low frustration tolerance and risk for aggression. The nursing diagnosis will be unique to the patient and set in the here and now.

Outcomes

Nursing outcomes (goals) will focus on anger management, emotional regulation, self-control, and safety for the patient. Concurrent or subsequent NCPs will need to address the pre– and post–acting out situations. Examples of goals might be that: incidents of angry, aggressive outbursts will be less frequent; the patient will seek out nurse for assistance early on when feelings of anger or agitation begin, to prevent escalation; and the patient will utilize anger control measures. Once identified, all outcomes require an evaluation date.

Planning

Planning interventions requires a sound assessment of history, present coping skills, and the patient's willingness and capacity to learn alternative and non-violent ways of handling angry feelings. In addition, the nurse needs to consider whether:
- The situation calls for:
  - Psychoeducational approaches to teach the patient new skills for handling anger
  - Immediate intervention to prevent overt violence (e.g., de-escalation techniques, restraint or seclusion, medications)
- The environment provides:
  - Privacy for the patient
  - Enough space for patients
  - A healthy balance between structured and quiet time
  - Adequate personnel to safely and effectively deal with potentially violent situations
- Staff skills call for:
  - Education in verbal de-escalation techniques
  - Education about positive and consistent approaches to patients
  - Education for appropriate use of restraints

Implementation

Ideally, intervention begins prior to any sign of escalation of anger. This intervention includes developing a trusting relationship with the patient by having numerous brief, non-threatening, non-directive interactions to get to know the patient. In certain settings (e.g., crisis units, emergency departments) episodes of patient anger and aggression can be predicted; therefore education and practice of verbal and non-verbal interventions with patients and staff are essential. Cultural competency is an essential part of staff education.

Health Teaching and Health Promotion

A nurse can model appropriate responses and ways to cope with anger, teach a variety of methods to appropriately express anger, and educate patients regarding coping mechanisms, identification of personal triggers, de-escalation techniques, and self-soothing skills to manage emotions. Skilled nurses can lead anger management, coping, and emotional awareness/regulation groups. Skills include removing themselves from a situation or taking a personal time out. Working with patients to explore their own psychological and somatic responses to anger or anger-provoking stimuli enhances self-awareness related to personal triggers and facilitates learning about how to intervene and exert self-management skills during these stressful events. Once trust is established between the nurse and patient, the nurse may begin to challenge discrepancies in what that person believes, says, or does. Challenges or the therapeutic use of assertiveness skills to present a reality check for the person and lead them to circumspection are essential for growth. To use this skill, it is vitally important that the nurse moderate tone of voice, non-verbal behaviours, and so forth so as not to appear judgemental or hostile in any way. The goal is to open communication and self-exploration in a non-threatening way.

Case Management

A multi-disciplinary approach is important for a patient with behavioural issues. Consistency and planning are key to the patient's success. Intervention strategies should be discussed during treatment team meetings and with the patient before implementation. The discharge plan may be composed of follow-up mental health care, anger management programs, and cognitive behavioural therapy.

Milieu Management

Behaviours rarely occur in a vacuum. A thorough, proactive examination of the environment is important when considering the potential for anger and aggression on a unit. It is hard to determine how the stimulation of any unit might affect someone whose anxiety is extremely high or who is delusional or confused.

Patient's ability to cope with their acute illness is confounded by unfamiliar environments full of unfamiliar and often unpredictable fellow patients. Frequent rounds on the unit are important as part of the ongoing assessment of the milieu and the patient's response to it.

Quiet rooms. If a patient is escalating but has enough self-control, a time-out in their room may be sufficient to enable the person to regain composure. Many inpatient psychiatric units, group homes, residential care facilities, and correctional centres offer a therapeutic quiet room. The room is partially lit and has relaxing music and comfortable furniture that promote feelings of security and safety. Individuals are free to avail themselves of this therapeutic space. However, in many institutions, quiet rooms are locked and used as seclusion rooms. The decision to lock the door is based on the patient's risk assessment and the discretion of the multi-disciplinary team.

Staff safety. Staff should all know which colleague is working with a potentially violent patient, keep an eye on the interaction, and be prepared to intervene if the situation escalates. At that time, other patients should be moved away from the incident, and the environment around the specific patient should be free from any object that could be used as a weapon. On psychiatric units, policies and procedures for working as a team in a critical incident of violence (or potential for violence) are in place. All staff should become familiar with the protocols. Discussing and rehearsing the protocols ensures confidence, safety, security, and trust.

De-escalation techniques. As the nurse determines a patient's emotional state, intervention begins. During this process, the nurse listens to the patient's story and acknowledges their needs. Summarizing what the patient has said demonstrates the nurse's empathy, compassion, and acceptance of the patient. Acceptance of the patient does not indicate an acceptance of aggressive or violent behaviour. It is important to clearly and simply state expectations for the patient's behaviour. In some situations the anger may not be resolved before the risk for violence arises.

Approaching an angry patient can be unnerving or frightening. The goal is to facilitate the expression of anger in an adaptive, non-violent manner.

When approaching the patient, the nurse will convey a calm, relaxed, open, non-threatening, and caring demeanour. The ability to maintain a calm exterior while feeling inner distress comes with experience.

> **BOX 23.4 Guide to De-Escalation Techniques**
>
> - Intervene as early as possible; alert team
> - Assess for personal safety; quick environmental scan
> - Assess the patient and the situation for stressors and stress indicators
> - Focus on the patient; active listening and eye contact
> - Establish what the patient considers to be needed
> - Maintain calmness for self and patient
> - Use a calm, clear tone of voice; appropriate eye contact
> - Speak clearly and concisely; short sentences only
> - Maintain the patient's self-esteem and dignity
> - Be factual
> - Remain honest; genuine, respectful
> - Maintain a large personal space
> - Stay in the here and now
> - Make the options clear

The nurse needs to pay attention to the environment. If the patient is in a state of low arousal, choose a quiet place to talk that is visible to other staff. This approach is most beneficial in helping a patient to regain control. If the patient is in a state of moderate arousal, pacing up and down a corridor together while the patient vents can be effective. The use of advanced communication skills to de-escalate the situation can help to dissipate pent-up energy fueled by the release of neurotransmitters and hormones. This technique is helpful when the patient is unable to use the flight response and may feel trapped. Box 23.4 offers some guidance for **de-escalation techniques.**

Personal space changes when the body and mind are in a heightened state of arousal. Patients in the pre-assaultive stage need much more space. Do not crowd the patient in or attempt to touch them. Allow the patient enough personal space so that you are not perceived as intrusive, but not so much space that the patient cannot speak in a normal voice. Always stay about 30 cm (1 foot) farther than the patient can reach with their arms or legs.

An agitated, angry, aggressive patient may invade the nurse's space physically and with verbal abuse and profanity. This means of communicating may be the only way the patient can express their feelings. As uncomfortable as this kind of communication may make someone feel, the nurse cannot take the patient's words personally or respond in kind (Pitts & Schaller, 2021). During an escalating situation is not the time to forbid the patient to communicate in this way or to end the conversation because of the patient's inappropriate word choices. Keeping the focus on the here and now and what needs to be done are priorities. The nurse should reflect that back in a calm tone during any barrage. The patient who is about to lose emotional control cannot be abandoned. For the protection of the patient and others, the nurse needs to remain engaged while a pre-planned crisis intervention begins to unfold. Even so, safety for the nurse is critical. Knowledge of crisis intervention techniques including staff safety plus the employer's policies prior to such a situation is of the utmost importance.

As escalation increases, the patient's ability to process stimuli decreases. The nurse should keep their voice audible but at a lower volume than the patient's. Eventually, the patient will match it and begin to listen more closely. The nurse will be sure to speak at an appropriate level and not whisper. Words must be chosen carefully, be spoken in short sentences, and be clear and concise, and the nurse must actively listen to the patient's responses and concerns. The use of open-ended statements and questions elicits the patient's thoughts. Punitive, threatening, accusatory, or challenging statements are avoided completely. They can too easily overwhelm.

Honest verbalization of the patient's options encourages the individual to assume responsibility for choices made. During the pre-assaultive stage, it may be strategic to give two options, such as "Do you want to go to your room or to the quiet room for a while?" Do not give more than two options at any time, to avoid overloading the patient's ability to process. Giving choice decreases the sense of powerlessness that often precipitates violence. This is quite appropriate in the anger stage, but not during the assaultive stage. In the pre-assaultive stage the patient's lack of clarity in thinking and poor decision making become key elements in the intervention. Therefore open-ended questions create too much confusion. The nurse might say, "Some quiet time in your room might help now," or "The quiet room is free." Again, the nurse's voice is calm and confident, with a tone that demonstrates that these statements to the patient are options, not directions.

In the assaultive stage seclusion, restraint, or pharmacological means of de-escalation may be necessary to ensure the safety of patients and staff. These measures should be used only when other interventions have failed. Canadian care facilities are mandated by policies that dictate the use of the least restrictive means to care for patients whenever possible. Nurses are also guided by position statements set out by their regulatory bodies.

> ⚡ **SAFETY TIP**
> Personal space changes when the body and mind are in a heightened state of arousal. Patients in the pre-assaultive stage need much more space. Do not crowd the patient in or attempt to touch them.

Engaging the angry or aggressive patient. Prior to engaging an angry or aggressive patient, the team must ensure that sufficient staff members are available for support. As everyone prepares, confrontation with the patient should be avoided. The technique of immediacy is used instead. If security personnel are called to stand by, they should stay in the background until they are asked to assist.

In a potentially volatile situation staff should not stand directly in front of the patient or in front of a doorway; this position could be interpreted as confrontational. Standing slightly off to the side is safer and more appropriate. The patient can be encouraged to have a seat. An angry person may sit. An aggressive person will not.

If a patient's behaviour begins to escalate, provide feedback: "You seem to be very angry." This reflective statement allows exploration of the patient's feelings and may lead to the early de-escalation of the situation. If the patient validates this, invite them to sit down and talk about it using a closed-ended statement, "Let's sit down and talk about it."

If any staff member believes that the aggression and violence are going to require additional help, a Code White can be called. In many hospitals nurses with experience dealing with anger, aggression, and violence and who have completed special training may be designated as Code White responders. In British Columbia this role may fall to the psychiatric nurse clinician in the emergency department. When a Code White is called, the Code White nurse attends and is met there by members of a trained Code White team. Upon arrival at the scene, the staff initiating the call defers to the expertise of the Code White nurse, who is supported in action by the Code White team.

Generally, the first staff member on the scene is the only person who should talk to the patient. That person takes the lead while other staff maintain an unobtrusive presence. They may be directed to call for additional help, prepare a seclusion room, gather restraints, or prepare to give medications.

Note: Code White policies and procedures are not in place in all jurisdictions nationally. The procedures may differ across jurisdictions. Refer to the Confederation of Nurses Unions website; their Violence Tool Kit offers a list of these and links to various guides (https://nursesunions.ca/

violence/). It is also important to check with the employer or institution regarding that institution's policies and procedures. In some instances the Code White team will not have a nurse as lead.

Pharmacological Interventions

When a patient is showing increased signs of anxiety or agitation that may forewarn anger, aggression, or violence, it is appropriate to offer antianxiety or antipsychotic medication to alleviate symptoms. When used in conjunction with psychosocial interventions and de-escalation techniques, these medications may prevent violent acting out. However, when dangerousness escalates and pharmacological restraint is needed, prn or stat medications are appropriate. Medications that are quick acting and easily administered in this type of situation (oral or intramuscular) are the best choices (Pitts & Schaller, 2021; Bak et al., 2019). Second-generation antipsychotics and benzodiazepines separately or in combination are commonly used. For patients who are psychotic, antipsychotic medication is the first priority. In an emergent situation medication orders should be received for stat and prn doses. Medications for Emergency Management of Agitated, Aggressive, or Violent Behaviour identifies medications of choice and indications. *Note:* Some medications are given concurrently for optimal therapeutic effect. See Chapter 11 for more information on psychotropic drugs.

> **MEDICATIONS FOR THE EMERGENCY MANAGEMENT OF AGITATED, AGGRESSIVE, OR VIOLENT BEHAVIOUR**
>
> **Combinations of fast-acting antipsychotics and antianxiety medications:** for moderate to severe, acute agitation; escalating violent behaviour
> - Haloperidol + lorazepam (Ativan) + benztropine (Cogentin)
> - Loxapine (Loxapac) + lorazepam (Ativan) + benztropine (Cogentin)
>
> **Antianxiety medications (Benzodiazepines):** for acute, mild to moderate agitation and anxiety; intoxicated or patients in acute withdrawal
> - Lorazepam (Ativan)
> - Diazepam (Valium)
>
> **First-generation antipsychotics:** for acute psychosis, agitation, aggression, disturbed, unpredictable behaviours
> - Haloperidol
> - Chlorpromazine
> - Loxapine (Loxapac) (*Note:* also indicated for acute mania)
>
> **Second-generation antipsychotics:** for acute psychosis, agitation, aggression, unpredictable behaviours
> - Risperidone
> - Olanzapine (Zyprexa, Zyprexa Zydis)
> - Zuclopenthixol acetate (Clopixol-Acuphase)
> - Ziprasidone (Geodon) (*Note:* also indicated for acute mania)
>
> **Antihistamine:** for acute agitation
> - Promethazine

Source s: Bak, M., Weltens, I., Bervoets, C., et al. (2019). The pharmacological management of agitated and aggressive behaviour: A systematic review and meta-analysis. *European Psychiatry, 57,* 78–100. https://doi.org/10.1016/j.eurpsy.2019.01.014; Pacciardi, B., Calcedo, A. A., & Messer, T., et al. (2019). Inhaled loxapine for the management of acute agitation in bipolar disorder and schizophrenia: Expert review and commentary in an era of change. *Drugs in R&D, 19,* 15–25. https://doi.org/10.1007/s40268-019-0262-3RE; Pitts, E., & Schaller, D. J. (2021, July 12). Violent patients. In *StatPearls [Internet].* Treasure Island: StatPearls Publishing. Retrieved from https://www.ncbi.nlm.nih.gov/books/NBK537281

It is the nurse's role to assess for appropriateness of prn medications. Many patients feel traumatized by the use of intramuscular injections; therefore the decision to use this route of administration needs to be determined by what is in the best interest of the patient and the speed with which effects of the medication are needed and what orders are available. Nurses must provide the patient with information about the medication, the reason it is being given, and potential adverse effects, even if the patient is out of control.

The long-term treatment of anger, aggression, and violence is based on treating the underlying psychiatric disorder. Selective serotonin reuptake inhibitors (SSRIs), lithium, anticonvulsants, benzodiazepines, atypical antipsychotics, and beta-blockers are all used successfully for specific patient populations. Clozapine is generally the medication of choice for persistent aggression and hostility in refractory schizophrenia (Cho et al., 2019; Patchan et al., 2018). For rage and severe, persistent agitation, anticonvulsants such as carbamazepine and gabapentin are often used (Alazawi & Bareham, 2018). Anger and aggression related to autism spectrum disorders may be reduced through the use of psycho-stimulants, but caution should be used in adults. Lithium provides some control for irritability, agitation, and aggression for those with intellectual disabilities (Loeks-Johnson & Power, 2020).

Physical Interventions

Use of restraints. Restraint is an intervention used to decrease the patient's ability to harm themselves or others. It is only used if the patient presents a clear and present danger to self or others. Restraints of any type should be used only when alternatives fail to protect the patient and others from harm. A policy of least restraint is best practice in Canada (PSEP-Canada, 2017). There are three different types of restraints (PSEP-Canada, 2017):

1. Environmental restraint: seclusion is an example of an environmental restraint. Movement is restricted to a defined area or locked room. The situation is temporary, the patient is alone, and there is no furniture or other amenities in the room.
2. Physical/mechanical restraints: any method whereby limbs or trunk are held down, that is, movement is restricted against the will of the patient (e.g., transfer belts, four-point restraints, Pinel or Posey restraints, locking geriatric chairs, strong sheets). In some jurisdictions, in an emergency situation, nurses are able to restrain prior to getting an order (BCCNM, 2022), for example, restraining a patient in the emergency room who is high on drugs or acutely psychotic and acting out. Nurses must be absolutely clear on their standards, rights, and obligations under their registration and other legislation prior to attempting this. Guidelines for the use of mechanical restraints are given in Box 23.5.
3. Chemical restraints: also known as pharmacological restraint, is achieved through the use of medications, with the sole intent of managing behaviour.

Comprehensive assessments of behaviours, patient's needs, and safety must be taken into account first. Alternatives should be sought, particularly with the elderly or cognitively impaired. Many precautions need to be taken legally and ethically by the nursing staff regarding the use of chemical restraints. The rationale for the use of chemical restraint must be clearly articulated in all documentation.

Use of seclusion. Prior to seclusion, a patient must be assessed for contraindications including pregnancy, chronic obstructive pulmonary disorder, head or spinal injury, seizure disorder, abuse, history of surgery or fracture, morbid obesity, and sleep apnea. Seclusion results in the removal of external stimuli by placing the patient in a locked private room. A patient can only be secluded or restrained with an order from a psychiatrist or physician in accordance with a provincial or territorial mental health act or other policy.

BOX 23.5 Guidelines for Use of Restraint or Seclusion

Indications for Use
- To protect the patient from self-harm
- To prevent the patient from assaulting others

Legal Requirements
- Multi-disciplinary involvement
- Appropriate health care provider's signature according to provincial and territorial law
- Patient advocate or relative notification
- Restraint or seclusion discontinuation as soon as possible

Documentation Describes
- Patient's behaviour leading to restraint or seclusion
- Nursing interventions used and the patient's responses (including least restrictive measures used prior to restraint or seclusion)
- Evaluation of the interventions used and patient's response

Plan of Care for Restraint Use or Seclusion Implementation
- Ongoing evaluations by nursing staff and appropriate health care providers
- Method of reintegration into the unit milieu
- Evidence of least restrictive measures used prior to restraint or seclusion
- Critical Incident or Unusual Occurrence Report form completed

Clinical Assessments
- Patient's mental state at time of restraint or seclusion (i.e., pre-assaultive, assaultive, post-assaultive)
- Physical examination for medical problems possibly causing behaviour changes
- Need for restraints or seclusion

Observation and Ongoing Assessment
- Staff in constant or close attendance
- Written record completed every 15 minutes
- Range of movement frequently assessed if limbs are restrained
- Vital signs monitored
- Circulation assessed: blood flow observed in hands or feet
- Observation to ensure that restraint is not rubbing or causing friction on skin
- Provision for nutrition, hydration, and elimination

Release Procedure
- Patient able to follow commands and stay in control
- Termination of restraints or seclusion
- Debriefing with patient

Staff work as a team when secluding a patient. The team leader briefly describes the rationale for seclusion and directs the team. One nurse prepares the seclusion room while others promote safety and privacy by clearing the area of onlookers, maintaining the patient's privacy and dignity. A nurse prepares prn or stat medication. Options are provided to the patient, including taking a time out, accepting medication orally, or walking with the nursing team into the seclusion room. When these options fail, the staff intervenes to physically restrain the patient and escort them into seclusion. The patient may be required to change into pyjamas and medication may be administered despite patient objections. One by one, team members back out of the room, locking the door behind them. Close or constant observation protocols are initiated per hospital policy. The patient remains in seclusion until assessed as being less at risk for harm to self or others.

Reintegration to the unit after restraint or seclusion occurs when the patient is assessed as being able to handle increasing amounts of stimulation. Reintegration should be gradual. If the process proves to be too much for the patient and increased agitation results, the individual is returned to the seclusion room or another quiet area, or restraints are reapplied. Prior to release from restraint or seclusion, patients must be able to follow directions and control behaviours. With restraints, a structured reintegration is the best approach. Begin by removing one of the four-point restraints, then another, and so on. Close observation of the patient is essential as the restraints are removed and for several hours afterward. If the patient is unable to manage their behaviour, further seclusion or restraint may be necessary. Following seclusion of a patient, the treatment team should debrief the incident and when seclusion is discontinued, the nurse and patient should also debrief.

Incidents that require the use of seclusion or restraints provoke anxiety for the staff and may trigger their stress responses. Skills in non-violent crisis intervention techniques are essential. Nurses should not be put into positions such as these without this additional training. Many health authorities, care facilities, and health institutions across Canada provide this training at the time of hiring and intermittently during employment.

Caring for Patients in General Hospital Settings

Patients with high anxiety related to hospitalization. Caring for hospitalized patients who exhibit signs of anxiety begins with listening to the patient's story and helping the patient to identify immediate goals. This kind of response can build rapport and reassure the patient. Mild anxiety can be moderated by the provision of comfort items before they are requested (beverage, deck of cards, access to TV). Interventions for anxiety might also include the use of distractions such as magazines, action comics, and video games. Generally, distractions that are colourful and do not require sustained attention work best, although the choice of distraction varies according to the patient's interests and abilities. Patients with a high level of baseline anxiety and limited coping skills are helped when their interactions with the treatment team are predictable. Visits by a chaplain or a volunteer may help by giving the patient more attention.

Anxiety can also be minimized by reducing ambiguity. This strategy includes clear and concrete communication. An interaction providing clarity about what the nurse can and cannot do is most usefully ended by offering something within the nurse's power to provide (i.e., leaving the patient with a "yes" or "I'll see what I can do about that."). When a patient is anxious, frustrated, angry, or fearful, pacing with the patient up and down the corridor can be a helpful strategy. Open communication and active listening while walking together are therapeutic.

Patients with healthy coping skills who are overwhelmed. A patient loses autonomy and control when hospitalized. This can cause a great deal of stress and distress. When this stress is combined with the uncertainty of illness, a patient may respond in ways that are not usual for them. A careful nursing assessment, with history and information from family members/significant others, helps evaluate whether responses are normal coping methods for the patient.

Spending one-to-one time with an overwhelmed patient is important to find a baseline to keep anxiety at a level that is manageable for them. Interventions for patients who generally have healthy coping strategies involve finding ways to support these in this environment or substitute similar means of dealing with the hospitalization. In stressful moments when the patient is struggling to cope or feeling overwhelmed, the nurse acknowledges the patient's distress, validates how understandable this is under the circumstances, and indicates a willingness to support and collaborate around coping. Validation and genuine caring also include making an apology to the patient when appropriate to alleviate anxiety and ensure the patient knows they are cared for. For example, when a promised intervention (e.g., changing a dressing by a certain time) has not been achieved or acknowledging the patient's response about the "horrible food" and assisting them in making tastier choices on the menu or asking if they would like to talk with the dietician are all helpful. All of these offer more autonomy to a person who is struggling to cope with the loss of personal power and control.

Any angry patient may be unable to temper this emotion sufficiently to problem-solve with their nurses; others may be unable to communicate the source of their anger. Often the nurse, knowing the patient and the context of the anger, can make an accurate guess at what emotion is behind the anger and help name it for the patient using a closed statement of reflection. Pausing momentarily to let the patient think about this and answer is an important therapeutic technique. Doing so can lead to a sense of being understood and dissipation of the anger. This results in a calmer discussion of the event or issue.

> **VIGNETTE**
>
> Jagwinder, a 21-year-old patient who had been in an automobile accident, was admitted to the medical unit with a pelvic fracture and is bedridden. Since admission, he has yelled at each nurse who walks by his room, using expletives to demand that the nurse enter and attend to his needs.
>
> **Intervention**
> The nurse assigned to the patient for the evening stops in his doorway after he yells at her and assertively states, "Jagwinder, it is inappropriate to yell and swear at the staff. If you would like our attention, please address us politely." She continues on her way, and Jagwinder is left to process the message, alone. He is unable to offer a retort or to engage the nurse in argument. He is initially angry and profane in response, but the nurse is not there to hear it and he is left unsatisfied. Should he repeat this behaviour on her next encounter with him, she will repeat her original message, consistently setting limits on his behaviour. She will not engage in conversation with him until he is prepared to act and speak appropriately. At each negative encounter, the patient is left to think about his behaviour. The nurse continues to care for him, but limits the aggressive, inappropriate behaviour. She explains this, offering the patient ways to get attention in an appropriate manner.
>
> **Response**
> Jagwinder eventually comes to realize how to get the attention he needs in a more appropriate manner. He gains insight and modifies his behaviour. His anger and frustration triggered by not getting his needs met immediately begin to dissipate. When the nurse meets with him, she engages him in the primary topic of his concern. He is overwhelmed by hospitalization and loss of personal control of his life. The source of his anger and behaviour have been found. Together they explore how to communicate his needs more effectively, more appropriately, and more assertively. They discuss his anger and frustration and explore his pattern of coping generally and how this might apply or be positively adapted while in hospital. Initially in the encounter, the nurse applied principles of behavioural therapy to her intervention strategies. Later, she used cognitive behavioural techniques.

Patients with marginal coping skills. Patients whose coping skills were marginal before hospitalization need a different set of interventions from those who have basically healthy ways of coping. They are poorly equipped to use alternatives when initial attempts to cope are unsuccessful or are found to be inappropriate. Such patients frequently manifest anxiety that moves quickly to anger and on to aggression. For some, anger and intimidation are primary coping strategies used to obtain short-term goals of control or mastery. For others, the anger occurs when their limited or primitive attempts at coping are unsuccessful, and alternatives are unknown. Fear, indignation, and arguing can be gratifying to many verbally abusive patients. For these patients, anger and violence are particular risks in inpatient settings. Marginalized coping may not be immediately apparent, and the nurse should watch for patterns and explore with the patient and their significant others. For patients with marginal coping skills, once anxiety is moderated, nursing interventions include teaching alternative behaviours and coping strategies.

Implementing appropriate interventions can be difficult when the nurse is feeling threatened. Remaining matter-of-fact with patients who habitually use anger and intimidation can be difficult, as they are often skillful at making personal and pointed statements. It is important to remember that patients do not know their nurses personally and thus have no basis on which to make judgements. It can be helpful for nurses to discuss their thoughts and feelings with other staff members or with the critical incident debriefing team.

Patients with marginal coping skills require information, consistency, and relationship building with staff while in hospital. Abusive, aggressive language and demanding behaviours can be highly disruptive to the staff and the unit. Intervention strategies include immediacy, consistency, role-modelling by the nurse, and teaching.

1. Leave the room as soon as the verbal abuse begins. Upon doing so, the patient is informed that the nurse will return in a specific amount of time (e.g., 20 minutes) if the situation is calmer. However, if the nurse is in the middle of a procedure and cannot leave immediately, they can break off conversation and eye contact, completing the procedure quickly and matter-of-factly before leaving the room. The nurse avoids chastising, threatening, or responding punitively to the patient.
2. Withdraw attention from the abuse. Withdrawal of attention to verbal or emotional abuse is successful only if a second intervention is also used. This step requires attending positively to, thus reinforcing, non-abusive communication by the patient. Interventions can include discussing non–illness-related topics, responding to requests, and providing emotional support, particularly when the patient is calm and approachable. This technique is quite effective when used in conjunction with the third strategy.
3. Schedule routine interactions. Patients who are verbally abusive may respond best to the predictability of routine. Give the patient the schedule. Routine provides nursing attention that is not contingent on the patient's behaviour; therefore it does not reinforce the abuse. Of course, the patient's illness or injury may sometimes require nursing visits for assessment or intervention outside the scheduled contact times. These visits can be carried out in a calm, brief, matter-of-fact manner.

Chemical dependence and marginal coping. there is a potential for aggression and violence for hospitalized patients with chemical dependence. They may be highly anxious about being cut off from the substance on which they depend. They also may have well-founded concerns that any physical pain will be inadequately addressed (Copeland, 2020). Many chemically dependent patients may see the source of their discomfort and anxiety as being outside themselves (i.e., external LOC) and therefore relief must come from an outside source (e.g., the nurse, medication). These patients exhibit severe frustration intolerance and can be quite verbally aggressive. Coping can include drug-seeking manipulative behaviours as well (Copeland, 2020). Anger and aggression can also be used in an attempt to manipulate staff to achieve immediate need gratification, even on a small scale. The provision of empathy, compassion, dignity, and an understanding of the patient's lived experience with addiction helps the nurse and other staff determine a course of action (see Chapter 18). Most hospitals have a withdrawal protocol that ensures that patients do not go through withdrawal without medication. Medication administration for chemically dependent patients needs to be provided promptly and consistently to communicate to patients that nurses can be trusted. Other than at medication times, time spent interacting with the patient is important to build a respectful, trusting relationship as well. Precautionary measures may be in place on the hospital unit to limit certain visitors in order to protect the sobriety or withdrawal. The facility may also have maintenance protocols for chemically dependent patients. These should all be explained and, if warranted, repeated respectfully to these highly anxious patients.

Caring for Patients in Inpatient Psychiatric Settings

Patients who are acutely psychotic. On a psychiatric unit, the potential for hostile aggression and violence is most often demonstrated by those who are acutely psychotic, in a manic phase, substance dependent, or being held under the authority of a mental health act.

In psychosis, cognitions are disturbed; misinterpretation of stimuli may occur and rational thoughts are skewed. Impulsivity may also be heightened and judgment impaired. Confusion, fear, paranoia, and misinterpretation of reality can all contribute to acts of violence. Responses may have some connection to reality or be based in hallucinations and/or delusions. Acting out with violence may be instrumental or reactive. For example, the psychotic patient may use violence to attempt to leave the unit for fear of being severely harmed or killed there. Implications for Nursing: a combination of an antipsychotic and a benzodiazepine are often given to help calm acutely psychotic patients and help with reducing thought distortions. Restraint or seclusion may be necessitated.

O'Reilly et al. (2019) suggest a link between moral cognition and violent acts by patients in psychosis. Generally, moral cognitions include thoughts about justice, standards, and what a person believes to be right and proper. These can be rooted in religion, culture, or society. For example, using a moral cognition approach, a patient who has very strong beliefs about gender and sexuality may spontaneously violently act out to protect themself from the perceived risk of rape.

There is a correlation between psychosis and violence, particularly in early psychosis. On top of that, the risk for violence by psychotic patients increases significantly when there is concurrent substance use (Lopez-Garcia et al., 2019; Moulin et al., 2018a, 2018b). Together, cognitive distortions, lack of insight, and emotional instability are heightened. For risk assessment, this is another reason why nurses need to know what a patient's delusions are and document them. Delusions can have triggers leading to violence (Ullrich et al., 2018) (see the Vignette about Ken).

> **VIGNETTE**
> Ken is a 32-year-old patient with a diagnosis of schizophrenia. He has lived in a group home for 10 years. His illness has been well-managed with medications and daily psychosocial programs. Admitted now to the psychiatric unit, Ken is experiencing an acute exacerbation of schizophrenia. His long-held delusion that the Canadian Security Intelligence Service is listening in on him because he has some intimate knowledge of nuclear weapons design has now overwhelmed him, preoccupying most of this thoughts. He is increasingly paranoid. Ken yells at the nurses and accuses them of being part of the conspiracy against him. He refuses medication because he believes that it will erase his knowledge about the secret weapon. He insists that he must remain alert, vigilant, and self-protective. Ken's impulsivity and aggression are escalating as his mental state deteriorates.

> **Implications for Nursing**
> A risk assessment was done on admission. Ken was determined to be at risk for violence. Protocols went into effect on the unit offering first a quiet room, prn medication, and reassuring Ken he is safe. Nurses will present reality of who they are and what is happening. Despite Ken's disturbed thinking, he is able to understand the potential for being secluded because he has been hospitalized before.
>
> **Intervention**
> When the nurse offers him a prn medication to settle, Ken makes the choice to take it rather than be "locked up." He reiterates that that room, too, is "bugged" and dangerous for him. He wants liquid medication.
>
> **Response**
> Ken examines and sniffs the oral prn medication. He asks if it is poison to kill him or some other hypnotic to erase his memory. Reassurance is given; reality is presented regarding his safety and the nurse's role. Ken's eyes bore into the nurse while he is listening, trying to judge the degree of truth. He starts to take the medication and then promptly throws it on the nurse. A Code White is called. Ken is taken to seclusion and given medication to settle.

Caring for Patients With Neurocognitive Disorders

Patients (or residents) with neurocognitive disorders are particularly at risk for acting aggressively, spontaneously, and dangerously. Risk factors may stem from delirium, dementia, or brain injury (see Chapter 17). Sometimes patients with dementia become frightened because they are confused. They may become increasingly agitated and even more aggressive. Implications for Nursing: distraction techniques are often helpful to distract the person from focusing on something that is triggering this emotional response. When confusion is the cause, try to have the individual focus on one thing, particularly something fairly plain but that the patient likes is therapeutic. If this is unsuccessful, prn of an antianxiety medication may help.

When suddenly and severely overwhelmed by the stimulus in the environment, a catastrophic reaction may happen. Extreme behaviours of screaming, swearing, punching, slapping, or banging are spontaneous and often quite violent. Implications for Nursing: to prevent this, adopting a calm and unhurried manner is the best approach at all times, as is reducing stimuli. Assessment of the patient will set the standard for whom multiple choices should not be given, because they, too, are overwhelming. Staff should never stand or stoop directly in front of patients with dementia but always stay slightly offside to avoid a sudden lashing out. A symbol or colour should appear on the patient/resident's chart to alert staff of the propensity for violence.

Evaluation

Evaluation of the NCP is essential for patients with a potential for anger, aggression, and violence. Evaluation provides information about the extent to which the interventions have achieved the outcomes. Results of the interventions are evaluated, documented, and the NCP is revised.

KEY POINTS TO REMEMBER

- Angry emotions and aggressive, violent actions are difficult targets for nursing intervention, and knowledge plus self-awareness of personal responses to these situations are essential.
- Nurses benefit from an understanding of how to intervene with an angry, aggressive, or violent patient.
- Understanding precipitating factors that can lead to an escalation of aggression facilitates care planning for individuals in a variety of situations.
- Psychosocial, cognitive, sociocultural, and biological theories provide explanations for anger and aggression.
- A patient's past aggressive behaviour is the most important indicator of future aggressive episodes. A variety of interventions are used to help patients de-escalate and maintain control, depending on their coping abilities, cognitive and mental status, and potential for violence.
- Administration of antipsychotics, mood stabilizers, and antianxiety medications may be indicated.
- Seclusion or restraints may be necessary to ensure safety for the patient and others on the unit.
- The nurse is expected to have a clear understanding of legislation, scope of practice, policies, protocols, practices, and legalities related to anger, aggression, and violence.

CRITICAL THINKING

1. Jennifer admits a 24-year-old man with a diagnosis of mania to an inpatient unit. She notes that the patient is irritable, has trouble sitting during the interview, and has a history of assault. Prioritizing care will include two of the following.
   a. Identifying appropriate responses the nurse can make to the patient.
   b. Risk assessment.
   c. Identifying at least three long-term outcomes to consider when planning care.
2. What are the two indicators for the use of seclusion or restraint rather than verbal interventions? Provide a rationale.
3. Enter into a debate on the use of restraint and seclusion with your clinical group or in class. Choose a side and defend it, even if you do not necessarily agree with it. Use these topics:
   a. There are always better alternatives to seclusion and restraint.
   b. Seclusion and restraint are underused—people who have tried to limit their use have gone too far.
   c. Using chemical restraint with medication is preferable to physical seclusion and restraint.
4. Jordan is a 24-year-old male prone to substance use. He likes to fight and initiate fights. He prides himself on his strength and aggressive personality. When he perceives another person is staring at him, according to theory, how is he likely to interpret this?

CHAPTER REVIEW

1. Which statement about violence in the workplace and nursing is accurate?
   a. Unless working in psychiatric or mental health settings, nurses are unlikely to experience patient violence.
   b. Almost two-thirds of nurses will experience violence in the workplace during their careers.
   c. Emergency, psychiatric, and step-down units have the highest rates of violence toward staff.
   d. Violence primarily affects inexperienced or unskilled staff who cannot calm their patients.
2. A patient describes himself as "always angry." What should the nurse assess for? **Select all that apply.**
   a. Pain
   b. History of violence
   c. Stomach ulcer

d. Hypertension
e. Mild or traumatic brain injury
3. Which statements by a patient indicate an increased risk for violence? **Select all that apply.**
   a. "People push me, but they can only push me so far."
   b. "I have a right to feel angry, and right now I am angry."
   c. "You are really stupid. I'd get better nursing care from a monkey."
   d. "A man has to do what a man has to do when somebody crosses him."
   e. "This is frustrating! I wish people would leave me alone! That's what would help me."
4. A nurse, Baljit, responds to a loud, angry voice coming from the day room. She finds Christopher pacing and shouting that he "isn't going to take this (expletive) anymore!" Which reaction by Baljit is likely to be helpful in de-escalating the situation with Christopher?
   a. Acts calm, quiet, and in control.
   b. States, "You are acting inappropriately and must calm yourself now."
   c. Matches the patient's volume level so that he is able to hear over his own shouting.
   d. Stands close to the patient so that she can intervene physically, if needed, to protect others.
5. Andrea, a patient, is anxiously waiting her turn to speak with a nurse. The nurse is very busy, however, and asks Andrea if she can wait a few minutes so she can finish her task. The nurse is distracted and forgets her promise temporarily. Forty-five minutes pass before the nurse remembers and approaches Andrea. On seeing the nurse, Andrea accuses the nurse of lying and refuses to speak with her. Choose the best therapeutic response.
   a. "You seem angry that I didn't speak with you when I promised I would."
   b. "Look, I'm sorry for being late, but screaming at me is not the best way to handle it."
   c. "You are too angry to talk right now. I'll come back in 20 minutes and we can try again."
   d. "Why are you angry? I told you that I was busy and would get to you soon as I could."

REFERENCES

Alazawi, D., & Bareham, J. (2018). Drugs of abuse: Gabapentinoids. *DOCTALK, 5*(2), 13–14. Retrieved from http://www.cps.sk.ca/iMIS/Documents/Newsletters/DOCTALK%20Vol%205%20Issue%202.pdf

Allen, J. J., & Anderson, C. A. (2017). Aggression and violence: Definitions and distinctions. In P. Sturmey (Ed.), *The Wiley handbook of violence and aggression* (Vol. 1). Wiley Online Library. https://doi.org/10.1002/9781119057574.whbva001

Baillien, E., Escartín, J., Gross, C., et al. (2017). Towards a conceptual and empirical differentiation between workplace bullying and interpersonal conflict. *European Journal of Work and Organizational Psychology, 26*(6), 870–881. https://doi.org/10.1080/1359432X.2017.1385601.

Bak, M., Weltens, I., Bervoets, C., et al. (2019). The pharmacological management of agitated and aggressive behaviour: A systematic review and meta-analysis. *European Psychiatry, 57*, 78–100. https://doi.org/10.1016/j.eurpsy.2019.01.014.

Bandura, A. (1973). *Aggression: A social learning analysis.* New York: Prentice Hall.

Barnett, L. (2016). *The "Spanking" Law: Section 43 of the Criminal Code.* Ottawa: Library of Parliament. Publication No. 2016-35-E. Retrieved from https://lop.parl.ca/staticfiles/PublicWebsite/Home/ResearchPublications/BackgroundPapers/PDF/2016-35-e.pdf.

British Columbia College of Nurses and Midwives (BCCNM). (2022). Registered Nurses: Learning resources. Restraints. https://www.bccnm.ca/RN/learning/consent/Pages/restraints.aspx

Beck, A. (1976). *Cognitive therapy and the emotional disorders.* New York: International Universities Press.

Beck, A., Emery, G., & Greenberg, R. (2005). *Anxiety disorders and phobias (15th anniversary ed.).* New York: Basic Books.

Boysan, M., & Kiral, E. (2016). An investigation into the interactions between positive and negative aspects of personality, perfectionism, coping, and locus of control: A latent profile analysis. *Sleep and Hypnosis: A Journal of Clinical Neuroscience and Psychopathology, 18*(2), 53–64. https://dx.doi.org/10.5350/Sleep.Hypn.2016.18.0116

Brodie, M. J., Besag, F., Ettinger, A. B., et al. (2016). Epilepsy, antiepileptic drugs, and aggression: An evidence-based review. *Pharmacological Reviews, 68*(3), 563–602. https://doi.org/10.1124/pr.115.012021

Brophy, J. T., Keith, M. M., & Hurley, M. (2017). Assaulted and unheard: Violence against healthcare staff. *New Solutions, a Journal of Environmental and Occupational Health Policy, 27*(4), 581–606. https://doi.org/10.1177/1048291117732301

Bushman, B. J. (2020). Aggression and violence. In R. Biswas-Diener, & E. Diener (Eds.), *Noba textbook series: Psychology.* DEF Publishers. Retrieved from https://noba.to/63vj7ykn

Canadian Nurses Association (CNA) & Canadian Federation of Nurses Unions (CFNU). (2015). *Joint position statement: Workplace violence and bullying.* Retrieved from https://nursesunions.ca/wp-content/uploads/2019/10/Workplace-Violence-and-Bullying_joint-position-statement.pdf

Caruso, G. D. (2017). *Public health and safety: The social determinants of health and criminal behavior.* ResearchersLinks Books.

Casey, B. (2019). *Violence facing health care workers in Canada. Report of the Standing Committee on Health.* House of Commons of Canada. Retrieved from https://www.ourcommons.ca/Content/Committee/421/HESA/Reports/RP10589455/hesarp29/hesarp29-e.pdf

Cassiello-Robbins, C., & Barlow, D. H. (2016). Anger: The unrecognized emotion in emotional disorders. *Clinical Psychology: Science and Practice, 23*(1), 66–85. https://doi.org/10.1111/cpsp.12139

Chester, D. S., DeWall, C. N., Derefinko, K. J., et al. (2016). Looking for reward in all the wrong places: Dopamine receptor gene polymorphisms indirectly affect aggression through sensation-seeking. *Social Neuroscience, 11*(5), 487–494. https://doi.org/10.1080/17470919.2015.1119191

Cho, W., Shin, W. S., An, I., et al. (2019). Biological aspects of aggression and violence in schizophrenia. *Clinical Psychopharmacology Neuroscience, 17*(4), 475–486. https://doi.org/10.9758/cpn.2019.17.4.475

Copeland, D. (2020). Drug-seeking: A literature review (and an exemplar of stigmatization in nursing). *Nursing Inquiry, 27*, e12329. https://doi.org/10.1111/nin.12329

Coyne, S. M., Nelson, D. A., Carroll, J. S., et al. (2017). Relational aggression and marital quality: A five-year longitudinal study. *Journal of Family Psychology, 31*(3), 282–293. https://doi.org/10.1037/fam0000274

Criminal Code of Canada (R.S.C., 1985, c. C-46). (2020a). *Uttering threats.* Justice Laws, Government of Canada, Section 264.1. Retrieved from https://laws-lois.justice.gc.ca/eng/acts/c-46/section-264.1.html.

Criminal Code of Canada (R.S.C., 1985, c. C-46). (2020b). *Assault.* Justice Laws, Government of Canada, Section 265.1. Retrieved from https://laws-lois.justice.gc.ca/eng/acts/c-46/section-265.html

Cristofori, I., Zhong, W., Mandoske, V., et al. (2016). Brain regions influencing implicit violent attitudes: A lesion-mapping study. *Journal of Neuroscience, 36*(9), 2757–2768. https://doi.org/10.1523/JNEUROSCI.2975-15

Dailey, N. S., Smith, R., Bajaj, S., et al. (2018). Elevated aggression and reduced white matter integrity in mild traumatic brain injury: A DTI study. *Frontiers in Behavioural Neuroscience, 12,* 118. https://doi.org/10.3389/fnbeh.2018.00118

Delhove, M., & Greitemeyer, T. (2021). Violent media use and aggression: Two longitudinal network studies. *The Journal of Social Psychology, 161*(6), 697–713. https://doi.org/10.1080/00224545.2021.1896465

Dutra, S. J., Siegle, G. J., Reeves, E. J., et al. (2016). Feeling without thinking? Anger provocation task predicts impaired cognitive performance in bipolar disorder but not major depression or healthy adults. *Cognitive Therapy and Research, 40,* 139–149. https://doi.org/10.1007/s10608-015-9734-0

Edmonson, C., & Zelonka, C. (2019). Our own worst enemies: The nurse bullying epidemic. *Nursing Administration Quarterly, 43*(3), 274–279. https://doi.org/10.1097/NAQ.0000000000000353

Ellis, A. (1973). *Humanistic psychotherapy: The rational-emotive approach.* New York: McGraw-Hill.

Ellis, A. (1990). *Anger: How to live with and without it.* New York: Citadel Press.

Falletta, E. (2017). Lateral violence in the workplace. *Nursing Ethics, On the Pulse.* Johns Hopkins Nursing. Retrieved from https://magazine.nursing.jhu.edu/2017/09/lateral-violence-workplace/

Fanning, J. R., & Coccaro, E. F. (2016). Neurobiology of impulsive aggression. In P. M. Kleepsies (Ed.), *The Oxford handbook of behavioral emergencies and crises.* New York: Oxford University Press. https://doi.org/10.1093/oxfordhb/978-19935277.001.0001.

Geniole, S. N., Bird, B. M., McVittie, J. S., et al. (2019). Is testosterone linked to human aggression? A meta-analytic examination of the relationship between baseline, dynamic, and manipulated testosterone on human aggression. *Hormones and Behavior, 123,* 104644. https://doi.org/10.1016/j.yhbeh.2019.104644

Geoffrion, S., Goncalves, J., Sader, J., et al. (2017). Workplace aggression against health care workers, law enforcement officials, and bus drivers: Differences in prevalence, perceptions, and psychological consequences. *Journal of Workplace Behavioral, 32*(3), 172–189. https://doi.org/10.1080/15555240.2017.1349611

Hango, D., & Moyser, M. (2018). *Harassment in Canadian workplaces. Insights on Canadian Society.* Statistics Canada Catalogue No. 75-006-X. Retrieved from https://publications.gc.ca/collections/collection_2018/statcan/75-006-x/75-006-2018-37-eng.pdf

Klasen, M., Wolf, D., Eisner, P. D., et al. (2019). Serotonergic contributions to human brain aggression networks. *Frontiers in Neuroscience, 13,* 42. https://doi.org/10.3389/fnins.2019.00042

Loeks-Johnson, A., & Power, D. (2020). What are the best treatments for intellectually disabled patients with aggression?. *Evidence-Based Practice, 23*(3), 21–22. https://doi.org/10.1097/EBP.0000000000000564

Lopez-Garcia, P., Ashby, S., Patel, P., et al. (2019). Clinical and neurodevelopmental correlates of aggression in early psychosis. *Schizophrenia Research, 212,* 171–176. https://doi.org/10.1016/j.schres.2019.07.045

Martínez-Monteagudo, M. C., Delgado, B., García-Fernández, J. M., et al. (2019). Cyberbullying, aggressiveness, and emotional intelligence in adolescence. *International Journal of Environmental Research and Public Health, 16,* 5079. https://doi.org/10.3390/ijerph16245079

Moulin, V., Alameda, L., Baumann, P. S., et al. (2018a). Three clinical risk profiles of violent behavior in a cohort of early psychosis patients. *L'encephale, 45*(3), 214–220. https://doi.org/10.1016/j.encep.2018.08.003

Moulin, V., Baumann, P., Gholamrezaee, M., et al. (2018b). Cannabis, a significant risk factor for violent behavior in the early phase psychosis. Two patterns of interaction of factors increase the risk of violent behavior: Cannabis use disorder and impulsivity; cannabis use disorder, lack of insight and treatment adherence. *Frontiers in Psychiatry, 9,* 294. https://doi.org/10.3389/fpsyt.2018.00294

O'Reilly, K., O'Connell, P., O'Sullivan, D., et al. (2019). Moral cognition, the missing link between psychotic symptoms and acts of violence: A cross-sectional national forensic cohort study. *BMC Psychiatry, 19,* 408. https://doi.org/10.1186/s12888-019-2372-4

O'Rourke, M., Wrigley, C., & Hammond, S. (2018). Violence within mental health services: How to enhance risk management. *Risk Management and Healthcare Policy, 11,* 159–167. https://doi.org/10.2147/RMHP.S131834

Pabian, S., Vandebosch, H., et al. (2016). (Cyber) bullying perpetration as an impulsive, angry reaction following (cyber) bullying victimisation? In M. Walrave, K. Ponnet, E. Vanderhoven et al. (Eds.), *Youth 2.0: Social media and adolescence: Part III* (pp. 193–209). Cham: Springer International Publishing. https://doi.org/10.1007/978-3-319-27893-3_11

Patchan, K., Vyas, G., Hackman, A. L., et al. (2018). Clozapine in reducing aggression and violence in forensic populations. *The Psychiatric Quarterly, 89*(1), 157–168. https://doi.org/10.1007/s11126-017-9521-z

Patient Safety Education Program (PSEP) Canada. (2017). *Module 13d: Mental health care: Seclusion and restraints: When all else fails. The Patient Safety Education Program—Canada. (PSEP—Canada) Curriculum.* PSEP—Canada and the Ontario Hospital Association (OHA). Retrieved from https://www.patientsafetyinstitute.ca/en/education/PatientSafetyEducationProgram/PatientSafetyEducationCurriculum/Documents/Module%2013d%20Seclusion%20and%20Restraint.pdf

Penney, S. R., Morgan, A., & Simpson, A. I. F. (2016). Assessing illness- and non–illness-based motivations for violence in persons with major mental illness. *Law and Human Behavior, 40*(1), 42–49. https://doi.org/10.1037/lhb0000155

Perelman School of Medicine. (2016, September 15). One in nine emergency room patients with injuries caused by violence will visit an ER again within two years, study finds. ScienceDaily.

Pitts, E., & Schaller, D. J. (2021, July 12). Violent patients. In *StatPearls [Internet].* Treasure Island: StatPearls Publishing. Retrieved from https://www.ncbi.nlm.nih.gov/books/NBK537281

Reichert, C. (2017). *Enough is enough—Putting a stop to violence in the health care sector—A discussion paper.* The Canadian Federation of Nurses Unions. Retrieved from https://nursesunions.ca/wp-content/uploads/2017/05/CFNU_Enough-is-Enough_June1_FINALlow.pdf

Rivara, F., Adhia, A., Lyons, V., et al. (2019). The effects of violence on health. *Overview—Violence, Health Affairs, 38*(10). https://doi.org/10.1377/hlthaff.2019.00480

Rotter, J. B. (1966). Generalized expectancies for internal versus external control of reinforcement. *Psychological Monographs: General and Applied, 80*(1), 1–28. https://doi.org/10.1037/h0092976

Schablon, A., Wendeler, D., Kozak, A., et al. (2018). Prevalence and consequences of aggression and violence towards nursing and care staff in Germany—A survey. *International Journal of Environmental Research and Public Health, 15*, 1247. https://doi.org/10.3390/ijerph15061274

Shubina, I. (2018). Locus of control and sense of happiness: A mediating role of self-esteem? In *Applied psychology readings* (pp. 1–16). Springer. https://doi.org/10.1007/978-981-10-8034-0_6

Standing Committee on Public Safety and National Security. (2016). *Healthy minds, safe communities: Supporting our public safety officers through a national strategy for operational stress injuries. Report of the Standing Committee on Public Safety and National Security 2016.* Government of Canada. https://www.parl.gc.ca/HousePublications/Publication.aspx?Mode=1&Parl=42&Ses=1&DocId=8457704&Language=E

Thomas, S. P. (2016). Aggression and violence: Perennial concerns for psychiatric-mental health nursing. *Issues in Mental Health Nursing, 37*, 443–445. https://doi.org/10.1080/01612840.2016.1187507

Ullrich, S., Keers, R., Shaw, J., et al. (2018). Acting on delusions: The role of negative affect in the pathway towards serious violence. *The Journal of Forensic Psychiatry & Psychology, 29*(5), 691–704. https://doi.org/10.1080/14789949.2018.1434227

Volicer, L., Citrome, L., & Volavka, J. (2017). Measurement of agitation and aggression in adult and aged neuropsychiatric patients: Review of definitions and frequently used measurement scales. *CNS Spectrums, 22*(5), 407–414. https://doi.org/10.1017/S1092852917000050

Wahab, W. A., Collinson, K., & Gross, D. W. (2019). Successful management of postictal violence with pindolol in temporal lobe epilepsy. *Epilepsy & Behavior Reports, 12*, 100346. https://doi.org/10.1016/j.ebr.2019.100346

Waller, G., & Reykos, B. (2019). Behavioral interventions in the treatment of eating disorders. *Psychiatric Clinics, 42*(2), 181–191. https://doi.org/10.1016/j.psc.2019.01.002

World Health Organization. (2002). *World report on violence and health: Summary.* Geneva: Author.

Zwelling, M. (2017). *The Vector Poll™—Canadian Federation of Nurses Unions membership poll on patient safety and working conditions: Summary of a poll conducted May 8–19, 2017.* Canadian Federation of Nurses Unions.

24

Interpersonal Violence: Child, Older Persons, and Intimate Partner Abuse

Robert J. Meadus
Originating US chapter by Margaret Jordan Halter

https://evolve.elsevier.com/Canada/Varcarolis/psychiatric/

OBJECTIVES

1. Differentiate anger, aggression, and interpersonal violence.
2. Identify nine types of violence: physical, sexual, psychological, emotional, spiritual, cultural, verbal abuse, financial abuse, and neglect.
3. Discuss the ecological model of violence in terms of etiology of violence (e.g., stresses on the perpetrator, vulnerable person, and environment that could escalate anxiety to the point at which abuse becomes the relief behaviour).
4. Compare and contrast three characteristics of a perpetrator with three characteristics of a vulnerable person.
5. Describe signs of escalating aggression and nursing interventions for de-escalation.
6. Describe four areas to assess when interviewing a person who has experienced violence.
7. Formulate four nursing diagnoses for the survivor of violence, and list supporting data from the assessment.
8. Write out a safety plan with the essential elements for a victim of intimate partner abuse.
9. Compare and contrast primary, secondary, and tertiary levels of intervention, giving two examples of intervention for each level.
10. Discuss three psychotherapeutic modalities that are useful in working with people experiencing violence.

KEY TERMS AND CONCEPTS

abuse
aggression
assault
crisis situation
cultural violence
ecological model
emotional violence
financial abuse
interpersonal violence
neglect
perpetrators
physical violence
primary prevention
psychological violence
safety plan
secondary prevention
sexual violence
spiritual (religious) violence
survivor
tertiary prevention
typology of interpersonal violence
verbal abuse
violence
vulnerable person

According to the World Health Organization (WHO) (Krug et al., 2002), interpersonal violence refers to violence between individuals and is subdivided into family and intimate partner violence (IPV) and community violence. The former category includes child abuse, IPV, and older persons abuse, whereas the latter is broken down into acquaintance and stranger violence and includes youth violence, assault by strangers, **violence** related to property crimes, and violence in workplaces and other institutions. Figure 24.1 illustrates this **typology of interpersonal violence**, identifying four modes of violence that we elaborate on further in this chapter as nine types of violence: physical, sexual, psychological, emotional, spiritual, cultural, verbal abuse, financial abuse, and neglect. **Interpersonal violence** includes child abuse, IPV, and older persons abuse and can involve all nine types of violence. Both acquaintance and stranger experiences of violence are described at the community level.

To be effective in working with victims, the nurse needs an understanding of the conditions for violence, the types of violence, and how the types of violence may be experienced. Fundamental to this entire discussion is self-understanding (see the Self-Assessment section later in the chapter).

CLINICAL PICTURE

Violence is defined by the WHO as "the intentional use of physical force or power, threatened or actual, against oneself, another person, or against a group or community, that either results in or has a high likelihood of resulting in injury, death, psychological harm, maldevelopment or deprivation" (WHO, 2017). The essential element of violence is power and control. Violence is used to establish and maintain power and control over another person and often reflects an imbalance of power between the victim and the abuser. In this way violence may be experienced through expressions of anger, but it is not caused by anger.

Anger can be understood as misunderstood and misaligned emotion that often follows fear, depression, stress, fatigue, or a perceived threat or personal attack. The situation that causes anger (for instance, the perceived threat) is not the problem; rather, the unhealthy response

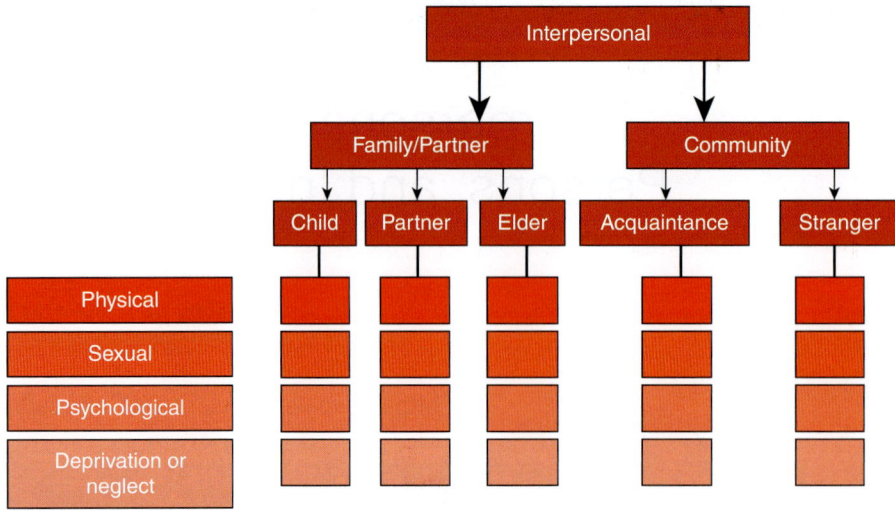

Fig. 24.1 Typology of interpersonal violence. (**Source:** Krug, E. G., Dahlberg, L. L., Mercy, J. A., et al. [Eds.]. [2002]. *World report on violence and health.* Geneva: World Health Organization. Retrieved from http://www.who.int/violence_injury_prevention/violence/world_report/en/.)

to anger is the problem (see Chapter 23 for more on anger and aggression). In How a Nurse Helped Me Rachel's reflection on receiving expert nursing care in a health crisis illustrates how understanding anger amid multiple vulnerabilities can make a difference to both patient experiences and health outcomes.

 HOW A NURSE HELPED ME

Maybe We Can Trust Each Other a Bit More: Understanding Anger Amid Multiple Vulnerabilities

I have diabetes and ended up with a number of problems with my circulation and then landed in hospital with severe pain in my left foot. Tests showed that the vessels to that foot were blocked. No surgery could fix it, so I just took medications, but that didn't always work out because I was in and out of housing and mostly living in the homeless shelter downtown. Then the medication didn't work and my foot slowly blackened, they called it necrotic. When they told me the foot should be amputated, that was the last straw. I just refused. Well, I should say I "lost it," nothing physical, just yelling, it was all I could do, I was so upset. I know they thought I was a problem on the ward; they ended up calling security to watch me like a prisoner or something. But, really, shouldn't we talk about options or at least try other things first? It is hard enough living downtown and trying to stay away from heroin, now they think I should do that with half a leg? But one of the nurses, Nadija, on the hospital ward spent time with me. She really asked about my day-to-day life and how unbalanced things had become for me over the past years without a stable home, money, or family. I will never forget that she really found out about how I was living in the street community. When she said, "It must be hard when your body is also turning on you," well, that was it exactly. My foot was like my family, not coming back. As soon as I thought about it that way, I could face the facts, though. I was able to think about what this would mean for me, for housing and getting around, and made an appointment with my social worker. Nadija said things would be okay, there would be changes, but there would be some help for me. I don't always trust the help out there, but am willing to try. And I didn't totally lose it in the hospital ward, so maybe we can all trust each other a bit more.

Further clarity is also needed concerning the terms *aggression, violence, abuse,* and *assault.* These may sometimes be used interchangeably, though there are particular distinctions regarding clinical and legal requirements and practices. For example, **abuse** is a term used for legal purposes to describe violence perpetrated against children and dependent adults, and the term **assault** is used to describe the intentional threat or application of force to another person (an assault can be physical or sexual in nature) (*Criminal Code*, 1985).

Understanding anger, aggression, cycles of violence, and interventions at multiple levels (individual, interpersonal, community, and societal) with an ecological perspective on violence enables mental health nurses to support patients experiencing relationship violence and to address prevention.

Aggression is an action or behaviour in response to misaligned anger that results in a verbal or physical attack. Aggression tends to be used synonymously with violence. However, aggression is not always inappropriate and is sometimes necessary for self-protection. On the other hand, violence is always an objectionable act that involves intentional use of force that results in, or has the potential to result in, injury to another person.

Effective nursing intervention becomes more difficult when patient anger becomes personal and is directed at the nurse or nursing student or when aggression interrupts functioning and threatens the safety of individuals or communities. In the clinical setting nursing interventions should ideally begin before anger and aggression become a problem. Anxiety is often the precipitant for negative feelings and behaviours. Assessing and responding to this anxiety can have extremely positive returns. Refer to Chapter 12 for interventions to reduce anxiety before it becomes a crisis (with crisis interventions discussed in more detail in Chapter 21).

Violence

Types of Violence

Nine types of violence have been identified: (1) physical, (2) sexual, (3) emotional, (4) psychological, (5) spiritual, (6) cultural, (7) verbal abuse, (8) financial abuse, and (9) neglect. The types of violence are defined in Table 24.1.

TABLE 24.1 Types of Violence

Physical violence	The infliction of physical pain or bodily harm (e.g., slapping, punching, hitting, choking, pushing, restraining, biting, throwing, burning).
Sexual violence	When a person is forced to unwillingly take part in sexual activity. Sexual violence against adults may be referred to as *rape*, or in legal terms as *sexual assault* (see Chapter 25).
Emotional violence	When someone says or does something to make a person feel belittled or worthless.
Psychological violence	When someone uses threats and causes fear in an individual to gain control.
Spiritual (or religious) violence	When someone uses an individual's spiritual beliefs to manipulate, dominate, or control that person.
Cultural violence	When an individual is harmed as a result of practices that are part their culture, religion, or tradition.
Verbal abuse	When someone uses language, whether spoken or written, to cause harm to an individual.
Financial abuse	The withholding of financial support or the illegal or improper exploitation of funds or other resources for one's personal gain.
Neglect	When someone has the responsibility to provide care or assistance for an individual but does not.

The nine types of violence are described in more detail below.

Physical violence. **Physical violence** may be experienced or perpetrated in a number of ways, including:
- Using physical force that results in pain, discomfort, or injury
- Hitting, pinching, hair-pulling, arm-twisting, strangling, burning, stabbing, punching, pushing, slapping, beating, shoving, kicking, choking, biting, force-feeding, or any other rough treatment
- Assault with a weapon or other object
- Threats with a weapon or other object
- Deliberate exposure to severe weather or inappropriate room temperatures
- Murder
- Medication abuse. Inappropriate use of medication, including:
  - Withholding medication
  - Not complying with prescription instructions
  - Overmedication or undermedication
- Restraints abuse:
  - Forcible confinement
  - Excessive, unwarranted, or unnecessary use of physical restraints
  - Forcing a person to remain in bed
  - Unwarranted use of medication to control a person (also called "chemical restraint")

Covert indicators of violence could include minor accidents, especially falls, and a series of minor complaints, such as low energy, fatigue, sleep problems, pain, swollen joints, sore muscles, faintness, dizziness, memory loss, difficulty concentrating, ringing in ears, indigestion, and appetite loss (Loxton et al., 2017; Lutgendorf, 2019). Overt signs of battering include bruises, scars, burns, and other wounds in various stages of healing, particularly around the head, face, chest, arms, abdomen, back, buttocks, and genitalia. Injuries that should arouse the nurse's suspicion are listed in Box 24.1.

If the explanation does not match the injury or if the patient minimizes the seriousness of the injury, abuse may be suspected. Ask directly, but in a non-threatening manner, if the injury has been caused by someone close to the patient. Observe the non-verbal response, such as hesitation or lack of eye contact, as well as the verbal response. Then ask specific questions such as "When was the last time it happened?" "How often does it happen?" "In what ways are you hurt?" Inconsistent explanations serve as a warning that further investigation is necessary. Vague explanations should alert the nurse to possible abuse ("She fell from a chair"; "The hot water was turned on by mistake"). The key to identification is a high index of suspicion.

BOX 24.1 Common Presenting Problems of Victims of Physical Violence

Emergency Department
- Bleeding injuries, especially to head and face
- Internal injuries, concussions, perforated eardrum, abdominal injuries, severe bruising, eye injuries, strangulation marks on neck
- Back injuries
- Broken or fractured jaw, arms, pelvis, ribs, clavicle, legs
- Burns from cigarettes, appliances, scalding liquids, acids
- Psychological trauma, anxiety, attacks of hyperventilation, heart palpitations, severe crying spells, suicidal tendencies
- Miscarriage

Ambulatory Care Settings
- Perforated eardrum, twisted or stiff neck and shoulder muscles, headache
- Depression, stress-related conditions (e.g., insomnia, violent nightmares, anxiety, extreme fatigue, eczema, loss of hair)
- Talk of having "problems" with spouse; describing person as very jealous, impulsive, or an alcohol or drug user
- Repeated visits with new complaints
- Bruises of various ages and specific shapes (fingers, belt)

Any Setting
- Signs of stress due to family violence: emotional, behavioural, school, or sleep problems and increase in aggressive behaviour
- Injuries in a pregnant woman
- Recurrent visits for injuries attributed to being "accident prone"

Non-specific bruising in older children is a common sign of abuse. Any bruises on an infant younger than 6 months of age should be considered suspicious. Non-accidental head injury formerly referred to as *Shaken baby syndrome*, one of the most serious types of child abuse, is the result of the brain moving in the opposite direction as the baby's head (Biswas & Shroff, 2021). A baby who has been shaken may present with respiratory problems, bulging fontanels, and central nervous system damage, resulting in seizures, vomiting, and coma.

Sexual violence. **Sexual violence** may be experienced or perpetrated in several ways, including but not limited to:
- Touching in a sexual manner without consent (i.e., kissing, grabbing, fondling)
- Forced sexual intercourse

- Forcing a person to perform sexual acts that may be degrading or painful
- Beating sexual parts of the body
- Forcing a person to view pornographic material; forcing participation in pornographic filming
- Using a weapon to force compliance
- Exhibitionism
- Making unwelcome sexual comments or jokes; leering behaviour
- Withholding sexual affection
- Denial of a person's sexuality or privacy (watching)
- Denial of sexual information and education
- Humiliating, criticizing, or trying to control a person's sexuality
- Forced prostitution
- Unfounded allegations of promiscuity or infidelity
- Purposefully exposing the person to human immunodeficiency virus (HIV) or other sexually transmitted infections

There are a variety of emotional and behavioural consequences of sexual violence, including depression, anxiety, eating disorders, suicide, aggression, chronic low self-esteem, and post-traumatic stress disorder (PTSD) (Kimber et al., 2020; Rivara et al., 2019). Childhood sexual abuse is a significant factor in the development of depression in many women (Adams et al., 2018). Girls are at higher risk for sexual abuse, although boys may be less likely to report it, and therefore sexual abuse of boys is less recognized and less treated (Manay & Collin-Vezina, 2021).

Emotional violence. Emotional violence occurs when someone says or does something to make a person feel belittled. It includes but is not limited to:
- Name-calling
- Blaming all relationship problems on the person
- Not allowing the person to have contact with family and friends
- Destroying possessions
- Humiliating or making fun of the person
- Recalling a person's past mistakes
- Expressing negative expectations
- Expressing distrust
- Telling a person that they are worthless or a burden

Emotional violence may exist on its own or as a result of co-occurring physical, sexual, or psychological violence or other forms of abuse. Emotional abuse has devastating effects on children. Although it is less obvious and more difficult to assess than physical violence, studies have shown that those who were emotionally abused as children show higher rates of anxiety, depression, interpersonal sensitivity, and dissociation (Public Health Agency of Canada, 2016).

Psychological violence. Psychological violence occurs when someone uses threats and causes fear in a person to gain control. It includes but is not limited to:
- Threatening to harm the person or their family if they leave
- Threatening to harm oneself
- Threats of violence
- Threats of abandonment
- Stalking or criminal harassment
- Socially isolating the person
- Not allowing access to a telephone
- Not allowing a competent person to make decisions
- Inappropriately controlling the person's activities
- Treating a person like a child or a servant
- Withholding important information
- Withholding companionship or affection
- Use of undue pressure to:
  - Sign legal documents
  - Not seek legal assistance or advice
  - Move out of the home
  - Make or change a legal will or beneficiary
  - Make or change an advance health care directive
  - Give money or other possessions to relatives or other caregivers
  - Do things the person does not want to do

Spiritual violence. Spiritual (religious) violence occurs when someone uses a person's spiritual beliefs to manipulate, dominate, or control the person. Spiritual violence includes but is not limited to:
- Not allowing the person to follow their preferred spiritual or religious tradition
- Forcing a spiritual or religious path or practice on another person
- Belittling or making fun of a person's spiritual or religious tradition, beliefs, or practices
- Using one's spiritual or religious position, rituals, or practices to manipulate, dominate, or control a person

Cultural violence. Cultural violence occurs when a person is harmed as a result of practices that are part of their culture, religion, or tradition (Adjei, 2018). It includes but is not limited to:
- Committing "honour" or other crimes against women in some parts of the world, where women especially may be physically harmed, shunned, maimed, or killed for:
  - Falling in love with the "wrong" person
  - Seeking divorce
  - Infidelity; committing adultery
  - Being raped
  - Practising witchcraft
  - Being older

Cultural violence may take place in some of the following ways:
- Lynching or stoning
- Banishment
- Abandonment of an older person at hospital by family
- Genital mutilation
- Rape-marriage
- Sexual slavery
- Murder

Verbal abuse. Verbal abuse occurs when someone uses language, whether spoken or written, to cause harm to a person. It includes but is not limited to:
- Expressing distrust
- Yelling
- Lying
- Name-calling
- Insulting, swearing
- Unreasonably ordering around

Financial abuse. Financial abuse occurs when someone controls a person's financial resources without the person's consent or misuses those resources. It includes but is not limited to:
- Not allowing the person to participate in educational programs
- Forcing the person to work in a certain job
- Refusing to let the person work outside the home or attend school
- Controlling the person's choice of occupation
- Illegally or improperly using a person's money, assets, or property
- Acts of fraud
- Taking funds from the person without permission for one's own use
- Misusing funds through lies, trickery, or controlling or withholding money
- Not allowing access to bank accounts, savings, or other income
- Requiring excessive detailed justification for all money spent
- Persuading the person to buy a product or give away money
- Selling the house or other possessions without permission
- Forging a signature on pension cheques or legal documents
- Misusing a power of attorney, an enduring power of attorney, or a legal guardianship

- Not paying bills
- Opening mail without permission
- Living in a person's home without paying fairly for expenses
- Destroying personal property

Neglect. Neglect is the failure to provide basic needs for a dependant. It can take several forms, including but not limited to:

- Failing to meet the needs of a person who is unable to meet those needs alone
- Abandonment in a public setting
- Not remaining with a person who needs help
- Physical neglect; disregarding necessities of daily living, including failing to provide adequate or necessary:
  - Nutrition or fluids
  - Shelter
  - Clean clothes and linens
  - Social companionship
- Failing to turn a bed-ridden person frequently to prevent stiffness and bedsores
- Medical neglect:
  - Ignoring special dietary requirements
  - Not providing needed medications
  - Not calling a physician; not reporting or taking action on a medical condition, injury, or problem
  - Not being aware of the possible negative effects of medications

Neglected children and older persons often appear undernourished, dirty, and poorly clothed. Neglect is also manifested by inadequate medical care, such as lack of immunizations or untreated medical conditions. Adults who were neglected in childhood are more likely to report current symptoms of anxiety, depression, somatization, psychosis, and hostility than those who were physically abused but did not suffer neglect (Inoue et al., 2021; Poole et al., 2017; Turner et al., 2019).

Cycle of Violence

Dr. Donald Dutton studied the relationship of borderline personality characteristics to the characteristics of both chronic and intermittent family abusers. Dutton (2007) identified three borderline personality characteristics: (1) an unstable sense of self with dependency and fear of abandonment, (2) unstable interpersonal relationships with manipulation, and (3) intense and impulsive behaviours, relating to the cycle of violence perpetrators use to control their partners.

The *cycle of violence*, first proposed by Walker (1979), includes three recurring phases of violence. These phases are characterized by periods of intense violence that tend to increase in severity and frequency, alternating with periods of safety, hope, and trust. Phase I of the borderline, or *cyclic*, personality consists of an internal buildup of tensions as a result of the abuser not knowing how to verbalize inner feelings of dysphoria. The abuser converts dysphoria into abuse through the assertion that it is the partner's fault for not being able to soothe the abuser's bad feelings (Dutton, 1998, 2007). The *tension-building stage* is characterized by relatively minor incidents, such as pushing, shoving, and verbal abuse. During this time, the victim often ignores or accepts the abuse for fear that more severe abuse will follow. Abusers then rationalize that their abusive behaviour is acceptable. As the tension escalates, both participants may try to reduce it. The abuser may try to reduce the tension through the use of alcohol or drugs, and the victim may try to reduce the tension by minimizing the importance of the incidents ("I should have had the house neater … dinner ready"). The abuser may become increasingly demanding. The splitting characteristics of borderline personality become evident, as the abuser sees the partner as "all bad," unloving, unfaithful, and malevolent (Dutton, 1998, 2007). During the *acute battering stage*, the unexpressed rage builds until the abuser with borderline personality releases the built-up tension through brutal beatings. Severe injuries can and do result, driving the victim further away and increasing the abuser's feelings of abandonment. Consequently, the abuser promises anything to get the victim back. The opposite side of splitting here becomes evident, as the abuser describes the victim as "all good" (Dutton, 1998, p. 96). This phase coincides with the *honeymoon stage*, which may be characterized by kindness and loving behaviours. The abuser, at least initially, feels remorseful and apologetic and may bring presents, make promises, and tell the victim how much they are loved and needed. The victim usually believes the promises, feels needed and loved, and drops any legal proceedings or plans to leave that may have been initiated during the acute battering stage.

Unfortunately, without intervention, the cycle will repeat itself. Over time, the periods of calmness and safety become briefer, and the periods of anger and violence increase. With each repetition of the pattern, the victim's self-esteem becomes more and more eroded. The victim either believes that the violence was deserved or accepts the blame for it. This self-blame can lead to feelings of depression, hopelessness, immobilization, and self-deprecation. Figure 24.2 illustrates the cycle of violence.

EPIDEMIOLOGY

Violence within families is among the most important Canadian public health issues and is therefore a significant nursing concern. The abusive behaviours exist within a context in which their purpose is to gain power and control and to induce fear. Abusive behaviour may involve one or more of the types of violence already described and may be inflicted on a child, an intimate partner, an older person, or other populations. While the true prevalence of child, older person, and intimate partner abuse is unknown (because of under-reporting and variability in reporting methods, instruments, sites, and reporters), it is clear that abuse is a significant problem. Notably during the COVID-19 pandemic Canada's Assaulted Women's Helpline and the Ontario Provincial Police reported a spike in domestic-related calls (Thompson, 2021). In April 2020 the Government of Canada provided additional funding of up to 40 million dollars to support services for survivors of violence throughout the provinces and territories. The funding included up to 4 million for sexual assault centres, 10 million for 46 emergency shelters for Indigenous women and their children, and 26 million distributed among Canada's domestic violence (DV) shelters (Moffitt et al., 2020).

Child Abuse

In 2016 the Public Health Agency of Canada estimated 85 440 substantiated child abuse investigations that year (14.19 investigations per 1 000 children). Thirty-four percent identified exposure to IPV as the primary type of abuse, and another 34% identified neglect as the over-riding concern, followed by physical abuse (20%), emotional abuse (9%), and sexual abuse (3%). There was some variation by age and sex in the incidence of investigated abuse, with rates being highest for infants. The rate of family-related sexual offences was more than four times higher for girls than for boys, and the rate of physical assault was similar for girls and boys (Statistics Canada, 2017). According to the Criminal Intelligence Service (Public Health Agency of Canada, 2016), 94% of substantiated investigations involved children whose primary caregiver was a biological parent, and 2% involved children whose primary caregiver was a parent's partner or an adoptive parent. Indigenous and Black children have been identified as a key group to examine because of concerns about their over-representation in the foster care system (Cénat et al., 2021; Pearce et al., 2021). The rate of substantiated child abuse investigations was four times higher in investigations involving Indigenous children than in those involving non-Indigenous children.

Fig. 24.2 The cycle of violence. (**Source:** Mayfield, C. [2016]. *Understanding the cycle of violence.* Retrieved from https://christymayfield.com/understanding-the-cycle-of-violence/)

Intimate Partner Violence

According to Statistics Canada (2021), 107 810 people in Canada were victims of IPV in 2019, representing just over a quarter (30%) of all victims of police-reported violent crime. Violence against spouses and dating partners in current and former relationships is referred to as *intimate partner violence (IPV)* or *domestic violence (DV)*. The definition of spouse includes current or former legally married, separated, divorced, and common-law partners, and the term *dating relationships* includes current or former partners as well as other intimate relationships (i.e., casual sexual relationships or encounters not considered to be committed relationships). In 2019 17% of all police-reported violent crime in Canada was the result of violence victimization from a dating partner, and over a quarter of intimate partner homicides were committed by a boyfriend or girlfriend (Conroy, 2021). Violence within dating relationships was more common than violence within spousal relationships, according to police-reported data. IPV was more likely to be perpetrated by current or former dating partners (36% of victims) than by current or former married or common-law spouses (29% of victims). Over half (53%) of the victims of violence were female, the large majority (79%) of victims of IPV were women. In 2019 the rate of police-reported IPV was 347 victims per 100 000 population with physical assault (75%) being the most common type of violence (Statistics Canada, 2021). Similar to the general crime data reported to police (Moreau et al., 2020), rates of IPV were highest in the prairies and territories. Nunavut had the highest rate of police-reported IPV in Canada (5 249 per 100 000 population), more than five times that of the highest provincial rate (Statistics Canada, 2021).

Women experienced a higher rate of IPV than men in every province and territory. In every province and territory in 2019 the rate of IPV increased from the previous year with the largest provincial increases noted in New Brunswick (NB), British Columbia (BC), and Newfoundland and Labrador (NL). Notably, in the provinces, the rate of IPV was 1.8 times higher in rural areas than urban areas (548 vs. 300 per 100 000), and this pattern was the same for women and men (Statistics Canada, 2021).

According to a report published by the Canadian Femicide Observatory for Justice and Accountability in 2020, 160 women were violently killed in Canada. In 90% of these cases (128) were committed by a current or former intimate partner (Dawson et al., 2020). According to police-reported data, between 2014 and 2019, there were 497 victims of intimate partner homicide, 8 in 10 (80%) of the victims were female. Most (75%) of the victims were killed by a current or former legally married or common-law spouse. About one quarter (26%, 125 victims) of IPV homicide between 2014 and 2019 were Indigenous (Statistics Canada, 2021).

According to Allen (2020), in Canada Indigenous women and girls experience the highest rates of violent and non-violent victimization of all population groups. Even though they are more at risk for spousal violence, many cultural barriers exist that inhibit them from seeking help. Factors reported were inaccessibility of supports and services, mistrust in police, the criminal justice system, and institutions intended to protect (National Inquiry into Missing and Murdered Indigenous Women and Girls, 2019). In many remote communities with Indigenous populations IPV is noted to be 10 times higher than those found in non-Indigenous communities (Allen, 2020). Similarly, Cotter (2021) in a survey report explored the experiences of visible minority women in Canada and IPV. The author found that among this population, Arab (40%), Black (42%), and Latin American women (47%) experienced higher rates of IPV since the age of 15 compared to the total visible minority population (29%).

Older Person Abuse

A recent large-scale 2015 Canadian survey uncovered that about 7.5% of older persons (approximately 695 248) were abused in the previous year. When neglect was added to psychological, physical, sexual, and financial abuse, this number increased to 8.2%, or 766 247 older Canadian persons. Survey respondents were, for the most part, relatively healthy adults in their sixties and early seventies, and very few were ill or identified as frail. Most common was psychological or emotional abuse, affecting 2.7% of older Canadians daily or almost daily and involving repeated criticism, yelling, or insults. Second most common was financial abuse, affecting 2.6% of older persons. Physical abuse was the third most common form of abuse of older persons, affecting 2.2% of older people. Fewer older Canadians reported that they were sexually assaulted, though 1.6% of survey respondents reported being sexually abused in the past 12 months. Finally, 1.2% of older persons were neglected a few times or more in the last year, typically by being denied assistance with housework and meals (Public Health Agency of Canada, 2017).

COMORBIDITY

Common long-term psychological and social effects of abuse include depression, suicidal ideation, chronic post-traumatic stress symptoms, dissociation, interpersonal disturbances, substance use, and revictimization (Adams et al., 2018; Rivara et al., 2019). Family violence is common in the childhood histories of juvenile offenders, runaways, violent criminals, prostitutes, and those who in turn are violent toward others. Exposure to abuse has been associated with decrements in children's optimal development in the areas of social behaviour, academic performance, physical health, and mental health (Public Health Agency of Canada, 2016).

Box 24.2 identifies some of the long-term effects of family violence.

ETIOLOGY

In any form anger, aggression, violence, and abuse profoundly affect individual mental health and well-being. The roots of all forms of violence are founded in the many types of inequality that continue to exist and grow in society, and ecological understanding of causation assists nurses in assessment and planning of interventions at multiple levels. The etiology of anger and aggression also provides a useful framework for mental health nursing practice (refer to Chapter 23).

The Ecological Model of Violence

The WHO adopted an "ecological model" in its *World Report on Violence and Health* to help understand the multi-level, multi-faceted nature of violence (Stewart & Vigod, 2017). As an analytical tool, the ecological model (Figure 24.3) recognizes and identifies personal history and characteristics of the victim or perpetrator, other family members, the immediate social context (often referred to as *community factors*), and the larger society. In contrast to simplistic explanations, the ecological model emphasizes that it is a *combination* of factors, acting at different levels, that influences the risk for and resiliency to violence and the potential for recurrence of abuse. The various factors relevant to the different levels of the ecological model are also affected by the context of the settings children interact with, in their home and family environment, at school, in institutions and workplaces, as well as in their community and broader society.

BOX 24.2 Long-Term Effects of Family Violence

- People involved in family violence are found to have a higher incidence of:
  - Depression
  - Suicidal feelings
  - Self-contempt
  - Inability to trust
  - Inability to develop intimate relationships in later life
- Victims of severe violence are also at higher risk for experiencing recurring symptoms of post-traumatic stress disorder (PTSD):
  - Flashbacks
  - Dissociation—out-of-body experiences
  - Poor self-esteem
  - Compulsive or impulsive behaviours (e.g., substance use, excessive spending, gambling, promiscuity)
  - Multiple somatic complaints
- Children who witness violence in their homes are at greater risk for developing behavioural and emotional problems throughout their lives.
- After the age of 5 or 6, children who witness violence at home show an indication of identifying with the aggressor and losing respect for the victim.
- Some mental and behavioural conditions are associated with childhood abuse or witnessing of abuse:
  - Depressive disorders
  - PTSD
  - Somatic complaints
  - Low self-esteem
  - Phobias (agoraphobia, social and specific phobias)
  - Anti-social behaviours
  - Potential for future child or intimate partner violence
- Adolescent victims or witnesses of abuse are more likely to have behavioural symptoms, such as:
  - Failing grades
  - Difficulty forming relationships
  - Increased incidence of theft, police arrest, and violent behaviours
  - Seductive or promiscuous behaviours
  - Running away from home

Environmental Factors

Violence and abuse occur across all segments of Canadian society. Whereas some risk factors may be unique to a particular type of violence, the various types of violence more commonly share a number of risk factors. Prevailing cultural norms, poverty, social isolation, and such factors as alcohol use, substance use, and access to firearms

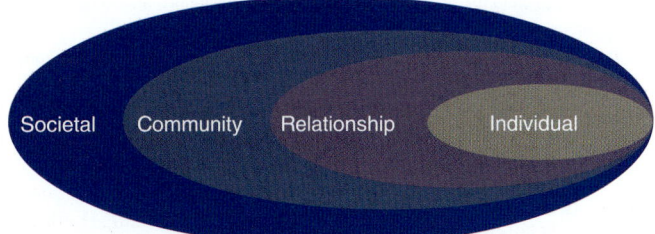

Fig. 24.3 The Ecological Model of Violence. (**Source:** Krug, E. G., Dahlberg, L. L., Mercy, J. A., et al. [Eds.]. [2002]. *World report on violence and health.* Geneva: World Health Organization. Retrieved from https://www.who.int/violence_injury_prevention/violence/world_report/en/)

are risk factors for more than one type of violence (Yakubovich et al., 2018).

The occurrence of abuse requires the following participants and conditions:
- A perpetrator
- Someone who, by age or situation, is vulnerable (e.g., child, woman, older person, mentally ill or physically challenged person)
- A crisis situation

Perpetrator

Perpetrators, those who initiate violence, often consider their own needs to be more important than anyone else's and look to others to meet their needs. The term *perpetrator* applies to any member of a household who is violent toward another member (e.g., children, siblings, same-sex partners, extended family members). Risk factors for those who may become abusive to their children are summarized in Box 24.3.

Control and power are acted out by perpetrators of abuse in all stages of the cycle of violence. The abuse of power and control is the foundational etiology of relationship violence (Figure 24.4 provides an example of IPV perpetrated by a man to a woman), with additional ecological risk and resiliency factors determining the typology. Because of extreme pathological jealousy, many perpetrators of relationship violence refuse to allow their partners to work outside the home; others demand that their partners work in the same place as they do so they can monitor activities and friendships. Many accompany their partners to and from all activities and forbid them to have personal friends or participate in recreational activities outside the home. Even after imposing such restrictions, perpetrators often accuse their partners of infidelity. Many perpetrators maintain their control and possessiveness by controlling the family finances so tightly that there is barely enough money for daily living. Typically, perpetrators believe in male supremacy, being in charge and being dominant. Messages of male dominance are reinforced via observations of the partner dyad, parent–child interactions, peer group experiences, and the influence of the media (Internet, television, movies, comics, computer games).

BOX 24.3 Characteristics of Abusive Parents

- A history of abuse, neglect, or emotional deprivation as a child
- Family authoritarianism: a commitment to raising children as they were raised by their own parents
- Low self-esteem, feelings of worthlessness, depression
- Poor coping skills
- Social isolation (may be suspicious of others): few or no friends, little or no involvement in social or community activities
- Involvement in a crisis situation: unemployment, divorce, financial difficulties
- Rigid, unrealistic expectations of child's behaviour
- History of severe mental illness
- Violent temper outbursts
- Looking to child for satisfaction of need for love, support, and reassurance (often unmet because of parenting deficits in family of origin)
- Projecting blame onto the child for parents' "troubles" (e.g., step-parent may project hostility toward new mate onto a child)
- Lack of effective parenting skills
- Inability to seek help from others
- Perception of the child as bad or evil
- History of drug or alcohol use
- Feeling of little or no control over life
- Low tolerance for frustration
- Poor impulse control

Culturally driven violence against women is a growing problem in Canada's immigrant communities (Okeke-Ihejirika et al., 2020). However, it is important to recognize that a wide variety of cultural norms in Canadian society dictate the dynamics of relationships between intimate partners and child-rearing practices. Learning about the cultural backgrounds of patients can assist health care providers in identifying risk factors and culturally appropriate interventions.

Vulnerable Person

The **vulnerable person** is an adult or child who, as a result of illness, physical condition, or experiences, is at greater risk than the general population for being harmed. The term **survivor** recognizes the recovery and healing process that follows victimization and does not have the connotation of passivity that *victim* has.

Child-bearing persons. Pregnancy may trigger or increase violence (Taillieu et al., 2020). The Public Health Agency of Canada (2016) reported the prevalence of abuse during pregnancy to be 5.7% to 6.6% based on two major studies done in Saskatoon and Toronto. A past history of abuse is one of the strongest predictors of abuse during pregnancy. Other risk factors include social instability (e.g., young, unmarried, failed to complete high school, unemployed, having an unplanned pregnancy), an unhealthy lifestyle (e.g., unhealthy diet, alcohol use, illicit drug use, emotional problems), and physical and psychological health problems (including prescription drug use). Incorporating intimate partner screening into routine pre-natal and post-natal care is recommended to identify families in need of support, and ultimately provide person-centred services to improve outcomes for women and their children (Taillieu et al., 2020).

Children. The Canadian Incidence Study (Public Health Agency of Canada, 2016) found that, in 46% of substantiated child abuse investigations, at least one child functioning issue was indicated. Academic difficulties were the most frequently reported functioning concern (23%), with 11% involving intellectual or developmental disabilities. The second most common functioning concern was depression, anxiety, or withdrawal (19%). Fifteen percent of cases involved child aggression, whereas 14% involved attachment issues. Eleven percent of investigations involved children experiencing attention-deficit disorder (ADD) or attention-deficit/hyperactivity disorder (ADHD). The increased risk for abuse could be due to the added stress of caring for a child with functioning difficulties as well as to the differences between the parents' expectations of their child and the reality of who the child is. Parental substance use is associated with an increase in the risk of exposure to both childhood physical and sexual abuse (Racine et al., 2021). As with relationship violence more broadly, the abuse of power and control and particular risks for child abuse are described in the Duluth model (Figure 24.5).

Older persons. Older person abuse is recognized as a serious problem in Canada. Risk factors for older person abuse include cognitive disability (e.g., Alzheimer's disease) or other mental illness, poor physical health, impairment in the activities of daily living (ADLs), dependency on the caregiver, isolation, stressful events, and a history of intergenerational conflict between the older person and the caregiver (Dominguez et al., 2020; Storey, 2020).

Crisis Situation

Anyone may be at risk for abuse in a **crisis situation**, crises of all kinds contribute to an increased risk for interpersonal violence. Refer to Chapter 21 for more on crisis and crisis intervention.

Fig. 24.4 The Duluth "Power and Control" Wheel. (**Source:** Redrawn from Domestic Abuse Intervention Project [Duluth, MN]. Retrieved from https://www.theduluthmodel.org/training/wheels.html)

APPLICATION OF THE NURSING PROCESS: INTERPERSONAL VIOLENCE

Assessment

General Assessment

It has been increasingly recommended that routine universal screening for both perpetrators and victims of violence be implemented within all manner of health care settings (Registered Nurses' Association of Ontario, 2005/2012; Zakrison et al., 2017). The nurse is often the first point of contact for people experiencing violence and thus is in an ideal position to contribute to prevention, detection, and effective intervention. Organizations need to develop policies that support nursing practice while considering the unique setting where the screening is to take place, patient needs, and outcomes (Paterno & Draughon, 2016).

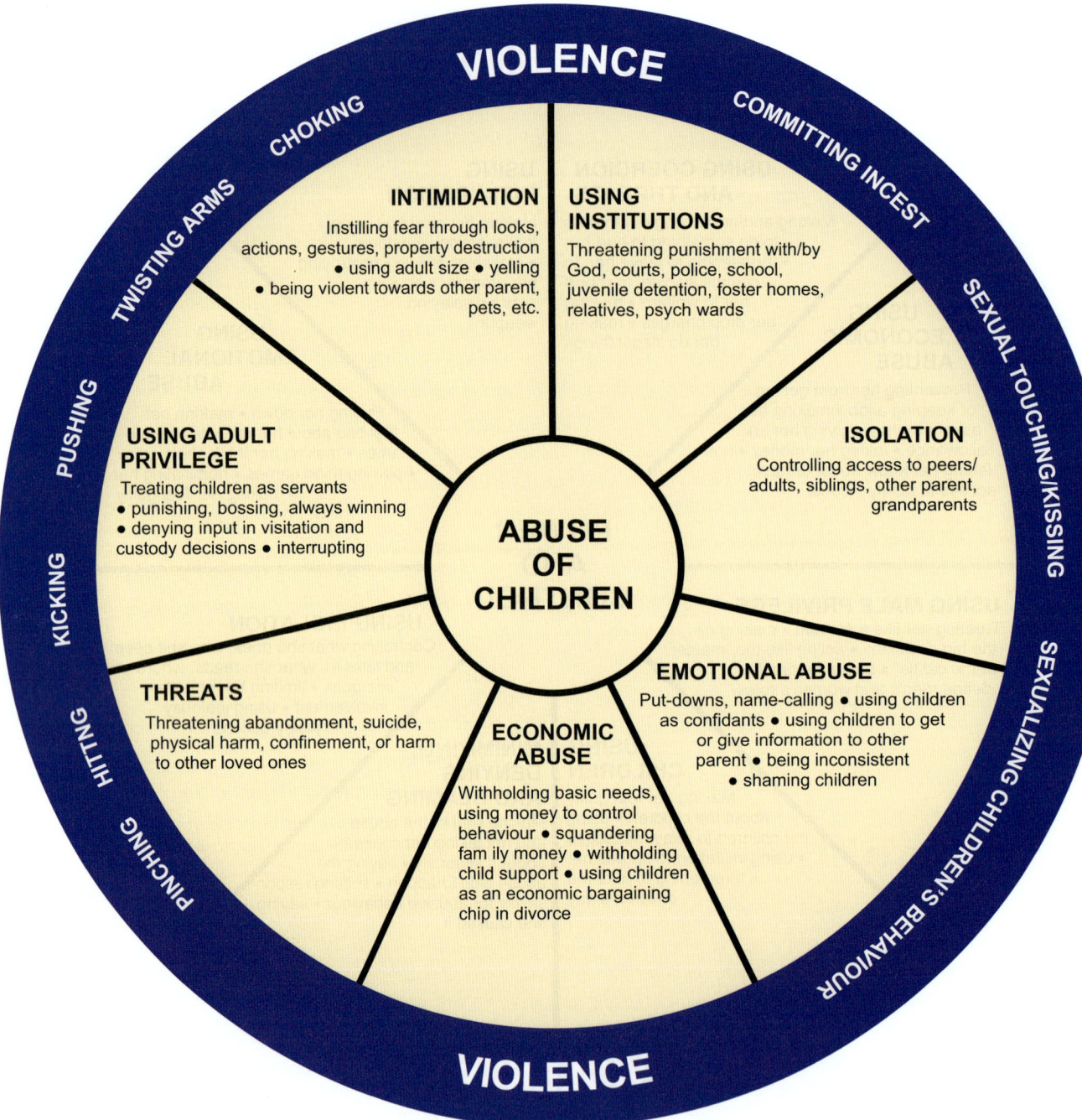

Fig. 24.5 The Duluth "Abuse of Children" Wheel. (**Source:** Redrawn from Domestic Abuse Intervention Project [Duluth, MN]. Retrieved from https://www.theduluthmodel.org/training/wheels.html)

ASSESSMENT GUIDELINES

Interpersonal Violence

During assessment and counselling, maintain an interested and empathetic manner. Assess the following:
- Presenting signs and symptoms of victims of abuse
- Potential indicators of vulnerable parents who might benefit from education and instruction in effective coping techniques
- Physical, sexual, or emotional abuse; neglect; and economic maltreatment of older persons
- Family coping patterns
- Patient's support system
- Drug or alcohol use
- Suicidal or homicidal ideas
- Post-traumatic stress

If the patient is a child or older person, identify the protective services in your province or territory that must be notified.

Effective programs to assess and intervene with violence target specific populations based on the risk and resiliency factors described as part of the clinical picture. Women are just one population considered at risk for violence and abuse (see Research Highlight box).

RESEARCH HIGHLIGHT

A Rural Shelter Adapting to Address the Changing Needs of Women Who Have Experienced Intimate Partner Violence

Problem
Intimate partner violence is recognized as a significant health problem, with shelters providing community-based solutions. Shelters in Canada are mandated to provide a safe place, protection planning, advocacy, and other critical services. However, the role of the shelter is shifting from an inpatient to outpatient focused care model. Women's shelters in rural settings provide services within a specific cultural context that may inhibit access to health and social services because of a lack of services. Identifying and adapting to supportive models and approaches to improve services is necessary to increase longer-term health outcomes and well-being of those experiencing violence.

Purpose of Study
This study explored how the shelter was changing and adapting to a new role of providing services to a rural population of women who had experienced IPV.

Methods
A qualitative case study approach based on a feminist, intersectional framework was used to examine the lived experiences of participants who were shelter service providers (n = 6) and women staying at or utilizing shelter services (n = 4). Each participant completed an audio-recorded semi-structured interview that was divided into four sections: demographics, current status of services, barriers/challenges, and strengths/success. The interviews were transcribed verbatim and thematic inductive content analysis was used to identify emergent themes.

Key Findings
The findings on the changing role of the shelter centered around three themes: filling gaps, case management, and system navigation. Filling gaps involved the need for the shelter to provide services left unaddressed by the current systems. This was envisioned as adaptation of strategies, through relationship building and community mobilization and delivery redesign. Case management was identified due to the increasing complexity of women's lives and health care needs. The final theme system navigation encompassed a new role for staff to help women effectively navigate the system of care services and help find new providers who understood the context of violence within the provision of care.

Implications for Nursing Practice
Nurses in all aspects of practice will be exposed to women who experience intimate partner violence. Nurses' knowledge of resources can facilitate patient referral to community agencies for help, thus reduce intimate partner violence rates. In addition, through provision of care, nurses will help women to manage healthcare and social services access, which leads to better health outcomes. It may be that these models of care will address the barriers and provide an integration of community services for those experiencing IPV.

Source: Mantler, T., & Wolfe, B. (2017). A rural shelter in Ontario adapting to address the changing needs of women who have experienced intimate partner violence: A qualitative study. *Rural and Remote Health, 17*, 1–13. https://doi.org/10.22605/RRH3987

Interview process and setting. Important and relevant information about the family situation can be incorporated into a routine health history process. Because many victims of violence do not disclose abuse the first time they are asked about it, nor do they recognize violence as a health issue, screening for violence among women and their families should occur not only on the initial health history but also each time the health history is updated (Registered Nurses' Association of Ontario, 2005/2012). For screening strategies, refer to Woman Abuse: Screening, Identification and Initial Response at http://rnao.ca/bpg/guidelines/woman-abuse-screening-identification-and-initial-response.

Screening tools use specific terminology that describes the *actions* of perpetrators of violence rather than general terminology such as "abuse." Therefore screening questions need to be clear, and examples of abusive behaviour may be needed to help the patient understand what constitutes abusive behaviour. There are validated tools that can be used in screening (e.g., the Abuse Assessment Screen [AAS], the Abuse Assessment Screen-Disability [AAS-D], the Woman Abuse Screening Tool [WAST]), or nurses can develop their own style, keeping in mind these principles (Registered Nurses' Association of Ontario, 2005/2012). The AAS, developed by the Nursing Research Consortium on Violence and Abuse (McFarlane et al., 2001), has been used extensively to assist in the routine identification of intimate partner abuse (Figure 24.6). More research does need to be conducted, however, on culturally sensitive screening, as well as on screening for male victims, and victims of IPV from the LGBTQ2 community (Arkins et al., 2016; Idriss-Wheeler et al., 2021).

Guiding principles for screening for abuse will assist the nurse in implementing effective interventions. The adapted mnemonic tool ABCD-ER, explained in Box 24.4, outlines the principles.

In the case of suspected child abuse or neglect, it is better to ask about methods of disciplining children rather than to use the words *abuse* or *violence*. Questions that are open-ended and require a descriptive response can be less threatening and elicit more relevant information than questions that are direct or can be answered with *yes* or *no* (see Chapter 10):

- What arrangements do you make when you have to leave your child alone?
- How do you discipline your child?
- When your infant cries for a long time, how do you get them to stop?
- What about your child's behaviour bothers you the most?

Areas to include in any abuse assessment (child, older person, IPV) include: (1) violence indicators, (2) levels of anxiety and coping responses, (3) family coping patterns, (4) support systems, (5) suicide potential, (6) homicide potential, and (7) drug and alcohol use. The vignette about Petra (later in this chapter) illustrates the key points in assessing a person in crisis at the initial interview, with suggested follow-up.

Maintaining accurate records. Documentation is an integral aspect of safe, effective nursing practice and must be comprehensive and legible and accurately reflect screening practice. For more information on documentation, refer to Chapter 7. According to the Registered Nurses' Association of Ontario (2005/2012), the health care record needs to include the following related to aggression and interpersonal violence:

- A safety check
- Direct quotations of what the victim describes
- Direct observations made by the nurse
- Referrals discussed and made, and information given

The record should be non-biased and contain direct observations by the nurse. Non-biased terms such as *chooses*, *declines*, or *patient states* are more appropriate than judgmental terms such as *alleges* or *victim*

1.	**Within the last year**, have you been hit, slapped, kicked, pushed, shoved, or otherwise physically hurt by someone?			YES	NO
	If YES, who? (Circle all that apply)				
	Intimate partner	Care provider	Health professional	Family member	Other
	Please describe: _____				
2.	**Within the last year**, has anyone forced you to have sexual activities?			YES	NO
	If YES, who? (Circle all that apply)				
	Intimate partner	Care provider	Health professional	Family member	Other
	Please describe: _____				
3.	**Within the last year**, has anyone prevented you from using a wheelchair, cane, respirator, or other assistive devices?			YES	NO
	If YES, who? (Circle all that apply)				
	Intimate partner	Care provider	Health professional	Family member	Other
	Please describe: _____				
4.	**Within the last year**, has anyone you depend on refused to help you with an important personal need, such as taking your medicine, getting to the bathroom, getting out of bed, bathing, getting dressed, or getting food or drink?			YES	NO
	If YES, who? (Circle all that apply)				
	Intimate partner	Care provider	Health professional	Family member	Other
	Please describe: _____				

Fig. 24.6 Abuse Assessment Screen. (**Source:** McFarlane, J., Hughes, R. B., Nosek, M. A., et al. (2001). Abuse Assessment Screen-Disability [AAS-D]: Measuring frequency, type, and perpetrator of abuse toward women with physical disabilities. *Journal of Women's Health & Gender-Based Medicine, 10,* 861–866. https://doi.org/doi:10.1089/152460901753285750. The publisher for this copyrighted material is Mary Ann Liebert, Inc. publishers.)

(Middlesex-London Health Unit, 2000). For example, it would be better to record "Patient states, 'My partner beat me'" (non-judgemental) than "Victim alleges they were assaulted by partner" (judgemental).

Referral services and secondary intervention would include more detailed documentation, such as (Middlesex-London Health Unit, 2000):
- Relevant health history
- History of abuse, including the first, worst, and most recent incident
- Where and when the abuse took place
- Name of and relationship to abuser
- Detailed description of injuries (e.g., a body map to indicate size, colour, shape, areas, and types of injuries, with explanations [see Figure 24.6] and photos, if taken)
- Physical evidence of sexual abuse, when possible
- All health care provided and information or referrals to resources provided

When no disclosure of abuse is made, the nurse should document "no disclosure to abuse screening."

Legal, ethical, and professional requirements guide the management of patient records, indicating that they must be carefully maintained (see Chapter 7). Policies and procedures concerning access to the patient's health information need to be developed as part of the screening protocol in all health care settings (Registered Nurses' Association of Ontario, 2005/2012). The patient needs to be informed prior to screening that the interaction will be documented, that the record will be kept confidential, and that it can serve as evidence should legal action be initiated. Even if intervention or legal action does not occur at this time, the record is begun, and the next provider will be aware of the problem and be in a better position to offer support. The vignette illustrates some of the issues related to assessment that are important for reporting and documentation related to a patient experiencing family violence.

BOX 24.4 The Mnemonic Tool ABCD-ER

A—Attitude and Approachability of the health care provider:
- Treat the patient with respect, dignity, and compassion.
- Be sensitive to differences in age, culture, language, ethnicity, and sexual orientation.
- State clearly that abuse is not the fault of the victim but the responsibility of the abuser.
- Reinforce that no one has the right to use physical, sexual, or emotional abuse to control another person's actions.
- Reinforce that physical and sexual abuse are against the law in Canada.
- Convey a non-threatening, non-judgmental stance in words, facial expressions, and body language.
- Express concern for the patient's safety.
- Acknowledge the strength the patient has shown in surviving abuse and disclosing it to you.
- Offer support.
- Avoid excessive criticism of the abuser.

B—Belief in the person's account of their own experience of abuse:
- Show by your words and your actions that you believe the patient's disclosure.
- Remember that the fear of not being believed silences many victims of abuse. Abusers may also convince victims that no one will believe them if they disclose the abuse.
- Help the patient to understand that most of us try to block out memories that are too painful to deal with. A patient disclosing retrospective abuse may not even be sure of exactly what happened or where it happened.
- Reassure and encourage the patient to have confidence in their own perceptions of the abuse.

C—Confidentiality is essential for disclosure:
- Interview in private, without the patient's partner or family members present.
- Use a professional interpreter if one is required, not a friend or family member.
- Tell the patient directly about the policies and procedures used in your practice or institution to protect patient confidentiality.
- Assure the patient that you will not release the information unless they give written permission.
- Outline the exceptions to this pledge of confidentiality: (1) where child abuse or neglect is in question; (2) where the health care provider has reason to fear for the safety of a third party; and (3) where a file is subpoenaed by a court order.
- Let the patient know that you are documenting the information disclosed so that it will help you provide appropriate medical services and referrals and so that it will be available to help the patient later if they should provide you with permission to share it.

D—Documentation:
- Document consistently and legibly.
- Distinguish between your observations and the patient's reports.
- Record information on the first, the worst, and the most recent abusive incident.
- If more than one person has abused the patient, distinguish between the abusers and the specific injuries or health effects of each incident.
- Indicate the frequency of abusive incidents, as well as any increase or decrease in frequency and seriousness.
- Avoid subjective statements and speculations that might undermine the patient's credibility.
- Use the patient's own words, in quotation marks, as frequently as possible.
- Use diagrams and photographs where possible to document physical injuries.

E—Education:
- Educate about abuse and its health effects.
- Help the patient to understand that they are not alone.
- Attempt to engage the patient in long-term continuity of care by offering appropriate referrals and follow-up.
- Know about available community resources and help the patient choose the services they need when ready to seek assistance.
- Display posters, brochures, and other available information about abuse in your office or institution.
- Provide the female patient with information about the abused women's helpline and the male patient with information about the crisis hotline.

R—Respect and Recognition:
- Respect the integrity and autonomy of the patient's life choices.
- Recognize that the patient must deal with the abuse at their own pace directed by their own decisions.
- Recognize that an abused person is an expert about their own abuse and abuser.
- Affirm the patient's strengths and survival skills.
- Do not try to tell the patient what to do but help them understand the options available; the patient must choose the options that will meet their own goals and priorities.
- Offer referrals to other specialized services and follow-up with you.
- Do not label the patient resistant or non-adherent if they decide not to accept your advice; make it clear you respect the patient's right to choose and will continue your support as their caregiver.
- Make sure any medications you offer to help the patient deal with stress or sleep problems do not impair the patient's ability to act appropriately on their own behalf.
- Help the patient to recognize that they cannot control the actions of others; the patient can choose only their own actions.

Source: Adapted from Middlesex-London Health Unit. (2000). *Task force on the health effects of woman abuse—Final report*. London: Author.

VIGNETTE

Petra is brought to the emergency department by ambulance in obvious distress with swollen eyes, lips, and nose, and lacerations to her face. She tells the nurse that her husband had been in bed asleep for hours before she joined him. On getting into bed, she attempted to redistribute the blankets. Suddenly he started punching her in the face and began to throw her against the wall. She called out to her 11-year-old son to call the police. The police arrived, called an ambulance, and took her husband, Dan, to jail. The nurse takes Petra to an individual examination room (to emphasize confidentiality) for a full assessment. She describes the relationship as "stormy" and "bad for a long time."

"Dan is always putting me down and yelling at me," she states. He started hitting her 5 years earlier when she became pregnant with her second and last child. The beatings have increased in intensity over the past year, and this emergency department visit is the fifth this year. Tonight is the first time she has ever called the police.

Petra has visibly lost control. Periods of crying alternate with periods of silence. She appears apathetic and depressed. The nurse remains calm and objective. After Petra has finished talking, the nurse explores alternatives designed to help her reduce the danger once she is discharged: "I'm concerned that you will be hurt again if you go home. What options do you have?" Acknowledging the escalating intensity of the violence, Petra is able to make arrangements with a shelter to take in her and her two children until after she has secured a restraining order. The nurse charts the abuse referrals. The keeping of careful and complete records helps to ensure that Petra will receive proper follow-up care and the documentation will assist her when and if she pursues legal action.

Self-Assessment

Self-reflection assists nurses in all areas of practice to identify the values and biases that underscore their approach and interventions in response to those experiencing abuse (Registered Nurses' Association of Ontario, 2005/2012). Strong negative feelings can cloud one's judgement and interfere with objective assessment and intervention, no matter how well we try to cover or deny personal bias. Common responses of health care providers to violence are listed in Table 24.2.

Since nursing is largely made up of women and women are more commonly the targets of abuse, it has been suggested that many nurses have experienced or are experiencing violence at the hands of their intimate partners (Registered Nurses' Association of Ontario, 2005/2012). Nurses need to become aware of their reactions by gaining insight into their own somatic signals of distress (Unrau et al., 2017). Supervision and multi-disciplinary team conferences can be especially helpful in clarifying reactions, neutralizing intense emotions, and reducing feelings of isolation and discomfort.

Level of Anxiety and Coping Responses

Non-verbal responses to the assessment interview can be indicative of the victim's anxiety level (see Chapter 12). Agitation and anxiety bordering on panic are often present in victims of violence. Abused individuals live under conditions of chronic stress, which can lead to health effects such as heart disease or heart attack, arthritis, fibromyalgia, asthma, stroke (Chandan et al., 2019; Peer et al., 2020), and cervical cancer (Alcala et al., 2017). Coping mechanisms to endure living in violent and terrifying situations may take the form of flawed beliefs or myths (Table 24.3).

TABLE 24.2 Common Responses of Health Care Providers to Violence

Response	Source
Anger	Anger may be felt toward the person responsible for the abuse, toward those who allowed it to happen, and toward society for condoning its occurrence through attitudes, traditions, and laws.
Embarrassment	The victim may be a symbol of something close to home: the nurse may have experienced abuse.
Confusion	One's view of the family as a haven of safety and privacy is challenged.
Fear	A small percentage of perpetrators are dangerous to others.
Helplessness	The nurse may want to do more, eliminate the problem, or cure the victim, perpetrator, or both.
Discouragement	Discouragement may result if no long-term solution is achieved.
"Blame the victim" mentality	Health care workers can get caught up in "blaming the victim" for behaviours they see as provoking the abuse. There is never an excuse for abuse, and no one has the right to hurt another person. "Blaming the victim" can occur when health care providers feel overwhelmed. Supervision is essential for therapeutic intervention.

TABLE 24.3 Myth Versus Fact: Interpersonal Violence

Myth	Fact
Ninety-five percent of intimate partner violence victims are women.	In statistical self-reports equal proportions of men and women reported being victims of spousal violence during the preceding 5 years, about 342 000 women and 418 000 men across the provinces (Statistics Canada, 2017).
The victim's behaviour often causes violence.	The victim's behaviour is *not* the cause of the violence. Violence is the perpetrator's pattern of behaviour, and the victim cannot learn how to control it.
Intimate partner abuse is a minor problem.	There is a *real* danger that victims may be killed by abusive partners.
Victims of intimate partner abuse could leave if they really wanted to.	Numerous factors influence a decision to stay or leave, including fear of injury or death, financial dependence, and welfare of children.
Interpersonal violence is most prevalent in poorly educated people from poor, working-class backgrounds.	Interpersonal violence occurs in all socioeconomic, religious, cultural, and educational backgrounds.
Family matters are private, and families should be allowed to take care of their own problems.	Intervention in interpersonal violence within families is justified; violence always escalates in frequency and intensity, can end in death, and is passed on to future generations.
Victims of violence tacitly accept the abuse by trying to conceal it, by not reporting it, or by failing to seek help.	When attempting to disclose their situation, many victims are met with disbelief, which discourages them from persevering.
Myths that victims commonly believe include: "I can't live without them." "If I hadn't done _____, it wouldn't have happened." "They will change." "I stay for the sake of the children."	These myths are coping mechanisms used to allay panic in a situation of random and brutal violence. They give the illusion of control and rationality.
Alcohol and stress are the major causes of physical and verbal abuse.	There are no excuses, violence is not acceptable behaviour. Aggression and violence are learned behaviours, not uncontrollable reactions. People are violent because they have acquired the belief that aggression is an acceptable and effective response to anger and a sense of lack of control.

Family Coping Patterns

Consistent with a view of the intergenerational nature of the conditions and contexts of trauma, all forms of violence occurring in families of origin are predictive of future relationship violence (Antle et al., 2019). Altering the pattern of violence against women can affect child abuse because the main predictor of violence toward children is violence toward their mothers. However, it is important for the nurse to be nonjudgmental and to assess family strengths as well as styles of coping and stressors. Attitudes about child-rearing and discipline, including how parents were disciplined as children, may provide insight into violence and abuse in the home.

Living with and caring for children and older persons can cause frustration, anger, and stress. If there is no relief, the caregiver may become overwhelmed, lose control, and abuse the child or the older person (Public Health Agency of Canada, 2016; Valimaki et al., 2020). Box 24.5 is a useful guide for assessing the risk for child or older person abuse in the home.

Support Systems

In the case of older person abuse risk factors include dependency on the caregiver for basic needs, isolation, limited or lack of access to support systems, and a history of intergenerational conflict between the older person and the caregiver (Pine & Steffen, 2019). Assessment of the support system is crucial to identification of risk and resiliency factors. Children's support system options are especially limited, as are those of people who are physically and mentally challenged. Assessment for support systems should focus on intrapersonal, interpersonal, and community resources (e.g., the school system for school-aged victims).

Suicide Potential

A suicide attempt may be the presenting symptom in the emergency department. With sensitive questioning conducted in a caring manner, the nurse can elicit the history of violence. A person experiencing violence may feel desperate to leave yet be trapped in a detrimental relationship, and suicide may seem like the only option. The threat of suicide may also be used by an emotionally abusive person in an attempt to manipulate the victim into caving in to demands ("Don't leave me or I'll kill myself"; "I took all my pills … . I said I would the next time you were late").

Often the means of attempted suicide is overdose with a combination of alcohol and other central nervous system depressants, or sleeping medications that have been prescribed in previous visits to physicians' offices, clinics, or emergency departments. Refer to Chapter 22 for more on suicide.

Homicide Potential

At a minimum, the nurse should inquire about the patient's current safety risks and possible safety strategies. Because victims of abuse often underestimate the risk, using a tool such as the Danger Assessment (Campbell et al., 2009) can be useful in helping victims to think about risk (for more information, see https://www.dangerassessment.org).

Individuals victimized by violence should be asked if they have ever felt like killing the perpetrator and, if so, whether they have the current desire and means to do so. If the answer is yes, intervention is required.

Drug and Alcohol Use

There is a high rate of co-occurrence of victimization and substance use among women (Radcliffe et al., 2019). A person experiencing violence may self-medicate with alcohol or other drugs as a way of escaping an intolerable situation. The drugs are usually central nervous system depressants (e.g., benzodiazepines) prescribed by physicians in response to the patient's presentation with vague complaints, which are often stress related (e.g., insomnia, gastrointestinal upsets, anxiety). The degree of intoxication can be determined by history, physical examination, and blood alcohol level. Refer to Chapter 18 for information on how to assess for a chronic alcohol or drug problem.

> **SAFETY TIP**
>
> Nurses working with the perpetrator either during home visitation or within a health facility should assess for potential violence, de-escalate the situation, and always have door access to exit safely and quickly.

Diagnosis

Nursing diagnoses are focused on the underlying causes and symptoms of family violence.

Table 24.4 lists potential nursing diagnoses for abuse.

The identification of desired outcomes and the design of nursing interventions that facilitate achieving those outcomes should be developed as much as possible in collaboration with the survivor and a primary support person. These outcomes should be continually

---

BOX 24.5 Factors to Assess During a Home Visit

For a Child
- Responsiveness to infant's signals
- Caregiver's facial expressions in response to infant
- Playfulness of caregiver with infant
- Nature of physical contact during feeding and other caretaking activities
- Temperament of infant
- Caregiver's history of harsh discipline or abuse as a child
- Parental attitudes:
  - Feelings of inadequacy as a parent
  - Unrealistic expectations of child
  - Fear of "doing something wrong"
  - Attribution of negative qualities to newborn
  - Misdirected anger
  - Continued evidence of isolation, apathy, anger, frustration
  - Adult conflict
- Environmental conditions:
  - Sleeping arrangements
  - Child management
  - Home management
  - Use of supports (formal and informal)
- Need for immediate services for situational (e.g., economics, child care), emotional, or educational information:
  - Information about hotlines, babysitters, homemakers, parent groups
  - Information about child development
  - Information about child care and home management services

For an Older Person
- Absence of or lack of access to basic necessities (e.g., food, water, medications)
- Unsafe housing
- Lack of or inadequate utilities, ventilation, space
- Poor physical hygiene
- Lack of necessary assistive devices (e.g., hearing aids, eyeglasses, wheelchair)
- Medication mismanagement (outdated prescriptions, unmarked bottles)

TABLE 24.4 Potential Nursing Diagnoses for Family Violence

Signs and Symptoms	Potential Nursing Diagnoses
Bruises, cuts, broken bones, lacerations, scars, burns, wounds in various phases of healing, particularly when explanations do not match injury or explanations are vague	Risk for injury Acute pain Chronic pain Risk for infection Impaired skin integrity Risk for post-traumatic stress
Isolation, fear, feelings of shame, low self-esteem, feelings of worthlessness, depression, feelings of helplessness	Powerlessness Ineffective coping Fear Risk for self-directed violence Chronic low self-esteem Situational low self-esteem Hopelessness Spiritual distress
Vaginal–anal bruises, sores, discharge, peritoneal pain, positive test results for sexually transmitted infections	Rape-trauma syndrome Risk for infection

TABLE 24.5 NOC Outcomes for Interpersonal Violence

Nursing Outcome and Definition	Short-Term and Intermediate Indicators
Abuse cessation: Evidence that the victim is no longer hurt or exploited	Evidence that physical abuse has ceased Evidence that emotional abuse has ceased Evidence that sexual abuse has ceased
Abuse recovery: Physical: Extent of healing of physical injuries due to abuse	Timely treatment of injuries Healing of physical injuries Resolution of physical health problems
Abuse recovery: Financial: Extent of control of monetary and legal matters following financial exploitation	Control of social security and pension income Protection of financial resources Control of withdrawal of money from account(s)
Abusive behaviour self-restraint: Self-restraint of abusive and neglectful behaviours toward others	Obtains needed treatment Controls impulses Discusses the abusive behaviour

NOC, Nursing Outcomes Classification.
Source: Data from Moorhead, S., Johnson, M., Maas, M. L., et al. (2013). *Nursing Outcomes Classification (NOC)* (5th ed.). St. Louis: Elsevier.

---

reassessed and revised as new information about the survivor's needs emerges. A comprehensive plan can also guide the actions of the multidisciplinary team.

Outcomes Identification

The *Nursing Outcomes Classification (NOC)* (Moorhead et al., 2018) identifies the following indicators for the outcome of *Abuse cessation,* defined as "evidence that the victim is no longer hurt or exploited":

- Physical abuse has ceased.
- Emotional abuse has ceased.
- Sexual abuse has ceased.
- Financial exploitation has ceased.

NOC offers other abuse-specific outcomes, including Abuse protection, Abuse recovery, Abuse recovery: Emotional, Abuse recovery: Financial, Abuse recovery: Physical, and Abuse recovery: Sexual. In addition, outcomes focused on improved coping, self-esteem, social support, and pain control, to name a few, are appropriate for these patients.

Table 24.5 provides some specific outcome criteria, along with short-term and intermediate indicators for victims of child, intimate partner, and older person abuse, as well as for the abuser.

Planning

Nurses and other health care workers encounter abuse frequently, not only in health care settings but also in their communities and families. Most hospitals and community centres provide protocols for dealing with child, intimate partner, or older person abuse, but these protocols may or may not meet all the needs of a given patient.

Unless the case is one of child abuse in which the child has been removed from the home, most interventions performed after necessary emergency care will take place within the community. Plans should centre on the patient's safety first. The nurse must ascertain whether the survivor is in danger for their life, either from suicide or homicide, and, if there are children involved, whether they are in danger (Jack et al., 2017).

Whenever it is possible or in the best interests of the patient, plans should be discussed with the patient. Planning should also take into consideration the needs of the abuser(s) (e.g., parents, caretakers, spouse, or partner), if they are willing to learn alternatives to abuse and violence.

Implementation

Interventions for those experiencing interpersonal violence are distinct from interventions for anger and aggression, though at times there may be overlapping concerns (reporting, debriefing, counselling, and so on). Anger management interventions concentrate on the distortions and misalignment of the expression of anger. In contrast, interventions for interpersonal violence focus on relationship power imbalances. Interventions for interpersonal violence are discussed below.

Reporting Abuse

There is no mandatory obligation to report abuse of a woman to the police. It is the woman's right to choose if she wishes to have police involvement, and she must consent to this involvement prior to the nurse's initiating contact with authorities (Registered Nurses' Association of Ontario, 2005/2012). According to provincial or territorial legislation, any suspected or actual cases of child abuse must be reported to the official social service agency. For example, under NL's *Children, Youth and Families Act* (2019), in accordance with section 11 every person in the province has a legal obligation to immediately report suspected abuse and neglect for children (under age 16) and youth (ages 16 and 17) to ensure children and youth are protected from harm.

Child witnesses to abuse may be reportable to the provincial or territorial social service agency, as proximity to such events can represent a condition of harm for the child (Registered Nurses' Association of Ontario, 2005/2012). Nurses are advised to consult their local social service agency to discuss individual situations, and all health care organizations need to have a protocol in place with their local social service agency.

The Canadian *Criminal Code* provides the legislation necessary to deal with physical, sexual, and financial abuse of older persons (Government of Canada, Department of Justice, 2021). In addition, provincial and territorial legislation addresses abuse and reporting. For example, some jurisdictions in Canada now enforce mandatory reporting of abuse of older persons, particularly of abuse in residential care facilities, but several others do not. Nova Scotia and NL have general mandatory reporting requirements in their adult protection legislation, placing a general social responsibility on all citizens to report suspected abuse or neglect. Alberta, Manitoba, and Ontario now have special legislation for the protection of persons in care, and laws in Prince Edward Island, NB, Saskatchewan, and BC provide for voluntary reporting for specific forms of abuse and neglect of older persons.

Elder abuse requires both intervention and prevention measures (Elder Abuse Prevention Ontario, 2021). Competency may be a consideration in a situation of older person abuse. Competent older persons have the right to self-determination. Unless the individual is found to be incompetent, help can be offered but cannot be forced on the person. In Canada there is no general test of competency. The definition of competency varies across legislations, institutions, agencies, and provinces and territories (McDonald & Collins, 2000). However, it can be generally defined as a person's ability to understand the situation they are in and the decisions that have to be made about that situation (McDonald & Collins, 2000). The legal determination of incompetency is a last resort because it dramatically changes the rights of an individual. For this reason, it is important that the least restrictive approaches be taken before attempting to have an older person declared incompetent.

Nurses must be cognizant of the cultural diversity of the populations with which they work (see Chapter 8). The term *cultural diversity* in this instance is used broadly and may be derived from one's race, ethnicity, class, religious or spiritual beliefs, age, ability, or sexual orientation (Registered Nurses' Association of Ontario, 2005/2012). The nurse must be aware of the cultural issues of those experiencing abuse, as such issues may affect the survivor's response to violence and to intervention. The nurse is responsible for developing a communication plan to make the survivor an informed partner in the provision of care. Nurses need to check their provincial practice standards for the provision of culturally sensitive care.

Counselling

Counselling includes crisis intervention measures. It is important to emphasize that people have a right to live without fear of violence, physical harm, or assault. Powerful statements such as "Abuse is never right "and "No one deserves to be abused" will display unconditional acceptance and positive regard (Reeves, 2015).

All individuals experiencing abuse should be counselled about developing a *safety plan*, a plan for a rapid escape when abuse recurs. Nurses should be aware that safety is never guaranteed, nor can the most detailed safety plan ensure that the violence will end (Registered Nurses' Association of Ontario, 2005/2012). The victim experiencing violence is ultimately the only one who can reliably predict the risks and the likelihood for further violence, and therefore the best plan is the victim's own plan, one that is viewed by the victim as achievable and one that the victim has a personal commitment to follow (Middlesex-London Health Unit, 2000). The nurse should suggest packing the items listed in Box 24.6 ahead of time. The packed bag should be kept in a place where the perpetrator will not find it.

If the abused person chooses to leave, shelters or safe houses are available in many communities in Canada. They are open 24 hours a day and can be reached through crisis hotline information numbers, hospital emergency departments, YWCA, diverse faith-based groups, or the local office of the National Council of Women of Canada.

BOX 24.6 Personalized Safety Guide

Suggestions for Increasing Safety While in the Relationship

- I will have important phone numbers available to my children and myself.
- I can tell _____ and _____ about the violence and ask them to call the police if they hear suspicious noises coming from my home.
- If I leave my home, I can go to (list four places) _____, _____, _____, or _____.
- I can leave extra money, car keys, clothes, and copies of documents with _____.
- If I leave, I will bring items _____ (e.g., identification, birth certificates, social insurance card, school and medical records, health insurance card, money, bank books, credit cards).
- To ensure safety and independence, I can keep my cellphone battery charged or have another phone available, open my own savings account, rehearse my escape route with a support person, and review my safety plan on _____ (date).

Suggestions for Increasing Safety When the Relationship Is Over

- I can change the locks and install steel or metal doors, a security system, smoke detectors, and an outside lighting system.
- I will inform _____ and _____ that my partner no longer lives with me and ask them to call the police if they are observed near my home or my children.
- I will tell people who take care of my children the names of those who have permission to pick them up. The people who have permission are _____, _____, and _____.
- I can tell _____ at work about my situation and ask _____ to screen my calls.
- I can avoid stores, banks, and _____ that I used when living with my battering partner.
- I can obtain a restraining order from _____. I can keep it on or near me at all times, as well as have a copy with _____.
- If I feel down and ready to return to a potentially abusive situation, I can call _____ for support or attend workshops and groups to gain support and strengthen my relationships with other people.

Important Phone Numbers

- Police _____
- Crisis hotline _____
- Family _____
- Friends _____
- Shelter _____

Besides offering protection for individuals and families in crisis, many of these shelters and safe houses offer important education, counselling, and transitional housing services. Patients should be given the number of the nearest available shelter, even if they decide for the present to stay with their partners. Referral phone numbers may be kept for years before the decision to call is made. Having the number and a contact person during that time contributes to thinking about options.

Case Management

Nurses working in outpatient and community mental health settings have the opportunity to coordinate community, medical, criminal justice, and social services to provide comprehensive assistance to families in crisis. Strategies must encompass needs for household necessities, child care, stability in providing basic needs, economic stability, physical and emotional safety, counselling, legal protection, career development or job training, education, ongoing support groups, and health care. Safe and affordable housing is often crucial to the person's ability to break free (Daoud et al., 2016). A nurse functioning in a case manager role can assist the patient in choosing the best options and coordinating the interventions of several agencies. Box 24.7 lists selected *Nursing Interventions Classification (NIC)* interventions for *Abuse protection support* for children, intimate partners, and older persons (Bulechek et al., 2013).

Milieu Management

Interventions are geared toward stabilizing the home situation and maintaining an abuse-free environment. Some mental health programs have caseworkers or clinicians who visit the home instead of requiring the family to go to the agency. Providing and maintaining a therapeutic environment in the home ideally involves three levels of help for abusive families:

1. Provides the family with economic support, job opportunities, and social services
2. Arranges social support in the form of a public health nurse, day care teacher, schoolteacher, social worker, respite worker, or any other potential contact person who has a good relationship with the family
3. Encourages and provides family therapy

Promotion of Self-Care Activities

Nurses can help victims of abuse to find hope and view themselves as "survivors," which emphasizes agency and choices, identifies strengths, and attributes more responsibility to them over aspects of their lives that are under their control (Flasch et al., 2017). Reimagining their own capacities to choose and act may empower survivors to find options and ultimately take steps to leave the abusive relationship. Czerny et al., (2018) found that women were able to promote the health of their families after leaving an abusive partner. Therefore offering hope, identifying strengths, and displaying confidence that the person can take care of themselves are important aspects of nursing care. Referrals regarding crisis counselling, emergency housing, or financial assistance, as well as legal and vocational counselling, should be made available to each patient. Referrals to parenting resources that explore alternative approaches to physical discipline of children in their care may also be appropriate.

Health Teaching and Health Promotion

Health teaching and health promotion include meeting with the individual, caregiver, and family to discuss the cycle of violence, associated risk factors, and situations that might trigger violence. Other nursing interventions can include teaching about healthy relationships and healthy sexuality, which may be especially important to children who have no role models.

Nurses who work on maternity units and in public health departments are often in a position to identify risk factors for abuse and initiate appropriate interventions, including education about effective parenting, caregiving, and coping techniques, as well as information

---

BOX 24.7 Interventions for Abuse Protection Support for Children, Intimate Partners, and Older Persons

Abuse Protection Support: Children

Definition of abuse protection support: children*:* Identification of high-risk, dependent child relationships and actions to prevent possible or further infliction of physical, sexual, or emotional harm, or neglect of basic necessities of life.
Activities[a]:
- Identify mothers who have a history of late (4 months or later) or no prenatal care.
- Identify parents who have had another child removed from the home or have placed previous children with relatives for extended periods.
- Identify parents with a history of domestic violence or a mother who has a history of numerous "accidental" injuries.
- Determine whether a child demonstrates signs of physical abuse, including numerous injuries in various stages of healing; unexplained bruises and welts; unexplained pattern, immersion, and friction burns; facial, spiral, shaft, or multiple fractures; unexplained facial lacerations and abrasions, and so on.
- Encourage admission of child for further observation and investigation as appropriate.
- Monitor parent–child interactions and record observations.
- Report suspected abuse or neglect to proper authorities in compliance with mandatory reporting laws.

Abuse Protection Support: Intimate Partners

Definition of abuse protection support: intimate partners*:* Identification of high-risk, dependent domestic relationships and action to prevent possible or further infliction of physical, sexual, or emotional harm or exploitation of a domestic partner.
Activities[a]:
- Screen for risk factors associated with IPV (e.g., history of domestic violence, abuse, rejection, excessive criticism, or feelings of being worthless and unloved; difficulty trusting others or feeling disliked by others; feeling that asking for help is an indication of personal incompetence; high physical care needs; intense family care responsibilities; substance use; depression; major psychiatric illness; social isolation; poor relationships between domestic partners; multiple marriages; pregnancy; poverty; unemployment; financial dependence; homelessness; infidelity; divorce; or death of a loved one).
- Document evidence of physical or sexual abuse using standardized assessment tools and photographs.
- Listen attentively to individual who begins to talk about own problems.
- Encourage admission to a hospital for further observation and investigation, as appropriate.
- Provide positive affirmation of worth.

Abuse Protection Support: Older Persons

Definition of abuse protection support: older persons*:* Identification of high-risk, dependent older person relationships and actions to prevent possible or further infliction of physical, sexual, or emotional harm; neglect of basic necessities of life; or exploitation.
Activities[a]:
- Identify older patients who perceive themselves to be dependent on caretakers due to impaired health status, functional impairment, limited economic resources, depression, substance use, or lack of knowledge of available resources and alternatives for care.
- Identify family caretakers who have a childhood history of abuse or neglect.
- Monitor patient–caretaker interactions and record observations.
- Report suspected abuse or neglect to proper authorities in compliance with mandatory reporting laws.

[a]Partial list.
Source: Adapted from Bulechek, G. M., Butcher, H. K., Dochterman, J. M., et al. (2013). *Nursing Interventions Classification (NIC)* (6th ed.). St. Louis: Mosby.

for nurturing healthy relationships. Information about these interventions should be shared with the patient's health care team for appropriate monitoring and follow-up in the community. Assessment of risk and resiliency factors is essential to the implementation of health-promoting activities. For example, parents who are at particular risk for abusing a child include:

- New parents whose behaviour toward the infant is rejecting, hostile, or indifferent
- Teenage parents who require special help in handling the baby, have difficulty discussing their expectations of caring for the child, or lack support systems
- Parents with cognitive deficits, for whom careful, explicit, and repeated instructions on caring for the child and recognizing the infant's needs are indicated
- Parents who grew up observing family violence (a significant risk factor for perpetuation of family violence)

Nurses can often recognize when children are at risk and make referrals to community resources, including emergency child care facilities, emergency telephone numbers, numbers of 24-hour crisis centres or hotlines, and respite programs for parents to have some relief from child care. Community and public health nurses can make home visits to identify risk factors for abuse in the crucial first few months of life, during which the style of parent–child interactions is established. See Box 24.5 for important factors for the community health nurse to assess during a home care visit. Such observations made by nurses in clinic and public health settings are fundamental in case finding and evaluation.

Prevention of Abuse

Primary prevention. **Primary prevention** consists of measures taken to prevent the occurrence of abuse. Identifying individuals and families at high risk, providing health teaching, and coordinating supportive services to prevent crises are examples of primary prevention. Specific strategies include (1) reducing stress, (2) reducing the influence of risk factors, (3) increasing social support, (4) increasing coping skills, and (5) increasing self-esteem. In particular, reducing the risk for the different forms of child abuse can contribute to reducing the repeated conditions and patterns of violence and abuse from generation to generation (Isobel et al., 2019). The most promising strategies for preventing child abuse include home visitation and parent education programs (Levey et al., 2017).

Community and public health nurses are in a unique position to assess family functioning in the home over time, which allows for assessment of changes (see Case Study and Nursing Care Plan 24.1). They are also in an excellent position to connect those at risk (such as people with addictions) to appropriate resources in the community that can meet their needs. All nurses can advocate for social policy change to improve the coordination of health, justice, and social services, thereby enhancing the health care response to abuse (Registered Nurses' Association of Ontario, 2005/2012).

Secondary prevention. **Secondary prevention** involves early intervention in abusive situations to minimize their disabling or long-term effects. Nurses can establish universal screening programs in all health care settings for individuals at risk, assist in treating any injuries resulting from abuse, and coordinate community referrals to provide continuity of care (Registered Nurses' Association of Ontario, 2005/2012). Stress, depression, low self-esteem, and social isolation can be addressed by providing supportive psychotherapy, psychoeducation, support groups, pharmacotherapy, and contact information for community resources. Caregiver burden can be reduced by arranging assistance in caregiving, nursing, or housekeeping or, if necessary, by placing the person in a different home or health care facility. For some, support through criminal proceedings may be important to prevent revictimization. Refer to the *Trauma-informed Practice Guide* from the BC Provincial Mental Health and Substance Use Planning Council (2013) at http://bccewh.bc.ca/wp-content/uploads/2012/05/2013_TIP-Guide.pdf. The Sheldon Kennedy Child Advocacy Centre, based in Calgary, Alberta, is another organization concerned with all levels of child abuse prevention, including community education and training to prevent revictimization and interrupt the potential cycle of violence from generation to generation. The vignette illustrates a successful secondary prevention effort.

> ### VIGNETTE
>
> George, aged 4 years, is brought to the physician's office by 25-year-old Asha, the child's nanny, with second-degree burns on his right hand. Asha is the nanny for George, his younger brother, Tyrone, aged 2, and older brother Logan, aged 6. Asha appears apprehensive and says she is very concerned. Asha tells the nurse that the children have told her in the past that their mother has threatened them with burning if they do not behave. George told her that his mother once held his hands on a cold stove element and told him that if he was bad, she would turn it on and burn him. Asha is shocked that George's mother would do such a thing, but at the same time, she says she feels guilty for "telling on Ms. J."
>
> Asha also states that the older brother, Logan, told her what happened to George but was afraid that if his mother found out, she would burn him also. Asha says she is aware that the mother hits the children, but she did not believe that anyone would burn her own child. The nurse reports the incident to the physician, and the mother is called and asked to come to the office. Meanwhile, the nurse asks Asha to stay with George while she examines him. George appears frightened and in pain.
>
> **Nurse:** "Tell me about your hand, George." *(George looks down and starts to cry.)* "It's okay if you don't want to talk about it, George."
> **George:** *(Does not look at the nurse and speaks softly.)* "My mommy burned my hand on the stove."
> **Nurse:** "Tell me what happened before that."
> **George:** "Mommy was mad because I didn't put my toys away."
> **Nurse:** "What does your mommy usually do when she gets mad?"
> **George:** "She yells mostly. Sometimes she hits us. Mommy is going to be so mad at Logan for telling."
> **Nurse:** "Tell me about the hitting."
> **George:** "Mommy hits us a lot since Daddy left." *(George starts to cry to himself.)*
>
> On examination, the nurse notices on George's right palm a ringed pattern of burns resembling the burner on an electric stove. There are blisters on his fingers. George appears well nourished and properly dressed. He is at his approximate developmental age except for some language delay. Because of the physical evidence and history, there is strong suspicion of child abuse. The provincial social service agency is notified, and the family situation is evaluated for possible placement of George in foster care. The initial evaluation concludes that there is no indication of serious potential harm to the child and that George should return home. The mother, who is initially defensive, starts to cry and states, "I can't cope with being alone, and I don't know where to turn."
>
> Nursing interventions centre on caring for George's immediate health needs, finding supports for the mother to help her cope with crises, providing a counselling referral for the mother to learn alternative ways of expressing anger and frustration, informing the mother of parents' groups, providing referrals to play groups or day care for the children to help increase their feelings of self-esteem and security, and providing a break and instruction in parenting for the mother.

Tertiary prevention. **Tertiary prevention**, which often occurs in mental health care settings, involves nurses facilitating the healing and rehabilitative process by counselling individuals and families, providing support for groups of survivors, and assisting survivors of violence to achieve their optimal level of safety, health, and well-being.

Examples of tertiary prevention include psychological therapies for abused children; screening and support services for victims of intimate partner, domestic, or family violence; and specific recognition of the needs of survivors of torture.

Advanced-Practice Interventions

Individual psychotherapy. The goals of individual therapy for a survivor are empowerment, the ability to recognize and choose productive life options, and the development of a solid sense of self. Survivors of abuse may choose individual therapy to address symptoms of depression, anxiety, somatization, or PTSD. Many of the psychological symptoms shown by women who have been abused can be understood as complex survival strategies and responses to violence. This constellation of symptoms, such as fear and a perceived inability to escape, has been referred to as battered woman syndrome in legal proceedings (Glancy et al., 2019).

Nurses must address the guilt, shame, and stigmatization experienced by survivors of abuse (dos Reis et al., 2017). It is helpful for nurses to understand that the patient's feelings and behaviours may reflect those of the grieving process since the survivor has experienced numerous losses as a result of the abusive relationship.

Programs for perpetrators of abuse are still associated with the justice system and are mandated interventions rather than voluntary and desirable community services for batterers. Although court-mandated treatment tends to be the most effective for perpetrators, it is critical that the DV movement make assistance for perpetrators of abuse more readily available so as to shift societal norms to encourage and promote voluntary help-seeking behaviours (Idriss-Wheeler et al., 2021). The perpetrator needs to seek help for issues concerning power and control. Refer to the Duluth model "Power and Control" wheel (Figure 24.4) and "Equality" wheel (Figure 24.7), which are standard frameworks for violence education.

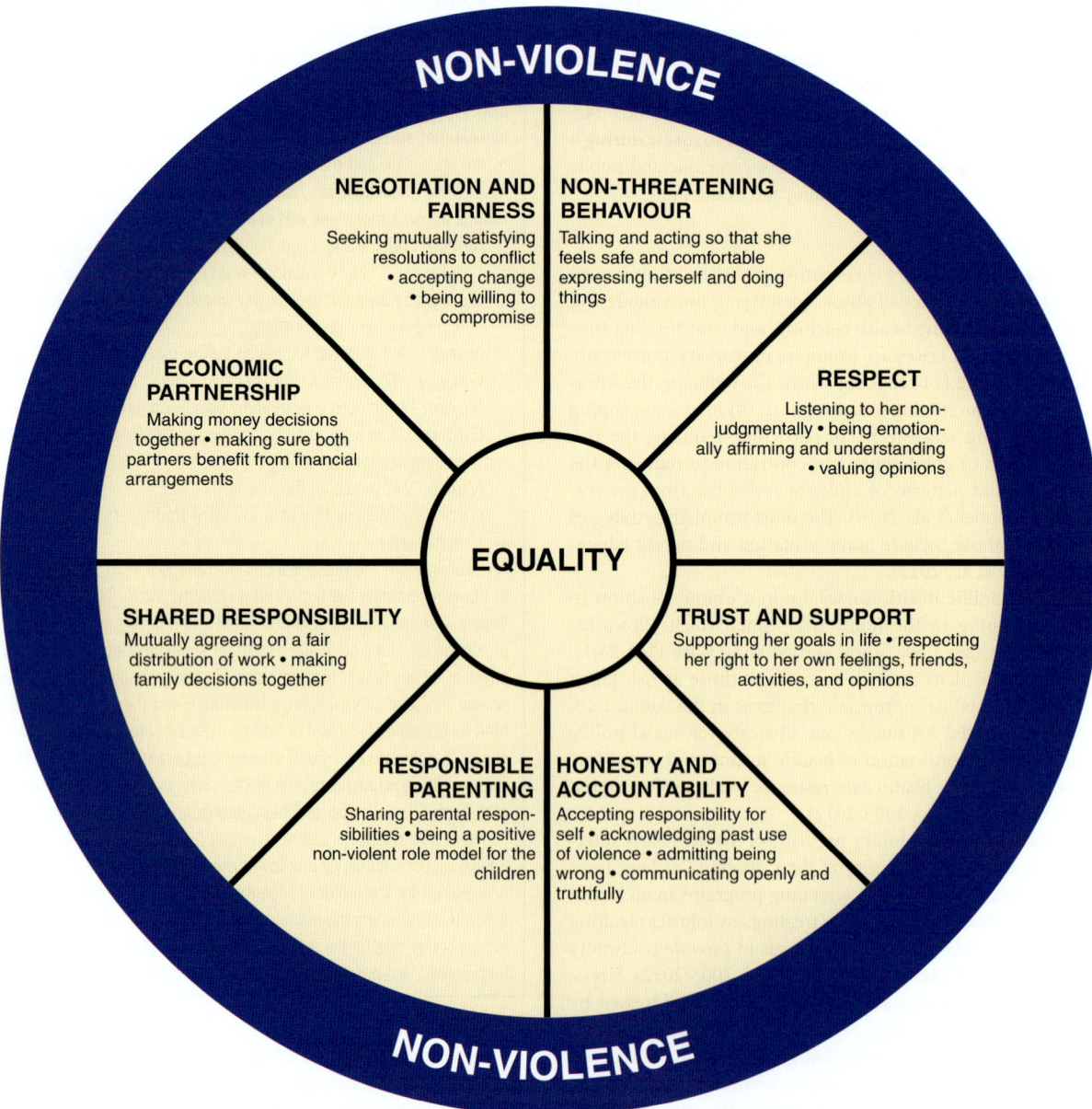

Fig. 24.7 The Duluth "Equality" Wheel. (**Source:** Redrawn from Domestic Abuse Intervention Project [Duluth, MN]. Retrieved from https://www.theduluthmodel.org/training/wheels.html.)

Nurses engaged in therapy with perpetrators of abuse have a duty to warn potential victims if they conclude that the perpetrator is a danger. Refer to Chapter 7 for a more detailed discussion of the duty to warn and the duty to protect.

Family psychotherapy. Because abuse is a symptom of a family in crisis, each member of the family system needs attention. Also, because change in one member of the family system affects the whole system, all members need support and understanding. Dialectical behavioural therapy (DBT) has been proven to be effective in treating individuals and families with histories of abuse by teaching emotion regulation, interpersonal skills, mindfulness, and distress tolerance skills (Bohus et al., 2019). Family or marital therapy should take place *only* if the perpetrator has had individual therapy and has demonstrated change as a result and if both parties agree to participate.

Expected outcomes are that the perpetrator will recognize destructive patterns of behaviour and learn alternative responses. Intermediate goals are that members of the family will openly communicate and learn to listen to each other. Refer to the Duluth model "Nurturing Children" wheel (Figure 24.8), which is a standard framework for the care of children in families with histories of abuse. Refer to Chapter 34 for a more detailed discussion of family therapy.

Group psychotherapy. Group therapy offers a powerful way to counter self-denigrating beliefs and to confront issues of secrecy and stigmatization while decreasing isolation, improving self-esteem, and

Fig. 24.8 The Duluth "Nurturing Children" Wheel. (**Source:** Redrawn from Domestic Abuse Intervention Project [Duluth, MN]. Retrieved from https://www.theduluthmodel.org/training/wheels.html)

increasing the potential for realistic problem solving (De La Rosa & Riva, 2021). Also, the therapeutic factor of universality, or the discovery that others have had similar experiences, may be beneficial, especially for child survivors. DBT has been used in groups with abusers to teach emotion regulation, interpersonal, mindfulness, and distress tolerance skills (Moore et al., 2018).

Emotion regulation skills are taught to manage intense labile moods, interpersonal skills are taught to develop assertiveness and problem-solving skills, mindfulness is taught for meditation, and distress tolerance skills are taught to learn how to tolerate and accept distress as a part of normal life (Horta Esper & Gherardi-Donato, 2019). Group therapy can help create a community of healing and restoration. Refer to Chapter 33 for a more detailed discussion of group therapy.

Evaluation

The failure of interventions with abusive families often is due to problems within the health, social, economic, and political systems. Nurses must act at all levels by lobbying for (1) better education about violence and abuse, (2) resources in health care settings to support more effective responses to violence and abuse, (3) better collaboration across all sectors, and (4) the development of policies on understanding the dynamics of violence in such areas as social assistance and child welfare (Ford-Gilboe et al., 2011). Nurses can play a powerful role in lobbying against factors that promote violence (such as media that depict violence, gender or racial inequity, and devaluing of older persons).

The evaluation of brief interventions can be based on whether the survivor acknowledges the violence, is willing to accept intervention, and removes themselves from the abusive situation. The ultimate outcome of long-term interventions and follow-up is to end the violence and to empower the survivor to lead a productive and safe life without the haunting memories of abuse. Because abuse is a symptom of a family in crisis, diagnosis, interventions, and evaluation should be carried out by a multi-disciplinary team that includes a physician, a nurse, a social worker, a lawyer, and perhaps a psychiatrist.

CASE STUDY AND NURSING CARE PLAN 24.1
Family Violence

Mrs. Tran, a recently widowed 84-year-old woman, moved into her son's apartment 3 months ago. She had been living in her third-floor walk-up in the city. Because of her declining health, crime in the neighbourhood, and the need to climb three flights of stairs, with her son Chien's encouragement, she went to live with him. He and his wife, Kim, who have been married for almost 20 years, have five children 6 to 18 years of age, all living in a rather cramped three-bedroom apartment.

Mrs. Tran is being cared for by a nurse from the Victorian Order of Nurses (VON), who monitors her blood pressure and adjusts her medication. Over a series of visits, the nurse, Ms. Grohl, notices that Mrs. Tran is looking unkempt, pale, and withdrawn. While taking her blood pressure, Ms. Grohl observes bruises on Mrs. Tran's arms and neck. When questioned about the bruises, Mrs. Tran appears anxious and nervous. She says that she slipped in the bathroom. Mrs. Tran becomes increasingly apprehensive and stiffens in her chair when her daughter-in-law, Kim, comes into the room to ask when the next visit will be. The nurse notices that Kim avoids eye contact with Mrs. Tran.

When the injuries are brought to Kim's attention, she responds by becoming angry and agitated, blaming Mrs. Tran for causing so many problems. She will not explain the reason for the change in Mrs. Tran's behaviour or the origin of the bruises to the nurse. She merely comments, "I have had to give up my job since my mother-in-law came here. It's been difficult and crowded ever since she moved in. The kids are complaining. We are having trouble making ends meet since I gave up my job. And my husband is no help at all."

Assessment

Self-Assessment

Ms. Grohl has worked in a number of situations with violent families, but this is the first time she has encountered older person abuse. She discusses her reactions with the other team members. She is especially angry at Kim, although she is able to understand the daughter-in-law's frustration. The team concurs with Ms. Grohl that there seems to be potential for positive change in this family. If abuse does not abate, more drastic measures will need to be taken and legal services contacted.

Objective Data	Subjective Data
Physical symptoms of violence (bruises, unkempt appearance, withdrawn attitude)	Mrs. Tran states she slipped in the bathroom, but physical findings do not support this explanation.
Stressful, crowded living conditions	Kim states, "It's been difficult and crowded ever since she moved in."
No eye contact between Mrs. Tran and her daughter-in-law	Mrs. Tran exhibits withdrawn and apprehensive behaviour in the presence of Kim.
Economic hardships leading to stress	
No support for the daughter-in-law from the rest of the family for care of Mrs. Tran	

Diagnosis

On the basis of the data, the nurse formulates the following nursing diagnoses:
1. *Risk for injury* related to increase in family stress, as evidenced by signs of violence

Supporting Data

- Statement by Mrs. Tran that she slipped in the bathroom, but physical findings do not support this explanation
- Physical symptoms of violence (bruises, unkempt appearance, withdrawn attitude)
- Stressful, crowded living conditions

2. *Ineffective coping* related to helplessness, as evidenced by inability to meet role expectations

CHAPTER 24 Interpersonal Violence: Child, Older Persons, and Intimate Partner Abuse

CASE STUDY AND NURSING CARE PLAN 24.1—cont'd
Family Violence

Supporting Data
- Unkempt, anxious, depressed
- Withdrawn and apprehensive behaviour
3. *Risk for other-directed violence* related to increased stressors within a short period, as evidenced by probable older person abuse and feelings of helplessness verbalized by the primary caregiver

Supporting Data
- Kim states, "It's been difficult and crowded ever since she moved in."
- No eye contact between Kim and Mrs. Tran
- Signs and symptoms of physical abuse on Mrs. Tran
- Kim says, "My husband is no help at all."
4. *Caregiver role strain* related to extreme feelings of being overwhelmed and feeling helpless

Supporting Data
- Family not helping with care of mother-in-law; burden of care on Kim
- Economic hardships, leading to stress when Kim gave up her job to care for Mrs. Tran

Outcomes Identification
Abuse cessation: Evidence that the victim is no longer hurt or exploited

Short-term indicators
- Evidence that physical abuse has ceased
- Evidence that emotional abuse has ceased

Planning
Ms. Grohl discusses several possible outcomes with members of her team, giving attention to the priority of outcomes and to whether they are realistic in this situation. She also plans to report the older person abuse to law enforcement and to work with Mrs. Tran, Kim, and the rest of the family to improve this situation for everyone.

Implementation
Mrs. Tran's plan of care is personalized as follows:
Nursing diagnosis: *Risk for injury* related to increase in family stress, as evidenced by signs of violence
Outcome: Abuse cessation

Short-Term Goal	Interventions	Rationale	Evaluation
1. On each visit made by the nurse, the patient will state that abuse has decreased, using a scale from 1 to 5 (1 being the least abuse).	1a. Follow provincial laws and guidelines for reporting older person abuse.	1a. Provides maximum protection under the law. Provides data for future use.	**Goal Met** Patient states that after family talked to the nurse and planned strategies, physical abuse no longer occurs.
	1b. Assess severity of signs and symptoms of abuse.	1b. Accurate charting (body map, pictures with permission, verbatim statements) helps follow progress and provides legal data.	
	1c. Do a careful home assessment to identify other areas of abuse and neglect. Identify community resources that could help the older person and caregivers.	1c. Check for inadequacy of food, presence of vermin, blocked stairways, medication safety issues, and so on—all indicate abuse and neglect.	
	1d. Identify community resources that could help the older person and caregivers to manage care at home.	1d. Determining the kinds of problems in the home and identifying available resources help with planning appropriate intervention.	
	1e. Discuss with patient factors leading to abuse and concern for safety.	1e. Allows for identification of family stressors and potential areas for intervention. Validates that situation is serious and increases patient's knowledge base.	

Continued

CASE STUDY AND NURSING CARE PLAN 24.1—cont'd
Family Violence

Short-Term Goal	Interventions	Rationale	Evaluation
2. Within 2 weeks, patient will be able to identify at least two supportive services to deal with emergency situations.	2. Discuss with patient supportive services such as crisis hotlines and 911 to call in case of emergency situations.	2. Maximizes patient's safety through use of support systems.	**Goal Met** Patient has been talking to two old friends she had stopped talking to because of shame and depression. She has called the crisis hotline once to get information on transportation to the older person centre in town.
3. Within 3 weeks, family members will be able to identify difficult issues that increase their stress levels.	3. Discuss with family members their feelings, and identify at least four areas that are most difficult for the various family members.	3. Listening to each family member and identifying unmet needs helps both family and nurse identify areas that require changing and appropriate interventions.	**Goal Met** Family members identify areas of increased stress, such as overwork, lack of free time, lack of privacy, and financial difficulties.
4. Within 3 weeks, family will seek out community resources to help with anger management, need for homemaker support, and other needs.	4. Identify potential community supports, skills training, respite places, homemakers, financial aids, and so on that might help meet family's unmet needs.	4. When stressed, individuals solve problems poorly and do not know about or cannot manage to organize outside help. Finances may be controlled by the perpetrator or become unmanageable in the crisis stages of abuse.	**Goal Met** The daughter-in-law is glad to get out of the house for anger management classes, and the son states he will try to take on more responsibility, but he often feels guilty and angry, too. Reluctantly, the son and his wife agree to try a support group with other caregivers in similar situations.

Evaluation

Eight weeks after Ms. Grohl's initial visit, Mrs. Tran appears well groomed, friendly, and more spontaneous in her conversation. She comments, "Things are better with my daughter-in-law." No bruises or other signs of physical violence are noticeable. She is considerably more outgoing and has even taken the initiative to contact an old friend. Mrs. Tran has talked openly to her son and daughter-in-law about stress in the family. Mrs. Tran says that she went for a walk when her daughter-in-law appeared tense and returned to find that the tension had lessened. Neither Mrs. Tran nor her family has initiated plans for alternative housing.

Moorhead, S., Swanson, E., Johnson, M., & Maas, M. (Eds.). (2018). *Nursing Outcomes Classification (NOC): Measurement of health outcomes* (6th ed.). St. Louis: Elsevier.

KEY POINTS TO REMEMBER

- Abuse can occur in any family and can be predicted with some accuracy by examining the risk and resiliency factors related to the characteristics of perpetrators, vulnerable people, and crisis situations in which violence is likely.
- Abuse can be physical, sexual, psychological or emotional, or economic or can be caused by deprivation or neglect.
- The cycle of violence includes three recurring phases of violence (tension building, acute battering, and honeymoon stages), which often increase in severity and frequency.
- Assessment includes identifying indicators of abuse, levels of anxiety, coping mechanisms, support systems, and suicide and homicide potential, as well as alcohol and drug use.
- Reporting abuse to the police is a matter of provincial legislation. Nurses should be aware that in cases involving abuse of adults, violence is something that competent adults must choose to self-report. Nurses are responsible for reporting abuse of children, dependent adults, and older persons to authorities, though the particular standards of reporting vary among provinces and territories. Awareness of these standards is the responsibility of the nurse.
- Interventions for victims or perpetrators of violence depend on the level of crisis and are focused on planning strategies to remove the individual and family members from violent situations and preventing abuse from recurring. Support and crisis intervention are key nursing interventions.

CRITICAL THINKING

1. A colleague who has witnessed a child being abused states, "I don't think it's any of our business what people do in the privacy of their own homes."
   a. What are you legally required to do?
   b. What are your ethical responsibilities?
2. Congratulations! You successfully convinced your colleagues to assess routinely for abuse. Now they want to know how to do it. How would you go about teaching them to assess for child abuse? Intimate partner abuse? Older person abuse?
3. Your health care organization's routine health screening form for adolescents, adults, and older persons has just been changed to include questions about family abuse. How would you respond to patients who indicate on this form that abuse occurs in their home?
4. Write out a safety plan that could be adopted by individuals who are being abused.
   a. Identify at least four referrals in your community for an abused person.

b. Identify two referrals in your community for a violent person, partner, or parent.
5. What would the nurse screen for when a young, visibly upset pregnant woman attends a prenatal outpatient clinic with multiple bruises on her upper arms?

CHAPTER REVIEW

1. A man becomes frustrated when his children cry repeatedly and he shoves his wife into the refrigerator. His wife explains to the neighbour, who witnessed this, that "I should have made the children go to bed earlier so they wouldn't be so cranky." This event is an example of:
   a. Masochism
   b. Emotional abuse
   c. Tension reduction
   d. Secondary prevention
2. Which statements about perpetrators and victims of abuse are accurate? **Select all that apply**.
   a. Approximately 40% of victims of intimate partner and family abuse are male.
   b. Abusive behaviour is usually the result of intoxication or stress.
   c. Perpetrators tend to respond best to treatment if it is court ordered.
   d. Victims do not report abuse because they tacitly are accepting of it.
   e. Victims of abuse stay in the relationship because they really do not want to leave.
   f. Disruptive behaviour may make older persons with dementia vulnerable to abuse.
3. A staff nurse, Chandra, is assisting a 30-year-old victim of domestic violence in the emergency department. The patient suffered numerous bruises and abrasions, is reluctant to be examined, seems very ashamed, and is very fearful that the Children's Aid Society will take custody of her young daughter, who has not been assaulted and is safe, if the police become involved. Which intervention is indicated?
   a. Report the assault to the police since reporting domestic violence is mandatory.
   b. Probe the patient for information to use as evidence in prosecuting the perpetrator.
   c. Press the patient to disrobe so that she can be examined for signs of hidden injuries.
   d. Guide and assist the patient to develop a safety plan for rapid escape should abuse recur.
4. Ms. Patel, a student nurse, is assigned to a patient recovering from injuries received during an episode of domestic violence, the third such assault for which she has received treatment. Ms. Patel left home at age 17 to escape an abusive father. Which statements about this situation are accurate? **Select all that apply**.
   a. Ms. Patel may be prone to blame the patient for her injuries and abuse.
   b. Ms. Patel's personal experiences give her special insight into the needs of this patient.
   c. Ms. Patel's experiences are likely to make her more empathic toward victims.
   d. Caring for victims of abuse will help Ms. Patel cope with her own abuse experiences.
   e. Ms. Patel may experience overwhelming anguish as a result of caring for abuse victims.
   f. Ms. Patel would likely benefit from clinical supervision related to caring for abuse victims.
5. Perpetrators of domestic violence tend to: **(Select all that apply)**
   a. Belong to lower socioeconomic groups and be poorly educated
   b. Have relatively poor social skills and have grown up with poor role models
   c. Believe that they, if male, should be dominant and in charge in relationships
   d. Force their mates to work and expect them to support the family
   e. Be controlling and willing to use force to maintain their power in relationships
   f. Prevent their mates from having relationships and activities outside the family

REFERENCES

Adams, J., Mrug, S., & Knight, D. C. (2018). Characteristics of child physical and sexual abuse as predictors of psychopathology. *Child Abuse & Neglect, 86,* 167–177. https://doi.org/10.1016/j.chiabu.2018.09.019

Adjei, S. B. (2018). "Correcting an erring wife is normal": Moral discourses of spousal violence in Ghana. *Journal of Interpersonal Violence, 33*(12), 1871–1892. https://doi.org/10.1177/0886260515619751

Alcala, H., Mitchell, E., & Keim-Malpass, J. (2017). Adverse childhood experiences and cervical cancer screening. *Journal of Women's Health, 26*(1), 36–43. Retrieved from https://www150.statcan.gc.ca/n1/pub/85-002-x/2020001/article/00013-eng.htm

Allen, M. (2020). *Crime reported by police serving areas where the majority of the population is Indigenous, 2018* (Catalogue no. 85-002-x). Juristat. Statistics Canada. Retrieved from https://www150.statcan.gc.ca/n1/pub/85-002-x/2020001/article/00013-eng.htm

Antle, B., Karam, E. A., Barbee, A. P., et al. (2019). Intergenerational transmission of intimate partner violence and its impact on adolescent relationship attitudes: A qualitative study. *Journal of Loss and Trauma, 25,* 1–21. https://doi.org/10.1080/15325024.2019.1634894

Arkins, B., Begley, C., & Higgins, A. (2016). Measures for screening for intimate partner violence: A systematic review. *Journal of Psychiatric and Mental Health Nursing, 23*(3–4), 217–235. https://doi.org/10.1111/jpm.12289

BC Provincial Mental Health and Substance Use Planning Council. (2013). *Trauma-informed practice guide*. Retrieved from http://bccewh.bc.ca/wp-content/uploads/2012/05/2013_TIP-Guide.pdf

Biswas, A., & Shroff, M. (2021). Abusive head trauma: Canadian and global perspectives. *Pediatric Radiology, 51,* 876–882. Retrieved from https://link-springer-com.que2a-proxy.mun.ca/article/10.1007%2Fs00247-020-04844-5

Bohus, M., Schmahl, C., Fydrich, T., et al. (2019). A research programme to evaluate DBT-PTSD, a modular treatment approach for complex PTSD after childhood abuse. *Borderline Personality Disorder and Emotion Dysregulation, 6,* 7. https://www.doi.org.10.1186/s40479-019-0099-y

Bulechek, G. M., Butcher, H. K., Dochterman, J. M., et al. (2013). *Nursing Interventions Classification (NIC)* (6th ed.). St. Louis: Mosby.

Campbell, J. C., Webster, D. W., & Glass, N. E. (2009). The danger assessment: Validation of a lethality risk assessment instrument for intimate partner femicide. *Journal of Interpersonal Violence, 24,* 653–674. https://doi.org/10.1177/0886260508317180

Cénat, J. M., Noorishad, P. G., Czechowski, K., et al. (2021). The seven reasons why Black children are overrepresented in the child welfare system in Ontario (Canada): A qualitative study from the perspectives of caseworkers and community facilitators. *Child and Adolescent Social Work Journal.* https://doi.org/10.1177/0886260519888515

Chandan, J. S., Thomas, T., Raza, K., et al. (2019). Intimate partner violence and the risk of developing fibromyalgia and chronic fatigue syndrome. *Journal of Interpersonal Violence, 36*(21–22), NP12279–NP12298. https://doi.org/10.1177/0886260519888515

Conroy, S. (2021). *Family violence in Canada: A statistical profile, 2019* (Catalogue no. 85-002-X). Juristat. Statistics Canada. Retrieved from https://www150.statcan.gc.ca/n1/daily-quotidien/210302/dq210302d-eng.htm

Cotter, A. (2021). *Intimate partner violence: Experiences of visible minority women in Canada, 2018* (Catalogue no. 85-002-x). Juristat. Statistics Canada. Retrieved from https://www150.statcan.gc.ca/n1/pub/85-002-x/2021001/article/00008-eng.htm

Criminal Code, R.S.C. (1985, *c. C-46). Assault.* Retrieved from https://laws-lois.justice.gc.ca/PDF/C-46.pdf

Czerny, A. B., Lassiter, P. S., & Lim, J. H. (2018). Post-abuse boundary renegotiation: Healing and reclaiming self after intimate partner violence. *Journal of Mental Health Counseling, 40*(3), 211–225. https://doi.org/10.17744/mehc.40.3.03

Daoud, N., Matheson, F. I., Pedersen, C., et al. (2016). Pathways and trajectories linking housing instability and poor health among low-income women experiencing intimate partner violence (IPV): Toward a conceptual framework. *Women and Health, 56*(2), 208–225. https://doi.org/10.1080/03630242.2015.1086465

Dawson, M., Sutton, D., Jaffe, P., et al. (2020). *One is too many: 10 years of domestic homicides in Canada: Canadian domestic homicide prevention initiative with vulnerable populations.* Canada Domestic Homicide Prevention Initiative-University of Guelph. Retrieved from http://www.CDHPI.ca

De La Rosa, S., & Riva, M. T. (2021). Relationship variables in group psychotherapy for women sexual trauma survivors. *The International Journal of Group Psychotherapy, 71*(1), 144–179. https://doi.org/10.1080/00207284.2020.1772072

Dominguez, S. F., Valiquette, J., Storey, J. E., Glorney, E., et al. (2020). Elder abuse detection and intervention: Challenges for professionals and strategies for engagement from a Canadian specialist service. *Journal of Forensic Nursing, 16*(4), 199–206. https://doi.org/10.1097/JFN.0000000000000301

Dos Reis, J. M., Lopes, M. H. B. M., Osis, M. J. D., et al. (2017). "It's much worse than dying": The experiences of female victims of sexual violence. *Journal of Clinical Nursing, 26*(15–16), 2353–2361. https://doi.org/10.1111/jocn.13247

Dutton, D. G. (1998). *The abusive personality.* New York: Guilford Press.

Dutton, D. G. (2007). *The abusive personality: Violence and control in intimate relationships* (2nd ed.). New York: Guilford Press.

Elder Abuse Prevention Ontario. (2021). *Elder abuse response guide.* Retrieved from https://eapon.ca/wp-content/uploads/2021/09/EAPO_ReponseGuideScreeningChart_2021.pdf

Flasch, P., Murray, C. E., & Crowe, A. (2017). Overcoming abuse: A phenomenological investigation of the journey to recovery from past intimate partner violence. *Journal of Interpersonal Violence, 32*(22), 3373–3401. https://doi.org/10.1177/0886260515599161

Ford-Gilboe, M., Varcoe, C., & Merritt-Gray, M. (2011). Intimate partner violence and nursing practice. In J. Humphrey, & J. C. Campbell (Eds.), *Family violence and nursing practice* (2nd ed.) (pp. 115–153). New York: Springer.

Glancy, G., Heintzman, M., & Wheeler, A. (2019). Battered woman syndrome: Updating the expert checklist. *International Journal of Risk and Recovery, 2*(2), 4–17. https://doi.org/10.15173/ijrr.v2i2.3820

Government of Canada, Department of Justice. (2021). *Legal definitions of elder abuse and neglect.* Retrieved from https://www.justice.gc.ca/eng/rp-pr/cj-jp/fv-vf/elder-aines/def/p212.html

Horta Esper, L., & Gherardi-Donato, E. C. S. (2019). Mindfulness-based interventions for women victims of interpersonal violence: A systematic review. *Archives of Psychiatric Nursing, 33*(1), 120–130. https://doi.org/10.1016/j.apnu.2018.09.003

Idriss-Wheeler, D., Hajjar, J., & Yaya, S. (2021). Interventions directed at men for preventing intimate partner violence: A systematic review protocol. *Systematic Reviews, 10*(161), 1–8. https://doi.org/10.1186/s13643-021-01712-7

Inoue, Y., Stickley, A., Yazawa, A., et al. (2021). Childhood adversities, late-life stressors and the onset of depressive symptoms in community-dwelling older adults. *Aging & Mental Health, 1,* 1–6. https://doi.org/10.1080/13607863.2021.1875190

Isobel, S., Goodyear, M., Furness, T., et al. (2019). Preventing intergenerational trauma transmission: A critical interpretive synthesis. *Journal of Clinical Nursing, 28*(7–8), 1100–1113. https://doi.org/10.1111/jocn.14735

Jack, S. M., Ford-Gilboe, M., Davidov, D., et al. (2017). Identification and assessment of intimate partner violence in nurse home visitation. *Journal of Clinical Nursing, 26*(15–16), 2215–2228. https://doi.org/10.1111/jocn.13392

Kimber, M., Gonzalez, A., & MacMillian, H. L. (2020). Recognizing and responding to child maltreatment: Strategies to apply when delivering family-based treatment for eating disorders. *Frontiers in Psychiatry, 11*(678), 1–10. https://doi.org/10.3389/fpsyt.2020.00678

Krug, E. G., Dahlberg, L. L., Mercy, J. A., et al. (2002). *World report on violence and health.* Geneva: World Health Organization. Retrieved from https://www.who.int/violence_injury_prevention/violence/world_report/en/

Levey, E. J., Gelaye, B., Bain, P., et al. (2017). A systematic review of randomized controlled trials of interventions designed to decrease child abuse in high-risk families. *Child Abuse & Neglect, 65,* 48–57. https://doi.org/10.1016/j.chiabu.2017.01.004

Loxton, D., Dolja-Gore, X., Anderson, A. E., et al. (2017). Intimate partner violence adversely impacts health over 16 years and across generations: A longitudinal cohort study. *PLoS One, 12*(6), e0178138. https://doi.org/10.1371/journal.pone.0178138

Lutgendorf, M. A. (2019). Intimate partner violence and women's health. *Obstetrics & Gynecology, 134*(3), 470–480. https://doi.org/10.1097/AOG.0000000000003326

Manay, N., & Collin-Vezina, D (2021). Recipients of children's and adolescents' disclosures of childhood sexual abuse: A systematic review. *Child Abuse & Neglect, 116,* 104192. https://doi.org/10.1016/j.chiabu.2019.104192

McDonald, L., & Collins, A. (2000). *Abuse and neglect of older adults: A discussion paper* (Catalogue no. H72-21/162-1998E). Retrieved from https://publications.gc.ca/collections/Collection/H88-3-30-2001/pdfs/violence/abuse_e.pdf

McFarlane, J., Hughes, R. B., Nosek, M. A., et al. (2001). Abuse Assessment Screen—Disability (AAS-D): Measuring frequency, type, and perpetrator of abuse toward women with physical disabilities. *Journal of Women's Health & Gender-Based Medicine, 10,* 861–866. https://publications.gc.ca/collections/Collection/H88-3-30-2001/pdfs/violence/abuse_e.pdf

Middlesex-London Health Unit. (2000). *Task Force on the Health Effects of Woman Abuse—Final report.* London: Author.

Moffitt, P., Aujla, W., Giesbrecht, C. J., et al. (2020). Intimate partner violence and COVID-19 in rural, remote, and Northern Canada: Relationship, vulnerability and risk. *Journal of Family Violence.* https://doi.org/10.1007/s10896-020-00212-x

Moore, K. E., Folk, J. B., Boren, E. A., et al. (2018). Pilot study of a brief dialectical behavior therapy skills group for jail inmates. *Psychological Services, 15*(1), 98–108. https://doi.org/10.1037/ser0000105

Moreau, G., Jaffray, B., & Armstrong, A. (2020). *Police-reported crime statistics in Canada, 2019* (Catalogue no. 85-002-x). Juristat. Retrieved from https://www150.statcan.gc.ca/n1/pub/85-002-x/2020001/article/00010-eng.htm

Moorhead, S., Johnson, M., Maas, M. L., et al. (2018). *Nursing Outcomes Classification (NOC)* (6th ed.). St. Louis: Elsevier.

National Inquiry into Missing and Murdered Indigenous Women and Girls. (2019). *Reclaiming power and place. The final report of the national inquiry into missing and murdered indigenous women and girls.* The National Inquiry. Retrieved from https://www.mmiwg-ffada.ca/wp-content/uploads/2019/06/Final_Report_Vol_1a-1.pdf

NL Children, Youth and Families Act. (2019). *Duty to report child and youth abuse and neglect.* Retrieved from https://www.gov.nl.ca/cssd/childprotection/report/

Okeke-Ihejirika, P., Yohani, S., Muster, J., et al. (2020). A scoping review on intimate partner violence in Canada's immigrant communities. *Trauma, Violence, & Abuse, 21*(4), 788–810. https://doi.org/10.1177/1524838018789156

Paterno, M. T., & Draughon, J. E. (2016). Screening for intimate partner violence. *Journal of Midwifery & Women's Health, 61*(3), 370–375. https://doi.org/10.1111/jmwh.12443

Pearce, M. E., Jongbloed, K., Pooyak, S., et al. (2021). The Cedar Project: Exploring the role of colonial harms and childhood maltreatment on HIV and hepatitis C infection in a cohort study involving young Indigenous people who use drugs in two Canadian cities. *BMJ Open, 11*, e042545. https://doi.org/10.1136/bmjopen-2020-042545

Peer, N., Abrahams, N., & Kengne, A.-P. (2020). A systematic review of the associations of adult sexual abuse in women with cardiovascular diseases and selected risk factors. *Global Heart, 15*(1), 65. https://doi.org/10.5334/gh.760

Pine, J., & Steffen, A. M. (2019). Intergenerational ambivalence and dyadic strain: Understanding stress in family care partners of older adults. *Clinical Gerontologist, 42*(1), 90–100. https://doi.org/10.1080/07317115.2017.1356894

Poole, J. C., Dobson, K. S., Pusch, D., et al. (2017). Anxiety among adults with a history of childhood adversity: Psychological resilience moderates the indirect effect of emotion dysregulation. *Journal of Affective Disorders, 217*, 144–152. https://dx.doi.org/10.1016/j.jad.2017.03.047

Public Health Agency of Canada. (2016). *The chief public health officer's report on the state of public health in Canada 2016: A focus on family violence in Canada.* Retrieved from http://www.healthycanadians.gc.ca/publications/department-ministere/state-public-health-family-violence-2016-etat-sante-publique-violence-familiale/alt/pdf-eng.pdf

Public Health Agency of Canada. (2017). *How you can identify abuse and help older adults at risk.* Retrieved from https://www.canada.ca/en/public-health/services/publications/health-risks-safety/how-identify-elder-abuse.html

Racine, N., Dimitropoulos, G., Hartwick, C., et al. (2021). Characteristics and service needs of maltreated children referred for mental health services at a child advocacy centre in Canada. *Journal of the Canadian Academy of Child and Adolescent Psychiatry, 30*(2), 92–103.

Radcliffe, P., Gadd, D., Henderson, J., et al. (2019). What role does substance use play in intimate partner violence? A narrative analysis of in-depth interviews with men in substance use treatment and their current female partner. *Journal of Interpersonal Violence, 36*(21–22), 10285–10313. https://doi.org/10.1177/0886260519879259

Reeves, E. (2015). A synthesis of the literature on trauma-informed care. *Issues in Mental Health Nursing, 36*(9), 698–709. https://doi.org/10.3109/01612840.2015.1025319

Registered Nurses' Association of Ontario. (2012). *Woman abuse: Screening, identification and initial response: Guideline Supplement.* Retrieved from https://rnao.ca/bpg/guidelines/woman-abuse-screening-identification-and-initial-response (Original work published 2005).

Russell. B. (2020). *Intimate partner violence and the LGBT+ community understanding power dynamics* (1st ed.). Springer International Publishing. https://doi.org/10.1007/978-3-030-44762-5

Rivara, F., Adhia, A., Lyons, V., et al. (2019). The effects of violence on health. *Health Affairs, 38*(10), 1622–1629. Retrieved from https://doi.org/10.1377/hlthaff.2019.00480

Statistics Canada. (2017). *Family violence in Canada: A statistical profile, 2015.* Retrieved from https://www150.statcan.gc.ca/n1/daily-quotidien/170216/dq170216b-eng.htm

Statistics Canada. (2021). *Section 3: Police-reported intimate partner violence in Canada, 2019.* Retrieved from https://www150.statcan.gc.ca/n1/pub/85-002-x/2020001/article/00010-eng.htm

Stewart, D. E., & Vigod, S. N. (2017). Mental health aspects of intimate partner violence. *Psychiatric Clinics of North America, 40*(2), 321–334. https://dx.doi.org/10.1016/j.psc.2017.01.009

Storey, J. E. (2020). Risk factors for elder abuse and neglect: A review of the literature. *Aggression and Violent Behavior, 50*, 1–13. https://doi.org/10.1016/j.avb.2019.101339

Taillieu, T. L., Brownridge, D. A., & Brownell, M. (2020). Screening for partner violence in the early postpartum period: Are we missing families most at risk of experiencing violence. *Canadian Journal of Public Health, 111*, 286–296. https://doi.org/10.17269/s41997-019-00266-5

Thompson, N. (2021). Reports of domestic, intimate partner violence continue to rise during the pandemic. *CBC.* Retrieved from https://www.cbc.ca/news/canada/toronto/domestic-intimate-partner-violence-up-in-pandemic-1.5914344

Turner, H.A., Vanderminden, J., Finkelhor, D., & Hamby, S. (2019). Child neglect and the broader context of child victimization. *Child Maltreatment, 24*(3), 265–274. https://doi.org/10.1177/1077559518825312

Unrau, M., Jakubec, S. L., & Jeske, S. (2017). Somatics education for crisis intervention training. *Arts & Health, 9*(1), 91–96. https://doi.org/10.1080/17533015.2016.1233122

Valimaki, T., Maki-Petaja-Leinonen, A., & Vaismoradi, M. (2020). Abuse in the caregiving relationship between older people with memory disorders and family caregivers: A systematic review. *Journal of Advanced Nursing, 76*, 1977–1987. https://doi.org/10.1111/jan.14397

Walker, L. E. (1979). *The battered woman* (2nd ed.). New York: Springer.

World Health Organization. (2017). *Health topics: Violence.* Retrieved from https://www.who.int/topics/violence/en/

Yakubovich, A., R., Stockel, H., Murray, et al. (2018). Risk and protective factors for intimate partner violence against women: Systematic review and meta-analyses of prospective-longitudinal studies. *American Journal of Public Health, 108*(7). https://doi.org/10.2105/AJPH.2018.304428

Zakrison, T. L., Ruiz, X., Gelbard, R., et al. (2017). Universal screening for intimate partner and sexual violence in trauma patients: An EAST multicenter trial. *Journal of Trauma & Acute Care Surgery, 83*(1), 105–110.

25

Sexual Assault

Erin Ziegler
Originating US chapter by Margaret Jordan Halter, Jodie Flynn

 https://evolve.elsevier.com/Canada/Varcarolis/psychiatric/

OBJECTIVES

1. Define sexual assault and aggravated sexual assault.
2. Describe the profiles of the survivor and the perpetrator of sexual assault.
3. Distinguish between the acute and long-term phases of the rape-trauma syndrome, and identify some common reactions during each phase.
4. Discuss a trauma-informed approach and describe three related practices.
5. Reflect on one's own thoughts and feelings and consider the myths about sexual assault and its impact on survivors.
6. Identify five areas to assess and six overall guidelines for nursing interventions related to sexual assault.
7. Discuss the long-term psychological effects of sexual assault.
8. Identify three outcome criteria that would signify successful interventions for a person who has suffered a sexual assault.

KEY TERMS AND CONCEPTS

aggravated sexual assault
blame
controlled style of coping
depersonalization
derealization
dissociative disorders
expressed style of coping
grounding techniques
intrusive thoughts
rape-trauma syndrome
secondary victimization
sexual assault
sexual assault nurse examiners
somatic therapies
vicarious trauma

In recent years accounts of individuals being sexually assaulted by multiple perpetrators have garnered international attention. College and university campus sexual assaults of men and women have become the focus of recent studies and interventions (Fedina et al., 2018; Voth Schrag, 2017). As many as one in four women will be sexually assaulted while obtaining a post-secondary education (Ending Violence Association of British Columbia, 2016). In Canada one in three women and one in eight men experience some form of sexual violence (Government of Ontario, 2021). In some of these cases further violation occurred through the display of electronic images of these assaults, and the resulting peer humiliation led to the hopelessness, desperation, and suicide of the victims. While horrific and extreme, these outcomes have reinforced the seriousness and life-threatening consequences of sexual violence. These accounts demonstrate some of the most contemptible violations that can be perpetrated by one human being on another. In this chapter we further explore the epidemiology, the consequences of, and the treatment approaches for sexual assault. **Sexual assault**, a legal term that refers to any sexual activity, physical or psychological, for which consent is not obtained or freely given, is also referred to as *sexual violence*. Sexual harassment and stalking, also criminal behaviours that are sexual in nature, are, however, not classified as assault. Sexual assault violates the sexual integrity of the victim and can result in a range of injury from no injury to serious injury. Using a weapon, threatening, or even endangering the life of the victim during a sexual attack are all defined as sexual assault (Government of Ontario, 2021).

Sex offenders may commit acts of sexual violence against children, which are considered sexual abuse (see Chapter 24). These offences are termed *sexual interference, invitation to sexual touching, incest,* and *sexual exploitation* in the criminal justice system. **Aggravated sexual assault** is another legal term that is used when, during a sexual assault, the life of the survivor is endangered or the assault results in injury (*Criminal Code*, 1985).

Regardless of the descriptor or legal framework of a sexual assault, it is an act of violence. A meta-analysis by Dworkin et al. (2017) found that a history of sexual assault significantly increased an individual's risk of developing a mental health illness. Sexual assault is not about sex but, rather, is an exertion of power and control over another individual. Children, older persons, women, and men can all be victims of sexual assault.

Nurses are often among the first to encounter patients who have been sexually assaulted and are instrumental not only in providing them with holistic care but also in helping to preserve evidence that could lead to prosecution of the perpetrator(s). It is essential that nurses be adequately informed about their roles and responsibilities with these patients.

Sexual assault is a multi-dimensional problem and calls for a public health approach that emphasizes the primary prevention of sexual violence (i.e., stopping it from occurring in the first place). Until recently, this approach has been relatively neglected in the field, with the majority of resources directed toward secondary or tertiary prevention (Mikton et al., 2017).

This chapter addresses issues surrounding sexual assault and the mental health impacts of this traumatic abuse of power and control. Throughout this chapter, survivors of sexual assault will be referred to using the female pronoun in recognition of the fact that women are significantly more frequently the victims of sexual assault. However, the principles discussed apply to anyone who has been sexually assaulted, male or female.

EPIDEMIOLOGY

Sexual assault is a topic people are reluctant to discuss because it is attached to much anguish, blame, shame, and desperation. The silence, however, has far-reaching impacts: it is estimated that more than 90% of sexual assaults in Canada go unreported. Nonetheless, more than 30 900 sexual assaults were reported nationwide in 2019 an increase of 7% from the previous year, according to Statistics Canada (2020a).

Everyone is at risk for sexual assault, it crosses all socioeconomic groups; ages, from infant to older persons; genders; sexual orientations; abilities; and cultural groups (Association of Alberta Sexual Assault Services, 2017). When compared to other traumatic events, sexual assault is associated with an increased risk of developing post-traumatic stress disorder (PTSD) with more severe symptoms (DiMauro & Renshaw, 2021).

Another important pattern of disease resulting from sexual assault is the concern for secondary victimization. **Secondary victimization** results when survivors experience further stress or trauma when seeking help through practices such as victim blaming, insensitive communication techniques, delays in care, disbelief, shame, stigmatization, or minimization of the experience by others (Greeson et al., 2016). Social reactions to sexual assault contribute to increased PTSD and revictimization for victims of sexual assault, making public mental health interventions an important area of program implementation (Ullman & Peter-Hagene, 2016). Because of the high rate of the above-mentioned patterns, understanding sexual assault and its effects, prevention, and treatment is an important mental health and public health concern.

The *Criminal Code* of Canada was amended in 1983 to replace the crimes of rape and indecent assault with three new sexual assault offences, focusing on the violent rather than sexual aspects of sexual assault. These changes were in keeping with the view that sexual assault is an abuse of power and control and reinforced that a spouse could be charged with sexual assault and that both males and females could be considered victims of sexual assault. Separate categories of sexual assault are identified based on the severity of the incident. Level 1 is a term that describes assault of a sexual nature that violates the sexual integrity of a person. Sexual assault with a weapon or causing bodily harm is considered level 2. A level 3 sexual assault is characterized by an assault that wounds, maims, disfigures, or endangers the life of another person (*Criminal Code*, 1985).

Of the almost 30 900 police-reported sexual assaults recorded in 2019, the majority (98%) were classified as level 1 sexual assault. Although the majority of sexual assaults are considered less severe forms (as opposed to aggravated sexual assault), this descriptor does not lessen the anguish experienced following any sexual assault.

The rate of sexual assault level 1 increased between 2018 and 2019, up 7% to 82 per 100 000 population. The rates of sexual assault level 2 also increased 6%, with a total of 525 incidents reported in 2019, or a rate of 1 per 100 000 population. In contrast, the rate of the most serious sexual assaults (aggravated sexual assaults) declined 22% in 2019, with 125 incidents (33 fewer than in 2018).

Police-reported sexual assaults of all levels increased in most provinces and territories between 2018 and 2019, with the exception of Nova Scotia (decreased 15%). The largest increases were reported in the Northwest Territories (58% increase), Yukon (53% increase), and British Columbia (24% increase) (Statistics Canada, 2020b). It is important to note that the number of sexual assaults reported by police is likely an underestimate of the true extent of sexual assault in Canada, as these types of offences often go unreported to police.

The rate of reported sexual assault among Indigenous people is 58 incidents per 1000 people, compared to 20 per 1000 among non-Indigenous people. Indigenous women are almost three times as likely to experience violent victimization (physical or sexual violence) than non-Indigenous women (Department of Justice Canada, 2017). The unique cultural and contextual circumstances of Indigenous victims of sexual assault must be better understood and met with effective responses to their particular needs (Du Mont et al., 2017). A report from the Chiefs of Ontario (2020) recommends using a culturally safe pathway for supporting First Nation communities to address sexual violence, including incorporating cultural practices, community healing, and using a restorative justice approach. Violence and sexual assault in Indigenous communities are unique from nation to nation, but share very complex issues involving historical trauma and childhood abuse that require multi-dimensional approaches, such as trauma and violence-informed practices (Lalonde et al., 2020). Culture (see Chapter 8) is an important consideration of services provided, and without attention, patients may experience secondary victimization.

Sexual minorities, those who identify as lesbian, gay, and bisexual are at an increased risk of sexual assault, with a rate that is triple that of heterosexual individuals. Furthermore, these individuals are more likely to sustain physical injuries due to the assault. Bisexual men and women experience sexual assault more frequently than gay and lesbian individuals. Transgender individuals are at a higher risk of sexual assault than cisgender individuals (Statistics Canada, 2020a). First Nations gender-diverse and two-spirit individuals also face higher rates of sexual assault. The Trans PLUSE study, a large Canadian study, found that 43% of participants who identified as two-spirit or Indigenous gender-diverse experience physical and sexual violence (Scheim et al., 2013).

Profile of Sexual Perpetrators

Females are statistically more likely to be sexually assaulted, and males are most likely to be the perpetrator or perpetrators. Police-reported data state that 98% of persons accused of sexual offences were male with a median age of 33. As mentioned, a large majority of reported sexual assaults were committed by a friend or acquaintance of the victim. Although we may think of the stranger lurking in the shadows in parking lots as the typical perpetrator, rape by a stranger is not typical: survivors typically know the person who sexually assaulted them. Two-thirds of all sexual assaults occurred on private property (Statistics Canada, 2017).

CLINICAL PICTURE

Relationships Between Victims and Perpetrators

The terms *intimate partner violence* and *spousal abuse* (see Chapter 24), *date rape*, *acquaintance rape*, and *drug-facilitated sexual assault* describe the relationship between the victim and perpetrator. In Canada spousal sexual assault became against the law in 1983. Whether it is spousal abuse or date rape, in such cases the perpetrator is known to, and presumably trusted by, the person who is sexually assaulted.

The psychological and emotional outcomes of sexual assault seem to vary depending on the level of intimacy and the relationship between the victim and the perpetrator. Sexual distress (including post-assault sexual problems such as dysfunction and pain) is more common among women who have been sexually assaulted by intimate partners; PTSD symptoms are common among those assaulted by someone they know; and fear and anxiety are more common in those assaulted by strangers. Depression has been found to be common among survivors, whether the perpetrators were known to them or not (Carter-Snell & Jakubec, 2013).

Drug-facilitated sexual assault has been increasingly recognized over the past 15 to 20 years. Many drugs, including alcohol (the most commonly used date rape drug), can be used alone or in combination to facilitate sexual assault (Table 25.1). Often these drugs are given to an unknowing victim. Once the drugs are ingested, victims lose their ability to ward off attackers, develop amnesia, and become unreliable witnesses. Because the symptoms mimic those of alcohol intoxication, survivors are not always screened for these drugs, resulting in underreporting of drug-facilitated sexual assault (Walsh et al., 2016). As nurses, we must remember that whether a person willingly or unwillingly consumes alcohol or drugs and is subsequently sexually assaulted, it is not the victim's fault. The *Criminal Code* (1985) states that consent cannot be given by a person who is unconscious or intoxicated.

Psychological Effects of Sexual Assault

Most people who are sexually assaulted suffer severe and long-lasting emotional trauma. Long-term psychological effects of sexual assault may include depression, suicide, anxiety, and fear; difficulties with daily functioning; low self-esteem; sexual dysfunction; and somatic complaints. Survivors of incest may experience a negative self-image, depression, eating disorders, personality disorders, self-destructive behaviour, and substance use. Reviews of the literature have summarized that timely intervention; trauma-informed approaches, such as having some control over the legal process; and the availability of positive support systems (both social and professional) provide resiliency to the psychological impacts of sexual assault (Carter-Snell & Jakubec, 2013).

Rape-Trauma Syndrome

Rape-trauma syndrome is a variant of PTSD and consists of an acute phase and a long-term reorganization process that occurs after an actual or attempted sexual assault. Each phase has separate symptoms, discussed below. See Chapter 12 for a more detailed discussion of PTSD.

Acute Phase

The acute phase of rape-trauma syndrome occurs immediately after the assault and may last 2 to 3 weeks. At this stage, patients usually are seen by emergency department personnel and, if available, the sexual assault nurse examiner (SANE), who is most involved in dealing with initial reactions. During this phase, there is a great deal of disorganization in the person's life, and somatic symptoms are common. This disorganization can be described in terms of impact, somatic, and emotional reactions (Box 25.1).

The survivor's most common initial reactions are shock, numbness, and disbelief. Outwardly, the person may appear self-contained and calm and may make remarks such as "It doesn't seem real" or "I don't believe this really happened to me." Sometimes, cognitive functions may be impaired, and the traumatized person may appear extremely confused and have difficulty concentrating and making decisions. Alternatively, the person may become hysterical or restless or may cry or even smile. These reactions to crisis are typical and may shift in presentation and reflect cognitive, affective, and behavioural disruptions resulting from the trauma.

TABLE 25.1 Drugs Associated With Date Rape

Drug, Alternative Names, and Status in Canada	Form, Mechanism of Action, and Onset	Effect on Victim	Overdose Symptoms and Treatment
Gamma-hydroxybutyrate (GHB) Also known as G, easy lay, liquid ecstasy, salty water, soap, cherry meth, and scoop Often made in illegal labs, resulting in the purity and strength of the final product being unpredictable	Liquid, white powder, or pill with a salty taste Schedule III central nervous system depressant A metabolite of gamma-aminobutyric acid (GABA) Onset within 5–20 minutes; duration, from 1 to 12 hours, is dose related	Produces relaxation, euphoria, and disinhibition Causes incoordination, confusion, deep sedation, and amnesia Tolerance and dependence exhibited by agitation, tachycardia, insomnia, anxiety, tremors, and sweating	*Symptoms:* Respiratory depression, seizures, nausea, vomiting, bradycardia, hypothermia, agitation, delirium, unconsciousness, and coma *Treatment:* Intubation for severe respiratory distress; atropine for bradycardia, and benzodiazepines for seizure activity; vomiting should be induced when possible
Rohypnol (flunitrazepam)[a] Also known as forget-me pill and roofies Mexico and other Latin American countries are the main illegal source of supply for North America	Pill that dissolves in liquids Schedule IV potent benzodiazepine; 10 times stronger than diazepam Impact is within 10–30 minutes and lasts 2–12 hours	More potent when combined with alcohol; causes sedation, psychomotor slowing, muscle relaxation, and amnesia Dependence and tolerance may develop	Overdose unlikely *Treatment:* Airway protection and gastrointestinal decontamination
Ketamine Also known as big K, kit-kat, Special K, wonk, and horsey P A rapid-acting anaesthetic drug used mainly by veterinarians and sometimes in human surgery	Liquid or a white powder An anaesthetic frequently used in veterinary practice; also a hallucinogenic substance related to phenylcyclohexyl piperidine (PCP) Onset within 30 seconds intravenously and 20 minutes orally; duration only 30–60 minutes; amnesia effects may last longer	Causes dissociative reaction, with a dream-like state leading to deep amnesia and analgesia and complete compliance of the victim May become confused, paranoid, delirious, combative, with drooling and hallucinations	*Treatment:* Airway maintenance and use of anti-cholinergics such as atropine and benzodiazepines

[a]Two other benzodiazepines, clonazepam (Clonapam) and alprazolam (Xanax), are also used. **Sources:** Data adapted from Burchum, J., & Rosenthal, L. (2019). *Lehne's pharmacology for nursing care* (10th ed.). Philadelphia: Elsevier; Health Canada. (2021). *Substance use.* Retrieved from https://www.canada.ca/en/health-canada/services/substance-use.html; U.S. Department of Health and Human Services. (2019). *Date rape drugs.* Retrieved from https://www.womenshealth.gov/a-z-topics/date-rape-drugs

BOX 25.1 Acute Phase of Rape-Trauma Syndrome

Impact Reaction

Expressed Style

Overt behaviours:
- Crying, sobbing
- Smiling, laughing, joking
- Agitation, anger, hysteria
- Volatility, lability, restlessness
- Confusion, incoherence, disorientation
- Tenseness

Controlled Style

Ambiguous appearances and reactions:
- Confusion, incoherence, disorientation, diminished alertness
- Lack of affective response
- Calm, subdued appearance
- Shock, numbness, confusion, freezing, disbelief
- Distractibility, difficulty making decisions

Somatic Reaction

Evidenced within first several weeks after a rape:
- Physical trauma
  - Bruises (breasts, throat, or back)
  - Soreness
- Skeletal muscle tension
  - Headaches
  - Sleep disturbances
  - Grimaces, twitches
- Gastrointestinal symptoms
  - Abdominal pains
  - Nausea
  - Loss of appetite
  - Diarrhea
- Genitourinary symptoms
  - Vaginal itching or discharge
  - Pain or discomfort

Emotional Reaction
- Fear of physical violence and death
- Denial
- Anxiety
- Shock
- Humiliation
- Fatigue
- Embarrassment
- Desire for revenge
- Self-blame
- Decreased self-esteem
- Shame
- Guilt
- Anger

Source: Adapted from Tannura, T. A. (2014). Rape trauma syndrome. *American Journal of Sexuality Education, 9*(2), 247–256. https://doi.org/10.1080/15546128.2014.883267; Burgess, A. W. (2018). Rape trauma syndrome. In P. Searles & R. J. Berger (Eds.), *Rape and society* (pp. 239–245). Routledge.

People who have experienced an emotionally overwhelming event may find it too painful to discuss. Examples of this response are found in statements such as "I don't want to talk about it" or "I just want to forget what happened." Behaviours that minimize the magnitude of the event include reluctance to seek medical attention and failure to follow up with legal counsel.

Long-Term Reorganization Phase

The long-term reorganization phase of rape-trauma syndrome occurs 2 or more weeks after the sexual assault. Nurses who care for survivors during the acute phase can help them anticipate and prepare for the reactions they are likely to experience during this later phase, which include the following:

- **Intrusive thoughts** of the sexual assault that break into the survivor's conscious mind both during the day and during sleep. These thoughts commonly include visions of violence toward the assailant, flashbacks (re-experiencing the traumatic event), or dreams with violent content contributing to insomnia, and incite emotions such as anger.
- Increased activity, such as moving, taking trips, changing telephone numbers, and making frequent visits to old friends. This activity stems from the fear that the assailant will return.
- Increased emotional lability, including intense anxiety, mood swings, crying spells, and depression.

Fears and phobias develop as a defensive reaction to the sexual assault. Typical phobias include the following:

- Fear of the indoors if the assault occurred indoors
- Fear of the outdoors if the assault occurred outdoors
- Fear of being alone (common for most women after an assault)
- Fear of crowds (women may believe that any person in the crowd might be a rapist)
- Fear of sexual encounters and activities

Many women experience acute disruption of their sex lives with their partners. Sexual assault is especially disruptive for those with no previous sexual experience.

As mentioned, the consequences of sexual assault may be severe, debilitating, and long term. Intervention and support for the survivor can help prevent some of the complications of anxiety, depression, suicide, difficulties with daily functioning and interpersonal relationships, sexual dysfunction, and somatic complaints.

APPLICATION OF THE NURSING PROCESS

A Trauma-Informed Approach

Trauma, such as a sexual assault, changes the world view of survivors so dramatically that it shifts the way they construct their sense of themselves and others. This trauma and the lasting effects then further inform other life choices and may guide the development of coping strategies that may help or hinder the growth and well-being of the patient. In this way, the impact of trauma may be felt throughout an individual's life in areas of functioning both related to and far removed from the trauma (Lalonde et al., 2020).

Using a trauma-informed approach in the care of patients who have experienced sexual assault appropriately responds to the deep and profound impact of trauma (see Chapter 21). This approach emphasizes the physical, psychological, and emotional safety of both patients and caregivers and creates opportunities for patients to rebuild a sense of control and empowerment. A trauma-informed approach can include a range of specific practices (Box 25.2).

> **BOX 25.2 Practices Used in a Trauma-Informed Approach**
>
> - Supporting patients in understanding the connections between their experience of trauma and their maladaptive or adaptive strategies for coping
> - Ensuring that patients have choices about and control over their treatment options
> - Using collaborative ways of determining needs and plans, and handling distress with sincere attempts to share power, decrease hierarchy, and build trust
> - Adapting screening and intake procedures so that patients are not required to disclose trauma before they are ready or to repeatedly tell their stories
> - Recognizing the range of emotional responses and symptoms that patients may experience, and identifying these as symptoms or adaptations to extreme life experiences rather than problem behaviours or extremes of personality
> - Facilitating the development and use of coping skills, culturally safe healing strategies, and mechanisms for personal empowerment (which may or may not involve seeking police or legal action or survivor's support)

Source: Adapted from Canadian Centre on Substance Abuse. (2014). *The essentials of trauma informed care.* Retrieved from https://www.ccsa.ca/sites/default/files/2019-04/CCSA-Trauma-informed-Care-Toolkit-2014-en.pdf

Assessment

Most sexual assault survivors do not report their sexual assault to the police, and few report it to doctors or nurses.

The Emergency Nurses Association (2017) position statement on care of sexual assault victims suggests the following interventions:

- Using a non-judgemental, empathic, and trauma-informed approach
- Rapidly assessing the needs and support required to prevent further trauma
- Treating and documenting injuries
- Providing a safe and private environment (e.g., limiting personnel to those health care providers examining the patient, a translator if needed, and a specially trained advocate if indicated and consented to by the patient)
- Assisting with or conducting the physical examination
- Collecting evidence, with appropriate documentation and technique
- Assessing for sexually transmitted infections (STIs) (including obtaining pertinent laboratory tests such as human immunodeficiency virus [HIV] testing, hepatitis profiles, and others) and provide prophylactic treatment
- Conducting pregnancy risk evaluation and provide emergency contraception
- Providing crisis intervention and arranging follow-up counselling

General Assessment

With consent, the SANE or nurse from the sexual assault response team (SART) should talk with the survivor, the family or friends who accompany the survivor, and the police to gather as much data as possible for assessing the crisis. The nurse then assesses the survivor's (1) level of anxiety, (2) coping mechanisms, (3) available support systems, (4) signs and symptoms of emotional trauma, and (5) signs and symptoms of physical trauma. Information obtained from the assessment is then analyzed, and nursing diagnoses are formulated.

Level of anxiety. A patient experiencing severe to panic levels of anxiety will not be able to problem-solve or process information. Providing support, reassurance, and appropriate therapeutic techniques can lower the patient's anxiety and facilitate mutual goal setting and the assimilation of information. Refer to Chapters 12 and 21 for more detailed discussions of the levels of anxiety and therapeutic interventions for crises.

Coping mechanisms. The same coping skills that have helped the survivor through other difficult problems in her lifetime will be used in adjusting to life after the sexual assault. In addition, new ways of getting through the difficult times may be developed for both the short-term and the long-term adjustment. Active and outwardly observable behavioural responses include crying; withdrawing; smoking; substance use; talking about the event; becoming extremely agitated, confused, disoriented, or incoherent; and even laughing or joking. These behaviours are examples of an **expressed style of coping** (see Box 25.1).

Cognitive coping mechanisms are the thoughts people have that help them deal with high anxiety levels. A positive cognitive response might be "At least I am alive and will get to see my children again." Not-so-positive responses may become generalized as a way to sum up the situation, "It's my fault this happened; my mother warned me about working in such a trashy place," and may develop into an ego-damaging refrain. If such thoughts are verbalized, the nurse will know what the survivor is thinking. If not, the nurse can ask questions such as "What are you thinking and feeling?" or "What can I do to help you in this difficult situation?" or "What has helped in the past?"

Available support systems. The availability, size, and usefulness of a survivor's social support system must be assessed. Often partners or family members do not understand the survivor's feelings about the sexual assault, and they may not be the best supports available. Pay careful attention to verbal and non-verbal cues from the survivor that may communicate the strength of her social network.

> **VIGNETTE**
>
> Sam, age 18, is brought to the emergency department by a concerned neighbour. She was found wandering aimlessly outside her house, sobbing and muttering, "He had no right to do that to me." Because of Sam's distraught appearance and her statement, the triage nurse suspects sexual assault and asks Sam if she would like to see the sexual assault nurse examiner (SANE). Sam agrees and is brought to a private area and introduced to the SANE, Ms. Davies. After respectful, non-judgemental questioning, Sam divulges that her boyfriend forced her to have sex with him. Following the assessment and treatment, plans for discharge are discussed. Sam has nowhere to go because her family is away, and she does not want anyone called. Her neighbour, MaiLin, told the nurse earlier that Sam can stay with her family.
>
> **Nurse:** "Earlier, your neighbour, MaiLin, told me that you are welcome to spend the weekend with her family."
> **Sam:** (loudly, sharply, with eyes wide) "Oh no, I couldn't do that."
> **Nurse:** "You don't like that idea?"
> **Sam:** (wringing a tissue in her hands, head hanging, voice soft) "I can't go in her house anymore."
> **Nurse:** "Something about being in that house disturbs you?"
> **Sam:** "MaiLin's husband, Don" (deep sigh, pause) "used to … uh … take advantage of me when I would babysit their children."
> **Nurse:** "Take advantage?"
> **Sam:** "Yes …" (sobbing) "He used to try to get me to have sex with him. He said he'd blame it on me if I told anyone."
> **Nurse:** "What a frightening experience that must have been for you."
> **Sam:** "Yes."
> **Nurse:** "I can see why you would not want to spend the night there. Let's explore other options."
>
> A suitable place to stay is finally arranged. Sam is given counselling referrals that will help her deal with the process of reorganization after this current rape experience. Her counsellor will explore her feelings about past sexual abuse she has suffered at the hands of her neighbour when she is ready.

Signs and symptoms of emotional trauma. Nurses work with sexual assault survivors most frequently in the emergency department soon after the sexual assault has occurred. Sexual assault is a psychological emergency and should receive immediate attention. Many emergency departments in urban areas provide the services of sexual assault nurse examiners specially trained to meet the needs of sexual assault survivors. They are trained to assess the extent of psychological and emotional trauma that may not be readily apparent, especially if the person uses the controlled style of coping, a contained response, during the acute phase of the rape trauma (see Box 25.1).

Whether a SANE or another nursing or medical professional is conducting the assessment and evidence collection, a patient history should be obtained and carefully recorded. When taking a history, the nurse determines only the details of the assault that will be helpful in addressing the immediate physical and psychological needs of the survivor. The nurse allows the survivor to talk at a comfortable pace; poses questions in non-judgemental, descriptive terms; and refrains from asking "why" questions. The survivor frequently finds relating the events of the sexual assault traumatic and embarrassing.

If suicidal thoughts are expressed, the nurse assesses what precautions are needed by asking direct questions, such as "Are you thinking of harming yourself?" and "Have you ever tried to kill yourself before or since this attack occurred?" If the answer is yes, the nurse conducts a thorough suicide assessment, as described in Chapter 22.

Signs and symptoms of physical trauma. It is essential that nurses provide psychological support while collecting and preserving legal evidence such as hair, skin, and semen samples that may be crucial for conviction of the perpetrator. The most characteristic physical signs of sexual assault are injuries to the face, head, neck, and extremities. Any physical injuries should be carefully documented, in both narrative and pictorial form using preprinted body maps, hand-drawn copies, or photographs. This assessment and all aspects must be conducted with the utmost respect for privacy and respect for the traumatic nature of the assault and potential for longer-term trauma and secondary victimization.

The nurse takes a brief gynecological history, including the date of the last menstrual period and the likelihood of current pregnancy, and assesses for a history of STIs. If the survivor has never undergone a pelvic examination, the steps of the examination will need to be explained. The nurse plays a crucial role in giving support and minimizing the trauma of the examination because the survivor may experience it as another violation of her body. Recognizing this, the nurse can explain the examination procedure in a way that will be reassuring and supportive. Allowing the survivor to participate in all decisions affecting care is essential to a trauma-informed approach and helps her to regain a sense of control over her life.

The survivor has the right to refuse either a legal or a medical examination. Consent forms must be signed before photographs are taken, a pelvic examination occurs, and any other procedures that might be needed to collect evidence and provide treatment are carried out. The correct preservation of body fluids and swabs is essential because DNA samples may identify the perpetrator. A shower and fresh clothing should be made available to the survivor as soon as possible after the examination and collection of specimens.

Prophylactic treatment for chlamydia, gonorrhea and trichomoniasis should be offered (Sachs et al., 2021). HIV and hepatitis B exposure can be a concern of sexual assault survivors. This concern should always be addressed, and the sexual assault survivor should be given the information needed to evaluate the likelihood of risk and offered testing. With this information, the person can make informed choice safer-sex practices until testing can be done.

Depending on circumstances, the risk for pregnancy should be considered along with treatment options. Emergency contraception may be offered and prescribed; a few options available are a pill and a copper intrauterine device (IUD) (Freedman, 2020).

All data are carefully documented, including verbatim statements by the survivor, detailed observations of emotional and physical status, and all results of the physical examination. All laboratory tests performed are noted, and findings are recorded as soon as they are available. One of the greatest concerns is that crucial evidence may be lost or overlooked. The Emergency Nurses Association (2018) position statement on forensic evidence collection underscores the role of the nurse in collecting and securing medical and legal evidence.

Self-Assessment

Nurses' attitudes influence the physical and psychological care received by sexual assault survivors. Knowing the myths and facts surrounding sexual assault can increase your awareness of your personal beliefs and feelings regarding sexual assault. If you examine personal feelings and reactions before encountering a sexual assault survivor, you will be better prepared to give empathic and effective care. Examining your feelings about pregnancy termination is also important, because a patient might choose to terminate a pregnancy that results from assault. Table 25.2 compares sexual assault myths and facts. Vicarious trauma, a term used to describe the disruptions in thinking and perspectives of those who are exposed to the stories of those who are traumatized, is of concern for healthcare practitioners working with sexual assault victims (Long, 2020). Supervision, reflection, and ongoing self-assessment are first steps to managing the effects of this trauma and burnout on nurses and on their nursing care.

ASSESSMENT GUIDELINES
Sexual Assault

1. Assess psychological trauma, and document the patient's verbatim statements.
2. Assess level of anxiety. If in a severe to panic level of anxiety, the patient will not be able to problem-solve or process information.
3. Assess physical trauma and document per institutional, provincial or territorial, and Royal Canadian Mounted Police (RCMP) protocols. Use a preprinted body map, and ask permission and obtain written consent to take photographs.
4. Assess the survivor's available support system. Often partners or family members do not understand the trauma of sexual assault, and they may not be the best supports to draw on at this time.
5. Identify community supports (e.g., crisis centres, support groups, therapists) that work in the area of sexual assault.
6. Encourage the patient to talk about the experience, but do not press the patient to tell.

Diagnosis

The nursing diagnosis *Rape-trauma syndrome* applies to the physical and psychological effects of a sexual assault. It includes an acute phase of disorganization of the survivor's lifestyle and a long-term phase of reorganization. The syndrome is manifested by post-traumatic features such as:

- Alterations in concentration
- Anger
- Dissociative amnesia
- Headache

TABLE 25.2 Myth Versus Fact: Rape

Myth	Fact
Rape is caused by lust or uncontrollable sexual urges and the need for sexual gratification.	Rape is an act of physical violence and domination that is not motivated by sexual gratification.
Only "bad" women get raped.	Women of all ages, cultural backgrounds, social classes, and sexual orientations are equally likely to become victims of sexual assault.
When a woman dresses provocatively, she's inviting sexual attention and "asking for it."	Suggesting that women provoke sexual assault by the way they dress transfers blame from the perpetrator to the victim. If a woman is sexually assaulted, it is NOT her fault. No one ever "asks" or deserves to be sexually assaulted regardless of how she dresses or behaves.
Rape only occurs outside and at night.	Many rapes occur during the day and in the victims' homes. Rape can and does occur anytime and anyplace.
Men cannot be sexually assaulted.	Men are sexually assaulted. Any man can be sexually assaulted regardless of size, strength, appearance, or sexual orientation.
Only homosexual men are sexually assaulted.	Heterosexual, gay, and bisexual men alike may all face the traumatic experience of sexual assault. Being sexually assaulted has nothing to do with your current or future sexual orientation.
Only homosexuals sexually assault other men.	Most men who sexually assault other men are heterosexual. This fact helps to highlight another reality that sexual assault is about violence, anger, and control over another person, not lust or sexual attraction.
Erection or ejaculation during sexual assault means "you really wanted it" or "enjoyed it" or consented to it.	Erection and ejaculation are physiological responses that may result from mere physical contact or even extreme stress. These responses do not imply that the victim wanted or enjoyed the assault and do not indicate anything about the victim's sexual orientation. Some rapists are aware how erection and ejaculation can confuse the sexual assault victim, manipulating their victims to the point of erection or ejaculation to increase their feelings of control and to discourage reporting of the crime.
It is impossible to sexually assault a man.	Young boys or adult males can be victims of rape or sexual assault.
Men do NOT experience the same degree of emotional pain associated with sexual assault as women. If a man experiences emotional pain, he should be able to deal with it.	All survivors may experience flashbacks, rage, depression, or anxiety when the traumatic experience is not acknowledged and treated. Survivors of trauma may turn to alcohol or drugs to cope with overwhelming feelings.

Sources: Created with data from https://well.wvu.edu/resources/sexual-violence/rape-myths; https://www.ontario.ca/page/dispelling-myths-about-sexual-assault; https://www.healthywa.wa.gov.au/Articles/A_E/Common-myths-about-sexual-assault; https://vsac.ca/myths/

- Irritability
- Nightmares

The vignette describing the response of a male student highlights some of the symptoms at different stages following sexual assault.

> **VIGNETTE**
> At a party, a male sexually assaults John, a 22-year-old university student. After John is brought to the emergency department by a friend, he describes feeling detached from his body. He cannot remember his surroundings during the assault: "It feels like it took place in a vacuum." He is agitated, irritable, and tells his friend to leave. John has difficulty concentrating on the examiner's questions. After a week, John still feels as though his mind is detached from his body. He reports having difficulty sleeping, nightmares, headaches, not being able to concentrate, and startling whenever anyone touches him.

Dissociative Disorders

Dissociative disorders occur after significant adverse experiences or traumas such as a sexual assault, and in these disorders, individuals respond to stress with a severe interruption of consciousness. Dissociation is an unconscious defence mechanism that protects the individual against overwhelming anxiety through an emotional separation. However, this separation results in disturbances in memory, consciousness, self-identity, and perception.

Patients with dissociative disorders have intact reality testing. This means that although the person may have flashbacks or images, these are triggered by current events, relate to the past trauma, and are not delusions or hallucinations. Mild, fleeting dissociative experiences are relatively common to all of us. For example, we say we are on "auto pilot" when we drive home from work and cannot recall the last 15 minutes before reaching the house.

These common experiences are distinctly different from the processes of pathological dissociation. Dissociation is involuntary and results in failure of the normal control over a person's mental processes and normal integration of conscious awareness. Dimensions of a memory that should be linked are not and are fragmented. For example, a person may be aware of a sound or smell, but these sensations would not be linked to the actual event itself, leaving the person fearful or confused. Dissociation causes people to experience a distressing fragmentation of consciousness and a sense of separation from themselves. Disturbances of perception, sensation, autonomic regulation, and movement are common for those who have suffered significant trauma because trauma is often stored physically in the body. In addition, the person may re-enact, as well as re-experience, trauma without consciously knowing why.

Symptoms of dissociation may be either positive or negative. Positive symptoms refer to unwanted additions to mental activity such as flashbacks. Negative symptoms refer to deficits such as memory problems or the ability to sense or control different parts of the body. Dissociation decreases the immediate subjective distress of the trauma and continues to protect the individual from full awareness of the disturbing event.

Dissociation can also be somewhat protective, for example, when a sexual assault victim from a small rural community or workplace regularly has contact with the perpetrator of the assault, or when a child is the victim of abuse by a close family member. This highlights the importance of attachments and relationships in allowing the child to grow socially, intellectually, and cognitively. If abuse or neglect has occurred, these memories become compartmentalized and often do not intrude into awareness until later in life when the person is in a stressful situation. Dissociative disorders include (1) depersonalization/derealization disorder, (2) dissociative amnesia, and (3) dissociative identity disorder.

Depersonalization/derealization disorder. Depersonalization/derealization disorder is found in both adolescents and adults, often in response to acute stress such as a sexual assault. In depersonalization the focus is on oneself. It is an extremely uncomfortable feeling of being an observer of one's own body or mental processes. In derealization the focus is on the outside world. It is the recurring feeling that one's surroundings are unreal or distant. The person may feel mechanical, dreamy, or detached from the body. Some people suffer episodes of these problems that come and go, whereas others have episodes that begin with stressors and eventually become constant. Patients describe these experiences as very distressing.

Outcomes Identification

The long-term outcome includes the absence of any residual symptoms after the trauma. The *Nursing Outcomes Classification (NOC)* identifies additional outcomes appropriate for the rape survivor: *Abuse protection*, *Abuse recovery: Emotional*, *Abuse recovery: Sexual*, *Coping*, *Personal resiliency*, *Sexual functioning*, and *Stress level* (Moorhead et al., 2018). Some of the suggested indicators for these outcomes include:

- Patient will demonstrate positive interpersonal relationships.
- Patient will demonstrate adequate social interactions.
- Patient will demonstrate healing of physical injuries.
- Patient will demonstrate evidence of appropriate opposite- or same-sex relationships.
- Patient will verbalize accurate information about sexual functioning.
- Patient will express comfort with body.
- Patient will express sexual interest.
- Patient will report increased psychological comfort.
- Patient will report a decrease in physical symptoms of stress.

Planning

Unless the survivor has sustained serious physical injury, treatment is offered, and the patient is released. However, because the ramifications of sexual assault are experienced for an extended time after the acute phase, the plan of care includes information for follow-up care. The survivor needs information about available community supports and how to access them. Nurses may also encounter sexual assault survivors in other settings when they are no longer in acute distress but still dealing with the aftermath of assault. Such settings include inpatient facilities, the community, and the home. A comprehensive plan of care addresses the continuing needs of the sexual assault survivor in any setting.

Implementation

The occurrence of sexual assault can be the most devastating experience in a person's life and constitutes an acute adventitious (unexpected) crisis. Comprehensive approaches to intervention address multiple levels and focus on leadership and policy, prevention, outreach, and interventions (Association of Alberta Sexual Assault Services, 2017).

BOX 25.3 Interventions for Rape-Trauma Syndrome

Definition of interventions for rape-trauma syndrome: Provision of emotional and physical support immediately following a reported sexual assault.

Activities

- Provide support person to stay with patient.
- Explain legal proceedings available to patient.
- Explain sexual assault protocol and obtain consent to proceed through protocol.
- Document whether patient has showered, douched, or bathed since incident.
- Document mental state, physical state (clothing, dirt, and debris), history of incident, evidence of violence, and prior gynecological history.
- Determine presence of cuts, bruises, bleeding, lacerations, or other signs of physical injury.
- Implement forensic evidence collection kit (e.g., label and save soiled clothing, vaginal secretions, and vaginal hair combings).
- Secure samples for legal evidence.
- Implement crisis intervention counselling.
- Offer medication to prevent pregnancy, as appropriate.
- Offer prophylactic antibiotic medication against sexually transmitted infection (STI).
- Discuss human immunodeficiency virus (HIV) post-exposure prophylaxis.
- Give clear, written instructions about medication use, crisis support services, and legal support.
- Offer follow-up services for STI results and counselling services.
- Document according to employer policy.

Source: Adapted from Butcher, H. K., Bulechek, G. M., Dochterman, J. M., et al. (Eds.). (2019). *Nursing Interventions Classification (NIC)* (7th ed.). St. Louis: Mosby.

Typical crisis reactions reflect cognitive, affective, and behavioural disruptions. For survivors to return to their previous level of functioning, it is necessary for them to fully mourn their losses, experience anger, and work through their fears. Box 25.3 provides *Nursing Interventions Classification (NIC)* interventions for rape-trauma syndrome (Butcher et al., 2019).

Counselling

The most effective approach for counselling in the emergency department or crisis centre is to provide non-judgemental care and optimal emotional support. Confidentiality is crucial. The most helpful things the nurse can do are to listen and to let the survivor talk. A survivor who feels understood is no longer alone and feels more in control of the situation. It is especially important to help the survivor and significant others to separate issues of vulnerability from blame, attachment of personal responsibility for the assault onto the victim. Although the person may have made choices that made her more vulnerable, she is not to blame for the sexual assault. She may, however, decide to avoid some of those choices in the future (e.g., walking alone late at night, using alcohol excessively). Focusing on one's behaviour (which is controllable) allows the survivor to believe that similar experiences can be avoided in the future.

In many rural and urban communities across Canada community-based organizations, health care providers, and grassroots organizations have brought forward concerns that the needs of survivors of sexual assault were not being met in emergency departments. Care provided was often delayed by long wait times, and nurses and physicians were not adequately trained to meet the unique needs of the survivor. Many communities have responded to these concerns. For instance, in 1984 Canada's first hospital-based sexual assault centre was opened at Women's College Hospital in Toronto. The mandate of such sexual assault and domestic violence treatment centres is to address the medical, emotional, social, forensic, and legal needs of women, men, and children who have been recently sexually assaulted or who are survivors of domestic abuse in a prompt, professional, and compassionate manner (Ontario Network of Sexual Assault/Domestic Violence Treatment Centres, n.d.). Since the first one was opened, similar sexual assault care centres have been introduced in many different formats throughout Canada, including individual centres serving vast rural communities. Other examples of regional sexual assault organizations include the Northern Society for Domestic Peace in Smithers, British Columbia, and the Avalon Sexual Assault Centre in Halifax, Nova Scotia.

If the survivor consents, involve supportive family or friends and discuss with them the nature and trauma of sexual assault, as well as the possible delayed reactions that may occur. One survivor expressed the aftermath of her assault as follows: "It takes a few days to hit you. It was bad. It was really rough for my husband. I needed to be reassured. I needed to be told that there was nothing I could have done to prevent it. Understanding helps."

Social support effectively moderates somatic symptoms and subjective health ratings. The survivor who is able to confide comfortably in one or two friends or family members, especially immediately after the assault, is likely to experience fewer somatic manifestations of stress. In many cases family and friends need support and reassurance as much as the survivor does. This is especially true for those from traditional cultures, particularly those cultures that believe that sexual assault brings shame to the entire family. The long-standing cultural myth that women are the property of men still prevents some people from empathizing with the woman's severe psychic injury and from being supportive. In these cases the woman is devalued instead.

Promotion of Self-Care Activities

When preparing the survivor for discharge, the nurse provides a printout of all referral information and follow-up instructions, detailing potential physical concerns and emotional reactions, legal matters, referrals to community agencies and counselling, and ways that family and friends can help. Providing this information in print is important because the amount of verbal information the patient can retain will likely be limited due to high levels of anxiety. Written material can be referred to repeatedly over time.

Follow-Up Care

The emotional state and psychological needs of the survivor should be reassessed by telephone or personal contact within 24 to 48 hours of discharge from the hospital. Repeat referrals should be made for resources or support services. Effective crisis intervention and continuity of care require outreach activities and services beyond the emergency medical setting.

Survivors may avoid seeking treatment from psychiatric mental health care providers because medical treatment is more socially sanctioned, and they are likely to be experiencing physical symptoms of stress. Thus the outpatient nurse can make a more focused assessment of stress-related symptoms, depression, or both and ascertain the need for mental health referral. Reporting symptoms and seeking medical treatment are adaptive coping behaviours and can be reinforced as such.

Follow-up visits should occur at least 2, 4, and 6 weeks after the initial evaluation; however, this frequency requires the consent of the survivor. At each visit, the survivor should be assessed for psychological progress, the presence of an STI, and pregnancy. Follow-up treatments for potential HIV exposure may also be administered if required. Case Study and Nursing Care Plan 25.1 describes the care of a patient who has been sexually assaulted.

CASE STUDY AND NURSING CARE PLAN 25.1
Sexual Assault

Jenna Smith is a 23-year-old Australian working at a Canadian ski hill hotel on a temporary work visa. One evening, when not on shift at the hotel, she goes out with some friends and workmates for a night of bowling and drinks at a club afterward. Later in the evening, Jenna is tired and ready to go home. A man, Ryan, who joined the group at the club, offers to take her home. She has seen Ryan at other parties before but does not know much about him, though he is fun to be around and is an acquaintance of one of her workmates. Not in the habit of going home alone with men she does not know, she hesitates. Their mutual friend, whom she trusts, encourages her to accept the ride, stating that he "seems like a nice man."

Ryan drives Jenna home. He then asks if he can come into her house to use the bathroom before driving the long distance back to his house. She reluctantly agrees and sits on the living room couch. After using the bathroom, Ryan sits next to Jenna and begins to kiss her and fondle her breasts. As she protests, Ryan becomes more forceful in his advances. Jenna is confused and frightened. She manages to get away from him briefly, but he begins grabbing, squeezing, and biting her. He tells her gruffly, "If you don't do what I say, I'll break your neck." She screams, but he proceeds to sexually assault her. Ryan becomes nervous that the noise will alert the neighbours and races out of the house.

A neighbour does in fact arrive just after Ryan flees. The neighbour calls the police and then brings Jenna to the local hospital emergency department for a physical examination, crisis intervention, and support. In the emergency department Jenna is visibly shaken. She keeps saying, over and over, "I shouldn't have let him take me home. I should have fought harder; I shouldn't have let him do this."

The nurse takes Jenna to a quiet cubicle. She does not want Jenna to stay alone and asks the neighbour to stay with her. The nurse then notifies the doctor and the SANE. When the nurse comes back, she tells Jenna that she would like to talk to her before the doctor comes. Jenna looks at her neighbour and then down. The nurse asks the neighbour to wait outside for a while and says she will call her later.

Jenna: "It was horrible. I feel so dirty."
Nurse: "You have had a traumatic experience. Do you want to talk about it?"
Jenna: "I feel so ashamed. I never should have let that man take me home."
Nurse: "You think that if you hadn't gone home with a stranger this wouldn't have happened?"
Jenna: "Yes ... I shouldn't have let him do it to me anyway. I shouldn't have let him rape me."
Nurse: "You mentioned that he said he would break your neck if you didn't do as he said."
Jenna: "Yes, he said that ... he was going to kill me. It was awful."
Nurse: "It seems you did the right thing in order to stay alive."

CASE STUDY AND NURSING CARE PLAN 25.1—cont'd

Sexual Assault

As the nurse continues to talk with her, Jenna's anxiety level seems to lessen. The nurse talks to Jenna about the kinds of experiences survivors may have after a sexual assault and explains that the reactions she might have 2 or 3 weeks from now are normal in these circumstances. The nurse continues to collect the necessary information. She says that the doctor will want to examine Jenna and explains the procedure to her. She then asks Jenna to sign a consent form. While preparing Jenna for examination, the nurse notices bite marks and bruises on both breasts. She also notes Jenna's lower lip, which is cut and bleeding. The nurse keeps detailed notes on her observations and draws a body map of the injuries. After the examination, Jenna is given clean clothes and a place to shower.

Assessment

Self-Assessment

The nurse has worked with sexual assault survivors before and has helped develop the hospital protocol. It took a while for her to be able to remain both neutral and responsive, because her own anger at perpetrators had initially interfered. She also remembers a time when a woman came in stating that she was assaulted but was so calm, smiling, and polite that the nurse initially did not believe her story. She had not at that point examined her own feelings or dealt with the popular societal myths regarding sexual assault. It was only later, when she had talked to more experienced health care personnel, that she learned that crisis reactions can seem bizarre, confusing, and contradictory.

The nurse learned that staying with the survivor, encouraging her to express her reactions and feelings, and listening are effective methods of reducing feelings of anxiety. Once the nurse learned through supervision and peer discussion to let go of her personal anger at the attacker and her ambivalence toward the survivor, her care and effectiveness improved greatly. All of this growth took time and support from more experienced nurses and other members of the health care team.

Objective Data	Subjective Data
Crying and sobbing	"He was going to kill me."
Bruises and bite marks on each breast	"It was horrible. I feel so dirty."
Lip cut and bleeding	"I shouldn't have let him rape me."
Sexual assault reported to the police	

Diagnosis

The nurse formulates the following diagnosis: *Rape-trauma syndrome.*

Supporting Data

- "I shouldn't have let him rape me."
- "He was going to kill me."
- Crying and sobbing.
- Bruises and bite marks on both breasts.
- Rape reported to the police.
- "It was horrible. I feel so dirty."

Outcomes Identification

Overall outcome: Abuse recovery: Emotional
Short-term indicator: Jenna will demonstrate appropriate affect for the situation.
Intermediate indicator: Jenna will demonstrate confidence. Short-term and intermediate outcome indicators are measured on a five-point Likert scale from 1 (none) to 5 (extensive).

Planning

The nurse plans to provide emotional and physical support to Jenna while she receives care in the emergency setting and to make sure that Jenna is aware of the importance of follow-up care.

Implementation

Jenna's plan of care is personalized as follows.

Short-Term Goal	Intervention	Rationale
1. Jenna will demonstrate appropriate affect by discharge from the emergency department.	1a. Remain neutral and non-judgemental, and assure survivor of confidentiality.	1a. Lessens feelings of shame and guilt and encourages sharing of painful feelings.
	1b. Do not leave survivor alone.	1b. Deters feelings of isolation and escalation of anxiety.
	1c. Allow patient negative expressions and behavioural self-blame while using reflective techniques.	1c. Fosters feelings of control.

Continued

CASE STUDY AND NURSING CARE PLAN 25.1—cont'd
Sexual Assault

Short-Term Goal	Intervention	Rationale
	1d. Assure survivor she did the right thing to save her life.	1d. Decreases burden of guilt and shame.
	1e. When anxiety level is down to moderate, encourage problem solving, choice, and power in decision making.	1e. Increases survivor's feeling of control in her own life. (When in severe anxiety, a person cannot problem-solve.)
	1f. Tell survivor of common reactions experienced by people in long-term reorganization phase (e.g., phobias, flashbacks, insomnia, increased motor activity).	1f. Helps survivor anticipate reactions and understand them as part of recovery process.
	1g. Explain emergency department procedure to survivor.	1g. Lowers anticipatory anxiety.
	1h. Explain physical examination.	1h. Allows for questions and concerns; survivor may be too traumatized and may refuse.
	1i. Stay with survivor during physical examination. A SANE can perform examination.	1i. Physical examination may be experienced as a second assault. Nurse provides comfort and support.

Evaluation

Jenna is able to express her feelings in the emergency department, as well as understand the feelings she may experience as she moves through the reorganization phase. The indicator is achieved at a level of 3 (moderate).

Advanced-Practice Interventions

Sexual assault nurse examiners. Internationally, forensic nursing is becoming a specialty, and the largest subspecialty of forensic nursing is caring for the sexual assault survivor. This role is filled by the SANE. Training to become a SANE requires knowledge and skill in the areas of testing and treatment for STIs; collection of forensic evidence; assessment of injuries; documentation; typical survivor responses and crisis intervention; collaboration with community agencies, such as police and women's shelters; and physical assessment and examination to determine the effects of the sexual assault (International Association of Forensic Nurses, 2021).

Survivors. Most of those who have been sexually assaulted are eventually able to resume their previous lifestyle and level of functioning after supportive services and crisis counselling. However, many continue to experience emotional trauma, including flashbacks, nightmares, fear, phobias, and other symptoms associated with the trauma and with the related PTSD (see Chapter 12). Some people who survive sexual assault may be susceptible to an acute stress response, dissociation, psychotic episode, or emotional disturbance so severe that hospitalization is required. Others whose emotional lives may be overburdened with multiple internal and external pressures may require individual psychotherapy.

Depression and suicidal ideation too frequently follow sexual assault. Depression is more common in those who do not disclose the assault to significant others because they have concerns about being stigmatized, have children living at home, or have a pending civil lawsuit. Any exposure to stimuli related to the traumatic event may activate a reliving of the traumatic state.

Evidence-based treatments include trauma-focused psychotherapy that may include components of exposure or cognitive restructuring and eye movement desensitization and reprocessing therapy. These modalities are often combined with anxiety management or stress reduction that focuses on alleviation of symptoms. Other helpful strategies include brief psychodynamic psychotherapy, imagery, relaxation techniques, and hypnosis. People who have been sexually assaulted are also likely to benefit from group therapy or support groups. These modalities may be particularly beneficial for survivors from cultures that are group oriented rather than individualistic and for women who derive much of their self-definition from cultural norms. Group therapy can make the difference between a person coming out of the crisis at a lower level of functioning and that person gradually adapting to the experience with an increase in coping skills.

Psychoeducation can benefit patients experiencing dissociative disorders following sexual assault or other traumatic events. There is a need to learn about these responses and to gain new coping skills and stress management to manage the symptoms that can be frightening. Normalizing experiences by explaining symptoms as adaptive responses to overwhelming events is important.

Grounding techniques promote awareness of in-the-moment real things and help counter dissociative episodes. For example, dissociation can be disrupted by stomping one's feet, taking a shower, holding an ice cube, exercising, deep breathing, or touching the upholstery on a chair. Patients can learn to keep a daily journal to increase awareness of feelings and to identify triggers to dissociation. If a patient has never written in a journal, the nurse should suggest beginning with a 5- to 10-minute daily writing exercise.

Somatic therapies or sensorimotor psychotherapy combines talk therapy with body-centred interventions and movement to address dissociative symptoms (Ogden et al., 2006). This therapy is based on the premise that the body, mind, emotions, and spirit are interrelated and that a change at one level results in changes in the others. Awareness, focusing on the present, and recognizing touch as a means of communicating are some of the principles of this therapy. During psychotherapy sessions, the patient describes current physical sensations. The goal is to safely disarm the pathological defence mechanism of dissociation and replace it with other resources, especially body awareness and mindfulness.

Perpetrators. As stated previously, sexual assault is an act of violence and an abuse of power and control. This abuse is not necessarily indicative of a particular mental health problem; however, psychotherapy is essential for perpetrators of sexual assault to gain consciousness and change behaviours. Unfortunately, most perpetrators do not acknowledge the need for behavioural change, and no single method or program of treatment has been found to be completely effective. The nurse's awareness of their own feelings and reactions will be crucial to avoid interference with the therapeutic process.

Evaluation

Sexual assault survivors are considered to be recovered if they are relatively free of any signs or symptoms of PTSD and dissociative disorders; that is, if they are

- Sleeping well, with very few instances of episodic nightmares or broken sleep
- Eating as they were before the assault (patients may respond to the crisis of rape by undereating or overeating)
- Calm and relaxed or only mildly suspicious, fearful, or restless
- Getting support from family and friends (some strain might still be present in relationships, but it should be minimal)
- Generally positive about themselves (on occasion, doubts about self-worth may occur)
- Managing stress adaptively, without dissociation and free from somatic reactions (if mild symptoms persist and minor discomfort is reported, the survivor should be able to talk about it and feel in control of the symptoms)
- Showing a return to pre–sexual assault sexual functioning and interest

In general, the closer the survivor's lifestyle is to the pattern that was present before the sexual assault, the more complete the recovery has been.

RESEARCH HIGHLIGHT

Can Virtual Environments Mediate Post-Traumatic Stress Disorder (PTSD) for Sexual Assault Victims?

Problem
Most women who are victims of sexual assault report a post-traumatic response in the days and weeks following the event. In most cases these manifestations fade away over time. Unfortunately, though, for about one quarter of victims of sexual assault, post-traumatic responses persist for months. Regardless, the effects can be disabling. Virtual reality has shown promising results in the treatment of PTSD for some traumatic experiences, but sexual assault has been understudied.

Purpose of Study
This study sought to examine the relevance and safety of a virtual environment intervention, allowing patients to be progressively exposed to a sexual assault scenario.

Methods
Thirty women (victims and non-victims of sexual assault) were randomly assigned in a counterbalanced order to two immersions in a virtual bar: a control scenario in which the encounter with the aggressor does not lead to sexual assault and an experimental scenario in which the participant is assaulted. Immersions were conducted in a fully immersive six-wall system. Questionnaires were administered, and psychophysiological measures were recorded. No adverse events were reported during or after the immersions.

Key Findings
Repeated-measures analyses of covariance revealed a significant time effect and significantly more anxiety and negative affect in the experimental scenario than in the control condition.

Implications for Nursing Practice
Given the safety of the scenario and its potential to induce emotions, it can be further tested to document its usefulness with sexual assault victims who suffer PTSD.

Source: Loranger, C., & Bouchard, S. (2017). Validating a virtual environment for sexual assault victims. *Journal of Traumatic Stress, 30*(2), 157–165. https://doi.org/10.1002/jts.22170

KEY POINTS TO REMEMBER

- Sexual assault is a common and often under-reported crime of violence in Canada.
- Females are far more likely to be survivors of sexual assault and tend to know their perpetrators. Sexual assault of males tends to be under-reported, owing to the humiliation and stigma attached to such victimization.
- Psychoactive substances play a major role in sexual assault, and alcohol is the most commonly used date rape drug. Other disinhibiting and amnesic substances also play a role in forcible sex acts.
- A sexual assault survivor experiences a wide range of feelings, which may or may not be exhibited to others.
- Feelings of fear, degradation, anger and rage, helplessness, and nervousness; sleep disturbances; disturbed relationships; flashbacks; depression; and somatic complaints are all common following sexual assault.
- The circumstances of the initial medical evaluation may be frightening and stressful. Police interrogation, repeated questioning by health care providers, and the physical examination itself all have the potential to add to the trauma of the sexual assault.
- The sexual assault nurse examiner (SANE) can serve to minimize repetition of questions and support the survivor as she goes through the entire ordeal.
- Survivors require long-term health care that can include counselling to minimize long-term effects of the sexual assault and assist in early return to a normal living pattern.
- Telephone and online resources are available to assist sexual assault survivors.

CRITICAL THINKING

1. Isaac, 18 years of age, is brutally beaten and sexually assaulted by a group of young men at a university party where Isaac was intoxicated and unconscious. After he regained consciousness, he tried to walk home but fell and was found semiconscious by a passerby and taken to the emergency department. Isaac has three large bruises around the occipital area of his head and several on his chest and buttocks. He has sustained a cracked rib, which he splints when walking. In assessment, he has a visible 2-cm anal tear and is wincing in pain that he states is an 8 out of 10. Ms. Lynkowski, a SANE, works with Isaac using the hospital's sexual assault protocol. Isaac appears stunned and confused and has difficulty focusing on what the nurse says. He states repeatedly, "This is crazy, this can't be happening . . . I can't believe this has happened to me . . . Oh, my God, I can't believe this."

    a. What areas of Isaac's assessment should be given highest priority by Ms. Lynkowski and her staff while he is in the emergency department?

    b. Chart the signs and symptoms of Isaac's physical and emotional trauma and verbatim statements in as much detail as you can.

    c. What are some of the pivotal issues that need to be addressed in terms of assessing Isaac's signs and symptoms of physical trauma? Although the risk of pregnancy is not present, what other real physical risks need to be assessed?

    d. What are some of the signs and symptoms of rape-trauma syndrome? Of the controlled style of coping?

    e. Identify the short-term outcome criteria for Isaac that ideally would be met before he leaves the emergency department.

    f. What information does Isaac need to have regarding potential signs and symptoms that may occur in the near future? Why is this important for him to understand at present?

g. Identify specific indicators that will be met if Isaac recovers with minimal trauma from the event. How would you evaluate these criteria?

CHAPTER REVIEW

1. The nurse is caring for a patient in the emergency department who was sexually assaulted just hours earlier. Which behaviours should the nurse expect if the patient was exhibiting controlled-style reactions?
   a. Shock, numbness
   b. Volatility, anger
   c. Crying, sobbing
   d. Smiling, laughing

2. The nurse is caring for a patient who has just been sexually assaulted. Which is the appropriate initial nursing response?
   a. "I will get you the number for the crisis intervention specialist."
   b. "May I get your consent to test you for pregnancy and HIV?"
   c. "You are safe here."
   d. "I need to look at your bruises and cuts."

3. A patient who has been sexually assaulted has chosen to accept pregnancy prophylaxis medication but states that she does not believe in abortion. What information can you, as a nurse, give that will help with her decision?
   a. "Emergency contraception is not an abortion pill and will not work if you are already pregnant. That is the reason we perform a pregnancy test."
   b. "Just take a few days to consider your options."
   c. "Here is the number to your local sexual health clinic. They can explain it to you."
   d. "I won't give you the pregnancy prophylaxis medication then."

4. The nurse is working at a telephone hotline centre when a sexual assault survivor calls. If the sexual assault survivor states that she is fearful of going to the hospital, what is the appropriate nursing response?
   a. "You don't need to go to the hospital if you don't want to."
   b. "I'm here to listen to you, and we can talk about your feelings."
   c. "Did you do something to make the other person attack you?"
   d. "Why are you afraid to seek medical attention?"

5. The nurse is caring for a patient who is in the long-term reorganization phase of rape-trauma syndrome. Which symptoms should the nurse anticipate? **Select all that apply.**
   a. Development of fear of locations that resemble the rape location
   b. Emergence of acceptance of the rape
   c. Dreams with violent content
   d. A shift from anxiety to calm
   e. Onset of phobia of being alone

REFERENCES

Association of Alberta Sexual Assault Services. (2017). *Sexual violence action plan*. Retrieved from https://aasas.ca/initiatives/sexual-violence-action-plan/

Butcher, H. K., Bulechek, G. M., Dochterman, J. M., et al. (2019). *Nursing Interventions Classification (NIC)* (7th ed.). St. Louis: Mosby.

Carter-Snell, C., & Jakubec, S. L. (2013). Exploring influences on women's mental health after interpersonal violence. *International Journal of Child, Youth and Family Studies, 1*, 72–99. Retrieved from http://journals.uvic.ca/index.php/ijcyfs/article/view/11844/3413

Chiefs of Ontario. (2020). *A discussion paper: Ending sexual violence and sexual exploitation in First Nations Communities*. Retrieved from http://chiefs-of-ontario.org/wp-content/uploads/2020/09/FORMATTED-FINAL-Ending-Sexual-Violence-and-Sexual-Exploitation-In-First-Nation-Communities-v4.pdf

Criminal Code. (1985). *Criminal Code (R.S.C., 1985, c. C-46): Assault*. Retrieved from https://laws-lois.justice.gc.ca/eng/acts/C-46/page-62.html

Department of Justice Canada. (2017). *Victimization of indigenous women and girls*. Retrieved from https://www.justice.gc.ca/eng/rp-pr/jr/jf-pf/2017/docs/july05.pdf

DiMauro, J., & Renshaw, K. D. (2021). Trauma-related disclosure in sexual assault survivors' intimate relationships: Associations with PTSD, shame, and partners' responses. *Journal of Interpersonal Violence, 36*(3–4), NP1986-2004NP. https://doi.org/10.1177/0886260518756117

Du Mont, J., Kosa, D., Macdonald, S., Benoit, A., & Forte, T. (2017). A comparison of Indigenous and non-Indigenous survivors of sexual assault and their receipt of and satisfaction with specialized health care services. *PloS One, 12*(11), e0188253. https://doi.org/10.1371/journal.pone.0188253

Dworkin, E. R., Menon, S. V., Bystrynski, J., et al. (2017). Sexual assault victimization and psychopathology: A review and meta-analysis. *Clinical Psychology Review, 56*, 65–81. https://doi.org/10.1016/j.cpr.2017.06.002

Emergency Nurses Association. (2017). Emergency Nurses Association position statements: Adult and adolescent sexual assault patients in the emergency care setting. Retrieved from https://www.nursingcenter.com/wkhlrp/Handlers/articleContent.pdf?key=pdf_01263942-201706000-00010

Emergency Nurses Association. (2018). Emergency Nurses Association position statement: Forensic evidence collection in the emergency care setting. *Journal of Emergency Nursing, 44*(3), 286–289. http://dx.doi.org/10.1016/j.jen.2018.03.010

Ending Violence Association of British Columbia. (2016). *Campus sexual violence: Guidelines for a comprehensive response*. Retrieved from http://endingviolence.org/wp-content/uploads/2016/05/EVABC_CampusSexualViolenceGuidelines_vF.pdf

Fedina, L., Holmes, J. L., & Backes, B. L. (2018). Campus sexual assault: A systematic review of prevalence research from 2000 to 2015. *Trauma, Violence and Abuse, 19*(1), 76–93. https://doi.org/10.1177/1524838016631129

Freedman, E. (2020). Clinical management of patients presenting following a sexual assault. *Australian Journal of General Practice, 49*(7), 406–411. https://doi.org/10.31128/AJGP-01-20-5199.

Government of Ontario. (2021). *Sexual violence*. Retrieved from https://www.ontario.ca/page/sexual-violence

Greeson, M. R., Campbell, R., & Fehler-Cabral, G. (2016). "Nobody deserves this": Adolescent sexual assault victims' perceptions of disbelief and victim blame from police. *Journal of Community Psychology, 44*(1), 90–110. https://doi.org/10.1002/jcop.21744

International Association of Forensic Nurses. (2021). *Sexual assault nurse examiners*. Retrieved from https://www.forensicnurses.org/page/aboutSANE

Lalonde, D., Tabibi, J., & Baker, L. (2020). Trauma- and violence - informed approaches: Supporting children exposed to intimate partner violence. Retrieved from http://www.vawlearningnetwork.ca/our-work/issuebased_newsletters/issue-31/LN-Issue-31-PT.pdf

Long, L. M. (2020). Rape medical advocates experiences with vicarious trauma, burnout and self-care. *Journal of Aggression,*

Maltreatment & Trauma, 29(4), 421–441. https://doi.org/10.1080/10926771.2019.1578315

Mikton, C. R., Tanaka, M., Tomlinson, M., et al. (2017). Global research priorities for interpersonal violence prevention: A modified Delphi study/Priorités mondiales de recherche pour la prévention de la violence interpersonnelle: Une étude delphi modifiée/Prioridades de investigación globales para la prevención de la violencia interpersonal: Un estudio de delphi modificado. *Bulletin of the World Health Organization, 95*(1), 36. https://doi.org/10.2471/BLT.16.172965

Moorhead, S., Johnson, M., Meridean, M. L., et al. (2018). *Nursing Outcomes Classification (NOC)* (6th ed.). St. Louis: Elsevier.

Ogden, P., Minton, K., & Pain, C. (2006). *Trauma and the body: A sensorimotor approach to psychotherapy*. New York: Norton.

Ontario Network of Sexual Assault/Domestic Violence Treatment Centres. (n.d.). *Our centres: Mandate*. Retrieved from https://www.sadvtreatmentcentres.ca

Sachs, C. J., Ladd, M., & Thomas B. (2021). *Sexual assault infectious disease prophylaxis*. Retrieved from https://www.ncbi.nlm.nih.gov/books/NBK482239/

Scheim, A. I., Jackson, R., James, L., et al. (2013). Barriers to well-being for Aboriginal gender-diverse people: Results from the Trans PULSE Project in Ontario, Canada. *Ethnicity and Inequalities in Health and Social Care, 6*(4), 108–120. https://doi.org/10.1108/EIHSC-08-2013-0010

Statistics Canada. (2017). *Police-reported sexual assaults in Canada 2009–2014: A statistical profile*. Retrieved from https://www150.statcan.gc.ca/n1/pub/85-002-x/2017001/article/54866-eng.htm

Statistics Canada. (2020a). *Police-reported crime statistics in Canada, 2019*. Retrieved from https://www150.statcan.gc.ca/n1/pub/85-002-x/2020001/article/00010-eng.htm

Statistics Canada. (2020b). *Experiences of violent victimization and unwanted sexual behaviour among gay, lesbian, bisexual and other sexual minority people, and the transgender population, in Canada 2018*. Retrieved from https://www150.statcan.gc.ca/n1/pub/85-002-x/2020001/article/00009-eng.htm

Ullman, S. E., & Peter-Hagene, L. C. (2016). Longitudinal relationships of social reactions, PTSD, and revictimization in sexual assault survivors. *Journal of Interpersonal Violence, 31*(6), 1074–1094. https://doi.org/10.1177/0886260514564069

Voth Schrag, R. J. (2017). Campus based sexual assaults and dating violence. *Affilia, 32*(1), 67. https://doi.org/10.1177/0886109916644644

Walsh, K., Zinzow, H. M., Badour, C. L., et al. (2016). Understanding disparities in service seeking following forcible versus drug- or alcohol-facilitated/incapacitated rape. *Journal of Interpersonal Violence, 31*(14), 2475–2491. https://doi.org/10.1177/0886260515576968

UNIT 6

Interventions for Distinct Populations

26. Sexuality and Gender

27. Disorders of Children and Adolescents

28. Psychosocial Needs of the Older Person

29. Recovery, Survivorship, and Public Mental Health Approaches

30. Psychological Needs of Patients With Medical Conditions

31. Care for the Dying and for Those Who Grieve

32. Forensic Psychiatric Nursing

26

Sexuality and Gender

Erin Ziegler

 https://evolve.elsevier.com/Canada/Varcarolis/psychiatric/

OBJECTIVES

1. Describe sexuality and gender and be able to differentiate between the two.
2. Examine the importance of nurses being knowledgeable about and comfortable discussing topics pertaining to sexuality and gender. Explore your personal values and biases.
3. Apply assessment techniques for sexual and gender history.
4. Develop a plan of care for individuals diagnosed with gender dysphoria.
5. Describe the unique mental health issues in the LGBTQI2S (lesbian, gay, bisexual, transgender, queer, intersex, and Two-Spirit) population.

KEY TERMS AND CONCEPTS

bisexual	gender non-conforming	non-binary
cisgender	heterosexual	queer
gay	homosexual	sexual orientation
gender	internalized homophobia	sexuality
gender dysphoria	intersex	transgender
gender identity	lesbian	Two-Spirit

Gender and sexuality impact all aspects of a patient's health and well-being. Everyday professional nursing practice requires us to engage in matter-of-fact discussions with patients on topics generally considered to be private. We perform head-to-toe assessments in which we inquire about everything from headaches and sore throats to difficulties urinating and problems with constipation. The realities of providing physical care necessitate becoming comfortable with several skills that relate to privacy and modesty, performing breast examinations, initiating urinary catheters, and inserting rectal medications.

Health promotion and disease prevention are key responsibilities for nurses. All nurses must assess a patient's sexuality and gender and be prepared to educate, dispel myths, assist with clarification, refer to appropriate care providers when indicated, and share resources. As a nursing student, you are introduced to complex aspects of sexuality and gender that should facilitate thoughtful discussion of the topic, make you aware of your personal belief systems, and help you consider the broader perspective of sexuality and gender as they exist in contemporary society. This chapter addresses two general categories, sexuality and gender, followed by an exploration of relevant mental health issues.

 HOW A NURSE HELPED ME

Coming Out

As a little girl, I grew up in a loving family. My mom and dad were always very supportive of me, encouraging me to "be who I want to be." They would frequently make comments such as "when you get married and have kids" and "marry a good guy, just like your father." In high school I had a few boyfriends, nothing serious. I moved away to go to university when I was 18. It was at school that I met Stephanie. Stephanie was great, funny, smart, and fun to be around. In fact, I wanted to spend all my time with her. Stephanie was gay. I started to think about what it would be like to be her girlfriend. These thoughts scared me. I had never had thoughts about my sexuality before. I just always assumed I would do what my parents said and marry a guy just like my father. But now, after meeting Stephanie, I began to question my sexuality.

I made an appointment to speak to the nurse at the health centre at school. I told the nurse all about my feelings and the thoughts that I was having. Over the course of a few meetings, the nurse helped me to explore my feelings and my sexuality. She provided me with guidance and resources, but most importantly she supported me. Through my conversations with the nurse, I began to feel comfortable with my sexuality. She also helped me by providing me with resources to come out to my family and friends. The nurse helped me to realize who I was and provided me with the necessary tools I needed to explain my sexuality to my family and friends.

CHAPTER 26 Sexuality and Gender

CONSIDERING CULTURE
Sexual Orientation and Gender Identity

When we think about culture, we often relate it to concepts such as language, ethnicity, and race. Yet culture can be an important consideration in our discussion of sexual orientation and gender identity. We live in a world where the idea of sexual relationships, marriage, and childbearing occur in the context of a monogamous male–female relationship. Having traditionally dominated the way that society is structured, these ideas have created a heteronormative culture, including particular language and expression, within Canadian society. Heteronormativity assumes that heterosexuality is the only sexual orientation or the norm and is often associated with homonegativity and homophobia. Homonegativity is the disapproval of homosexuality, where homophobia is fear, aversion, or hatred toward homosexuality. Heteronormativity remains prevalent, but unacknowledged and can be a source of structural harms for LGBTQ2 patients. It is important to move beyond these traditional notions of sexuality and recognize that sexual orientation and gender identity can be diverse. Lesbian, gay, bisexual, transgender, and queer issues are increasingly visible in our society. As nurses, we must recognize the dominance of our heterosexual culture and its shaping of our own values and beliefs when providing care for all patients.

Sources: Davis-Delano, L., Morgan, E. M., Gillard, A., et al. (2018) When heterosexuality is questioned: Stifling suspicion through public displays of heterosexual identity. *Journal of Homosexuality, 65*(13), 1683–1708. https://doi.org/10.1080/00918369.2017.1387465; Searle, J. (2019). Queer phenomenology, the disruption of heteronormativity, and structurally responsive care. *Advances in Nursing Science, 42*(2), 109–122. https://doi.org/10.1097/ANS.0000000000000258

SEXUALITY

Sexuality is the way that people experience and express themselves as sexual beings. **Sexual orientation** is a person's sexual identity in relation to the gender to which they are attracted. An individual's sexual orientation can be said to be heterosexual, homosexual, or bisexual. Sexual orientation is biological; people are born heterosexual, homosexual, or bisexual. People who identify as **heterosexual** are sexually attracted to people of the opposite sex. Those who identify as **homosexual** are sexually attracted to people of the same sex. Homosexuality can be further classified as **gay** and **lesbian**. Men who are sexually attracted to men often use the term *gay* to describe their sexual orientation, whereas women who are sexually attracted to women may use the term *lesbian*. *Gay* may be used interchangeably by both men and women to describe their sexual orientation. People who are attracted to both men and women use the term **bisexual** to describe their sexual orientation. **Queer** is often used as an umbrella term for individuals who do not identify as heterosexual. Statistics Canada (2015) reported that 1.7% of Canadians between the ages of 18 and 59 identified as gay or lesbian, whereas 1.3% of Canadians in the same age group identified as bisexual.

In this chapter exploration of nursing care related to sexuality is for people who identify as homosexual or bisexual. To provide competent and compassionate nursing care to individuals who identify as homosexual or bisexual, it is important to also understand the acronyms used to describe this population. Acronyms such as LGBT (lesbian, gay, bisexual, and transgender), LGBTQ (lesbian, gay, bisexual, transgender, and queer), and LGBTTIQQ2SA (lesbian, gay, bisexual, transsexual, transgender, intersex, queer, questioning, Two-Spirit, and allies) have been used in the media, popular culture, and literature. Recently, the term *allies* was added to the community. *Allies* is a term used to describe someone who is supportive of LGBTQI2S people. It encompasses non-LGBTQI2S allies as well as those within the LGBTQI2S community who support each other. Although LGBTQI2S is the generally accepted acronym in Canada, this text will use LGBTQ2 as the government-sanctioned term to describe this population.

GENDER

When we inquire about the birth of a new infant, one of the first things we want to know is whether the baby is a boy or a girl. Actually, we are asking about the sex of the child (i.e., whether its chromosomes are XX or XY). Sometimes the gender of the individual is not known. Intersex is a set of medical conditions that features a congenital anomaly of the reproductive system or genitals. **Intersex** individuals are born with chromosomes, external genitalia, or internal reproductive systems that are not considered either male or female. However, biological assignment does not determine whether individuals think of themselves as male or female. **Gender** refers to a person's identity and social classifications, often based on masculine or feminine qualities and traits. Cultural influences can influence expectations about attributes or behaviours specific to gender. Gender roles and inequality can have an impact of social determinates of health. **Gender identity** refers to one's sense of self as male or female. Gender identity can be classified as cisgender or transgender. **Cisgender** refers to one's gender identity being aligned with the gender assigned at birth. A cisgender female is a person who was born female, identifies as female, and uses feminine pronouns such as *she* and *her*. **Transgender** refers to an incongruence in a person's gender identity with the gender assigned at birth. A transgender male is a person who was born female, identifies as male, and may use male pronouns such as *him* and *he* (Bourns, 2019). Recent estimates suggest that 0.6% of adults identify as transgender, which is approximately 200 000 transgender adults in Canada (Giblon & Bauer, 2017). **Gender non-conforming** individuals have a gender expression that does not conform to traditional social and cultural gender norms of male and female. Individuals whose gender identity is not male or female, who identify as no gender, as a gender other than male or female, or as more than one gender may use the term **non-binary** to describe their gender (James et al., 2016). **Two-Spirit** is used by some Indigenous people to describe their gender, sexual, or spiritual identity and refers to a person who embodies both a male and a female spirit. Two-Spirit encompasses the Indigenous views of gender roles, including the sexual and gender diversity in Indigenous communities (Trans Care BC, 2021).

Transgender is included within the acronym LGBTQ2, which represents a sexual and gender minority. However, it is very important to distinguish that lesbian, gay, bisexual, and queer are related to sexual orientation, whereas transgender is related to gender identity. The sexual orientation of transgender individuals can be heterosexual, lesbian, gay, bisexual, or queer. As with cisgender people, sexual orientation should never be assumed. When asking a patient about sexual activities, avoid asking questions such as "Do you have a boyfriend?" or "In the last 6 months, how many women have you had sex with?" Such questions assume heterosexuality. For patients who do not identify as heterosexual, these types of questions may cause the patient to not fully disclose or discuss anything further, as they may feel that you are not open or may pass judgement. Instead, when asking about sexual activity or sexuality, make general statements such as "Do you have sex with men, women, or both?" By asking this question, the nurse is opening the door for further discussion and letting the patient know that sexuality is not an issue and that they can feel comfortable having these conversations.

VIGNETTE

Casey self-identifies as male. He uses male pronouns and has a masculine appearance. His family and friends are accepting and supporting of his transition. Casey still gets nervous in certain social situations and worries about his safety. His main concerns are having to use the men's washroom and showing his identification, which still has the name Cassandra and a female gender marker. What if someone questions or challenges him? What if this is not safe for him? For this reason, Casey tries his best to avoid anywhere he must show identification and using public washrooms.

Casey gets sick and needs to go to the clinic. He arrives at a new medical clinic to meet with the nurse. When he arrives, the first thing he notices is the large Safe Space poster on the door and in the reception area. He meets with the nurse, who right away asks him what name and pronouns he uses. The nurse advises him that the clinic is a safe space and has gender-neutral washrooms for everyone's use. Because of these actions, Casey feels comfortable using this clinic and is able to talk with the nurse about his transition goals.

GENDER DYSPHORIA

Gender dysphoria is the distress experienced by an individual when their gender identity and their gender assigned at birth are incongruent. Gender dysphoria, as outlined in the *Diagnostic and Statistics Manual of Mental Disorders*, fifth edition (*DSM-5*), is a medical diagnosis often required prior to initiation of transgender medical or surgical transition. However, there has been great debate about the use of and appropriateness of using a psychiatric diagnosis with transgender individuals, within both the medical and the transgender communities. It is important to be aware of the potential for stigmatization of transgender individuals when the diagnosis of gender dysphoria is perceived as a psychiatric illness (Bourns, 2019). Diagnostic criteria for gender dysphoria in children, adolescents, and adults are listed in the DSM-5: Criteria for Gender Dysphoria.

DSM-5
Criteria for Gender Dysphoria

Gender Dysphoria in Children

A. A marked incongruence between one's experienced or expressed gender and assigned gender, of at least 6 months' duration, as manifested by at least six of the following (one of which must be Criterion A1):
  1. A strong desire to be of the other gender or an insistence that one is the other gender (or some alternative gender different from one's assigned gender).
  2. In boys (assigned gender) a strong preference for cross-dressing or simulating female attire; in girls (assigned gender) a strong preference for wearing only typical masculine clothing and a strong resistance to wearing typical feminine clothing.
  3. A strong preference for cross-gender roles in make-believe play or fantasy play.
  4. A strong preference for the toys, games, or activities stereotypically used or engaged in by the other gender.
  5. A strong preference for playmates of the other gender.
  6. In boys (assigned gender) a strong rejection of typically masculine toys, games, and activities and a strong avoidance of rough-and-tumble play; in girls (assigned gender) a strong rejection of typically feminine toys, games, and activities.
  7. A strong dislike of one's sexual anatomy.
  8. A strong desire for the primary and/or secondary sex characteristics that match one's experienced gender.

B. The condition is associated with clinically significant distress or impairment in social, school, or other important areas of functioning.

Gender Dysphoria in Adolescents and Adults

A. A marked incongruence between one's experienced or expressed gender and assigned gender, of at least 6 months' duration, as manifested by at least two of the following:
  1. A marked incongruence between one's experienced or expressed gender and primary and/or secondary sex characteristics.
  2. A strong desire to be rid of one's primary and/or secondary sex characteristics because of a marked incongruence with one's experienced or expressed gender (or in adolescents, a desire to prevent the development of the anticipated secondary sex characteristics).
  3. A strong desire for the primary and/or secondary sex characteristics of the other gender.
  4. A strong desire to be of the other gender (or some alternative gender different from one's assigned gender).
  5. A strong desire to be treated as the other gender (or some alternative gender different from one's assigned gender).
  6. A strong conviction that one has the typical feelings and reactions of the other gender (or some alternative gender different from one's assigned gender).

B. The condition is associated with clinically significant distress or impairment in social, occupational, or other important areas of functioning.

Specify if:
With a disorder of sex development (e.g., a congenital adrenogenital disorder such as 255.2 [E25.0] congenital adrenal hyperplasia or 259.50 [E34.50] androgen insensitivity syndrome).
Coding note: Code the disorder of sex development and gender dysphoria.
Specify if:
Post-transition: The individual has transitioned to living full-time in the desired gender (with or without legalization of gender change) and has undergone (or is preparing to have) at least one cross-sex medical procedure or treatment regimen, namely, regular cross-sex hormone treatment or gender reassignment surgery confirming the desired gender (e.g., penectomy, vaginoplasty in a natal male; mastectomy or phalloplasty in a natal female).

Source: Modified from American Psychiatric Association. (2013). *Diagnostic and statistical manual of disorders* (5th ed., pp. 452–453). Washington, DC: Author.

GENDER INCONGRUENCE

To further depathologize transgender identities, the updated *International Classification of Diseases*, 11 Revision (ICD-11) renamed and moved the diagnosis *Gender Incongruence* from the mental health section to the section on sexual health. Unlike the DSM, there is no criteria for significant impairment and distress. The move to the sexual health section further supports that gender identity is not a mental health condition. The aim of the updated ICD-11 diagnosis is to ensure transgender individuals have access to gender-affirming health care. Gender-affirmative healthcare includes medical, social, psychological, and/or behavioural healthcare that is supportive and affirming of someone's gender identity. Diagnostic criteria for gender incongruence are listed in ICD-11: Gender Incongruence.

ICD-11
Criteria for Gender Incongruence

Gender Incongruence of Childhood
In pre-pubertal children the criteria include a marked incongruence between an individual's experienced/expressed gender and the assigned sex. This incongruence includes: a strong desire to be a different gender than the assigned sex; a strong dislike on the child's part of their sexual anatomy or anticipated secondary sex characteristics, and/or a strong desire for the primary and/or anticipated secondary sex characteristics that match the experienced gender; and make-believe or fantasy play, toys, games, or activities and playmates that are typical of the experienced gender rather than the assigned sex. The incongruence must be present for about 2 years. Note that gender variant behaviour and preferences alone are not a basis for assigning the diagnosis.

Gender Incongruence of Adolescents or Adults
In adolescents and adults the diagnosis is characterized by marked and persistent incongruence between an individual's experienced gender and the assigned sex. This incongruence often leads to a desire to "transition," in order to live and be accepted as a person of the experienced gender, through hormonal treatment, surgery or other health care services to make the individual's body align, as much as desired and to the extent possible, with the experienced gender. The diagnosis is not assigned prior to the onset of puberty. Gender variant behaviour and preferences alone are not a basis for assigning the diagnosis; there must be a desire to prevent the development of the anticipated secondary sex characteristics in adolescents or to be rid of the secondary sex characteristics in adults.

Source: World Health Organization. (2019). *ICD-11- International classification of diseases for mortality and morbidity statistics*. Retrieved from https://icd.who.int/icd11refguide/en/index.html

CLINICAL PICTURE

Gender incongruence in children includes expressions of a desire to be the opposite sex. Some children insist that they *are* the opposite sex and ask their families to call them by another name. Adolescents may dread the appearance of secondary sexual characteristics. Individuals may seek hormones or surgery as part of their gender transition.

EPIDEMIOLOGY

There are approximately 25 million transgender individuals worldwide, with 0.6% of the adult population identifying as transgender. Rates for adolescents are higher than for adults, with 1.2 to 4% reporting a gender incongruence (Becker et al., 2017; Bonifacio, 2019; Eisenberg et al., 2017). Specific Canadian data on the prevalence of transgender individuals are lacking. Statistics Canada currently collects gender data for only two categories: male and female, while acknowledging that gender may change over time and the life course (Statistics Canada, 2019).

NURSING CARE FOR TRANSGENDER INDIVIDUALS

Nurses have a role in providing care and support for transgender individuals. Nurses can help individuals in seeking social support, using healthy coping behaviors, and acknowledging and accepting gender identity.

ADVANCED INTERVENTIONS

Pharmacological

Pharmacological interventions in childhood and adolescents may be used to delay puberty and to give youth and their families more time to make decisions about transitioning. Hormonal suppression can prevent the development of secondary sex characteristics which can improve self-esteem and body image. Adolescents and adults may choose to take hormones to help them in their transition. Transmasculine transitions can include the use of testosterone. The testosterone allows for more muscle development, facial and body hair, clitoral enlargement, amenorrhea, and increased sex drive. Transfeminine individuals may take estrogen and anti-androgens. These medications cause body fat redistribution, reduction in facial and body hair, breast growth, and loss of spontaneous erections and testicular volume.

Surgical

Gender-affirming surgery may be the ultimate goal for some transgender individuals, although it is important to note that not all transgender individuals have surgery. Surgical options for transgender women individuals include the removal of the penis (penectomy) and testes (orchiectomy) and the addition of a vagina (vaginoplasty). Some transgender women individuals also choose to have facial feminization surgery, including tracheal shaving, to have more feminine facial features as well as breast augmentation. For transgender men, surgical procedures may include the removal of the breasts (mastectomy) and chest re-contouring, removal of the uterus (hysterectomy) and ovaries (oophorectomy), and the construction of a neopenis (phalloplasty).

APPLICATION OF THE NURSING PROCESS

Assessment

Self-Assessment

Despite a learned fearlessness when it comes to addressing other intimate issues, nurses, as well as other health care providers, may often find the topic of sexuality and gender a source of discomfort. Nurses have a role in providing patients with support, education, and information, and by conducting a complete assessment, nurses will gather the information necessary to help their patients. Patients need and want access to non-judgmental and accurate education about gender, sexuality, and sexual health (Fennell & Grant, 2019). For LGBTQ2 individuals, meeting a new nurse involves a decision if they are going to reveal their sexual orientation or gender identity (Manzer et al., 2018). As a nurse, it is important for you to bring up the topic of sexuality and gender when assessing your patients. By you starting the conversation, you provide a clear message that it is okay for your patients to talk about these issues and that it is a safe space for them. Assess in yourself where you may have hesitancy or discomfort and seek supervision and support to begin patient care with skill and compassion.

Remembering your position as a professional and addressing the topics in a tone and manner appropriate will increase your comfort, along with the patients'. Nurses can set the comfort level for discussion and foster opportunities to address feelings and concerns. Further, letting the patient know why you are asking such personal questions increases openness and cooperation. For example, you can say, "I am going to ask you some questions now that relate to your sexuality and gender. Your sexual health is important to your overall physical and emotional health."

Perhaps the most helpful consideration is that assessing sexuality and gender identity is part of holistic nursing care. Your role and responsibility are to assist the patient in dealing with responses to illness or the treatment of the illness. Understanding your patient's concerns, acknowledging any discomfort or distress, and providing useful feedback will enhance your professional abilities to care for your patient and perhaps even improve self-understanding.

ASSESSMENT GUIDELINES
Sexuality and Gender Assessments

1. The interviewer should reflect on their own personal biases and judgmental attitudes that could block open discussion of sexuality and gender.
2. A sexuality or gender assessment should be conducted in a setting that allows privacy and eliminates distractions.
3. Although note taking may be necessary for the beginner, it can be distracting to the patient and interrupt the flow of the interview. When note taking is necessary, it should be unobtrusive and kept to a minimum.
4. Good eye contact, relaxed posture, and friendly facial expressions communicate openness and receptivity on the part of the nurse and facilitate the patient's comfort.

General Assessment

It is important to perform a comprehensive assessment, including a health history. When assessing a patient, ask questions about gender and sexuality as a routine part of the health history. With some patients, a sexual or gender history may come up as part of the discussion initiated by the patient. However, the more likely scenario is that the nurse will need to start the conversation. Before bringing up the topic of sex, sexuality, or gender, it is extremely important to explain to the patient why you are asking these questions and that you ask all your patients these questions. Patients may ask why you are asking these questions, and it is important to provide them with answers that will further facilitate discussion. For example, if a patient asks why you are asking about their sexuality, you could say, "Your sexuality and sexual health are important aspects of your overall health and important to discuss."

When talking to patients about gender and sexuality, it is extremely important to avoid making assumptions. Making heterosexist and gender assumptions could jeopardize the nurse–patient relationship. For example, you are doing an initial assessment on a new female patient, and you want to know about her sexual history. If you ask the question, "Do you have a boyfriend?" you are assuming that this patient identifies as heterosexual. If the patient identifies as lesbian, she may answer "no." Not only could this affect the nurse–patient relationship, but it could also cause you to miss key points from her health history. Instead, you could ask, "Do you have a partner?" *Partner* is a gender-neutral term and is appropriate to use when questioning all patients to avoid assumptions. Similarly, to avoid assumptions when asking about sexual activity, you should ask, "Do you have sex with men, women, or both?" Your comfort in asking questions openly like this can support the helping relationship and facilitate a stronger assessment. Nurses can effectively obtain a complete sexual history using the algorithm in Box 26.1. Assessing gender can be approached along the same lines. When meeting a new patient, introduce yourself with your pronoun and ask which gender pronoun the patient uses. Introducing yourself this way normalizes that people may identify in any number of ways and reduces stigma for transgender and gender non-conforming individuals. By asking these questions, you will be able to effectively communicate and assess your patients without making assumptions.

BOX 26.1 Algorithm for Taking a Sexual History

Set the Stage
- Bring up the sexual history as part of the overall history
- Explain that you ask these questions of all patients
- Ensure confidentially

Begin With Three Screening Questions
- Have you been sexually active in the last year?
- Do you have sex with men, women, or both?
- How many people have you had sex with in the last year?

Multiple Partners, New Partners
- Ask about
  - Partners
  - STI/HIV protection
  - Substance abuse
  - Sexual function and satisfaction
  - History of STIs
  - Other concerns

Long-Term Monogamous Partner
- Ask about
  - Pregnancy plans/protection
  - Trauma/violence
  - Sexual function and satisfaction
  - Other concerns

Not Sexually Active
- Ask about
  - Past partners
  - Any questions or concerns

Follow up as appropriate
- Counselling and education
- Referral
- STI or HIV testing

HIV, Human immunodeficiency virus; *STI*, sexually transmitted infection.
Source: Makadon, H., & Goldhammer, H. (2015). Taking a sexual history and creating affirming environments for lesbian, gay, bisexual, and transgender people. *The Journal of the Mississippi State Medical Association, 56*(12), 358–362.

Planning

Planning nursing care for patients may occur as part of care in any setting in which the patient seeks treatment for any of a variety of conditions. Once the assessment is completed, priority nursing diagnoses are developed and implemented in collaboration with the patient.

Implementation

All nurses need to be able to facilitate a discussion about sexuality and gender with the patient. To be a facilitator, the nurse must be nonjudgmental, have basic knowledge of sexuality and gender, and be able to conduct a basic assessment. Once the assessment is completed, the nurse may have the knowledge, skills, and judgement to address the patient's sexual health concern. Or the nurse may need to know when and to whom to refer the patient. Depending on the nature of the problem, the patient may require a referral to a professional such as a nurse practitioner, physician, social worker, psychologist, or psychiatrist.

RESEARCH HIGHLIGHT
Nursing Students' Knowledge, Attitude, Understanding, and Cultural Competence

Problem
A critical element of nursing education is the development of awareness and knowledge regarding diverse populations. Historically LGBTQ2 (lesbian, gay, bisexual, transgender, and queer) individuals have faced stigmatization accessing healthcare. LGBTQ2 older persons experience the same challenges as the general population but may also encounter unique barriers that can negatively influence their quality of life. Improved cultural competence among nurses is needed to provide care that better meets the needs of the LGBTQ2 community.

Purpose of Study
This study sought to develop undergraduate nursing students' knowledge of terminology, using inclusive language, and the historical and social contexts of older LGBTQ2 persons.

Methods
A convenience sample of 42 third year undergraduate nursing students was accessed in this study. Participants completed a survey prior to and following implementation of a case study learning activity exploring a family experience with a transgender older person. Students also provided narrative feedback on the educational intervention.

Key Findings
- Through a case study learning experience, students gained knowledge and understanding of the nurses' role encouraging inclusiveness and access to healthcare, advocating for vulnerable populations, and addressing specific health concerns for transgender older persons.
- The case study experience increased student knowledge and critical thinking regarding discrimination and aging.
- The education initiative facilitated understanding of the unique health needs for LGBTQ2 older persons.

Implications for Nursing Practice
Education sessions can improve attitudes and knowledge in LGBTQ2 healthcare. To promote nursing competence in providing health care to the LGBTQ2 population, undergraduate nursing curriculum must incorporate focused and facilitated case study learning experiences.

Source: Henriquez, N., Hyndman, K., & Chachula, K. (2019). It's complicated: Improving undergraduate nursing students' understanding family and care of LGBTQ older adults. *Journal of Family Nursing*, 25(4), 506–532. https://doi.org/10.1177/1074840719864099

PROVIDING SAFE AND INCLUSIVE NURSING CARE

Nurses need to create safe, inclusive, and gender-affirming healthcare environments for LGBTQ2 individuals. Nurses can demonstrate an inclusive and non-judgmental practice by using appropriate terminology, and asking about sexual orientation, gender identity, pronouns, and preferred names for all patients. If not already in place, nurses can advocate for a safe and gender-affirming healthcare space or "safe space." Implementing a safe space in an organization can include training for staff, ensuring all employees are committed to providing an inclusive environment, having gender-affirming policies, making medical forms more inclusive of gender identity and sexual orientation, and having gender-neutral washrooms. Visual cues such as a rainbow flag or a poster showing LGBTQ2 people and families also help to create a safe space.

MENTAL HEALTH ISSUES IN THE LGBTQ2 POPULATION

Clinical Picture

In the first part of this chapter we examined the concepts of sexuality and gender. We now turn our attention to mental health issues within the LGBTQ2 population. Mental health literature has demonstrated an increased incidence of alcohol and drug use, depression, self-harm, suicide, low self-esteem, and eating disorders in the LGBTQ2 population. The higher risk for mental health issues is thought to be related to health disparities in the LGBTQ2 population. Health disparities in this population may include discrimination, prejudice, social stigma, and living in a heterosexist and homophobic environment (Hafeez et al., 2017; Valdiserri et al., 2018). Stigma and discrimination have a variety of negative effects on people. Experiences of stigma and discrimination may increase an individual's internalized homophobia. **Internalized homophobia** is an individual's discomfort and internal conflict as a result of their own homosexuality. Features of internalized homophobia include negative attitudes, feelings of shame, embarrassment, anger, exclusion, and hopelessness and a discomfort with disclosing sexual orientation. Internalized homophobia is related to increased risk for depression (Yolaç & Meriç, 2021).

Depression

Depression is a highly prevalent, chronic illness with significant impact on quality of life. Identifying as lesbian, gay, or bisexual does not directly correlate with a higher risk for developing depression when compared to the heterosexual population. However, risk factors, including discrimination and homophobia, can increase the risk for depression within this population. Recent literature demonstrates an increased risk for depression in individuals who identify as bisexual, whereas individuals who identify as lesbian or gay have similar rates of depression when compared to the heterosexual population (Li et al., 2016; Scott et al., 2016). Increased stress may be associated with a greater risk for depression in bisexual individuals, even when compared to gay and lesbian individuals. Increased rates of stress and depression in bisexual individuals can be related to experiencing discrimination and bisexual invisibility, a lack of bisexual-affirmative support (Ross et al., 2018), and internalized biphobia (Taylor et al., 2019). Bisexual women are more likely to have worse mental health outcomes compared to heterosexual and homosexual women and bisexual men (Ross et al., 2018). Two-Spirit individuals are likely to experience higher rates of depression related to racism, homophobia, transphobia, heteronormativity, and intergenerational trauma (Hunt, 2016). A lack of access to culturally appropriate services for Two-Spirit individuals may further impact their mental health.

The transgender population experiences high rates of depression and negative mental health outcomes when compared to cisgender, lesbian, gay, and bisexual individuals. The lifetime prevalence of depression within the transgender population is reported to be as high as 50% to 67% (Carmel & Erickson-Schroth, 2016). This increased risk is related to transphobia, gender discrimination, or abuse. Rates of depression significantly improve when transgender individuals begin their social and medical transition. The use of feminizing or masculinizing hormones is associated with a theoretical risk for depression, as well as for mania and aggression. However, evidence also suggests that use of the gender-affirming hormones improves quality of life and reduces depression. Transgender individuals who are experiencing an acute mental health decompensation should not be started on hormone therapy until their mental health status has stabilized. Transgender individuals already on hormone therapy, however, should not have their hormones discontinued because of an acute episode or hospitalization. The discontinuation of hormones may result in worsening the patient's mood.

Self-Harm and Suicide

It is a critical component of the nurse's role to assess patients and screen for risks for self-harm or suicidal ideation (refer also to Chapter 22). Self-harm involves the intentional act of causing personal injury to the body without the intent of suicide. Self-harm acts include cutting or burning the skin, hair pulling (trichotillomania), and ingestion of harmful substances or objects. Self-harm is most common in adolescents and young adults. Although of concern in the general population, rates of self-harm, suicide attempts, and death by suicide are alarming in the LGBTQ2 population. Jackman et al. (2016) reviewed the rates of self-harm in the LGBTQ2 population compared to the heterosexual population and found a prevalence of self-harm in the LGBTQ2 population as high as 47%, relative to prevalence in the heterosexual group of 15%. Within the LGBTQ2 population, they found that those who identified as bisexual or transgender were more likely to engage in acts of self-harm than those who identified as lesbian or gay. The Canadian Trans Youth Health Survey (TYHS) collected data from 923 transgender and gender-diverse youth living in Canada. Three-quarters of transgender youth in the study had reported engaging in self-harm behaviours in the past year (Veale et al., 2017). Individuals with intersex variations also experience high rates of self-harm. In a study of 176 participants with an intersex variation 42% had thought about self-harm and 26% had engaged in self-harm behaviours (Jones, 2016).

Statistics on death by suicide in the LGBTQ2 community are not available, as sexual orientation is often not recorded. Therefore it is assumed that data on LGBTQ2 suicide are, ultimately, underestimated. A systematic review by Salway Hottes et al. (2016) affirmed that those who identify as lesbian, gay, and bisexual were more likely than heterosexual individuals to attempt suicide. Rates of suicidal ideation and suicide attempts in the transgender adult population range from 25% to 76% (Carmel & Erickson-Schroth, 2016). A large study in Ontario found that 35% of transgender adults seriously considered suicide and 11% had made a suicide attempt within the last year (Bauer et al., 2015). The TYHS found that transgender youth had five times the risk of suicidal ideation and two-thirds of study participants had considered suicide in the past year (Veale et al., 2017). The intersex population also experience high rates with 60% having thoughts about suicide, and 19% having attempted suicide in the past (Jones, 2016). Two-Spirit individuals are at greater risk for suicide than heterosexual Indigenous individuals due to isolation, rejection, and homophobia (Hunt, 2016).

> **VIGNETTE**
>
> Ryan is a 19-year-old man who presents to the emergency department for the second time in a few weeks with superficial cuts to his forearm. He is seeing the nurse for his initial assessment. Ryan has been cutting his arm since the age of 15 at an average frequency of about once every 2 weeks. He states that doing so gives him relief from feelings of guilt and despair, which can become intense at times. He denies any episodes of low mood. The nurse starts to explore Ryan's feelings and asks him about his life, including his schooling, friends, sexual relationships, and sexual orientation. Ryan tells the nurse that no one has ever asked him about his sexuality before, and he feels comfortable telling the nurse that he identifies as bisexual. Through further discussion, Ryan discloses that his cutting is related to his feelings around his sexual orientation and fear around acceptance.

Substance Use

Substance use in the LGBTQ2 population has been reported at rates two to four times that in the general population. Substance use in the LGBTQ2 population, including use of alcohol, tobacco, and drugs, has been well documented. LGBTQ2 individuals may use substances for the same reason as heterosexual individuals, but there also are some culturally specific reasons that may account for the higher rates of use in the LGBTQ2 population. Coping with stigma, discrimination, and trauma may be a cause of substance use. Substance use may be used to cope with stresses associated with coming out, homophobia, transphobia, or internalized homophobia.

Within the LGBTQ2 community, there may be some cultural acceptance of substance use. Historically, discrimination against the LGBTQ2 population caused there to be a lack of safe spaces for socialization. Bars, nightclubs, and parties are considered safe places for LGBTQ2 individuals to socialize, establishing social networks and patterns that include people who use substances and triggers for substance use. There is a perceived normality of substance use in LGBTQ2 communities, which increases the risk of addiction in this population (Abdulrahim et al., 2016).

Smoking in the LGBTQ2 population is documented in the literature with rates as high as 59% for youth and 50% for adults. Use of electronic vapor products is also increased in this population, with 17.5% of lesbian, gay, and bisexual youth currently using, compared to 13.2% of heterosexual youth (Kann et al., 2018). In the transgender population smoking is reportedly as high as one in three individuals (Buchting et al., 2017). Alcohol and drug use within the LGBTQ2 community is shown to be higher than that in the general population. Bisexual adults engage in a significantly higher rate of heavy drinking compared to lesbian and gay adults, almost double the rate of heterosexual adults (Gonzales et al., 2016). A Canadian study found that bisexual women were five times more likely to use cannabis relative to heterosexual women (Robinson et al., 2016). Gay men have higher rates of cannabis and illicit drug use compared to heterosexual men (Schuler et al., 2018). LGBTQ2 populations also experience rates of use and misuse of prescription pain relievers and opioids (National LGBT Health Education Center, 2018). Substance use within the transgender population is also high, about 2.5 to 4 times the rates of the general population (Day et al., 2017; James et al., 2016). Transgender individuals have reported high substance use rates to deal with negative experiences, transphobia, and depression.

Evaluation

Evaluation of patients with mental health disorders related to gender dysphoria or discrimination and social factors related to sexual orientation or gender identity is based, in part, on determining whether the outcomes for the presenting problem were achieved. Respectful, frank, and open communication is central to this practice, as a part of both the general therapeutic relationship (see Chapter 9) and the nursing process related to any specific sexuality concerns or gender dysphoria.

■ KEY POINTS TO REMEMBER

- Sexual orientation is a person's sexual identity in relation to the gender to which they are attracted. An individual's sexual orientation is described as heterosexual, homosexual, or bisexual.
- Gender identity refers to one's sense of self as male or female.
- Health care workers are often uncomfortable asking questions related to sexuality and gender. Providing professional and holistic care requires that nurses include this vital area of assessment.
- There are distinctions between biological sex and gender identity. Gender dysphoria is the strong and persistent feeling of

unease about one's maleness or femaleness. Gender incongruence is a marked incongruence between an individual's experienced/expressed gender and the assigned sex.
- Health disparities in the LGBTQ2 population are linked to higher rates of depression, self-harm, suicide, and substance use.

CRITICAL THINKING

1. To understand your own beliefs, answer these questions:
    a. Are you comfortable with your own sexuality? Are you comfortable with those who have a sexual orientation different from your own?
    b. Are you comfortable with your gender? Are you comfortable with those you identify as transgender, non-binary or gender non-conforming?
    c. What factors have influenced your beliefs and values regarding sexuality and gender?
    d. How could you be helpful to someone who is questioning their sexuality or gender?
2. Kyle, a 14-year-old transgender male, was admitted to the adolescent psychiatric mental health unit for depression and self-harm. He has asked to be referred to as Kyle, and gets very upset if anyone, including family members and staff, uses his previous name or female pronouns. What further information do you need from Kyle to complete a gender assessment? As a nurse, how can you advocate for Kyle on your unit and with Kyle's family?
3. As a nurse, you are constantly encountering adolescents who are misinformed about sexuality. What information would you include in a teaching session that would help adolescents acquire a greater understanding of sexuality?

CHAPTER REVIEW

1. A 27-year-old patient states that she is confused about her sexuality. Which response is most likely to be therapeutic?
    a. "What does your boyfriend think of this?"
    b. "Tell me more about what is confusing you."
    c. "Tell me about your sexual activities."
    d. "This is a common problem, which you shouldn't worry about right now."
2. Matthew, a 21-year-old male, is meeting with the nurse for support and counselling. Matthew is questioning his sexuality. Which of the following are realistic short-term outcomes for Matthew? **Select all that apply.**
    a. Matthew displays a clear sense of his sexual orientation.
    b. Matthew accepts a negative self-image of his sexuality.
    c. Matthew develops healthy coping skills.
    d. Matthew shows comfort with his sexual orientation.
3. A young patient tells you that, somehow, he feels that he should not be a man, that inside he is a woman. This is likely an example of:
    a. Confusion
    b. Gender dysphoria
    c. Borderline personality disorder
    d. Intersex
4. Farah is the nurse assigned to work with Mr. Roberts, a transgender male on a step-down unit. Farah is anxious at the prospect of working with Mr. Roberts and spends only the briefest periods of time possible responding to his needs. What are the best descriptions of what is occurring here? **Select all that apply.**
    a. Farah is failing to maintain professional objectivity because of her values and beliefs about this patient's decisions and behaviour.
    b. Farah is experiencing a common negative response to a situation about which she has limited knowledge and little understanding.
    c. Nurses have a right to have personal feelings about social issues, and as long as Mr. Roberts' minimal care needs are addressed, Farah is within her rights to respond in this way.
    d. Farah may be having difficulty looking beyond Mr. Roberts' gender issues and, as a result, is failing to see or respond to him simply as a person.

REFERENCES

Abdulrahim, D., Whiteley, C., Moncrieff, M., et al. (2016). Club drug use among lesbian, gay, bisexual and trans people. Novel Psychoactive Treatment UK Network (NEPTUNE). Retrieved from https://ecom.ngo/wp-content/uploads/2018/01/neptune-club-drug-use-among-lgbt-people.pdf

Bauer, G., Scheim, A., Pyne, J., et al. (2015). Intervenable factors associated with suicide risk in transgender persons: A respondent driven sampling study in Ontario, Canada. *BMC Public Health, 15*, 525–540. https://doi.org/10.1186/s12889-015-1867-2

Becker, I., Ravens-Sieberer, U., Ottová-Jordan, V., et al. (2017). Prevalence of adolescent gender experiences and gender expression in Germany. *The Journal of Adolescent Health: Official Publication of the Society for Adolescent Medicine, 61*(1), 83–90. https://doi.org/10.1016/j.jadohealth.2017.02.001

Bonifacio, J. H., Maser, C., Stadelman, K., et al. (2019). Management of gender dysphoria in adolescents in primary care. *CMAJ: Canadian Medical Association Journal, 191*(3), E69–E75. https://doi.org/10.1503/cmaj.180672

Bourns, A. (2019). *Guidelines for gender-affirming primary care with trans and non-binary patients.* Retrieved from https://www.rainbowhealthontario.ca/wp-content/uploads//woocommerce_uploads/2019/12/Guidelines-FINAL-Dec-2019.pdf

Buchting, F. O., Emory, K. T., Scout, et al. (2017). Transgender use of cigarettes, cigars, and e-cigarettes in a national study. *American Journal of Preventive Medicine, 53*(1), e1–e7. https://doi.org/10.1016/j.amepre.2016.11.022

Carmel, T., & Erickson-Schroth, L. (2016). Mental health and the transgender population. *Journal of Psychosocial Nursing, 54*(12), 44–48. https://doi.org/10.3928/02793695-20161208-09

Day, J. K., Fish, J. N., Perez-Brumer, A., et al. (2017). Transgender youth substance use disparities: Results from a population-based sample. *The Journal of Adolescent Health: Official Publication of the Society for Adolescent Medicine, 61*(6), 729–735. https://doi.org/10.1016/j.jadohealth.2017.06.024

Eisenberg, M. E., Gower, A. L., McMorris, B. J., et al. (2017). Risk and protective factors in the lives of transgender/gender nonconforming adolescents. *The Journal of Adolescent Health: Official Publication of the Society for Adolescent Medicine, 61*(4), 521–526. https://doi.org/10.1016/j.jadohealth.2017.04.014

Fennell, R., & Grant, B. (2019). Discussing sexuality in health care: A systematic review. *Journal of Clinical Nursing, 28*, 3065–3076. https://doi.org/10.1111/jocn.14900

Giblon, R., & Bauer, G. (2017). Health care availability, quality, and unmet need: A comparison of transgender and cisgender residents in Ontario, Canada. *BMC Health Services Research, 17*(283). https://doi.org/10.1186/s12913-017-2226-z

Gonzales, G., Przedworski, J., & Henning-Smith, C. (2016). Comparison of health and health risk factors between lesbian, gay, and bisexual adults and heterosexual adults in the United States: Results from the National Health Interview Survey. *JAMA*

Hafeez, H., Zeshan, M., Tahir, M. A., et al. (2017). Health care disparities among lesbian, gay, bisexual, and transgender youth: A literature review. *Cureus, 9*(4), e1184. https://doi.org/10.7759/cureus.1184

Hunt, S. (2016). *An introduction to the health of Two-Spirit people: Historical, contemporary and emergent issues*. Prince George: National Collaborating Centre for Aboriginal Health. Retrieved from https://www.nccih.ca/docs/emerging/RPT-HealthTwoSpirit-Hunt-EN.pdf

Jackman, K., Honig, J., & Bockting, W. (2016). Nonsuicidal self-injury among lesbian, gay, bisexual and transgender populations: An integrative review. *Journal of Clinical Nursing, 25*, 3438–3453. https://doi.org/10.1111/jocn.13236

James, S. E., Herman, J. L., Rankin, S., et al. (2016). *The report of the 2015 U.S. Transgender Survey*. Retrieved from https://www.transequality.org/sites/default/files/docs/USTS-Full-Report-FINAL.PDF

Jones, T. (2016). The needs of students with intersex variations. *Sex Educations, 16*(6), 1–17. https://doi.org/10.1080/14681811.2016.1149808

Kann, L., McManus, T., Harris, W., et al. (2018). Youth risk behavior surveillance—United States, 2017. *Surveillance Summaries, 67*(SS-8), 1–114. https://dx.doi.org/10.15585/mmwr.ss6708a1

Li, G., Pollitt, A., & Russell, S. (2016). Depression and sexual orientation during young adulthood: Diversity among sexual minority subgroups and the role of gender nonconformity. *Archives of Sexual Behaviors, 45*(3), 697–711. https://doi.org/10.1007/s10508-015-0515-3

Manzer, D., O'Sullivan, L., & Doucet, S. (2018). Myths, misunderstandings, and missing information: Experiences of nurse practitioners providing primary care to lesbian, gay, bisexual, and transgender patients. *The Canadian Journal of Human Sexuality, 27*(2), 157–170. https://doi.org/10.3138/cjhs.2018-0017

National LGBT Health Education Center. (2018). *Addressing opioid use disorder among LGBTQ populations*. Boston: Fenway Institute. Retrieved from https://www.lgbtqiahealtheducation.org/wp-content/uploads/2018/06/OpioidUseAmongLGBTQPopulations.pdf

Robinson, M., Sanches, M., & MacLeod, M. A. (2016). Prevalence and mental health correlates of illegal cannabis use among bisexual women. *Journal of Bisexuality, 16*(2), 181–202. https://doi.org/10.1080/15299716.2016.1147402

Ross, L. E., Salway, T., Tarasoff, L. A., et al. (2018). Prevalence of depression and anxiety among bisexual people compared to gay, lesbian, and heterosexual individuals: A systematic review and meta-analysis. *The Journal of Sex Research, 55*(4–5), 435–456. https://doi.org/10.1080/00224499.2017.1387755

Salway Hottes, T., Bogaert, L., Rhodes, A. E., et al. (2016). Lifetime prevalence of suicide attempts among sexual minority adults by study sampling strategies: A systematic review and meta-analysis. *American Journal of Public Health, 106*, e1–e12. https://doi.org/10.2105/AJPH.2016.303088

Schuler, M. S., Rice, C. E., Evans-Polce, R. J., et al. (2018). Disparities in substance use behaviors and disorders among adult sexual minorities by age, gender, and sexual identity. *Drug and Alcohol Dependence, 189*, 139–146. https://doi.org/10.1016/j.drugalcdep.2018.05.008

Scott, R., Lasiuk, G., & Norris, C. (2016). The relationship between sexual orientation and depression in a national population sample. *Journal of Clinical Nursing, 25*, 3522–3532. https://doi.org/10.1111/jocn.13286

Statistics Canada. (2015). *Canadian Community Health Survey*. Retrieved from https://www23.statcan.gc.ca/imdb/p2SV.pl?Function=getSurvey&SDDS=3226

Statistics Canada. (2019). *Gender of person*. Retrieved from https://www23.statcan.gc.ca/imdb/p3Var.pl?Function=DEC&Id=410445

Taylor, J., Power, J., Smith, E., et al. (2019). Bisexual mental health: Findings from the "who am I study". *Australian Journal of General Practice, 48*(3), 138–144. https://doi.org/10.31128/AJGP-06-18-4615

Trans Care BC. (2021). *Gender-affirming care for trans, Two-Spirit, and gender diverse patients in BC: A primary care toolkit*. Retrieved from http://www.phsa.ca/transcarebc/Documents/HealthProf/Primary-Care-Toolkit.pdf

Valdiserri, R. O., Holtgrave, D. R., Poteat, T. C., et al. (2018). Unraveling health disparities among sexual and gender minorities: A commentary on the persistent impact of stigma. *Journal of Homosexuality, 66*(5), 571–589. https://doi.org/10.1080/00918369.2017.1422944T

Veale, J. F., Watson, R. J., Peter, T., et al. (2017). Mental health disparities among Canadian transgender youth. *The Journal of Adolescent Health: Official Publication of the Society for Adolescent Medicine, 60*(1), 44–49. https://doi.org/10.1016/j.jadohealth.2016.09.014

Yolaç, E., & Meriç, M. (2021). Internalized homophobia and depression levels in LGBT individuals. *Perspectives in Psychiatric Care, 57*, 304–310. https://doi.org/10.1111/ppc.12564

27

Disorders of Children and Adolescents

Cheryl L. Pollard

 https://evolve.elsevier.com/Canada/Varcarolis/psychiatric/

OBJECTIVES

1. Explore factors contributing to child and adolescent mental health disorders, and develop intervention strategies for this population.
2. Explain characteristics associated with resiliency.
3. Identify characteristics of positive mental health and development in children and adolescents.
4. Discuss holistic assessment of a child or adolescent.
5. Explore areas in the assessment of suicide for children and adolescents.
6. Compare and contrast at least six treatment modalities for children and adolescents.
7. Describe clinical features and behaviours of at least three child and adolescent mental health disorders.
8. Formulate three nursing diagnoses, stating patient outcomes and interventions for each.

KEY TERMS AND CONCEPTS

assent
attention-deficit/hyperactivity disorder
bibliotherapy
conduct disorder
consent
dissent
mutual storytelling
neurodevelopmental disorders
oppositional defiant disorder
pica
play therapy
principle of least restrictive intervention
rumination disorder
temperament
therapeutic games

Mental health and well-being are essential components to healthy child development. Many children and adolescents may struggle with a disabling mental illness, but most of these illnesses go unnoticed and unidentified (Ng et al., 2021). Until *Changing Directions, Changing Lives: The Mental Health Strategy for Canada* was released by the Mental Health Commission of Canada (MHCC) in 2012, the mental health needs of young people in Canada had not received much attention.

Mental health disorders in children and adolescents are associated with disturbances in psychological, physiological, academic, and social functioning. The economic, social, and personal costs to society associated with childhood- and adolescent-onset mental health disorders are tremendous because the illness occurs during important developmental periods, has frequent recurrences, and persists into adulthood (World Health Organization, 2018). Stigma and misconceptions can cause patients and families to attempt to conceal the conditions or even limit help seeking professional care (United Nations, 2020). The MHCC also reports that stigma, a silent public health epidemic, can be addressed through "contact-based education" (Livingston, 2020), that is, through meeting and talking with people and families who experience mental health problems.

Childhood and adolescence are distinct developmental periods during which significant changes in physical, cognitive, and social functioning occur. As such, childhood is defined in terms of early (1–4 years) and middle childhood (5–10 years), whereas adolescence is described in terms of the subphases of early (11–14 years), middle (15–17 years), and late (18–21 years) (Hagan et al., 2017). Important mental health disorders that can occur in children and adolescents include mood disorders, anxiety disorders, schizophrenia, and substance use. Anxiety and depression as they relate to this age group are discussed in this chapter. These disorders, as well as the others discussed in this chapter, are more difficult to diagnose in younger children because of limited language skills and cognitive and emotional development. In addition, children undergo more rapid psychological, neurological, and physiological changes over a briefer period than adults do. The rapidity and complexity of this development must be taken into consideration during assessment for mental health disorders. Clinicians and parents often wait to see whether symptoms are the result of a developmental lag or trauma response that will eventually correct itself; therefore intervention may be delayed, for instance, until the child reaches school age. Usually, a number of factors influence a child's or adolescent's mental health, so a variety of interventions are needed to improve psychological, social, physical, educational, and spiritual well-being.

Meeting the mental health needs of youth and their families is a challenge for the nurse because need is steadily increasing while funding and access to care are decreasing and existing services remain fragmented or lacking in many communities. Considering all of the developmental changes and associated vulnerabilities and resiliencies that occur during childhood and adolescence, it is clear that this is an optimal time to target prevention and intervention.

This chapter describes the nurse's role in assessment and interventions for selected mental health disorders, as well as broad treatment modalities that are implemented through the nursing process with this population and their families. For more information related to family interventions, refer to Chapter 34.

EPIDEMIOLOGY

One in five children and adolescents in Canada suffers from a major mental illness that causes significant impairments at home, at school, with peers, and in the community. Some of these mental health disorders have a likelihood of recurrence and chronicity in young adulthood; in fact, 80% of adults with mental illness experienced problems in childhood or early adolescence. Epidemiology data suggest that approximately 13% of Canadian children and youth may be experiencing a mental health disorder at any given time (Scaini et al., 2020; Wiens et al., 2020). It is estimated that two-thirds of young people with mental health problems are not receiving needed services. Suicide ranks as the second leading cause of death for youth ages 10 to 19 years, and suffocation was the predominant means of committing suicide among young Canadians. Suicide rates in Canada are increasing among female youth but decreasing among male children and adolescents (DeMaso & Walter, 2020).

Suicide is a significant problem for some Indigenous youth whose communities lack the necessary protective benefits and appropriate sources of support, including professional and nonprofessional help. It is reported that Indigenous youth have a suicide rate that is five to six times greater than that of non-Indigenous youth (Pollack et al., 2016).

The Canadian government's recognition of childhood and adolescent mental health problems and efforts toward identifying effective treatments were reported in the Senate report *Out of the Shadows at Last* (Standing Senate Committee on Social Affairs, Science and Technology, 2006). Based on a key recommendation of this Senate committee, the MHCC was formed and, in close consultation with people living with mental health problems and illnesses, families, stakeholder organizations, governments, and experts, identified child and youth mental health services as a critical component to improving the mental health outcomes of Canadians. However, barriers to assessment, treatment, prevention, and early intervention remain, including:

- Lack of clarity about conditions for screening children
- Lack of coordination among multiple systems
- Lack of resources and long wait times for services
- Shortage of mental health care providers
- Lack of a child and youth mental health framework

More research is needed to understand the reasons for the underuse and early termination of mental health care services, and funding is needed to improve access to and coordination among existing resources to provide programs for these young people (Angeles & Roberton, 2020).

COMORBIDITY

Children and adolescents with mental health disorders often meet the criteria for more than one diagnostic category. Attention-deficit/hyperactivity disorder (ADHD), a prominent comorbid condition, occurs in 90% of individuals with juvenile-onset bipolar disorder, 90% of children with oppositional defiant disorder, and 50% of those with conduct disorder. Childhood depression has a high incidence of comorbidity: 20% to 80% of children with depression have conduct or oppositional disorders, 30% to 75% have anxiety disorders, and 5% to 60% display symptoms of ADHD (Charach & Andrews, 2019). Multiple services are often needed by those with coexisting diagnoses, such as special education evaluation and services, after-school services, family counselling, and behaviour management.

RISK FACTORS

Mental illness can become serious or severe and persistent if early detection and effective intervention are not implemented. A child with a parent with depression is at risk for developing an anxiety disorder, mood disorder, conduct disorder, or substance use disorder.

RESEARCH HIGHLIGHT

"Objectively Terrifying": A Qualitative Study of Youth's Experiences of Transitions Out of Child and Adolescent Mental Health Services at Age 18

Problem
Mental health issues presenting in childhood will often persist into adulthood. Services that bridge care options for adolescents and adults are very limited. The discontinuity of care during this transitional time leave youth vulnerable to deteriorating mental health outcomes.

Purpose of Study
The purpose of this research study is to explore the transition-related knowledge and experiences of youth prior to and after transition.

Methods
The principles of participatory action research were used to guide a longitudinal follow-up study of 22 youth, ages 16 to 19, who were discharged from two Canadian child and adolescent mental health programs. Semistructured interviews were used to gather information about their personal transition-related experiences.

Key Findings
There were six common experiences among the participants. (1) Shifting awareness of the meaning of "transition." Participants reported feeling nervous when the concept of transition shifted from an abstract concept to an inevitable reality. (2) Ready or not to transition. Feeling both ready and not ready to transition from one care provider to another was described as a common experience. (3) Mixed reactions to transitional age of 18 years. The arbitrary nature of 18 being a "cut off" age for services was frustrating for many as the decision to discontinue services was not related to needs but only to age. (4) Lack of information, preparation, and involvement in the transition planning process. The majority of the pretransition participants felt uninformed, disconnected, and confused about the process. Transition meetings were described as uninformative, vague, and offered very little direction. (5) Confusion around roles and responsibilities within the transition process. Participants described the system as opaque. It was not clear who was responsible for what parts of the transitions. This resulted in participants feeling terrified because there really didn't seem to be a "plan." (6) Concerns over transition gaps leading to poor mental health outcomes. Those who were concerned that there would be gaps in services worried that they would not have the needed supports available once they turned 18 years.

Implications for Nursing Practice
Continuity during the transition process is a critical factor in reducing transition-related worries and distress. Each youth needs an individualized transition plan based on their unique developmental needs. Transition best practices involve codesigning transition plans with the youth and caregivers.

Source: Cleverley, K., Lenters, L., & McCann, E. (2020). "Objectively terrifying": A qualitative study of youth's experiences of transitions out of child and adolescent mental health services at age 18. *BMC Psychiatry, 20*(1), 1–11. https://doi.org/10.1186/s12888-020-02516-0

The parent's inability to model effective coping strategies can lead to learned helplessness, the creation of anxiety or apathy, and an inability to master the environment. A child with a conduct disorder may develop an antisocial personality disorder. In fact, two-thirds of youth in the juvenile justice system have one or more diagnosable mental health disorders (Charach & Andrews, 2019).

Children who have been abused or neglected are at great risk for developing emotional, intellectual, and social problems as a result of their traumatic experiences (Scaini et al., 2020). Exposure to intimate partner violence and neglect are two of the most prevalent forms of child abuse in Canada. According to Statistics Canada (2021), at least 30% of Canadians have experienced physical or sexual abuse by an adult prior to the age of 15. This study also found that males experienced physical abuse more commonly than females. However, females experienced sexual abuse more frequently than males. While boys are also sexually abused, the numbers are under-reported due to shame and stigma. The nurse must understand that sexual abuse ranges from fondling to forcing a child to observe or participate in lewd acts to sexual intercourse. All instances of sexual abuse are devastating to a child who lacks the mental capacity or emotional maturation to consent to this type of a relationship.

Witnessing violence is traumatizing and results in an increased risk for depression, anxiety, nightmares, intrusive thoughts, hypervigilance, aggressive and delinquent behaviour, drug use, academic failure, and low self-esteem. Children who have been abused also are at risk for identifying with the aggressor, and they may act out, bully others, become abusers in adulthood, or otherwise develop dysfunctional patterns in close interpersonal relationships.

There are more than 430 active gangs in Canada (Northcott, 2018). Many adult members began their gang involvement as children to get respect, money, protection, or to fit in. Approximately 20% of gangs in Canada are Indigenous (Northcott, 2018). Indigenous youth also join gangs to escape poverty and obtain the necessities of life (Goodwill & Giannone, 2017). Youths ages 11 to 13, a time of particular vulnerability, are solicited to become gang members because their decision-making capacities are limited, and they may look up to older peers for status and belonging. Gang members often inflict violence on others, including vandalism, theft, and aggression. Many end up in the juvenile court system, where they exhibit mental health problems that may remain untreated.

All Canadian provinces and territories have child protection legislation, and all instances of suspected abuse of a minor child are required to be reported to the local child protection services. Further, in 2001 the Government of Canada passed legislation that came into effect in 2008 to help protect youth from non-exploitative sexual activity by raising the age of consent for sexual activity from 14 to 16 years (Parliament of Canada, 2017). This legislation brought the age of consent in line with that of other countries such as the United States and Australia. Depending on the province or territory, a *child* is defined as a young person up to age 16 to 19, and the age of majority is 18 or 19 years. Box 27.1 discusses the decision-making terms *consent*, *assent*, and *dissent* as they relate to children.

It is important for nurses working in youth detention, school, and community settings to assess for post-traumatic stress disorder (PTSD) and the safety of the environment for young people who have been traumatized or who have experienced abuse or a history of violence. Interventions should focus on teaching coping skills to deal with trauma, supporting efforts to achieve socially appropriate goals, and facilitating integration into healthy social support systems. Chapter 24 provides more information on interpersonal violence.

> **BOX 27.1 Including the Child in Health Care Decision Making**
>
> Nurses working with children and youth need to recognize the young person's right to self-determination and participation in decision making related to health care and research. **Consent** is an expression of autonomy. It represents a person's capacity to understand information and to voluntarily act on this information. For example, a person may give consent (agree) to participate in a research study, or they may withhold consent (refuse) to participate in a particular health care treatment. Provincial and territorial legislation stipulates the age of majority—the age at which a person may give their own consent. Although not legally binding, including the child in the decision-making process shows respect for the child and gives the child a sense of ownership about what is happening. Despite children lacking the capacity to consent, they still may be able to express their wishes in a meaningful way (*assent* or *dissent*). **Assent** refers to the child's agreement to participate; **dissent** indicates a child's refusal to participate in the suggested health care or research study (Lambert & Glacken, 2011). Including the child in health care decision making supports the child's growth and development. However, a disagreement between the child and the legally recognized decision maker (i.e., parent or guardian) creates complex ethical dilemmas for members of the health care team. In these situations, requesting an ethics consult, often provided by a clinical ethicist, is appropriate.

Source: Lambert, V., & Glacken, M. (2011). Engaging with children in research: Theoretical and practical implications of negotiating informed consent/assent. *Nursing Ethics, 18*(6), 781–801.

ETIOLOGY

Mental illness in children and adolescents, as in adults, is caused by multiple factors, and distinguishing among the genetic, psychosocial, and environmental factors makes diagnosis challenging. Increasing numbers of children are born with or develop disordered brain function related to malnutrition, human immunodeficiency virus (HIV) infection, fetal alcohol syndrome, drug addiction, and brain injury. In addition, they are exposed to environmental stressors in the family, school, peer group, or community that have an impact on their social, emotional, cognitive, psychological, and spiritual development (Lawrence et al., 2019).

The degree of a child's vulnerability to mental illness changes over time. The resilience of the child and the presence of positive environmental factors (e.g., parental role models, a healthy school environment) enable a child to learn and adapt. Positive influences can decrease vulnerability to mental health disorders or improve functioning to the fullest possible level if a disorder exists.

Biological Factors
Genetic
Hereditary factors are implicated in a number of mental health disorders, including autism, bipolar disorders, schizophrenia, attention-deficit problems, and intellectual developmental disorder. Because not all genetically vulnerable children develop mental health disorders, it is assumed that resilience and a supportive environment are key factors in avoiding the development of mental health disorders. According to DiBlasi, and colleagues (2020), suggest that both autism spectrum disorders (ASD) and suicidal behaviour may have a direct genetic link.

Brain Development and Biochemicals

Dramatic changes occur in the brain during childhood and adolescence, including a declining number of synapses (they peak at age 5), myelination of brain fibres, changes in the relative volume and activity level in different brain regions, and interactions of hormones. Myelination increases the speed of information processing, improves the conduction speed of nerve impulses, and enables faster reactions to occur. Maturation of the cortex of the brain occurs most rapidly during childhood but continues until well after puberty. The teen years are also marked by changes in the frontal and prefrontal cortex regions, leading to improvements in executive functions, organization and planning skills, and inhibiting responses (Machinskaya et al., 2020). These changes, including cerebellum maturation and hormonal changes, reflect the emotional and behavioural fluctuations characteristic of adolescence. Early adolescence is typically characterized by low emotional regulation and intolerance for frustration; emotional and behavioural control usually increase over the course of adolescence.

Alterations in neurotransmitters have also been implicated as playing a role in causing child and adolescent disorders. Decreased norepinephrine and serotonin levels are related to depression and suicide, and elevated levels are related to mania and pathological fear. Abnormalities in dopamine receptors and dopamine transporters are implicated in ADHD, certain addictions, and schizophrenia (Schatzberg, 2017).

Temperament

Temperament is the style of reacting and regulating responses. Varying temperaments are present in infants, are modified by maturation, and develop in the context of the social environment (Rothbart, 2011). All people have temperaments, and the fit between the child's and the parent's temperament is critical to the child's development. The parent's role in shaping that relationship is of primary importance, and, when needed, the nurse can teach parents ways to modify their behaviours to improve interactions with their children. If there is incongruence between parent and child temperament and the parent is unable to respond positively to the child, there is a risk for insecure attachment, developmental problems, and future mental health disorders.

Early childhood temperament and behaviour traits (e.g., traits such as shyness, aggressiveness, and rebelliousness) influence substance use in adulthood (Lahat et al., 2012). External risk factors for such abuse include substance use among peers, parental drug use, and involvement in legal problems such as truancy or vandalism. Researchers have also identified childhood protective factors that shield some children from drug use, including self-control, parental monitoring, academic achievement, anti–drug use policies, and strong neighbourhood attachment (Goodwill & Giannone, 2017).

Resilience

Most children with risk factors for the development of mental illness develop normally. The term *resilience* has been used to denote the relationship between a child's constitutional endowment and success negotiating stressful environmental factors. Studies have shown that a resilient child has the following characteristics (Cicchetti, 2010):
- Adaptability to changes in the environment
- Ability to form nurturing relationships with other adults when the parent is not available
- Ability to distance self from emotional chaos
- Good social intelligence
- Good problem-solving skills

Family stability in the face of poverty and adversity can also have a stabilizing effect. The nurse's role is to identify and foster these qualities to prevent at-risk children from developing emotional and mental problems.

Environmental Factors

External factors in the environment can either support or put stress on children and adolescents and shape their development. To a greater degree than adults, young people are vulnerable in an environment in which systems (e.g., schools, court systems) and people (e.g., parents, counsellors) have power and control. During childhood, the main context is the family. Parents model behaviour and provide the child with a view of the world. If parents, or another caregiver, are abusive, rejecting, or overly controlling, the child may suffer detrimental effects. The child is unable to progress through their developmental milestones. A number of familial risk factors correlate with childhood psychiatric disorders, including severe marital discord, low socioeconomic status, large families and overcrowding, parental criminality, parental mental health disorders, and foster care placement.

Cultural Factors

Children and youth in ethnic minority groups may be at risk for a variety of mental health problems. As with all children, economics, service availability, cultural beliefs, values, and attitudes of health care providers affect help seeking. Because of the lack of same-culture role models, children in some minority groups experience increased risk. Differences in the cultural expectations of family and peers, presence of stresses, and lack of support within the dominant culture may have profound effects on these children and increase the risk for mental, emotional, and academic problems. Nurses working with children and adolescents from diverse backgrounds require an increased awareness of their own biases, as well as the patient's needs. The social and cultural context of the patient and family, including factors such as age, ethnicity, gender, sexual orientation, world view, religiosity, and socioeconomic status, should be taken into consideration when assessing and planning care.

CHILD AND ADOLESCENT PSYCHIATRIC MENTAL HEALTH NURSING

Child and adolescent psychiatric mental health nurses use evidence-informed knowledge to provide care that is responsive to the patient's and family's specific problems, strengths, personality, sociocultural context, and preferences.

Although the number of young people with acute mental illness in our society is increasing, inpatient and residential treatment time among this population has steadily decreased. Treatment for children often consists of brief hospitalization followed by interventions conducted in a wide spectrum of community support settings, including day treatment programs, partial hospitalization programs, clinics, schools, and psychiatric home care. To be considered eligible for inpatient hospitalization, the child or adolescent typically must be an imminent danger to self or others. In short-term inpatient facilities the nurse has less time to form a therapeutic relationship with the child and family, making it more difficult to facilitate lasting behavioural changes. Residential and group home facilities for long-term placement are more difficult to secure because availability is often scarce, the cost is high, and consistent evidence of their effectiveness in reducing symptoms and improving long-term functioning is lacking (Chambers et al., 2020).

As psychiatric care moved from inpatient facilities to the community, child and adolescent psychiatric mental health nurses became an integral part of these programs. Advanced-practice registered nurses, including clinical nurse specialists, nurse counsellors, and nurse practitioners, have established outpatient practices, school-based primary prevention, and other innovative treatment programs for young

CONSIDERING CULTURE
Hostility Toward LGBTQ2 Adolescents

How do nurses contribute to changing the social culture from intolerance to acceptance? Lesbian, gay, bisexual, transgender, queer, intersex, and Two-Spirited (LGBTQ2) adolescents are not a specific cultural group; however, these individuals live within communities that have developed characteristics and attitudes in others that can manifest as discrimination and prejudice.

On October 18, 2011, in Ottawa A.Y. Jackson High School student Jamie Hubley, 15 years of age, committed suicide. Jamie, who was openly gay, reported on his blog months before he died that he suffered continuous and constant bullying because of his sexuality. According to his father, an Ottawa city councillor, Jamie had been bullied throughout elementary school and into high school (Woods, 2011). At the time of his suicide, he was experiencing depression and receiving care from health care providers. Reaction to Jamie's death was brought forward in the House of Commons by members of Parliament, highlighting the need for bullying and other forms of intolerance toward others to end. This event illuminates the difficulties that schools and communities may have in coping with the needs of youth with emotional and behavioural difficulties and can open dialogue for nurses about how to increase community readiness to work with LGBTQ2 youth.

Statistics on hate crimes in Canada indicate that about 16% are related to sexual orientation, and two thirds of those crimes are marked by violence (Allen, 2015). Teenagers and children as young as 10 years of age may experience feelings of identification with or sexual attraction to the same gender. Young people often disclose these feelings to friends, and they may be met with social rejection, anger, ridicule, bullying, and violence. Studies have shown that LGBTQ2 youth are at risk for a variety of negative outcomes, including dramatically increased suicidality, mental health problems, high-risk behaviours, poorer school outcomes, and homelessness. Externally, LGBTQ2 youth are subject to higher rates of violence and victimization than heterosexual youth are.

A nursing diagnosis that may apply is *Readiness for enhanced community coping* related to adapting and problem solving to meet the demands or needs of the community (in this case the school) for the management of current stressors. Better community adapting and problem solving would lead to improved communication among community members and larger organizations. In addition to providing counselling for LGBTQ2 youth, nurses could play a key role in:

- Educating schools and parents about the needs of LGBTQ2 youth in an effort to change attitudes
- Helping the community to apply for and obtain funds for additional programs for LGBTQ2 youth
- Encouraging communication and collaboration among community members on these issues
- Serving as advocates for LGBTQ2 youth

In its landmark document, *Changing Directions, Changing Lives: The Mental Health Strategy for Canada*, the Mental Health Commission of Canada (2012) identified this population as a priority. Stemming from one of the six key strategic directions was a recommendation for increased services and more knowledge and understanding among the public and among health care providers about the impact of discrimination and stigma for LGBTQ2 individuals.

Sources: Allen, M. (2015). *Police-reported hate crime in Canada, 2013*. Ottawa: Statistics Canada; Mental Health Commission of Canada. (2012). *Changing directions, changing lives: The mental health strategy for Canada*. Calgary: Author; Woods, M. (2011, October 18). Bullied son of Ottawa city councillor commits suicide. *Toronto Star*. Retrieved from https://www.thestar.com/news/canada/2011/10/18/bullied_son_of_ottawa_city_councillor_commits_suicide.html

---

people. Research on interventions for young people at risk for developing mental illness is also being carried out in non-traditional settings such as homeless shelters, group homes, and mentoring programs, as well as online.

Assessing Development and Functioning

A child or adolescent with mental illness is one whose progressive personality development and functioning is hindered or arrested due to biological, psychosocial, or spiritual factors, resulting in functional impairments. In comparison, a child or adolescent who does not have a mental illness matures with only minor regressions, coping with the stressors and developmental tasks of life. Learning and adapting to the environment and bonding with others in a mutually satisfying way are signs of mental health (Box 27.2). The degree of mental health or illness can be viewed on a continuum, with one's level on the continuum changing over time. Many mental illnesses are chronic but can be managed effectively with evidence-informed treatments.

Data Collection

Methods of collecting data include interviewing, screening, testing (neurological, psychological, intelligence), observing, and interacting with the child or adolescent. Histories are taken from multiple sources, including parents, other caregivers, the child or adolescent, and other adults, such as teachers, when possible. Structured questionnaires and behaviour checklists can be completed by parents and teachers. A genogram can document family composition, history, and relationships (see Chapter 34). Numerous assessment tools are available, and with education, nurses can use them to effectively monitor symptoms and behavioural changes.

BOX 27.2 Characteristics of a Mentally Healthy Child or Adolescent

- Trusts others and sees their world as being safe and supportive
- Correctly interprets reality—makes accurate perceptions of the environment and their ability to influence it through actions (e.g., self-determination)
- Behaves in a way that is developmentally appropriate and does not violate social norms
- Has a positive, realistic self-concept and developing identity
- Adapts to and copes with anxiety and stress using age-appropriate behaviour
- Can learn and master developmental tasks and new situations
- Expresses self in spontaneous and creative ways
- Develops and maintains satisfying relationships

The observation–interaction part of a mental health assessment begins with a semistructured interview in which the nurse meets with the child or adolescent alone and asks about the home environment, parents, and siblings and the school environment, teachers, and peers. In this format the young person is free to describe current problems and give information about their own developmental history. Play activities, such as games, drawings, and puppets, are used for younger children who cannot respond to a direct approach. The initial interview is key to observing interactions among the child, caregiver, and siblings (if available) and to building trust and rapport. The nurse needs to be cognizant of being nonthreatening in approach and using language appropriate to the young person's cognitive capabilities and verbal skills.

> **SAFETY TIP**
>
> When preparing to conduct an assessment of a child, and their support systems, the nurse will estimate the developmental age of the child and select age-appropriate activities prior to beginning the assessment. Generally, two to three potential activities are identified and selected based on the interests of the child and the reasons the child and their support systems are requesting services. Removing extra "toys" or other activity supplies from view will help decrease potential distractions and can minimize behavioural management if the child is engaging in activities that are not directly related to the assessment. Put away all items that you do not need available during the assessment.

Assessment Data

The types of data collected to assess mental health depend on the setting, the severity of the presenting problem, and the availability of resources. Employer policies determine which data are collected, but a nurse should be prepared to make an independent judgement about what to assess and how to assess it. In all cases a physical examination is part of a complete assessment for serious mental health problems. Box 27.3 identifies essential assessment data.

Developmental assessment. The developmental assessment provides information about the child or adolescent's maturational level. These data are then reviewed in relation to the child's chronological age to identify developmental strengths or deficits. The Denver II Developmental Screening Test is a popular assessment tool. For adolescents, tools may be tailored to specific areas of assessment, such as neuropsychological, physical, hormonal, and biochemical. One tool that can be used to assess risk is the Youth Risk Behavior Survey for children and adolescents.

Abnormal findings in the developmental and mental status assessments may be related to stress and adjustment problems or to more serious disorders. Children may outgrow a difficulty, but nurses need to evaluate behaviours indicative of stress or minor regressions, as well as those indicative of more serious psychopathology, and identify the need for further evaluation, intervention, or referral. Stress-related behaviours or minor regressions may be handled by working with parents or caregivers. However, as young people develop maladaptive coping behaviours and use these behaviours over time, they are at risk for developing mental health disorders. Serious psychopathology requires evaluation by an advanced-practice nurse in collaboration with clinicians specializing in child and adolescent health.

Mental status examination. Assessment of the mental status of children and youth is similar to that of adults. It provides information about the mental state at the time of the examination and identifies problems with thinking, feeling, and behaving. Broad categories to assess include safety, general appearance, socialization, activity level, speech, coordination and motor function, affect, manner of relating, intellectual function, thought processes and content, and characteristics of play. It is also important to obtain information not only from the child or adolescent but also from others (e.g., parents, teachers, health care providers) who have been involved with the young person.

BOX 27.3 Types of Assessment Data

History of Present Illness
- Chief complaint
- Development and duration of problems
- Help sought and results
- Effect of problem on child's life at home and school
- Effect of problem on family and siblings' lives

Developmental History
- Pregnancy, birth, neonatal data
- Developmental milestones
- Description of eating, sleeping, and elimination habits and routines
- Attachment behaviours
- Types of play
- Social skills and friendships
- Sexual activity
- Spiritual beliefs

Developmental Assessment
- Psychomotor skills
- Language skills
- Cognitive skills
- Interpersonal and social skills
- Academic achievement
- Behaviour (response to stress, to changes in environment)
- Problem-solving and coping skills (impulse control, delay of gratification)
- Energy level and motivation
- Self-concept
- Drug and alcohol use

Neurological Assessment
- Cerebral functions
- Cerebellar functions
- Sensory functions
- Reflexes

Note: Functions can be observed during developmental assessment and while playing games involving a specific ability (e.g., "Simon says touch your nose").

Medical History
- Review of body systems
- Traumas, hospitalizations, operations, and child's response
- Illnesses or injuries affecting central nervous system
- Medications (past and current)
- Allergies

Family History
- Illnesses in related family members (e.g., seizures, mental health disorders, drug and alcohol use, diabetes, cancer)
- Background of family members (occupation, education, social activities, religion)
- Family relationship (separation, divorce, deaths, contact with extended family, communication, support system)

Mental Status Assessment
- General appearance
- Activity level
- Coordination and motor function
- Affect
- Speech
- Manner of relating
- Intellectual functions
- Thought processes and content
- Risk assessment
- Characteristics of play

Risk assessment. Suicide is a leading cause of death in adolescence (Statistics Canada, 2022); therefore assessment of suicidality is an essential nursing skill. Some children and youths make idle threats about killing themselves, but to determine the cause of the distress and the risk for violence, the nurse must use active listening when interacting with any young person expressing the wish to hurt self or others. The number-one predictor of suicidal risk is a past suicide attempt. Areas to explore when assessing suicidal risk include:

- Past and current suicidal thoughts, threats, or attempts
- Existence of a plan, lethality of the plan, and accessibility of any necessities for carrying out the plan
- Feelings of hopelessness; changes in level of energy
- Circumstances, state of mind, and motivation
- Viewpoints about suicide and death (e.g., Has a family member or friend attempted suicide?)
- Depression and other moods or feelings (e.g., anger, guilt, rejection)
- History of impulsivity, poor judgement, or decreased decision making
- Drug or alcohol use
- Prescribed medications and any recent adherence issues

Additional questions may be asked of teens, including those about risk-taking and acting-out behaviours, artwork with a violent theme, interests in music or books with morbid themes, and recent changes in behaviour or social life (e.g., eating, sleeping, isolating, loss of a relationship).

Assessing the lethality of a young child's suicide plan is complicated by the distorted concept of death, immature ego functions, and an immature understanding of lethality. For instance, a child who is highly suicidal may believe that a few aspirin will cause death. The incorrect judgement about the lethality does not diminish the seriousness of the intent. Another child simply seeking attention may threaten to jump off a bridge, believing that this action would not be fatal. Some teens may make a pact to kill themselves or become upset after a friend has committed suicide or died accidentally (Stewart et al., 2020). Early intervention is essential, and parents need to understand that suicidal thoughts or self-harming behaviour (e.g., burning, cutting, reckless driving, binge drinking) must be taken seriously and evaluated by mental health care providers as an emergency. Suicide prevention among children and youths is also reflected in several of the strategic directions in *Changing Directions, Changing Lives: The Mental Health Strategy for Canada* (MHCC, 2012).

Cultural factors. Mental health care providers recognize the importance of culture in evaluating psychiatric disorders, especially when working with families. The *Diagnostic and Statistical Manual of Mental Disorders, fifth edition (DSM-5)*, identifies culture-bound syndromes of mental illness that are not diagnostic categories in Western medicine (see Chapter 8). Sensitivity to cultural influences in mental illness is a necessity to show respect for cultural preferences in providing individualized care and to avoid behaviour stereotyping and incorrect assessment. A translator should be used if there are any issues with understanding and communicating with the child, youth, or their guardians.

General Interventions

The interventions described in this section can be used by nurses in a variety of clinical and non-clinical settings. Many of the modalities can encompass activities of daily living, learning activities, multiple forms of play and recreational activities, and interactions with adults and peers.

Family Therapy

The family is seen as critical to improving the function of a young person with a psychiatric illness; therefore family counselling is often a key component of treatment used by nurses. There are many models of family therapy (see Chapter 34), but the focus of all models is on promoting, improving, and maintaining family functioning. Following assessment, the nurse works with family members to identify specific goals and provides education on ways to achieve the goals for the family or subunits within the family (e.g., parental, sibling). Homework assignments are often used for family members to practise newly learned skills outside the therapeutic environment.

In addition to therapy involving a single family, multiple-family therapy provides useful interaction for participants to learn how other families solve problems and build on strengths, develop insight and improve judgement about their own family, learn and practise new information, and develop lasting and satisfying relationships with other families (Wright & Leahey, 2019).

Group Therapy

Nurses use group therapy as an integral component of their practice to promote therapeutic change among children and adolescents. Group therapy (see Chapter 33) for younger children takes the form of play to introduce ideas and work through issues. For pre-school and grade school children, it combines play, learning skills, and talk about the activity. The child learns social skills by taking turns and sharing with peers. For adolescents, group therapy involves learning skills and talking, focusing largely on peer relationships and working through specific problems. Adolescent group therapy might use a popular media event or personality as the basis for a group discussion. Groups can be used effectively to deal with specific issues in a young person's life (e.g., bereavement, depression, physical abuse, substance use, dating, chronic illnesses such as juvenile diabetes). When designing the groups, the nurse must take into consideration the child's or youth's age to determine the most appropriate pedagogy.

Behavioural Therapy

Behavioural therapy involves rewarding desired behaviour to reduce maladaptive behaviours. In a healthy relationship a child's developmentally appropriate behaviours are validated by a significant adult (*operant conditioning*). Behaviour management in psychiatry is classified according to the level of restrictiveness and intrusiveness. To ensure that the civil and legal rights of individuals are not violated, and effective treatment is provided, techniques are selected according to the **principle of least restrictive intervention**. This principle requires that more restrictive interventions be used only after less restrictive interventions to manage the behaviour have been attempted. Intrusive techniques (such as physical restraints) are implemented to manage behaviour and maintain safety only when very severe or dangerous behaviours (i.e., those that may result in injury to the patient or others) are exhibited.

Most child and adolescent treatment settings use a behaviour modification program to motivate and reward age-appropriate behaviours. Points are used to obtain a specific reward, which can be part of the system or be negotiated on an individual or group basis. One popular method is the point or level system, in which points are awarded for desired behaviours and increasing levels of privileges can be earned. The value for specific behaviours and privileges for each level are spelled out, and points earned each day are recorded. Older youth can be made responsible for keeping their own point sheet and for requesting points for their behaviours. Children who work on individual behavioural goals (e.g., seeking help in problem solving) can earn additional points.

Cognitive Behavioural Therapy

As discussed in Chapter 4, cognitive behavioural therapy (CBT) is an evidence-informed treatment approach based on the premise that negative and self-defeating thoughts lead to psychiatric pathology and that learning to replace these thoughts with more accurate appraisals results in improved functioning. Children experiencing mood and anxiety symptoms may also benefit from CBT.

Milieu Management

Milieu management is the mechanism for structuring inpatient, residential, and day treatment programs. The nurse collaborates with other health care providers in structuring and maintaining the therapeutic environment to achieve the following:

- Provide physical and psychological security
- Promote growth and mastery of developmental tasks
- Ameliorate mental health disorders and promote well-being

The physical milieu for inpatient or residential care is designed to provide a safe, comfortable place to live, play, and learn, with areas for both private time and group activity. There may be a gym, outdoor playground, swimming pool, recreational facilities, and even pets. A daily schedule sets the structure for what activities will occur (e.g., school, therapy sessions, outings, family or home visits). The nurse and multidisciplinary team share and articulate a philosophy regarding how to provide physical and psychological security, promote personal growth, and work with problematic behaviours. This philosophy is reflected in the policies of the facility and is typically written in a handbook given to patients and families upon admission. The child or adolescent's behaviour, emotions, and cognitive processes are the focus of the therapeutic interventions in the milieu. The therapeutic factors operating in the milieu's structure, activities, and interactions with staff are listed in Box 27.4.

Seclusion and restraint. Hospitalized patients are often a high risk to themselves, and effective use of prevention strategies for dangerous behaviour begins at intake. Nurses have an important role in the promotion of a culture of patient safety through assessment and intervention. Promoting a therapeutic environment for all patients involves the following (De Hert et al., 2011):

- Actively engaging the patient and family in treatment planning to avoid the use of seclusion or restraint
- Maintaining adequate staffing patterns with motivated staff experienced in working with patients who have been violent, abused, or both
- Accurately assessing the acuity of the individuals and group make-up of the unit
- Using positive and less restrictive alternatives (e.g., de-escalation strategies, time-space interviews)

Although policymakers and advocates lobbied for a reduction or elimination of seclusion and restraint use over the past decade, a majority of inpatient treatment centres for children and adolescents report using such practices (Green-Hennessy & Hennessy, 2015). Evidence on the use of locked seclusion and physical restraint in managing dangerous behaviour suggests that both are psychologically harmful and can be physically harmful. Deaths have resulted, primarily by asphyxiation due to physical holds during restraints (Eblin, 2019). However, at times a child's behaviour is so destructive or dangerous that physical restraint or seclusion is needed. All nurses who might be involved in therapeutic holding or physical restraint of children and adolescents must receive education and training to decrease the risk for injury to themselves and the child. This intervention requires prompt, firm, non-retaliatory protective restraint that is gentle and safe. Children are released as soon as they are no longer dangerous, usually after a few minutes, and most facilities strive to avoid all intensive interventions that restrict movement, such as holds and restraints.

The decision to restrain or seclude a child is made by the nurse who is working with the patient. A physician, nurse practitioner, or another advanced-level practitioner must authorize this action, either at the same time or after the fact. All patients in seclusion or restraints must be monitored constantly. Vital signs, including pulse and blood pressure, and range of motion in extremities must be monitored every 15 minutes. Hydration, elimination, comfort, and other psychological and physical needs should also be monitored. The patient's family should be informed of any incident of seclusion or restraint, and they should be encouraged to discuss the event with their child and reinforce the treatment plan to reduce the likelihood of future incidents.

Debriefings with staff after the incident help to strengthen the nurse–patient relationship, which may have been disrupted, and also enable staff to learn from the event to prevent it from happening in the future. Debriefings are important to determine if injury has occurred and identify whether the situation could have been avoided by using less restrictive alternatives. Research emphasizes the need for further reduction and eventual elimination of the use of restraints and seclusion as best practice in the clinical specialty of child and adolescent mental health (Eblin, 2019).

Quiet room. A unit may have an unlocked *quiet room* for a child who needs an area with decreased stimulation for regaining and maintaining self-control. Variations on the quiet room include the *feelings room*, which is carpeted and supplied with soft objects that can be punched and thrown, and the *freedom room*, which contains items for relaxation and meditation, such as music and yoga mats. The child is encouraged to express freely and work through feelings of anger or sadness in privacy and with staff support. When a child has difficulty being in touch with or expressing feelings, staff members provide practice sessions and act as role models.

Time out. Asking or directing a child or adolescent to take a *time out* from an activity is another method for intervening to halt disruptive behaviours or encourage self-control. It has been reported to be a less restrictive alternative to seclusion (Eblin, 2019). Taking a time out may require going to a designated room or sitting on the periphery of an activity until self-control is regained and the episode is reviewed with a staff member. The child's individual behavioural goals are considered in setting limits on behaviour and using time-out periods. If they are overused or used as an automatic response to a behavioural infraction, time-outs lose their effectiveness.

Mind–Body Therapies

Mind–body therapies have been used in Western society for years as a treatment modality for a variety of physical and psychological disorders. These approaches focus on interactions between the mind and the body, using the mind to affect physical reactions and promote emotional health. Hypnotherapy, guided imagery, meditation, music therapy, and yoga have been shown to be effective for children and youth with mental health problems such as phobias, self-harming behaviour, anxiety, and eating disorders (Govindan et al., 2020).

BOX 27.4 Therapeutic Factors in the Milieu

- Safe, therapeutic environment with roles, boundaries, and limits
- Reduction of stressors
- Structure for coping with stress
- Ability to express feelings without fear of rejection or retaliation
- Availability of emotional support and comfort
- Assistance with reality testing and support for weak or missing ego functions
- Interventions for impulsive, aggressive, or inappropriate behaviours
- Opportunities for learning and testing new adaptive behaviours and mastering developmental tasks
- Consistent, constructive feedback from trained and supportive adult staff
- Reinforcement of positive behaviours and development of self-esteem
- Corrective emotional experiences
- Availability of role models for making healthy identifications and positive attachments
- Opportunities to develop peer relationships and practise handling peer pressure
- Opportunities to be spontaneous and creative
- Opportunities to explore issues related to self-esteem and identity formation

> **INTEGRATIVE THERAPY**
> **Yoga for Adolescents**
>
> Low self-esteem contributes to feelings of depression, suicide, teen pregnancy, and other health-related problems of adolescence. To live a healthy and safe life, teens need to feel good about themselves and be confident. This study involved a 20-session mindful yoga curriculum. The curriculum used the acronym *Be BOLD—Breathe, Observe, Let it go, and Do it again*. Sessions were provided to junior and senior high school students for 50 minutes three times a week for 7 weeks. Each session concluded with an affirmation of respect to self and others. Benefits of the program included decreased alcohol use, improved relationships, and improved attention spans.
>
> Before teaching yoga, the nurse must assess for any physical limitation to yoga, obtain parental consent, and encourage children to progress safely, listening to their bodies and not forcing movements that might be painful.

Source: Fishbein, D., Miller, S., Herman-Stahl, M., et al. (2016). Behavioral and psychophysiological effects of a yoga intervention on high-risk adolescents: A randomized control trial. *Journal of Child and Family Studies, 25*(2), 518–529. https://doi.org/10.1007/s10826-015-0231-6

Play Therapy

Play is often described as the work of childhood through which the child learns to master impulses and adapt to the environment. A choice of play materials can be offered to the child to aid self-expression, assess developmental and emotional status, determine diagnosis, and institute therapeutic interventions. Clinicians can also use imaginary or pretend play with young children to gain an understanding of their world (Yanof, 2013). Melanie Klein (1955) and Anna Freud (1965) were the first to use play as a therapeutic tool in their psychoanalysis of children in the 1920s and 1930s. Axline (1969) identified the guiding principles of **play therapy**, which are still used by mental health care providers:

- Accept the child as they are and follow the child's lead.
- Establish a warm, friendly relationship that helps the child to express feelings.
- Recognize the child's feelings and reflect them back so that the child can gain insight into the behaviour.
- Accept the child's ability to solve personal problems.
- Set limits only to provide reality and security.

The many forms of play therapy can be used individually or in groups. The term *play therapy* usually refers to a one-to-one session the therapist has with a child in a playroom. Most playrooms are equipped with a range of developmentally appropriate toys, including art supplies, clay or play dough, dolls and dollhouses, hand puppets, toys, building blocks, and trucks and cars. The dolls, puppets, and dollhouse provide the child with opportunities to act out conflicts and situations involving the family, work through feelings, and develop more adaptive ways of coping. The following vignette shows how play therapy can help a child cope with a significant loss.

> **VIGNETTE**
> Hannah, a 6-year-old, begins having nightmares and refusing to go to school after her grandmother, who was also her babysitter, dies. Her parents do not let her attend the funeral, thinking it will upset her. Hannah becomes fearful and preoccupied with the death. In play sessions she repeatedly uses dolls to act out her grandmother's hospitalization, death, and funeral. She then pretends to bury her grandmother in a small, coffinlike box. Her parents have told Hannah that "Grandma has gone to heaven." Hannah demonstrates the concept by removing "Grandma" from the box and placing her high up on a bookshelf in the playroom, looking down on the rest of the doll family.

Mutual storytelling. **Mutual storytelling** is a psychodramatic technique developed by Gardner (1971) to help young children express themselves verbally. The child is asked to make up a story with a beginning, middle, and ending. At the end of the story, the child is asked to state the lesson or moral of the story. The nurse determines the psychodynamic meaning of the story and selects one or two of its important themes. Using the same characters and a similar setting, the nurse retells the story, providing a healthier resolution. The lesson of the story is also reformulated to help the child become consciously aware of the better resolution. If the child has trouble starting a story, the nurse can assist by beginning the story with "Once upon a time in a faraway land there lived a …" and then asking the child to continue. After the child has identified the main characters, the nurse may need to keep prompting with comments such as "and then …" until the story is completed. The story can be recorded as audio or video, which allows for a review to reinforce the learning. A similar technique called multi-sensory storytelling is used with children and youth. This approach involves a combination of verbal and sensory technology (games, storytelling, video, computer animation) with an emphasis on sensory experience and social engagement (Hettiarachchi et al., 2020).

Therapeutic games. The use of therapeutic games is ideal for children who have difficulty talking about their feelings and problems. Playing a game with a child facilitates the development of a therapeutic alliance and provides an opportunity for conversation. The game might be as simple as checkers, but specific **therapeutic games** are more effective in eliciting children's fears and fantasies. Gardner (1979) developed a series of therapeutic games for children, one of which, Board of Objects, can be used with children 4 to 8 years of age. The game pieces are small items (people, animals, various objects) that are placed on a checkerboard. The players roll coloured dice. If a red side lands face up, the player selects an object. To get a reward chip, the player must say something about the object; if the player tells a story about the object, they get two reward chips. The child's statement or story can be used in a therapeutic interchange (e.g., to communicate empathy or make a statement suggesting a more adaptive way to cope with a difficult situation). In the end the player with the most chips (usually the child) wins.

A board game appropriate for latency-age children (6 to 12 years) is Gardner's (1986) Talking, Feeling, and Doing Game. The player throws dice to advance their playing piece along a pathway of different-coloured squares. Depending on the colour landed upon, the player draws a talking, feeling, or doing card, which gives instructions or asks a question. A reward chip is given when the player responds appropriately. For example, a feeling card might read, "All the girls in the class were invited to a birthday party except one. How did she feel?" If this game is played with more than one child, the nurse can elicit additional responses and engage the whole group in the therapeutic interchange. The nurse may stack the deck to make sure that cards relating to the child's problems will be selected.

Bibliotherapy. **Bibliotherapy** involves using literature for children or adolescents to help the child express feelings in a supportive environment, gain insight into feelings and behaviour, and learn new ways to cope with difficult situations. When children listen to or read a story, they unconsciously identify with the characters and experience a catharsis of feelings. The books selected by the nurse should reflect the situations or feelings the child is experiencing. It is important to assess not only the needs of the child but also the child's readiness for the particular topic and the child's level of understanding. A children's librarian has access to a large collection of stories and knows which books are written specifically to help children deal with particular subjects; however, the nurse should read the book first to be sure that the content is age appropriate and fits with the treatment plan and be prepared to discuss it with the patient. Whenever possible, the nurse consults with the family to make sure the books do not violate the family's belief systems. A choice of several books is offered, and a book is never forced on the child.

Therapeutic drawing. Many children and adolescents love to draw and paint and will spontaneously express themselves in the artwork. Their drawings capture the thoughts, feelings, and tensions they may not be able to express verbally, are unaware of, or are denying. For some, however, this modality may be too threatening or not engaging. Children and adolescents can be encouraged to draw themes, such as people, families, themselves, or more abstract themes, such as feelings. To use this modality, the nurse needs to be familiar with the drawing capabilities expected of children at particular developmental levels, and additional training is recommended. In the next vignette the art therapist and the nurse use a family art session to identify family dynamics and begin interventions.

> **VIGNETTE**
>
> Yotam, an intelligent 15-year-old with obsessive-compulsive behaviours and severe insecurity, lives with his parents and younger sister. In an art session all family members are given a paper on an easel and asked to draw themselves and the other members of the family. Yotam draws his parents and sister as being the same size and standing together shoulder to shoulder. He draws himself as a tiny figure in a box that appears to be suspended in space. When questioned, he reports feeling as though he were trapped in a falling elevator and disconnected from the family.
>
> The family is surprised that he feels isolated (he is a normal size in their drawings). After completing a series of drawings and discussing them, the family is asked to draw a joint picture that requires them to work together. The picture they draw shows a smiling family standing by a house near a tree and a fence. The picture suggests that the family does view Yotam as separate and different, for although he is standing beside the family, he is placed behind the fence. This observation is discussed, and as an intervention, the family is given the task of finding ways to make Yotam feel included.

Psychopharmacology. Due to the lack of safety and efficacy data on many medications, they are not used as the first line of defence in the treatment of children and youth with mental health disorders. Medicating children typically works best when combined with another treatment such as CBT (Schatzberg, 2017). Medications that target specific symptoms can make a real difference in a family's ability to cope and in quality of life, and they can enhance the child or adolescent's potential for growth. The Medication Treatment box lists some child and adolescent disorders and identifies some of the medications used in the treatment of these disorders.

NEURODEVELOPMENTAL DISORDERS

Neurodevelopmental disorders (NDDs) are a complex group of diseases that cause abnormal functions of the brain or central nervous system. Children and youth with these types of disorders show impairment in language, speech, learning, memory, and motor skills that can bring enduring, lifelong disability. These attributes inhibit the child's ability to participate in age-appropriate activities and introduce the need for specific programs for the child and family. A population-based study reported that 5% of Canadian children had a disability, and, of these, 74% were classified as NDDs (Mâsse et al., 2013). The disorders discussed in this section of the chapter are some of the most common child and adolescent NDDs.

Intellectual Disabilities

Impairment in children that includes deficits in problem solving, reasoning, judgement, communication, self-care activities, and social participation may indicate a potential intellectual developmental disorder (intellectual disability). The child may experience mild to profound levels of impairment.

Communication Disorders

Communication disorders occur during the early developmental period of the child and are manifested by difficulty in language skills acquisition, which affects academic achievement, social achievement, and self-care activities. The main indicators of this condition are speech and language disorders, which affect a child's ability to communicate. The child has speech-related deficits in both expressive and receptive ability, which may be evident by the inability to make vocal sounds or a disturbance in fluency. As a result, the child may stutter. The child has little or no vocabulary growth, limiting the ability to initiate or maintain engagement with others (Carlsson et al., 2013). Nurses who work in a variety of settings have knowledge of appropriate developmental milestones and can serve as an important resource for children and families in early identification and referral.

Autism Spectrum Disorder

ASD is a complex neurobiological and developmental disability that is evident during the first 3 years of a child's life. However, few children are diagnosed before reaching school age. The prevalence of ASD is 1 in 66 children and youth (Autism Society Canada, 2021; Government of Canada, 2018). This disorder affects the normal development of the brain in social interaction and communication skills. People with ASD typically have difficulties in verbal and non-verbal communication, social interactions, and leisure or play activities. These communication difficulties can include delays in babbling, echolalia (the pathological repeating of another's words), and non-meaningful sentences. Severity is determined by the level of communication impairments and repetitive, stereotyped behaviours (Mazurek et al., 2019).

Twin studies have demonstrated that ASD is due to strong genetic effects, with variation in symptomatology influenced in part by non-shared environmental factors (Castelbaum et al., 2020; Tick et al., 2016). Autism is three times more common in boys than in girls, though a gender bias in diagnostic criteria is notable (Loomes et al., 2017). It has no racial, ethnic, or social boundaries and is not influenced by family income, educational levels, or lifestyles.

Although there is currently no universally recommended screening program for detecting ASD, Autism Society Canada (2021) has advocated for screening to be made available in Canada. Early diagnosis, identification, and intervention for children with ASD are critical to promoting better developmental outcomes for affected children and their families (Mazurek et al., 2019). Unfortunately, many families who have a child with ASD may not know it. Often symptoms are first noticed when the infant fails to be interested in others or to be socially responsive through eye contact and facial expressions. Some children show improvement during development, but puberty can be a turning point toward either improvement or deterioration.

Severity levels of ASD are rated as level 1, or requiring support in areas of social and communication functioning; level 2, which requires substantial support for functioning; and level 3, requiring very substantial support. Without intensive intervention, individuals with severe ASD may not be able to live and work independently, and only about one-third achieve partial independence with restricted interests and activities. Managing the care of a child with ASD can be very stressful for parents and families. It is important for nurses to support and educate families in the provision of health care services that are critical in assessment, detection, and intervention for these young children. Nurses from a variety of practice settings may be involved in providing care and must use a family-centred approach.

MEDICATION TREATMENT OF CHILD AND ADOLESCENT DISORDERS AND SYMPTOMS

Disorder or Symptom	Type of Medication	Examples and Comments
Neurodevelopmental disorders	Antipsychotics	Risperidone (Risperdal) reduces hyperactivity, fidgetiness, and labile affect.
		Olanzapine (Zyprexa) reduces hyperactivity, social withdrawal, use of language, and depression.
Autism spectrum disorder	Antipsychotics	Haloperidol (Haldol) can reduce irritability and labile affect.
	Propranolol hydrochloride	Propranolol hydrochloride (Inderal) reduces rage outbursts, aggression, and severe anxiety.
	Selective serotonin reuptake inhibitors (SSRIs)	Clomipramine (Anafranil) may help treat anger and compulsive behaviour.
Attention-deficit/hyperactivity disorder (ADHD)	Stimulants	Methylphenidate hydrochloride (Ritalin, Biphentin)
		Amphetamine (Adderall XR)
		Both improve symptoms of ADHD.
	Antidepressants	Nortriptyline hydrochloride (Aventyl)
		Bupropion hydrochloride (Wellbutrin)
		Fluoxetine hydrochloride (Prozac)
		All produce improvements in issues of hyperactivity, attention, and global functioning.
	α-Adrenergic agonists	Clonidine hydrochloride (Catapres) can be used for aggressiveness, impulsivity, and hyperactivity in patients with ADHD.
Conduct disorders	Antipsychotics	Risperidone decreases aggression.
	Stimulants	Methylphenidate decreases antisocial behaviours.
	Antidepressants	Bupropion improves symptoms of conduct disorder.
	Mood stabilizers	Carbamazepine (Tegretol) and lithium both have demonstrated efficacy in decreasing aggression.
	α-Adrenergic agonists	Clonidine hydrochloride may help with impulsive and disordered behaviours.
Panic and school phobia	SSRIs	Citalopram (Celexa), fluoxetine, and paroxetine (Paxil) decrease symptoms of anxiety.
	Tricyclic antidepressants (TCAs)	Imipramine (Tofranil) is commonly used.
Obsessive-compulsive disorder (OCD)	SSRIs	Fluoxetine hydrochloride and paroxetine (Paxil) decrease symptoms of anxiety.
	TCAs	Clomipramine decreases symptoms of anxiety.
	Atypical anxiolytics	Buspirone hydrochloride (Bustab) is used as adjunct treatment for refractory OCD.
Separation anxiety disorder	TCAs	Imipramine decreases symptoms of anxiety.
	SSRIs	Fluoxetine hydrochloride decreases symptoms of anxiety.
Social phobia	TCAs	Imipramine decreases symptoms of anxiety.
	Anxiolytics	Buspirone hydrochloride decreases symptoms of anxiety.
Post-traumatic stress disorder (PTSD)	Atypical antipsychotics	Risperidone is used to control the flashbacks and aggression in PTSD.
Insomnia	Antihistamines	Diphenhydramine (Benadryl) causes the adverse effect of mild sedation.
Major depression and dysthymia	SSRIs	Fluoxetine is effective in decreasing depressive symptoms.
	TCAs	No significant differences have been found between responses to TCAs and placebo.
	Atypical antidepressants	Venlafaxine (Effexor XR): One small study reported no difference between venlafaxine and placebo.
Psychotic symptoms	Antipsychotics	Quetiapine (Seroquel) and risperidone are effective in reducing positive psychotic symptoms.

Source: Adapted from Schatzberg, A. F. (2017). *Textbook of psychopharmacology: DSM-5 ed.* Arlington: American Psychiatric Association Publishing.

The core presenting symptoms of ASD (Autism Society Canada, 2021) include:
- Persistent deficits in social communication and interaction (with wide-ranging social-emotional expression and response difficulties, such as disinterest and difficulties in developing and maintaining social relationships).
- Restricted and repetitive patterns of behaviour, interests, or activities (with wide-ranging symptoms such as stereotyped movements including arm flapping or rocking, insistence on sameness, difficulties with transition, and preoccupations with specific sensations like touch or sound).

These symptoms are present early in the developmental period, are not explained by other communication or intellectual disabilities, and impair daily functioning in the child.

Attention-Deficit/Hyperactivity Disorder

Children with attention-deficit/hyperactivity disorder show an inappropriate degree of inattention, impulsiveness, and hyperactivity, all of which interfere with functioning or development. Some children can have attention-deficit disorder without hyperactivity (ADHD-inattentive type). Pre-schoolers with ADHD exhibit excessive gross motor activity that becomes less pronounced as the child matures. The disorder is most often detected when the child has difficulty adjusting to elementary school. Attention problems and hyperactivity contribute to low frustration tolerance, temper outbursts, labile moods, poor school performance, peer rejection, and low self-esteem (Tarver et al., 2015).

For a diagnosis of ADHD, symptoms must be present in at least two settings (e.g., at home and school). Children with ADHD often meet the diagnostic criteria for more than one mental health disorder. They may also be diagnosed as having oppositional defiant disorder or conduct disorder. Presenting symptoms of ADHD include:

- Inattention
  - Has difficulty paying attention during tasks (especially those requiring sustained attention) or play, even if they are enjoyable activities
  - Has difficulty listening, even with prompts and redirection
  - Is easily distracted, loses things, and is forgetful in daily activities
  - Does not pay attention to social cues
- Hyperactivity
  - Fidgets, climbs, is unable to sit still or play quietly
  - Acts as if "driven by a motor" and is constantly "on the go"
  - Talks excessively
- Impulsivity
  - Blurts out answers before the question has been completed
  - Has difficulty waiting for own turn or being patient
  - Interrupts, intrudes in others' conversations and games

ADHD in adults is now well established as a recognized disorder (Centre for Addiction and Mental Health, 2022), with a prevalence of 4.4% (Canadian Attention Deficit Hyperactivity Disorder Resource Alliance [CADDRA], 2020). Most adults who seek out a referral for assessment do so after the diagnosis of their own child or someone they know well (CADDRA, 2020). Adults with ADHD may present with a primary complaint that is an associated symptom, such as procrastination, disorganization, lack of motivation, insomnia, rage attacks, or labile moods (CADDRA, 2020). Adult ADHD represents a significant health care need requiring physician and nursing education, the establishment of services within the health care system, and appropriate research on treatment and service delivery. The latest practice guidelines published by the CADDRA are available online at https://adhdlearn.caddra.ca/.

Specific Learning Disorder

Specific learning disorder (SLD) in children is identified during the school-aged years and varies in severity from mild to moderate to severe. One prominent feature is impairment in academic skills such as reading (dyslexia), mathematics (dyscalculia), and written expression (dysgraphia) acquisition. The prevalence of this disorder is 5% to 15% among school-aged children, and it is more common in males than in females (Peterson & Pennington, 2012). SLD is lifelong, so early assessment, intervention, and support are important for the child and the family. Nurses are instrumental in teaching parents and children how to manage and live with the disorder. Also, ongoing assessment will involve other professionals with expertise in the areas of SLD and psychological and cognitive assessment.

Children and youth with SLD may require accommodation in school and their work environment. Individuals with an SLD are at higher risk of not graduating high school, college, or university and also have more difficulty maintaining steady employment. The Learning Disabilities Association of Canada, an important advocacy group, provides education and support to families, teachers, and health care providers. Many children and their families receive assistance through provincial and territorial school-based services and also through a disability tax credit offered by the federal government to reduce the long-term impact of the SLD.

Motor Disorders

Motor coordination is important for children as they negotiate their world. Developmental coordination disorder is diagnosed before 5 years of age when the acquisition of motor skills or coordination is below what is expected for young children achieving motor milestones such as sitting, crawling, or walking. These disorders present in the early developmental period, interfering with gross motor and fine motor skills. These disorders are chronic and cause impairment in activities of daily living.

Two prevalent motor disorders are *stereotypic movement disorder* and *Tourette's disorder (TD)*. Stereotypic movement disorder is demonstrated by repetitive and stereotypic motor behaviour (e.g., body rocking, head nodding, hand shaking, waving). These movements are usually seen in young children during the first 3 years of life, and behaviours may occur many times during the day and last seconds, minutes, or longer. The stereotypic self-injury behaviours (e.g., head banging, self-biting, eye poking) may persist for years. The repetitive motor behaviour interferes with social, academic, or other daily activities (Mackenzie, 2017). In assessment the nurse needs to be aware that simple stereotypic movements are common in infancy and childhood (e.g., rocking) but usually resolve with age.

Interventions focus on changing behaviour, promoting safety, and preventing injury. In extreme situations medication may also be used. Protective clothing (e.g., helmet, gloves) may be recommended for children who are prone to self-harm behaviour, as well as behaviour modification techniques including distraction and replacement.

TD usually presents itself before 18 years of age. The disorder is characterized by the presence of multiple motor tics (sudden, repetitive motor movements) and one or more vocal tics that repeat many times throughout the day. Tic disorders typically begin between 4 and 6 years of age, and diagnosis is based on the presence of motor or vocal tics or both for more than 1 year. Tics are classified as either simple (e.g., eye blinking, grunting) or complex (e.g., sexual or obscene gestures [copropraxia]). A child or adolescent with tics may experience impairment in social and academic relationships as a result of feeling ashamed and self-conscious and of being ridiculed or bullied by peers (Muth, 2017). Other symptoms associated with TD are obsessions, compulsions, hyperactivity, distractibility, and impulsivity.

Prevalence estimates in school-aged children range from 3 to 8 per 1000, with males more commonly affected than females (Aldred & Cavanna, 2015). The disorder is usually permanent, but periods of remission may occur, and symptoms often diminish during adolescence and sometimes disappear by young adulthood. About 90% of people with TD have a comorbid disorder (Aldred & Cavanna, 2015). Common comorbidities include ADHD; obsessive-compulsive disorder; and depressive, bipolar, or substance use disorders.

The Canadian guidelines for the treatment of tic disorders support the use of behavioural therapy, particularly habit-reversal therapy and exposure and response prevention, for both adults and children. Pharmacological treatment is recommended only if tics are distressing and interfering with daily activities (Pringsheim et al., 2012). The use of deep brain stimulation or transcranial magnetic stimulation as treatment options is not recommended. Due to a lack of evidence to support their effectiveness, these treatments are considered experimental and are recommended only for adults in severe cases (Steeves et al., 2012).

APPLICATION OF THE NURSING PROCESS

Assessment

Assessment is the first stage of the nursing process. Assessing for developmental milestones, child–parent relationship, and mental status is critical when initiating care for patients with NDDs.

ASSESSMENT GUIDELINES
Neurodevelopmental Disorders

- Assess for developmental delays, uneven development, or loss of acquired abilities. Use baby books and diaries, photographs, films, or videotapes.
- Assess the quality of the parent–child relationship for evidence of bonding, anxiety, tension, and quality of caregiver–child temperaments.
- Be aware that children with behavioural and developmental problems are at risk for abuse and be knowledgeable about community programs providing support services for parents and children, including parent education, counselling for parents and children, and after-school programs.

ASSESSMENT GUIDELINES
Attention-Deficit/Hyperactivity Disorder (ADHD)

- Observe for level of physical activity, attention span, talkativeness, frustration tolerance, impulse control, and the ability to follow directions.
- Assess social skills, friendship history, problem-solving skills, and school performance. Academic failure and poor peer relationships lead to low self-esteem, depression, and further acting out.
- Assess for associated comorbidities, such as depression.

Diagnosis

The child with an NDD has severe impairments in social interactions and communication skills, often accompanied by stereotypical behaviour, interests, and activities. The stress on the family can be severe, owing to the chronic nature of the disorder. The severity of the impairment is evident in the degree of responsiveness to or interest in others, the presence of associated behavioural problems (e.g., head banging), and the ability to bond with peers. Table 27.1 lists potential nursing diagnoses.

Outcomes Identification

Nursing Outcomes Classification (NOC) (Moorhead et al., 2018) identifies a number of outcomes appropriate for the child with an NDD. Table 27.2 presents examples of *NOC* outcomes and supporting indicators that target developmental competencies and coping skills.

TABLE 27.1 Potential Nursing Diagnoses for Disorders of Childhood and Adolescence

Signs and Symptoms	Nursing Diagnosis
Lack of responsiveness or interest in others, lack of empathy, or unwillingness to share	Impaired social interaction Risk for impaired parent or child attachment
Severe behaviour problems, creating stress on family members	Risk for caregiver role strain Interrupted family processes Chronic sorrow Spiritual distress
Lack of cooperation or imaginative play with peers	Activity intolerance
Disruptive, hostile behaviour, leading to difficulty in making or keeping friends	Situational low self-esteem
Language delay or absence, stereotyped or repetitive use of language	Impaired verbal communication
Inability to feed, bathe, dress, or toilet self at age-appropriate level	Delayed growth and development
Head banging, face slapping, hand biting	Risk for trauma
Catastrophic reactions (e.g., severe temper tantrums, rage reactions)	Risk for other-directed violence
Impulsiveness, anger, and aggression	Risk for self-mutilation
Thoughts or verbalizations regarding self-harm	Risk for self-directed violence
Frequent disregard for bodily needs	Self-care deficit (bathing, dressing, feeding, and toileting) Risk for situational low self-esteem
Conflict with authority, refusal to comply with requests	Powerlessness Readiness for enhanced power
Failure to follow age-appropriate social norms	Ineffective coping
Blaming of others for problems or for causing the child's/youth's actions	Defensive coping Impaired individual resilience
Fear of being separated from parent (e.g., going to school or to a party)	Anxiety Relocation stress syndrome
Depression	Stress overload Spiritual distress
Refusal to attend school	Ineffective coping Readiness for enhanced parenting
Inability to concentrate, withdrawal, difficulty in functioning, feeling down, change in vegetative symptoms	Risk for suicide
Re-experiences of past trauma (dreams, illusions, flashbacks)	Post-trauma syndrome Rape-trauma syndrome
Fear of objects, people, or situations	Anxiety

TABLE 27.2 NOC Outcomes for Neurodevelopmental Disorders

Nursing Outcome and Definition	Intermediate Indicators	Short-Term Indicators
Child development: 3 Years: Milestones of physical, cognitive, and psychosocial progression by 3 years of age	Speech understood by strangers	Gives own first name
Child development: 4 Years: Milestones of physical, cognitive, and psychosocial progression by 4 years of age	Engages in creative play	Draws person with three parts
Child development: 5 Years: Milestones of physical, cognitive, and psychosocial progression by 5 years of age	Follows simple rules of interactive games with peers	Recognizes most letters of the alphabet
Communication: Expressive: Expression of meaningful verbal or non-verbal messages	Directs messages appropriately	Uses spoken language; vocal
Play participation: Use of activities by a child from 1 year through 11 years of age to promote enjoyment, entertainment, and development	Expresses emotions during play activities	Expresses satisfaction with play activities

NOC, Nursing Outcomes Classification.
Source: Moorhead, S., Swanson, E., Johnson, M., et al. (2018). *Nursing Outcomes Classification (NOC): Measurement of health outcomes* (6th ed.). St. Louis, MO: Elsevier.

Implementation

Currently, two therapies reported to be effective interventions for ASD are applied behavioural analysis and intensive behavioural intervention. These therapies are expensive, not available in all provinces and territories, and not routinely publicly funded. However, the federal government offers a variety of income support for individuals with autism and their parents through the *Income Tax Act* and Canada Pension Plan Disability Benefits (Standing Senate Committee on Social Affairs, Science and Technology, 2007). These supports are usually insufficient to meet the demands of individuals with autism and their families.

Treatment plans include behaviour management plans with a reward system and education of parents for providing structure, rewards, consistency in rules, and expectations at home in order to shape and modify behaviour and foster the development of socially appropriate skills. It is important that the nurse recognize and capitalize on the individual's and family's strengths and incorporate them into the plan of care. Pharmacological agents such as risperidone (Risperdal), clomipramine (Anafranil), and desipramine are used with some success in conjunction with ongoing psychiatric medication management.

Interventions for ADHD include administration of pharmacological agents for the inattention and hyperactive-impulsive behaviours, behaviour modification, family counselling, and play therapy for young children. As the child ages, special education programs to address the academic difficulties and CBT may also be appropriate. Children and teens in specialized programs (e.g., day treatment programs) may receive additional services, such as recreational or art therapy.

Paradoxically, the mainstay of treatment for ADHD is the use of psychostimulant medications. Responses to these medications can be dramatic and can quickly increase attention and task-directed behaviour while reducing impulsivity, restlessness, and distractibility (Burchum & Rosenthal, 2018). Methylphenidate (Ritalin) is the most widely used psychostimulant because of its safety and simplicity of use. However, there is a risk for abuse and misuse. Unfortunately, the medication has gained a reputation as a street drug. A common adverse effect of stimulant ADHD medications is insomnia (Burchum & Rosenthal, 2018). To combat this effect, treating with the minimal effective dose is essential, as is administering the medication no later than 1600 hours. Other adverse effects include headache, abdominal pain, and lethargy. Growth retardation secondary to appetite suppression has been associated with the use of stimulants, although studies have provided contradictory findings.

A non-stimulant serotonin–norepinephrine reuptake inhibitor (SNRI), atomoxetine (Strattera), is approved for childhood and adult ADHD. Although not as effective in improving symptoms as the stimulants, this medication eliminates the risk for abuse. Therapeutic responses develop slowly, and full improvement may take up to 3 weeks (Burchum & Rosenthal, 2018). The most common adverse effects are gastrointestinal disturbances, reduced appetite, weight loss, dizziness, fatigue, and insomnia. It may also cause a small increase in blood pressure and heart rate. Rarely, serious allergic reactions occur.

The dosing schedule of stimulant and non-stimulant medications is important. Medication preparations vary in their onset of action and duration of action, so dosing may be only once a day (in the morning) or up to three times a day. Because once-a-day dosing is easier and avoids the uncertainty and potential stigma of taking medications at school, long-acting medications tend to be more attractive. See Medication Treatment of Patients with ADHD for a summary of the Canadian-approved medications used to treat ADHD.

DISRUPTIVE, IMPULSE CONTROL, AND CONDUCT DISORDERS

Oppositional Defiant Disorder

Oppositional defiant disorder is a recurrent pattern of negativistic, disobedient, hostile, defiant behaviour toward authority figures without going so far as to seriously violate the basic rights of others (Winther et al., 2013). Children with this disorder exhibit persistent stubbornness and argumentativeness, limit testing, unwillingness to give in or negotiate, touchiness and quick annoyance, and refusal to accept blame for misdeeds. The behaviours lead to significant impairment in home or social relationships and school or occupational functioning. Children and adolescents with oppositional defiant disorder justify their behaviour as a response to unreasonable demands or situations.

This disorder is usually evident before 8 years of age and, until puberty, is more common in males; after that point, the prevalence is equal for males and females. This disorder may vary in severity from mild to moderate to severe, and the severity is determined by the symptoms and setting (e.g., at home, at school, with peers, at work). Symptoms may be confined to only one setting (mild), be present in at least two settings (moderate), or appear in three or more settings (severe). Children and youth with this diagnosis have an increased risk for

MEDICATION TREATMENT OF PATIENTS WITH ADHD

Classification	Trade Name	Indications	Duration	Schedule
Methylphenidate hydrochloride	Ritalin	Ages 6–12	3–5 hours	2 or 3 times a day
Extended or sustained release	Ritalin SR	Ages 6–12	6–8 hours	1 or 2 times a day
	Biphentin	Ages 6 and older	10–12 hours	Once a day
	Concerta	Ages 6–65	Up to 14 hours	Once a day
Dextroamphetamine sulphate *Short acting*	Dexedrine	Ages 3–16	4–6 hours	2 or 3 times a day
Intermediate acting	Dexedrine Spansule SRC	Ages 6–16	6–10 hours	1 or 2 times a day
Lisdexamfetamine dimesylate	Vyvanse	Ages 6–12	10–12 hours	Once a day
Amphetamine mixture *Extended release*	Adderall XR	Ages 6 and older	10–12 hours	1 or 2 times a day
Atomoxetine hydrochloride *Extended release*	Strattera	Ages 6–65	24 hours	Once a day

Source: Adapted from Burchum, J., & Rosenthal, L. (2018). *Lehne's pharmacology for nursing care* (10th ed.). Philadelphia: Saunders; Riddle, M. A. (2021). *Pediatric psychopharmacology for primary care* (3rd ed.). Elk Grove Village: American Academy of Pediatrics; Schatzberg, A. F. (2017). *Textbook of psychopharmacology: DSM-5 ed.* Arlington: American Psychiatric Association Publishing.

problems (e.g., antisocial behaviour, impulse control issues, substance use, anxiety, depression) as they transition to adulthood (Burke, 2012).

Conduct Disorder

Conduct disorder is characterized by a persistent pattern of antisocial behaviour in which children and adolescents have no concern for the rights of others and a disregard for appropriate societal norms or rules. Children with this disorder also display callous–unemotional traits (e.g., lack of empathy or guilt, shallow affect) (American Psychiatric Association, 2013) and bullying, threatening, or intimidating behaviour. It is one of the most frequently diagnosed disorders of childhood and adolescence, and the behaviours associated with conduct disorder are commonly observed within settings frequented by this population (e.g., school, home, community). Complications associated with conduct disorder are academic failure, school suspensions and dropouts, juvenile delinquency, substance misuse and dependency, and juvenile court involvement. Psychiatric disorders that frequently coexist with conduct disorder are anxiety, depression, ADHD, learning disabilities, and substance dependency.

There are four types of conduct disorder: (1) aggression toward people and animals, (2) property destruction, (3) theft, and (4) serious violations of rules. There are two subtypes of conduct disorder, child onset and adolescent onset, both of which can occur in mild, moderate, or severe forms. Predisposing factors are ADHD, oppositional child behaviours, parental rejection, inconsistent parenting with harsh discipline, early institutional living, chaotic home life, large family size, absent parent, caregiver who misuses alcohol, antisocial and drug-dependent family members, and association with delinquent peers.

Childhood-onset conduct disorder occurs prior to age 10 years and is found mainly in males who are physically aggressive, have poor peer relationships, show little concern for others, and lack feelings of guilt or remorse. These children frequently misperceive others' intentions as hostile and believe that their aggressive responses are justified. Violent children also often display antisocial reasoning, such as "He deserved it," when rationalizing aggressive behaviours (Frick, 2012). Children with childhood-onset conduct disorder attempt to project a strong image, but they actually have low self-esteem. They also display limited frustration tolerance, irritability, and temper outbursts. Individuals with childhood-onset conduct disorder are more likely to have problems that persist through adolescence and, without intensive treatment, develop antisocial personality disorder in the adult years.

In *adolescent-onset conduct disorder* youths tend to act out misconduct with their peer group (e.g., early onset of sexual behaviour, substance abuse, risk-taking behaviours). Males are apt to fight, steal, vandalize, and have discipline problems in school, whereas girls tend to lie, be truant, run away, abuse substances, and engage in prostitution. The male-to-female ratio is not as high as for the childhood-onset type, indicating that more girls become aggressive during this period of development (Thornton et al., 2013).

Bullying

Bullying, as a concept, is broadly defined in terms of behaviour and its impact on those who are bullied. Globally, the occurrence of child and adolescent bullying in society has become a universal concern and is recognized as a major public health problem. Children and youth with disruptive behaviour, impulse control, or conduct disorder may display aggressive behaviour toward others. Bullying is identified as an abuse of power that involves three components: harm, repetition, and unequal power. It is manifested in several ways, often called *physical* (e.g., hitting, kicking), *verbal* (e.g., threats, derogatory remarks or names), *relational* (e.g., social exclusion, spreading of rumours), and *cyberbullying* (i.e., bullying carried out online or through social media).

Children who are victims of bullying experience low self-esteem, see themselves as socially incompetent, have more physical health problems, may go through depression, and may experience suicidal ideation. Research has also reported that the bullies themselves are more prone to substance misuse and to becoming involved in antisocial behaviours as teens and adults (Armitage, 2021).

Nurses should be aware that children who are being bullied may not report problems unless asked directly (Carpenter & Hubbard, 2014). It is imperative that nurses and parents or other caregivers be knowledgeable of specific signs that may indicate bullying. Sleep disturbances, unexplained cuts or bruises, tearfulness, requesting to change schools, fear of walking to and from school, and self-harm behaviours are behaviours that are symptomatic of being bullied. Nurses play an important role in detecting early symptoms and signs through assessment and screening and need to work with the patient, family, and members of the school system to offset difficulties for these children and adolescents. A great resource for bullied children and their families is a government website that aims to stop bullying called Bullying Canada at https://www.bullyingcanada.ca/.

APPLICATION OF THE NURSING PROCESS

Assessment
When clinicians are assessing for the presence of a behavioural disorder, it is important to gather information from the perspective of the child and from that of the parent or guardian. Determining how the child and parent interact with each other as well as how the child interacts with peers, extended family, and authority figures yields valuable assessment data.

Diagnosis
Children and adolescents with oppositional defiant disorder or conduct disorder display disruptive behaviours that are impulsive, angry or aggressive, and often dangerous. They are often in conflict with others, do not follow rules, do not follow age-appropriate social norms, and have inappropriate ways of meeting their needs. Refer to Table 27.1 for potential nursing diagnoses.

Outcomes Identification
NOC identifies a number of outcomes appropriate for the child experiencing hyperactivity, severe inattention, or difficulty controlling their own impulses. These symptoms are most commonly seen in children with the NDD ADHD and in children who have any of the disruptive, impulse control, and conduct disorders (e.g., oppositional defiant disorder, conduct disorder, intermittent explosive disorder). Table 27.3 lists a sampling of NOC outcomes and supporting indicators that target hyperactivity, impulse self-control, the development of self-identity and self-esteem, positive coping skills, and family functioning.

Implementation
Interventions for severe oppositional defiant and conduct disorders focus on correcting the faulty personality (ego and superego) development, which includes firmly entrenched patterns such as blaming others and denial of responsibility for actions. Children and adolescents with

---

ASSESSMENT GUIDELINES

Disruptive, Impulse Control, and Conduct Disorders
- Assess the quality of the relationship between the child or adolescent and parents or caregivers for evidence of bonding, anxiety, tension, and quality of fit between temperaments, all of which can contribute to the development of disruptive behaviours.
- Assess parents' or caregivers' understanding of growth and development, effective parenting skills, and handling of problematic behaviours; a lack of knowledge and poor parenting contribute to the development of these problems.
- Assess cognitive, psychosocial, and moral development for lags or deficits because immaturity in developmental competencies results in disruptive behaviours.
- Assess for involvement in the justice system, which may suggest a lack of impulse control or a disregard for the rights of others.
- Assess parenting practices for rules, roles, and responsibilities in the family, relationships with siblings and extended family, history of conflict, and presence of support system (e.g., extended family members, clergy, after-school program).
- Assess the school history for problems and strengths in school, grades, occupational goals, disciplinary problems, and placements.

Oppositional Defiant Disorder
- Identify issues that result in power struggles and triggers for outbursts; note when they begin and how they are handled.

- Assess the child's or adolescent's view of their own behaviour and its impact on others at home, at school, and with peers. Explore feelings of empathy and remorse.
- Explore how the child or adolescent can exercise control and take responsibility, problem-solve for situations that occur, and plan to handle things differently in the future. Assess barriers to change, motivation to change, and potential rewards to engage the patient.

Conduct Disorder
- Assess the seriousness, types, and initiation of disruptive behaviour and how it has been managed.
- Assess anxiety, aggression and anger levels, motivation, and the ability to control impulses.
- Assess moral development, problem solving, belief system, and spirituality for the ability to understand the impact of hurtful behaviour on others, to empathize with others, and to feel remorse.
- Assess the ability to form a therapeutic relationship and engage in honest and committed therapeutic work leading to observable behavioural change (e.g., signing a behavioural contract, drug testing, living according to "house rules").
- Assess for substance use (past and present).

TABLE 27.3 NOC Outcomes for Attention-Deficit/Hyperactivity Disorder and Disruptive, Impulse Control, and Conduct Disorders

Nursing Outcome and Definition	Intermediate Indicators	Short-Term Indicators
Hyperactivity level: Severity of patterns of inattention and impulsivity in a child from 1 year through 17 years of age	Inappropriate aggressive behaviour decreases	Active listening
Impulse self-control: Self-restraint of compulsive or impulsive behaviours	Self-control maintenance without supervision	Identification of harmful impulsive behaviours
Self-esteem: Personal judgement of self-worth	Expression of feelings about self-worth	Acceptance of self-limitations
Coping: Personal actions to manage stressors that tax an individual's resources	Reports of psychological comfort increase	Identification of effective coping patterns
Family normalization: Capacity of the family system to maintain routines and develop strategies for optimal functioning when a member has a chronic illness or disability	Maintenance of usual parenting expectations for affected child; help sought from a health care provider as appropriate	Acknowledgment of impairment and its potential to alter family routines

NOC, Nursing Outcomes Classification.

Sources: Data from Ackley, B., Ladwig, G., Makic, B. F., et al. (2019). *Nursing diagnosis handbook: An evidence-based guide to planning care* (12th ed.). St. Louis: Mosby; Moorhead, S., Swanson, E., Johnson, M., et al. (2018) *Nursing Outcomes Classification (NOC): Measurement of health outcomes* (6th ed.). St. Louis: Elsevier.

these disorders also must generate more mature and adaptive coping mechanisms and prosocial goals, a process that is gradual and cannot be accomplished during short-term treatment. In the case of conduct disorder inpatient hospitalization for crisis intervention, evaluation, and treatment planning, as well as transfer to therapeutic foster care, a group home, or long-term residential treatment, is often needed. Oppositional youths are generally treated on an outpatient basis, using individual, group, and family therapy, with much of the focus on parenting issues.

Unfortunately, studies indicate that many children who are simply placed in group homes and in some residential programs do not maintain improvements following discharge. However, intensive programs such as multi-systemic therapy and therapeutic foster care and the use of interprofessional, community-based treatment teams for children with serious emotional and behavioural disturbances have been found to improve outcomes and reduce offences over the long term (Cleverley et al., 2020). These types of programs are more promising in improving positive adjustment, decreasing negative behaviours, and improving family stability. Unfortunately, many of these types of resources are limited to youth under the age of 18 years. Active case management strategies are required to assist youth transitioning into the adult system.

To control the aggressive behaviours, a wide variety of pharmacological agents have been tried, including antipsychotics, lithium, anticonvulsants, and antidepressants, with limited effect (Calles, 2011). CBT is used to change the pattern of misconduct by fostering the development of internal controls and working with the family to improve coping and support. The development of problem solving, conflict resolution, empathy, and social skills is an important component of the treatment program.

Families are actively engaged in therapy and given support in using parenting skills to provide nurturance and set consistent limits. They are taught techniques for behaviour modification, monitoring medication for effects, collaborating with teachers to foster academic success, and setting up a home environment that is consistent, structured, and nurturing and that promotes the achievement of normal developmental milestones. If families are abusive, drug dependent, or highly disorganized, the child may require out-of-home placement. The following nursing interventions are helpful when working with parents and caregivers:

- Explore the impact of the child's behaviours on family life and the impact of the other members' behaviour on the child.
- Assist the immediate and extended family to access available and supportive individuals and systems.
- Discuss how to make home a safe environment, especially in regard to weapons and drugs; attempt to talk separately to family members whenever possible.
- Discuss realistic behavioural goals and how to set them; problem-solve potential problems.
- Teach behaviour modification techniques. Practise the techniques through role-play with the parents in different problem situations that might arise with their child.
- Give support and encouragement as parents learn to apply new techniques.
- Provide education about medications.
- Refer parents or caregivers to a local self-help group.
- Advocate for special education services if needed.

Techniques for managing disruptive behaviours are listed in Box 27.5.

BOX 27.5 Techniques for Managing Disruptive Behaviours

Behavioural contract: A verbal or written agreement between the patient and nurse or other parties (e.g., family, treatment team, teacher) about behaviours, expectations, and needs. The contract is periodically evaluated and reviewed and typically coupled with rewards and other contingencies, both positive and negative.

Counselling: Verbal interactions, role-playing, and modelling to teach, coach, or maintain adaptive behaviour and provide positive reinforcement. It is most effective for motivated youth and those with well-developed communication and self-reflective skills.

Modelling: A method of learning behaviours or skills by observation and imitation that can be used in a wide variety of situations. It is enhanced when the modeller is perceived to be similar (e.g., age, interests) and attending to the task is required.

Role-playing: A counselling technique in which the nurse, the patient, or a group of youngsters act out a specified script or role to enhance the understanding of that role, learn and practise new behaviours or skills, and practise specific situations. It requires well-developed expressive and receptive language skills.

Planned ignoring: When behaviours are determined by staff not to be dangerous but are attention seeking, they may be ignored. Additional interventions may be used in conjunction (e.g., positive reinforcement for on-task actions).

Use of signals or gestures: Use a word, a gesture, or eye contact to remind the child to use self-control. To help promote behavioural change, this technique may be used in conjunction with a behavioural contract and a reward system. An example is placing your finger to your lips and making eye contact with a child who is talking during a quiet drawing activity.

Physical distance and touch control: You could move closer to the child for a calming effect, perhaps putting an arm around the child (with permission). Evaluate the effect of this, because some children may find such an action more agitating and may need more space and less physical closeness. This technique also may involve putting the nurse or a staff member between certain children who have a history of conflict.

Redirection: A technique used following an undesirable or inappropriate behaviour to engage or re-engage an individual in an appropriate activity. It may involve the use of verbal directives (e.g., setting firm limits), gestures, or physical prompts.

Additional affection: Giving a child planned emotional support for a specific problem or engaging in an enjoyable activity. It can be used to redirect a child away from an undesirable activity as well. This might be involvement in an activity, such as a game of basketball or working on a puzzle. This shows acceptance of the child while ignoring the behaviour and can increase rapport in the nurse–patient relationship.

Use of humour: Use well-timed, appropriate kidding about some external, non-personal (to the child) event as a diversion to help the child save face and relieve feelings of guilt or fear.

Clarification as intervention: Breaking down a problem situation that a child experiences can help the child understand the situation, other people's roles, and their own motivation for the behaviour. This technique can be done verbally or using worksheets, depending on the age and functional level of the child.

Restructuring: Changing an activity in a way that will decrease the stimulation or frustration (e.g., shorten a story, change to a physical activity). Restructuring requires flexibility and planning in advance to have an alternative in mind in case the activity is not going well.

Limit setting: Giving direction, stating an expectation, or telling a child what to do or where to go. Limit setting should be done firmly, calmly, without judgement or anger, preferably in advance of any problem behaviour occurring and consistently when in a treatment setting among multiple staff members. An example is "I would like for you to stop turning the light on and off."

Simple restitution: Refers to a procedure in which an individual is required or expected to correct the adverse environmental or relational effects of their misbehaviour by restoring the environment to its prior state, making a plan to correct their actions with the nurse, and implementing the plan (e.g., apologizing to the persons harmed, fixing the chairs that are upturned). Simple restitution is not punitive in nature, and there are typically additional activities involved (e.g., counselling).

Physical restraint: Therapeutic holding to control and protect the child from their own impulses to act out and hurt self or others.

ANXIETY DISORDERS

The developmental period of childhood through adolescence poses many challenges. As a result, an anxiety disorder, such as separation anxiety disorder, specific phobia, social anxiety disorder, or adjustment disorder, may develop. Separation anxiety disorder and generalized anxiety disorder (GAD) are discussed in more detail below.

The prevalence of anxiety disorders is higher than virtually all other mental health disorders of childhood and adolescence (Dozois & Mental Health Research Canada, 2020). Not all anxiety is abnormal in childhood or adolescence, and a number of fears are a part of normal development. Young people may worry about grades, peer problems, or family issues. Anxiety becomes problematic when the child or adolescent fails to move beyond the fears associated with a particular problem or when the anxiety interferes with functioning over an extended period of time.

There is evidence of genetic contributions to anxiety disorders (Shimada-Sugimoto et al., 2015). However, genetic predisposition does not mean that a disorder will develop. From a prevention standpoint, early intervention and support can be effective. Cognitive theorists propose that anxiety is the result of dysfunctional efforts to make sense of life events.

The physiological, behavioural, and cognitive characteristics of anxiety in youth are clinically similar to those in adults. Selective serotonin reuptake inhibitors (SSRIs) have demonstrated efficacy for the treatment of childhood social anxiety disorder (Burchum & Rosenthal, 2018).

Separation Anxiety Disorder

Children and adolescents with separation anxiety disorder become excessively anxious when separated from or anticipating separation from their home or parental figures. The fear or anxiety in children is usually persistent and excessive and results in impairment in social, academic, or occupational functioning. Separation anxiety disorder is recognized as one of the most common anxiety disorders in childhood and may develop after a significant stress, such as the death of a relative or pet, an illness, a move or change in schools, or a physical or sexual assault. The prevalence in children is estimated to be 4%, with a higher incidence among females. It is common in first-degree biological relatives of an affected individual, and the incidence may be higher in children whose mothers have a panic disorder. Although remission rates are high, the disorder can persist and lead to panic disorder with agoraphobia. A depressed mood often accompanies the anxiety.

Characteristics of separation anxiety disorder identified in this population are:
- Excessive distress when separated or anticipating separation from home or parental figures
- Excessive worries one will be lost, that parents will be harmed, or that the home will be violated or damaged
- Fear of being home alone or in situations without significant adults
- Refusal to sleep unless near a parental figure or refusal to sleep away from home
- Refusal to attend school or other activities without parents
- Physical or somatic symptoms of anxiety

Generalized Anxiety Disorder

The child or youth with GAD has excessive worry or anxiety over routine activities such as school, family, or sports. The individual finds it difficult to control the worry and experiences physiological symptoms such as headache, muscle tension, sleep disturbance, fatigue, difficulty concentrating, heart palpitations, and restlessness. This disorder occurs in about 10% of children and adolescents, with an average age of onset of about 8.5 years. Children with GAD tend to need and seek reassurance about all performance activities or other things they are worried about. In considering a diagnosis, a complete assessment is recommended to rule out other explanations for symptoms that may not be related to anxiety (Jarrett et al., 2015).

APPLICATION OF THE NURSING PROCESS

Assessment

Children generally report their experiences of anxiety honestly but may be a bit hesitant to elaborate on their worries. The clinician needs to use a sensitive and caring approach with an anxious child.

> **ASSESSMENT GUIDELINES**
> *Anxiety Disorders*
>
> - Assess the quality of the parent–child relationship for evidence of anxiety, conflicts, and quality of fit between their temperaments.
> - Assess relationships among other family members.
> - Observe parent–child interactions to determine patterns.
> - Assess for recent stressors and their severity, duration, and proximity to the child.
> - Assess parent or caregiver understanding of developmental norms, parenting skills, and handling of problematic behaviours.
> - Assess the child's developmental level and determine whether regression has occurred.
> - Assess for symptoms of anxiety and coping style.
>
> **Separation Anxiety Disorder**
>
> Assess the child's previous and current ability to separate from parents or caregivers. (The separation or individuation process may not be completed, or the child may have regressed.)

Diagnosis

The chief characteristic of anxiety disorders is disabling anxiety. Refer to Table 27.1 for potential nursing diagnoses.

Outcomes Identification

NOC identifies a number of outcomes appropriate for children with an anxiety disorder. The two most relevant outcomes focus on decreasing the anxiety level of the child or adolescent and increasing the child's ability to control anxiety (Table 27.4).

Implementation

The nursing interventions for an anxious child or adolescent include:
- Help prevent the child or adolescent from experiencing panic levels of anxiety by acting as a parental surrogate, providing a safe environment, and providing for biological and psychosocial needs.
- Accept regression, but give emotional support and praise to enable progression, healing, and reintegration into activities of daily living.
- Increase self-esteem and feelings of competence in the ability to perform, achieve, and influence the present and future.
- Help the child or adolescent to accept and work through traumatic events without the use of cognitive distortions or unrealistic fears.
- Teach and practise positive self-talk and reframing to reduce cognitive distortions.
- Teach coping skills (e.g., deep breathing, counting to 10, exercise, guided imagery, listening to music, distraction) to manage feelings.

Children and adolescents with anxiety disorders are most often treated on an outpatient basis, using CBT techniques in individual,

TABLE 27.4 NOC Outcomes for Anxiety Disorders

Nursing Outcome and Definition	Intermediate Indicator	Short-Term Indicator
Anxiety level: Severity of manifested apprehension, tension, or uneasiness arising from an unidentifiable source	School achievement and performance in activities of daily living	Problem behaviours (e.g., avoidance) with peers, family members, or other community members
Anxiety self-control: Personal actions to eliminate or reduce feelings of apprehension, tension, or uneasiness from an unidentifiable source	Controls anxiety response and demonstrates return of basic problem-solving skills	Monitors intensity of anxiety

NOC, Nursing Outcomes Classification.

Source: Data from Ackley, B., Ladwig, G., Makic, B. F., et al. (2019). *Nursing diagnosis handbook: An evidence-based guide to planning care* (12th ed.). St. Louis: Mosby; Moorhead, S., Swanson, E., Johnson, M., et al. (2018). *Nursing Outcomes Classification (NOC): Measurement of health outcomes* (6th ed.). St. Louis: Elsevier.

group, or family therapy. Medications such as antidepressants, anxiolytics, and beta-blockers are also used. Cognitive therapy focuses on the underlying fears and concerns, and behaviour modification is used to shape behaviour and reinforce self-control behaviours. Children who refuse to start school are introduced gradually into the school environment, with a supportive adult present for part of the day. When adolescents develop school phobia, the goal is to return them to the classroom at the earliest possible date and give parents support in setting limits on truancy.

Refer to the Medication Treatment box for a summary of medications used in the treatment of childhood and adolescent clinical and developmental disorders.

OTHER DISORDERS OF CHILDREN AND ADOLESCENTS

Depressive Disorders and Bipolar and Related Disorders

The most frequently diagnosed mood disorders (disorders whose primary symptoms are related to changes in mood) in children and adolescents are major depressive disorder, persistent depressive disorder, and bipolar I or II disorder. Symptoms of depressive or bipolar disorders in young people may be similar to the symptoms in adults (see Chapters 13 and 14), with feelings of sadness, pessimism, hopelessness, and anhedonia (inability to experience happiness); social withdrawal; and suicidal ideation. Children may have somatic complaints, be critical of themselves and others, and feel unloved. Adolescents may have psychomotor agitation or retardation and hypersomnia (Maughan et al., 2013). Both children and adolescents often manifest irritability leading to aggressiveness. They are less likely than adults to have psychotic symptoms.

Factors associated with child and adolescent depression are physical and sexual abuse or neglect; homelessness; parental problems, including marital discord, death, divorce or separation, or separation from parents; learning disabilities; chronic illness; and conflicts with others, such as peers. The complications of depression are school failure and dropout, substance abuse, sexual acting out, pregnancy, running away, illegal behaviour, and suicide.

Post-Traumatic Stress Disorder

Children exposed to traumatic events such as receiving acute injuries from accidents or witnessing significant harm to others may develop a trauma- or stressor-related disorder. After an assessment for personal exposure to an extreme traumatic stressor, further information is needed about any evidence of internalized or externalized symptoms. These symptoms may include anxiety, dissociative symptoms, emotional re-experience of the trauma, and avoidance. It is also important to explore the child's understanding of the meaning of the event and feelings of safety and security. Children whose symptoms last longer than 1 month will be diagnosed with PTSD, a disorder that can occur at any age. Young children may engage in repetitive play in which themes of the traumatic event are expressed. The child may experience frightening dreams without recognizable content. Younger children with PTSD tend to exhibit behaviours indicative of internalized anxiety. In older children and adolescents the anxiety is more often externalized. There may be comorbid disorders such as depression and anxiety and behaviours such as self-mutilation, depending on the severity and longevity of the trauma that precipitated the PTSD (Hornor, 2013).

Feeding and Eating Disorders

Feeding and eating disorders include pica, rumination disorder, and avoidant/restrictive food intake disorder. Anorexia nervosa and bulimia nervosa, which also can occur in childhood and adolescence, are described in detail in Chapter 16. **Pica** is the persistent eating of non-nutritive substances without an aversion to eating food. Infants and toddlers may eat paint, plaster, string, or cloth. This behaviour is frequently associated with an intellectual disorder. **Rumination disorder** is the repeated regurgitation and rechewing of food without apparent nausea, retching, or gastrointestinal problems. In avoidant/restrictive food intake disorder the child fails to eat adequate amounts of food, despite availability, and there is no medical condition or intellectual disability. However, because the child fails to gain weight or undergoes a significant weight loss, they can develop nutritional problems that lead to developmental delays.

Interventions for these disorders include working with the family to provide a safe and well-monitored environment that prohibits placing unsafe items in the child's mouth and ensures removal of unsafe items; working with associated care providers (e.g., pediatricians, nutritionists); and providing praise and support for parents and caregivers as they manage the child's behaviour.

KEY POINTS TO REMEMBER

- One in five children and adolescents in Canada suffers from a major mental illness that causes significant impairments at home, at school, with peers, and in the community.
- Factors known to affect the development of mental and emotional problems in children and adolescents include genetic influences, biochemical (pre-natal and post-natal) factors, temperament, psychosocial developmental factors, social and environmental factors, and cultural influences.
- The characteristics of a resilient child include an adaptable temperament, the ability to form nurturing relationships with surrogate parental figures, the ability to distance the self from emotional chaos in parents and family, and good social intelligence and problem-solving skills.

- Children experience a number of psychiatric disorders. The most commonly diagnosed child psychiatric disorders are anxiety disorders, depressive disorders, bipolar and related disorders, and impulse control disorders.
- Treatment of childhood and adolescent disorders requires a multimodal approach in almost all instances, and family involvement is seen as critical to improvement in outcomes.
- Nurses can be important advocates for children with severe emotional and behavioural disorders.
- Cognitive behavioural therapies, social skills groups, family therapy, parent training in behavioural techniques, and individual therapy focused on self-esteem issues have been found useful.
- Skills training may focus on a variety of areas, depending on the child's or adolescent's presenting symptoms, and require an individualized assessment to determine each child's need.

CRITICAL THINKING

1. Owen, a 4-year-old boy, has been diagnosed with a neurodevelopmental disorder (NDD): autism.
    a. Describe the specific behavioural data you would find on assessment in terms of (1) communication, (2) social interactions, (3) behaviours and activities.
    b. Name at least three realistic outcomes for a child with an NDD.
    c. Which interventions are the most important for a child with an NDD? Identify at least six.
    d. What kinds of support should the family receive?
2. Natasha is a 7-year-old girl in grade 2 who has been diagnosed with attention-deficit/hyperactivity disorder (ADHD).
    a. What clinical behaviours might she be exhibiting at home and in the classroom? Give behavioural examples for her (1) inattention, (2) hyperactivity, and (3) impulsivity.
    b. Identify at least six intervention strategies one might use for Natasha, including medication management.
    c. Describe the concept of time out.
3. Saed is an 8-year-old boy who has been diagnosed with conduct disorder.
    a. Explain to one of your classmates his probable behaviours in terms of (1) aggression toward others, (2) destruction of property, (3) deceitfulness, and (4) violation of rules.
    b. What are three outcomes for this child? What is the overall prognosis for children with this disorder?
    c. What are four ways you could support Saed's parents? Where could you refer this family within your own community?
4. Jasmine is a 16-year-old who is attending an appointment with her nurse-therapist at the local community health clinic. Jasmine has been diagnosed with depression.
    a. Based on current research, what themes would you expect to hear as Jasmine describes her experiences of depression?
    b. As you complete a mental status exam, what area of assessment is essential?

CHAPTER REVIEW

1. The nurse is assessing a teenage patient for suicidal risk. Which patient response requires immediate further nursing assessment?
    a. "The idea of death really scares me."
    b. "I smoked only one time in my life."
    c. "My mom keeps a bunch of pills in her nightstand."
    d. "I've never tried to kill myself before."
2. The nurse meets with the parents of a child diagnosed with conduct disorder. What advice from the nurse is most appropriate?
    a. "Use time out as a way to control any unacceptable behaviour."
    b. "Ignore his head banging. He is just trying to get attention."
    c. "Allow the child to come up with a list of play activities."
    d. "Encourage the child to talk when he is around others."
3. The nurse is caring for a 9-year-old patient who will be entering a freedom room. Which activity should the nurse anticipate the child would engage in?
    a. Listening to a CD
    b. Throwing pillows
    c. Sitting in the periphery of the room
    d. Punching soft objects
4. A 7-year-old male who has not met earlier normal expectations in cognitive and language development and who has difficulty establishing friendships with other schoolchildren develops a fascination with the water fountain in his neighbourhood. Which condition should the nurse anticipate?
    a. Intellectual developmental disorder
    b. Major depressive disorder
    c. Tourette's disorder
    d. Autism spectrum disorder
5. The school nurse is assessing Than, who has been coming to the office over the past week with cuts and bruises for treatment. What must the nurse include in his assessment?
    a. Assess for suicidal ideation
    b. Offer professional advice about his reasons for the visits
    c. Question Than directly about bullying
    d. Anticipate the need for an anxiolytic

https://evolve.elsevier.com/Canada/Varcarolis/psychiatric/

REFERENCES

Aldred, M., & Cavanna, A. E. (2015). Tourette syndrome and socioeconomic status. *Neurological Sciences, 36*(9), 1643–1649. https://doi.org/10.1007/s10072-015-2223-0

American Psychiatric Association. (2013). *Diagnostic and statistical manual of mental disorders* (5th ed.). Arlington: Author.

Angeles, L. C., & Roberton, J. (2020). Empathy and inclusive public safety in the city: Examining LGBTQ2+ voices and experiences of intersectional discrimination. *Women's Studies International Forum, 78*(2020), 1–12. https://doi.org/10.1016/j.wsif.2019.102313

Armitage, R. (2021). Bullying in children: Impact on child health. *BMJ Paediatrics Open, 5*, e000939. https://doi.org/10.1136/bmjpo-2020-000939

Autism Society Canada. (2021). *Autism explained: What is autism?* Retrieved from https://autismcanada.org/autism-explained/

Axline, V. (1969). *Play therapy*. New York: Ballantine Books.

Burchum, J., & Rosenthal, L. (2018). *Lehne's pharmacology for nursing care* (10th ed.). Philadelphia: Saunders.

Burke, J. D. (2012). An affective dimension within oppositional defiant disorder symptoms among boys: Personality and psychopathology outcomes into early adulthood. *Journal of Child Psychology and Psychiatry, 53*(11), 1176–1183. https://doi.org/10.1111/j.1469-7610.2012.02598.x

Calles, J. L., Jr. (2011). Psychopharmacologic control of aggression and violence in children and adolescents. *Pediatric Clinics of North America, 58*, 73–84. https://doi.org/10.1016/j.pcl.2010.11.002

Canadian Attention Deficit Hyperactivity Disorder Resource Alliance (CADDRA). (2020). *Canadian ADHS practice guidelines: CAP-Guidelines* (4th ed.). Retrieved from https://www.caddra.ca/wp-content/uploads/CADDRA-Guidelines-4th-Edition_-Feb2018.pdf

Carlsson, L. H., Norrelgen, F., Kjellmer, L., et al. (2013). Coexisting disorders and problems in preschool children with autism spectrum disorders. *Scientific World Journal, 2013*, 213979. https://doi.org/10.1155/2013/213979

Carpenter, L. M. & Hubbard, G. B. (2014). Cyberbullying: Implications for the psychiatric nurse practitioner. *Journal of Child and Adolescent Psychiatric Nursing, 27*(3), 142–148. https://doi.org/10.1111/jcap.12079

Castelbaum, L., Sylvester, C. M., Zhang, Y., et al. (2020). On the nature of monozygotic twin concordance and discordance for autistic trait severity: A quantitative analysis. *Behaviour Genetics, 50*, 263–272. https://doi.org/10.1007/s10519-019-09987-2

Centre for Addiction and Mental Health. (2022). *Adult ADHD screening and assessment*. https://www.camh.ca/en/professionals/treating-conditions-and-disorders/adult-adhd/adult-adhd---screening-and-assessment

Chambers, R. M., Crutchfield, R. M., Willis, T. Y., et al. (2020). "Be supportive and understanding of the stress that youth are going through": Foster care alumni recommendations for youth, caregivers and caseworkers on placement transitions. *Children & Youth Services Review, 108*, 104644. https://doi.org/10.1016/j.childyouth.2019.104644

Charach, A., & Andrews, D. (2019). *Suicidal ideation and behaviour*. Retrieved from https://www.cps.ca/en/documents/position/suicidal-ideation-and-behaviour.

Cicchetti, D. (2010). Resilience under conditions of extreme stress: A multilevel perspective. *World Psychiatry, 9*(3), 145–154.

Cleverley, K., Lenters, L., & McCann, E. (2020). "Objectively terrifying": A qualitative study of youth's experiences of transitions out of child and adolescent mental health services at age 18. *BMC Psychiatry, 20*(1), 1–11. https://doi.org/10.1186/s12888-020-02516-0

De Hert, M., Dirix, N., Demunter, H., et al. (2011). Prevalence and correlates of seclusion and restraint use in children and adolescents: A systematic review. *European Child and Adolescent Psychiatry, 20*(5), 221–230. https://doi.org/10.1007/s00787-011-0160-x

DeMaso, D. R., & Walter, H. J. (2020). Psychopharmacology. In R. M. Kliegman, J. St. Geme, & N. J. Blum et al. (Eds.), *Nelson textbook of pediatrics* (21st ed.). Elsevier.

DiBlasi, E., Kirby, A. V., Gaj, E., et al. (2020). Brief report: Genetic links between autism and suicidal behavior—A preliminary investigation. *Journal of Autism & Developmental Disorders, 50*(10), 3525–3530. https://doi.org/10.1007/s10803-020-04419-1

Dozois, D. J. A., & Canada, Mental Health Research (2020). Anxiety and depression in Canada during the COVID-19 pandemic: A national survey. *Canadian Psychology/Psychologie canadienne, 62*(1), 136–142. https://doi.org/10.1037/cap0000251

Eblin, A. (2019). Reducing seclusion and restraints on the inpatient child and adolescent behavioral health unit: A quality improvement study. *Journal of Child & Adolescent Psychiatric Nursing, 32*(3), 122–128. https://doi.org/10.1111/jcap.12248

Freud, A. (1965). *Normality and pathology in childhood: Assessments of development*. New York: International Universities Press.

Frick, P. J. (2012). Developmental pathways to conduct disorder: Implications for future directions in research, assessment, and treatment. *Journal of Clinical Child & Adolescent Psychology, 41*(3), 378–389. https://doi.org/10.1080/15374416.2012.664815

Gardner, R. A. (1971). *Therapeutic communication with children: The mutual story-telling technique*. New York: Jason Aronson.

Gardner, R. A. (1979). Helping children cooperate in therapy. In J. D. Noshpitz, & S. I. Harrison (Eds.), *Basic handbook of child psychiatry: Therapeutic interventions* (pp. 414–432). New York: Basic Books.

Gardner, R. A. (1986). The talking, feeling and doing game. In C. E. Schaefer, & S. E. Reid (Eds.), *Game play: Therapeutic use of childhood games* (pp. 41–72). New York: Wiley.

Goodwill, A., & Giannone, Z. (2017). From research to practice: Bridging the gaps for psychologists working in indigenous communities affected by gangs. *Canadian Psychology, 58*(4), 345–353. https://doi.org/10.1037/cap0000091

Government of Canada. (2018). *Autism prevalence among children and youth in Canada: 2018 report of the National Autism Spectrum Disorder (ASD) Surveillance System*. Retrieved from https://www.canada.ca/en/public-health/services/publications/diseases-conditions/infographic-autism-spectrum-disorder-children-youth-canada-2018.html

Govindan, R., Kommu, J., & Bhaskarapillai, B. (2020). The effectiveness of nurses implemented music add-on therapy in children with behavioral problems. *Indian Journal of Psychological Medicine, 42*(3), 274–280. https://doi.org/10.4103/IJPSYM.IJPSYM_240_19

Green-Hennessy, S., & Hennessy, K. (2015). Predictors of seclusion or restraint use within residential treatment centers for children and adolescents. *Psychiatric Quarterly, 86*(4), 545–554. https://doi.org/10.1007/s11126-015-9352-8

Hagan, J. F., Shaw, J. S., & Duncan, P. M. (2017). *Bright futures: Guidelines for health supervision of infants, children, and adolescents* (4th ed.). Elk Grove Village: American Academy of Pediatrics.

Hettiarachchi, S., Walisundara, D. C., & Ranaweera, M. (2020). The effectiveness of a multisensory traditional storytelling programme on target vocabulary development in children with disabilities accessing English as a second language: A preliminary study. *Journal of Intellectual Disabilities*. https://doi.org/10.1177/1744629520961605. Advance online publication.

Hornor, G. (2013). Posttraumatic stress disorder. *Journal of Pediatric Health Care, 27*(3), e29–e38. https://doi.org/10.1016/j.pedhc.2012.07.020

Jarrett, M., Black, A., Rapport, H., et al. (2015). Generalized anxiety disorder in younger and older children: Implications for learning and school functioning. *Journal of Child & Family Studies, 24*(4), 992–1003. https://doi.org/10.1007/s10826-014-9910-y

Klein, M. (1955). The psychoanalytic play technique. *American Journal of Orthopsychiatry, 25*, 223–237.

Lahat, A., Pérez-Edgar, K., Degnan, K. A., et al. (2012). Early childhood temperament predicts substance use in young adults. *Translational Psychiatry, 2*(9), e157. https://doi.org/10.1038/tp.2012.87

Lawrence, P., Murayama, K., & Creswell, C. (2019). Systematic review and meta-analysis: Anxiety and depressive disorders in offspring of parents with anxiety disorders. *Journal of the American Academy of Child & Adolescent Psychiatry, 58*(1), 46–60. https://doi.org/10.1016/j.jaac.2018.07.898

Livingston, J. D. (2020). *Structural stigma in health-care contexts for people with mental health and substance use issues: A literature review*. Ottawa: Mental Health Commission of Canada.

Loomes, R., Hull, L., & Mandy, W. (2017). What is the male-to-female ratio in autism spectrum disorder? A systematic review and meta-analysis. *Journal of the American Academy of Child and Adolescent Psychiatry, 56*(6), 466–474. https://doi.org/10.1016/j.jaac.2017.03.013

Machinskaya, R. I., Zakharova, M. N., & Lomakin, D. I. (2020). Brain regulatory functions in adolescents with signs of deviant behavior. An interdisciplinary analysis. *Human Physiology, 46*(3), 264–280. https://doi.org/10.1134/S0362119720030111

Mackenzie, K. (2018). Stereotypic movement disorders. *Seminars in Pediatric Neurology, 25*, 19–24. https://doi.org/10.1016/j.spen.2017.12.004

Mâsse, L. C., Miller, A. R., Shen, J., et al. (2013). Patterns of participation across a range of activities among Canadian children with neurodevelopmental disorders and disabilities. *Developmental Medicine & Child Neurology, 55*(8), 729–736. https://doi.org/10.1111/dmcn.12167

Maughan, B., Collishaw, S., & Stringaris, A. (2013). Depression in childhood and adolescence. *Journal of the Canadian Academy of Child and Adolescent Psychiatry, 22*(1), 35–40.

Mazurek, M. O., Lu, F., Macklin, E. A., et al. (2019). Factors associated with DSM-5 severity level ratings for autism spectrum disorder. *Autism : The International Journal of Research and Practice, 23*(2), 468–476. https://doi.org/10.1177/1362361318755318

Mental Health Commission of Canada. (2012). *Changing directions, changing lives: The mental health strategy for Canada.* Calgary: Author.

Moorhead, S., Johnson, M., Maas, M., et al. (2018). *Nursing Outcomes Classification (NOC)* (6th ed.). St. Louis: Mosby.

Muth, C. C. (2017). Tics and Tourette syndrome. *JAMA, 317*(15), 1592. https://doi.org/10.1001/jama.2017.0547

Ng, S. H., Tan, N. J. H., Luo, Y., et al. (2021). A systematic review of youth and teen mental health first aid: Improving adolescent mental health. *Journal of Adolescent Health, 69*(2), 199–210. https://doi.org/10.1016/j.jadohealth.2020.10.018

Northcott, P. (2018). Just the facts: Gangs. *Gazette Magazine, 80*(3). Retrieved from https://www.rcmp-grc.gc.ca/en/gazette/gangs

Parliament of Canada. (2017). *Canada's legal age of consent to sexual activity.* Ottawa: Author. Retrieved from https://lop.parl.ca/sites/PublicWebsite/default/en_CA/ResearchPublications/201724E

Peterson, R. L., & Pennington, B. F. (2012). Developmental dyslexia. *Lancet, 379*(9830), 1997–2007. https://doi.org/10.1016/S0140-6736(12)60198-6

Pollack, N., Mulay, S., Valcour, J., et al. (2016). Suicide rates in Aboriginal communities in Labrador, Canada. *American Journal of Public Health, 106*(7), 1309–1315. https://doi.org/10.2105/AJPH.2016.303151

Pringsheim, T., Doja, A., Gorman, D., et al. (2012). Canadian guidelines for the evidence-based treatment of tic disorders: Pharmacotherapy. *Canadian Journal of Psychiatry, 57*(3), 133–143.

Rothbart, M. K. (2011). *Becoming who we are.* New York: The Guilford Press.

Scaini, S., Centorame, G., Lissandrello, F., et al. (2020). The role of genetic and environmental factors in covariation between anxiety and anger in childhood. *European Child & Adolescent Psychiatry, 30*(4), 607–617. https://doi.org/10.1007/s00787-020-01543-2

Schatzberg, A. F. (2017). *Textbook of psychopharmacology: DSM-5 ed.* Arlington: American Psychiatric Association Publishing.

Shimada-Sugimoto, M., Otowa, T., & Hettema, J. M. (2015). Genetics of anxiety disorders: Genetic epidemiological and molecular studies in humans. *Psychiatry and Clinical Neurosciences, 69*(7), 388–401. https://doi.org/10.1037/t07557-000

Standing Senate Committee on Social Affairs, Science and Technology. (2006). *Out of the shadows at last: Transforming mental health, mental illness and addiction services in Canada.* Retrieved from https://www.parl.gc.ca/39/1/parlbus/commbus/senate/com-e/soci-e/rep-e/rep02may06-e.htm.

Standing Senate Committee on Social Affairs, Science and Technology. (2007). *Pay now or pay later: Autism families in crisis.* Retrieved from https://www.parl.gc.ca/Content/SEN/Committee/391/soci/rep/repfinmar07-e.htm.

Statistics Canada. (2021). *Family violence in Canada: A statistical profile 2019.* Retrieved from https://www150.statcan.gc.ca/n1/daily-quotidien/210302/dq210302d-eng.htm.

Statistics Canada. (2022). *Leading causes of death, total population, by age group.* Retrieved from https://www150.statcan.gc.ca/t1/tbl1/en/tv.action?pid=1310039401.

Steeves, T., McKinlay, B. D., Gorman, D., et al. (2012). Canadian guidelines for the evidence-based treatment of tic disorders: Behavioural therapy, deep brain stimulation, and transcranial magnetic stimulation. *Canadian Journal of Psychiatry, 57*(3), 144–151.

Stewart, S. L., Celebre, A., Hirdes, J. P., et al. (2020). Risk of suicide and self-harm in kids: The development of an algorithm to identify high-risk individuals within the children's mental health system. *Child Psychiatry & Human Development, 51*(6), 913–924. https://doi.org/10.1007/s10578-020-00968-9

Tarver, J., Daley, D., & Sayal, K. (2015). Beyond symptom control for attention-deficit hyperactivity disorder (ADHD): What can parents do to improve outcomes. *Child: Care, Health & Development, 41*(1), 1–14. https://doi.org/10.1111/cch.12159

Thornton, L. C., Frick, P. J., Crapanzano, A. M., et al. (2013). The incremental utility of callous-unemotional traits and conduct problems in predicting aggression and bullying in a community sample of boys and girls. *Psychological Assessment, 25*(2), 366–378. https://doi.org/10.1037/a0031153

United Nations. (2020). *The sustainable development goals report.* New York: Author.

Wiens, K., Bhattarai, A., Pedram, P., et al. (2020). A growing need for youth mental health services in Canada: Examining trends in youth mental health from 2011 to 2018. *Epidemiology and Psychiatric Sciences, 29*(e115), 1–9. https://doi.org/10.1017/S2045796020000281

Winther, J., Carlsson, A., & Vance, A. (2013). A pilot study of a school-based prevention and early intervention program to reduce oppositional defiant disorder/conduct disorder. *Early Intervention in Psychiatry, 8*(2), 181–189. https://doi.org/10.1111/eip.12050

World Health Organization. (2018). *Mental health: Strengthening our response.* Geneva: Author.

Wright, L. M., & Leahey, M. (2019). *Nurses and families: A guide to family assessment and intervention* (6th ed.). Philadelphia: F. A. Davis.

Yanof, J. A. (2013). Play technique in psychodynamic psychotherapy. *Child and Adolescent Psychiatric Clinics of North America, 22*(2), 261–282. https://doi.org/10.1016/j.chc.2012.12.002

28

Psychosocial Needs of the Older Person

Cheryl L. Pollard
Originating US chapter by Margaret Jordan Halter, Leslie A. Briscoe

🛜 https://evolve.elsevier.com/Canada/Varcarolis/psychiatric/

OBJECTIVES

1. Discuss facts and myths about aging.
2. Describe mental health disorders that may occur in older persons.
3. Analyze how ageism may affect attitudes and willingness to care for older persons.
4. Explain the importance of a comprehensive geriatric assessment.
5. Describe the role of the nurse in different settings of care.
6. Discuss the importance of pain assessment and identify three tools used to assess pain in older persons.

KEY TERMS AND CONCEPTS

adult support program
ageism
caregiver burden
medication reconciliation

The aging of the population is a global phenomenon that is occurring at a record-breaking rate, especially in developing countries around the world. In 2015 the number of Canadians aged 65 years and older exceeded the number of Canadian children aged 0 to 14 years (Statistics Canada, 2015). The Canadian economy, as well as health and social services, is affected by this marked increase in the proportion of older persons in the population. Among older persons, the fastest-growing subgroups are minorities, the poor, and those aged 85 years and older. Of the G7 countries, the United States (15%) and Canada (16.1%) have the lowest proportions of persons aged 65 years and older. Conversely, Japan's population is among the oldest in the world, with the highest proportion of persons aged 65 years and older (26%) among the G7 countries (Statistics Canada, 2015).

Providing "person-centered nursing care in partnership with persons experiencing a mental health condition and/or addiction, along the continuum of care and across the lifespan" (Canadian Association of Schools of Nursing [CASN] & Canadian Federation of Mental Health Nurses [CFMHN], 2017, p. 14) is an essential competency for nurses. As nurses therapeutically engage with older persons with mental illness or addiction, they must also demonstrate professional responsibility and accountability to recognize and reduce the detrimental impact of these attitudes (CASN & CFMHN, 2017).

The chapter begins with a summary of the major developmental theories relevant to providing mental health care to an aging population. This is followed by a brief discussion highlighting mental health issues related to aging. As people age, distinguishing between psychiatric and physical symptoms can be even more challenging than with the general adult population. Pain is one area where an overlap of symptoms can make assessment and treatment less straightforward, particularly if there are also cognitive impairments. Therefore the assessment of pain in individuals with a major neurocognitive disorder is presented. The chapter concludes with a discussion of the nursing care of older persons.

DEVELOPMENTAL THEORIES OF AGING

An outline of some major developmental theories of aging is provided in Box 28.1. Although these theories provide the framework for formulating appropriate nursing interventions for caring for older persons, there is no specific theory that encompasses all developmental stages.

In addition to dealing with the developmental milestones associated with aging, as people live longer, they are more likely to deal with chronic illness and disability. Statistics indicate that women generally outlive men. This disparity has significant ramifications for society at large and for the health care system in particular. Women constitute the largest proportion of older persons, use health care services more frequently than men, and seek services earlier. Most provincial governments recognize an impending crisis as health care costs soar, resources dwindle, and the baby boomers age (Statistics Canada, 2015).

Chronological age is considered an arbitrary indicator of function because there are significant variables that contribute to the capabilities of adults. Surveys focusing on how older persons see themselves reveal that nearly half of people age 65 years and older consider themselves to be middle-aged or young. There is a significant difference between a person who is 65 years old and a person who is 90 years old. Imagine this same age range in younger people. A person who is 25 years old has different experiences and expectations than a person who is 50 years old.

Aging is accompanied by increased rates of medical and psychiatric illnesses. This increase is brought about in part by increasingly stressful life events (e.g., the loss of a spouse, family members, and independence) and comorbid illness. Polypharmacy also contributes to health problems, especially since there is a gradual reduction in renal, hepatic, and gastric function, all of which are needed to metabolize and degrade medications.

Aging is a complex psychological and physical process. Box 28.2 provides some facts and myths about aging that influence how society perceives the older person.

BOX 28.1 Major Theories of Aging

Biological
Aging is influenced by molecular, cellular, or physiological systems and processes.
- *Gene theory:* Harmful genes become active in later life.
- *Error theory:* Error in protein synthesis results in impaired cellular function.
- *Free radical theory:* Reactive molecules damage DNA.
- *Wear-and-tear theory:* Internal and external stressors harm cells.
- *Programmed aging theory:* Biological or genetic clock plays out on genes.
- *Neuroendocrine theory:* There is neurohormonal regulation of life until death.
- *Immunological theory:* Immune system diversifies with age.

Psychological
- *Kohlberg's theory:* Crises and turning points in adult life are moral dilemmas.
- *Piaget's theory:* Cognitive operations in youth influence aging.
- *Erikson's theory:* Integrity is built on morality and ethics.
- *Bandura's theory:* Self-efficacy is essential for longevity.
- *Sullivan's theory:* Interpersonal responses influence behaviour.
- *Freud's theory:* Control of instinctual responses decreases with age.
- *Psychobiological theory:* Neurotransmitters modulate behaviours, emotions, and thoughts.
- *Dialectical theory:* Crises and transitions release positive and negative forces that lead to developmental progress.
- *Behavioural theory:* Learning determines the organization of behaviour.

Psychosocial
- *Maslow's theory:* Self-actualization and the evolution of developmental needs occur as the individual ages.
- *Disengagement theory:* Mutual withdrawal occurs between the aging person and others.
- *Activity theory:* Actions, roles, and social pursuits are important for satisfactory aging.
- *Continuity theory:* Life satisfaction and activity are expressions of enduring personality traits.

Source: Touhy, T. A., & Jett, K. F. (Eds.). (2016). *Ebersole & Hess' toward healthy aging: Human needs and nursing response* (9th ed.). St. Louis: Mosby.

BOX 28.2 Facts and Myths About Aging

Facts
- The senses of vision, hearing, touch, taste, and smell decline with age.
- Muscular strength decreases with age. Muscle fibres atrophy and decrease in number.
- Regular sexual expressions are important to maintain sexual capacity and effective sexual performance.
- At least 50% of restorative sleep is lost as a result of the aging process.
- Older persons are major consumers of prescription drugs because of the high incidence of chronic diseases in this population.
- Older persons have a high incidence of depression.
- Many individuals experience difficulty when they retire.
- Older persons are prone to become victims of crime.
- Older widows appear to adjust better than younger ones.

Myths
- Most adults past the age of 65 have dementia.
- Sexual interest declines with age.
- Older persons are unable to learn new tasks.
- As individuals age, they become more rigid in their thinking and more set in their ways.
- The aged are well off and no longer impoverished.
- Most older persons are infirm and require help with daily activities.
- Most older persons are socially isolated and lonely.

CONSIDERING CULTURE
Aging and Frailty in First Nations Communities

By 2031 the population of First Nations people in Canada is expected to increase by 40%. The majority of this growth will occur with those 60 years and older. Within this population there are increased risks for many age-related chronic conditions as compared to other populations in Canada. The onset of diseases such as diabetes, renal disease, and dementia often strike this population at an earlier age than other populations within Canada. As the First Nations peoples age, the health management needs related to these chronic conditions increase. First Nations peoples also report a higher than the average number of barriers to accessing needed health care services. Frailty in non-Indigenous populations represents a syndrome of decreasing physiological resilience resulting in a decrease in physiological reserve, decreased ability to resist environmental stressors and an increased risk for functional decline. However, what does "frailty" mean for First Nations people and communities? To understand this concept from an Indigenous perspective, it is imperative that data be used in ways that reflect Indigenous conceptions of health and well-being, respect First Nations governance of data, and promote culturally safe health and supportive care. This is one of the first steps to improve health outcomes for older First Nations people and to plan for the future.

The most common chronic health conditions among older First Nations people are high blood pressure, arthritis, and type 2 diabetes. Many experience multiple comorbidities. The conditions most often associated with frailty within Indigenous communities are arthritis and chronic back pain. Unlike the other Canadian populations, frailty did not show the same age-related prevalence patterns. Frailty increased between the ages of 35 to 44 and 55 to 64. However, past the age of 65, there were insubstantial declines. These findings reflect a population that assesses themselves as having a high level of wellness despite living with many chronic conditions. This paradox is created for non-Indigenous Canadian people as First Nations peoples' meanings of aging, frailty, and age-related wellness are inconsistent with non-Indigenous populations. Findings suggest that the deficit-based understandings of health are inconsistent with Indigenous models of well-being, which are based on balance, strengths, and resilience. This has significant consequences on the planning and delivery of supportive services and ongoing management of chronic conditions within First Nations communities.

Source: First Nations Information Governance Centre & Walker, J. D. (2020). Aging and frailty in First Nations communities. *Canadian Journal on Aging, 39*(2), 133–144. Retrieved from https://muse.jhu.edu/article/756390

MENTAL HEALTH ISSUES RELATED TO AGING

Changing Directions, Changing Lives: The Mental Health Strategy for Canada (Mental Health Commission of Canada, 2012) has made several recommendations that relate to mental health issues in Canada's aging population. These strategies include identifying and treating mental illnesses early, decreasing age discrimination, and helping older persons to continue to engage in meaningful activities.

Late-Life Mental Illness

Older persons who develop late-life mental illness are less likely than young adults to be accurately diagnosed and receive mental health treatment. Psychiatric issues such as depression, memory loss, and prolonged grieving are not a normal part of aging and should be diagnosed and treated. Treating psychiatric disorders prolongs the individual's ability to remain independent and increases their ability to take the lead in personal decision making.

Depression

Depression is not a normal part of aging and is often under-identified because of comorbid medical conditions. Depression is often confused with a neurocognitive disorder, and delirium is often misdiagnosed as a neurocognitive disorder. A careful, systematic assessment is necessary to properly distinguish among the three.

This assessment must determine:
- Onset of mental-status change and course of illness
- Level of consciousness
- Attention span

All three illnesses are treatable if properly identified. Delirium and major neurocognitive disorders are discussed in significantly more detail in Chapter 17; therefore they are not discussed further in this chapter. Chapter 17 also provides more information on distinguishing among depression, dementia, and delirium.

Selective serotonin reuptake inhibitors (SSRIs) are the first-line treatment for depression; this category of drug is often helpful if anxiety, worry, or rumination is problematic. If pain or diabetic neuropathy is a comorbid condition, serotonin–norepinephrine reuptake inhibitors (SNRIs) are often prescribed. Tricyclic antidepressants (TCAs) are used for those with chronic pain. Treatment-resistant depression can be treated with psychostimulants such as methylphenidate (Concerta); such monoamine oxidase inhibitors (MAOIs) are older treatments but remain effective.

Depression and suicide risk. Death by suicide is a significant consideration when working with Canadians between the ages of 80 and 84 years. Within this category, men are at the highest risk of taking their own life. The factors that affect the risk for suicide within this demographic are mental illness and addictions, personality factors, medical illness, negative life events, difficult transitions, lack of social support, and functional impairment (Van Orden & Deming, 2017). Approximately 70% of people who commit suicide suffer from depression. Early identification of and treatment for depression therefore are key measures for suicide prevention. Other factors that can lead to suicide are feelings of hopelessness, uselessness, and despair. For older persons, suicide may be seen as a final gesture of control at a stage when independence is at risk or activities are limited. Severe medical illness, functional disability, alcohol abuse, history of suicide attempts, comorbid anxiety, and psychotic depression are added risk factors for suicide (Szanto, 2017). Unlike younger persons, whose suicidal gestures may be a cry for help, older persons more frequently have a real desire to die.

Even though the suicide rate among older persons is high, suicide in this group is probably under-reported. Suicide is often not listed on the death certificate, even if it is suspected. The numbers also do not reflect those who passively or indirectly die by suicide by abusing alcohol, starving themselves, overdosing or mixing medications, stopping life-sustaining medications, or simply losing the will to live. Unfortunately, primary care providers continue to under-recognize and under-treat depression; many are slow to refer older persons to mental health care providers despite evidence that treatment of depression is cost effective and decreases the amount of health care expenditures used (Van Orden & Deming, 2017). Review Chapter 22 for an in-depth discussion of suicide.

Anxiety Disorders

Disabling anxiety disorders are twice as prevalent as dementia and four to eight times as common as major depressive disorders. Again, accurate diagnosis of the anxiety disorder is difficult. The most common sources of anxiety are phobias and generalized anxiety disorder (Kishita & Laidlaw, 2017). One unique anxiety-related problem in older persons is the fear of falling. Its impact on keeping individuals homebound is similar to agoraphobia because fear of falling results in activity restriction (Denkinger et al., 2015). Comorbid conditions, including depression, bipolar disorder, dementia, and alcoholism, may contribute to anxiety.

Psychosocial risk factors for anxiety include childlessness, low socioeconomic status, and having experienced trauma. Other risk factors include being female, being single, and having multiple medical conditions. Protective factors include social support, spiritual beliefs, physical activity, cognitive stimulation, and having coping strategies. Anxiety disorders may have been present earlier in life, but they did not significantly impair functioning. Once the stress of aging, retirement, loss, or physical frailty occurs, the previous coping strategies may no longer be effective. Older persons with anxiety often have physical complaints or describe fears of illness.

Treatment for anxiety disorders typically includes an SSRI. Antianxiety medications are also used, but they should be used cautiously since they may result in confusion, oversedation, and paradoxical agitation. Anxiety disorders are discussed in greater detail in Chapter 12.

Substance Use Disorders

People of any age can abuse any type of substance. Regardless of age, substance use has social, psychological, and physical consequences. Almost 80% of Canadians consume alcohol at least once a year (Canadian Centre on Substance Use and Addiction, 2017). Although heavy drinking tends to decline with age, it continues to be a serious problem that can create particular difficulties for older persons. The risk factors for heavy drinking among older persons are being male and single, having less than a high school education, having a low income, and smoking (Sorrell, 2017). Identifying alcohol and substance use is often difficult because personality and behavioural changes frequently go unrecognized in older persons.

The stressful or reactive factors that precipitate late-onset substance use are often related to environmental conditions and may include retirement, widowhood, and loneliness. These stressors in the older person, who may have retired, may not drive, and may be isolated from family and friends, are often greater than the problems faced by the middle-aged adult, who has to manage a job or career and care for a family and household. Work and family responsibilities may help keep a potential alcoholic from drinking too much. Once these demands are gone and the structure of daily life is disrupted, there is little impetus to remain sober. Another factor that may lead to late-onset substance use is chronic pain. Chronic pain is discussed in more detail later in this chapter.

Caution is required when medicating the older person who abuses alcohol or other substances. Central nervous system toxicity from psychoactive medications increases with aging. Ingestion of antidepressants or tranquillizers can be particularly harmful because their effect is further potentiated by alcohol. The toxicity of other drugs (e.g., acetaminophen) is enhanced by alcohol and by the age-related decrease in clearance (Burchum & Rosenthal, 2018).

Whenever there is a suspicion or indication that an older person is abusing alcohol, the health care provider should conduct a screening test. The CAGE-AID screening tool (Wagenaar et al., 2001) (Box 28.3) and the MAST-G (Box 28.4) are instruments commonly used to assess high-risk drinking in older persons.

Signs of alcohol abuse in younger individuals (e.g., alcohol-induced pancreatitis or liver disease, blackouts, major trauma) occur infrequently in older persons. Instead, the older person who abuses alcohol displays vague geriatric syndromes of contusions, malnutrition, self-neglect, depression, and falls (Sorrell, 2017). Diarrhea, urinary incontinence, decreased functional status, failure to thrive, and apparent dementia may also be present. Although confusion and disorientation

> **BOX 28.3 CAGE-AID Screening Tool**
>
> **C**—Have you ever felt you ought to **C**ut down on your drinking (drug use)?
> **A**—Have people **A**nnoyed you by criticizing your drinking (drug use)?
> **G**—Have you ever felt bad or **G**uilty about your drinking (drug use)?
> **E**—Have you ever had a drink (used drugs) first thing in the morning (**E**ye-opener) to steady your nerves or get rid of a hangover?
> **AID**—**A**dapt to **I**nclude **D**rugs.
>
> One positive answer indicates a possible problem; two positive answers indicate a probable problem.

Source: Ewing, J. A. (1984). Detecting alcoholism: The CAGE questionnaire. *Journal of the American Medical Association, 252*(14), 1905–1907. Copyright © 1984 American Medical Association. All rights reserved.

in an older patient are often associated with dementia or Alzheimer's disease, they could be caused by other factors, including alcohol abuse. Assessment of these conditions is necessary to differentiate the normal physiological changes of aging from those caused by excessive drinking.

Although the older person with alcohol or substance use issues is difficult to treat, the prognosis for a person who has lived to this point without recourse to substances, and their use being precipitated by losses and stressors, is excellent. This individual often responds very positively to a recovery program, especially if it is accompanied by environmental interventions. It is important that health care providers recognize this recovery potential. Treatment plans should emphasize social therapies. Older people respond well to emotional and social support, and family therapy should be encouraged (Sorrell, 2017). Group therapy with other middle-aged and older persons with alcoholism, as well as self-help groups like Alcoholics Anonymous, can also be effective. Nurses can be pioneers in the developing need for substance use rehabilitation focused on older persons. Refer to Chapter 18 for more information on treatment approaches for people with a substance use disorder.

Trauma

Older persons are also susceptible to the effects of psychological trauma. Chapter 24 discusses interpersonal violence in more detail. Refer to Chapter 25 for more information on the consequences of sexual assault.

> **BOX 28.4 MICHIGAN ALCOHOLISM SCREENING TEST—GERIATRIC VERSION (MAST-G)**
>
> Please answer "Yes" or "No" to each question by marking the line next to the question. When you finish answering the questions, please add up how many "Yes" responses you checked, and put that number in the space provided at the end.
>
> 1. After drinking, have you ever noticed an increase in your heart rate or beating in your chest? ____ Yes ____ No
> 2. When talking to others, do you ever underestimate how much you actually drank? ____ Yes ____ No
> 3. Does alcohol make you sleepy so that you often fall asleep in your chair? ____ Yes ____ No
> 4. After a few drinks, have you sometimes not eaten or been able to skip a meal because you didn't feel hungry? ____ Yes ____ No
> 5. Does having a few drinks help you decrease your shakiness or tremors? ____ Yes ____ No
> 6. Does alcohol sometimes make it hard for you to remember parts of the day or night? ____ Yes ____ No
> 7. Do you have rules for yourself that you won't drink before a certain time of the day? ____ Yes ____ No
> 8. Have you lost interest in hobbies or activities you used to enjoy? ____ Yes ____ No
> 9. When you wake up in the morning, do you ever have trouble remembering part of the night before? ____ Yes ____ No
> 10. Does having a drink help you sleep? ____ Yes ____ No
> 11. Do you hide your alcohol bottles from family members? ____ Yes ____ No
> 12. After a social gathering, have you ever felt embarrassed because you drank too much? ____ Yes ____ No
> 13. Have you ever been concerned that drinking might be harmful to your health? ____ Yes ____ No
> 14. Do you like to end an evening with a nightcap? ____ Yes ____ No
> 15. Did you find your drinking increased after someone close to you died? ____ Yes ____ No
> 16. In general, would you prefer to have a few drinks at home rather than go out to social events? ____ Yes ____ No
> 17. Are you drinking more now than in the past? ____ Yes ____ No
> 18. Do you usually take a drink to relax or calm your nerves? ____ Yes ____ No
> 19. Do you drink to take your mind off your problems? ____ Yes ____ No
> 20. Have you ever increased your drinking after experiencing a loss in your life? ____ Yes ____ No
> 21. Do you sometimes drive when you have had too much to drink? ____ Yes ____ No
> 22. Has a doctor or nurse ever said they were worried or concerned about your drinking? ____ Yes ____ No
> 23. Have you ever made rules to manage your drinking? ____ Yes ____ No
> 24. When you feel lonely, does having a drink help? ____ Yes ____ No
>
> **TOTALS:** ____ **Yes** ____ **No**

Scoring: A score of 3 points or less is considered to indicate no alcoholism; a score of 4 points is suggestive of alcoholism; a score of 5 points or more indicates alcoholism.

Source: Blow, F., Brower, K., Schulenberg, J. E., et al. (1992). The Michigan Alcoholism Screening Test–Geriatric Version: A new elderly specific screening instrument. *Alcoholism: Clinical and Experimental Research, 16*, 372. Michigan Alcoholism Screening Test-Geriatric Version (MAST-G). © The Regents of the University of Michigan, 1991.

RESEARCH HIGHLIGHT

Implementing Volunteer-Navigation for Older Persons With Advanced Chronic Illness (Nav-CARE): A Knowledge to Action Study

Problem
Older persons are at the highest risk for experiencing multiple complex illnesses that lead to increased experiences of social isolation and poor quality of life.

Purpose of Study
The goals of this knowledge-to-action study was to better understand the factors that influenced the implementation of Nav-CARE (Navigation—Connecting, Accessing, Resourcing, Engaging) in eight diverse Canadian contexts.

Methods
Nav-CARE is a public health community approach intervention designed to better support older persons living with advanced chronic illness through the use of specially trained volunteers who visit frail individuals living at home to provide social support and facilitate connections to resources. Participants were recruited from hospice societies across urban and rural sites in British Columbia, Alberta, and Nova Scotia. Data were collected through semistructured qualitative individual and group interviews with stakeholders (e.g., hospice society directors and board members, volunteer coordinators, volunteers, healthcare providers, Nav-CARE advisory committee members) at baseline, midpoint, and conclusion of the intervention. Additional information was collected from email and phone correspondence with coordinators and other leaders, regular coordinator teleconferences, and through volunteer mentoring sessions conducted via teleconference.

Key Findings
- There is a complementary role for volunteers within hospice outreach programs to support individuals earlier in their disease trajectory.
- Stakeholders identified that Nav-CARE was an opportunity to de-medicalize chronic disease care, specifically palliative care.
- Organizational capacity and community connectedness and volunteer preparation and mentorship were key factors affecting Nav-CARE implementation.
- The underutilization of volunteers is attributed to the misunderstanding of the role that volunteers can play in improving the quality of life of patients and their families.

Implications for Nursing Practice
- There is a potential to challenge and change public perceptions that hospice care is only for those who are imminently dying.
- With an improved relationship with home care, there is an important gap that could be filled within the public healthcare system that addresses the relational needs of individuals with chronic disease.
- Leveraging the social capital within communities is a public health approach that can be used to improve the health of the very frail.
- The results of the study focus on non-Indigenous notions of frailty and the needs of those imminently dying. Utilization of these findings within Indigenous peoples must be done with caution and reinterpretation of the results using an Indigenous world view of frailty, aging, and disease.

Source: Pesut, B., Duggleby, W., Warner, G., et al. (2020). Implementing volunteer-navigation for older persons with advanced chronic illness (Nav-CARE): A knowledge to action study. *BMC Palliative Care, 19*(1), 1–16. https://doi.org/10.1186/s12904-020-00578-1

Caregiver Burden

Another phenomenon with the aging population is the increase in caregiver burden. Although there is not a consistent definition of caregiver burden, most researchers and clinicians view this concept as the physical, psychological, emotional (e.g., increased depression, increased stress, increased fatigue), social, and financial (e.g., increased costs associated with caring, decreased work hours) stresses that individuals experience as a result of providing care (Parmar et al., 2020). A common scenario is the two-income family in the middle of raising children and planning for their future retirement that is now faced with aging parents in need of help. Shorter lengths of stay for hospitalization, limited home care options, and complicated procedures to access care have increased the need for adult children to advocate for and provide care to aging parents. Unfortunately, this scenario is different for older persons who have lived with a chronic mental illness. Schizophrenia and bipolar disorders take a toll on family members and intimate relationships, and it is not uncommon for those with severe mental illness to have no family support available as they age. Grown children may be estranged because of a parent's frequent hospitalization, poor parenting ability, or paranoid symptoms. The support system of those aging with chronic mental illness often becomes case managers, community nurses, and mental health care providers.

Access to Care

The disparity of mental health services in Canada has led to a complicated and fragmented system of care (Mental Health Commission of Canada, 2014). Nurses may feel powerless to change shortfalls in the health care system; however, they can take advantage of their numbers and the respect given to the profession to be strong advocates for improving health care.

Access to care is also affected by the availability of financial resources. Although every Canadian has access to all medically necessary services, regardless of ability to pay, "all medically necessary services" is typically interpreted within an illness- or disease-focused paradigm. As a result, health promotion activities and many factors associated with the social determinants of health, for example, housing, are not included within the delivery of "all medically necessary services." People therefore are individually responsible for the costs associated with meeting their overall health care needs.

Ageism

In Western culture growing older is not viewed as a privilege, and old age does not tend to confer a revered social status on those who have attained it. Ageism has been defined as a bias against older people because of their age. It is based on erroneous beliefs that older persons are unattractive, unintelligent, asexual, unemployable, and senile. Ageism affects the quality of health care this population receives. For example, most older people present with several comorbid conditions, yet the Canadian health care system is organized into single diagnostic specialties (e.g., psychiatry, endocrinology, hematology, surgery). This division poses the risk that patients with diagnoses in several areas may not receive the best possible care because of the complexity of their presentation.

Ageism is not limited to the way the young view the old, though; it can also be exhibited by older persons themselves. Indeed, the attitudes of older persons toward their contemporaries, particularly those with mental health disabilities, are often negative—perhaps because the threat of contagion by association with the frail and infirm raises feelings of vulnerability. Ageism differs from other forms of discrimination in that it cuts across gender, race, religion, and socioeconomic status to reach the majority of those over age 65.

Ageism and Public Policy

The results of ageism can be observed in every level of society. Financial and political support for programs for older persons is difficult to obtain. The needs of this population often are addressed only after those of younger, albeit smaller, population groups. However, the Canadian Association for Retired Persons, a powerful lobbying group, is fighting to change this trend.

Ageism and Drug Testing

Clinical drug trials often exclude people over the age of 65 on the assumption that they already take multiple medications or have an existing chronic illness. Information about medications for the general population has to be generalized for older persons, and appropriate (generally lower) doses may not have been tested or even be available (Shepherd et al., 2015).

DISTINGUISHING BETWEEN PSYCHIATRIC AND PHYSICAL SYMPTOMS

Older persons are the fastest growing segment of the world's population. As people age, there is an increased incidence and prevalence of pain. The pain that older persons experience may be related to many medical conditions, such as arthritis, peripheral vascular disease, diabetic neuropathy, or musculoskeletal disease. Like many mental health disorders, pain may be under-reported and incorrectly believed to be a normal part of the aging process. Pain and mental health problems affect an older person's sense of well-being and quality of life.

Pain

Pain is often associated with depression (Hung et al., 2017). There are three categories of depressive symptoms: emotional (mood, motivation, apathy, anxiety), cognitive (concentration, memory), and physical (insomnia, fatigue, headache, and pain). When experiencing pain, your emotional, cognitive, and physical functioning can also be affected. Pain can lead to increased stress, delayed healing, decreased mobility, disturbances in sleep, decreased appetite, and agitation with accompanying aggressive behaviours. Nurses must be able to determine what the presenting symptoms are related to in order to make an accurate nursing diagnosis and an effective treatment plan.

Principles of Pain Management

Assessment tools. When pain is suspected, the nurse begins with a physical assessment for the origins of the pain and assesses characteristics of the pain itself. To aid older persons who may have sensory deficits or cognitive impairments, simply worded questions and simple drawings may be necessary. The Wong-Baker FACES Pain Rating Scale (Figure 28.1) is an assessment instrument currently in use. The FACES scale shows facial expressions on a scale from 0 (a smile) to 5 (crying grimace). Respondents are asked to choose the face that depicts the pain they feel.

The present pain intensity rating from the McGill Pain Questionnaire (Powell et al., 2015) is another tool accepted for use with older patients. Patients are asked to respond by selecting the description (from "no pain" [0] to "excruciating pain" [5]) that they believe identifies the pain they feel.

The Pain Assessment in Advanced Dementia scale is used to evaluate the presence and severity of pain in patients with advanced dementia who no longer have the ability to communicate verbally (Figure 28.2). The scale evaluates five domains: breathing, negative vocalization, facial expression, body language, and consolability (Box 28.5). The score guides the caregiver in the appropriate pain intervention.

Barriers to accurate pain assessment. There are a number of beliefs and misconceptions that may interfere with appropriate assessment and treatment. Older persons may believe that pain is a punishment for past behaviours, an inevitable part of aging, indicative of pending death, related to serious illness, or a sign of weakness. External obstacles include inadequate assessment by health care providers, complicated clinical presentation, assumptions by health care providers that pain is part of aging, and communication deficits due to cognitive impairment.

Changes in behaviour may indicate pain and should be assessed, especially in people who have difficulty verbally communicating their needs (e.g., those with dementia). Unlike younger adults, older persons may understate their pain using words such as *discomfort, hurting,* or *aching.* Multiple painful problems may occur together, making it difficult to differentiate new pain from pre-existing pain. Sensory impairments, memory loss, dementia, and depression can add to the difficulty of obtaining an accurate pain assessment. An interview with family members, caregivers, or friends is vital.

Pain treatment

There are three essential features of treating pain:

1. Do a thorough assessment and establish an accurate diagnosis.
2. Recognize that pain reduction, rather than the complete elimination of pain, may be the treatment goal.
3. Treat symptoms of coexisting disorders, such as depression, anxiety, or other physical conditions, that exacerbate the pain.

Pharmacological pain treatments. The cause of the pain should be addressed along with treatment of the pain itself. Pain should be managed with pharmacological or alternative measures. Pharmacological pain management relies on the use of prescription and nonprescription medications, frequently based on the recommendation of the health care provider. These include analgesics, opioid analgesics, and adjuvant medications. When administering and teaching patients about these types of medication, information should be provided about their potentially addictive nature. Consultation with a pain-management specialist is often helpful with chronic pain syndromes. Some

Fig. 28.1 Wong-Baker FACES Pain Rating Scale. (**Source:** Hockenberry, M. J., & Wilson, D. [2013]. *Wong's essentials of pediatric nursing* [9th ed.]. St. Louis: Mosby. Used with permission. Copyright Mosby.)

	0	1	2	Score
Breathing Independent of vocalization	Normal	Occasional laboured breathing; short period of hyperventilation	Noisy, laboured breathing; long period of hyperventilation; Cheyne-Stokes respirations	
Negative Vocalization	None	Occasional moan or groan; low-level speech with a negative or disapproving quality	Repeated troubled calling out; loud moaning or groaning; crying	
Facial Expression	Smiling or inexpressive	Sad; frightened; frown	Facial grimacing	
Body Language	Relaxed	Tense; distressed pacing; fidgeting	Rigid; fists clenched; knees pulled up; pulling or pushing away; striking out	
Consolability	No need to console	Distracted or reassured by voice or touch	Unable to console, distract, or reassure	
			TOTAL	

Fig. 28.2 Pain Assessment in Advanced Dementia (PAINAD) Scale. (**Source:** Reprinted from Warden, V., Hurley, A. C., & Volicer, L. [2003]. Development and psychometric evaluation of the pain assessment in advanced dementia [PAINAD] scale. *Journal of the American Medical Directors Association, 4*[1], 9–15. Copyright 2003, with permission from Elsevier.)

considerations for pharmacological pain management in older persons are listed in Box 28.6.

As an individual ages, the body's ability to eliminate drugs via the kidney decreases. Nurses must be aware of this change, which can result in overdosing. On the other hand, fear of narcotic overmedication, which can cause respiratory depression and falls, may lead the nurse to give out less pain medication to older persons than is needed for effective treatment (Burchum & Rosenthal, 2018). It is critical for nurses to evaluate the effectiveness of pain interventions at regular intervals and to be attentive to behavioural changes or verbal responses that indicate that the patient is experiencing pain. It is a common misconception that the ability to perceive pain decreases with aging. No physiological changes in pain perception in older persons have been demonstrated. In fact, older persons may feel pain even more keenly than younger persons do. Careful and continuing assessments and an understanding of pain physiology are necessary for effective pain management of older persons.

In older persons it is important to perform a systematic review of current medication use, known as medication reconciliation. **Medication reconciliation** is the process of developing the most accurate list possible of all medication a patient is taking. This list should include drug name, dose, frequency, and route. The purpose of this process is to reduce adverse incidents, side effects, and potentially lethal combinations.

Assessing the use of multiple medications (polypharmacy) includes prescription, over-the-counter drugs, and herbal agents. Adverse drug reactions or negative responses to drugs are common among older persons. Older persons are at greater risk for these events due to multiple medical problems and memory issues that may result in taking too little or too much medication. Renal and liver impairment affect excretion and are associated with dose-related adverse reactions.

Metabolic changes and decreased drug clearance compound the risk of drug–drug interactions. Adverse drug reactions occur in one in four adult hospitalizations (Jennings et al., 2020). The American Geriatrics Society (2019) recently updated the criteria for and list of potentially inappropriate medications for older persons. Many psychiatric medications appear on the list, including benzodiazepines, anticholinergics, antipsychotics, antidepressants, anti-epileptics, and antiparkinson drugs. Nurses must be diligent in reviewing older persons' medication lists for completeness.

Prescribing cascades happen when drug-induced symptoms are treated with another drug. The health care provider may assess the side effect of the first drug as part of the original medical problem or a new one. Prescribing cascades are particularly problematic and complicated. One of the most common examples is when a person begins anti-parkinson therapy for symptoms brought about by antipsychotics. Anti-parkinson drugs may bring about new and dangerous symptoms such as delirium and orthostatic hypotension. Anti-cholinesterase inhibitor drugs used to treat dementia (e.g., donepezil, rivastigmine, galantamine) may cause urinary incontinence and diarrhea. These symptoms may result in a prescribing cascade with use of an anticholinergic such as oxybutynin, which can cause cognitive dulling and confusion.

Pharmacists have begun to play a critical role in reviewing and advising on matters of prescribing for the older person. The American Geriatrics Society (2019) has updated the Beers List and Criteria, which was developed in 1991 to identify inappropriate medications for the older person. Jennings et al. (2020) identify how polypharmacy

BOX 28.5 The Five Elements of the Pain Assessment in Advanced Dementia (PAINAD) Scale

1. Breathing
   Normal breathing is effortless breathing characterized by quiet, rhythmic respirations.
   Occasional laboured breathing is characterized by episodic bursts of harsh, difficult, or wearing respirations.
   Short period of hyperventilation is characterized by intervals of rapid, deep breaths lasting a short period of time.
   Long period of hyperventilation is characterized by excessive rate and depth of respirations lasting a considerable time.
   Cheyne-Stokes respirations are characterized by rhythmic waxing and waning of breathing from very deep to shallow respirations with periods of apnea.
2. Negative Vocalization
   None is characterized by speech or vocalization that has a neutral or pleasant quality.
   Occasional moan or groan: Occasional moaning is characterized by mournful or murmuring sounds, wails, or laments. Occasional groaning is characterized by louder than usual inarticulate involuntary sounds, often abruptly beginning and ending.
   Low-level speech with negative or disapproving quality is characterized by muttering, mumbling, whining, grumbling, or swearing in a low volume with a complaining, sarcastic, or caustic tone.
   Repeated, troubled calling out is characterized by phrases or words being used over and over in a tone that suggests anxiety, uneasiness, or distress.
   Loud moaning or groaning: Loud moaning is characterized by mournful or murmuring sounds, wails, or laments in a much louder than usual volume. Loud groaning is characterized by louder than usual inarticulate involuntary sounds, often abruptly beginning and ending.
   Crying is characterized by an utterance of emotion accompanied by tears. There may be sobbing or quiet weeping.
3. Facial Expression
   Smiling or inexpressiveness: Smiling is characterized by upturned corners of the mouth, brightening of the eyes, and a look of pleasure or contentment. Inexpressiveness refers to a neutral, at ease, relaxed, or blank look.
   Sad is characterized by an unhappy, lonesome, sorrowful, or dejected look. Eyes may be teary.
   Frightened is characterized by a look of fear, alarm, or heightened anxiety. Eyes may appear wide open.
   Frowning is characterized by a downward turn of the corners of the mouth. Increased facial wrinkling in the forehead and around the corners of the mouth may appear.
   Facial grimacing is characterized by a distorted, distressed look. The brow is more wrinkled, as is the area around the mouth. Eyes may be squeezed shut.
4. Body Language
   Relaxed is characterized by a calm, restful, mellow appearance. The person seems to be taking it easy.
   Tense is characterized by a strained, apprehensive, or worried appearance. The jaw may be clenched.
   Distressed pacing is characterized by activity that seems unsettled. There may be a fearful, worried, or disturbed element present. The rate may be faster or slower.
   Fidgeting is characterized by restless movement. Squirming about or wiggling in the chair may occur. The person might be hitching a chair across the room. Repetitive touching, tugging, or rubbing body parts can also be observed.
   Rigid is characterized by stiffening of the body. The arms and/or legs are tight and inflexible. The trunk may appear straight and unyielding (exclude contractures).
   Fists clenched is characterized by tightly closed hands. They may be opened and closed repeatedly or held tightly shut.
   Knees pulled up is characterized by flexing the legs and drawing the knees upward toward the chest (exclude contractures).
   Pulling or pushing away is characterized by resistiveness upon approach or to care. The person is trying to escape by yanking or wrenching themself free or by shoving you away.
   Striking out is characterized by hitting, kicking, grabbing, punching, biting, or other forms of personal assault.
5. Consolability
   No need to console is characterized by a sense of well-being. The person appears content.
   Distracted or reassured by voice or touch is characterized by a disruption in the behaviour when the person is spoken to or touched. The behaviour stops during the period of interaction, with no indication that the person is at all distressed.
   Unable to console, distract, or reassure is characterized by the inability to soothe the person or stop a behaviour with words or actions. No amount of verbal or physical comforting will alleviate the behaviour.

Scoring: (See Figure 28.3 for point allocation.)
0–1 = No significant pain
2–3 = Mild to moderate pain
4–6 = Moderate to severe pain
7–10 = Severe to very severe pain

Source: Lane, P., Kuntupis, M., MacDonald, S., et al. (2003). A pain assessment tool for people with advanced Alzheimer's and other progressive dementias. *Home Healthcare Nurse, 21*(1), 36.

---

affects the older person. There are nine negative clinical consequences of inappropriate drug use:
1. Increased health care costs
2. Adverse drug reactions
3. Drug interactions
4. Non-adherence
5. Decline in functional status
6. Increased cognitive impairment
7. Increased falls
8. Increased urinary incontinence
9. Increased risk for malnutrition

Common problems associated with medication include confusion, which can be caused by anti-cholinergics, anti-histamines, and benzodiazepines. Psychosis has been linked to levodopa, steroids, and even cholesterol-lowering medications. Depressive symptoms have been linked with α-adrenergic agonists and opiates.

Non-pharmacological pain treatments. Non-pharmacological treatments for pain include vagal nerve stimulation, exercise, hydrotherapy, heat and cold packs, chiropractics, and transcutaneous electrical nerve stimulation. Yoga, biofeedback, hypnosis, acupuncture, massage, shiatsu, reiki, guided imagery, reflexology, and therapeutic touch are integrative therapies for managing pain. Herbal remedies include cayenne, capsaicin, ginger extract, echinacea, kava kava, and willow bark. It is important to ask older persons if they are using any alternative treatments for pain relief. Pain-management education is important for both the patient and caregivers. The key to successful pain management lies in the application of a variety of techniques that the patient must learn and practise.

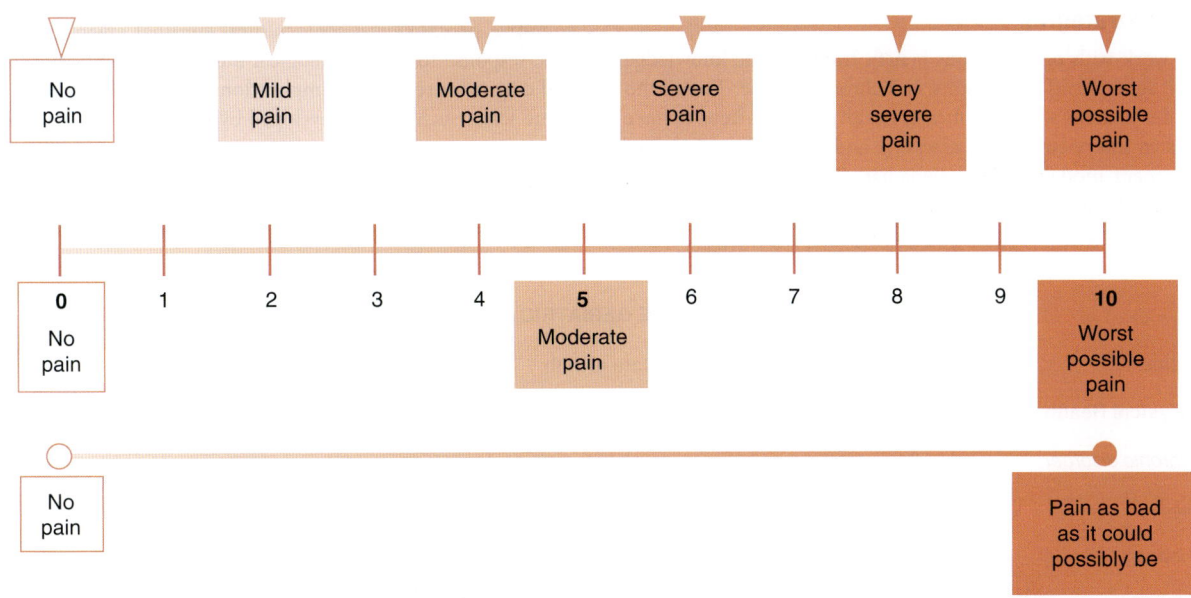

Fig. 28.3 Visual analogue scales used in the management of cancer pain. (**Source:** Jacox, A., Carr, D. B., Payne, R., et al. [1994]. *Management of cancer pain [Clinical Practice Guideline No. 9, AHCPR Publication No. 94-0952].* Rockville: U.S. Department of Health and Human Services, Public Health Service, Agency for Health Care Policy and Research.)

BOX 28.6 Tips for Pharmacological Pain Management in Older Persons

- Remember that many older persons receive pain medication less often than younger adults because their pain is often considered a natural part of aging. As a result, many older persons receive inadequate pain relief.
- Safe administration of analgesics is complicated because of possible interactions with drugs used to treat certain chronic disorders, as well as because of nutritional alterations and altered pharmacokinetics in older persons.
- Analgesics reach a higher peak and have a longer duration of action in older persons than in younger individuals. Start with one-fourth to one-half the adult dose, and titrate up carefully.
- Give oral analgesics around the clock at the beginning. Administer on an as-needed basis later on, as indicated by the patient's pain status.
- If acute confusion occurs, assess for other contributing factors before changing the medication or stopping analgesic use. Confusion in post-operative patients has been found to be associated with unrelieved pain rather than with opiate use.
- Acetaminophen is an effective analgesic in older persons. Although there is an increased risk of end-stage renal disease with long-term use, it does not produce the gastrointestinal bleeding seen with non-steroidal anti-inflammatory drugs (NSAIDs).
- Analgesics and adjuvants, such as anti-cholinergics and pentazocine, may produce increased confusion in older persons. NSAIDs can have the same effect during their initial period of administration.
- Opiates have a greater analgesic effect and longer duration of action than non-opioid analgesics. Avoid the use of meperidine, whose active metabolite may stimulate the central nervous system and lead to confusion, seizures, and mood alterations. If this drug is selected, do not use it for more than 48 hours. Avoid intramuscular administration in the older person because of tissue irritation and poor absorption. Morphine is a safer choice than meperidine because its duration of action is longer, so a smaller overall dose is required.
- Assess bowel function daily, because constipation can be a frequent adverse effect of opiates.

Source: Lehne, R. A. (2013). *Pharmacology for nursing care* (8th ed.). St Louis: Elsevier.

NURSING CARE OF OLDER PERSONS

Nurses encounter older persons in a variety of settings, and in each of these settings, the nurse is responsible for applying the nursing process to the individual patient's situation.

Studies suggest that because nursing students are not given enough information about older persons and often are not exposed to older patients, they may hold ageist views when they begin their nursing careers. Such biases have significant implications for practice, education, and research (Dahlke et al., 2020). It is important for all nurses to gain a better understanding of the aging process. Adequate theory and principles of practice are needed to provide safe and excellent care for older persons. The Canadian Gerontological Nursing Association (2019) has developed practice standards to define the uniqueness and scope of gerontological nursing. The standards are organized into six categories: (1) physiological health, (2) optimizing functional health, (3) responsive care, (4) relationship care, (5) health system, and (6) safety and security.

Positive attitudes toward older persons and their care need to be instilled during basic nursing education. Education programs must include:

- Information about the aging process
- Discussion of attitudes relating to the care of older persons
- Sensitization of participants to their patients' needs
- Exploration of the dynamics of nurse–patient and staff–patient interactions
- Respect for older patients and appreciation of their wisdom and life experience

Assessment Strategies

Nurses who work with older persons benefit from specific knowledge about normal aging, drug interactions, and chronic disease. Those who work with older patients who have mental health problems need to have specific skills in interviewing and assessing and special knowledge of effective treatment modalities. The Canadian Gerontological Nursing Association (2019) has recommended a comprehensive geriatric assessment, which includes the following areas: physiological, functional, cognitive, psychological, sociocultural, spiritual, environmental, risk factors, response to pharmacological intervention and drug use patterns, and diagnostic results and implications related to treatment. Visual analogue scales such as that developed by Jacox et al. (1994) can be used in the assessment and evaluation of management strategies for cancer pain.

Specific assessment questions should also be asked regarding pain in older persons. Figure 28.4 shows what is considered in a comprehensive geriatric assessment.

COMPREHENSIVE GERIATRIC ASSESSMENT									
Name:			Date of birth:				Gender:		
Physical Health									
Chronic disorder									
Vision	Adequate	Inadequate	Eyeglasses:	Y	N		Needs evaluation		
Hearing	Adequate	Inadequate	Hearing aids:	Y	N				
Mobility	Ambulatory:	Y	N	Assistive device:					
	Falls:	Y	N				Needs evaluation		
Nutrition	Albumin:		TLC:		HCT:				
	Weight:		Weight loss or gain:	Y	N		Needs evaluation		
Incontinence	Y	N	Treatment:			Y	N	Needs evaluation	
Medications	Total number:		Reviewed & revised:			Y	N		
	Adverse effects/allergy:								
Screening	Cholesterol:		TSH:			B12:		Folate:	
	Colonoscopy:	Date:				N/A			
	Mammogram:	Date:				N/A			
	Osteoporosis:	Date:				N/A			
	Pap smear:	Date:				N/A			
	PSA:	Date:				N/A			
Immunization	Influenza:	Date:							
	Pneumonia:	Date:							
	Tetanus:	Date:				Booster:			
Counselling	Diet	Exercise	Calcium			Vitamin D			
	Smoking	Alcohol	Driving			Injury prevention			
Mental Health									
Dementia	Y	N	MMSE score:		Date:		Cause (if known):		
Depression	Y	N	GDS score:		Date:		Treatment:	Y	N
Functional Status									
ADL	Bathing:	I	D	Dressing:	I	D	Toileting:	I	D
	Transferring:	I	D	Feeding:	I	D	Continence:	Y	N

Fig. 28.4 Comprehensive geriatric assessment. *ADL*, Activities of daily living; *B12*, vitamin B_{12}; *D*, dependent; *GDS*, Geriatric Depression Scale; *HCT*, hematocrit; *I*, independent; *MMSE*, Mini-Mental State Examination; *N*, no; *PSA*, prostate-specific antigen; *TLC*, total lymphocyte count; *TSH*, thyroid-stimulating hormone; *Y*, yes.

A thorough assessment, including a physical assessment and diagnostic testing, must precede any treatment or diagnosis of a mental illness in older persons. Common tests include thyroid, kidney, and liver function; complete blood count; comprehensive metabolic panel; vitamin B_{12}, folic acid, and therapeutic drug levels; urinalysis; syphilis serology; B-type natriuretic peptide; and computed tomography of the head. A review of current medications and possible adverse reactions or drug–drug interactions must also occur (Burchum & Rosenthal, 2018). Confusion can be caused by anti-cholinergics, anti-histamine, and benzodiazepines. Psychosis has been linked to steroids and even to cholesterol-lowering medications, and depression has been linked to beta-blockers, α-adrenergic agonists, and opiates. Serious medical conditions such as cancer, anemia, diabetes, infections, electrolyte imbalance, malnutrition, dehydration, and cardiac disease can manifest in symptoms such as fatigue or anorexia before more specific physical manifestations occur. Nurses are in a unique position to advocate for and coordinate appropriate medical evaluation for older persons.

An examination and interview of an older person conducted in unfamiliar surroundings can produce anxiety. Unlike younger patients, who may be comfortable discussing personal issues, such as family conflicts, feelings of sadness, sexual practices, finances, and bodily functions, older persons may view such topics as private or taboo and be uncomfortable discussing them. It is important to respect these feelings while reviewing essential history by doing the following:

- Conducting the interview in a private area
- Introducing oneself and asking the patient what they would like to be called (use of the first name is rarely appropriate unless one is invited to use it)
- Establishing rapport and putting the patient at ease by sitting or standing at the same level as the patient
- Ensuring that lighting is adequate and noise level is low in recognition of the fact that hearing and vision may be impaired
- Using touch (with permission) to convey warmth while at the same time respecting the patient's comfort level with personal touch
- Summarizing the interaction, inviting feedback and questions, and thanking the patient for giving their time and information

Assessment of the cognitive, behavioural, and emotional status of the older person is very important in managing the nursing care of the patient and is particularly vital for detecting dementia, delirium, and depression, whose prevalence increases with age (Prince et al., 2015). The Geriatric Depression Scale (Short Form) (Box 28.7) is a subjective questionnaire (Sheikh & Yesavage, 1986), and the Cornell Scale for Depression in Dementia is an objective screening tool for caregivers to help identify the presence of depressive symptoms (Alexopoulos et al., 1988). The periodic repetition of these assessments serves to evaluate the effectiveness of intervention.

It is also essential to assess for suicidal thoughts and suicidal intent by asking specific questions:

- Have you ever thought about killing yourself?
- Have you ever felt that life is not worth living?
- Have you ever tried to hurt yourself in the past?

Thoughts of harming others also must be assessed. Interventions for the prevention of suicide in older persons are discussed in greater depth later in this chapter. Also see Chapter 22 for a more detailed discussion of suicide assessment and intervention.

Older person abuse is another area to explore during a nursing assessment and is discussed in depth in Chapter 24. Questions about being hit, pushed, kicked, and slapped are important, but it is also imperative to inquire about care being withheld. Not being fed, cleaned, helped, or cared for are critical issues. Asking initially, "How are you being treated at home?" or "Are you afraid of anyone?" may encourage further exploration. Financial exploitation is another issue that is difficult to uncover. Older persons may feel ashamed or embarrassed to admit that they have been taken advantage of by family, friends, or strangers. Box 28.8 provides helpful interview techniques to use with older persons.

BOX 28.7 Geriatric Depression Scale (Short Form)

1. Are you basically satisfied with your life?	Yes/No
2. Have you dropped many of your activities and interests?	Yes/No
3. Do you feel that your life is empty?	Yes/No
4. Do you often get bored?	Yes/No
5. Are you in good spirits most of the time?	Yes/No
6. Are you afraid that something bad is going to happen to you?	Yes/No
7. Do you feel happy most of the time?	Yes/No
8. Do you often feel helpless?	Yes/No
9. Do you prefer to stay at home rather than go out and do new things?	Yes/No
10. Do you feel you have more problems with memory than most?	Yes/No
10. Do you think it is wonderful to be alive now?	Yes/No
12. Do you feel pretty worthless the way you are now?	Yes/No
13. Do you feel full of energy?	Yes/No
14. Do you feel that your situation is hopeless?	Yes/No
15. Do you think that most people are better off than you are?	Yes/No

Source: Sheikh, J. I., & Yesavage, J. A. (1986). Geriatric Depression Scale (GDS): Recent evidence and development of a shorter version. In T. Brink (Ed.), *Clinical gerontology: A guide to assessment and intervention*. New York: The Haworth Press.

BOX 28.8 Making the Interview More Effective

- Gather preliminary data before the session, and keep questionnaires relatively short.
- Ask about often-overlooked problems, such as difficulty sleeping, incontinence, falling, depression, dizziness, and loss of energy.
- Pace the interview to allow the patient to formulate answers; resist the tendency to interrupt pre-maturely.
- Use yes-or-no or simple-choice questions if the person has trouble coping with open-ended questions.
- Begin with general questions such as "How can I help you most at this visit?" or "What's been happening?"
- Be alert for information about the patient's relationships with others, thoughts about families or co-workers, typical responses to stress, and attitudes toward aging, illness, occupation, and death.
- Assess mental status for deficits in recent or remote memory, and determine if confusion exists.
- Be aware of all medications the patient is taking, and assess for adverse effects, efficacy, and possible drug interactions.
- Determine how fast the condition of the patient has been changing to assess the extent of the patient's concerns.
- Include the family or significant other in the interview process for added input, clarification, support, and reinforcement.

Intervention Strategies

Certain psychotherapeutic methods are especially useful for older persons:

- Applying crisis intervention techniques (see Chapter 21)
- Providing empathic understanding and active listening
- Encouraging ventilation of feelings and normalizing emotional responses
- Re-establishing emotional equilibrium when anxiety is moderate to severe
- Providing health education and explaining alternative solutions
- Assisting in the use of problem-solving approaches
- Allowing adequate time to process information
- Ensuring that hearing aids are working or using an amplifier to facilitate good communication

An older person may require acute inpatient mental health care for signs and symptoms of severe psychiatric conditions, such as non-dementia psychiatric illnesses, major depression with suicidal thoughts, bipolar disorder, and schizophrenia. Just as in the general adult population, with the shift to community-based service delivery models, the number of patients with psychiatric illnesses treated on an inpatient basis is declining. Regardless of the person's age, inpatient treatment is recommended when the patient is at high risk for self-harm (whether intentional or unintentional) or poses a risk for harm to other people.

Specialized geropsychiatric units provide a comprehensive and specialized approach to care. These units use a multi-disciplinary approach to assessment, treatment planning, implementation, and evaluation of care. Ideally, the team consists of a geriatric psychiatrist, geriatrician, social worker, nurses, a pharmacist, psychologist, dietitian, occupational therapist, physiotherapist, and other specialists as indicated. Nurses play the major role in providing continuous care from admission to discharge.

Psychosocial Interventions

The basic-level nurse uses counselling skills to assist the patient in talking about present problems, examining their present situation, looking at alternatives, and planning for the future. Sometimes counselling is provided through group therapy, which helps to decrease the sense of disorientation and isolation. Remotivation therapy (Box 28.9) and reminiscence therapy are also appropriate interventions for the basic-level nurse. Remotivation therapy is a form of group therapy that promotes self-esteem, awareness, and socialization and relates to the creation of engagement and interest in life, such as in a person's daily activities, talents, hobbies, environment, and social relationships with family and friends (Araújo & Ribeiro, 2015).

The advanced-practice nurse may provide individual or group psychotherapy to older persons with depression. Groups are useful because they can diminish social isolation and loneliness and help the members understand that they are not alone in their situation. Group members can learn creative ways to improve their mood and increase the quality of life (Yalom, 2005). Table 28.1 outlines the purpose, format, and desired outcomes for each type of psychotherapeutic group. Individual therapies, specifically cognitive behavioural, interpersonal, and psychodynamic therapy, are also useful. The best outcomes result from combining some kind of therapy with medication. Primary care providers therefore must acquire the skills to enable sensitive assessment for depression and suicide risk and must be knowledgeable about methods of intervention. Collaboration with other mental health care providers is best practice.

BOX 28.9 Example of Remotivation Session (Bodies of Water)

Step 1: Climate of Acceptance

The leaders personally welcomed each participant as they arrived at the group session. After the leaders introduced themselves, each group member made a self-introduction. The leader used a calendar to orient the members to the date and time of the current remotivation session. The theme for session four was introduced by the leader as "Bodies of Water—Rivers, Lakes, and Oceans." All group members had some familiarity with bodies of water because of their residence in Seattle.

Step 2: Creating a Bridge to Reality

The world globe was used as a visual aid to stimulate discussion on bodies of water. The leader asked questions such as "How are bodies of water formed from glaciers?" Pictures of glaciers, rivers, and lakes were shown.

The leader read poems about tide pools, seashells, and fishing written by anonymous grade-school children. Discussion was stimulated by the leader's asking, "What can we do at the ocean?" Visual aids and props were provided for direct sensory stimulation. Some examples of these aids and props were (1) different types of seashells, (2) fishing tackle and bait, (3) suntan lotion, (4) sun hat, and (5) sunglasses.

An anonymous author's poem about fishing was read to the group, followed by recorded music with lyrics about fishing experiences.

Step 3: Sharing the World We Live in

Group discussion focused on jobs related to bodies of water. Topics the participants discussed in regard to self or others included crabbing, clamming, shrimping, and fishing. Visual aids, such as pictures of river rafting, canoeing, scuba diving, and sailing, stimulated further discussions of past related experiences involving bodies of water.

Step 4: An Appreciation of the World of Work

This time was used for the members to think about work in relation to others. More experiences in past work roles, as well as hobbies and pastimes, were discussed. The group then participated in singing a familiar old song, "Love Letters in the Sand," written in 1931 by J. Fred Coots and revived in 1957, when sung by Pat Boone.

Step 5: Climate of Appreciation

The leaders thanked the group members individually for coming to the group and sharing their experiences. The next remotivation session theme and meeting date were announced prior to terminating the session.

Group Response to Session Four

Most members of the group appeared to enjoy discussing their experiences in relation to bodies of water. Many members recalled fishing and boating experiences. Other members expressed interest in this topic by their non-verbal participation in touching and smelling some physical props and observation of visual aids. All but two participants touched the seashells and smelled the fish eggs. One lady in the group stood up and modelled the sun hat and glasses, while a man demonstrated how to reel in the line on a fishing pole. Several participants remarked on how beautiful the pictures of the glaciers were. All but a couple of group members sang to the recorded lyrics on fishing. One member stood up and danced to the music while many others clapped to her movements.

Source: Araújo, L., Ribeiro, O. (2015). Remotivation therapy. In: Pachana N. (Ed.), *Encyclopedia of geropsychology*. Springer. https://doi.org/10.1007/978-981-287-080-3_269-1; Reprinted with permission from SLACK Incorporated: Janssen, J. A., & Giberson, D. L. (1988). Remotivation therapy. *Journal of Gerontological Nursing, 14*(6), 31–34.

TABLE 28.1 Useful Group Therapy Modalities for Older Persons

Remotivation Therapy	Reminiscence Therapy (Life Review)	Psychotherapy
Purpose of Group		
Resocialize regressed and apathetic patients. Reawaken interest in the environment.	Share memories of the past. Increase self-esteem. Increase socialization. Increase awareness of the uniqueness of each participant	Alleviate psychiatric symptoms. Increase ability to interact with others in a group. Increase self-esteem. Increase ability to make decisions and function more independently
Format		
Groups are made up of 10–15 people. Meetings are held once or twice a week. Meetings are highly structured in a classroom-like setting. Group uses props. Each session discusses a particular topic. See Box 28.9 for the five basic steps used in each session.	Groups are made up of 6–8 people. Meetings are held once or twice weekly for 1 hour. Topics include holidays, major life events, birthdays, travel, and food.	Group size is 6–12 members. Group members should share similar: • Problems • Mental status • Needs Groups should be mixed (both men and women). Group meets at regularly scheduled times (certain number of times a week, specific duration of session) and place.
Desired Outcomes		
Increases participants' sense of reality. Offers practice of health roles. Realizes more objective self-image.	Alleviates depression in institutionalized older persons. Through the process of reorganization and reintegration, provides avenue by which members: • Achieve a new sense of identity • Achieve a positive self-concept	Decreases sense of isolation. Facilitates development of new roles and re-establishes former roles. Provides information for other types of groups. Provides group support for effecting changes and increasing self-esteem.

Source: Touhy, T. A., & Jett, K. F. (Eds.). (2016). *Ebersole & Hess' toward healthy aging: Human needs and nursing response* (9th ed.). St. Louis: Mosby.

Pharmacological Interventions

Evidence about the biology of mental illness and the discovery of new psychotropic medications have expanded the role of the geropsychiatric nurse. Nurses play a vital role in monitoring, reporting, and managing medication adverse effects such as acute dystonia, akathisia, pseudoparkinsonism, neuroleptic malignant syndrome, serotonin syndrome, and anti-cholinergic effects. Physical assessment of response to medication is also important and includes monitoring vital signs, pain, laboratory work, elimination (bowel and bladder), changes in gait, prevention of falls, and neurological checks when appropriate. The nurse assesses for underlying medical problems. Often patients with chronic persistent mental illnesses, such as schizophrenia, misinterpret or do not report visceral cues, pain, and vital symptoms of illness. As a result, the nurse needs to be vigilant to assess and appropriately treat these symptoms.

Health Teaching and Health Promotion

The nurse provides health teaching to both patient and caregiver on a variety of issues, including the nature of the patient's illness, symptom management, maintenance of safety, self-care strategies, management of medications (see Patient and Family Teaching: Medication Safety), coping skills, steps necessary for recovery, and resources that will support recovery. When information is printed, providing a large-print version is often helpful.

Promotion of Self-Care Activities

Hospitalization may result in regression that ranges from needing assistance to requiring total care in accomplishing the activities of daily living. A goal for nurses is to encourage the patient to regain independence in the realm of personal care. Hospitalization may be an

PATIENT AND FAMILY TEACHING
Medication Safety

- Learn about your medicines:
  - Read medicine labels and package inserts, and follow the directions.
  - If you have questions, ask your doctor or other health care providers.
- Talk to your team of health care providers about your medical conditions, health concerns, and all the medicines you take (both prescription and over-the-counter), as well as dietary supplements, vitamins, and herbal supplements.
  - The more they know, the more they can help.
  - Do not be afraid to ask questions.
- Keep track of adverse effects or possible drug interactions, and let your doctor know right away about any unexpected symptoms or changes in the way you feel.
- Make sure to go to all doctor appointments and to any appointments for monitoring tests done by your doctor or at a laboratory.
- Use a calendar, pillbox, or something to help you remember what medications you need to take and when.
- Write down information your doctor gives you about your medicines or your health condition.
- Take a friend or relative to your doctor's appointments if you think you need help to understand or remember what the doctor tells you.
- Have a "medicine checkup" at least once a year.
  - Go through your medicine cabinet to get rid of old or expired medicines.
  - Ask your doctor or pharmacist to go over all the medicines you now take. Remember to include all over-the-counter medicines, vitamins, dietary supplements, and herbal supplements you take.
- Keep all medicines out of the sight and reach of children.

opportunity for the patient to receive much-needed assessment of the skin, feet, hair, mouth, and perineal areas. These assessments can often uncover hidden infections, unhealed wounds, and growths that may otherwise have been missed and lead to needed medical attention.

Milieu Management

The major roles of the nurse in terms of milieu management are to assist the patient in adjusting to the environment, keep the patient safe at all times (e.g., make sure roommates are compatible, call lights are within reach, patients at risk for falling are placed close to the nurses' station), minimize the adverse effects of hospitalization on functional capacity (e.g., encourage patients to walk and to do so as independently as possible), provide reality orientation, and engage in therapeutic communication with the patient. It helps to know that reorienting a patient is not always therapeutic, especially if the patient has dementia and reorientation causes agitation. Using distraction techniques is often the intervention of choice.

Another vital aspect of milieu management is the prevention and reduction of agitation by maintaining a visible presence on the unit and anticipating the patient's needs. Crisis intervention techniques may be used if an agitated patient does not respond to redirection or verbal attempts to de-escalate agitation. As a crisis situation unfolds, staff response will largely determine the outcome, and a well-trained crisis team improves these outcomes. The crisis team leader is usually a nurse for several reasons:

- Nurses provide professional care 24 hours a day, 7 days a week, and have detailed knowledge of patients.
- The nurse is aware of the patient's medical condition.
- The nurse is able to guide the team and help prevent injury of a patient who needs physical restraint but has osteoporosis.

After the crisis has been de-escalated, the team leader, the team, and other patients (as indicated) help to restore a sense of safety and calm. As the agitated patient gains control, it is important to help the individual ease back into the milieu with dignity.

Care Settings

As discussed in Chapter 3, the mental health system has increasingly become focused on the goal of community living rather than institutional living, but resources necessary to meet this goal have been chronically underfunded. Patients who would benefit from residential care are often moved from the most structured environment (inpatient care) to unstructured and unsupervised living situations in the community.

Long-Term Care Facilities

Some long-term care settings provide specialized psychiatric mental health care, but most do not. There are many of the entry-to-practice competencies directly related to providing mental health care. The emphasis placed on tasks and interventions associated with these competencies varies by educational program.

> ⚡ **SAFETY TIP**
>
> As you work with patients exhibiting behavioural symptoms such as neglect of personal hygiene, omitting prescribed medication, or refusing to participate in other care activities, it is key to understand why these behaviours are present. Ask yourself: Are these behaviours related to the patient exercising their autonomy? Are these negative symptoms related to schizophrenia? A consequence of a lack of insight? Understanding why these behaviours are present will provide help to deliver care that is relevant to the patient and deliver it in a way that does not escalate behavioural symptoms further.

Clinicians may believe that patients who refuse personal hygiene, medication, or wound care are exercising their right to refuse care rather than recognizing the negative symptoms of schizophrenia. Nurses who accept these refusals may inadvertently contribute to a patient's deterioration.

A geriatric psychiatric unit can be a stabilizing environment for a person with severe mental illness who thrives within the structure of a therapeutic environment. Providing a documented plan of care and intervening when behavioural symptoms increase are as important as monitoring and intervening when a resident has signs of infection. Specialized geropsychiatric units provide a comprehensive and specialized approach to care. These units use a multi-disciplinary approach to assessment, treatment planning, implementation, and evaluation of care. Ideally the team consists of registered nurses, geriatric psychiatrists, geriatricians, social workers, pharmacists, psychologists, dietitians, occupational therapists, and physiotherapists.

There now is much greater awareness of and focus on the use of non-pharmacological interventions for the treatment of agitation, wandering, confusion, yelling, and aggression. Medications often deemed "unnecessary" are generally antipsychotics, antianxiety medications, and sedatives. Patients with a history of depression, schizophrenia, obsessive-compulsive disorder, generalized anxiety disorder, or bipolar disorder need ongoing treatment to prevent relapse and re-emergence of symptoms. Nurses can play an important role in advocating for psychiatric evaluation and intervention to assist with (1) managing medications, (2) monitoring and documenting behavioural changes, (3) notifying the physician of behavioural changes, and (4) planning care for the needs of those residents with mental illness.

Should the services provided within a long-term care setting be required, the move may often trigger a sense of loss for both the patient and the caregiver. Family members of people admitted to long-term care will often go through a grieving process as they accept the changing needs of their loved ones. Many family members describe feeling guilty despite knowing that they can no longer care for their loved one at home. Nurses are in an excellent position to support both the person admitted and the caregivers in taking on a less physically demanding role but remaining involved in providing care.

Partial Hospitalization

Partial hospitalization, or an acute psychiatric day hospital program, is sometimes recommended for ambulatory patients who do not need 24-hour nursing care but require and would benefit from intensive, structured psychiatric treatment. Health services provided in these programs include symptom monitoring and management, medication education and management, relapse and stress prevention, and problem solving of health maintenance issues to enable the patient to adapt to active functioning in the community. The nurse also reviews with the team, in collaboration with the patient and family or caregiver, additional referrals for needed services (e.g., Meals on Wheels, transportation services, church activities, home care services).

Day Treatment Programs

Multi-purpose centres for older persons provide a broad range of services, including (1) health promotion and wellness programs; (2) health screening; (3) social, educational, and recreational activities; (4) meals; and (5) information and referral services. For those in need of nursing care and custodial care services, an **adult support program** is an appropriate choice. There are three types of adult support programs: (1) social care, (2) adult health or medical treatment programs, and (3) maintenance care. In each type older persons are cared for during the day and stay in a home environment at night. The boundaries of these programs blend and overlap. All three models are meant to provide a safe, supportive, and non-threatening environment and fulfill a vital function for older persons and their families. The programs allow older persons to continue their present living arrangements and maintain their social ties to the community; they also relieve families of the burden of 24-hour-a-day care for older person dependants. If institutionalization becomes necessary, adult day care staff can work with patients and their families to assess the situation and make recommendations for placement.

Behavioural Health Home Care

Older persons typically prefer that the continuum of services be delivered in the least restrictive setting, which is usually their homes. Home-based behavioural health care is particularly recommended to assist the homebound older person in adjusting to and managing illness and disability either before or after hospitalization. It is often the role of the behavioural health home care nurse to help a person affected by a cognitive brain disorder or a severe and persistent mental illness to remain in the home or to facilitate a transfer to a temporary or permanent facility, if necessary. Local home care agencies can assist with providing nursing and rehabilitation services; home health care aide services to provide assistance with activities of daily living; homemaking services, such as housekeeping and meal preparation (although many provincial health care plans do not cover homemaking costs); or a combination of services. The goal of all of these services is to increase the older person's ability to live independently.

The target population for behavioural health home care includes older persons who need help with activities of daily living, have behavioural issues related to their physical illness, or have an enduring mental illness. Nursing services are usually provided by a basic-level practitioner, a certified generalist nurse in community health or home health care, or an advanced-practice registered nurse certified in adult psychiatric mental health nursing.

Respite Care

Family caregivers are at great risk for burnout. Respite care is designed to allow caregivers to have a break for a specific number of days. During this time, the patient is admitted to a nursing facility for a planned number of days. Family can then go on vacation, travel, or just have a needed break from caregiving. Respite care can also be provided in the home as well.

Community-Based Programs

The hazards of institutionalization are numerous: increased risk for health care–associated infections, which may result in increased mortality; injuries occurring due to initial disorientation to a new setting; and patients developing learned helplessness and losing interest in self-care activities. (Chapter 2 provides a historical overview of deinstitutionalization.) There also may be fewer opportunities for socialization in an institutional setting. In contrast, community-based programs aim to promote the older person's independent functioning and reduce the stress on the family system.

Community-based programs that provide specialized case-management services assist older persons with coordination of care and assistance (e.g., Meals on Wheels, transportation). Constant assessment of the changing needs of older persons requires frequent contact and rapid intervention when they become sick or need additional services. Hospitalization can be averted if aggressive and skilled case management is in place, and nurses are uniquely qualified to fulfill the role of case manager.

Older persons living in the community may still be driving, which can become a safety concern for caregivers, family, and the public. If there is evidence that the older person can no longer safely drive a vehicle (e.g., failing visual acuity, hearing loss, memory deficits, impaired mobility, movement disorders such as Parkinson's disease), or if there have been frequent small collisions, it is appropriate to notify the provincial or territorial ministry of motor vehicles for a driving evaluation to determine the older person's capacity for the safe operation of a vehicle.

KEY POINTS TO REMEMBER

- The older persons population continues to increase exponentially.
- The increase in the number of older persons poses a challenge not only to nurses but also to the entire health care system to be prepared to respond to the special needs of this population.
- Attitudes toward older persons are often negative, reflecting ageism—a bias against older persons based solely on age.
- Ageism is found at all levels of society and even among health care providers and can affect the quality of care of older patients.
- Nurses who care for older persons in various settings may function at different levels. All should be knowledgeable about the process of aging and be cognizant of the differences between normal and abnormal aging changes.
- Older persons face increasing problems of substance use and suicide.
- Adequate pain assessment is important, and the nurse must bear in mind that older persons tend to understate their pain. Sufficient pain medication should be administered and drugs should be carefully titrated.
- Nurses working with mentally ill patients must know psychotherapeutic approaches relevant to the older person. Advanced-practice nurses may offer psychotherapy groups geared toward the special needs of this population.

CRITICAL THINKING

1. Mr. Abbott has received treatment for alcohol withdrawal. He is a very quiet, religious man who refuses to eat, does not sleep at night, admits to thoughts of desperation, and wishes he could die. He also confides that he attempted suicide when his wife died 5 years earlier, which is when he started drinking heavily.
   a. What cultural considerations may be helpful to know about religious people's response to depression?
   b. Which depression assessment tool is appropriate to use in assessing the severity of Mr. Abbott's condition? Explain your answer.
2. Mrs. Bélanger is 75 years old and lives with her daughter's family. She has moderate to advanced Alzheimer's disease. Although Mrs. Bélanger's family wants to keep her at home for as long as possible, they are overwhelmed by her needs and by being unable to leave her alone. What community placements might be best for Mrs. Bélanger? Explain your answer.
3. How should the nurse frame the multi-generational effects of historical trauma among Indigenous people in Canada? Useful frameworks should describe the trauma in terms of connectedness, collectivity, and relationships.

CHAPTER REVIEW

1. The nurse is caring for an older person. Which symptom should the nurse recognize as a normal part of aging?
   a. Depression
   b. Memory loss
   c. Situational grieving
   d. Dementia

2. The nurse is caring for an older person with depression. Which nursing response is appropriate when the patient's daughter asks, "Will he ever stop acting like this?"
    a. "I'm sorry, your father will likely be in this state from now on."
    b. "Although older persons have a high incidence of depression, it is treatable and your father will improve on the antidepressants."
    c. "Depression is caused by infections or electrolyte imbalances, and the damage is permanent."
    d. "A benzodiazepine will help alleviate the depression."
3. The nurse is caring for an older person with pain. What is one myth about pain held by health care providers?
    a. Pain is an inevitable part of aging.
    b. Older persons may understate their pain using words such as *discomfort, hurting,* or *aching*.
    c. Dementia and depression can add to the difficulty of obtaining an accurate pain assessment.
    d. An interview with family members, caregivers, or friends is vital.
4. An older person experiencing pain states that she is going to use kava kava, which she has heard provides pain relief. Which nursing response is appropriate?
    a. "Kava kava is an appropriate herb to use for pain relief."
    b. "Older persons should not use herbal preparations."
    c. "Willow bark would be a better herbal supplement to use."
    d. "Are you using any other treatments for pain relief?"

https://evolve.elsevier.com/Canada/Varcarolis/psychiatric/

REFERENCES

Alexopoulos, G. S., Abrams, R. C., Young, R. C., et al. (1988). Cornell scale for depression in dementia. *Biological Psychiatry, 23*, 271–284. https://doi.org/10.1016/0006-3223(88)90038-8

Araújo, L. & Ribeiro, O. (2015). Remotivation therapy. In: N. Pachana (Ed.), *Encyclopedia of geropsychology*. Springer. https://doi.org/10.1007/978-981-287-080-3_269-1

Burchum, J., & Rosenthal, L. (2018). *Lehne's pharmacology for nursing care* (10th ed.). Philadelphia: Saunders.

By the 2019 American Geriatrics Society Beers Criteria® Update Expert Panel. (2019). American Geriatrics Society 2019 Updated AGS Beers Criteria® for Potentially Inappropriate Medication Use in Older Adults. *Journal of the American Geriatrics Society, 67*(4), 674–694. https://doi.org/10.1111/jgs.15767

Canadian Association of Schools of Nursing (CASN) & Canadian Federation of Mental Health Nurses (CFMHN). (2017). *Entry-to-practice mental health and addiction competencies for undergraduate nursing education in Canada*. Ottawa: CASN.

Canadian Centre on Substance Use and Addiction. (2017). *Canadian drug summary*. Ottawa, ON: Author.

Canadian Gerontological Nursing Association. (2019). *Gerontological Nursing Standards of Practice and Competencies 2019* (4th ed.). Toronto, Canada: CGNA.

Dahlke, S., Davidson, S., Kalogirou, M. R., et al. (2020). Nursing faculty and students' perspectives of how students learn to work with older people. *Nurse Education Today, 93*, 104537. https://doi-org.ezproxy.macewan.ca/10.1016/j.nedt.2020.104537

Denkinger, M. D., Lukas, A., Nikolaus, T., et al. (2015). Factors associated with fear of falling and associated activity restriction in community-dwelling older adults. *The American Journal of Geriatric Psychiatry, 23*(1), 72–86.

Hung, M., Bounsanga, J., Voss, M. W., et al. (2017). The relationship between family support: Pain and depression in elderly with arthritis. *Psychology, Health & Medicine, 22*(1), 75–86. https://doi.org/10.1080/13548506.2016.1211293

Jacox, A., Carr, D. B., Payne, R., et al. (1994). *Visual analogue scales used in the management of cancer pain. Management of Cancer Pain (Clinical Practice Guideline No. 9, AHCPR Publication No. 94-0952)*. Rockville: U.S. Department of Health and Human Services, Public Health Service, Agency for Health Care Policy and Research.

Jennings, E. L. M., Murphy, K. D., Gallagher, P., et al. (2020). In-hospital adverse drug reactions in older adults; prevalence, presentation and associated drugs—A systematic review and meta-analysis. *Age & Ageing, 49*(6), 948–958. https://doi.org/10.1093/ageing/afaa188

Kishita, N., & Laidlaw, K. (2017). Cognitive behaviour therapy for generalized anxiety disorder: Is CBT equally efficacious in adults of working age and older adults?. *Clinical Psychology Review, 52*(1), 124–136. https://doi.org/10.1016/j.cpr.2017.01.003

Mental Health Commission of Canada. (2012). *Changing directions, changing lives: The mental health strategy for Canada*. Calgary: Author.

Mental Health Commission of Canada. (2014). *Addressing the mental health needs of Canadians*. Ottawa: Presentation at HealthPartners.

Parmar, J., Anderson, S., Duggleby, W., et al. (2020). Developing person-centred care competencies for the healthcare workforce to support family caregivers: Caregiver centred care. *Health & Social Care in the Community, 29*(5), 1327–1338. https://doi.org/10.1111/hsc.13173

Powell, M., Corbo, V., Fonda, J., et al. (2015). Sleep quality and re-experiencing symptoms of PTSD are associated with current pain in U.S. OEF/OIF/OND/veterans with and without mTBIs. *Journal of Traumatic Stress, 28*(4), 322–329. https://doi.org/10.1002/jts.22027

Prince, M., Wimo, A., Guerchet, M., et al. (2015). *World Alzheimer report 2015: The global impact on dementia: An analysis of prevalence, in cadence, cost and trends*. London: Alzheimer's Disease International.

Sheikh, J. I., & Yesavage, J. A. (1986). Geriatric Depression Scale (GDS): Recent evidence and development of a shorter version. In T. Brink (Ed.), *Clinical gerontology: A guide to assessment and intervention*. New York: The Haworth Press.

Shepherd, V., Nuttall, J., Hood, K., et al. (2015). Setting up a clinical trial in care homes: Challenges encountered and recommendations for future research practice. *BioMedCentral Research Notes, 8*(1), 1–4. https://doi.org/10.1186/s13104-015-1276-8

Sorrell, J. M. (2017). Substance use disorders in long-term care settings: A crisis of care for older adults. *Journal of Psychosocial Nursing and Mental Health Services, 55*(1), 24–27. https://doi.org/10.3928/02793695-20170119-08

Statistics Canada. (2015). *Canada's population estimates: Age and sex, July 1, 2015*. Retrieved from https://www.statcan.gc.ca/daily-quotidien/150929/dq150929b-eng.htm

Szanto, K. (2017). Cognitive deficits: Underappreciated contributors to suicide. *The American Journal of Geriatric Psychiatry, 25*(6), 630–632. https://doi.org/10.1016/j.jagp.2017.02.012

Van Orden, K., & Deming, C. (2017). Late-life suicide prevention strategies: Current status and future directions. *Current Opinion in Psychology, 22*(8), 79–83. https://doi.org/10.1016/j.copsyc.2017.08.033

Wagenaar, D., Mickus, M., & Wilson, J. (2001). Alcoholism in late life: Challenges and complexities. *Psychiatric Annals, 31*(11), 665–672.

Yalom, I. D. (2005). *The theory and practice of group psychotherapy* (5th ed.). Cambridge: Basic Books.

29

Recovery, Survivorship, and Public Mental Health Approaches

Sonya L. Jakubec

 https://evolve.elsevier.com/Canada/Varcarolis/psychiatric/

OBJECTIVES

1. Discuss the effects of serious mental illness on daily functioning, interpersonal relationships, and quality of life.
2. Describe rehabilitation, recovery, human rights, and population health approaches to living with serious mental illness.
3. Describe three common problems associated with serious mental illness.
4. Discuss five evidence-informed practices for the care of the person with serious mental illness.
5. Explain the role of the nurse in the care of the person with serious mental illness.
6. Develop a nursing care plan for a person with serious mental illness.

KEY TERMS AND CONCEPTS

community treatment orders
institutionalized
population health approaches
population mental health
psychoeducation

recovery
rehabilitation
social skills training
stigma

supported-employment model
supportive psychotherapy
survivorship
vocational rehabilitation

The term *mental illness* encompasses a wide range of human illness experience, from acute and time-limited reactions to stress to severe disruptions in cognitive functioning. The terms *serious mental illness* (SMI) and *biologically based mental illness* refer to a small but significant group of mental illnesses. In Canada there is no uniform definition of SMI or *serious and persistent mental illness* (SPMI), but many Canadian researchers and clinicians use SMI to refer to schizophrenia, mood disorders, and other psychotic disorders. SMI is a significant health care challenge, the leading cause of disability in Canada. It is estimated that by the time Canadians reach age 40 that one in two Canadians will have had, or have, a mental illness, with the majority of people reporting SMI also enduring other comorbid chronic health conditions (Centre for Addiction and Mental Health, 2021b). SMIs can be chronic or recurrent. Some patients experience remissions interrupted by exacerbations of varying lengths; the remissions may be essentially symptom-free but in most cases involve some degree of residual symptoms. Other patients experience illness as a chronic and sometimes deteriorating experience, during which symptoms wax and wane but never remit.

People with SMI are at risk for multiple physical, emotional, and social problems: they are more likely to be victims of crime, be medically ill, have undertreated or untreated physical illnesses, die prematurely, be homeless, be incarcerated, be unemployed or underemployed, engage in substance use, live in poverty, and report loneliness as well as lower quality of life and social satisfaction than persons without such illnesses. Social support matters in terms of outcomes for people with SMI, and in their recovery and social functioning and there is some evidence that greater loneliness predicts poorer outcomes (Wang et al., 2018).

The impairments associated with SMI, along with related factors such as poverty, stigma, unemployment, and inadequate housing, can significantly affect quality of life. While these factors, increasingly described as social determinants of mental health, have a tremendous impact on people, the necessary social and political interventions are still placed well in the background, eclipsed by the largely individual treatment focus of interventions for SMI (Alegría et al., 2018). A human rights and population health approach is advocated for by the Canadian Public Health Association (CPHA), with position statements that include consideration of the mental wellness implications of social determinants, including early childhood education and care, racism, and public health governance (CPHA, 2021).

SERIOUS MENTAL ILLNESS ACROSS THE LIFESPAN

SMI occurs in persons of any gender, age, culture, or geographical location. However, the population of people currently living with SMIs can be separated into two groups that have had different experiences with the mental health care system: (1) those old enough to have experienced long-term institutionalization, and (2) those young enough to have been hospitalized only for acute care during exacerbations of their disorders.

Older Persons

Until the second half of the twentieth century, most psychiatric inpatient treatment took place in large institutions uniquely dedicated to the care of the severely mentally ill. During this time, psychiatric hospitals were the long-term residences for many people (see Chapter 2). Medical paternalism, in which the health care provider made all decisions for patients with SMIs, was a pervasive philosophical stance at that time. Thus many patients became **institutionalized** (i.e., they became dependent on the services and structure of institutions and unable to function independently outside such institutions). It was difficult to distinguish whether behaviours were the result of the disease process or altered responses that resulted from institutionalization. Opportunities for recovery were hampered both by the limited treatments of the day, the rampant stigmatization and institutionalization.

Some of today's older persons with SMI have experience with this system of care. They have learned that they are expected to accept the treatment team's decisions. Today's emphasis on patient-centred care, which requires the patient to express their opinions and wishes, challenges some older persons who grew up in the paternalistic institutions of the past.

It was between 1960 and 1980 that all Canadian provinces began to make changes in the inpatient treatment of SMI by closing beds in large mental hospitals and opening inpatient units in general hospitals. The 1990s heralded further deinstitutionalization of psychiatric services as the total number of inpatient days for mental health care in psychiatric hospitals and general hospitals declined (Spagnolo, 2014). Advances towards more empowering and less paternalistic approaches have origins in the **survivorship** movement. Referencing a survival experience, not of illness but of the psychiatric system, the movement arose from the shift from institutionalization and people resisting institutionalization and traditional psychiatric treatment (Adame et al., 2017).

> **VIGNETTE**
> At the age of 19, Marian was admitted to a facility that cares for people with serious mental illnesses (SMI). Now 79, and with the exception of living in a group home between age 32 and 34, Marian has been an inpatient at the SMI facility. Marian's symptoms have been stable, so the treatment team begins to discuss discharge and Marian accepts their recommendation that she no longer needs inpatient treatment. Discharged to a community supportive-living home, Marian spends long periods sitting in front of the living room window, just watching. Marian does not ask to go out into the garden she watches for so many hours. Indeed, it is rare that Marian asks for anything, including snacks or recreational activities. The caregivers work with Marian for several months to support self-awareness, the identification of needs of the moment, and ways to articulate or act on those needs. There is a major celebration on the day Marian walks into the kitchen and makes a peanut butter sandwich, following that sequence of identifying hunger, interest in food, this particular food, and taking action to make the sandwich. Seemingly small, a positive shift from some of the dependency caused by the institutionalization is truly significant for Marian.

Younger Adults

People young enough never to have been institutionalized usually do not experience the passivity and dependency such conditions set up for residents. However, treatment via a series of shorter-term hospitalizations has given them limited experience with formal treatment and has contributed to some patients not truly believing serious or persistent illness exists. Individuals who do not understand that they are ill, perhaps because of the impairment of the illness itself (poor insight, possibly related to *anosognosia*), face other challenges, including longer-term hospitalizations. Overcoming these challenges and building capacities for successful community life outside of hospital are specific treatment goals that need concentrated support. Without these supports, young adults with SMI are at particular risks for unemployment, housing instability, as well legal and social difficulties. For some people with SMI, specific supported housing is central to successful community living (Lequin et al., 2021). Even young adults with minor symptoms of SMI risk functional impairment, and preventative care and support for age-appropriate social functioning is recommended (Romanowska et al., 2020).

> **VIGNETTE**
> After graduating from high school, Christopher enlists in the armed forces and serves for 5 years. Following that time, Christopher settles in Nova Scotia and takes a job in a security firm. In a first psychotic break Christopher becomes paranoid and threatening at work and is hospitalized briefly. Upon discharge, Christopher refuses aftercare and will not take medication. Difficulties mount as Christopher leaves the security job and moves to another city, knowing no one, having no supports. For the next 15 years, Christopher works intermittently, is homeless off and on, and drinks heavily when money is available. Hospitalized only once for threatening others, Christopher consistently resists follow-up care or recommendations, showing no insight into the illness. One day, Christopher simply disappears.

DEVELOPMENT OF SERIOUS MENTAL ILLNESS

SMI has much in common with chronic physical illness: the original problem increasingly overwhelms and erodes basic coping mechanisms and increases the use of compensatory processes. As the disorder extends beyond the acute stage, more and more of the neighbouring systems are involved. For example, a person with schizophrenia may experience disturbed thought processes and social skills, which cause interactions with others to become increasingly awkward and anxiety provoking for both parties. This awkwardness, in turn, results in others becoming increasingly hesitant to interact with the affected person and in the affected person's self-esteem weakening.

REHABILITATION VERSUS RECOVERY: TWO MODELS OF CARE

For many years, the concept of **rehabilitation**, which focused on managing patients' deficits and helping patients learn to live with their illnesses, dominated psychiatric care. Staff directed the treatment and concentrated on helping patients function in their daily roles. Advocates for improved mental health care and people with SMI (many of whom prefer to call themselves *consumers* to emphasize the choices they have, or seek to have, over their treatment, or *survivors* to indicate a separation from or survival of the formal psychiatric system) have increasingly sought a different treatment approach.

The recovery model developed out of the consumer and survivorship movement. Recovery is one of several identified patient-reported outcomes of treatment for psychotic illnesses (schizophrenia and bipolar disorder) (McKenzie et al., 2021). The **recovery** model is patient- or consumer-centred, involves active partnership with care providers, and is integrated within broader social and political agendas (Garverich et al., 2021; Sánchez, 2020). It is a hopeful, empowering, strengths-focused model whereby staff assist the consumer in achieving the highest quality of life possible. This model of care encourages a high degree of patient independence and self-determination, focusing on achieving goals of the patient's choosing and leading increasingly productive and meaningful lives (Sánchez, 2020). The emphasis is on the person and the future rather than on the illness and the present.

Although it has been suggested that the recovery philosophy has been slower to take hold in Canada than in other countries (Mulvale & Bartram, 2015), the Mental Health Commission of Canada (MHCC, 2015) identified recovery as central to mental health care reform. According to the MHCC, a recovery-oriented system creates the possibility for people with severe mental illness to gain more control over their lives and make choices about treatments while being supported by professionals, families, and other people who are significant in their lives. Systems of recovery increasingly involve new technology, and the use and potential of mobile and computer devices to support recovery is discussed in the Research Highlight box.

ISSUES CONFRONTING PEOPLE WITH SERIOUS MENTAL ILLNESS

Establishing a Meaningful Life

Finding meaning in life and establishing goals can be difficult for people living with SMI, particularly if they also experience poor self-esteem or apathy. Patients may struggle with the possibility that they may never be the person they once were or expected to be. Finding a way to "reset" one's goals so that meaning can be found in new ways (e.g., helping others, volunteering, exploring new routines, establishing or re-establishing friendships, or simply surmounting a significant illness) is important to achieving a satisfactory quality of life and avoiding despair.

People who cannot work or attend school have a significant amount of time to occupy. If these people do not own a car or have easy access to public transit, lack money for movies or other pastimes, are afraid to go outside, or do not have enough confidence to join peers, options can be very limited. Further, imagine the energy and effort it takes to build sufficient confidence to overcome poor self-esteem or enduring stigma, let alone address systemic barriers such as transportation, basic income, and housing. After the energy required to manage personal and systemic barriers, there may be little remaining to engage in meaningful activities. Advocates of social determinants of mental health seek enhanced capabilities and guaranteed income or living wage strategies, stress the value of stable access to housing, safe transportation, and guaranteed income as a starting place for a meaningful life with mental illness (Kerman & Sylvestre, 2020; Pender, 2021).

Comorbid Conditions

Physical Disorders

One of the strategic directions of the MHCC is to achieve an "increase (in) the life expectancy of people living with severe mental illnesses" (MHCC, 2012, p. 129). People with SMI are at greater risk for co-occurring physical illnesses and die pre-maturely (on average, 15 years pre-maturely for women and 20 years for men). Furthermore, the conditions of this pre-mature mortality are increasingly understood to result from a combination of socioeconomic, health care, and clinical risk factors, and not from higher rates of suicide (Wynaden et al., 2016).

Contributing domains including individual factors, such as failing to provide for their own health needs; policy and systemic issues such as barriers to access or payment required for community home care or psychological services; and other community-wide and social obstacles, such as professional culture, stigma, or stereotyping (Stefancic et al., 2021; Wynaden et al., 2016).

Depression and Suicide

Persons with SMI may experience a profound sense of loss. This loss can lead to acute or chronic grief, which, along with the chronicity of the illness and its demands and impact on daily life, can contribute to despair, depression, and, in the case of people experiencing schizophrenia, a lifetime risk for suicide 20 times higher than the general population (Zaheer et al., 2020). It is estimated that many more people with SMI engage in self-harming behaviours, which are strongly associated with substance use (Dharmawardene & Menkes, 2017).

Substance Use

People who experience SMI are at much higher risk for substance use than people in the general population (McKee, 2017). A person who

> ## RESEARCH HIGHLIGHT
> ### Using Mobile and Computer Devices to Support Recovery for People With SMI
>
> **Problem**
> Mental health recovery refers to an individual's experience of gaining a sense of personal control, striving towards one's life goals, and meeting one's needs. The capacity to recover can, and must be supported as part of care in the community, and the use of mobile and computer devices is one tool to support recovery capacities of people with SMI. Although people with SMI own and use electronic devices for general purposes, knowledge of their current use and interest in future use for supporting mental health recovery remains limited.
>
> **Purpose of Study**
> This study aimed to identify the smartphone, tablet, and computer apps that persons with SMI used or wanted to use to support their recovery.
>
> **Methods**
> This pilot study employed surveys to gather the perspectives and experiences of a convenience sample of 63 mental health service recipients with SMI. The survey assessed current use and interest in mobile and computer devices to support recovery.
>
> **Key Findings**
> Listening to music (60%), accessing the internet (59%), calling (59%), and texting (54%) people were the top functions currently used by participants on their device to support their recovery. Participants expressed interest in learning how to use apps for anxiety/stress management (45%), mood management (45%), monitoring mental health symptoms (43%), cognitive behavioral therapy (40%), sleep (38%), and dialectical behavior therapy (38%) to support their recovery.
>
> **Implications for Nursing Practice**
> The people with SMI surveyed predominantly used general functions such as listening to music and calling friends to support recovery. Nevertheless, they reported interest in trying more specific illness-management apps. Further study into ways and means apps can be applied to support service providers and people with SMI in building recovery should be further explored.
>
> **Source:** Noel, V. A., Acquilano, S. C., Carpenter-Song, E., et al. (2019). Use of mobile and computer devices to support recovery in people with serious mental illness: Survey study. *JMIR Mental Health*, *6*(2), e12255. https://doi.org/10.2196/12255

experiences both a mental health disorder and a substance use disorder is said to have a *concurrent disorder*. People with mental illnesses are twice as likely to have a substance use problem compared to the general population. It is estimated that 20% of people with a mental illness have a concurrent disorder, and the rate may be as high as 50% for people with schizophrenia. Similarly, those with substance use problems are three times as likely to have a mental illness as the general population. It is estimated that more than 15% of those with substance use disorders have a comorbid mental illness (Centre for Addiction and Mental Health, 2021b).

Substance use may be a form of self-medication, countering the dysphoria or other symptoms caused by illness or its treatment (e.g., the sedation caused by one's medications). Nicotine use has always been higher among those with SMI and is not declining as it has been in the general population, with many patients with SMI less responsive to smoking cessation programs than the general population (DeAtley et al., 2020). Substance use contributes to comorbid physical health problems, reduced quality of life, potential overdose or poisoning incarceration, relapse, and reduced effectiveness of medications (Centre for Addiction and Mental Health, 2021a, 2021b).

Social Problems

Stigma

Stigma has been described as negative attitudes or behaviours toward a person or group based on a belief that they possess negative traits (Gaebel et al., 2017). The MHCC (2012) reported that stigma and discrimination of all kinds "are the major reasons that mental health issues have remained in the shadows for so long" (pp. 22–23). Stigma stems from a lack of understanding of mental illness that causes others to make assumptions about those with SMI. Stigma can result in discrimination and cause shame, anger, and further isolation (Patten et al., 2016). Self or internalized stigma is associated with poor outcomes in patients with SMI, with over 30% of patients experiencing high levels of self-stigma (Dubreucq et al., 2021). Meeting and talking with someone with an SMI can help the general public to reduce their stigmatizing behaviours and attitudes toward people with SMIs. A recovery approach, group therapy, and peer support activities have all been found to combat self-stigma (Drapalski et al., 2021; Dubreucq et al., 2021).

Isolation and Loneliness

Social isolation and loneliness are concerns of many people with chronic illnesses, not just those with SMI (Leigh-Hunt et al., 2017). Stigma reduces the social contact of persons with SMI, and individual factors such as poor self-image, poverty (which interferes with recreational and social activities), passivity, and impaired hygiene may also interfere with relationships. Romantic relationships and opportunities for sexual expression, usually desired among persons with SMI just as in any population, are also affected by isolation (and often by sexual dysfunction from medications). Community connection and service access has been strengthened through technology and social networking opportunities while at the same time increasing social pressure and stigma (Naslund et al., 2019). Highlighting the importance of social connectedness, definitions of community for people with SMI were found by Pahwa and colleagues to encompass a structural aspect of people and places; a functional aspect of socializing, helping and receiving resources; and an experiential aspect of shared struggles and experiences, finding safety, and identifying with others (Pahwa et al., 2021).

Victimization

Stereotypes would have us believe that people with SMI are more likely to be violent than people who do not have mental illness. However, the reverse is actually true: mentally ill people are more likely to be victims of violence than perpetrators of it (Centre for Addiction and Mental Health, 2020). Sexual assault or coerced sexual activity also commonly occurs within this vulnerable population. Impaired judgement, impaired interpersonal skills (e.g., unknowingly acting in ways that might provoke others, such as standing too close or not leaving when told to), passivity, poor self-esteem, dependency, residence in high-crime neighbourhoods, and an appearance of vulnerability may contribute to this significant problem.

Economic Challenges

Unemployment and Poverty

Most people derive at least part of their identity and sense of value from the work they do. Many people with SMI would like to work, but symptoms such as cognitive slowing or disorganization interfere with obtaining or succeeding at work. According to the MHCC (2017), between 70% and 90% of people with SMI are unemployed, and 50% of those with SMI do not receive sufficient income from their disability entitlements. It can be difficult to find an employer open to hiring a person with SMI, and laws to prevent discrimination do not guarantee a job. Further, workplaces are sites that must address social determinants of mental health with physically and psychologically safe environments that enable people to be and stay well (Compton & Shim, 2020). Among many workplace mental health initiatives, the MHCC has developed a free online training program about psychological health and safety in the workplace (Canadian Centre for Occupational Health and Safety, 2021), see the Evolve resources for more information.

Atypical antipsychotic medications can be extremely expensive. Each province administers its own prescription drug plan, and patients with SMI may be able to obtain coverage under these plans. However, not every medication is covered. Because people with SMI are less likely to be employed, they are less likely to have employee health benefits to cover the additional costs of medication if they are not supported by a disability benefit. In addition to the challenges of obtaining pharmacological treatment, in many cases those with SMI do not have health benefits available to cover treatment from other non-publicly paid mental health care providers (e.g., psychologists), which may be a significant barrier to mental health treatment in Canada (Dezetter et al., 2015). On their own, community mental health programs and social support programs cannot sufficiently address the conditions of poverty in which many people with SMI find themselves. Advocates for universal basic income and widespread social justice directives and chance take up these challenges (Sylvestre et al., 2018).

Housing Instability

Even though stable, safe, and affordable housing is very important for people living with SMI, homelessness is unfortunately prevalent (Kerman et al., 2018). Many people with SMI have limited funds, which equates to limited options for housing. Obtaining an affordable apartment may require one to live far from needed resources (e.g., stores, health care centres, support persons) or in unsafe neighbourhoods. An episode of behaviour deemed inappropriate could lead to eviction and a negative reputation among landlords, closing doors to future housing. Living with family can produce interpersonal strains and conflict about patient behaviour (e.g., non-adherence, impaired self-care), which in turn often lead to estrangement and loss of housing with family.

Symptoms can cause behaviour that leads to police arrest. For example, one patient asked a store clerk if he could pay him later for a bottle of pop and, thinking concretely, mistook the clerk's sarcastic "Oh, sure" as genuine approval, only to leave with the pop and find himself charged with theft an hour later. A single bad decision caused an arrest that could leave the person ineligible for housing subsidies or public housing. Even with a subsidy, however, waiting lists can be up to 2 years long. Finding and keeping good housing can be very challenging for these patients.

Caregiver Burden

Caregivers, particularly family members, provide important support for people with SMI. However, coping with the persistent and challenging needs of people with SMI can be extremely challenging and requires significant emotional, physical, and, at times, financial resources. Caregivers also age, become ill, and may require care themselves, depleting their ability to provide support for the person with SMI. When caregivers are no longer able to provide the needed support for the person with SMI, a very difficult adjustment can result, leading to crises such as homelessness, conflict between caregiver and patient, and even exacerbation of the SMI symptoms.

Treatment Issues

Non-adherence

At any point in time, nearly half of all people with mental illness are not receiving treatment or are non-adherent to treatment, thereby potentially increasing the likelihood of relapse (Velligan et al., 2017). Most health care providers address this problem with medication education, but patients faced with repetitive medication groups and exhortations to take medications often become more resistant rather than insightful. Other obstacles, such as adverse effects, drug costs, interruptions in treatment, and rotating treatment providers, increase the risk for non-adherence and threaten stability and prognosis. The underlying shame from stigma, self-stigma, and cultural beliefs also plays an important role in non-adherence (Albassam et al., 2017). Box 29.1 describes nursing interventions that promote adherence.

Anosognosia

Many people assume that people with mental illness who do not understand that they are mentally ill must be in denial (i.e., they know they are ill but cannot accept it). Although denial is a possibility, another is *anosognosia* (ă-nō′sog-nō′sē-ă), the inability to recognize one's deficits due to one's illness. Anosognosia is a lack of awareness of neurological and neuropsychological deficits associated with frontotemporal-parietal damage, observed in some patients with dementia or who have had a stroke. There is some evidence linking the phenomenon to the core pathophysiology of schizophrenia, which justifies extension of the construct of anosognosia to schizophrenia-related insight deficits. What is known is that individuals who do not understand that their positive symptoms are illness related will find it difficult to recognize that they have an illness. Others may believe or hope that the illness will go away on its own (Little, 2021). People who do not perceive themselves to be mentally ill are unlikely to seek or accept treatment. It can take months or years for a person with SMI to acknowledge having a mental illness. The best approach of mental health nurses should be empathic, supportive, and focused on harm reduction rather than punitive (Weiden, 2016).

It is important for mental health nurses to listen and assess carefully where there may be high risk or potential for harm to self or others and to build a trusting helping relationship to support safety and optimal recovery. For others, who are functioning and may simply hold understandings of their distress or preferences that differ from the medical approach to treatment, assessment and support must be provided through building trust and understanding.

Medication Adverse Effects

Psychotropic medications, especially antipsychotic medications, can produce a range of distressing adverse effects, from involuntary movements to increased risk for diabetes. Some adverse effects are treatable; others may diminish over time or can be compensated for via behavioural changes (e.g., changing position slowly to reduce dizziness from hypotension). Addressing adverse effects in an evidence-informed, humble, and honest manner is essential to gaining an understanding of a patient's situation and struggles with diagnosis, treatment, and adverse effects. While newer medications have fewer adverse effects and people increasingly respond well to medication, psychiatric drugs can sometimes induce or exacerbate illness or create new problems, and adverse effects are a key reason for non-adherence (Lincoln et al., 2016).

Some people with schizophrenia may pursue alternative treatments or select to refrain from long-term psychiatric medication use. Some patients with strong support networks and insight into potential triggers of relapse fare better than others, but it is the work of careful and attentive professionals to ensure that those who are most at risk for non-adherence are supported and that their safety is secured.

The approach of motivational interviewing is suggested as a way to explore the acceptance and commitment of individuals and to assess readiness for participating more actively in the treatment. Motivational interviewing can also be employed to develop strategies for obstacles specific to symptoms of schizophrenia, such as cognitive deficits and negative symptoms with associated motivational problems (Yıldız & Aylaz, 2020). Research Highlight: Motivational Interviewing and Medication Adherence describes recent research validating this approach. Regardless of therapeutic strategies or approaches, a strong helping relationship can support understanding and perhaps a realistic and sustained treatment that can promote equilibrium and recovery and maximize quality of life (Dobber et al., 2018). See Chapter 9 for more on the therapeutic relationship and Chapter 11 for a detailed discussion of antipsychotic medications.

Treatment Inadequacy

It has been suggested that there are significant gaps between the quality of mental health care provided and optimal care (Treichler et al., 2021). Often discontinuation of treatment is precipitated by poor treatment response and inadequate follow-up or fragmented care. Patients must be informed and diligent in ensuring that they are receiving the most effective treatment, and agencies and staff must be diligent in updating their programs and practice. A strong therapeutic alliance and commitment to a recovery model are pivotal in staying the course

---

BOX 29.1 Interventions to Improve Adherence to Treatment

- Select treatments and dosages that are most likely to be effective and well tolerated by each patient.
- Actively manage adverse effects to avert or minimize patient distress, which could result in non-adherence.
- Simplify treatment regimens to make them more acceptable and understandable to the patient (e.g., once-a-day dosing instead of twice-daily dosing).
- Tie treatment adherence to achieving the patient's goals to increase motivation. Point out and reinforce improvements, connecting them to treatment adherence.
- To improve patient insight and motivation, provide **psychoeducation** (an approach to care that emphasizes helping a person to gain the knowledge necessary to manage the illness) about SMI and the role of treatment in recovery. Take care not to assume that non-adherence means that the patient does not understand. There are many reasons for non-adherence; applying psychoeducation when the problem is something other than a lack of knowledge is unlikely to succeed.
- Assign consistent, committed caregivers who have (or are skilled at building) positive therapeutic bonds with the patient and who will be able to work with the patient for extended periods of time.
- Involve the patient in support groups with members who have greater insight and first-hand experience with illness and treatment—people whose viewpoints the patient may be more likely to accept.
- Provide culturally safe, trauma-informed care. Cultural beliefs and practices (e.g., suspicious attitudes or traumatic histories with health care and authority figures, valuing self-sufficiency or privacy above health care) can be a barrier to therapeutic relationships and result in rejection of treatment.
- Carefully monitor medication decreases or changes to control adverse effects and improve the therapeutic effect.
- When other interventions have not been successful, use medication monitoring, long-acting forms of medication (depot injections or sustained-release formats), motivational interviewing, and other techniques as indicated to increase adherence.
- Never reject, blame, or shame the patient when non-adherence occurs. Instead, label it as simply an issue for continuing focus, and work toward harm reduction.

SMI, Serious mental illness. **Sources:** Weiden, P. J. (2016). Redefining medication adherence in the treatment of schizophrenia: How current approaches to adherence lead to misinformation and threaten therapeutic relationships. *The Psychiatric Clinics of North America, 39*(2), 199.

RESEARCH HIGHLIGHT
Motivational Interviewing and Medication Adherence

Problem
Non-adherence to antipsychotic medication is common among patients and contributes to high relapse rates. Little is known, however, about interventions to support medication adherence.

Purpose of Study
This study was designed to test and evaluate the effectiveness of an adherence therapy for outpatients with schizophrenia spectrum disorders, based on a motivational interviewing approach over a 6-month follow-up period.

Methods
A single-blind, randomized controlled trial with a repeated-measures, two-parallel-groups design was conducted using a random sample of 114 participants with schizophrenia spectrum disorders in one community psychiatric nursing service. After pre-test, the participants were randomly assigned to either an eight-session course of motivational interviewing treatment plus usual care or usual psychiatric care alone (n = 57 per group). The main outcomes, including medication adherence, symptom severity, insight into treatment, hospitalization rate, and functioning, were measured at baseline and 1 to 3 times in the 6 months after intervention.

Key Findings
A total of 110 participants completed this trial, with an attrition rate of 3.5%. Results indicated that the treatment participants reported significantly greater improvements in their insight into illness or treatment, psychosocial functioning, symptom severity, number of rehospitalizations, and medication adherence over a 6-month follow-up, when compared with usual care.

Implications for Nursing Practice
Motivational interviewing approaches for people with schizophrenia can be effective to reduce symptom severity and rehospitalizations and to improve medication adherence, functioning, and insight into illness or treatment over a medium-term (6 months) period of follow-up.

Source: Chien, W. T., Mui, J. H. C., Cheung, E. F. C., et al. (2015). Effects of motivational interviewing-based adherence therapy for schizophrenia spectrum disorders: A randomized controlled trial. *Trials, 16*(1), 270. https://doi.org/10.1186/s13063-015-0785-z

and persevering through setbacks, ineffective treatments, and patient choices (Browne et al., 2021).

Residual Symptoms

Residual symptoms are those that do not improve completely or consistently with treatment. They can be very frustrating, and patients may feel that these symptoms mean they will not get better or that treatments are not working (promoting helplessness and hopelessness). The patient may then discontinue treatment, worsening the illness. Residual symptoms can also cause or worsen associated issues (e.g., inappropriate social behaviour and impulsiveness that can add to stigmatization and isolation). Psychoeducation about both symptoms and treatment has been found to be effective in reducing stigma related to aspects of treatment (Choe et al., 2016).

Relapse, Chronicity, and Loss

The majority of patients with SMI face the possibility of relapse even when adhering to treatment, which may contribute to hopelessness and helplessness. Living with SMI paradoxically requires more effort and emotional resources from people who are less able to cope with such demands. Each relapse can cause loss of relationships, employment, and housing, adding that much more loss to the patient's life and making discharge planning significantly more complicated.

RESOURCES FOR PEOPLE WITH SERIOUS MENTAL ILLNESS

Comprehensive Community Treatment

Community services, particularly for those with SMI, have been described as fragmented and inefficient, with the blurring of responsibility among agencies, programs, and levels of government (Flood & Bryan, 2017). Ideally, the community-based mental health care system provides comprehensive, coordinated, and cost-effective (from the perspective of the government) care for the patient with mental illness; however, great chasms exist between the ideal and the actual (Treichler et al., 2021). Interventions at the individual, family, community, and societal or political levels must all be part of the complex coordination of all levels of prevention for those with SPMI.

The overall goal of community psychiatric treatment is to improve the patient's ability to function independently in the community. Community services vary according to local needs and resources. Patients sometimes find that needed services are not locally available or have long wait lists, and they may have difficulty identifying the best programs for their needs amid the maze of agencies and services. When people with SMI are unable to access community-based services, including stable housing, they experience poorer quality of life and are often forced to rely on institution-based care (Harrison et al., 2020; Kerman & Sylvestre, 2020).

Community Services and Programs

A case-management program is a comprehensive service provided by a multi-disciplinary team. The team coordinates the patient's overall care, brokers access to services, and provides psychosocial education, guidance, and support (Dieterich et al., 2017). Case managers can provide medication monitoring, wherein they observe and facilitate the patient's use of medications. Intensive case management has been strongly linked to improved consumer engagement, psychological functioning, and adaptation to the demands of everyday living

> **VIGNETTE**
>
> After 3 years of living on his own, Christopher (who uses the pronouns he/him) returns home to his parents. He is soon arrested for threatening a police officer with a steel pipe, is found "not criminally responsible," and is released on the condition that he receive psychiatric treatment. Because of his history of non-adherence, he goes to a clinic and receives intramuscular depot medication. He is also enrolled in a day program and is assigned a case manager, who helps him apply for income assistance and refers him to a group home when his aging parents state that he can no longer live with them. Because Christopher wants to work, referral is made to a supported-employment program. A job with a park trail maintenance team is assigned, and Christopher stays in that job for the next 5 years. When the requirements of the conditional release are completed, Christopher continues in treatment and continues working nearly full time with another park maintenance team who value all his experience and skills. He met a volunteer in the park with whom he now has a supportive relationship. Because the illness is now stabilized, Christopher's medication is changed to an oral atypical antipsychotic that treats both his positive and negative symptoms of schizophrenia very effectively. Also supporting the recovery plan, Christopher continues to receive the structure and social support of the group home living situation. On many days, Christopher and his family would say he is not just stable, but recovered!

(Fink-Samnick, 2021). Assertive community treatment (ACT), discussed later in this chapter, is one model of case management. Other community services and programs that may be available include social skills training, crisis intervention services, emergency psychiatric services, and community outreach programs.

Substance Use Treatment

A variety of services exist for those who have a concurrent diagnosis of SMI and substance use disorders. Therapeutic and rehabilitative services, including medical and psychosocial assessment, detoxification, crisis intervention, and medication administration such as methadone clinics and safe consumption sites. Most clinicians endorse treatment that is integrated (i.e., delivered by a single provider rather than split between a mental health agency and a drug or alcohol agency), using personnel with dual areas of expertise, though this standard has not yet been met in some settings (Centre for Addiction and Mental Health, 2021b). See Chapter 18 for a detailed discussion of treatment settings for patients with substance use disorders and concurrent disorders.

EVIDENCE-INFORMED TREATMENT APPROACHES

Assertive Community Treatment

ACT is an approach to caring for the person with severe mental illness in the community. ACT teams provide multi-disciplinary, comprehensive, and, in some cases intensive treatment services. The ACT model of care is a structure of treatment and rehabilitative and supportive services that enhance the ability of the person with SMI to live successfully in the community. ACT serves individuals who have not been able to successfully manage their illnesses in traditional outpatient or rehabilitation services. Key principles of ACT include maintaining small patient-to-staff ratios, engaging in a proactive approach, and establishing highly individualized treatment plans. ACT has been shown to improve symptoms of SMI and reduce inpatient admissions, incarceration, and homelessness among persons with mental illness in phased transition to less assertive care as needed, for both urban and rural communities, and during the COVID-19 crisis (Law et al., 2021; LeFebvre et al., 2018).

Cognitive Behavioural Therapy and Meta-cognitive Therapy

Cognitive behavioural therapy (CBT) has been shown to be effective in helping patients with SMI to cope with symptoms such as auditory hallucinations or hypomania, to address defeating beliefs and self-stigma,

> **SAFETY TIP**
>
> **Safety on the Streets During COVID-19**
>
> The COVID-19 pandemic has highlighted the reality that most patients receiving ACT live in deep poverty, many dwelling in "tent cities," homeless, or in cycles of unstable housing in Canadian cities where disability benefits cannot afford even basic shared accommodations. The safety of ACT teams and shelter staff was also illuminated during the pandemic. This highlights the ongoing need for systemic level advocacy for the safety and social justice to improve income and increase housing opportunities, and ensure sufficient community and clinical supports during and post-pandemic.
>
> **Source:** Mental Health Commission of Canada. (2021). *COVID-19, mental wellness, and the homelessness workforce*. Ottawa: Mental Health Commission of Canada. Retrieved from https://www.mentalhealthcommission.ca/wp-content/uploads/drupal/2021-07/covid_mental_wellness_homelessness_workforce_eng.pdf

> **VIGNETTE**
>
> Christopher, now age 50, has schizophrenia. He has lived in a group home since his late twenties. He has been stable for the past 10 years and has had a steady girlfriend for the past 3 years. He announces that he wants to move out on his own and maybe get married. Despite respectful disagreement from his nurse therapist, he finds himself a room to rent. Over the next 2 months, his mental status remains stable: he is polite, quiet, and guarded as usual. However, his psychiatrist, who weighs him monthly, notices that he has lost 10 kg. Christopher cannot identify any change in his eating habits, and he is referred to his primary care provider for an evaluation. He does not follow up with the primary care provider, and over the next 4 weeks, he loses another 5 kg. Christopher's nurse therapist calls his work supervisor, who reports that Christopher is behaving differently: he is talking out loud to himself, becoming more isolated, and, one morning, smelled of alcohol. She is supportive of Christopher and hopes he will get treatment. At his next clinic appointment, the psychiatrist and therapist discuss these changes and recommend that Christopher go into the partial hospital program for medication re-evaluation. He reluctantly agrees, denying that he has any problem.

and to contemplate recovery (Kukla et al., 2021; Leopold et al., 2020). The cognitive component of CBT focuses on patterns of thinking and "self-talk" (i.e., what one says to oneself internally). It identifies cognitive distortions and guides patients to substitute more effective forms of thinking. The behavioural component of CBT uses natural consequences and positive reinforcers to shape the person's behaviour in a more positive or adaptive manner. While research suggests that many with schizophrenia experience deficits in metacognition, and that while these deficits are tied to poorer treatment outcomes, metacognitive and insight-oriented therapy, may support personally meaningful recovery if matched with engaged patients and trained therapists and in some self-direct reflective, insight activities (Lysaker et al., 2018).

Family Support and Partnerships

Families and significant others can face considerable stresses related to the mental illness of a loved one and may suffer as a result of insufficient empathy and understanding (Brown & Weisman de Mamani, 2018). Having sound family support and partnerships is one of the strongest predictors of recovery; treatment is enhanced and conflict is reduced when treatment providers work as empathic partners with both patients and their significant others. Family members themselves need support to be able to serve in roles they identify as unique from other social or community supports. The roles are identified as support directly to the person in terms of material or physical needs, support for individuals to remain autonomous, support to participate in community, support to manage health, and day-to-day living support (Chronister et al., 2021). The Canadian Mental Health Association (CMHA) partners with a variety of public and private agencies to provide family support programs that are tailored to the specific needs of a community or region. Provincial branches of the CMHA serve as an excellent source of information, support, and practical guidance for patients and their significant others.

Social Skills Training

Social skills training focuses on the teaching of a wide variety of social and activities of daily living (ADLs) skills. People with SMI often have social deficits that cause functional impairment; for example, those unable to respond assertively may respond aggressively instead. Complex interpersonal skills, such as negotiating or resolving a conflict, are broken down into subcomponents, which are then taught in a step-by-step fashion. This therapy has been found to be beneficial for enhanced recovery and in supporting housing stability (Gabrielian et al., 2019; Isaacs et al., 2019).

Supportive Psychotherapy and Peer Support

Although definitions vary, supportive psychotherapy is generally understood to be an approach that stresses empathic understanding, a non-judgemental attitude, and the development of a therapeutic alliance (Winston et al., 2020). Supportive psychotherapy has been shown to enhance the therapeutic alliance and improve long-term recovery prospects in patients with SMI (Battaglia, 2020). Numerous examples of peer support programs also exist for people with SMI (Fuhr et al., 2014). While few formal studies of impact exist, the sense of purpose and opportunity to give and receive understanding from a shared experience are well documented (Chien et al., 2019).

> **VIGNETTE**
>
> Christopher attends the partial hospital program for 4 weeks. In the first week the nurse calls the therapist to report that he is severely paranoid: he will not eat or drink out of any open containers and is observed spitting out his pills. His medication is changed to a quickly disintegrating tablet form. He attends groups that focus on education about medication, chronic illness, substance use, and healthy habits. He begins to eat normally, gaining 2 kg in 2 weeks. Finally, he admits that he had not taken any medication since he moved out of his group home.
>
> The discharge plan is referral to the psychosocial program again for structure and case management to assist him with finding a new home, medical care, and eventual return to work, with a biweekly medication injection and supportive group therapy. Over the next 3 months, Christopher gradually returns to his baseline level of functioning. His case manager finds him another group home with his previous caregiver. He returns to work 2 days per week and attends the day program 3 days per week. Christopher never is able to identify the trigger for his relapse, but his nurse therapist now observes his physical status more closely and inquires specifically about his work and social activities at each session.

Vocational Rehabilitation and Related Services

Vocational rehabilitation and related services vary widely but can include vocational training, financial support for attaining employment, or supported-employment services. Like most people, those with SMI want to feel as though they contribute and therefore want to be engaged in meaningful employment (Reid et al., 2020). The benefits of employment (or volunteer work) are enhanced self-esteem, improved organizational abilities, and increased socialization and income.

Vocational rehabilitation programs using a clubhouse model, in which patients jointly run their own business, such as a coffee shop or housekeeping service, teach all members to perform a job in order to make the business work. Such programs have led to the supported-employment model, which has been shown to be one of the most effective evidence-informed interventions for helping people with SMI to achieve employment. The model includes rapid job placement, on-the-job support, and provision of a job coach who is linked to the mental health team (Suijkerbuijk et al., 2017).

OTHER POTENTIALLY BENEFICIAL SERVICES OR TREATMENT APPROACHES

While not yet evidence-informed practices, research to date supports the use of the following services and treatment approaches.

Consumer-Run Programs

The CMHA and other organizations offer training that enables consumers to assist peers in the recovery process. Consumer-run programs range from informal "clubhouses," which offer socialization, recreation, and sometimes other services, such as educational programs, to competitive businesses, which are often part of a vocational rehabilitation program.

Wellness and Recovery Action Plans

Wellness and recovery action plans and similar programs are psycho-educational programs that empower and train patients in skills that promote recovery and prepare them to deal with stressors and crises (Petros & Solomon, 2020). Training focuses on daily maintenance plans (i.e., things that must be done and resources needed to maintain wellness), identification and management of triggers that could provoke a relapse, early identification of impending relapse, and crisis plans (i.e., plans for managing crises or impending relapse). Typically, a wide variety of useful tools, templates, and techniques are provided, and the programs lead to developing practical and concrete action plans for promoting recovery.

Exercise

Exercise holds many benefits for persons with SMI, including improved activity tolerance and ability to cope with symptoms, reduced anxiety and depression, enhanced self-esteem, weight control or loss (important for patients with weight-related comorbidities, such as diabetes and hypertension), as well as key social and community connectedness needs (Quirk et al., 2017; Snethen et al., 2021).

NURSING CARE OF PATIENTS WITH SERIOUS MENTAL ILLNESS

Nurses encounter patients with SMI in a variety of inpatient and community settings. All roles and techniques used by psychiatric mental health nurses in inpatient psychiatric settings also apply in the community and other settings.

Assessment Strategies

Important assessments include:
- Signs of risk to self or others (suicidality or homicidality)
- Depression or hopelessness
- Signs of relapse (especially increased impulsivity or paranoia, diminished reality testing, increased delusional thinking or command hallucinations)
- Inadequate attention to proper nutrition, adequate clothing or medical care, and carelessness while driving, smoking, or cooking (e.g., leaving pots on the stove and becoming distracted or falling asleep)
- Signs of treatment non-adherence or impending relapse (early detection and correction of relapse reduces its intensity and duration and prevents hospitalization, loss of housing, arrest, and loss of entitlements)
- Physical health problems, such as brain tumours or drug toxicity, that can cause psychiatric symptoms and be mistaken for mental illness or relapse
- Comorbid illnesses (ensuring that the patient provides appropriate self-care and receives adequate health care)

Table 29.1 lists potential nursing diagnoses that apply to the patient with SMI. Table 29.2 lists examples of specific nursing outcomes.

Intervention Strategies

Basic nursing interventions for patients with SMI include:
- Empowering the patient by involving them in goal setting and treatment selection increases the likelihood of treatment adherence and success.
- Emphasizing quality-of-life issues conveys an interest in the person (rather than in the illness) and reflects the patient's best interests (rather than the staff's preferences).

TABLE 29.1 Potential Nursing Diagnoses for the Patient With Serious Mental Illness

Signs and Symptoms	Nursing Diagnoses
Speaking too softly to be heard	Communication, impaired verbal
Verbalization incongruent with the setting	Social interaction, impaired
Silence in groups or withdrawal when approached	Social isolation
Failure to keep appointments	Non-adherence
Admitted missing of medication or observed return of symptoms	
Self-negating verbalization	Chronic low self-esteem
Fear of trying new things or situations	Powerlessness
Non-assertiveness or passivity	
Distortion of patient's health problem, often denial	Disabled family coping
Neglect of other members of family	Caregiver role strain
Excessive concern for and supervision of patient	

TABLE 29.2 NOC Outcomes Related to Serious Mental Illness

Nursing Outcome and Definition	Intermediate Indicators	Short-Term Indicators
Self-care: Instrumental activities of daily living (IADL): Ability to perform activities needed to function independently in the home or community, with or without assistive device	Manages medications Manages money	Shops for groceries Prepares meals Uses phone Travels on public transportation
Family coping: Family actions to manage stressors that tax family resources	Uses available social support Cares for needs of all members	Involves family members in decision making Establishes family priorities Plans for emergencies

NOC, Nursing Outcomes Classification.
Source: Moorhead, S., Johnson, M., Maas, M. L., et al. (2018). *Nursing Outcomes Classification (NOC): Measurement of health outcomes* (6th ed.). St Louis: Mosby.

- Developing and maintaining relationships are keys to overcoming anosognosia and achieving treatment adherence. People with SMI often require extended periods of working with staff to form these connections.
- Supportive psychotherapy aids in maintaining therapeutic rapport and helps the patient to maintain positive self-esteem and cope effectively.
- Impaired reality testing is the hallmark of SMI and contributes to hallucinations and delusional thinking. Encouraging the patient to seek independent information on whether experiences are real or not can help the patient to identify these experiences as part of the illness and respond accordingly.
- SMIs predispose people to isolation due to stigma, impaired social skills, and social discomfort. Isolation contributes to loneliness and reduces access to support. Activities that increase skill and comfort with interaction, reduce aloneness, or provide opportunities for socialization (especially with supportive persons and positive role models, such as other patients who are further along in recovery) contribute to improved functioning and a higher quality of life.
- Support groups such as the Schizophrenia Society of Canada expose the patient to members who "have been there." In addition to providing support and socialization opportunities, such groups often have practical suggestions for issues and problems that patients and significant others face. Involvement in support groups is often empowering for the patient.
- Education and reinforcement are essential, since SMI may result in impaired judgement, desperation for connectedness, or other vulnerabilities that increase the risk for victimization, sexually transmitted infections, and undesired pregnancies.
- Care for the whole person is especially important with SMI patients, who have higher burdens of physical illness, poorer hygiene and health practices, less access to effective medical treatment, and more pre-mature mortality than the general population. Exercise has also been found to reduce cardiometabolic risk, negative symptoms, and cognitive deficits, which often go untreated in patients with SMI (Firth et al., 2015).
- Involving people with co-occurring substance use in Alcoholics Anonymous or Narcotics Anonymous and other services for people with concurrent disorders is important, since substance use rates are high in SMI populations, and misuse increases relapse and interferes with recovery.

Box 29.2 outlines two relevant *Nursing Interventions Classification (NIC)* interventions for the management of SMI (Butcher et al., 2019).

BOX 29.2 NIC Interventions for Serious Mental Illness Self-Care Assistance: IADL

Definition of self-care assistance: IADL*:* Assisting and instructing a person to perform instrumental activities of daily living (IADL) needed to function in the home or community

Activities:
- Instruct individual on appropriate and safe storage of medications.
- Instruct individual on alternative methods of transportation (e.g., buses and bus schedules, taxis, city or county transportation for disabled people).
- Assist individual in establishing methods and routines for cooking, cleaning, and shopping.

Family Support
Definition of family support*:* Promotion of family values, interests, and goals
Activities[a]:
- Listen to family concerns, feelings, and questions.
- Accept the family's values in a non-judgemental manner.
- Identify congruence between patient, family, and health professional expectations.

[a]Partial list.
NIC, Nursing Interventions Classification.
Source: Butcher, H. K., Bulechek, G. M., Dochterman, J. M., et al. (2019). *Nursing Interventions Classification (NIC)* (7th ed.). Elsevier.

Evaluation

Identified outcomes serve as the basis for evaluation. Each *Nursing Outcomes Classification (NOC)* outcome has a built-in rating scale (immediate, short-term, and potentially long-term indicators) that helps the nurse to measure improvement.

CURRENT ISSUES

Population Health & Social Justice Approaches

Public and population mental health is the state of psychological and emotional well-being at the population level and among different groups of people. Interventions that can support mental well-being at this scale require social system and policy level implementation. The intersection of social justice and human rights with public health and population mental health approaches is established, although, as yet, minimally resourced and implemented, internationally (Hoffman et al., 2016). Actions taken at the community and systems levels, such as anti-racism policy, and income supports, are none-the-less having positive effects at the personal level. The challenge is to translate this potential into consistent, effective, and measurable actions by all levels of government to meet the needs of all living in Canada (CPHA, 2021).

Involuntary Treatment

Involuntary treatment involves treatment mandated by a court and delivered without the patient's consent. Traditionally, this situation involved involuntary inpatient admissions, but beginning in the 1990s, provinces began to experiment with community treatment orders (CTOs), which provide mandatory treatment in a less restrictive setting than involuntary psychiatric settings. It has been suggested that implementation of a CTO may be preferable to involuntary hospitalization and support some aspects of recovery within treatment (Francombe Pridham et al., 2018). Challenges exist with implementation; for example, the renewal process has been found to be overly complicated and conflicts between and among colleagues about the process are widespread. Further, a recovery-oriented approach requires a trusting therapeutic relationship and the coercion inherent in the CTO process can interrupt the trust building, development, and ongoing relationship so vital to recovery. Detrimental effects on therapeutic relationships have been described in Canada and elsewhere in relation to CTOs (Corring et al., 2018a, 2018b; McMillan et al., 2019). Despite some of the challenges of mandated treatment, it was found in Quebec that the average time the patients with SMI spent in the community and outside the hospital was significantly longer under a CTO, and the duration of hospitalizations was decreased (Frank et al., 2020). On balance, the value and benefits for supporting stable medication and supervision are described by professional practitioners as worthwhile, with future evaluation and procedural modifications desired (Corring et al., 2018a, 2018b). Mindful of the potential challenges and harms, nurses can work with a harm reduction focus, focus on patient goals in relation to CTO processes, and engage with patients to maintain trust when CTOs are part of the care they provide (McMillan et al., 2019).

Criminal Offences and Incarceration

In Canada the number of incarcerated offenders with mental illness continues to increase and the transition from incarceration to community mental health care can prove challenging (Murphy et al., 2018). Trauma, the physically or emotionally harmful or threatening experiences that have long-term effects on functioning and well-being, is common among offenders, especially those who engage in self-injurious behaviour (Martin et al., 2017). Research from Correctional Services Canada (2015) over several years shows that 75% of female offenders in the criminal justice system had a lifetime or current mental illness and over 67% of offenders with a mental health disorder meet the criteria for at least one other mental health disorder (Brown et al., 2018). People with SMI may commit crimes out of desperation, impaired judgement, or impulsivity; most often they are non-violent crimes, such as disorderly conduct. Police may also become involved with patients who seem unable to care for themselves and cannot be persuaded to accept treatment but who do not meet the criteria for involuntary treatment (usually imminent danger to self or others). Consider a patient with impaired judgement who does not dress adequately for cold weather and spends time in laundromats and libraries for warmth, causing disruption. When expelled, the individual is at risk for hypothermia. In such cases the risk to self may not be "imminent," and therefore hospitalization may not be possible. Loved ones or police may then seek arrest simply to get the person off the street for their own safety.

Many advocates for people with mental illness feel that incarceration, even if considered "for the patient's safety," is ultimately harmful. Imprisonment can lead to victimization, increased hopelessness, relapse due to increased stress and isolation, or overstimulation. Also, mental health care in correctional settings is usually both expensive and inadequate, and a criminal record can reduce future access to housing or employment important to recovery. Advocates instead seek diversion from jail to clinical care (Centre for Addiction and Mental Health, 2020). Two interventions to achieve this end are:

1. Educating police so they can identify mental illness, distinguish it from criminal intent, and connect persons with SMI to help instead of jailing them.
2. Establishing mental health courts that are designed to intercept persons whose crimes are secondary to mental illness and that feature specially trained officials with the authority to order treatment instead of imprisonment.

KEY POINTS TO REMEMBER

- Patients with SMI suffer from multiple impairments in thinking, feeling, and interacting with others.
- The course of SMI involves exacerbations and remissions, as do many chronic medical illnesses.
- Coordinated, comprehensive community services help the SMI patient to function at their optimal level.
- People with SMI often suffer complications due to insufficient housing, non-adherence to treatment, comorbid medical or substance use problems, and the stigma of mental illness.
- The family and support systems play a major part in the care of many persons with SMI and should be included as much as possible in planning, education, and treatment activities.
- The recovery model stresses hope, strengths, quality of life, patient involvement as an active partner in treatment, and eventual recovery.
- Public and population mental health represents the state of psychological and emotional well-being at the population level and among different groups of people. Interventions at the social system and policy level can support mental wellness on this scale.

CRITICAL THINKING

1. John Yang, age 42, concurrently diagnosed with schizophrenia and alcohol and marijuana misuse, is brought to the clinic by his mother, Mrs. Yang. During this initial assessment, Mrs. Yang reports that she has been caring for her son at home since he was 15 years old; however, since recently moving to town, she is at a loss about what is available in the community. John has been prescribed haloperidol

(Haldol), but Mrs. Yang says that he rarely takes it because of muscle rigidity and sexual adverse effects. They have tried many of the traditional antipsychotic drugs without success.
   a. Given your understanding of the problems faced by a person with a severe mental illness, what are some areas of John's life you might want to explore in your assessment? Consider relationships, employment history, cognitive abilities, social skills, and behaviour. How would knowledge in these areas help your long-term planning?
   b. After you assess John's medication history, how can you be an advocate in terms of his non-adherence to traditional antipsychotics? What are some of the obstacles to adherence for a person with a concurrent disorder? What approach or change in treatment would offer the best chance of success?
   c. Of the resources mentioned in this chapter, which might be appropriate for John?
   d. Identify three basic aims of psychoeducation for John and his mother.
   e. What would recovery mean to John?
2. You are doing your clinical practicum course in a psychiatric inpatient unit where many of the patients are diagnosed with schizophrenia. Although you had been apprehensive about this course, you are surprised to realize that patients respond well to you and that you are fascinated by this specialty area and may consider it as a career. A fellow student remarks, "You must be crazy yourself to want to work with these people."
   a. What social problem is represented by this student's remark?
   b. Identify other social prejudices that have been significant problems in Canada. What responses were effective in reducing and eliminating their impact?
3. During your mental health rotation, you notice that there are several patients with other chronic physical illnesses. When assessing a person with serious mental illness (SMI), why is it important to include a comprehensive physical assessment?
4. Competitive employment is an important factor in recovering from a psychotic episode. Identify the factors related to work that contribute to its importance in recovering from mental illness.

CHAPTER REVIEW

1. A patient with schizophrenia does not feel that they need medication because "there is nothing wrong with me." This response is most likely an example of:
   a. Denial
   b. Projection
   c. Anosognosia
   d. Paranoid ideation
2. Sarah, a young woman with schizophrenia who has struggled with hygiene and other activities of daily living, has been on a 4-hour pass from the inpatient psychiatric unit. She is tearful and reports that when she sat down on the bus to return to the hospital, the woman she sat next to immediately moved to another seat. Which responses would most likely be therapeutic? **Select all that apply.**
   a. Acknowledge Sarah's distress, and remind her that dinner will be ready in 30 minutes so that she has time to settle in before eating.
   b. State, "You sound discouraged. Sometimes people who do not understand mental illness can be hurtful," and offer to sit with her.
   c. Advise Sarah that the woman's behaviour was simply rude and can be ignored because it is something people with mental illness have to get used to.
   d. Suggest to Sarah that perhaps her hygiene would benefit from improvement, and offer to help her improve her hygiene so that others will be less likely to reject her.
3. Christopher is a 25-year-old male who has been hospitalized three times for exacerbations of schizophrenia. Each time he was discharged, he became homeless and relapsed. Typically, he is very disorganized, does not spend his money responsibly, loses his housing when he does not pay the rent, and, in turn, cannot be located by his case manager, leading to treatment non-adherence and relapse. Which response would be most therapeutic in this situation?
   a. Advise Christopher that if he does not pay his rent, he will be placed in a group home instead of independent housing.
   b. Discuss with Christopher the option of having a guardian who will ensure that the rent is paid and that his money is managed to meet his basic needs.
   c. Suggest to Christopher's prescribing clinician that he be prescribed a long-acting injectable form of antipsychotic medication to address the issue of treatment non-adherence.
   d. Encourage Christopher's case manager to hold him responsible for the outcomes of his poor decisions by allowing such periods of homelessness to serve as a natural consequence.
4. Pia has experienced repeated episodes of severe depression and mania. These episodes and related hospitalizations have disrupted her full-time employment and created discord within her marriage. She argues with the outpatient staff about medications, does not believe that she has a mental illness, and, although she takes her medications while hospitalized, stops taking them after discharge. She will be discharged in 2 weeks. Which intervention is most likely to increase her adherence to medications?
   a. Advise Pia that she will be assigned to new outpatient staff to reduce the conflicts she is experiencing with her current providers.
   b. Explain to Pia that the medications will help her and that all medications have adverse effects she can learn to live with in time.
   c. Involve Pia in a medication education group that will help her learn the types and names of psychotropic medications, their purpose, and possible adverse effects.
   d. Explore with Pia her perceptions of the medications and her experiences with them, and guide her to connect the use of the medications with achieving her goals.
5. Which interventions would be appropriate to promote recovery for persons with serious mental illness (SMI) who live in the community? **Select all that apply.**
   a. Meet regularly with the patients, and encourage them to make steady progress toward complete independence.
   b. Introduce patients to others with similar illnesses, and encourage participation in social activities with peers.
   c. Support the development of advance directives and involvement in social and employment activities run by other patients.
   d. Use public transportation to take patients to a museum, and share a nutritious dinner with them at an inexpensive restaurant.
   e. Instruct them to develop written plans that identify resources to maintain stability and steps to take when faced with unusual stressors.
   f. Over time, guide the patients to identify and switch to sources of support outside the family to reduce dependence on their loved ones as their primary support resource.

https://evolve.elsevier.com/Canada/Varcarolis/psychiatric/

REFERENCES

Adame, A. L., Morsey, M., Bassman, R., et al. (2017). A brief history of the psychiatric survivor movement. In A. L. Adame, M. Morsey, & R. Bassman, et al. (Eds.), *Exploring identities of psychiatric survivor therapists* (pp. 33–53). London: Palgrave Macmillan. https://doi.org/10.1057/978-1-137-58492-2_2

Albassam, A., Ameen, A., Chiappetta, V., et al. (2017). The impact of shame and cultural beliefs on mental illness and treatment adherence: A case report. *European Psychiatry, 41*(S1), S511. https://doi.org/10.1016/j.eurpsy.2017.01.660

Alegría, M., NeMoyer, A., Falgàs Bagué, I., et al. (2018). Social determinants of mental health: Where we are and where we need to go. *Current Psychiatry Reports, 20*(11), 1–13. https://doi.org/10.1007/s11920-018-0969-9

Battaglia, J. (2020). *Doing supportive psychotherapy*. American Psychiatric Association Publishing.

Brown, G. P., Stewart, L. A., Rabinowitz, T., Boudreau, H., & Wright, A. J. (2018). Approved and off-label use of prescribed psychotropic medications among federal Canadian inmates. *Canadian Journal of Psychiatry, 63*, 683–691. https://doi.org/10.1177/0706743718773734

Brown, C. A., & Weisman de Mamani, A. (2018). The mediating effect of family cohesion in reducing patient symptoms and family distress in a culturally informed family therapy for schizophrenia: A parallel-process latent-growth model. *Journal of Consulting and Clinical Psychology, 86*(1), 1–14. https://doi.org/10.1037/ccp0000257

Browne, J., Wright, A. C., Berry, K., et al. (2021). The alliance-outcome relationship in individual psychosocial treatment for schizophrenia and early psychosis: A meta-analysis. *Schizophrenia Research, 231*, 154–163. https://doi.org/10.1016/j.schres.2021.04.002

Butcher, H. K., Bulechek, G. M., Dochterman, J. M., et al. (2019). *Nursing Interventions Classification (NIC)* (7th ed.). Elsevier.

Canadian Centre for Occupational Health and Safety. (2021). *Being a mindful employee: An orientation to psychological health and safety in the workplace (free online course)*. Retrieved from https://www.ccohs.ca/products/courses/mindful_employee/

Canadian Public Health Association. (2021). *Advocacy/position statements: A public health approach to population mental wellness*. Retrieved from https://www.cpha.ca/public-health-approach-population-mental-wellness

Centre for Addiction and Mental Health. (2020). *Mental health and criminal justice policy framework*. Retrieved from https://www.camh.ca/-/media/files/pdfs-public-policy-submissions/camh-cj-framework-2020-pdf.pdf

Centre for Addiction and Mental Health. (2021a). *Mental illness and addictions: Facts and statistics*. Retrieved from https://www.camh.ca/en/driving-change/the-crisis-is-real/mental-health-statistics

Centre for Addiction and Mental Health. (2021b). *Concurrent disorders*. Retrieved from https://www.camh.ca/en/health-info/mental-illness-and-addiction-index/concurrent-disorders

Chien, W. T., Clifton, A. V., Zhao, S., et al. (2019). Peer support for people with schizophrenia or other serious mental illness. *The Cochrane Database of Systematic Reviews, 2019*(4), CD010880. https://doi.org/10.1002/14651858.CD010880.pub2

Choe, K., Sung, B., Kang, Y., et al. (2016). Impact of psychoeducation on knowledge of and attitude toward medications in clients with schizophrenia and schizoaffective disorders. *Perspectives in Psychiatric Care, 52*(2), 113–119. https://doi.org/10.1111/ppc.12106

Chronister, J., Fitzgerald, S., & Chou, C. C. (2021). The meaning of social support for persons with serious mental illness: A family member perspective. *Rehabilitation Psychology, 66*(1), 87–101. https://doi.org/10.1037/rep0000369

Compton, M. T., & Shim, R. S. (2020). Why employers must focus on the social determinants of mental health. *American Journal of Health Promotion, 34*(2), 215–219. https://doi.org/10.1177/0890117119896122c

Correctional Services Canada. (2015). *Research results—Mental health*. Retrieved from http://www.csc-scc.gc.ca/publications/005007-3030-eng.shtml

Corring, D., O'Reilly, R. L., Sommerdyk, C., et al. (2018a). What clinicians say about the experience of working with individuals on community treatment orders. *Psychiatric Services, 69*(7), 791–796. https://doi.org/10.1176/appi.ps.201700492

Corring, D., O'Reilly, R., Sommerdyk, C., et al. (2018b). What families have to say about community treatment orders (CTOs). *Canadian Journal of Community Mental Health, 37*(2), 1–12. https://doi.org/10.7870/cjcmh-2018-008

DeAtley, T., Denlinger-Apte, R. L., Cioe, P. A., et al. (2020). Biopsychosocial mechanisms associated with tobacco use in smokers with and without serious mental illness. *Preventive Medicine, 140*, 106190. https://doi.org/10.1016/j.ypmed.2020.106190

Dezetter, A., Duhoux, A., Menear, M., et al. (2015). Reasons and determinants for perceiving unmet needs for mental health in primary care in Quebec. *The Canadian Journal of Psychiatry, 60*(6), 284–293. https://doi.org/10.1177/070674371506000607

Dharmawardene, V., & Menkes, D. B. (2017). Violence and self-harm in severe mental illness: Inpatient study of associations with ethnicity, cannabis and alcohol. *Australasian Psychiatry, 25*(1), 28–31. https://doi.org/10.1177/1039856216671650

Dieterich, M., Irving, C. B., Bergman, H., et al. (2017). Intensive case management for severe mental illness. *The Cochrane Database of Systematic Reviews, 1*, CD007906

Dobber, J., Latour, C., de Haan, L., et al. (2018). Medication adherence in patients with schizophrenia: A qualitative study of the patient process in motivational interviewing. *BMC Psychiatry, 18*(1), 135. https://doi.org/10.1186/s12888-018-1724-9

Drapalski, A. L., Lucksted, A., Brown, C. H., et al. (2021). Outcomes of ending self-stigma, a group intervention to reduce internalized stigma, among individuals with serious mental illness. *Psychiatric Services, 72*(2), 136–142. https://doi.org/10.1176/appi.ps.201900296

Dubreucq, J., Plasse, J., & Franck, N. (2021). Self-stigma in serious mental illness: A systematic review of frequency, correlates, and consequences. *Schizophrenia Bulletin, 47*(5), 1261–1287. https://doi.org/10.1093/schbul/sbaa181

Fink-Samnick, E. (2021). The social determinants of mental health: Definitions, distinctions, and dimensions for professional case management: Part 1. *Professional Case Management, 26*(3), 121–137. https://doi.org/10.1097/NCM.0000000000000497

Firth, J., Cotter, J., Elliott, R., et al. (2015). A systematic review and meta-analysis of exercise interventions in schizophrenia patients. *Psychological Medicine, 45*(7), 1343–1361. https://doi.org/10.1017/S0033291714003110

Flood, C. M., & Bryan, T. (2017). Fragmented law & fragmented lives: Canada's mental health care system. In J. A. Chandler, & C. M. Flood (Eds.), *Law and mind: Mental health law and policy in Canada (Ottawa Faculty of Law Working Paper No. 2020-33)*. Toronto: LexisNexis. Retrieved from https://ssrn.com/abstract=3662667

Francombe Pridham, K., Nakhost, A., Tugg, L., et al. (2018). Exploring experiences with compulsory psychiatric community treatment: A qualitative multi-perspective pilot study in an urban Canadian context. *International Journal of Law and Psychiatry, 57*, 122–130. https://doi.org/10.1016/j.ijlp.2018.02.007

Frank, D., Fan, E., Georghiou, A., et al. (2020). Community treatment order outcomes in Quebec: A unique jurisdiction. *Canadian Journal of Psychiatry, 65*(7), 484–491. https://doi.org/10.1177/0706743719892718

Fuhr, D. C., Salisbury, T. T., De Silva, M. J., et al. (2014). Effectiveness of peer-delivered interventions for severe mental illness and depression on clinical and psychosocial outcomes: A systematic review and meta-analysis. *Social Psychiatry and Psychiatric Epidemiology, 49*(11), 1691–1702. https://doi.org/10.1007/s00127-014-0857-5

Gabrielian, S., Hamilton, A. B., Gelberg, L., et al. (2019). Identifying social skills that support housing attainment and retention among homeless persons with serious mental illness. *Psychiatric Services, 70*(5), 374–380. https://doi.org/10.1176/appi.ps.201800508

Gaebel, W., Rössler, W., & Sartorius, N. (2017). *The stigma of mental illness: End of the story?*. Cham: Springer.

Garverich, S., Prener, C. G., Guyer, M. E., et al. (2021). What matters: Factors impacting the recovery process among outpatient mental health service users. *Psychiatric Rehabilitation Journal, 44*(1), 77–86. https://doi.org/10.1037/prj0000407

Harrison, M., Roy, A. S., Hultqvist, J., et al. (2020). Quality of life outcomes for people with serious mental illness living in supported accommodation: Systematic review and meta-analysis. *Social Psychiatry and Psychiatric Epidemiology, 55*(8), 977–988. https://doi.org/10.1007/s00127-020-01885-x

Hoffman, S. J., Sritharan, L., & Tejpar, A. (2016). Is the UN convention on the rights of persons with disabilities impacting mental health laws and policies in high-income countries? A case study of implementation in Canada. *BMC International Health and Human Rights, 16*(1), 28. https://doi.org/10.1186/s12914-016-0103-1

Isaacs, A. N., Beauchamp, A., Sutton, K., et al. (2019). Unmet needs of persons with a severe and persistent mental illness and their relationship to unmet accommodation needs. *Health & Social Care in the Community, 27*(4), e246–e256. https://doi.org/10.1111/hsc.12729

Kerman, N., & Sylvestre, J. (2020). Surviving versus living life: Capabilities and service use among adults with mental health problems and histories of homelessness. *Health & Social Care in the Community, 28*(2), 414–422. https://doi.org/10.1111/hsc.12873

Kerman, N., Sylvestre, J., Aubry, T., et al. (2018). The effects of housing stability on service use among homeless adults with mental illness in a randomized controlled trial of housing first. *BMC Health Services Research, 18*(1), 190. https://doi.org/10.1186/s12913-018-3028-7

Kukla, M., Strasburger, A. M., Salyers, M. P., et al. (2021). Psychosocial outcomes of a pilot study of work-tailored cognitive behavioral therapy intervention for adults with serious mental illness. *Journal of Clinical Psychology, 77*(3), 488–495. https://doi.org/10.1002/jclp.23048

Law, S., Guan, I., Beder, M., et al. (2021). Further adaptations and reflections by an assertive community treatment team to serve clients with severe mental illness during COVID-19. *Community Mental Health Journal, 57*(7), 1227–1229. https://doi.org/10.1007/s10597-021-00855-0

LeFebvre, A. M., Dare, B., Farrell, S. J., et al. (2018). Transitions from assertive community treatment among urban and rural teams: Identifying barriers, service options, and strategies. *Community Mental Health Journal, 54*(4), 469–479. https://doi.org/10.1007/s10597-017-0162-3

Lequin, P., Golay, P., Herrera, F., et al. (2021). Recovering the capacity to live outside of a psychiatric hospital: Impact of a specialized inpatient program. *Psychiatric Quarterly, 92*(2), 751–759. https://doi.org/10.1007/s11126-020-09846-y

Leigh-Hunt, N., Bagguley, D., Bash, K., et al. (2017). An overview of systematic reviews on the public health consequences of social isolation and loneliness. *Public Health (London), 152*, 157–171. https://doi.org/10.1016/j.puhe.2017.07.035

Leopold, K., Bauer, M., Bechdolf, A., et al. (2020). Efficacy of cognitive-behavioral group therapy in patients at risk for serious mental illness presenting with subthreshold bipolar symptoms: Results from a prespecified interim analysis of a multicenter, randomized, controlled study. *Bipolar Disorders, 22*(5), 517–529. https://doi.org/10.1111/bdi.12894

Lincoln, T. M., Jung, E., Wiesjahn, M., et al. (2016). The impact of negative treatment experiences on persistent refusal of antipsychotics. *Comprehensive Psychiatry, 70*, 165–173. https://doi.org/10.1016/j.comppsych.2016.07.009

Little, J. D. (2021). In schizophrenia, are lack of capacity and lack of insight more usefully understood as anosognosia? *Australasian Psychiatry: Bulletin of the Royal Australian and New Zealand College of Psychiatrists, 29*(3), 346–348. https://doi.org/10.1177/1039856220975296

Lysaker, P. H., Hamm, J. A., Hasson-Ohayon, I., et al. (2018). Promoting recovery from severe mental illness: Implications from research on metacognition and metacognitive reflection and insight therapy. *World Journal of Psychiatry, 8*(1), 1–11. https://doi.org/10.5498/wjp.v8.i1.1

Martin, M. S., Viau-Deschênes, C., & Yogarajah, T. (2017). *Trauma-informed care for offenders who engage in chronic self-injurious behaviour: A rapid evidence assessment*. Ottawa: Correctional Service of Canada. R-388. Retrieved from https://www.csc-scc.gc.ca/research/r-388-en.shtml

McKee, S. A. (2017). Concurrent substance use disorders and mental illness: Bridging the gap between research and treatment. *Canadian Psychology, 58*(1), 50. https://doi.org/10.1037/cap0000093

McKenzie, E., Matkin, L., Sousa Fialho, L., et al. (2021). Developing an international standard set of patient-reported outcome measures for psychotic disorders. *Psychiatric Services*. https://doi.org/10.1176/appi.ps.202000888

McMillan, J., Lawn, S., & Delany-Crowe, T. (2019). Trust and community treatment orders. *Frontiers in Psychiatry, 10*, 349. https://doi.org/10.3389/fpsyt.2019.00349

Mental Health Commission of Canada (MHCC). (2012). *Changing directions, changing lives: The mental health strategy for Canada*. Calgary: Author.

Mental Health Commission of Canada (MHCC). (2015). *Guidelines for recovery-oriented practice*. Retrieved from https://mentalhealthcommission.ca/wp-content/uploads/2021/05/MHCC_Recovery_Guidelines_2016_ENG.pdf

Mental Health Commission of Canada (MHCC). (2017). *Discussion paper: Reducing employment barriers for people living with a mental illness: Using evidence-based practices to inform Canada's mental health and employment policy framework*. Retrieved from https://www.mentalhealthcommission.ca/wp-content/uploads/drupal/2018-04/FPT_Discussion_Paper_eng.pdf

Mulvale, G., & Bartram, M. (2015). No more "us" and "them": Integrating recovery and well-being into a conceptual model for mental health policy. *Canadian Journal of Community Mental Health, 34*(4), 31.

Murphy, Y., Ali, F., & Fischer, B. (2018). *Health and service access challenges for correctional offenders with mental health and* substance use problems in transition from incarceration to community: A literature review. Ottawa: Correctional Service of Canada. Research Report R-398. Retrieved from https://www.csc-scc.gc.ca/research/r-398-en.shtml

Naslund, J. A., Aschbrenner, K. A., McHugo, G. J., et al. (2019). Exploring opportunities to support mental health care using social media: A survey of social media users with mental illness. *Early Intervention in Psychiatry, 13*(3), 405–413. https://doi.org/10.1111/eip.12496

Pahwa, R., Smith, M. E., Kelly, E. L., et al. (2021). Definitions of community for individuals with serious mental illnesses: Implications for community integration and recovery. *Administration and Policy in Mental Health and Mental Health Services Research, 48*(1), 143–154. https://doi.org/10.1007/s10488-020-01055-w

Patten, S. B., Williams, J. V. A., Lavorato, D. H., et al. (2016). Perceived stigma among recipients of mental health care in the general Canadian population. *The Canadian Journal of Psychiatry, 61*(8), 480–488. doi:10.1177/0706743716639928

Pender, V. B. (2021). Addressing social determinants of mental health. *Psychiatric News, 56*(7). https://doi.org/10.1176/appi.pn.2021.7.42

Petros, R., & Solomon, P. (2020). Examining factors associated with perceived recovery among users of wellness recovery action plan. *Psychiatric Rehabilitation Journal, 43*(2), 132–139. https://doi.org/10.1037/prj0000389

Quirk, H., Crank, H., Harrop, D., et al. (2017). Understanding the experience of initiating community-based physical activity and social support by people with serious mental illness: A systematic review using a meta-ethnographic approach. *Systematic Reviews, 6*(1), 214. https://doi.org/10.1186/s13643-017-0596-2

Reid, C., Clark, N., Landy, A., et al. (2020). The lived experience of recovery: The role of health work in addressing the social determinants of mental health. *Canadian Journal of Community Mental Health, 38*(4), 1–17. https://doi.org/10.7870/cjcmh-2019-018

Romanowska, S., MacQueen, G., Goldstein, B. I., et al. (2020). Social and role functioning in youth at risk of serious mental illness. *Early Intervention in Psychiatry, 14*(4), 463–469. https://doi.org/10.1111/eip.12872

Sánchez, J. (2020 December). Predicting recovery in individuals with serious mental illness: Expanding the International Classification of Functioning, Disability, and Health (ICF) framework. *Rehabilitation Counseling Bulletin.* https://doi.org/10.1177/0034355220976835

Snethen, G., Brusilovskiy, E., McCormick, B. P., et al. (2021). The relationship between community participation and physical activity among individuals with serious mental illnesses. *Mental Health and Physical Activity, 20*, 100381. https://doi.org/10.1016/j.mhpa.2021.100381

Spagnolo, J. (2014). Improving first-line mental health services in Canada: Addressing two challenges caused by the deinstitutionalization movement. *Healthcare Quarterly, 17*(4), 41.

Stefancic, A., Bochicchio, L., Svehaug, K., et al. (2021). "We Die 25 Years Sooner": Addressing physical health among persons with serious mental illness in supportive housing. *Community Mental Health Journal, 57*(6), 1195–1207. https://doi.org/10.1007/s10597-020-00752-y

Suijkerbuijk, Y. B., Schaafsma, F. G., van Mechelen, J. C., et al. (2017). Interventions for obtaining and maintaining employment in adults with severe mental illness, a network meta-analysis. *The Cochrane Database of Systematic Reviews, 9*, CD011867. https://doi.org/10.1002/14651858.CD011867.pub2

Sylvestre, J., Notten, G., Kerman, N., et al. (2018). Poverty and serious mental illness: Toward action on a seemingly intractable problem. *American Journal of Community Psychology, 61*(1–2), 153–165. https://doi.org/10.1002/ajcp.12211

Treichler, E. B. H., Evans, E. A., & Spaulding, W. D. (2021). Ideal and real treatment planning processes for people with serious mental illness in public mental health care. *Psychological Services, 18*(1), 93–103. https://doi.org/10.1037/ser0000361

Velligan, D. I., Sajatovic, M., Hatch, A., et al. (2017). Why do psychiatric patients stop antipsychotic medication? A systematic review of reasons for nonadherence to medication in patients with serious mental illness. *Patient Preference and Adherence, 11*, 449–468. https://doi.org/10.2147/PPA.S124658

Wang, J., Mann, F., Lloyd-Evans, B., et al. (2018). Associations between loneliness and perceived social support and outcomes of mental health problems: A systematic review. *BMC Psychiatry, 18*(1), 156–156. https://doi.org/10.1186/s12888-018-1736-5

Weiden, P. J. (2016). Redefining medication adherence in the treatment of schizophrenia: How current approaches to adherence lead to misinformation and threaten therapeutic relationships. *The Psychiatric Clinics of North America, 39*(2), 199.

Winston, A., Rosenthal, R. N., & Roberts, L. W. (2020). *Learning supportive psychotherapy : An illustrated guide* (2nd ed.): American Psychiatric Association Publishing.

Wynaden, D., Heslop, B., Heslop, K., et al. (2016). The chasm of care: Where does the mental health nursing responsibility lie for the physical health care of people with severe mental illness?. *International Journal of Mental Health Nursing, 25*(6), 516–525. https://doi.org/10.1111/inm.12242

Yıldız, E., & Aylaz, R. (2020). How counseling based on acceptance and commitment therapy and supported with motivational interviewing affects the perceptions of treatment motivation in patients diagnosed with schizophrenia: A qualitative study. *Journal of the American Psychiatric Nurses Association, 27*(5), 390–404. https://doi.org/10.1177/1078390320945380

Zaheer, J., Olfson, M., Mallia, E., et al. (2020). Predictors of suicide at time of diagnosis in schizophrenia spectrum disorder: A 20-year total population study in Ontario, Canada. *Schizophrenia Research, 222*, 382–388. https://doi.org/10.1016/j.schres.2020.04.025

30

Psychological Needs of Patients With Medical Conditions

Cheryl L. Pollard

 https://evolve.elsevier.com/Canada/Varcarolis/psychiatric/

OBJECTIVES

1. Assess a person with a general medical condition and a psychiatric condition.
2. Formulate a nursing diagnosis appropriate for an individual with a non-psychiatric and psychiatric diagnosis.
3. Consider the impact of stress on general medical conditions.
4. Describe two psychosocial interventions that would be appropriate for a patient with a non-psychiatric and psychiatric diagnosis.
5. Explain the importance of nurses being knowledgeable about and comfortable discussing topics pertaining to the relationship between non-psychiatric and psychiatric illnesses.
6. Identify two instances in which a consultation with a psychiatric consultation liaison nurse might have been useful for your medical–surgical patients.

KEY TERMS AND CONCEPTS

coping skills
holistic approach

psychiatric consultation liaison nurse
stigmatized persons with medical conditions

There are two separate though related classifications of the relationship between physical conditions and psychological factors: (1) somatic symptom disorders, distressing somatic symptoms with abnormal thoughts, feelings, and behaviours in response to these symptoms, (discussed in Chapter 12) and (2) the influence of psychological factors or psychiatric disorders on non-psychiatric disorders. The latter more fully recognizes the relationships among health, health care, the determinants of health, and well-being.

This chapter helps to prepare nurses to use a **holistic approach**, which addresses both the psychological and the physiological needs of patients. Despite the unfortunate reality that the health care delivery system is fragmented for people with both medical and mental health problems, psychiatric mental health nurses must provide holistic care for patients with physical illnesses, and nurses who work outside of psychiatric settings must be aware of the influence of psychological factors and psychiatric disorders on the course of general medical conditions and plan for care accordingly.

PSYCHOLOGICAL FACTORS AFFECTING MEDICAL CONDITIONS

Psychological factors have been found to influence a variety of physical illnesses. The presence of psychiatric disorders along with general medical conditions increases the length of patient stays and also may negatively affect care outcomes (Wu et al., 2017). As a result of the interrelationships between psychiatric and medical comorbidities, collaboration among providers of primary health care and mental health care can lead to more accurate diagnoses and effective treatments.

Hans Selye (1956) was the first to introduce the concept of stress into the fields of medicine and physiology. Stress can lead to changes in physical and mental health in many ways (see Chapter 5). Cannon's (1914) identification of the fight-or-flight response and Selye's description of the general adaptation syndrome provided insight into the biological and molecular reactions to stressors in the sympathetic nervous system, the hypothalamic–pituitary–adrenal axis, and the immune system. Researchers have continued to increase our understanding of the basic physiological responses to stress (see Chapter 5), and there is deep interest in improving both the outcomes and the efficiency of health care delivery.

Without conflating health with well-being, a key determinant of health is how individuals promote self-care, cope with challenges, develop self-reliance, solve problems, and make choices. The psychological impact of medical illness can be severe and can account for a higher rate of disruption in functional ability than just the medical illness alone would indicate.

Among the most common psychological responses to physical illness are depression, anxiety, substance use, denial, hopelessness, and anger. A psychological condition, however, may supersede or be comorbid with a medical condition. In general, individuals with medical disorders and psychological symptoms have poorer outcomes than those with the same medical disorders but without psychological problems (Wu et al., 2017). Table 12.7 identifies some common medical conditions, such as cardiovascular disease, ulcers, cancer, and headaches, that are negatively affected by stress and would benefit from stress reduction and support. However, anyone experiencing a serious medical condition needs a variety of psychological supports and may benefit from learning new coping skills.

> **RESEARCH HIGHLIGHT**
> *When Fear of Cancer Recurrence Becomes a Clinical Issue*
>
> **Problem**
> Cancer is a life-threatening illness. Cancer survivors with low levels of fear of recurrence may be motivated to take care of their health and follow the advice of their health care team. However, when this fear escalates and is difficult to manage, it is associated with anxiety and depression and tends not to decrease over time. As a result, these cancer survivors experience a lower quality of life and impaired physical, social, occupational, and cognitive functioning.
>
> **Purpose of Study**
> Currently, there is no agreed-upon definition of the fear of cancer recurrence or agreement on when this phenomenon becomes "clinical" and should be a focus of treatment. The goal of this study was to investigate the potential hallmarks of clinical fear of cancer recurrence.
>
> **Methods**
> After receiving ethics approval, semistructured interviews were conducted with cancer survivors of both genders, of various cancer types, and who experienced a range of fear of cancer recurrence severity. Study participants met the following inclusion criteria: (1) had been diagnosed with breast, prostate, lung, or colorectal cancer; (2) had received treatment from the Ottawa Hospital Cancer Centre within the last 13 years; (3) were under 85 years of age to help ensure that participants did not have significant cognitive deficits; and (4) were able to comprehend and speak English. Forty interviews were completed. The analysis reflected this combination of approaches, as the interviews were analyzed with an understanding of the features of clinical fear of cancer recurrence, such as intrusive thoughts, impairment in functioning, the role of coping strategies, intolerance of uncertainty, and triggers of fear of cancer recurrence.
>
> **Key Findings**
> The nine most commonly reported features associated with clinical fear of cancer recurrence were death-related thoughts; feeling alone; experiencing fear of cancer recurrence–related thoughts and imagery that lasted 30 minutes or more; experiencing fear of cancer recurrence–related thoughts and imagery that were daily, recurrent, and difficult to control; experiencing more fear of cancer recurrence–related thoughts as time goes on; feeling certain that the cancer will return; experiencing distress; impairment in functioning; and intolerance of uncertainty. Participants experiencing non-clinical and clinical fear of cancer recurrence reported similar coping strategies and triggers of fear of cancer recurrence, thereby suggesting that the simple occurrence of coping strategies or triggers of fear of cancer recurrence may not indicate clinical fear of cancer recurrence.
>
> **Implications for Nursing Practice**
> While features of clinical fear of cancer recurrence such as intrusive thoughts, distress, and impact on functioning found in this analysis confirmed previous fear of cancer recurrence research, other features including death-related thoughts, feeling alone, and belief that the cancer will return spontaneously emerged from the interviews. The participants' descriptions of cancer-specific fear and worry suggest that fear of cancer recurrence is a distinct phenomenon related to cancer survivorship, despite its similarity to psychological disorders (e.g., anxiety, depressive disorders). Although a distinct phenomenon, nurses should consider using cognitive reframing and thought monitoring techniques, which may help those who believe that a cancer recurrence will inevitably happen by reframing thoughts to include the idea that the return of cancer is only one possible outcome. The "feeling alone" symptom may respond to therapeutic techniques that establish a connection with others who have had similar experiences, including social support, therapy, or self-help groups. Future research investigating the construct of fear of cancer recurrence and the distinguishing features of clinical fear of cancer recurrence across a range of cancer types and genders is required.

Source: Mutsaers, B., Jones, G., Rutowski, N., et al. (2016). When fear of cancer recurrence becomes a clinical issue: A qualitative analysis of features associates with clinical fear of cancer reoccurrence. *Support Care Cancer, 24*(10), 4207–4218. https://doi.org/10.1007/s00520-016-3248-5

Caregivers of those with a chronic illness also experience psychological sequelae. Often this includes depression and anxiety. HealthPartners (2015) reports that 20% of caregivers experience depression as a result of their caregiving responsibilities. Many caregivers attempt to balance their caregiving responsibilities with other family duties while continuing to work.

PSYCHOLOGICAL RESPONSES TO SERIOUS MEDICAL CONDITIONS

The diagnosis of a medical problem or condition is stressful for nearly everyone. However, the degree of stress depends on the person's perception of the illness. People's questions can be many and varied when they find themselves faced with a serious medical problem:
- Will I be disfigured?
- Will I have a long-term disability?
- Will I be able to function as a wife or husband, parent, and member of society?
- Will I be able to continue to work?
- Will I suffer pain?
- Will I be stigmatized?

When strong emotional supports and social ties are not available, other questions may arise:
- How will I cope?
- How will this affect my life?
- Will I retain a reasonable quality of life?

Depression

A strong body of evidence suggests that depression is more common in patients with physical disorders, particularly in those with multiple physical disorders. The Mental Health Commission of Canada (2014) suggests that up to 50% of people living with a chronic illness also suffer from depression. People with a chronic medical condition are three times as likely to experience depression than those without one. Often depression is masked by the medical condition itself and goes unrecognized and thus untreated. For example, uremic symptoms in patients who have renal disease may mask the somatic and neurovegetative symptoms of depression. Just a few of the medical illnesses that typically are associated with depression are cancer, human immunodeficiency virus (HIV), COVID-19 disease and the pandemic context generally (Government of Quebec, 2021), diabetes, hypertension, and stroke.

If not recognized and treated, depression can affect the severity of the medical disorder, increase personal distress, impair functioning, and interfere with adherence to a prescribed medical regimen. Patients with depression have been found to be three times more likely to be non-adherent to medical treatment than are patients without depression (Volpato et al., 2017). This is because people with depression are often less motivated, or able, to follow self-care regimens. They may have poor diet, neglect exercise routines, smoke, overindulge in substances, all of which take away from recovery (HealthPartners, 2015). However, people with medical conditions who are treated for co-occurring depression often experience improvement in their overall medical condition, show better adherence to recommendations for general medical care, and experience a better quality of life.

> **VIGNETTE**
> Candace is a single 30-year-old head administrative paralegal who recently arrived in emergency with nausea, vomiting, and abdominal pain. She reports having no energy, a lack of interest in her usual hobbies, and difficulty concentrating. She states, "I feel very scared and alone. I don't know where I would get the money to live if I need to miss work." These observations were reported to the nurse practitioner. After a thorough assessment and medical workup, it is determined that Candace has pre-renal acute renal failure and depression.

Anxiety

Acute anxiety can influence a person's coping capacity, defensive structure, adaptive capacity, and resilience. Illnesses that evoke sympathetic nervous system responses, such as nervousness, insomnia, breathlessness, palpitations, jitteriness, high blood pressure, and high cholesterol, are complicated when the individual also has a comorbid anxiety disorder. Anxiety leads to heightened awareness of physical symptoms, as well as to physiologically caused medical symptoms because of increased muscle tension and autonomic nervous system and hypothalamic–pituitary–adrenal axis dysregulation. Recognizing treatable anxiety disorders that are highly concurrent with medical comorbid conditions, for example, cancer, chronic illnesses, and infectious diseases such as COVID-19 (Huda et al., 2021; Stafford et al., 2021), is important in alleviating distress and improving the course of the illness.

Verbalization can be an effective outlet for anxiety. However, the ability to effectively communicate one's feelings may be compromised by cultural expectations, disability, or lack of a listener. A sense of helplessness often accompanies anxiety in the person who feels a loss of control over events, such as when awaiting surgery or undergoing invasive treatments. In this case defence mechanisms (e.g., denial, regression) may be used with greater frequency, or compulsive behaviours may surface. Unreasonable requests of caregivers (e.g., demanding that the nurse sit with a patient throughout the night) may be a cover for feelings of inadequacy.

> **VIGNETTE**
> Pat is 19 years old. He has been diagnosed with Crohn's disease. He knows that there is no known cure for his illness. He belongs to an online "Gutsy Peer Support Group." The bloating, nausea, cramping, and loss of appetite he experiences are constant. Sometimes the symptoms are better, and sometimes they are worse. Final exams are approaching, and Pat always finds exams stressful. When he is stressed, the symptoms always get worse. He finds it hard to concentrate when he is always worrying about having to go to the bathroom.
> The nurse at student counselling services talks to Pat about the power of the mind–body connection. The nurse works with Pat to explore practical ways of managing the urgency of his diarrhea, nausea, and cramping during the exams. Stress-management practices are taught to help him cope with stress in a helpful and empowering way. Assertiveness techniques are also practised to reduce the chances of becoming overcommitted and overscheduled, as it is difficult to feel healthy when one is drained and overwhelmed.

Possible nursing diagnoses for Pat in the vignette include:
- *Risk for ineffective coping* related to high levels of anxiety that are interfering with his ability to study.
- *Ineffective role performance* related to diagnosis of Crohn's disease as evidenced by fatigue and lack of energy.

Substance Use

Long-term abuse of various substances can lead to a variety of medical complications; for example, alcohol use is associated with hepatic conditions, marijuana use with lung disease, cocaine use with cardiac toxicity, and ecstasy (3,4-methylenedioxymethamphetamine or MDMA) use with neurotoxicity (e.g., problems with memory, reasoning, impulse control). However, patients who are diagnosed with serious medical conditions often turn to alcohol or other substances to cope with overwhelming feelings of hopelessness, fear, anxiety, depression, or pain.

Thus health care providers need to be diligent in their initial assessments and identify any co-existing or resulting psychological responses or disorders. In most cases of physical illness the focus is on the complaints of physical symptoms, and minimal attention is given to the psychological responses of the patient.

Grief and Loss

Serious medical illnesses are nearly always accompanied by grief. As well, any type of treatment or procedure intended to treat a physical illness that creates a major permanent change is accompanied by feelings of loss. The dynamics involved in coping with these feelings are similar to those in a person who is dealing with their own impending death or the death of a loved one. The person must grieve for the loss, just as the dying person must work through confusion and darkness until a degree of acceptance and relative peace is achieved. Negotiating the loss of physical well-being involves moving through feelings of frustration, vulnerability, and sadness to become a whole person once again. This journey encompasses both spiritual and emotional changes and, for this reason, requires spiritual assessment of the patient, as well as a focus on psychosocial issues.

> **VIGNETTE**
> Candace's kidney damage continues. Her kidneys have failed, and she is being treated with hemodialysis. She has been complaining of frequent tension headaches and occasional stomach upsets before her treatment appointments. The hemodialysis nurse has always been impressed by Candace's patience and compliant attitude despite her debilitating illness, which has robbed her of a normal family life. For this reason, the nurse suspects that Candace's physical complaints could be a way of dealing with her emotions, so the nurse makes a point to spend more time with Candace to allow her to talk about her frustrations. Candace expresses anger and some feelings of hopelessness. She resents others who are healthy, including the people who care for her. Frequent opportunities to verbalize these feelings gradually result in the lessening of her somatic complaints and a decrease in her sense of powerlessness and isolation.

Possible nursing diagnoses for Candace in the vignette above include:
- *Hopelessness* related to chronic illness as evidenced by verbal comments and feelings of resentment toward others who are healthy.
- *Ineffective individual coping* related to chronic illness as evidenced by expressions of anger and feelings of hopelessness.

Denial

Bodily changes affect individuals' identities in important ways, and some chronically ill patients work very hard at maintaining their pre-illness identity, sometimes to the detriment of their health. Common responses to the initial symptoms of illness, the diagnosis, and functional limitations and impairments evoke the complicated process of denial, acceptance, and adaptation (although not necessarily in that order). Denial, an unconscious defence mechanism, may be evident when the diagnosed person and the family seem to have little knowledge or interest in learning about the condition or define the illness as acute rather than chronic. Nurses and other health care providers may actually foster such beliefs by withholding information about the meaning and likely consequences of a particular problem. Initial illness crises support explanations of the illness as acute and can be so overwhelming for patients and families as to prevent consideration of a long-term course of illness.

As symptoms and acute crises repeat over time, individuals begin to accept the chronicity of their illnesses and the effects of the illnesses on their daily lives. People begin to experience their bodies as altered and come to think of illness as real in ways that allow them to relate symptoms to the changes in their lives. They compare their present condition with that of the past, weighing the risks of continuing their regular activities and activity levels and then adapting those activity levels. Patients may feel estranged from the persons they have become, betrayed by their own bodies, or guilty for not meeting standards of activity levels, functioning, and appearance. Patients can also distance themselves from their illness, diagnosis, and body, objectifying their symptoms as a way of coping.

> **VIGNETTE**
> After a car accident, Katya is being assessed by the triage nurse in the emergency department for possible injuries. She complains of a slight headache and dizziness but denies having any other pain or symptoms. Katya is preoccupied with ensuring that her 2-year-old son, who was also in the car, is being examined, so she denies her own need for medical attention. Katya's blood pressure is 86/50 mm Hg, and her body posture indicates that she is guarding her abdomen. These observations are reported to the examining physician immediately because they indicate possible internal bleeding and danger of shock. Katya is eventually taken to the operating room so that the bleeding may be stopped.

Possible nursing diagnoses for Katya in the vignette include:
- *Acute pain* related to recent car accident as evidenced by headache, dizziness, and body posture indicating she is guarding her abdomen.
- *Anxiety* related to concern for her child as evidenced by being preoccupied with seeing her 2-year-old son.

Fear of Dependency

Responses to being dependent may be exhibited as an inability to accept warmth, nurturing, or tenderness from caregivers or as a refusal to accept treatment or medical advice. This reaction is strongest in those who have unmet dependencies and those who have had negative experiences when seeking help in the past. Anger may mask acute embarrassment over being in a dependent position or may be used by the patient who feels the need to project an independent image. Others are fearful of not having their dependency needs met and do not express any negative feelings to caregivers. These people strive to be "good" patients out of fear that they will be abandoned if they are perceived to be difficult. Suppressed anxiety or anger, however, could be exhibited through increased somatic complaints.

A possible nursing diagnosis for Rebecca in the vignette is:
- *Anxiety* related to recent change in health status as evidenced by impaired concentration and palpitations.

> **VIGNETTE**
> Rebecca, a 25-year-old with multiple sclerosis, worked as a home attendant until she fractured her leg and sustained a severe elbow injury when a patient she was assisting fell on her. The resultant disabilities and flare-up of her multiple sclerosis have prevented her from resuming her job as a home attendant. Prior to this incident, she was independent, hard working, self-supporting, and able to manage a mild anxiety disorder through cognitive reframing and controlled breathing. Her injuries forced her to apply for financial support and rely on her boyfriend for assistance with transportation and care of her apartment. She began to experience shortness of breath, palpitations, and impaired concentration.

HUMAN RIGHTS ABUSES OF STIGMATIZED PERSONS WITH MEDICAL CONDITIONS

Some consumers of health care and some health care providers have voiced the need to examine human rights abuses in the health care system, specifically the inadequate care of people who are stigmatized by health care providers. These **stigmatized persons with medical conditions** are assumed by health care providers to be bad, disgusting, or even just unusual and often include those who have mental illnesses, those who are HIV positive, and those who have undergone transgender surgeries or treatments. The abuses that many of these patients endure can result in inadequate care and lead to undue stress, worsening of physical illness, and even death. By making assumptions about these patients, health care workers fail to acknowledge and understand that these patients' psychosocial issues are similar to those of other patients and that the same nursing interventions for anger, anxiety, and grief are applicable. Examples of human rights abuse include:
- Failure to fully investigate somatic complaints made by emergency department patients with a history of psychiatric illness
- Avoidance of contact with, or refusal to care for, persons who are stigmatized, which results in worsening illness or death
- Hastily labelling with a psychiatric diagnosis and giving a prescription of antipsychotic drugs to persons who are experiencing normal emotional responses (e.g., sadness, anger) to chronic physical illness
- Inappropriate psychiatric admission of persons who are on medical units or in nursing homes, based on the financial needs of the institution or on the staff's inability to manage emotional responses to physical illness or the aging process

Such situations may occur more frequently to individuals who lack family support or the personal resources to advocate for themselves (e.g., those from lower socioeconomic classes, newly arrived immigrants, those living socially "unacceptable" lifestyles). The key to increasing awareness of human rights issues in psychiatric mental health care may be the integration of these concepts into nursing curricula. Humanitarian values are at the very heart of our profession and practice. Nurses are in a unique position to advocate for equal patient treatment, but many hesitate to confront employers about violations of basic patient rights, fearing reprisal. A committee composed of nurses and other hospital employees could be formed to review such cases and make recommendations to the hospital administration. In this age of managed care and cuts to hospital budgets upholding human rights is one of nursing's greatest challenges.

APPLICATION OF THE NURSING PROCESS

Assessment

Assessment of patients is a complex process that requires careful and complete documentation. Assessment should begin with the collection of data about the nature, location, onset, character, and duration of the symptom or symptoms. A thorough medical, emotional, and psychosocial history is also essential. Assessment of nutrition, fluid balance, and elimination needs should be a high priority in patients with complaints relating to gastrointestinal distress, diarrhea, constipation, and anorexia.

Psychosocial Assessment

Psychosocial factors are relevant to the course of an illness, and the way a person thinks and feels can have a profound effect on how the disease progresses. Struggling with illness evokes a range of difficult emotions, such as fear, anger, sadness, confusion, and guilt. Patients may feel overwhelmed and alone, whereas family members may feel helpless and at a loss emotionally. The elements of a thorough psychosocial assessment are described in detail in Chapter 10.

ASSESSMENT GUIDELINES
Psychological Needs of Patients With Medical Conditions

1. Assess for nature, location, onset, characteristics, and duration of the physical and psychological symptoms.
2. Assess the patient's ability to meet basic needs and quality of life.
3. Determine availability and capacity of social supports.
4. Assess risks to safety and security needs of the patient, including self-harm and suicide, as a result of all symptoms.
5. Assess for substance use (i.e., prescription and non-prescription medication, alcohol consumption, nicotine, and caffeine consumption).
6. Explore the patient's cognitive style and ability to communicate feelings and needs.
7. Determine current level of psychological symptoms (mild, moderate, severe, or panic).
8. Perform a psychosocial assessment. Always ask the person, "What is going on in your life that may be contributing to your health issues?" The patient may identify a problem that should be addressed by counselling (e.g., stressful marriage, recent loss, stressful job or school situation).
9. Remember that culture can affect how psychological symptoms are manifested.

SAFETY TIP

Pain, and other causes of physical and emotional discomfort, affect how patients respond to stressful situations. Responses can vary from agitation, frustration, and irritability to withdrawal. When approaching a patient, the nurse will make introductions and state the intent of the interaction. Patients will respond and engage more when they are not in pain.

Quality of life assessment. For interventions to be most effective, the nurse must understand how a person's medical condition affects their quality of life. For example, how is the medical illness affecting the ability to function in the home, at work, or in school? How are the patient's feelings about the illness (e.g., depression, anxiety, hopelessness) affecting their relationships and ability to function? There are a number of quality of life assessment tools, ranging from self-assessment rating scales to lengthy questionnaires. Different organizations use different tools. One example of an assessment tool is the World Health Organization's (2012) Quality of Life–BREF (WHOQOL-BREF), which can be used to examine an individual's perceptions about quality of life in the context of culture, value systems, and personal goals, standards, and concerns. The development of this tool was based on statements made by patients from a variety of cultures and with a range of diseases. This tool is available in English and French. The most useful assessment tool is a simple one: ask the patient how the illness or disease is affecting the quality of their life.

Coping skills. Assessing how a patient has dealt with adversity in the past provides information about the person's coping skills available for use now and in the future. Health care providers can also support the patient in gaining additional coping skills that may help them to better manage a serious medical or surgical situation.

A person who has a life-threatening disease or chronic illness often deals with distressing physical adverse effects and changes in body image. For example, a patient who is given a colostomy to avoid death from cancer or ulcerative colitis is left with complex emotional and physical issues. The patient must learn techniques for dealing with not only the stoma but also the lifelong consequences and their effects on body image, appearance, and relationships. Concerns such as the following may arise:
- Will my partner still be attracted to me?
- Will I continue to be interested in sexual relationships?

Breast cancer survivors, for example, have been helped by camaraderie with other survivors who openly share their techniques for dealing with appliances or prostheses. Other survivors can also show patients how to respond to well-intended but probing or embarrassing questions. People who have previously travelled the same path are the best resources for helping those newly diagnosed to establish how to manage inevitable questions about their illness.

Table 30.1 highlights some of the characteristics that allow people to cope well and some of the characteristics that may be changed or improved through psychosocial interventions or cognitive behavioural approaches.

Social and spiritual support. Medical conditions initially may elicit strong support from friends and family, but as time wears on, this support may begin to wane. Knowing who is there for the patient will be helpful in planning for later interventions. Does the patient have sufficient social supports (e.g., family, friends, elders, religious or spiritual help) to enable them to share thoughts and feelings? Would the patient benefit from a medical support group?

Nurses and other health care workers are becoming increasingly aware of the role that spirituality or religion plays in many patients' lives and its importance as a source of peace. Support from a priest, pastor, rabbi, or an other religious leader may be indicated, especially in a case of spiritual distress. Beliefs and practices are forces that promote resilience; practising healthy coping depends on the capacity to create meaning.

Self-Assessment

Nurses and other health care providers can find it difficult to work with individuals who have strong emotional reactions. They feel more confident dealing with patients' physical needs. Many worry that they may say something wrong and make the patient more upset. However, connection, mutuality, vulnerability, and respect are used to establish a therapeutic relationship, wherein teaching, coaching, and modelling are most effective.

It is helpful for health care providers, no matter the setting, to discuss emotional reactions to patients in conferences with other members of the health care team. Sharing these feelings facilitates critical reflections and helps the clinician to develop an awareness of countertransference issues that will negatively affect patient care.

TABLE 30.1 Assessment of Coping Skills

Effective Coping Skills	Ineffective Coping Behaviours
Has optimistic attitude (sees glass as half full)	Has pessimistic attitude (sees glass as half empty)
Confronts the issues; acts accordingly	Minimizes critical health status or signals
Seeks information; gets guidance	Shows tendency to escape or withdraw
Shares concerns; finds consolation	Blames someone or something else
Has capacity for healthy denial	Denies as much as possible; shows prolonged denial
Redefines the situation, reviews alternatives, examines consequences	Feels things are hopeless, were meant to be; has attitude of "What's the use?"
Constructively uses distractions: keeping busy; maintaining positive emotional ties with family, friends, community	Withdraws; broods; is overwhelmed with self-pity, anger, envy, guilt about having caused the illness

Diagnosis

Patients will present with many different diseases, illnesses, and disorders. *Ineffective coping, powerlessness, interrupted family processes,* and *self-care deficit* are frequently diagnosed. Causal statements might include:
- Suppression of feelings
- Caregiver burnout
- Inability to meet role expectations
- Dependence on others
- Inability to meet basic care needs

Outcomes Identification

Some of the *Nursing Outcomes Classification (NOC)*–recommended outcomes related to anxiety include *Anxiety self-control, Anxiety level, Stress level, Coping, Social interaction skills,* and *Symptom control* (Moorhead et al., 2018). Additional outcomes may be developed through a shared decision-making process that helps the patient and the nurse to see concrete evidence of progress. The following are examples of possible outcomes:
- Patient will identify ineffective coping patterns.
- Patient will make realistic appraisal of strengths and weaknesses.
- Patient will assertively verbalize feelings such as anger, shame, or guilt.

Planning

Because patients with primary non-psychiatric disorders are rarely admitted to psychiatric care settings for treatment, treatment is initiated in other settings. In primary care settings providers are generally less confident about managing psychological symptoms. Because of the frequency of comorbidities between non-psychiatric and psychiatric illnesses in primary care, an integrated model of care among mental health and medical clinicians is essential. In an ideal situation a multi-disciplinary team of clinicians would include an advanced-practice nurse who could provide consultation to health care providers outside of psychiatry.

The following are some highlights that can help the nurse plan necessary interventions. When working with someone who is medically ill, it is important to know if the person has any of the following:
- Someone who can share their concerns and who cares for them
- Friends and supports in the community
- Any coexisting conditions that could negatively affect adjustment to the illness, the course of the illness, adaptation to the illness, or ability to heal (e.g., depression; personality disorder; substance use; compulsive behaviours such as gambling, eating, or cybersex)
- Risky health behaviours (e.g., sedentary lifestyle, smoking, engaging in unsafe sex practices, using alcohol or drugs)
- A cultural view of health and illness that helps or impedes the process of seeking adequate care

Implementation

People who have a medical condition are vulnerable to a variety of psychosocial stresses. These influences affect lifestyle choice through at least five areas: personal life skills, stress, culture, social relationships and belonging, and a sense of control. Interventions that support the creation of supportive environments will enhance the capacity of individuals to make healthy lifestyle choices in a world where many choices are possible. As a result, how individuals cope with these stresses may be the difference between living with an acceptable quality of life and giving in to despair, withdrawal, helplessness, or hopelessness.

Nurses are in a position to assess and understand patients' psychosocial stressors, identify needed coping skills, and teach stress-management techniques (for more information, refer to Chapters 5 and 12). Nurses can play an important role not only in providing and managing patients' immediate medical care but also in helping patients to improve their ability to cope and increase their quality of life during the course of a chronic medical illness.

Health Teaching and Health Promotion

The type and depth of teaching is determined by the information the patient already understands about their illnesses and coping strategies. The Patient and Family Teaching box provides guidelines for teaching patients and their families about how to adapt to a major medical illness.

Coping Skills

Effective coping skills are healthier ways of looking at and dealing with illness (e.g., assertiveness training, cognitive reframing, problem-solving skills, social supports). They are many and varied and can be taught. A nurse is in a key position to assess patients' ability to cope, educate patients about coping skills, or provide referrals to patients to learn healthier ways of looking at and dealing with illness. Consider referring the patient for instruction in a variety of relaxation techniques, such as meditation, guided imagery, or breathing exercises, or teach the patient such techniques yourself. Behavioural techniques are useful, and nurses with special training can offer their patients progressive muscle relaxation or biofeedback. Relaxation techniques, stress management, and supportive education should be part of the care of the patient with a medical condition, regardless of the medical diagnosis. Other beneficial approaches include cognitive behavioural psychotherapy, guided imagery, biofeedback, acupressure, and psychodynamic psychotherapy.

Although medical procedures may extend or promote life, they often take a toll on the patient's physical state because of the high degree of anxiety they evoke. Research has shifted the focus from patients' knowledge of the disease and its treatment to their confidence and skills in managing their condition. Interventions now support patients and their support systems being active participants in managing their

PATIENT AND FAMILY TEACHING
Coping With a Major Medical Illness

- **Learn all you can about your illness.** Understanding your options can help keep your anxiety at manageable levels. Knowing what choices are available can help you feel more in control.
- **Practise healthy behaviours.** Good sleep hygiene, diet, and exercise are good practices that promote well-being. Neglecting healthy behaviours can result in increased pain, irritability, and fatigue. Improper nutrition also compromises our immune system.
- **Take advantage of support groups that help you manage your medical condition.** Sharing and listening to the experiences of people who have or are facing similar issues can be comforting. Support groups can provide you with information, help you learn how to handle difficult situations related to your illness, reduce isolation, and offer a safe place to share difficult thoughts and feelings.
- **Consider entering psychotherapy.** Illnesses affect us mentally and physically. Seeking professional assistance to develop coping strategies can result in better pain control, better coping skills, and even longer survival in some situations.
- **Find a way to express your feelings.** Acknowledging thoughts and feelings can help your nervous system relax. For example, putting experiences into words (e.g., writing them down, keeping a journal). Doing anything creative, writing poetry or prose, painting or making collages, playing an instrument or singing, is a powerful tool in working with the feelings of fear, anger, and loss that are stirred up by illness.
- **Communicate with your health provider.** Seek additional help if you become depressed, demoralized, anxious, or panicky or have unremitting pain. There are approaches (e.g., acupuncture, acupressure, biofeedback) that can give people control over their physiological responses and reduce the need for higher doses of medication.

condition (Hillebregt et al., 2017). The following have all been shown to affect a patient's recovery positively:

- Educating the patient regarding the specific medical treatment
- Referring the patient to community support groups (or systems)
- Teaching patients more effective coping skills that take into consideration patients' values, preferences, and lifestyle
- Focusing on a patient's strengths and reinforcing coping skills that work (e.g., prayerfulness, participation in hobbies, relaxation techniques)

Advanced-Practice Interventions

When working as part of non-psychiatric multi-disciplinary teams, the advanced-practice nurse is often referred to as a **psychiatric consultation liaison nurse** (PCLN). Within this role, the PCLN functions as a consultant to other nurses in managing psychological concerns and symptoms of psychiatric disorders and also works directly with patients as a clinician to help them deal more effectively with physical and emotional problems. The PCLN is a resource for members of a nursing staff who feel unable to intervene therapeutically with a patient who presents a management problem or has problems that impede care. The PCLN first meets with the nurse who initiated the consultation and then reviews the patient's medical records, talks with the physicians, and interviews the patient. After the patient interview, the PCLN discusses the assessment and suggestions for care with the referring nurse.

Evaluation

Interventions are determined to be effective when patients remain safe, new coping strategies have improved quality of life, and stress is handled more adaptively. Evaluation of patients with comorbid disorders is a simple process when measurable behavioural outcomes have been written clearly and realistically.

KEY POINTS TO REMEMBER

- There is irrefutable evidence that psychiatric disorders and psychological responses influence general medical conditions.
- A bidirectional effect exists between physical and emotional states of health. Physical illnesses are often accompanied by a spectrum of emotional responses, particularly anxiety and depression. Likewise, adverse emotional states often increase the severity of physical symptoms.
- The holistic philosophy of nursing dictates that all nurses, regardless of their roles or specialties, assess patients' psychosocial needs as well as their strengths.
- Health care personnel in the medical and mental health communities recognize the need to target both the psychological and the physical problems of a patient to increase adherence to the care regimen, maximize the quality of life, and promote healing.
- Understanding a patient's psychosocial needs and knowing when to intervene and where to refer the patient are essential for the nurse who practises holistic care and more effectively promotes health.
- Identifying the existence of depression, anxiety, and substance use and getting the patient treatment can help promote a positive outcome of the medical disorder and improve the patient's quality of life.
- A holistic approach to patient care includes assessment of physical, psychosocial, social, and spiritual needs.
- A growing concern about patients is the state of their spiritual lives. Including this dimension in the holistic nursing assessment allows nurses to see inner strengths in their patients that might be overlooked when using a more traditional approach.
- The psychiatric consultation liaison nurse is a nurse clinician who is in the key position of being able to help other health care personnel look at their patients in a holistic manner and help those who care for these patients understand non-medical issues that are impeding medical progress.

CRITICAL THINKING

1. Marie Vaudrie is a 45-year-old woman who has had a partial hysterectomy. Although she is asymptomatic and has a normal physical examination, her laboratory results indicate that she is HIV positive. Marie was unaware that her boyfriend of 2 years was engaging in unprotected sex with men. She and her ex-husband have been divorced for 5 years but maintain a good relationship and share custody of their three teenage children. Marie has a supportive extended family and several close friends, and she belongs to a church. After her diagnosis, Marie is encouraged to talk about her feelings and see a therapist. Marie states, "I will be able to do everything I did before. I feel healthy." The nurse has several concerns, including Marie's focus on self-care, her acceptance and understanding of her HIV-positive status, and her willingness to disclose her status to sexual or intimate partners.
   a. How would you evaluate Marie's social support system?
   b. What other information about Marie's situation would be helpful in your assessment (e.g., cultural beliefs about illness)?
   c. What recommendations or referrals could you make to Marie, and how would you approach her with these recommendations? Would you include contact data for any medically related or HIV-related support groups in the information you would give her?
2. Discuss how you would approach the physician regarding Marie's need to be evaluated for depression. What are some of the compelling reasons why depression (and any co-existing mental condition) should be treated in any and all seriously ill medical patients?

3. What cognitive behavioural coping skills have proven useful for a patient who is HIV positive?
4. What important areas should the nurse assess with an Indigenous woman with a past history of intimate partner violence who is attending an outpatient clinic and expressing a fear that she may be HIV positive?

CHAPTER REVIEW

1. Which statement about the psychological impact of medical illnesses is accurate?
   a. An experience of grief and loss is not typical of most serious medical illnesses.
   b. Depression is a significant issue in more than 60% of persons with cancer or heart disease.
   c. Psychological responses to medical illnesses can delay recovery but do not worsen the outcome.
   d. Patients often have significant concerns regarding the impact a medical illness can have on their ability to function.
2. While taking the vital signs of a patient about to undergo surgery, you notice that she is tearful. When asked, she tells you that her mother had the same surgery and later died of a post-operative infection. Which response is most likely to be therapeutic?
   a. Ask the patient if she would like to speak with the chaplain before surgery.
   b. Reassure the patient that she has an excellent surgeon and that complications for her surgery are rare.
   c. State, "Surgery can be very frightening," and sit down next to the patient to convey your availability to talk.
   d. State, "Many people become anxious before surgery, but this is a normal reaction. You will be fine."
3. An older adult male with heart disease feels both angry and guilty about his illness, blaming himself for becoming obese and inactive and feeling anger toward tobacco and fast-food companies. He presented in the emergency department today 4 hours after the onset of unrelenting chest pain, reporting that it "didn't hurt that much" and that, given his prior experiences with chest pain, he "did not think it would matter much" whether he came in quickly or tried to "wait it out." Now awaiting the results of his electrocardiogram (ECG), he is reading magazines and talking about the likelihood that a new stent will once again give him a new lease on life. Based on this information, how well would you expect this patient to be able to cope with his illness?
   a. Poorly
   b. Inadequately
   c. Adequately
   d. Exceptionally
4. A nurse on a medical–surgical unit is admitting a patient with a history of bipolar disorder and alcohol abuse. Which action would be most appropriate for ensuring that this patient receives the best possible nursing care?
   a. Consult with the psychiatric consultation liaison nurse regarding assessment skills and interventions likely to benefit this patient.
   b. Review online, textbook, or journal resources pertaining to the patient's mental health and substance abuse disorders.
   c. Consult more experienced colleagues and the head nurse for tips on assessing and caring for persons with comorbid psychiatric disorders.
   d. Focus primarily on the patient's physical health needs, and refer the patient for outpatient psychiatric care at discharge if the patient requests it.
5. Which statements about persons with mental illness who present with serious medical conditions are most accurate? **Select all that apply.**
   a. Such patients are at higher risk for receiving inadequate care, owing to failure to fully assess somatic complaints.
   b. Patients who have both a medical and a mental illness tend to receive more care and more costly care because of their concurrent disorders.
   c. Staff are more likely to minimize their time with such patients compared to medically ill patients without mental illness.
   d. Such patients risk being admitted to psychiatric settings instead of needed medical–surgical units, owing to staff's anxiety about caring for them.
   e. Emotional responses to medical conditions may be mistakenly attributed to psychiatric illness rather than being addressed as normal responses to medical conditions.

https://evolve.elsevier.com/Canada/Varcarolis/psychiatric/

REFERENCES

Cannon, W. B. (1914). The emergency function of the adrenal medulla in pain and the major emotions. *American Journal of Physiology, 33*, 356–372.

Government of Quebec. (2021). Stress, anxiety and depression associated with COVID-19. Retrieved from https://publications.msss.gouv.qc.ca/msss/fichiers/2019/19-210-14WA.pdf

HealthPartners. (2015). *Chronic disease and mental health report.* Ottawa: Author.

Hillebregt, C. F., Vlonk, A. J., Bruijnzeels, M. A., et al. (2017). Barriers and facilitators influencing self-management among COPD patients: A mixed methods exploration in primary and affiliated specialist care. *International Journal of Chronic Obstructive Pulmonary Disease, 12*, 123–133. https://doi.org/10.2147/COPD.103998

Huda, N., Shaw, M. K., & Chang, H.-J. (2021). Psychological distress among patients with advanced cancer: A conceptual analysis. *Cancer Nursing, 45*(2): 487–503. https://doi.org/10.1097/NCC.0000000000000940

Mental Health Commission of Canada. (2014). *Addressing the mental health needs of Canadians.* Ottawa: Presentation at HealthPartners.

Moorhead, S., Johnson, M., Maas, M., et al. (2018). *Nursing Outcomes Classification (NOC)* (6th ed.). St. Louis: Mosby.

Selye, H. (1956). *The stress of life.* New York: McGraw-Hill.

Stafford, O., Berry, A., Taylor, L. K., et al. (2021). Comorbidity and COVID-19: Investigating the relationship between medical and psychological well-being. *Irish Journal of Psychological Medicine, 38*(4), 272–277. https://doi.org/10.1017/ipm.2021.37

Volpato, E., Banfi, P., & Pagnini, F. (2017). A psychological intervention to promote acceptance and adherence to non-invasive ventilation in people with chronic obstructive pulmonary disease: Study protocol of a randomized controlled trial. *Trials, 18*(59), 1–9. https://doi.org/10.1186/s13063-017-1802-1

World Health Organization. (2012). *World Health Organization Quality of Life—BREF.* Retrieved from https://www.who.int/publications/i/item/WHO-MSD-MER-Rev-2012-02

Wu, J., Suk, K., Dekker, R., et al. (2017). Prehospital delay, precipitants of admission, and length of stay in patients with exacerbation of heart failure. *American Journal of Critical Care, 26*(1), 62–69. https://doi.org/10.4037/ajcc2017750

31

Care for the Dying and for Those Who Grieve

Sonya L. Jakubec

 https://evolve.elsevier.com/Canada/Varcarolis/psychiatric/

OBJECTIVES

1. Compare and contrast specific goals of end-of-life care inherent in the hospice palliative care model with those of the medical model.
2. Analyze the effects of specific interventions nurses can implement when working with a dying person and their family and loved ones.
3. Analyze how the Four Gifts of Resolving Relationships (forgiveness, love, gratitude, and farewell) can be used to help people respond to a dying loved one.
4. Explain the distinction between the terms *grief* and *mourning* as presented in this chapter and how the effectiveness of a holistic approach can be beneficial to the person.
5. Differentiate among some of the characteristics of typical bereavement and complicated grieving.
6. Explain how various models of understanding grieving (dual process, four tasks of mourning) can enhance your care of those who grieve.
7. Discuss at least five guidelines for dealing with catastrophic loss, and identify appropriate support for someone in acute grief.

KEY TERMS AND CONCEPTS

anticipatory grief
bereavement
complicated grief
disenfranchised grief
Four Gifts of Resolving Relationships
grief
hospice palliative care
mourning
palliative care
prolonged grief

Caring for patients who have terminal illnesses or are near death due to other conditions challenges and rewards nurses in deep and personal ways. In caring for people who are dying nurses may grow personally, both by accepting their patients' deaths and by developing a richer understanding of their own mortality. Nurses also have an opportunity to bring dignity to the dying and help shape an enduring positive memory for family members and caregivers. At times of crisis (e.g., traumatic death such as death by suicide), mental health nurses may work closely as witnesses and companions in the grief process of those surviving.

Nurses continue to provide care for dying patients primarily in medical institutions, despite evidence supporting care in the home and the overwhelming wish of most Canadians to die at home, surrounded by loved ones (Mondor et al., 2020). Although 60% of Canadian deaths occur in hospital (Canadian Institute for Health Information, 2021), alternatives for community-based palliative care and grief support are emerging across the country. Patient-centred **palliative care** is an inter-disciplinary and collaborative effort aimed at relieving pain and suffering and involving various health care providers at all levels of interventions (Canadian Hospice Palliative Care Association, 2021) in which nurses play an integral and important role. In addition to using the necessary assessment and management skills, nurses are often the entry point into the system for patients and their families.

Health care providers in all settings (home, residential care, street, shelter, hospital or intensive care unit, palliative care unit or hospice) must be advocates for people with life-limiting illnesses and their often-overburdened caregivers. The Canadian hospice palliative care treatment model (Canadian Hospice Palliative Care Association, 2013) and the advance care planning national framework (Canadian Hospice Palliative Care Association, 2020) provide tools that promote patient- and family-centred care for people facing potentially life-threatening situations. The tools support basic human rights, including having control over decisions affecting health and living situations; having advance directives (such as instructions to suspend or withhold curative efforts) completed and followed; and receiving excellent palliative care that promotes optimum comfort.

HOSPICE PALLIATIVE CARE

In 1967 in response to a system in which dying people were often neglected, isolated, and left to die in pain, Dame Cicely Saunders, a nurse, social worker, and physician, established St. Christopher's Hospice in London, England. Dame Cicely received universal recognition as the founder of the modern hospice movement. Central to her work was an aggressive pursuit of effective pain management that contributed to optimal quality of life (Clarke, 2010).

During the same period, in the United States, Dr. Elisabeth Kübler-Ross, also a nurse, began actively listening to the terminally ill. In her ground-breaking work, Kübler-Ross (1969) identified distinctive phases, or cycles, in people's responses to terminal illness: denial, anger, bargaining, depression, and acceptance. Kübler-Ross also realized that personal growth actually accelerated in the last stages of life. Encouraged by the work of Kübler-Ross, those working with the dying adapted the St. Christopher's comprehensive model, and the interprofessional care team evolved to include a physician, a nurse, a social worker, a pastor or chaplain, and an aide.

The term *palliative care* was coined in the mid-1970s by Canadian physician Balfour Mount, who was inspired by the work of Kübler-Ross and Dame Cicely Saunders (McGill University, 2021). Like those before him, Dr. Mount found that treatments for the terminally ill were abysmally inadequate, so he set up a hospital-based palliative care unit at the Royal Victoria Hospital in Montreal, taking the name *palliative* from its meaning, "to improve the quality of something." Dr. Balfour is known as "the father of palliative care," an approach that evolved into a pan-Canadian movement, with goals of relieving suffering and improving quality of life for those who are living with or dying from an illness (Canadian Hospice Palliative Care Association, 2021). This movement eventually led to the development of the Canadian Hospice Palliative Care Association (CHPCA), established in 1991, which is the national voice for hospice palliative care (HPC) in Canada. HPC is defined as whole-person health care aimed at relieving suffering and improving quality of life rather than aimed at a cure (Canadian Hospice Palliative Care Association, 2021).

Death is a natural and inevitable part of life. Using an interdisciplinary approach, the national HPC model is appropriate for patients and families of all ages living with or at risk for developing a life-threatening illness of any kind or magnitude, for whom HPC may complement therapy or be the total focus of care (Canadian Hospice Palliative Care Association, 2021). The goals of HPC are to address all needs (physical, psychological, social, cultural, spiritual, and practical), prepare for and manage self-determined life closure and the dying process, and help with coping with loss and grief during illness and bereavement (Canadian Hospice Palliative Care Association, 2021). Historically, the terms *hospice* and *palliative care* were often used interchangeably; however, the CHPCA has brought the two terms together to form HPC. One of the central themes of HPC in Canada is the belief that each of us has the right to die pain-free and with dignity (Canadian Hospice Palliative Care Association, 2021).

Quality palliative care is identified as a human right in a growing collection of studies and global action items (Clark et al., 2018; LeBarron & Galassi, 2019; Mason et al., 2020). Although palliative care is widely available to all Canadians, regardless of age or diagnosis, access to high-quality integrated care is not the same across the county. Despite the progressive move toward an integrated, streamlined system, many Canadians, unlike Mr. Spence, are still dying without adequate supports (Canadian Hospice Palliative Care Association, 2010). Among the reasons for this lack of supports are geography, lack of patient-centred care, lack of knowledge and policy leadership, discrimination, and funding. Although HPC grew from the concept of caring for the dying, it is now used to guide care at any point during an acute, chronic, or life-threatening illness or bereavement (Canadian Hospice Palliative Care Association, 2013).

Palliative care is a philosophy of care as opposed to a treatment or place of treatment. Because Canadians are living longer with chronic health conditions, bringing this philosophy into being through access to quality care is necessary at earlier points in the continuum of life, not just at the end of life. Patients can receive HPC in hospital, at home, in community care homes (e.g., long-term care), or in hospice programs. Respite beds are also available in some centres. Innovative programs in Ottawa, Toronto, Calgary, Victoria, and Thunder Bay to provide palliative care to structurally vulnerable populations, particularly people experiencing homeless, have emerged over the past decade, highlighting a number of systemic challenges. These programs also demonstrate the challenges of merging complex street-level care and harm reduction with palliative care principles to address structural vulnerability (Stajduhar & Mollison, 2018). Several factors need to be considered when determining the best place for providing care, such as personal choice, a balance between patient and family needs, and the availability of resources to meet those needs (Giesbrecht et al., 2018; Stajduhar et al., 2019).

Regardless of the setting, the HPC approach is interprofessional and cross-sector in nature. In addition to access to health care providers, this approach also requires spiritual care, volunteer services, bereavement services, medical equipment, medications, and supplies related to the illness. A personalized plan of care is developed with the patient, reflected in the care, and regularly reviewed and updated.

VIGNETTE

Del Spence was diagnosed with amyotrophic lateral sclerosis (ALS) at the age of 52. Del lived at home until caregiving overwhelmed his family, resulting in admission to a care centre for the past 9 months. At this time, Del is almost completely paralyzed and uses a letter board with a head-mounted laser pointer to communicate. A warm smile and a pleasant gaze enable Del's communication and connection with family and professional caregivers as well as numerous friends who visit often. Shooting leg pain, alongside increasing difficulty with swallowing and breathing, is increasingly impairing Del's quality of life. Despite being barely able to eat, he has refused a feeding tube. The staff feel helpless. How can they just stand by while Del starves to death? Will Del starve to death? One of the aides has decided to quit working with Del because this concern of "not doing everything possible" has become so emotionally difficult for her.

An HPC referral was made. A nurse and social worker visited the care facility and offered practical help and guidance for staff, patient, and family in treating Del. They explored with Del what to expect as ALS progresses. Comfort-oriented medication and non-pharmacological care were reviewed, and Del was offered as many choices as possible. Emotional, spiritual, and educational support were offered to the family and staff concerning the course of the illness, anticipatory grieving, and ways of using the remaining time to meet goals and nurture relationships. Del, assisted by his family and an HPC volunteer, chose to work on a memoir about the illness and its impact on their personal growth and discoveries.

⚡ SAFETY TIP

Safety in HPC Is Everyone's Concern, Everywhere!

Ways of improving safety in HPC must be considered as part of everyday mental health nursing practice. This is particularly important in light of the variety of locations of HPC and predominance of care at home and non-professional caregivers providing care. Safety tips to remember:

1. Safety is everyone's concern. All providers, including family/friend caregivers, must be supported in the provision of safe care as an integral part of quality end-of-life care.
2. Safety involves more than the consideration of errors, mortality, and serious morbidity; it also involves considering minimizing suffering for patients and family/friend caregivers.
3. Palliative care environments, like other medical environments are not necessarily safe. Home environments have less structure to maintain safety; additional consideration is needed and can extend and support quality of life and reduce suffering for both patients and caregivers.
4. Seeking blame for errors does not solve any problems. Safety issues are system issues. Ongoing reflection, review, and resolving safety concerns circle back to being everyone's concern

Source: Based on Librach, S. L. (2021). *To err is human: Is patient safety an issue in palliative care?* Retrieved from https://www.virtualhospice.ca/en_US/Main+Site+Navigation/Home/For+Professionals/For+Professionals/The+Exchange/Current/To+Err+Is+Human_+Is+Patient+Safety+an+Issue+in+Palliative+Care_.aspx

NURSING CARE AT THE END OF LIFE

End-of-life (EOL) care is a term that describes care to assist people as they progress through the final stage of dying, then continues until death and into family bereavement and care of the body. It is provided across all settings of the continuum of care to relieve suffering and improve the quality of living until death (Canadian Nurses Association, Canadian Hospice Palliative Care Association, Canadian Hospice Palliative Care Nurses Group, 2015, p. 2).

Hospice Palliative Care Nursing

Although nurses are educated to provide holistic care, few are prepared to deal with the death and dying trajectory they will ultimately face at some point in their careers. The Canadian Association of Schools of Nursing (CASN, 2011) developed entry-to-practice competencies and indicators for registered nurses. Post-education competencies for nurses and interprofessional practitioners also provide guidance and shape HPC practice in Canada (BC Centre for Palliative Care, 2019b). The Canadian Network of Palliative Care for Children and Canadian Hospice Palliative Care Association (2021) also established competencies for pediatric palliative care. Again, these competencies emphasize interprofessional practice and holistic approaches to care that include family, community, cultural, and spiritual components of care that are discussed in more detail in this chapter.

In addition to providing practical care, nurses need to demonstrate enhanced communication, coordination, and management skills; self-care; and the ability to attend to the compassion and dignity needs of those suffering loss. Nurses working in HPC settings should ideally pursue additional certification and can support compassionate community care through volunteer training as well as death doula training (Rawlings et al., 2021). Nurses also work collaboratively in EOL care, with the interprofessional team and alongside community supports such as death doulas who, like the care provided by birth doulas during the pregnancy and birthing process, support a person during the dying process. This support is specific to family needs, beliefs, and desires, as well as making connections to culture and Indigenous values (End of Life Doula Association of Canada, 2021; Gaspard et al., 2021).

The Art, Presence, and Caring of Nursing

Caring for patients at the end of life requires a shift in professional expectations. It involves not only curing but also healing concepts of care (Chochinov, 2016; Walshe et al., 2018), the demand for genuine human presence toward the patient while using evidence-informed knowledge, the management of pain and symptom control, and other technical aspects of care. "Whole-person care" involves seeing the patient first as a human being while being attentive to all aspects of suffering. The Canadian Hospice Palliative Care Association (2006) developed gold standards for nurses providing HPC and EOL care, with the following five dimensions of nursing to help guide their work in any setting.

- **Valuing**—believing in the intrinsic value of others, in the value of life, and that death is a natural process
- **Connecting**—establishing a therapeutic relationship with the person and the family through making, sustaining, and closing the relationship
- **Empowering**—providing care that is empowering for the person and the family
- **Doing for**—providing care based on best practice in pain and symptom management, coordination of care, and advocacy
- **Finding meaning**—helping the person and family to find meaning in their lives and their experiences of illness

To work towards these standards, two essential skills you can practise are listening and observing (see Chapters 9 and 10). Reflect back to the speaker what you heard by restating or summarizing the message. Observe the patient's non-verbal communications. Do you sense well-being? Sorrow? Suffering? Ask the patient and family open-ended questions such as:

- Would you tell me what this is like for you?
- How do you see your condition right now?
- Where do you see things going?
- Are you worried about anything?
- What would be important for you?
- What are you hoping for?

Practise staying silent and giving the patient or family member all the time needed to respond. Offer a reassuring touch. The nurse can invite and permit the patient to discover new dimensions of their own experiences, bringing greater meaning at the end of life or in grief and loss.

Assessment for Spiritual Issues

Spirituality, the dimension of human experience that can provide meaning for life, is integral to EOL care. Conducting a comprehensive spiritual assessment is important to understanding how a patient's spirituality may enhance comfort. Time spent with the patient and family and genuine expressions of compassion (Sinclair et al., 2021) are considered essential for successful spiritual care assessment and outcomes. Although no one approach is validated for assessment of spirituality in palliative care (Perry et al., 2021; Steinhauser et al., 2020), assessment can be guided by tools such as FICA (measuring faith or belief, importance of spirituality and individual's spiritual community, and interventions to address spiritual needs) (Puchalski, 2007) or HOPE (sources of hope, organized religion, spiritual practices, and effects on health) (Anandarajah & Hight, 2001). Regardless of the tool used, it is important to use unbiased, open language and ensure appropriate timing in the relationship, having already established trust and rapport as a companion and witness in the palliative experience (Chochinov, 2016). Some examples of questions are: Tell me how you are doing spiritually. What gives your life meaning? What role do your beliefs play in regaining your health? Spiritual caring is a vital part of holistic care and can be interwoven with the nurse's daily work through the process of self-awareness, empathy, and commitment to EOL care (Lormans et al., 2021). In addition to thoroughly assessing connections to a specific religion, nurses can become skilled at listening for the patient's intrinsic spirituality. For many patients, religion and spiritual practices provide context, community, and comfort when facing EOL challenges.

Awareness and Sensitivity of Cultural Contexts

Spiritual and cultural contexts and care are often inextricably intertwined. Although it is impossible for the nurse to know all things about all cultures, it is imperative as professionals to be aware of the need to explore cultural practices that affect care at all times across the health care continuum (see Chapter 8). Canada is a multi-cultural nation, but in particular, it has a growing older person Indigenous population (Webkamigad et al., 2020). As Indigenous people age, they suffer even higher burdens of chronic disease and illness than do non-Indigenous Canadians. In addition, many Indigenous people live in rural communities, which often do not have the same access to health care services (palliative care among these) as their urban counterparts (Caxaj et al., 2018; Schill & Caxaj, 2019). Like so many people, the majority of Indigenous people living in remote communities would prefer to die at home. However, unlike many others, they are not often given this opportunity, due to a lack of services and resources (Caxaj et al., 2018; Gaspard et al., 2021). In addition to this difference, even when HPC is available, this care is often not safe for or sensitive to Indigenous or other cultures. The Canadian Virtual Hospice (2021) developed a curriculum for health care providers that is inclusive of culturally sensitive and appropriate protocols for providing support to Indigenous families in need of HPC services. Many cultural practices of Indigenous persons (e.g., respect for elders, the special gifts of elders, the role of sacred items and ceremonies) are rooted in culture and grounded in spirituality (Canadian Virtual Hospice, 2021). Research on palliative care for Indigenous communities is a priority (see Research Highlight box).

RESEARCH HIGHLIGHT
First Nations Communities and Palliative Care

Problem
In Canada there is a growing need to develop community-based, culturally appropriate palliative care for Indigenous people living in First Nations communities. The public health approach to palliative care, which emphasizes community-based initiatives, is especially relevant in First Nations communities because care is shaped by the particular social and cultural context. A public health approach to palliative care is concerned with educational strategies that strengthen communities' capacity to care for people as they die.

Purpose of Study
This project aimed to assess and address local palliative care educational needs to improve community capacity in palliative care.

Methods
A three-phase participatory action research (PAR) process with four First Nations communities in Canada was conducted over a 6-year period (2010 to 2016): (1) focus groups, interviews, and surveys to assess community-specific needs and resources; (2) recommendations were developed to guide the PAR; (3) educational resources were created to address the identified educational needs. These resources were implemented incrementally over 4 years with an ongoing process evaluation and revisions to the resources.

Key Findings
The palliative care educational needs of patients, families, community members, and internal and external health care providers were assessed. A wide and comprehensive range of educational resources were created to address palliative care learning needs. A culturally appropriate palliative care resource workbook was developed and is available for use by other Indigenous people and communities.

Implications for Nursing Practice
This public health palliative care approach offers implementation strategies for education relevant to Indigenous communities that can guide communities and nurses. A model for nurses and communities is available for conducting a culturally appropriate assessment of educational needs, creating recommendations, facilitating development, and implementation of educational resources in the community to improve community capacity in palliative care.

Source: Prince, H., Nadin, S., Crow, M., et al. (2019). "If you understand you cope better with it": The role of education in building palliative care capacity in four First Nations communities in Canada. *BMC Public Health, 19*(1), 768. https://doi.org/10.1186/s12889-019-6983-y

Palliative Symptom Management

Excellent symptom management is a hallmark of HPC nursing (BC Centre for Palliative Care, 2019a). The patient or substitute decision maker has the right to be informed and make decisions about all aspects of care, including the right to a dignified and comfortable death (Canadian Hospice Palliative Care Association, 2013; Canadian Nurses Association, 2017a). Nurses can offer a wide spectrum of interventions to alleviate symptoms, guided by patients' own reports and careful assessment. The most commonly reported EOL symptoms are pain, constipation, dyspnea, fatigue, depression, and delirium (National

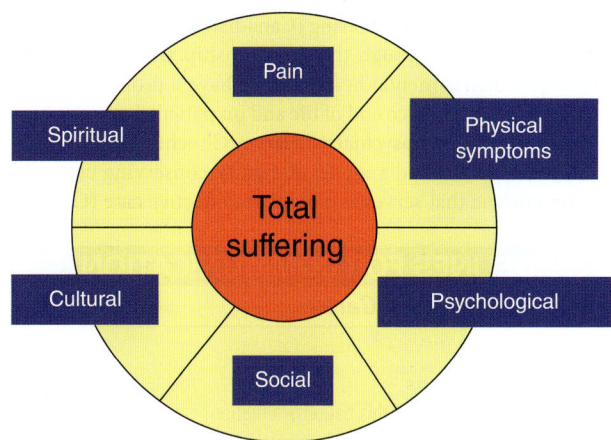

Fig. 31.1 Woodruff's total suffering model. (**Source:** Woodruff, R. [2004]. Palliative medicine: Evidence-based symptomatic and supportive care for patients with advanced cancer [4th ed.]. New York: Oxford University Press.)

Institute for Health and Care Excellence, 2021). It is gratifying to relieve pain or nausea or to give patients control over bowel medications and breathing treatments. For symptoms such as worry, fear, sadness, and low energy, however, better approaches might include education, normalization, counselling, integrative therapies (e.g., massage, music), and stress-reduction practices. Music therapy has been found to produce beneficial effects for quality of life, management of distress, and treatment satisfaction (Warth et al., 2021).

Each symptom should be assessed individually. Treatable, reversible, and temporary conditions can be mistakenly attributed to the terminal diagnosis. For example, if a patient reports feeling depressed, it is important not to assume that the feelings are due to the dying process. If the patient becomes short of breath, confused, or lethargic, it is essential to rule out causes such as medication effects, dehydration, delirium, pneumonia, urinary tract infections, and constipation before attributing the symptom to terminal decline.

Care of the patient and family can be viewed through the lens of Roger Woodruff's total suffering model (Figure 31.1). This model can also be used to describe guidelines when caring for the dying (Box 31.1). The use of such a model can help guide the practice of nurses throughout the nursing process when working with palliative care patients.

The Importance of Effective Communication

Nurses need excellent communication skills when working in all settings, at all times, and with all members involved in the HPC experience (Matzo & Sherman, 2018). Nurses have a role even at the beginning of the EOL continuum. The value of simply asking patients and their families, "Do you have any concerns?" followed by strong encouragement to seek out their support system while waiting for news cannot be understated.

During stressful periods, two factors seem to make things more bearable: (1) the ability to have, or believe one can have, some control over the situation and (2) the ability to predict changes. Information and education from nurses can improve a family's sense of control. Information should be conveyed slowly, given repeatedly, written down, and reviewed often. People tend to need several reiterations of information when under stress (see Chapters 5, 12, and 21). Effective communication skills are at the heart of developing a therapeutic relationship, assessing the patient, and providing holistic care to the patient and family. A strong therapeutic relationship will guide discussions and decision making for patients and families in times of loss (see Chapter 9). In addition, effective communication helps to decrease distress and total pain and suffering (Canadian Hospice Palliative Care Association, 2009b). Through their relationship and communication practices, psychiatric mental health nurses have a profound influence on how patients experience end of life and on patients' sense of dignity. Canadian palliative care psychiatrist Harvey Chochinov and colleagues have developed and tested a model of dignity-conserving care with an ABCD mnemonic that serves as a guide for effective care (Chochinov, 2007). Guidelines for Communication: Dignity-Conserving Care highlights practical approaches in more detail.

The balance of kindness and respect through empathy and information is always at the front of the mind in care of the dying. The following vignette illustrates the confusion and misery that can result from lack of information, the desire to take control of one's life situation, and the inadequacy of the term *dying* to describe living with a terminal disease.

GUIDELINES FOR COMMUNICATION
Dignity-Conserving Care

Attitudes
Reflective Questions
- How would I be feeling in this patient's situation?
- What is leading me to draw those conclusions?
- Have I checked whether my assumptions are accurate?
- Am I aware of how my attitude toward the patient may be affecting them?
- Could my attitude toward the patient be based on something to do with my own experiences, anxieties, or fears?
- Does my attitude as a nurse enable or disenable me to establish open and empathic professional relationships with my patients?

Actions to Be Taken
- Consciously and routinely make these questions a part of your reflection on the care of each and every patient
- Discuss attitudes in regular clinical supervision and debriefings
- Embrace learning opportunities and experiences that challenge and question your attitudes and assumptions as they might affect patient care
- Support the acknowledgement and discussion of these issues with others in the workplace to support a growing culture of dignity-conserving care

Behaviours
General Disposition
- Treat contact with patients as you would any potent and important clinical intervention
- Professional behaviours toward patients must always include respect and kindness
- Lack of curative options should never rationalize or justify a lack of ongoing patient contact

Assessment Practices
- Always ask the patient's permission to engage in any clinical assessment or intervention
- Always ask the patient's permission to include others in the assessment or interventions
- Although assessment and interventions may be part of routine care, it is rarely routine for the patient, so always, as much as possible, take time to set the patient at ease and show that you have some appreciation for what they are about to go through (e.g., "I know this might feel a bit uncomfortable"; "I'm sorry that we have to do this to you"; "I know this is an inconvenience"; "This should only hurt for a moment"; "Let me know if you feel we need to stop for any reason"; "Asking these questions again is necessary because …")
- Limit conversations with patients during medical interventions (aside from providing them with instruction or encouragement) until they have dressed or been covered appropriately and are rested

Facilitating Communication
- Demonstrate to your patient that they have your full and complete attention
- Always invite the patient to have people from their support network present, particularly when you plan to discuss complex or "difficult" information
- All personal issues should be raised in ways that respect the patient's need for privacy
- When speaking with the patient, try to be seated at a comfortable distance for conversation, at the patient's eye level when possible
- Offer patients and families repeated explanations as requested
- Present information free of jargon, using only language that the patient will understand
- Ask if the patient has questions and allow time for questions to arise and be recalled

Compassion
Getting in touch with one's own feelings requires the consideration of human life and experience, through a number of avenues, such as:
- Reading and discussing stories and novels and experiencing films, theatre, expert talks, and art that portray the depth and despair of the human condition
- Reflecting on the personal stories that accompany illness
- Experiencing some degree of identification with those who are ill or suffering—be with your vulnerability

Ways to Show Compassion
- An understanding look
- A gentle touch on the shoulder, arm, or hand
- Honest communication, spoken or unspoken, that acknowledges the person beyond their illness

Dialogue
Acknowledging Personhood
- "This must be frightening for you."
- "I can only imagine what you must be going through."
- "It's natural to feel pretty overwhelmed at times like these."

Knowing the Patient
- "What should I know about you as a person to help me take the best care of you that I can?"
- "What are the things at this time in your life that are most important to you or that concern you most?"
- "Who else (or what else) will be affected by what's happening with your health?"
- "Who should be here to help support you?" (friends, family, spiritual or religious support network, etc.)
- "Who else should we get involved at this point, to help support you through this difficult time?" (psychosocial services, group support, chaplaincy, complementary care specialists, etc.)

Psychotherapeutic Approaches
- Dignity therapy
- Meaning-centred therapy
- Life review/reminiscence

Source: Adapted from Chochinov, H. M. (2007). Dignity and the essence of medicine: The A, B, C, and D of dignity conserving care. *BMJ, 335*(7612), 184–187. https://doi.org/10.1136/bmj.39244.650926.47

BOX 31.1 Guidelines When Caring for the Dying

Pain—Remember that patients' pain is what they say it is, and they have the right to have their pain needs met effectively, using the simplest route. Reassure them that you will provide relief from their pain to help decrease their anxiety.

Physical—Intervene quickly to manage symptoms that may affect other organ systems (e.g., nausea, constipation or diarrhea, incontinence, air hunger, inadequate nutrition) in order to promote and maintain the highest level of comfort possible.

Psychological—Keep patients and their families informed about the disease and its symptoms. Invite them to deal with their emotions, acknowledging the losses and changes in their lives. Practise the art of presence and caring through active listening, genuine empathy, and personal sharing.

Social—Many people at the end of life are afraid of dying alone and need reassurance that they are not alone. Promote this sense of security by verbalizing this reassurance, and demonstrate it by responding to their needs quickly and spending time with them. Provide companionship for them by supporting their visitors, engaging in conversations with them and their families, and providing privacy when appropriate or when requested.

Cultural—Ask questions to discover the person's cultural background and meaningful practices used during end-of-life care to promote a peaceful journey. Explore appropriate language used (are there any taboo words?), and inquire about whom to share information with first. Explore the role of the family in care, and explore care practices other than science-based medicine, such as alternative medicines or other therapies.

Spiritual—By asking appropriate questions, offer the opportunity to patients to discuss what is meaningful in their lives, such as relationships, any faith or spiritual practices they use to keep themselves calm, and who or what they turn to when dealing with the challenges of life. Exploring spirituality can offer the opportunity to assess and promote effective coping skills based on past behaviours.

VIGNETTE

Susan, a 74-year-old divorced woman who lives alone and uses the pronouns she/her, is told by her doctor that she is dying of liver cancer. Upon hearing that she cannot be cured, she assumes that she will die in a few days or weeks. She goes home, settles all her affairs, calls everyone she cares about and says goodbye, accepts hospice care, and begins to await death. As weeks and then months go by, Susan feels betrayed by her doctor, embarrassed to be alive, unsure how to behave, and uncomfortable with her friends and relatives. She has time to begin worrying about how her death will be, how much control she will lose, and how she can afford care at the end. She is confused and even disoriented by the unexpected apparent improvement in her symptoms.

Susan shares her feelings with the nurse. The nurse educates Susan about her cancer and how to interpret her symptoms. The HPC team addresses her emotions and needs in many ways. They encourage her to take a trip she had postponed and to begin seeing friends again. They educate her on the concept of "living with terminal illness" rather than dying from it. Susan needs to learn new approaches to living meaningfully with an uncertain future. When Susan finally enters the end stage of her disease, she is comfortable and cared for by her relatives at home.

Anticipatory Grief

Patients and families can experience grief in advance of loss, known as **anticipatory grief**, when they receive a life-limiting diagnosis or when they are threatened with loss of ability to function independently, loss of identity, and changes in role definition (Rogalla, 2020). Future loss is mourned as people acknowledge the importance of the impending loss, adjust their lives to accommodate the intervening time, and anticipate how their futures will be altered by the loss. Sensitive communication and support can help family members process this information (Overton & Cottone, 2016). The experience of anticipatory grief varies by individual, family, and culture (Box 31.2). Nurses can help patients and loved ones understand that their feelings are common and assist them with developing coping strategies and with redefining their roles within the family and in the outside world (Matzo & Sherman, 2018). Nurses must also remind those in their care to keep in mind that, although they are experiencing loss, there is always hope.

As with all types of grieving, nurses need to recognize that people can experience symptoms of grief physically, cognitively, emotionally, socially, and spiritually (Canadian Hospice Palliative Care Association, 2008) and intervene appropriately.

The Four Gifts of Resolving Relationships

An important role of the nurse during EOL care is to invite families to accept the dying of their loved one and say goodbye. Taking the opportunity to say goodbye has been correlated with more positive bereavement outcomes, something taken for granted that was illuminated during the COVID-19 pandemic (Selman et al., 2021). The **Four Gifts of Resolving Relationships** is one means of opening conversations about the coming separation. The concept of the Four Gifts was interpreted from the writings of Elisabeth Kübler-Ross and used with her permission by Beverly Ryan of the Hospice of the Twin Cities in Minnesota. In her workshops for the terminally ill Dr. Kübler-Ross witnessed many couples and families shift from being distant, cold, or angry to becoming warm, loving, and close. Kübler-Ross observed that this change resulted from a predictable sequence of communications, which were later formulated into the Four Gifts. People often intuitively recognize the gifts as processes they have already been experiencing. Perhaps these processes are innate within human relationships, but anxiety, sorrow, and denial can obstruct their expression.

The nurse can describe the Four Gifts in simple terms and encourage families and patients to express them in their own ways. The gifts, namely, forgiveness, love, gratitude, and farewell, can work for both giver and receiver. When given with sincerity and simplicity, they can precipitate a healing shift in relationships.

Forgiveness. The first step in forgiveness is to admit to wrongs and hurts experienced in the relationship. The intention is to forgive, seek forgiveness, and release the hurt so that healing can occur. Sometimes a face-to-face encounter is not possible (e.g., when the patient is sedated, comatose, or experiencing dementia), and sometimes it is not advisable (e.g., when it would cause more distress than it would relieve). Reconciliation requires two people who wish to heal a broken relationship. Forgiveness is a one-sided act, which can be given unilaterally.

BOX 31.2 Signs of Anticipatory Grief

- Feelings of emptiness or of being lost
- A sense of being numb and fatigued
- A feeling of unreality and disbelief
- Periods of weeping or raging
- The desire to run away from the situation
- The need to protect the patient from suffering or death by overseeing every detail of care
- Worry about the future and the unknown
- Anger at the patient, health care providers, or both
- Pronounced clinging to or dependency on the patient or other family members
- Fear of going crazy

Granting forgiveness does not mean condoning or accepting a truly injurious or abusive action. It does not make a wrong right. What it does is signal a desire to let go of blame and anger, to release one's own heart from the chains of resentment. As such, it is a gift to the one who offers forgiveness, whether reconciliation is possible or not.

Love. The second gift is to express love to each other. Many adult children wish to hear their parent say, "I love you, and I am proud of you." Between spouses, in some long-term marriages, these words have faded away to be replaced by daily togetherness and the practical caring of a shared life. It is not uncommon in bereavement for survivors to regret that they did not hear or say the words "I love you" and long for that final recognition of the relationship's value. Ultimately, the message we need to hear at the end of life is that we are loved for being who we are, not for what we have done or achieved.

Gratitude. Expressions of love naturally flow into gratitude for what each has been in the other person's life. People look back over life together and remember the good times and the tough times. They can take out photograph albums, show videotapes, reminisce, and listen again to favourite stories. It is especially gratifying to acknowledge the things that were taken for granted. Parents or caregivers may never have been thanked for going to work every day for 30 or 40 years, caring for the home, or offering nurturance, support, or guidance. Similarly, acknowledgement of the love and attention of caregivers or dependants can be important expressions of gratitude. Many exhausted caregivers weep when they are told they really are doing a good job and are appreciated.

Farewell. Many people say they hate goodbyes because they bring up feelings of grief at the finality of parting. Also, it is awkward to say goodbye before someone is actually leaving. It may appear to be rushing the person or even causing the departure. Yet when the final separation of death awaits us, the act of saying goodbye is deeply appropriate and meaningful. In cases when there is no chance to say goodbye, or when the opportunity to say goodbye is not taken, survivors may express long-term regret. The words or gestures used do not matter as long as the meaning is adequately expressed.

In the preceding vignette Trent did not rehearse, resist, or complicate the Four Gifts but used the sequence to express the full range of feelings. This story illustrates how simple and natural this process can be. Many families need no encouragement to forgive, cherish, thank, and release a loved one. The Four Gifts can be a helpful contribution, however, to families whose members are overwhelmed, cling to false hope, or are emotionally reticent.

Self-Care

As front-line medical caregivers, nurses are educated to help patients get better, stronger, and more independent. Supporting patients at the end of life, as they grow weaker, sicker, and ultimately die, can be overwhelming, challenging the nurse's sense of competency and professionalism. The demands inherent in EOL nursing lead to increased vulnerability to emotional attachments and compassion fatigue. These experiences, along with daily exposure to grief and dying, require nurses to practise conscious self-care in both their professional and their private lives. Health care providers naturally grow attached to some patients and may experience both anticipatory grieving and bereavement. To maintain emotional balance and health, it is essential to rely on the support of others and practise good self-care. This is a journey that promotes greater self-understanding, wisdom, and compassion (Worden, 2018). The multi-disciplinary team approach of supportive supervision is helpful in this process.

Caring for patients who are dying and those who grieve can bring up personal reactions, which may be triggered by a patient who is younger than the nurse, one who resembles a significant person in the nurse's own life, one who is experiencing symptoms reminiscent of other difficult deaths, or one who offends the nurse's sense of fairness or acceptability. Workplace conditions such as complex caseloads, rapid turnover in office staff, several losses in a short period, or too many demands for on-call time or overtime can intensify a nurse's vulnerability to feeling overwhelmed. Box 31.3 provides guidelines to help the health care provider maintain emotional health when working with death and the dying.

VIGNETTE

Trent is a 28-year-old person with developmental disabilities and bipolar disorder. Dan is Trent's father and is dying of end-stage liver failure. Trent takes a short bus trip in order to see Dan for the last time as Trent lives in a group home in a smaller community 1 hour away and has not seen Dan and extended family for many months. Unfortunately, on the previous visit, Trent forgot to bring a regular medication, which exacerbated a hypomania, and the resulting behaviour caused Trent's family distress and ultimately avoidance of Trent altogether. The HPC nurse tells Trent that Dan is dying and explains the Four Gifts. Trent sadly enters Dan's bedroom and sits on the bed. Trent explains, "Dad, I know you are going to die, and I want you to know that I am so sorry for the ways I have acted and the trouble I have caused. Please forgive me, Dad. You have always looked out for me, and I shouldn't have gone off my meds. I love you, Dad. You've never given up on me. Thank you for finding me the place where I live and people to love me and look after me. Thanks for being my Dad. I know I have to say goodbye. I promise I will keep taking my meds so I will behave right. I promise I'll listen to my counsellors and have a good life. I love you so much, Dad. Goodbye." He weeps with his father, who holds him for a little while. Trent leaves Dan's room with a tear-streaked face, knowing this will be their last moments together, and the last moments of Dan's life. Painful as it is, Trent feels complete. The important things were spoken with courage and Dan and Trent have nothing left unsaid. There is nothing else to do, say, or be in this moment.

BOX 31.3 Guidelines for Self-Care When Caring for the Dying

1. Remind yourself that what is happening to your patients and their families is not happening to you. This is their life drama right now but not your own.
2. When you notice that you are having a particularly strong emotional reaction, either positive or negative (counter-transference), take it as a signal to explore your deeper issues or needs by talking with a trusted friend, counsellor, or colleague.
3. Protect your private life by practising time management, avoiding working outside of normal hours, protecting your pager or telephone number, and taking regular days off and vacations.
4. Clearly state what you can and cannot do for your patients so that your human and professional limitations are known up front.
5. Practise humility. There is much you can do, but there is also much that is unknown and unknowable.
6. Do your own mourning when your heart is touched and you need to acknowledge the importance of others in your life. Even after a person has died, you can honour the relationship you had in your memory. Attend funerals or create grieving rituals when someone you felt close to dies.
7. Create a healthy, balanced private life by releasing stress. Working with patients who are dying creates stresses at many levels. The challenge is to work them into your busy schedule and stay on course. Foremost among these methods are regular exercise, a balanced diet, adequate rest, vacations, fun and laughter, loving and accepting relationships, and a connection to higher meaning in life.

NURSING CARE FOR THOSE WHO GRIEVE

Loss is part of the human experience, and grieving is the response that enables people to accept and reconcile the loss and adapt to change. We grieve the commonplace losses in our lives, be they loss of a relationship (e.g., divorce, separation, death, abortion); health (e.g., a body function or part, mental or physical capacity); friendship, status, or prestige; security (e.g., occupational, financial, social, cultural); or a dream. Other normal losses include changes in circumstances, such as retirement, promotion, marriage, and aging. These losses can promote growth through adaptation or may result in apathy, anger, and resentment.

Losing a significant person through death is a major life crisis. Long-term relationships deeply bond us to each other, shaping our world and our identity in it. Their loss can diminish aspects of our own self-concept and tear apart our assumptive world. Grief is experienced holistically, affecting us emotionally, cognitively, spiritually, and physically. Those who grieve sometimes describe the death of a loved one as an amputation.

GRIEF REACTIONS, BEREAVEMENT, AND MOURNING

Grief encompasses all of an individual's reactions to loss and is defined as sorrow experienced in anticipation of, during, and after a loss (Canadian Hospice Palliative Care Association, 2013). Normal grief reactions include depressed mood, insomnia, anxiety, poor appetite, loss of interest, guilt, dreams about the deceased, and poor concentration. Psychological states include shock, denial, and yearning or searching for the deceased. **Bereavement**, derived from the Old English word *berafian*, meaning "to rob," is the period of grieving following a death. **Mourning** refers to things people do to cope with their grief, including shared social expressions of grief, such as attending funerals and other ceremonies or rituals, as well as participating in bereavement groups. Everyone grieves, but not everyone engages in the work of mourning. The length of time, degree, and rituals for mourning are often typically determined by cultural, religious, and familial factors. Despite a wide variation in experiences of duration and intensity, grief becomes a serious physical and mental health concern for relatively few people (Gray, 2014).

The study of human grief and bereavement has evolved over the past 40 years. Research examines questions such as: What constitutes normal, healthy grieving? What are predictors of complicated grief? What interventions, if any, benefit different populations of grieving people? When is medication useful for the bereaved person? What is the impact of losses on family systems? What are cultural mediators of delivering grief support? How does complicated or unresolved grief affect public and private health care usage? What are best practices to intervene in special types of loss, such as traumatic loss, genocidal loss, societal loss, and wartime loss?

Types of Grief

Grief is a multi-faceted, deeply personal human response to loss. The time it takes to grieve is individual and unique to each person. Even each family member affected grieves differently. Many variables, such as how the death occurred, coping skills, previous losses, other life stressors, and support systems, affect how people grieve. The nature of the relationship with the person who has died is of particular importance (Mortell, 2015). Nurses are in a position to provide appropriate assessment to help differentiate disenfranchised grief, anticipatory grief, and complicated grief from the normal grieving process (Canadian Nurses Association, Canadian Hospice Palliative Care Association, & Canadian Hospice Palliative Care Nurses Group, 2015).

Disenfranchised grief can occur when losses are not always openly acknowledged, supported, or recognized as significant, such as a loss through suicide, the loss of a friend, the loss of a pet, or the grief of someone thought incapable of grieving (e.g., a child, a person with dementia). A sense of isolation can occur, and nurses need to recognize the grief as real and intervene by acknowledging the loss, supporting feelings, and encouraging the person grieving to reach out to supportive networks. Disenfranchised grief has numerous psychological components that can create the conditions for dysregulation and confusion and that have been associated with complicated grief (McNutt & Yakushko, 2013).

Nurses also need to recognize when grief becomes **complicated grief**, a term applied to grief that remains unresolved and is thought to affect between 3% and 25% of those who grieve. With complicated grief, bereavement symptoms can at times evolve into other mental health concerns, such as substance use or chronic depression (Shear et al., 2013). Taken together, these grief presentations warrant careful assessment and appropriate levels of psychiatric mental health nursing intervention (Mortell, 2015).

In the past there was debate about how best to recognize and manage more severe reactions to grief, with some supporting the need to consider complicated grief a separate entity under the *Diagnostic and Statistical Manual of Mental Disorders (DSM-5)* and others arguing the need to stop trying to pathologize varied grief experiences (Boelen & Smid, 2017; Stroebe et al., 2017). The *DSM-5* has addressed this debate and cautions clinicians to differentiate normal grieving from a mental health diagnosis of major depressive or adjustment disorder, following clear criteria for these distinct disorders. The goal is to ensure that those who need intervention receive an accurate diagnosis.

With appropriate supports, patients should be allowed to experience grief as a normal process of life in their own unique and personal way. Nurses should also consider *Chronic sorrow*, the presence of enduring lifelong feelings of grief, as a potential nursing diagnosis (Alligood, 2018).

> **VIGNETTE**
>
> On a large, extended-family picnic, Mr. and Mrs. Doiron's youngest child was accidentally crushed by the tires of a relative's truck as it backed up. The 3-year-old died in her mother's arms on the way to the hospital. Many family members, including the older siblings of the toddler, witnessed the event. After 6 months, the Doiron family was still in chaos and shock. Mrs. Doiron, especially, was unable to resume normal responsibilities. Her husband had returned to work and did his best to support her. The surviving children were exhibiting behavioural problems. The Doirons sought out a grief counsellor and attended support groups. The mixture of horror, shock, anger, disbelief, grief, and senselessness that engulfed them complicated their mourning. Gradually, some of the feelings softened, and the family began to regain some stable routines. After 2 years, Mrs. Doiron had progressed to the point of organizing support networks in her daughter's name for parents whose children had suffered similar deaths.

Nurses are expected to identify those at risk for complicated grief and differentiate between grief and depression (Canadian Hospice Palliative Care Association, 2009a), intervening in timely and appropriate ways, such as providing counselling and coordinating referrals.

Assessment may include validated screening inventories for depression and other specific grief measures such as the Brief Grief Questionnaire and Inventory of Complicated Grief (Igarashi et al., 2021). Identification of risk factors that can complicate grieving is another place to begin the assessment and would include a number of factors, such as:

- Heavy emotional dependence on the deceased
- Unresolved conflicts between the bereaved person and the deceased
- Young age of the deceased (often the most profound loss) or of the bereaved person
- Lack of a surviving meaningful relationship or support system
- A history of losses
- A lack of sound coping skills
- A death that was associated with a cultural stigma (e.g., acquired immune deficiency syndrome [AIDS], suicide)
- A death that was unexpected or associated with violence (e.g., murder, suicide)
- A history of depression, drug or alcohol use, or other psychiatric illness

Prolonged depression is the most common response to unresolved grief, and assessment of mood should follow the practices described in Chapter 13. Disturbances in mood are associated with biological changes in the body during stress-related depressive illness. Some examples are electrolyte disturbance, nervous system alterations, and faulty regulation of the autonomic nervous system. Always assess the potential for suicide.

Table 31.1 identifies common grief experiences and describes the pathological intensification of these phenomena that indicates the need for psychotherapy.

Models for understanding grief are being clinically tested and refined so that health care systems can understand grieving, best use limited health care resources, and relieve suffering whenever possible.

Theories

The psychoanalytic model of grieving posits a distinct psychological process that involves disengaging strong emotional ties from a significant relationship and reinvesting those ties in a new and productive direction. This process requires engaging in "grief work" that is thought to progress through predictable stages and phases. Since Kübler-Ross's ground-breaking work with the dying in the 1960s, her phases of denial, anger, bargaining, depression, and acceptance (Kübler-Ross, 1969) have been identified by many with the stages of grieving. Other models of grieving emphasize dual processes of coping with bereavement stressors, the potential for personal growth and coping skills, and adaptive tasks (Stroebe et al., 2017).

The goals of mourning have evolved from "doing the grief work, getting over it, and moving on with life." Many now regard mourning as a complex, individual, culturally embedded process of accepting the death, confronting the painful experience of grief, constructing an identity and a life in a transformed environment, and finding an enduring relationship with the deceased, based not on physical presence but on accurate memory. Depending on many factors, this process can take many months to a number of years. Our losses transform our lives, and we are never quite the same person again. Over time, people move from pain defining who they are, and constant pre-occupation with their loss, to living with the residual pain and forever carrying the memory of the loved one.

Dual Process Model of Coping With Bereavement

Bereavement is an enormously challenging life stressor (Table 31.2). Healthy adaptation is crucial for long-term health and re-engagement in life. In a review of the dual process model (DPM) Stroebe and colleagues (2017) identify adaptive versus maladaptive coping activities using three central constructs: loss-oriented coping, restoration-oriented coping, and oscillation. The DPM attempts to address inadequacies in the "grief work" concept, such as a lack of specificity about grief stressors, cultural bias, the favouring of intuitive or female expressions of grief over instrumental styles (Stroebe et al., 2017), and the discounting of the value of denial and distraction in grieving.

Using the DPM as a guide, Stroebe and colleagues (2017) identified *loss-oriented stressors*, which include concentrating on the loss experience, feeling the pain of grief, remembering, and longing. *Restoration-oriented stressors* re-engage the mourner with the outer world, as in overcoming loneliness (seeking social support), mastering skills and

TABLE 31.1 Common Experiences During Grief and Their Pathological Intensification

Phenomenon	Typical Response	Pathological Intensification
Dying	Emotional expression and immediate coping with the dying process	Avoidance; feeling of being overwhelmed, dazed, confused; self-punitive feelings; inappropriately hostile feelings
Death and outcry	Outcry of emotions with news of the death and turning to others for help or isolating self with self-soothing	Panic; dissociative reactions, reactive psychoses
Warding off (denial)	Avoidance of reminders and social withdrawal, focusing elsewhere, emotional numbing, not thinking of implications to self or of certain themes	Maladaptive avoidance of confronting the implications of death, drug or alcohol use, promiscuity, fugue states, phobic avoidance, feeling of being dead or unreal
Re-experience (intrusion)	Intrusive experiences, including recollections of negative experiences during relationship with the deceased, bad dreams, reduced concentration, compulsive re-enactments	Flooding with negative images and emotions; uncontrolled ideation, self-impairing compulsive re-enactments, night terrors, recurrent nightmares, distraught feelings resulting from the intrusion of anger, anxiety, despair, shame, or guilt; physiological exhaustion resulting from hyperarousal
Working through	Recollection of the deceased and a contemplation of self with reduced intrusiveness of memories and fantasies and with increased rational acceptance, reduced numbness and avoidance, more "dosing" of recollections, and a sense of working through it	Feeling of inability to integrate the death with a sense of self and continued life; persistent warding-off of themes that may manifest as anxious, depressed, enraged, shame-filled, or guilty moods and psychophysiological syndromes
Completion	Reduction in emotional swings and a sense of self-coherence and readiness for new relationships; ability to experience positive states of mind	Failure to complete mourning, which may be associated with inability to work or create or to feel emotion or positive states of mind

Source: Horowitz, M. J. (1990). A model of mourning: Change in schemas of self and others. *Journal of the American Psychoanalytic Association, 38*(2), 297–324. https://doi.org/10.1177/000306519003800202. Copyright © 1990 by SAGE. Reprinted by Permission of SAGE Publications.

TABLE 31.2 Phenomena Experienced During Bereavement

Symptoms	Examples
Sensations of Somatic Distress The bereaved person may experience tightness in the throat, shortness of breath, sighing, mental pain, or exhaustion; food may taste like sand; things may feel unreal. Pain or discomfort may be identical to the symptoms experienced by the dead person. Normally, symptoms are brief.	A woman whose husband died of a stroke complains of weakness and numbness on her left side.
Pre-occupation With the Image of the Deceased The bereaved person brings up, thinks about, and talks about numerous memories of the deceased. The memories are positive. This process goes on with great sadness. The idealization of the deceased lets the bereaved person relive the gratifications associated with the deceased and helps resolve any guilt they feel concerning the deceased. The bereaved person may also take on many of the mannerisms of the deceased through identification—identification serves the purpose of holding on to the deceased. Pre-occupation with the dead person can continue for many months before it lessens.	A man whose wife recently died states, "I just can't stop thinking about my wife. Everything I see reminds me of her. We picked up this seashell on our honeymoon. I remember every wonderful moment we had together. The pain is so great, but the memories just keep coming." His friends notice that when he talks, his hand gestures and expressions are like those of his recently deceased wife.
Guilt The bereaved person reproaches themself for real or fancied acts of negligence or omissions in the relationship with the deceased.	"I should have made him go to the doctor sooner." "I should have paid more attention to her, been more thoughtful."
Anger The anger the bereaved person experiences may not be toward the object that gives rise to it. Often the anger is displaced onto the medical or nursing staff. Other times, it is directed toward the deceased. The anger is at its height during the first month but is often intermittent throughout the first year. The overflow of hostility disturbs the bereaved person, resulting in the feeling that they are "going insane."	"The doctor didn't operate in time. If he had, Mary would be alive today." "How could he leave me like this … how could he?"
Change in Behaviour: Depression, Disorganization, Restlessness The bereaved person may exhibit marked restlessness and an inability to organize their behaviour. A depressive mood during routine activities is common, decreasing as the year passes and the intensity of the grief declines. Absence of depression is more abnormal than its presence. Loneliness and aimlessness are most pronounced 6–9 months after the death.	Six months after her husband died, Mrs. Faye states, "I just can't seem to function. I have a hard time doing the simplest tasks. I can't be bothered with socializing. I feel so down … so, so empty."
Reorganization of Behaviour Directed Toward a New Object or Activity Gradually, the bereaved person renews their interest in people and activities. The grieving thus releases them from one interpersonal relationship, and new ones are free to take its place.	Twenty months after her husband's death, Mrs. Faye tells a friend, "I'll be away this weekend. I am going fishing with my brother and his friend. This is the first time I've felt like doing anything since Harry died."

roles once performed by the deceased person, finding a new identity, and facing many practical details of life. By identifying specific coping activities on both sides of the model, the nurse can strengthen a grieving person's skills and reinforce positive meanings.

Both orientations assert that denial, avoidance, and distraction from grief are beneficial, as long as they are not excessive. The process of alternating between the two spheres of coping results in the third construct called *oscillation*, wherein confronting and avoiding various stressors of bereavement are an indication of healthy adaptation. However, a prolonged moving back and forth between these poles can be seen as an indication of complicated grieving (Stroebe et al., 2017).

Four Tasks of Mourning

Many theorists who have studied the grief process, including George Engel, Colin Parkes, Erich Lindemann, John Bowlby, and J. William Worden, have identified similar, commonly experienced psychological and behavioural phenomena, including:

- Shock and disbelief
- Sensation of somatic distress
- Preoccupation with the image of the deceased
- Guilt
- Anger
- Change in behaviour (e.g., depression, disorganization, restlessness)
- Reorganization of behaviour directed toward a new object or activity

Worden organizes aspects of mourning into four tasks: (1) accept the reality of the loss, (2) experience the pain of grief, (3) adjust to an environment without the loved one (externally, internally, and spiritually), and (4) relocate and memorialize the loved one. He emphasizes that every loss must be assessed according to mediating factors such as the nature of the person who died, the nature of the attachment, the circumstances of the death, personality factors, family history, social circumstances, and concurrent changes resulting from the death (Worden, 2018). His model can be readily understood by the mourner as empowering and hopeful and serves as a specific guide for the nurse providing counselling or therapy.

Helping People Cope With Loss

The majority of people who suffer bereavement are resilient and integrate experiences of loss into their lives. There are, however, known risk and resiliency factors for mental health problems associated with grief. Some risk factors cannot be changed (e.g., gender, unexpected death) or might be difficult to change (e.g., a negative change in finances), but it is important to identify those risk factors that can be ameliorated with appropriate interventions. Some people who are grieving are resilient, and limited counselling support, focusing on grief education, normalizing of experiences, and skilled supportive presence, seems to be helpful for them. A deeper understanding of the grief process can provide reassurance for those grieving (Worden, 2018). Most importantly, social support is also instrumental in natural helping through the grief process and can be supported with multiple levels of intervention (Cacciatore et al., 2021; Hoy, 2016). Other helpful interventions include writing letters (both to and from the deceased), performing simple rituals and ceremonies, "dosing" times of grieving throughout the day or week, working on projects to memorialize the deceased (e.g., planting a tree, creating a website), walking and time in nature, and planning ahead for holidays and anniversary dates. Table 31.3 provides guidelines for helping people to grieve, and the Guidelines for Communication box offers advice for communicating with a person suffering a profound loss.

Box 31.4 offers guidelines that can help people and their families to cope with bereavement.

CURRENT TOPICS AND FUTURE DIRECTIONS

Medical Assistance in Dying (MAiD) Legislation

The Supreme Court of Canada has decriminalized MAiD, and existing international legislation sets out that (until 2023) if mental illness is the only life limiting illness, MAiD is not permitted. The legislation (also discussed in Chapter 22) provides the legal framework for the process, with mental health and competency parameters for assessment built into the law. The role of psychiatric mental health professionals will continue to evolve in key related areas of capacity assessment, the perception of suicide, and the assessment of suffering. These are opportunities for the development of new skills in EOL care, particularly in addressing goals of care (Coyle et al., 2015), in mediating institutional challenges to provide compassionate interprofessional care (Pesut et al., 2020), addressing family caregivers' needs for support and information (Hales et al., 2019), as well as supporting both access to MAiD and palliative care for people with structural vulnerabilities (Wright

GUIDELINES FOR COMMUNICATION WITH A BEREAVED PERSON

Situation	Sample Response
When you sense an overwhelming sorrow	"This must hurt terribly."
When you hear anger in the bereaved person's voice	"I hear anger in your voice. Most people go through periods of anger when their loved one dies. Are you feeling angry now?"
If you discern guilt	"Are you feeling guilty? This is a common reaction many people have. What are some of your thoughts about this?"
If you sense a fear of the future	"It must be scary to go through this."
When the bereaved person seems confused	"This can be a bewildering time."
In almost any painful situation	"This must be very difficult for you."

Source: *Good intentions* by Duke Robinson. Copyright © 1996 by Reverend Andrew (Duke) Robinson. By permission of Grand Central Publishing. All rights reserved.

TABLE 31.3 Guidelines for Helping People in Acute Grief

Intervention	Rationale
Give your full presence: Use appropriate eye contact, attentive listening, and appropriate touch.	Talking is one of the most important ways of dealing with acute grief. Listening patiently helps the bereaved person express all feelings, even ones they feel are "negative."
	Appropriate eye contact helps to convey that you are there and are sharing the person's sadness.
	Suitable human touch can express warmth and nurture healing. Inappropriate touch can leave a person confused and uncomfortable.
Be patient with the bereaved person in times of silence. Do not fill silence with empty chatter.	Sharing painful feelings during periods of silence is healing and conveys your concern.
Know about and share with the bereaved person information about the phenomena that occur during the normal mourning process because they may concern some people (e.g., intense anger at the deceased, guilt, symptoms the deceased had before death, unbidden floods of memories). Give the bereaved person support during the occurrence of these phenomena and a written handout to refer to.	Although the knowledge will not eliminate the emotions, it can greatly relieve a person who is thinking that there is something wrong with having these feelings.
Encourage the support of family and friends. If no supports are available, refer the person to a community bereavement group. (Bereavement groups are helpful even when a person has many friends or much family support.)	Friends can help with routine matters, for example: • Bringing food into the house • Making phone calls • Driving to the funeral home • Taking care of the bereaved person's children or other family members
Offer spiritual support and referrals when needed.	Dealing with an illness or catastrophic loss can cause the most profound spiritual anguish.
When intense emotions are in evidence, show understanding and support (see Guidelines for Communication box).	Empathic words that reflect acceptance of a bereaved individual's feelings are healing.

> **BOX 31.4 Coping with Grief and Loss**
>
> As part of coping, people need to accept our full range of human emotions and know that they are all completely normal. A few things to support coping include:
>
> - Acknowledge the loss
> - Learn about grief and coping through reading or listening about the process and emotions
> - Connect with others and seek social support
> - Turn to their faith for further coping for people who find that helpful
> - Search for a meaning by celebrating the life or experiences lost. Volunteering with or creating foundations or charities related to the loss has also helped some people move through the grieving process
> - Join a support group to talk about the pain and suffering of the loss and the emotions experienced.
>
> Focus on daily living tasks, routines and a healthy lifestyle. Engage in self-care such as trying to eat healthy meals and at regular times; engage in some daily exercise (even walking for 15 minutes can be beneficial—especially outside); engage in careful sleep hygiene despite the insomnia that may be experienced; and refrain from unhealthy coping, such as with nicotine, caffeine, excessive eating, or substance use.

Source: Adapted from Centre for Addiction and Mental Health. (2022). Coping with loss and grief. https://www.camh.ca/en/camh-news-and-stories/coping-with-loss-and-grief

& Shaw, 2019). A national nursing framework for MAiD has been developed by the Canadian Nurses Association (2017b) with updates forthcoming. Certainly, future case studies and other research will lead to new guidelines in capacity assessment, suicide and suffering assessment, and support for professional caregivers in the process (Brooks, 2019) as well as to new areas of therapy and intervention broadly in the field of death and dying.

Palliative Care for Patients With Dementia

The incidence of Alzheimer's disease and related dementias in Canada continues to grow at a staggering rate (Alzheimer Society, 2021), and is a trend that is expected to continue. It is difficult to determine survival or time until death, often leaving those with dementia to die without appropriate palliative care services or, as some researchers suggest, to receive aggressive interventions to the detriment of their quality of life (Broady et al., 2018). As with other chronic illnesses, HPC should be considered at the time of a dementia diagnosis and assessed regularly for changes in status. Enhanced educational opportunities for nurses and other caregivers about the unique elements of palliative dementia care are essential to promote increased comfort and enhanced quality of life for this population.

People with advanced dementia experience significant impairments in insight, language, and judgement, limiting their ability to communicate unmet needs and desires. Difficult behaviours such as irritability or refusal to cooperate with care are often a form of communication, indicating discomfort in body, mind, or spirit. Caregivers who use an anticipatory approach to care can frequently prevent or reduce behaviours that result when a person with dementia is unable to communicate important unmet needs. Caregivers must remember to focus on the person, rather than the disease, and recognize the numerous opportunities that arise with every interaction to affirm the meaning of the individual's life, uphold dignity, and provide pleasurable sensory and spiritual experiences. The goal is to create meaningful connections for these patients. One effective method for customizing care that honours the unique preferences and lifelong interests of the patient is to use some form of life story process (Gridley et al., 2020). This abbreviated biography guides and informs care to enhance the patient's enjoyment of life's simple pleasures. Dignity therapy is another approach suited to older persons and to adults with dementia at end of life (Martínez et al., 2017).

Best practice recommendations for palliative care in dementia are to ensure that people with advanced dementia are included in the provision of palliative care; they remain in familiar surroundings whenever possible; restraint-free policy and staff education programs are developed; and quality of EOL experiences for those with dementia and their families are evaluated (Palmer et al., 2020). More specifically, it is also important to address health care decisions for those with advanced dementia, such as resuscitation, hospitalizations, antibiotics, and nutrition and hydration. Health care providers should (1) identify the patient's goals for care and consider educating the family to minimize aggressive medical interventions, (2) eliminate medications that may detract from safety or quality of life, and (3) proactively manage issues such as pain and depression. Families and friends spend a significant amount of time, finances, and emotions caring for a loved one with dementia. It is important to recognize and support the role of family caregivers as they navigate the day-to-day challenges and cope with many losses.

Areas for Future Discovery

We are emerging from a time when many people who are grieving have been pathologized and treated with psychotropic drugs for depression, anxiety, and sleep disorders (Worden, 2018). On one end of the spectrum, grief has been overlooked by many health care providers as a possible underlying contributor to their patients' presenting problems (Stroebe et al., 2017). Alongside these patterns, however, populations around the world are experiencing mass death and loss as a result of the uncovered truths of Indigenous genocide (Methot, 2019), the opioid epidemic (BC Centre on Substance use, 2018), COVID-19 pandemic (Simon et al., 2020), and as a consequence of the global climate emergency (Aylward et al., 2021). Through these experiences, we have as a global society "cracked open" the meaning and required professional and community responses to grief (Selman, 2021). The classification of *prolonged grief* disorder, characterized by severe and disabling, chronic grief, in light of the multiple and overlapping global crises, will warrant further exploration (Rosner et al., 2021). Current diagnostic categories intend to address the issues of overdiagnosis and underdiagnosis; however, the classification system can never stand in for compassion and genuinely meeting patients and families with a shared humanity (Nakajima, 2018). Internationally, grief recovery models are being adapted to diverse cultures to assist traumatized people, especially children and youth, in beginning to heal and re-engage with life, hope, and the future as a result of the COVID-19 pandemic (Killikelly et al., 2021). There is a growing urgency for practitioners to become knowledgeable about and skilled at supporting human mourning in all health care settings. The realization of full human health and happiness may depend on it.

KEY POINTS TO REMEMBER

- The HPC movement offers compassionate care for those who are dying. HPC focuses on patients' physical and emotional comfort and offers holistic support for people who are dying and their families.
- More hospitals are offering palliative expertise for EOL care, but in many hospitals conflict continues to exist between the wishes of people who are dying and their families and the medical model of treatment that focuses on the prolongation of life.

- In working with HPC patients nursing goals include providing physical, emotional, cultural, and spiritual support and helping with adjustments in lifestyle and relationships. Nurses need to understand the value of providing a caring human presence even in the face of helplessness.
- People with dementia may exhibit challenging behaviours during EOL care that may communicate discomfort in mind, body, or spirit. Care should focus on providing meaningful connections with patients and between family members and patients.
- Those who work with people who are dying need to maintain their own emotional health. EOL care is usually delivered by multidisciplinary teams so that no one discipline bears too much responsibility. Nurses need to learn to draw on team support, protect their private lives by setting clear personal boundaries, and recognize their human and professional limitations.
- Providing timely and ongoing information about the disease and its effects and about physical and psychological signs of death can help the family deal with anticipatory mourning.
- Health care workers involved in the care of the dying can teach families communication skills, such as the Four Gifts of Resolving Relationships, that will help them to express love, share memories, say goodbye, and provide a sense of peace.
- Family members may experience anticipatory grief, and it is helpful for them to understand that this grief is normal, although difficult.
- Common phenomena are evident during the experience of grief, and mourning is greatly influenced by cultural norms. However, everyone's experience of grieving is shaped by many mediating factors, such as the relationship to the person who died and the capacities of the mourner.
- Indicators of the potential for complicated grief include social isolation, extensive dependency on the deceased person, unresolved interpersonal conflicts, loss of a child, violent and senseless death, and catastrophic loss.
- Grief work is successful when the relationship to the deceased person has been restructured, energy is available for new relationships and life pursuits, and the mourner can remember realistically both the pleasures and the disappointments of the lost relationship. Outcomes for successful grief work have been identified.

CRITICAL THINKING

1. George is dying of pancreatic cancer. George's spouse and adult children are asking about using HPC services. Help George's family to make an informed decision by comparing and contrasting the HPC model of care with the medical model of care for someone who is dying.
2. How can you use the Four Gifts of Resolving Relationships in working with the families of dying people in your practice of nursing? Do you think you would find this tool useful for a personal family member in the future?
3. What are some concrete ways in which you can help another person to cope with a loss? Identify specific components in the following areas:
   a. How can you let the person tell their story, and what is the potential therapeutic value of doing so?
   b. Avoiding banal (overused or trite) advice, what are some things you might say that could offer comfort? Use the guidelines in Table 31.3 and the Guidelines for Communication box to describe how you would help a person who is suffering a profound loss.
4. What practices would demonstrate a culturally safe and sensitive approach for Indigenous people in Canada seeking palliative care?

CHAPTER REVIEW

1. The nurse is caring for a patient who is grieving. The patient has stated that they are angry they have been diagnosed with terminal cancer. Which behaviour should the nurse anticipate next as the patient reconciles their anger?
   a. Denial that they have cancer
   b. Depression over the diagnosis of cancer
   c. Acceptance that cancer is their reality
   d. Begging God to remove the cancer from their body
2. The nurse is planning hospice palliative care for a dying patient. Which outcome is most appropriate?
   a. Patient will regain health
   b. Patient will remain pain-free
   c. Patient will not fear death
   d. Patient will decline all medications
3. Which patient statement regarding spirituality would require further nursing teaching?
   a. "I am not religious, so therefore I am not spiritual."
   b. "Death scares me."
   c. "My family is what gives my life meaning."
   d. "I believe in a higher power."
4. The nurse identifies that a patient is experiencing complicated grief related to the loss of their spouse. Which evaluation finding would indicate that a treatment plan is appropriate? The patient:
   a. No longer thinks of their spouse
   b. Copes without the need for a support system
   c. States that they should have taken their spouse to the doctor more often
   d. Laughs occasionally with their grandchildren
5. The nurse is caring for a patient whose partner, with whom they were having a secret affair, died suddenly after a myocardial infarction. The patient had told no one about the affair, so no friends or family were aware that they had experienced this significant loss. How should the nurse document the patient's grieving?
   a. Disenfranchised grief
   b. Dysfunctional grief
   c. Maladaptive grief
   d. Normal bereavement

 https://evolve.elsevier.com/Canada/Varcarolis/psychiatric/

REFERENCES

Alligood, M. R. (2018). *Nursing theorists and their work* (9th ed.). Philadelphia: Elsevier.

Alzheimer Society. (2021). *About dementia*. Retrieved from https://www.alzheimer.ca/en/About-dementia

Anandarajah, G., & Hight, E. (2001). Spirituality and medical practice: Using the HOPE questions as a practical tool for spiritual assessment. *American Family Physician, 63*(1), 81–88. Retrieved from http://www.aafp.org/afp/2001/0101/p81.pdf

Aylward, B., Cooper, M., & Cunsolo, A. (2021). Generation climate change: Growing up with ecological grief and anxiety. *Psychiatric News, 56*(6). https://doi.org/10.1176/appi.pn.2021.6.20

BC Centre for Palliative Care. (2019a). *BC interprofessional palliative symptom management guidelines*. Retrieved from https://bc-cpc.ca/wp-content/uploads/2019/10/ColourFullPrintOct16_2019.pdf

BC Centre for Palliative Care. (2019b). *Interprofessional palliative competency framework*. Retrieved from https://bc-cpc.ca/publications/competency-framework/

BC Centre on Substance Use. (2018). *Gone too soon: Navigating grief and loss as a result of substance use*. Retrieved from https://www.bccsu.ca/wp-content/uploads/2018/11/Grief_Handbook.pdf

Boelen, P. A., & Smid, G. E. (2017). Disturbed grief: Prolonged grief disorder and persistent complex bereavement disorder. *BMJ (Online), 357*, j2016. https://doi.org/10.1136/bmj.j2016

Broady, T. R., Saich, F., & Hinton, T. (2018). Caring for a family member or friend with dementia at the end of life: A scoping review and implications for palliative care practice. *Palliative Medicine, 32*(3), 643–656. https://doi.org/10.1177/0269216317748844

Brooks, L. (2019). Health care provider experiences of and perspectives on medical assistance in dying: A scoping review of qualitative studies. *Canadian Journal on Aging, 38*(3), 384–396. https://doi.org/10.1017/S0714980818000600

Cacciatore, J., Thieleman, K., Fretts, R., et al. (2021). What is good grief support? Exploring the actors and actions in social support after traumatic grief. *PLoS One, 16*(5), e0252324. https://doi.org/10.1371/journal.pone.0252324

Canadian Association of Schools of Nursing. (2011). *Palliative and end-of-life care: Entry-to-practice competencies and indicators for registered nurses*. Retrieved from http://casn.ca/wp-content/uploads/2014/12/PEOLCCompetenciesandIndicatorsEn1.pdf

Canadian Hospice Palliative Care Association. (2006). *The pan-Canadian gold standard for palliative home care*. Ottawa: Author. Retrieved from http://www.chpca.net/media/7652/Gold_Standards_Palliative_Home_Care.pdf

Canadian Hospice Palliative Care Association. (2009a). *Canadian hospice palliative care nursing standards of practice*. Ottawa: Author. Retrieved from https://www.chpca.ca/product/hospice-palliative-care-nursing-standards-of-practice-download/

Canadian Hospice Palliative Care Association. (2009b). *Nursing competencies case examples*. Ottawa: Author. Retrieved from https://www.virtualhospice.ca/Assets/Canadian%20Hospice%20Palliative%20Care%20Nursing%20Competencies%20Case%20Examples-Revised%20Feb%202010_20100211150854.pdf

Canadian Hospice Palliative Care Association. (2010). *Policy brief on hospice palliative care: Quality end-of-life care? It depends on where you live and where you die*. Ottawa: Author. Retrieved from https://www.chpca.ca/wp-content/uploads/2019/12/HPC_Policy_Brief_-_Systems_Approach_-_June_2010.pdf

Canadian Hospice Palliative Care Association. (2013). *A model to guide hospice palliative care*. Retrieved from https://www.chpca.ca/wp-content/uploads/2019/12/norms-of-practice-eng-web.pdf

Canadian Hospice Palliative Care Association. (2020). *Advance care planning in Canada: A pan-Canadian framework*. Retrieved from https://www.advancecareplanning.ca/wp-content/uploads/2020/06/ACP-Framework-EN-Updated.pdf

Canadian Hospice Palliative Care Association. (2021). *Hospice palliative care: Defining hospice palliative care*. Ottawa: Author. Retrieved from https://www.chpca.ca/about-hpc/

Canadian Institute for Health Information. (2021). *Your health system: Hospital deaths*. Retrieved from https://yourhealthsystem.cihi.ca/hsp/inbrief?lang=en#!/indicators/005/hospital-deaths-hsmr/;mapC1;mapLevel2;/

Canadian Network of Palliative Care for Children, & Canadian Hospice Palliative Care Association. (2021). *Canadian pediatric palliative care nursing competencies*. Retrieved from https://www.chpca.ca/wp-content/uploads/2021/03/PediatricPalliativeCareNursingCompetencies_Jan2021.pdf

Canadian Nurses Association, Canadian Hospice Palliative Care Association, Canadian Hospice Palliative Care Nurses Group. (2015). *Joint position statement: The palliative approach to care and the role of the nurse*. Retrieved from https://www.virtualhospice.ca/Assets/A%20Palliative%20Approach%20to%20Care%20and%20the%20Role%20of%20the%20Nurse_20151001151135.pdf

Canadian Nurses Association. (2017a). *Code of Ethics for Registered Nurses*. Ottawa: Author. Retrieved from https://hl-prod-ca-oc-download.s3-ca-central-1.amazonaws.com/CNA/2f975e7e-4a40-45ca-863c-5ebf0a138d5e/UploadedImages/documents/Code_of_Ethics_2017_Edition_Secure_Interactive.pdf

Canadian Nurses Association. (2017b). *National nursing framework on medical assistance in dying in Canada*. Retrieved from https://www.virtualhospice.ca/Assets/cna-national-nursing-framework-on-maidEng_20170216155827.pdf

Canadian Virtual Hospice. (2021). *Living my culture*. Retrieved from http://livingmyculture.ca/culture/

Caxaj, C. S., Schill, K., & Janke, R. (2018). Priorities and challenges for a palliative approach to care for rural indigenous populations: A scoping review. *Health & Social Care in the Community, 26*(3), e329–e336. https://doi.org/10.1111/hsc.12469

Chochinov, H. M. (2007). Dignity and the essence of medicine: The A, B, C and D of dignity conserving care. *British Medical Journal, 335*, 184–187.

Chochinov, H. M. (2016). Health-care provider as witness. *Lancet, 388*(10051), 1272–1273. https://doi.org/10.1016/S0140-6736(16)31668-3

Clark, J., Barnes, A., & Gardiner, C. (2018). Reframing global palliative care advocacy for the sustainable development goal era: A qualitative study of the views of international palliative care experts. *Journal of Pain and Symptom Management, 56*(3), 363–370. https://doi.org/10.1016/j.jpainsymman.2018.06.009

Clarke, D. (2010). Dame Cicely biography. *Cicely Saunders International*. Retrieved from https://www.cicelysaundersfoundation.org/about-us/dame-cicely-biography

Coyle, N., Manna, R., Shen, M. J., et al. (2015). Discussing death, dying, and end-of-life goals of care: A communication skills training module for oncology nurses. *Clinical Journal of Oncology Nursing, 19*(6), 697–702. https://doi.org/10.1188/15.CJON.697-702

End of Life Doula Association of Canada. (2021). *Let's start the conversation. Providing personalized end of life care: Advocacy, community awareness and support*. Retrieved from https://endoflifedoulaassociation.org/

Gaspard, G., Gadsby, C., & Mallmes, J. (2021). Indigenous end-of-life doula course: Bringing the culture home. *International Journal of Indigenous Health, 16*(2), 151–165. https://doi.org/10.32799/ijih.v16i2.33230

Giesbrecht, M., Stajduhar, K., Mollison, A., Pauly, B., Reimer-Kirkham, S., McNeil, R., & Rose, C. (2018). Hospitals, clinics, and palliative care units: Place-based experiences of formal healthcare settings by people experiencing structural vulnerability at the end-of-life. *Health and Place, 53*, 43–51

Gray, B. (2014). The use of rituals, primarily related to grief, in a hospital setting: How are they helpful and how can they be most effective?. *Critical Horizons, 2*(2), 165–177. https://doi.org/10.1558/hscc.v2i2.23838

Gridley, K., Birks, Y., & Parker, G. (2020). Exploring good practice in life story work with people with dementia: The findings of a qualitative study looking at the multiple views of stakeholders. *Dementia, 19*(2), 182–194. https://doi.org/10.1177/1471301218768921

Hales, B. M., Bean, S., Isenberg-Grzeda, E., et al. (2019). Improving the medical assistance in dying (MAID) process: A qualitative study of family caregiver perspectives. *Palliative & Supportive Care, 17*(5), 590–595. https://doi.org/10.1017/S147895151900004X

Hoy, W. G. (2016). *Bereavement groups and the role of social support: Integrating theory, research, and practice.* New York: Routledge/Taylor & Francis Group.

Igarashi, N., Aoyama, M., Ito, M., et al. (2021). Comparison of two measures for complicated grief: Brief Grief Questionnaire (BGQ) and Inventory of Complicated Grief (ICG). *Japanese Journal of Clinical Oncology, 51*(2), 252–257. https://doi.org/10.1093/jjco/hyaa185

Killikelly, C., Smid, G., Wagner, B., et al. (2021). Responding to the new *International Classification of Diseases-11* prolonged grief disorder during the COVID-19 pandemic: A new bereavement network and three-tiered model of care. *Public Health, 191,* 85–90. https://doi.org/10.1016/j.puhe.2020.10.034

Kübler-Ross, E. (1969). *On death and dying.* New York: Macmillan.

LeBarron, V., & Galassi, A. (2019). Global palliative care. In B. R. Ferrell, & J. A. Paice (Eds.), *Oxford textbook of palliative nursing* (5th ed.) (pp. 867–876). New York: Oxford University Press.

Lormans, T., de Graaf, E., van de Geer, J., et al. (2021). Toward a socio-spiritual approach? A mixed-methods systematic review on the social and spiritual needs of patients in the palliative phase of their illness. *Palliative Medicine, 35*(6), 1071–1098. https://doi.org/10.1177/02692163211010384

Martínez, M., Arantzamendi, M., Belar, A., et al. (2017). "Dignity therapy," a promising intervention in palliative care: A comprehensive systematic literature review. *Palliative Medicine, 31*(6), 492–509. https://doi.org/10.1177/0269216316665562

Mason, S., Paal, P., Elsner, F., et al. (2020). Palliative care for all: An international health education challenge. *Palliative & Supportive Care, 18*(6), 760–762. https://doi.org/10.1017/S1478951520000188

Matzo, M., & Sherman, D. W. (2018). *Palliative care nursing: Quality care to the end of life* (5th ed.). New York: Springer.

McGill University. (2021). *Palliative care McGill: Balfour Mount.* Retrieved from https://www.mcgill.ca/palliativecare/portraits-0/balfour-mount

McNutt, B., & Yakushko, O. (2013). Disenfranchised grief among lesbian and gay bereaved individuals. *Journal of LGBT Issues in Counseling, 7*(1), 87–116. https://doi.org/10.1080/15538605.2013.758345

Methot, S. (2019). *Legacy: Trauma, story and Indigenous healing.* ECW Press.

Mondor, L., Wodchis, W., & Tanuseputro, P. (2020). Persistent socioeconomic inequalities in location of death and receipt of palliative care: A population-based cohort study. *Palliative Medicine, 34*(10), 1393–1401. https://doi.org/10.1177/0269216320947964

Mortell, S. (2015). Assisting clients with disenfranchised grief: The role of a mental health nurse. *Journal of Psychosocial Nursing and Mental Health Services, 53*(4), 52–57. https://doi.org/10.3928/02793695-20150319-05

Nakajima, S. (2018). Complicated grief: Recent developments in diagnostic criteria and treatment. *Philosophical Transactions. Biological Sciences, 373*(1754), 20170273. https://doi.org/10.1098/rstb.2017.0273

National Institute for Health and Care Excellence. (2021). *Managing symptoms for an adult in the last days of life.* Retrieved from https://pathways.nice.org.uk/pathways/end-of-life-care-for-people-with-life-limiting-conditions#path=view%3A/pathways/end-of-life-care-for-people-with-life-limiting-conditions/managing-symptoms-for-an-adult-in-the-last-days-of-life.xml&content=view-index

Overton, B. L., & Cottone, R. R. (2016). Anticipatory grief: A family systems approach. *The Family Journal, 24*(4), 430–432. https://doi.org/10.1177/1066480716663490

Palmer, J. A., Smith, A. M., Paasche-Orlow, R. S., et al. (2020). Research literature on the intersection of dementia, spirituality, and palliative care: A scoping review. *Journal of Pain and Symptom Management, 60*(1), 116–134. https://doi.org/10.1016/j.jpainsymman.2019.12.369

Perry, K. R., King, H. A., Parker, R., et al. (2021). Coordinating assessment of spiritual needs: A cross-walk of narrative and psychometric assessment tools used in palliative care. *Journal of Health Care Chaplaincy, 59*(2), 1–14. https://doi.org/10.1080/08854726.2021.1904653

Pesut, B., Thorne, S., Schiller, C. J., et al. (2020). The rocks and hard places of MAiD: A qualitative study of nursing practice in the context of legislated assisted death. *BMC Nursing, 19*(1), 12. https://doi.org/10.1186/s12912-020-0404-5

Puchalski, C. M. (2007). Spirituality and the care of patients at the end-of-life: An essential component of care. *OMEGA: Journal of Death and Dying, 56*(1), 33–46.

Rawlings, D., Davies, G., & Tieman, J. (2021). Compassionate communities—What does this mean for roles such as a death doula in end-of-life care?. *Public Health, 194,* 167–169. https://doi.org/10.1016/j.puhe.2021.02.038

Rogalla, K. B. (2020). Anticipatory grief, proactive coping, social support, and growth: Exploring positive experiences of preparing for loss. *Omega: Journal of Death and Dying, 81*(1), 107–129. https://doi.org/10.1177/0030222818761461

Rosner, R., Comtesse, H., Vogel, A., et al. (2021). Prevalence of prolonged grief disorder. *Journal of Affective Disorders, 287,* 301–307. https://doi.org/10.1016/j.jad.2021.03.058

Schill, K., & Caxaj, S. (2019). Cultural safety strategies for rural Indigenous palliative care: A scoping review. *BMC Palliative Care, 18*(1), 21. https://doi.org/10.1186/s12904-019-0404-y

Selman, L. (2021). Covid grief has cracked us open: How clinicians respond could reshape attitudes to bereavement—An essay by Lucy Selman. *BMJ (Online), 374,* n1803. https://doi.org/10.1136/bmj.n1803

Selman, L. E., Sowden, R., & Borgstrom, E. (2021). Saying goodbye" during the COVID-19 pandemic: A document analysis of online newspapers with implications for end of life care. *Palliative Medicine, 35*(7), 1277–1287. https://doi.org/10.1177/02692163211017023

Shear, M. K., Ghesquiere, A., & Glickman, K. (2013). Bereavement and complicated grief. *Current Psychiatry Reports, 15*(11), 1–7. https://doi.org/10.1007/s11920-013-0406-z

Simon, N. M., Saxe, G. N., & Marmar, C. R. (2020). Mental health disorders related to COVID-19–related deaths. *JAMA: The Journal of the American Medical Association, 324*(15), 1493–1494. https://doi.org/10.1001/jama.2020.19632

Sinclair, S., Hack, T. F., MacInnis, C. C., et al. (2021). Development and validation of a patient-reported measure of compassion in healthcare: The Sinclair Compassion Questionnaire (SCQ). *BMJ Open, 11*(6), e045988. https://doi.org/10.1136/bmjopen-2020-045988

Stajduhar, K. I., & Mollison, A. (2018). *Too little, too late: How we fail vulnerable Canadians as they die and what to do about it.* Victoria: University of Victoria Institute on Aging & Lifelong Health. Retrieved from https://www.uvic.ca/research/groups/peol/assets/docs/too-little-too-late.pdf

Stajduhar, K., Mollison, A., Giesbrecht, M., et al. (2019). "Just too busy living in the moment and surviving": Barriers to accessing health care for structurally vulnerable populations at end-of-life. *BMC Palliative Care, 18*(11). https://www.doi.org/10.1186/s12904-019-0396-7

Steinhauser, K., King, H., Parker, R., et al. (2020). Developing a spiritual assessment tool for palliative care (GP791). *Journal of Pain and Symptom Management, 60*(1), P299. https://doi.org/10.1016/j.jpainsymman.2020.04.218

Stroebe, M., Stroebe, W., Schut, H., et al. (2017). Grief is not a disease but bereavement merits medical awareness. *Lancet, 389*(10067), 347–349. https://doi.org/10.1016/S0140-6736(17)30189-7

Walshe, C., Preston, N., & Johnston, B. (2018). *Palliative care nursing: Principles and evidence for practice* (3rd ed.). Open University Press.

Warth, M., Koehler, F., Brehmen, M., et al. (2021). "Song of Life": Results of a multicenter randomized trial on the effects of biographical music therapy in palliative care. *Palliative Medicine, 35*(6), 1126–1136. https://doi.org/10.1177/02692163211010394

Webkamigad, S., Rowe, R., Peltier, S., et al. (2020). Identifying and understanding the health and social care needs of Indigenous older adults with multiple chronic conditions and their caregivers: A scoping review. *BMC Geriatrics, 20*(1), 145. https://doi.org/10.1186/s12877-020-01552-5

Worden, J. W. (2018). *Grief counseling and grief therapy: A handbook for the mental health practitioner* (5th ed.). Springer.

Wright, A. C., & Shaw, J. C. (2019). The spectrum of end of life care: an argument for access to medical assistance in dying for vulnerable populations. *Medicine, Health Care, and Philosophy, 22*(2), 211–219. https://doi.org/10.1007/s11019-018-9860-z

32

Forensic Psychiatric Nursing

Lisa-Marie Forcier, Eric MacMullin

 https://evolve.elsevier.com/Canada/Varcarolis/psychiatric

OBJECTIVES

1. Define forensic nursing, forensic psychiatric mental health nursing, and correctional nursing.
2. Identify the functions of forensic nurses.
3. Describe three sub-specialties of forensic nursing.
4. Identify three roles of psychiatric mental health nurses in the specialty of forensic nursing.
5. Describe clinical competencies associated with forensic psychiatric mental health nursing.
6. Compare and contrast the roles of forensic psychiatric mental health nurses and correctional nurses.
7. Describe the health care needs of incarcerated individuals.
8. Discuss the challenges or issues associated with being a nurse in a correctional facility.

KEY TERMS AND CONCEPTS

correctional nursing
forensic nursing
forensic psychiatric mental health nurses
forensics
index offence
Indigenous
not criminally responsible (NCR)
post-traumatic stress disorder (PTSD)
recidivism

Several high-profile incidents involving people with mental illness and criminal activity, police shootings, and suicides in prison have brought increased attention to the relationship of the mental health and criminal justice systems in Canada and elsewhere. Although the vast majority of people living with mental health and addictions conditions rarely come into contact with the criminal justice system, there is an over-representation of people with serious mental health issues in Canadian courts and correctional/remand facilities. (Canadian Mental Health Association, 2021). Societal factors such as access to treatment, substance use, poverty, inadequate housing, and trauma all increase risk. There are also instances when mental illnesses cause people to behave in ways that can lead to a criminal justice response, sometimes resulting in an arrest or apprehension. Whatever the reason, the over-representation of people with mental illness in the criminal justice system is often referred to as the "criminalization" of mental illness. This criminalization of people with mental illness can be viewed through a social justice lens for clinical practice so that individuals receive the support, care, and treatment they need and to which they are entitled (Centre for Addiction and Mental Health, 2020; Scannell, 2018).

In many respects, it is not surprising that there is such a high incidence of antisocial personality disorder in corrections populations, both in institutions and in the community. Clinically, the disorder is characterized by behaviours that involve failure to conform to social norms that constitute grounds for arrest, such as rule breaking, deceitfulness, impulsivity or failure to plan ahead, irritability and aggressiveness, and disregard for the safety of self or others (refer to Chapter 19 for more on personality disorders). By definition, the majority of people in the criminal justice system meet many of these criteria, and related history of trauma. However, much of the concern about over-representation relates to those with a serious mental health disorder, primarily schizophrenia or other types of psychosis, for whom social-ecological issues, rather than specific pathology, are key contributing factors in their criminal involvement (Mental Health Commission of Canada, 2020).

Another concern is the over-representation of Indigenous people in the Canadian criminal justice system as both victims and offenders. The rate of violent victimization among Indigenous people was more than double that among non-Indigenous people (163 incidents per 1000 people vs. 74 per 1000). In particular, in 2014 Indigenous females had an overall rate of violent victimization that was double that of Indigenous males and close to triple that of non-Indigenous females. When controlling for various risk factors, Indigenous males were no more at risk for violent victimization than their non-Indigenous counterparts (Department of Justice Canada, 2017).

The over-representation of Indigenous peoples is also observed within the custody of Canadian correctional services. In the provinces and territories in 2018 to 2019 Indigenous females accounted for 42% of female custody admissions, while Indigenous males accounted for 28% of male custody admissions. Indigenous adults represented three-quarters (75%) of admissions to custody in Manitoba and Saskatchewan. The highest proportion of Indigenous adults live in these two provinces, representing 16% of the population in Manitoba and 14% of the population in Saskatchewan (Statistics Canada, 2020). Gutierrez et al. (2013) note that Indigenous offenders are more likely than non-Indigenous offenders to have experienced historical and intergenerational trauma, poverty, family violence, and substance use in their home environment, and as children, they were more likely to have been involved with child welfare services. According to Dr. Ivan Zinger, with the Office of the

Correctional Investigator, as of early 2021, individuals of Indigenous ancestry represented approximately 30% of the total inmate population (Government of Canada, 2020). Refer to Chapter 8 for more on the impact of culture on mental health and trauma-informed practice.

A number of other factors have contributed to the over-representation of all people with mental health problems in the criminal justice system, including the deinstitutionalization of people challenged by mental illness without adequate community mental health services, a lack of affordable housing, and inadequate income-support programs. These factors increase the vulnerability of individuals with mental illnesses, leading to greater victimization of this population. The media often portray individuals living with mental illness as violent and unpredictable; however, the reality is that people who have a mental illness are much more likely to be the victims of violence than are people in the general population. In fact, one in four individuals with a mental illness is likely to be a victim of violence in a given year. Experiencing victimization intensifies feelings of anxiety and vulnerability and can lead to an exacerbation of one's illness and a lower quality of life (Canadian Mental Health Association, 2021).

At times, people experiencing mental illness, crisis, or the effects of substance use have interactions that result in violent encounters with police. Improving interactions between people with mental illness and the police requires adhering to best practices in this area, such as specialized training for police officers and employing the least restrictive and forceful measures. In addition, mobile crisis teams and accessible community-based mental health and social services are also needed (Kara, 2014). Collaborative intersectoral collaboration among criminal justice and mental health systems is necessary. No one sector can be solely responsible for dealing with the response.

Demonstration of procedural systems in police interactions with persons experiencing mental health crises (and other marginalized groups) has the potential to profoundly change the nature of these police encounters. If people with mental illness and others perceive that they are treated fairly by police and in a procedural manner with decency and respect they are more likely to acknowledge the legitimacy of police authority and cooperate with investigations or arrests if necessary. If, however, persons with mental illness experience a police interaction in which they believe they are not treated according to procedures, they are more likely to resist authority (Kara, 2014).

This increased risk for victimization continues during incarceration. Both male and female inmates with a mental illness are more likely than other inmates to have been physically assaulted by their peers or correctional staff. In addition, individuals with a mental illness may be more likely to engage in acts of self-harm while incarcerated. Self-harm behaviour among federal inmates is increasing, as individuals struggle with a stressful and often dehumanizing environment and limited assistive services. Among those incarcerated in Canada, death by suicide is reported to be seven times greater than the national average (Centre for Addiction and Mental Health, 2020).

Mental health support must not end when a person is released from incarceration, however. The transition back into society is difficult for many individuals, who often receive little to no support in obtaining housing, employment, and other services upon their release. Transition and reintegration programs are, as yet, not well evaluated, and few best practices are identified (Centre for Addiction and Mental Health, 2020). Individuals with a mental illness who have been involved in the criminal justice system tend to have higher rates of homelessness, difficulty adhering to treatment, lower rates of social support, and greater incidence of substance use in comparison to other adults with a mental illness (Simpson et al., 2013). Without adequate services and a treatment plan in place, the likelihood of further victimization and **recidivism** (the tendency of people previously justice involved to be re-exposed to the criminal justice system) among this population is high. Mental health care in the criminal justice system serves, in this way, as a crime prevention strategy.

Canada's National Crime Prevention Strategy (NCPS) is based on the premise that well-designed interventions can have a positive influence on behaviours: by addressing risk factors associated with offending, crimes can be reduced or prevented. Successful interventions have been shown to reduce not only victimization but also the social and economic costs that result from criminal activities and the costs related to processing cases in the criminal justice system. The Government of Canada has focused on key project areas in the crime prevention strategy, with evidence-informed interventions and evaluations currently being expanded across the country (Public Safety Canada, 2015). Box 32.1 outlines the key elements of the NCPS.

Forensics (an abbreviation derived from *forensic science*) is an umbrella term that refers to legal issues and/or working with the courts. In recent years nurses formalized a broad category called **forensic nursing**, which brings together components of traditional nursing care and legal issues to serve victims of violence and individuals who have committed acts that have brought them into contact with the criminal justice system. In this chapter we explore a variety of roles that nurses assume within the legal system, identify competencies and challenges associated with the forensic nursing role, and profile the priority health care needs of patients who have committed an offence.

FORENSIC NURSING

Forensic nursing is the application of nursing science to public or legal proceedings and the combination of the forensic and biopsychosocial aspects of health care in the scientific investigation of trauma or death of victims and perpetrators of abuse, violence, criminal activity, and traumatic accidents (International Association of Forensic Nurses, 2022). Unlike most nursing specialties, forensic nursing includes several different but interrelated areas of nursing practice: *forensic nurse examiners* work with sexual assault survivors; *forensic nurse death investigators* work with the deceased; *forensic psychiatric mental health nurses* work with mentally ill offenders; *clinical forensic nurses* work with victims of interpersonal violence; *forensic correctional nurses* work with offenders; and *forensic geriatric* or *pediatric nurses* work with victims of abuse and neglect (Kent-Wilkinson, 2009, 2010). Forensic nurses provide direct services to victims of crime and individuals who have committed crimes; consultation services to colleagues in nursing-, medical-, and law-related agencies; and expert court testimony in cases of trauma or questioned death, adequacy of service delivery, and specialized diagnoses of specific conditions related to nursing. Forensic nurses also work with families or significant others and the community (International Association of Forensic Nurses, 2022), for instance, in the death investigation and care of survivors of a workplace fatality (Harris, 2017).

> **BOX 32.1 Key Project Areas of Canada's National Crime Prevention Strategy**
>
> - Bullying
> - Substance use
> - Youth gangs
> - Offender reintegration
> - Indigenous crime prevention
> - School-based crime prevention
>
> **Source:** Public Safety Canada. (2015). *Crime prevention information, project descriptions and summaries.* Retrieved from https://www.publicsafety.gc.ca/cnt/cntrng-crm/crm-prvntn/tls-rsrcs/nfrmtn-dscrptns-smmrs-en.aspx

The International Association of Forensic Nurses (IAFN), formed in 1992 by 74 nurses, most of whom were sexual assault nurse examiners (SANEs), represents nurses whose practice overlaps with key areas of forensic science and law. The group currently represents nurses who are forensic nurse generalists, SANEs, forensic psychiatric nurses, death investigators, coroners, correctional nurse specialists, and those in other forensic nursing specialties that continue to evolve (International Association of Forensic Nurses, 2022). The American Nurses Association (ANA) officially recognized forensic nursing as a specialty practice area in 1995 and combined efforts with the IAFN to develop the *Scope and Standards of Forensic Nursing* in 1997 and updated it in 2015 (American Nurses Association & International Association of Forensic Nurses, 2017). *While these standards may be useful guidelines for forensic nursing practice, they may not be directly applicable in Canada. Each provincial or territorial practice site and the federal Correctional Service of Canada (CSC) has unique guidelines that nurses in Canada must follow.*

The goals of the IAFN (2016) are paraphrased as follows:
- To incorporate primary prevention strategies into nurses' work at every level in an attempt to eliminate violence
- To establish and improve standards and ethics for forensic nursing practice
- To promote and encourage the exchange of ideas and the transmission of knowledge among members and related disciplines
- To create and facilitate educational opportunities for forensic nurses and related disciplines

Although the Canadian Nurses Association (CNA) has endorsed psychiatric mental health nursing as a specialty area of practice and offers certification for nurses who meet the criteria, it has not yet recognized forensic nursing as a distinct specialty area of practice.

Education

In 2001 certification in forensic nursing became available for the subspecialty of SANEs. At the same time, the IAFN called for the incorporation of forensic content at all levels of nursing education. In Canada, however, many nurses are involved in forensic nursing without having any specialized training. Some topics relevant to forensic nursing may be covered at the undergraduate level as part of psychiatric mental health nursing or community nursing courses; however, more often, forensic nursing is taught as a certificate program following the completion of a basic nursing program or as a course at the post-graduate level, where the core fundamentals of nursing are already established. Canada was the first in the world to offer an online forensic studies certificate program; however, there are no specific forensic nursing master's or doctoral programs currently available (Kent-Wilkinson, 2009, 2010). A master of nursing program with the specialty of forensic nursing is offered at the University of Saskatchewan. The Canadian Forensic Nurses Association (CFNA, 2022) maintains a list of forensic related courses and programs on their website, https://forensicnurse.ca.

Roles and Functions

In forensic nursing it is not the role of the forensic nurse to make a decision as to guilt or innocence or to determine whether a victim is being candid in their reporting of what happened. The roles of the forensic nurse centre on the identification of victims; creation of appropriate treatment plans; and collection, documentation, and preservation of potential evidence. The forensic nurse possesses expertise in assessment and treatment roles related to competency, risk, and danger. Forensic nurses are educated in nursing science and may have taken additional courses in theories of violence and victimology and legal issues, enabling them to objectively assess the circumstances of the case.

An understanding of both the victim and the offender enhances evidence collection. Forensic nurses may apply medical–surgical knowledge to the care of victims and offenders, and they may function in a legal role as they collect evidence, testify in court, or collaborate with law practitioners with relation to a forensic patient.

Nurse Examiner or Sexual Assault Nurse Examiner

The SANE was the first specialized forensic role for nurses that required advanced education. The largest group of self-identified forensic nurses, SANEs are nurses who seek training in the care of adult and pediatric victims of sexual assault (*SANE-A* and *SANE-P*, respectively).

The IAFN has established clear guidelines for the preparation of SANEs and provides SANE certification for nurses, although not all nurses who work in this capacity have certification. The training is

---

RESEARCH HIGHLIGHT

Survivors' Satisfaction With Nurse-Led Sexual Assault and Domestic Violence Care

Problem
Respect for confidentiality and an ethical responsibility not to retraumatize victims of sexual assault challenge the ability to conduct research or evaluation on survivors' experiences and satisfaction with services. As a result, little is known about the impact of comprehensive nursing-led, hospital-based sexual assault and domestic violence treatment programs.

Purpose of Study
The study sought out the views and opinions of survivors of sexual assault on their experiences with nurse-led sexual assault care in Ontario.

Methods
This study surveyed patients or guardians who presented to 30 of 35 of Ontario's Sexual Assault/Domestic Violence Treatment Centres on seven key domains: presentation characteristics, patient characteristics, assailant characteristics, assault characteristics, health consequences, service use, and satisfaction with services.

Key Findings
Participation rates were high, with 1484 people participating in the study, 96% of whom were women or girls. Participants were mostly White (75.3%), 12 to 44 years old (87.8%), and living with family (69.6%); 97.9% of patients used at least one service. The most commonly used service was assessment and/or documentation of injury (84.8%), followed by on-site follow-up care (73.6%). Nearly all of the patients or guardians reported that they received the care needed (98.6%) and rated the overall care as excellent or good (98.8%). Most (95.4%) stated that the care had been provided in a sensitive manner. Concerns about and recommendations to improve care expressed by a small proportion of patients or guardians focused on broader systemic and institutional issues of long wait times, negative attitudes of emergency department staff, issues of privacy and confidentiality, and difficulty with accessing services.

Implications for Nursing Practice
Based on their findings, recommendations for cross-training and attention to broader systemic issues can be made. The high uptake and overwhelmingly positive evaluation of services provided by Ontario's Sexual Assault/Domestic Violence Treatment Centre programs confirm the value of nursing-led, hospital-based care in the aftermath of sexual assault and domestic violence. Ongoing evaluation of such services will ensure the best care possible for this patient population.

Source: Du Mont, J., Macdonald, S., White, M., et al. (2014). Client satisfaction with nursing-led sexual assault and domestic violence services in Ontario. *Journal of Forensic Nursing, 10*(3), 122.

relatively brief: the course is typically 5 days and 40 contact hours and is available online or in a classroom setting. The course may also include a clinical component. Currently 7 of the 10 provinces in Canada offer SANE programs.

Nurses recognize the need to provide consistent care for all victims; therefore nurses and leaders in many communities in Canada have set standards for educating the public on sexual assault prevention techniques and establishing comprehensive care for victims through sexual assault response teams (SARTs), which use a multi-disciplinary model in providing care. SANEs are involved in the formation of SARTs in many communities across Canada. Along with SANEs, members of a SART may include representatives from the health department, police services, advocacy groups, the local department of children and family services, crown attorneys' offices, local hospitals, victim assistance programs, and other service areas, as pertinent (Adams & Hulton, 2016). The multi-disciplinary approach provides a standard of care that includes expert care in the acute setting, advocacy for the acute and long-term needs of the victim, and referral for counselling for survivors to decrease long-term effects resulting from the assault. The Research Highlight box describes the findings of a research study on survivors' satisfaction with nurse-led sexual assault and domestic violence care in Ontario.

Nurse Coroner or Death Investigator

This forensic nursing subspecialty is recognized internationally as having its historical roots in Alberta. Passage of the *Fatalities Inquiries Act* led to the formation of the Medical Examiners' Office in 1977 in Alberta. Subsequently, the medical examiner system for investigation of all deaths (unnatural, unexpected, or unexplained) was adopted, and nurses were hired as death investigators or medical examiner nurse investigators (Constantino et al., 2013). Currently, the medical examiner system operates in Alberta, Manitoba, Nova Scotia, and Newfoundland. Other provinces have a coroner system or a combination of both system types (Kent-Wilkinson, 2009, 2010). Over the years, registered nurses have also held the position of coroner in some territories and provinces. This nursing role involves assessing the deceased through understanding, discovery, preservation, and use of evidence.

As a representative of the medical examiner's or coroner's office, the forensic nurse death investigator is in charge of the body at a scene and works in collaboration with police services and other officials involved in the case. This nurse interviews witnesses, collects evidence, and documents findings. The nurse may also notify the next of kin of the death (Baumann & Stark, 2015). Such nurses are able to expand the role of the coroner and improve services provided to families, health care agencies, and communities by employing the basic principles of holistic nursing care.

The Forensic Mental Health System in Canada

An increasing number of individuals struggling with mental illness and living in the community without adequate mental health services and resources are coming into contact with the law. This phenomenon is frequently referred to as the *criminalization of the mentally ill*. According to Stall (2013), the psychiatric deinstitutionalization movement, which started in the 1960s, and changes to civil law that rendered involuntary treatment and hospitalization more difficult (both part of the movement toward the promotion of the self-determination of individuals with mental illness) have contributed to the criminal justice system becoming the new entry point to mental health services for many individuals with mental illness. Peternelj-Taylor and Panosky (2013) point to the continuing lack of adequate mental health policies for individuals living with chronic mental illness and the lack of community-based services, resulting in a fragmented mental health care system.

The Canadian forensic mental health system provides mental health services (inpatient and community) to individuals who have a mental illness and have come into contact with the justice system. Although health care in Canada receives financial support from the federal government and the *Criminal Code* dictates some degree of consistency, the forensic mental health systems in the provinces and territories have evolved separately because the Constitution grants each jurisdiction authority over health matters (Library of Parliament, 2013). The provincial and territorial forensic mental health systems therefore reflect the uniqueness of each jurisdiction, including geography, climate, existing services, population needs, and available resources and expertise.

FORENSIC PSYCHIATRIC NURSING

Forensic psychiatric mental health nurses "seek the truth about when, what, where, how and who in a traumatic or catastrophic event" (Zalon et al., 2013, p. 3). Devnick (2010, p. 48) describes forensic mental health nursing as multi-faceted, calling for the balancing of competing philosophies of caring and containment; inciting contradictory emotions in response to trauma; and the complex skills of collaborating with inter-disciplinary health, legal, and security staff in the management of clinical interventions to address potentially dangerous behaviours. This specialty requires skills in psychiatric mental health nursing assessment, evaluation, and treatment of forensic patients diagnosed with a mental illness.

Evidence collection is central to the role of the forensic psychiatric nurse. For example, evidence is collected by a careful evaluation of a forensic patient's mental status at the time of an offence. This evaluation aids in determining the individual's fitness to stand trial and may later influence the sentence. Forensic psychiatric nurses may spend considerable time with an accused individual collecting evidence and carefully documenting the interaction and dialogue. In this capacity the role of the forensic psychiatric nurse is not to determine guilt or innocence but to provide assessment data that can help make a final diagnosis within the multi-disciplinary forensic team (Emergency Nurses Association, 2018; Scannell, 2018).

Roles and Functions

The role of the forensic psychiatric nurse formally began in Canada in the 1970s, when mentally disordered offenders were separated from the general inmate population and forensic psychiatric services were provided federally by CSC. The role subsequently evolved with the establishment of forensic psychiatric inpatient units (Kent-Wilkinson, 2009, 2010). The role has continued to evolve, and forensic psychiatric nurses may now function as forensic nurse examiners, expert witnesses, and consultants to the criminal justice system, law enforcement, or health care agencies. These roles may involve providing nursing services to forensic patients and victims of violence, expert court testimony, and services to a Crown attorney or defence lawyer.

Roles of the forensic psychiatric nurse may be examined in relationship to the settings in which the nurse is employed. The forensic psychiatric nurse, as a member of an interprofessional team, may work on a forensic assessment unit in a mental health facility, conducting court-ordered evaluations of criminal responsibility and court-ordered treatment to determine if individuals are fit to stand trial, or may work on a forensic rehabilitation unit providing treatment, care, and rehabilitation for patients who have been found to be unfit or not criminally responsible (NCR) on account of mental health disorder.

Canadian law specifies that a person cannot be tried for a criminal offence if, because of a mental health disorder, they are unable to provide a defence. The *Criminal Code* defines "unfit to stand trial" as unable on account of a mental health disorder to conduct a defence at any stage of the proceedings before a verdict is rendered or to instruct counsel to do so and, in particular, unable on account of mental illness to:

1. understand the nature or object of the proceedings,
2. understand the possible consequences of the proceedings, or
3. communicate with counsel. (*Criminal Code R.S.C.*, 1985, c. C-46, s. 2)

It is the accused individual's capacity *at the time of trial* that is in question in determining fitness to stand trial. The court may decide that an individual found unfit to stand trial is to be treated for the purpose of making the individual fit to do so. Before rendering this decision, the court must be satisfied, based on medical evidence, that the proposed treatment is likely to make the individual fit to stand trial and that without treatment, the individual is likely to remain unfit; that any potential harm associated with the treatment does not outweigh the anticipated benefits; and that the specified treatment is the least restrictive and least intrusive given the circumstances. Then every 2 years, until the person is either acquitted or tried, a review board holds a hearing to determine if the person has become fit to stand trial (Department of Justice Canada, 2015a). Although there continues to be much debate, Canadian law currently requires only that individuals be able to provide a factual account to their lawyers, not necessarily an analytical or rational analysis.

Criminal responsibility refers to the mental state of a defendant at the time of the offence. A person is **not criminally responsible** if they have a mental health disorder that makes them unable to judge the nature or quality of the criminal act or to understand that the act was wrong at the time it was committed (*Criminal Code R.S.C.*, 1985, c. C-46, s. 16). Merely having a mental health disorder does not automatically exempt a person from criminal responsibility. The courts make the decision based on a thorough legal and psychiatric review to determine the person's state at the time of the offence. If the person is tried, the verdict will then be guilty, not guilty, or NCR on account of mental health disorder.

A literature review of the role of the forensic psychiatric mental health nurse identified a series of competencies (Box 32.2).

The forensic psychiatric nurse must be highly skilled in interpersonal communications and able to develop collegial relationships with those in other disciplines. The ability to be self-reflective and objective is also critical (Sekula & Amar, 2016).

One of the most challenging aspects of forensic psychiatric nursing is balancing the custodial role with the therapeutic role. The forensic psychiatric nurse must be able to look beyond the **index offence** (the serious and recorded criminal act that brought the accused to a Review Board) and see forensic patients as human beings with specific needs (Dhaliwal & Hirst, 2016).

Forensic psychiatric nursing appeals to a particular type of nurse, one who thrives in a stimulating intellectual environment, seeks out opportunities to apply clinical skills to complex legal problems, and enjoys pushing the limits of traditional boundaries. Because of the value placed on tradition by the nursing profession, the forensic psychiatric nurse is sometimes viewed with skepticism in nursing and with caution in the legal system. These responses must be met with professionalism by forensic psychiatric nurses in their practice, research, and education.

Correctional Nursing in Canada

The number of incarcerated individuals (both men and women) in Canada has decreased by 7% in custody and 5% in community over recent years. In Canada in 2018 to 2019 there were 368 821 admissions to provincial/territorial correctional services, with 14 548 admissions to federal correctional services (Statistics Canada, 2020). Incarcerated individuals are significantly more likely than those in the general public to have infectious diseases, chronic health conditions such as diabetes, cardiovascular conditions, and asthma, as well as to experience mental illness and substance use disorders (Kouyoumdjian et al., 2016).

Offenders are guaranteed the right to treatment as well as the right to refuse treatment (Department of Justice Canada, 2015b). Therefore correctional facilities are required to provide "adequate and reasonable" health services to inmates, either directly or through community-based health services organizations. **Correctional nursing** is defined by the location of the work or the legal status of the patient rather than by the role or functions being performed by the nurse. In fact, the role of nurses in correctional settings involves all aspects of nursing practice, including emergency care, medication administration, comprehensive mental and physical health assessments, infection control, health teaching, provision of treatments such as wound care, management of

---

BOX 32.2 Competencies Associated With the Role of a Forensic Psychiatric Mental Health Nurse

Specific Task-Oriented Areas
- Safety and security
- Assessment and management of risk
- Monitoring of patients and their property
- Management of violent and aggressive behaviour
- Therapies
- Practical skills (e.g., first aid)
- Escorting patients within and outside of the secure environment
- Visitor-related issues (e.g., observation, communication)
- Management of hostage situations and other security breaches
- Report writing

Knowledge
- Mental health and criminal justice systems
- Appreciation of physical, legal, emotional, and spiritual consequences of being legally detained
- Mental health wellness and illness
- Public attitudes, moral values, ignorance and stigma, empowerment, and paternalism

Skills
- Self-awareness, reflection, and honesty
- Therapeutic use of self
- Clinical risk assessment and management
- Planning of therapeutic interventions
- Development and maintenance of independent living skills
- Facilitation of meaningful relationships
- Help in the identification of behavioural boundaries and the development of self-control
- Addressing of socially unacceptable behaviours

Personal Qualities (Values and Attitudes)
- Ability to be non-judgmental (e.g., ensuring that principles of equality, fairness, and confidentiality are maintained)
- Ability to be detached (i.e., not personalizing negative events)
- Ability to appear calm and relaxed (i.e., never being threatening)
- Understanding and setting boundaries in therapeutic relationships
- Ability to make decisions effectively

Source: Adapted from Bowering-Lossock, E. (2006). The forensic mental health nurse: A literature review. *Journal of Psychiatric & Mental Health Nursing, 13,* 780–785. https://doi.org/10.1111/j.1365-2850.2006.00993.x. Copyright © 2006, John Wiley and Sons.

acute and chronic mental and physical illnesses, and collaboration with other health care providers (American Nurses Association, 2020).

As mentioned, today's inmates experience a disproportionately greater number of chronic illnesses and infectious diseases than the general population. Treatment and services for inmates with mental health challenges are a significant part of the job for nurses working in correctional facilities. Research from the CSC over several years shows that 62% of incoming female offenders in the criminal justice system required further mental health evaluation. For incoming male offenders, 50% required further mental health assessment, and 40% of male offenders met the criteria for a current mental illness diagnosis other than substance use or antisocial personality disorder (CSC, 2015). Lifetime substance use was particularly notable for male and female offenders. The rate of mental illness among offenders is several times higher than the rate of mental health disorders in the general Canadian population.

Correctional nurses provide care for many individuals with serious mental illness who are caught in a cycle of homelessness, psychiatric facilities, and prison. Unfortunately, only some will end up being admitted to either a regional hospital or a regional mental health treatment centre, where they can receive comprehensive psychiatric mental health services. Frequently, these individuals instead become incarcerated as a result of psychiatric emergencies that generally include threats made to others. Because psychiatric resources to help manage such emergencies are scarce, these individuals often end up in prison instead of a hospital. Once they are in a correctional facility, their psychiatric condition often worsens because of the lack of adequate psychiatric intervention and the trauma of incarceration.

Another issue that must be considered in the treatment of those who are incarcerated is substance use and abuse. In Canada some 80% of offenders serving prison sentences of 2 years or more have faced challenges with drugs, alcohol, or both (CSC, 2015). Drug courts, mandatory drug treatment, and drug or alcohol treatment within correctional facilities have all been shown to decrease the likelihood of recidivism and to increase the likelihood of abstinence from drugs or alcohol after release.

Because of the impacts of mental health and addiction problems on recidivism and on resource allocation, policymakers and legislators are beginning to recognize the importance of providing treatment for individuals who are incarcerated. In Canada the *Corrections and Conditional Release Act S.C. 1992 c. 20* (2019) references the fact that inmates receiving mental health treatment alongside correctional programming (in prison and in the community) demonstrate functional improvement. The correctional setting, however, is not conducive to the intensive therapy required to adequately treat mental health issues; therefore the needs of the vast majority of people with mental illnesses or concurrent disorders in the correctional system are not appropriately addressed.

There are more than 700 nurses at the CSC working in a variety of settings, including correctional remand, psychiatric assessment, prison facilities, regional hospitals, mental health treatment centres, and Indigenous healing lodges (Box 32.3). They can specialize in a wide range of areas, from mental health disorders to substance use to chronic care (CSC, 2013). Alongside drug and alcohol treatment interventions, nurses working with incarcerated patients with mental illness employ biological treatments as well as psychoeducation, cognitive behavioural therapies, and other integrative therapies to promote coping (for instance, yoga therapy, which has a strong evidence base for this population) (Maruca & Shelton, 2016).

The CSC has recognized that correctional nurses face a number of challenges, including a high level of stress associated with the correctional environment, demanding work hours, caring for individuals who have a substance use disorder, and concerns for personal safety expressed by family and friends. In response to these challenges the CSC

> **BOX 32.3 Types of Health Care Settings in the Correctional Service of Canada**
>
> **Institutional Health Units (Ambulatory Care Centres)**
> Every CSC institution has a health services centre with varying hours of operation based on factors such as level of security and proximity to community services. The primary care providers in these units are nurses. Each institution provides a variety of routine and emergency psychology services to offenders.
>
> **CSC Regional Hospital**
> Each region has a hospital located within the compound of a multi-level or maximum security level institution that provides more specialized or comprehensive health care services on a 24-hour basis. Services include but are not limited to post-operative care, trauma care, observation, dialysis, palliative care, and any condition requiring 24-hour nursing services.
>
> **CSC Reception Centre**
> Each region has at least one reception centre that conducts the CSC standardized admission process (both health and security) for all newly sentenced federal offenders. The admission process involves various health assessments, such as a mental status assessment, comprehensive health assessment, and tuberculosis assessment.
>
> **CSC Regional Treatment Centre (Mental Health)**
> An inpatient mental health treatment facility is located in each region to provide treatment to inmates with psychiatric disorders that are too severe to allow them to remain in the general inmate population.

has implemented extensive education and training for newly hired nurses as well as for those who have been working in corrections for a number of years (CSC, 2013).

Correctional nurses perform psychiatric mental health nursing role functions, including completing comprehensive mental status examinations and implementing psychiatric care plans. The vignette illustrates a challenging situation facing a nurse working in the health services centre of a correctional facility.

> **VIGNETTE**
> Suzanne is a 45-year-old woman incarcerated at a federal institution in the general inmate population. She was convicted of assault with a deadly weapon following a confrontation with another incarcerated individual. Her psychiatric diagnoses include major depression and **post-traumatic stress disorder (PTSD)** (resulting from severe abuse in her childhood and from an intimate partner during her early twenties). Although she is not on a locked forensic unit, she is being treated with medication and being seen by one of the institution's nurses for medication management.
>
> While watching television in the common area one morning, Suzanne attacked a fellow inmate for no apparent reason, screaming and clawing at anyone who approached her. The staff was unable to control her physically. She was placed in solitary confinement with mechanical restraints; these actions did nothing to control her screaming. She was seen by the nurse on call, who reported that Suzanne was having a flashback related to her PTSD. The solitary confinement and mechanical restraints were only worsening these flashbacks. The staff and the nurse were facing a common dilemma in correctional health care: custody versus caring. While the nurse was focused on the needs of the individual inmate, the correctional staff was focused on the goals of the correctional facility related to custody of violent offenders and protection of the environment. The successful correctional treatment team seeks to balance the two sides of this debate: creating an environment in which the potential rehabilitation of offenders is possible without compromising the compulsory "punitive" aspects of incarceration.

KEY POINTS TO REMEMBER

- Forensic nursing is an emerging specialty area of practice that combines elements of traditional nursing, forensic science, and criminal justice.
- The IAFN was established in 1992 as the professional association representing this specialty internationally.
- Forensic nurses fulfill a variety of roles, including that of sexual assault nurse examiner, nurse coroner or death investigator, forensic psychiatric mental health nurse, and correctional nurse.
- Incarcerated individuals have higher rates of serious and chronic physical and mental illnesses than the general population.

CRITICAL THINKING

1. How would you describe the nurse–patient relationship in forensic nursing? In what ways does it differ from the nurse–patient relationship in other areas of nursing?
2. Respect is an essential component of any therapeutic nurse–patient relationship; however, nurses often find it challenging to respect patients who have committed serious offences. Is it possible for nurses working in a forensic or correctional setting to respect every patient? Explain your answer.

CHAPTER REVIEW

1. Which statement regarding forensic nursing is accurate?
   a. Forensic nurses must all be prepared at the doctoral level.
   b. Forensic nurses perform only sexual assault examinations.
   c. Forensic nurses may participate in death investigations.
   d. Forensic psychiatric mental health nurses work only in correctional facilities.
2. What is one of the most challenging aspects of forensic psychiatric nursing?
   a. Working independently instead of as a member of an interdisciplinary team
   b. Balancing the custodial role with the therapeutic role
   c. Spending time in maximum security settings
   d. Determining the guilt or innocence of forensic patients
3. What does it mean for an individual to be found unfit to stand trial?
   a. The individual is unable to understand the court proceedings.
   b. The individual has a life-threatening physical illness.
   c. The individual has a chronic mental illness.
   d. The individual does not demonstrate insight into their mental illness.
4. Which type of patients would a correctional nurse typically see?
   a. Students
   b. Police officers
   c. Teachers
   d. Inmates
5. The nurse is caring for an incarcerated patient. Based on an understanding of the health profile of incarcerated individuals, what health care challenge may the nurse most anticipate working on with this patient?
   a. Drug or alcohol issues
   b. Autoimmune diseases
   c. Eating disorders
   d. Anxiety

https://evolve.elsevier.com/Canada/Varcarolis/psychiatric/.

REFERENCES

Adams, P., & Hulton, L. (2016). The sexual assault nurse examiner's interactions within the sexual assault response team: A systematic review. *Advanced Emergency Nursing Journal, 38*(3), 213–227. https://doi.org/10.1097/TME.0000000000000112

American Nurses Association. (2020). *Correctional nursing: Scope and standards of practice* (3rd ed.). Washington, DC: Nursebooks.org.

American Nurses Association, & International Association of Forensic Nurses. (2017). *Forensic nursing: Scope and standards of practice* (2nd ed.). Silver Spring: Nursesbooks.org.

Baumann, R., & Stark, S. (2015). The role of forensic death investigators interacting with the survivors of death by homicide and suicide. *Journal of Forensic Nursing, 11*(1), 28–32. https://doi.org/10.1097/JFN.0000000000000058

Bowering-Lossock, E. (2006). The forensic mental health nurse: A literature review. *Journal of Psychiatric & Mental Health Nursing, 13*, 780–785. https://doi.org/10.1111/j.1365-2850.2006.00993

Canadian Forensic Nurses Association. (2012). *About*. https://forensicnurse.ca/about/

Canadian Mental Health Association. (2021). *Myths about mental illness*. Retrieved from https://cmha.ca/documents/myths-about-mental-illness

Centre for Addiction and Mental Health. (2020). *Mental health and criminal justice policy framework*. Retrieved from https://www.camh.ca/-/media/files/pdfs—public-policy-submissions/camh-cj-framework-2020-pdf.pdf

Constantino, R. E. B., Crane, P. A., & Young, S. E. (2013). *Forensic nursing: Evidence-based principles and practice*. Philadelphia: F. A. Davis Co.

Correctional Services of Canada (CSC). (2013). *Careers at CSC—Nurses*. Retrieved from https://www.csc-scc.gc.ca/careers/003001-1301-eng.shtml

Correctional Services of Canada (CSC). (2015). *Research results—Mental health*. Retrieved from https://www.csc-scc.gc.ca/publications/005007-3030-eng.shtml

Corrections and Conditional Release Act, S.C. 1992, c. 20. (2019). Retrieved from https://laws-lois.justice.gc.ca/eng/acts/c-44.6/

Criminal Code R.S.C., 1985, c. C-46. (2022). Retrieved from https://laws-lois.justice.gc.ca/eng/acts/c-46/

Department of Justice Canada. (2015a). *The review board systems in Canada: An overview of results from the mentally disordered accused data collection study*. Retrieved from https://www.justice.gc.ca/eng/rp-pr/csj-sjc/jsp-sjp/rr06_1/p1.html

Department of Justice Canada. (2015b). *Canada's system of justice*. Retrieved from https://www.justice.gc.ca/eng/csj-sjc/just/img/courten.pdf

Department of Justice Canada. (2017). *Indigenous overrepresentation in the criminal justice system: JustFacts*. Retrieved from https://www.justice.gc.ca/eng/rp-pr/jr/jf-pf/2017/jan02.html

Devnick, B. R. (2010). *The forensic mental health nurse: Confusion, illusion, or specialization? A scoping literature review*. Master's thesis, University of Victoria, DSpace University of Victoria Repository. Retrieved from https://dspace.library.uvic.ca/bitstream/handle/1828/4092/Devnick_Betty_MN_2010.pdf?sequence=1

Dhaliwal, K., & Hirst, S. (2016). Caring in correctional nursing: A systematic search and narrative synthesis. *Journal of Forensic Nursing, 12*(1), 5.

Emergency Nurses Association. (2018). Forensic evidence collection in the emergency care setting. *Journal of Emergency Nursing, 44*(3), 286–289. Retrieved from https://forensicnurses.org/page/WhatisFN

Government of Canada. (2020). Office of the Correctional Investigator: Indigenous people in federal custody surpasses 30%—Correctional Investigator issues statement and challenge. Retrieved from https://www.oci-bec.gc.ca/cnt/comm/press/press20200121-eng.aspx

Gutierrez, L., Wilson, H. A., Rugge, T., et al. (2013). The prediction of recidivism with aboriginal offenders: A theoretically informed meta-analysis. *Canadian Journal of Criminology and Criminal Justice, 55*(1), 55–99. https://doi.org/10.3138/cjccj.2011.E.51

Harris, C. (2017). Forensic nursing provides closure in workplace fatality. *Journal of Forensic Nursing, 13*(1), 35–38. https://doi.org/10.1097/JFN.0000000000000137

International Association of Forensic Nurses. (2022). *Forensic nursing*. Retrieved from https://www.forensicnurses.org/?page=WhatisFN

Kara, F. B. (2014). Police interactions with the mentally ill: The role of procedural justice. *Canadian Graduate Journal of Sociology and Criminology, 3*(1), 79–94.

Kent-Wilkinson, A. E. (2009). An exploratory study of forensic nursing education in North America: Constructed definitions of forensic nursing. *Journal of Forensic Nursing, 5*(4), 201–211. https://doi.org/10.1111/j.1939-3938.2009.01055.x

Kent-Wilkinson, A. E. (2010). Forensic psychiatric/mental health nursing: Responsive to social need. *Issues in Mental Health Nursing, 31*(6), 425.

Kouyoumdjian, F., Schuler, A., Matheson, F. I., et al. (2016). Health status of prisoners in Canada: Narrative review. *Canadian Family Physician/Médecin de Famille Canadien, 62*(3), 215.

Library of Parliament. (2013). *The federal role in health and health care*. Retrieved from https://lop.parl.ca/sites/PublicWebsite/default/en_CA/ResearchPublications/201191E

Maruca, A. T., & Shelton, D. (2016). Correctional nursing interventions for incarcerated persons with mental disorders: An integrative review. *Issues in Mental Health Nursing, 37*(5), 285.

Mental Health Commission of Canada. (2020). *Mental health and the criminal justice system: "What we heard"—evidence summary*. Retrieved from https://www.mentalhealthcommission.ca/wp-content/uploads/drupal/2020-08/mental_health_and_the_law_evidence_summary_report_eng.pdf

Peternelj-Taylor, C., & Panosky, D. (2013). Advancing forensic correctional nursing. *Journal of Forensic Nursing, 9*(1), 1.

Public Safety Canada. (2015). *Crime prevention information, project descriptions and summaries*. Retrieved from https://www.publicsafety.gc.ca/cnt/cntrng-crm/crm-prvntn/tls-rsrcs/nfrmtn-dscrptns-smmrs-en.aspx

Scannell, M. J. (2018). *Fast facts about forensic nursing: What you need to know*. Springer Publishing Company.

Sekula, K., & Amar, A. F (2016). Forensic mental health nursing. In A. F. Amar, & L. K. Sekula (Eds.), *A practice guide to forensic nursing: Incorporating forensic principles into forensic practice* (pp. 1–15). Indianapolis: Sigma Theta Tau International.

Simpson, A. I. F., McMaster, J. J., & Cohen, S. N. (2013). Challenges for Canada in meeting the needs of persons with serious mental illness in prison. *Journal of the American Academy of Psychiatry and the Law Online, 41*(4), 501.

Stall, N. (2013). Imprisoning the mentally ill. *CMAJ: Canadian Medical Association Journal—Journal de l'Association Medicale Canadienne, 185*(3), 201–202. https://doi.org/10.1503/cmaj.109-4390

Statistics Canada. (2020). *Adult correctional statistics 2018/2019*. Retrieved from https://www150.statcan.gc.ca/n1/pub/85-002-x/2020001/article/00016-eng.htm

Zalon, M. L., Constantino, R. E., & Crane, P. A (2013). Fundamentals of contemporary forensic nursing practice, education and research. In R. E. B. Constantino, P. A. Crane, & S. E. Young (Eds.), *Forensic nursing: Evidence-based principles and practice* (pp. 2–26). Philadelphia: F. A. Davis Co.

UNIT 7

Advanced Intervention Modalities

33. Therapeutic Groups

34. Family Interventions

35. Integrative and Complementary Therapies

33

Therapeutic Groups

Cheryl L. Pollard
Originating US chapter by Donna Rolin, Emily Fowler

 https://evolve.elsevier.com/Canada/Varcarolis/psychiatric/.

OBJECTIVES

1. Identify basic concepts related to group work.
2. Describe the phases of group development.
3. Define task and maintenance roles of group members.
4. Discuss the therapeutic factors that operate in all groups.
5. Discuss four types of groups commonly led by nurses.
6. Describe a group intervention for (1) a member who is silent or (2) a member who is monopolizing the group.

KEY TERMS AND CONCEPTS

conflict
group
group content
group norms
group process
group psychotherapy
group themes
group work
psychoeducational groups
self-help groups
support groups
therapeutic factors

We all live among and interact with groups throughout our lives. We are born into a family group and grow up with various peer groups, such as those at school, at work, within religious or spiritual affiliations, and so on. As adults, we establish our own family group. A **group** consists of two or more people who come together for the purpose of pursuing common goals, interests, or both. A group's progress and outcomes are influenced by the group's characteristics, including:

- Size
- Defined purpose
- Degree of similarity among members
- Rules
- Boundaries
- Content (what is said in the group)
- Process (underlying dynamics among group members)

Box 33.1 defines terms related to types of groups and group work. **Group work** is a method whereby individuals with a common purpose come together and benefit by giving and receiving feedback within the context of group life.

There are advantages and disadvantages of group therapies for people living with mental illness. Advantages include:

- Engaging multiple people in treatment at the same time, thereby saving costs
- Enabling participants to benefit from the feedback not only of the nurse leader but also of peers, who may possess a unique understanding of the issues
- Providing a relatively safe setting to try out new ways of relating to other people and practising new communication skills
- Promoting a feeling of belonging

Disadvantages include:

- Time constraints in which an individual member may feel cheated of floor time, particularly in large groups
- Concerns that private issues may be shared outside the group
- Disruptive member behaviour during an emotionally vulnerable point

Not everyone benefits from group treatment. People who are acutely psychotic, acutely manic, or intoxicated experience difficulty interacting in groups and may interfere with other members' ability to remain focused on group goals and process. Foundational group therapy processes, group functions, and leadership in groups are overviewed in this chapter. Specific interventions delivered in groups such as insight-oriented psychotherapy and cognitive behavioural and supportive therapies are highlighted, bearing in mind that, for many group therapies, advanced skill and training is essential for effective and safe nursing practice.

THERAPEUTIC FACTORS COMMON TO ALL GROUPS

Irvin D. Yalom & Leszcz, 2020, one of the most noted researchers on group psychotherapy, is credited with identifying the factors that make groups therapeutic (Box 33.2). **Therapeutic factors** are aspects of the group experience that facilitate therapeutic change. For example, as group members begin to share life experiences, feelings, and concerns, they may recognize for the first time that they are not "alone in the world"—their experiences may be more universal than they initially thought, allowing them to connect with others. Yalom calls this factor *universality*—the recognition that other people feel the same way or have had the same experiences. Recognizing universality can provide a validation of the person's experiences and, subsequently, a profound sense of relief. Different therapeutic factors operate at different phases of a group, and during the initial phase, the leader may role-model several behaviours, such as instilling hope and imparting information. Just as with other types of treatment, each person's response to a group is highly individualized, based on past experiences and level of participation.

PLANNING A GROUP

Planning a group should include developing a description of its specific characteristics, for example:

> **BOX 33.1 Terms Central to Therapeutic Groups**
>
> **Terms Describing Group Work**
> **Group content**—all that is said in the group
> **Group process**—the dynamics of interaction among the members (e.g., who talks to whom, facial expressions, body language)
> **Group norms**—expectations for behaviour in the group that develop over time and provide structure for members (e.g., starting on time, not interrupting)
> **Group themes**—members' expressed ideas or feelings that recur and have a common thread. (The leader can clarify a theme to help members recognize it more fully.)
> **Conflict**—open disagreement among members. (Positive conflict resolution within a group is key to successful outcomes.)
>
> **Terms Describing Types of Groups**
> **Heterogeneous group**—a group in which there is a range of differences among members
> **Homogeneous group**—a group in which all members share central traits (e.g., men's group, group of people with bipolar disorder)
> **Closed group**—a group in which membership is restricted; no new members are added when others leave
> **Open group**—a group in which new members are added as others leave
> **Subgroup**—an individual or a small group that is isolated within a larger group and functions separately. (Members of a subgroup may have greater loyalty, more similar goals, or more perceived similarities to one another than they do to the larger group.)

> **BOX 33.2 Therapeutic Factors in Groups**
>
> **Instillation of hope**—The leader shares optimism about group treatment, and members share their improvements.
> **Universality**—Members realize that they are not alone in their problems, feelings, or thoughts.
> **Imparting of information**—Participants receive formal teaching by the leader or advice from peers.
> **Altruism**—Members feel a reward from giving support to others.
> **Corrective recapitulation of the primary family group**—Members repeat patterns of behaviour in the group that they learned in their families; with feedback from the leader and peers, they learn about their own behaviour.
> **Development of socializing techniques**—Members learn new social skills based on feedback from others.
> **Imitative behaviour**—Members may copy behaviour from the leader or peers and can adopt healthier habits.
> **Interpersonal learning**—Members gain insight into themselves based on feedback from others. This process is complex and occurs later in the group, after trust is established.
> **Group cohesiveness**—This powerful factor arises in a mature group, when each member feels connected to the other members, the leader, and the group as a whole; in a cohesive group, members can accept positive feedback and constructive criticism.
> **Catharsis**—Intense feelings, as judged by the member, are shared.
> **Existential resolution**—Members learn to accept painful aspects of life (e.g., loneliness, death) that affect everyone.
>
> Source: Data from Yalom, J. D., & Leszcz, M. (2020). *The theory and practice of group psychotherapy* (6th ed.). New York: Basic Books.

- Name and objectives of the group
- Common concerns or diagnoses of members
- Group schedule (frequency, times of meetings, etc.)
- Descriptions of leader's and members' responsibilities
- Methods or means of evaluating outcomes of the group

Planning and structure are especially important when group leaders are likely to change (e.g., in inpatient settings, where staffing patterns change) or when several groups are running at the same time with a common goal (e.g., in a research study).

PHASES OF GROUP DEVELOPMENT

All groups go through developmental phases similar to those identified for individual therapeutic relationships (see Chapter 9). In each phase the group leader has specific roles and challenges to address in support of positive interaction, growth, and change.

In the *orientation phase* the group leader's role is to structure an atmosphere of respect, confidentiality, and trust. The purpose of the group is stated, and members are encouraged to get to know one another. Group rules such as confidentiality or avoidance of potentially inflammatory topics such as politics are reviewed. Initially, members may be overly silent or overbearing because they have not yet established trust with one another. Therapeutic interaction is supported when the group leader points out similarities between members, encourages them to talk directly to each other rather than to the leader, and reminds members about ground rules for respectful interaction.

In the *working phase* the group leader's role is to encourage a focus on problem solving consistent with the purpose of the group. As group members begin to feel safe within the group, conflicts may be expressed, which should be viewed by the group leader as a positive opportunity for group growth. It is important for the leader to guide and support conflict resolution. Through the successful resolution of conflicts, group members are empowered to develop confidence in their problem-solving abilities and better support one another in their individual efforts to grow and change.

In the *termination phase* the group leader's role is to encourage members to reflect on the progress they have made and identify post-termination goals. Members may experience feelings of loss or anger about the group ending; at times, these feelings can be directed toward other group members or the leader. It is important to openly address such feelings as part of the group's work toward successful termination.

Evaluation and follow-up are fundamental aspects of a therapeutic group. Objective measures are an important way to demonstrate group effectiveness. Questionnaires can be helpful in refining what patients found helpful. The Therapeutic Factors Inventory-19 (Joyce et al., 2011) is a questionnaire that asks patients to identify which of the therapeutic factors were present in therapy. The Group Questionnaire (Burlingame, 2010) is another tool that evaluates the climate, cohesion, empathy, and alliance of the group. Regardless of the scale or instrument used, group leaders should evaluate all groups to determine if goals set in the planning phase were accomplished and to re-evaluate or re-design future groups.

GROUP MEMBER ROLES

We each have a unique style of interacting with others, and we gravitate toward specific comfort zones within groups. Consider your own behaviours within groups. You may tend to sit back and mainly observe, giving your opinion only after careful consideration. Or perhaps you feel that it is important to keep everyone moving in a common direction or to help maintain order and actively urge people to continue working. The way we behave in groups is a function of our innate personalities, our socialization, and the specific context of the group.

Studies of group dynamics have identified informal roles that group members often assume and that may or may not be helpful in the group's development. The classic descriptive categories for these roles are *task*, *maintenance*, and *individual* roles (Benne & Sheats, 1948). Task roles serve to keep the group focused on its main purpose and get the work done. Maintenance roles function to help each person feel worthwhile and create a sense of group cohesion. Individual roles have nothing to do with helping the group but instead relate to specific personalities, personal agendas, and a desire to have needs met by shifting the group's focus to them. Awareness of roles can assist the group leader in identifying behaviours that need to be confronted or reinforced. Table 33.1 describes the informal roles of group members.

GROUP LEADERSHIP

Nurse as Group Leader

Psychiatric mental health nurses are involved in a variety of therapeutic groups in acute care and long-term treatment settings. Nurses are able to provide strong leadership skills in a variety of basic groups, such as activity, psychoeducational, task, and support groups, and, with support, they may co-lead more advanced groups, such as cognitive behavioural therapy or counselling groups. More complex skills are necessary for leading psychotherapy groups, and only advanced-practice nurses or nurse therapists are qualified to lead these and other specialized groups. The interaction patterns within the specialized groups are often very complex and require a greater degree of interactional analysis than more basic groups. A clear theoretical framework may be used to structure the group interaction analysis. Table 33.2 describes several theoretical frameworks commonly used in group work.

Responsibilities

The group leader has multiple responsibilities in initiating, maintaining, and terminating a group.

The first responsibility is to determine the purpose, parameters, and membership of the group. Will the group be open, accepting new members regularly, or closed to new members after it begins? How often will the group meet, where, and for how long? It is also advisable in many instances to choose a co-leader to help facilitate the group and, especially on inpatient units, one or more observers.

The leader and co-leader should base the selection of group members on clear criteria, depending on the type of group. Group members need to have a certain degree of cognitive functioning in order to participate in an insight-oriented psychotherapy group.

The styles of group leadership vary depending on the type of group and on the stage of group development. For example, the leader is often most direct in the orientation phase. During this phase, the structure, size, composition, purpose, and timing of the group are defined.

TABLE 33.1 Informal Roles of Group Members

	Role	Function
Task roles	Coordinator	Tries to connect various ideas and suggestions
	Elaborator	Gives examples and follows up meaning of ideas
	Energizer	Encourages group to make decisions or take actions
	Evaluator	Measures the group's work against a standard
	Information giver	Shares facts or own experience as an authority figure
	Information seeker	Tries to clarify the group's values
	Initiator–contributor	Offers new ideas or a new outlook on an issue
	Opinion giver	Shares opinions, especially to influence group values
	Orienter	Notes the progress of the group toward goals
	Procedural technician	Supports group activity by distributing papers, arranging seating, etc.
	Recorder	Keeps notes and acts as the group's memory
Maintenance roles	Compromiser	In a conflict yields to preserve group harmony
	Encourager	Praises and seeks input from others
	Follower	Agrees with the flow of the group
	Gatekeeper	Monitors the participation of all members to keep communication open
	Group observer	Keeps records of different aspects of group process and reports to the group
	Harmonizer	Tries to mediate conflicts between members
	Standard setter	Verbalizes standards for the group
Individual roles	Aggressor	Criticizes and attacks others' ideas and feelings
	Blocker	Disagrees with group issues; oppositional
	Dominator	Tries to control other members of the group with flattery or interruptions
	Help seeker	Asks for sympathy of group excessively
	Playboy	Acts uninterested in group process
	Recognition seeker	Seeks attention by boasting and discussing achievements
	Self-confessor	Verbalizes feelings or observations unrelated to group
	Special-interest pleader	Advocates for a special group, usually with own prejudice or bias

Source: Data from Benne, K., & Sheats, P. (1948). Functional roles of group members. *Journal of Social Issues, 4*, 41–49. https://doi.org/10.1111/j.1540-4560.1948.tb01783.x

TABLE 33.2 Theoretical Foundations for Group Therapy

Theory	Concepts	Role of Therapist
Psychodynamic/psychoanalytic	Applies Freud's concepts of psychoanalysis to individual members and to the group itself; focus is on unconscious conflicts and transference; goal is insight	Helps members to recognize unconscious conflicts and encourages peer feedback
Interpersonal	Applies Sullivan's theories about interpersonal learning; focus is on understanding how current relationships repeat early significant relationships; goal is to rebuild individual's personality	Helps to reduce anxiety and encourages members to validate feelings and thoughts with each other
Communication	Applies a systems model, holding that the whole (group) is greater than the sum of its parts (members); focus is on subgroups and communication, both verbal and nonverbal; goal is to learn clear, congruent communication skills	Helps point out confusing or contradictory messages; acts as a role model for clear communication
Group process	Analyzes the group with a focus on individual roles and group patterns of behaviour (phases, norms, etc.); goal is to resolve authority and intimacy issues	Helps develop a mature group in which members trust each other and give supportive feedback
Existential/gestalt	Applies theories of Maslow and Rogers to encourage individuals to develop to full potential; focus is on the here and now to increase members' awareness of feelings; goal is self-actualization, in which individual takes full responsibility for choices	Helps focus members on here-and-now experiences to promote self-learning; promotes emphasis on the "what" of behaviours, not the "why"
Cognitive behavioural	Applies concepts of learning theory and Ellis's cognitive therapy; focus is on behaviour and thinking patterns, with the group used to reinforce adaptive behaviour and extinguish maladaptive patterns; usually time limited; goal is to change behaviour or thinking patterns	Helps develop a trusting group in which members give supportive feedback to reinforce healthier behaviour; may provide formal teaching, including homework assignments

Sources: Data from Dies, R. (1992). Models of group psychotherapy: Sifting through confusion. *International Journal of Group Psychotherapy, 42*(1), 1–17; Scheidlinger, S. (1997). Group dynamics and group psychotherapy revisited: Four decades later. *International Journal of Group Psychotherapy, 47*(2), 141–159.

Task and maintenance functions may be discussed and demonstrated. During the working phase, the leader facilitates communication and ensures that meetings begin and end on time. In the termination phase the leader ensures that each member summarizes individual accomplishments and gives positive and negative feedback regarding the group experience.

Maintenance of cultural safety for individual members is a key responsibility of the group leader. The leader initially sets a foundation for open communication by defining the importance of mutual respect and rules for group conduct. As group members begin to engage with one another, the leader's sensitivity to issues that may have a cultural basis can be pivotal in facilitating efforts to maintain open communication and mutual respect.

Diversity may exist in many forms, including racial, ethnic, economic, and sexual orientation. Encouraging members to share and explore their cultural foundations and beliefs promotes genuine communication and provides the group with the opportunity to share similarities and differences in an environment of mutual respect.

Consider the example of a woman who came to group after seriously harming herself. She remained silent and withdrawn until the leader encouraged her to explore her feelings about the group. The woman revealed that she "wasn't smart like everyone else" and that she was "basically just trailer trash." Other group members began to share their similarities and differences in backgrounds, with a focus on their common needs, fears, and insecurities. When this woman finished the group, she acknowledged having learned an important lesson: she could give and get help from people she saw as different from her, and not everyone would treat her as though she was "less than them."

Styles of Leadership

There are three main styles of group leadership, and a leader selects the style that is best suited to the therapeutic needs of a particular group, the therapeutic needs of the group are determined by the type of group and by the stage of group development. The *autocratic leader* exerts control over the group and does not encourage much interaction among members. For example, staff leading a community meeting with a fixed, time-limited agenda may tend to be more autocratic. In contrast, the *democratic leader* supports extensive group interaction in the process of problem solving. Psychotherapy groups most often employ this leadership style. In this style the leader and co-leader take a facilitative role, redirecting questions or issues to group members rather than providing answers or solutions. A *laissez-faire leader* allows the group members to behave in any way they choose and does not attempt to control the direction of the group. In a creative group such as an art or horticulture group the leader may choose a laissez-faire style.

In any group the leader must be thoughtful about communication techniques since these can have a tremendous impact on group content and process. Table 33.3 describes communication techniques frequently used by group leaders. It is also important to note that inpatient groups have significant differences from outpatient groups (Table 33.4), and consequently the role of the leader must be adapted accordingly.

Clinical Supervision

Clinical supervision, sometimes referred to as *peer supervision* or *clinical consultation*, is important for group leaders, as it provides feedback about performance and enhances the professional growth of the nurse. Transference and counter-transference issues occur in groups just as in individual treatment (see Chapter 4), and a more objective input supports a focus on therapeutic goals. Feedback related to the functioning of the group and the leadership style being used can also help further develop the skills related to respect and engagement. Another strategy used to support group leader development is co-leadership. Co-leadership is a common practice and has several benefits, including (1) providing training for less experienced staff, (2) allowing for immediate feedback between leaders after each session, and (3) offering two role models for teaching communication skills to members.

TABLE 33.3 Group Leader Communication Techniques

Technique	Example
Giving information—provides resources and information that support treatment goals	"Antidepressants may take as long as 4 weeks or more to show real therapeutic effects."
Clarification—asks group members to expand and clarify what they mean	"What do you mean when you say 'I can't go back to work'?"
Confrontation—encourages group members to explore inconsistencies in their communication or behaviour	"Jane, you're saying 'nothing's wrong,' but you're crying."
Reflection—encourages group members to explore and expand on feelings (rather than on thoughts or events)	"I noticed you're clenching your fists. What are you feeling right now?" "It sounds like that really upset you."
Summarization—closes a discussion or group session by pointing out key issues and insights	"We've talked about different types of cognitive distortions, and everyone identified at least one irrational thought that has influenced their own behaviour in a negative way. In the next group, we'll explore some strategies for correcting negative thinking."
Support—gives positive feedback and acknowledgement	"It took a lot of courage to explore those painful feelings. You're really working hard on resolving this problem."

TABLE 33.4 Comparison of Outpatient and Inpatient Groups

Outpatient Groups	Inpatient Groups
The group has a stable composition.	The group is rarely made up of the same members for more than one or two meetings.
Members are carefully selected and prepared.	Members are admitted to the group with little prior selection or preparation.
The group is homogeneous with regard to ego function.	The group has a heterogeneous level of ego function.
Motivated, self-referred people make up the group; therapy is growth oriented.	Members are ambivalent, and often therapy is compulsory; therapy is relief oriented.
Treatment proceeds as long as required: it may continue for 1–2 years.	Treatment is limited to the hospital period, with rapid member turnover.
The boundary of the group is well maintained, with few external influences.	Whatever happens on the unit affects the group.
Group cohesion develops normally, given sufficient time in treatment.	There is no time for cohesion to develop spontaneously; group development is limited to the initial phase.
The leader allows the process to unfold; there is ample time to set up group norms.	The group leader structures time and is not passive.
Members are encouraged to avoid extra-group contact.	Members eat, sleep, and live together outside of the group; extra-group contact is endorsed.

Source: Adapted from Mackenzie, K. R. (1997). *Time-managed group psychotherapy: Effective clinical applications.* Washington: American Psychiatric Press.

 SAFETY TIP

Transference and counter-transference issues can be significant obstructions to building a therapeutic alliance with your patient. Openly reflecting on the interaction patterns can help understand the impact of these psychodynamic constructs on the therapeutic relationship and ways to mitigate the negative effects of psychological phenomena.

Group Observation

In some groups it is useful, and even essential, to assign staff as observers. In some cases the use of an observer may occur for the purpose of clinical supervision. Another reason would be for staff to observe how group members interact and then share their observations with the leaders in order to assess and plan for modifications to the group or individual patient care plans. In inpatient groups or day programs, there may be concern about patients leaving the group in a fragile emotional state; one role of the observer is to maintain safety. The observer follows and tends to the needs of any group member who left the session before it was over.

It is useful for the group observer to monitor not just content but also process, that is, not only *what* is talked about but *how* it is talked about. A simple method is to draw a diagram of who is sitting where and, while observing, draw lines between members to indicate who speaks to whom. This diagram can give instant feedback as to patterns of behaviour in group members.

Ethical Issues in Group Therapy

The Canadian Nurses Association (2017) provide the definition for professional ethical conduct for registered nurses. The nurse group leader has an ethical obligation to inform participants of risks and benefits of group participation (informed consent). They must also discuss both confidentiality and exceptions to confidentiality. Because a group contains individuals who are not bound by a professional code of ethics, there is no way to guarantee confidentiality. Other topics the group leader must address are, "Who is free to leave the group?" and "What are the rules about group members socializing outside the group?"

A member is only removed from the group as a last resort. One obvious reason is if one member were to become violent or aggressive toward another member. This would necessitate temporary or permanent removal. Other reasons that might require temporary or permanent removal from the group include (1) a member who is consistently unwilling or unable to participate or (2) a member who violates the agreements created for group membership.

Group leaders should obtain appropriate training or credentialing to practise and must work within their regulatory body's defined scope of practice. The best way to help patients is for the group leader to consistently follow the ethical guidelines and professional standards of practice.

To protect the integrity of the group therapy process, nurse clinicians should use evidence-based practice. Staying current with research helps nurse clinicians to select the best therapeutic modality for the target group audience. Evidence-based practice helps ensure that the therapeutic group maximizes benefit and minimizes harm.

Basic Groups

Psychoeducational Groups

Psychoeducational groups aim to increase knowledge or skills about a specific subject and allow members to communicate emotional concerns. These groups may be time limited or may be supportive for long-term treatment. Generally, written handouts or audiovisual aids are used to focus on specific teaching points. Nurses are prepared to teach a variety of health subjects.

Medication education. The most common psychoeducational group led by a nurse is the medication education group. These groups are designed to teach patients about their medications, answer their questions, and prepare them for self-management. When patients have concerns about taking medications, it is often the group members themselves who are in the position to respond to these questions: "Yes, I got a dry mouth when I first started taking that, but it got better. Hang in there." Box 33.3 outlines an example of a medication education group protocol, and Figure 33.1 provides a means of evaluating the effectiveness of this type of nursing intervention.

Health education. Nurses also frequently lead health education groups, including groups on sex education. For instance, people who have used poor judgement in sexual behaviour because of mental illness are at high risk for sexually transmitted infections.

Family education. Nurses may also facilitate family psychoeducational groups, usually as part of an interdisciplinary team. Individual relapse rates decrease significantly when families are educated about mental illness, treatments, and recovery, as well as strategies for interacting with an ill family member and managing crises. Family psychoeducation is a recognized evidence-informed practice in psychosocial rehabilitation (Niemelä et al., 2016).

Concurrent disorders. Concurrent disorder groups integrate learning about co-existing mental illnesses and substance use. Since treatment issues for people with a concurrent disorder can be complex, group leaders must have demonstrated competency in both mental health and chemical dependence treatment. The goal is to engage people in treatment and decrease their use of substances or to maintain recovery in a supported process (Fogger & Lehmann, 2017). Research has shown that combined treatment for people with serious mental illness produces improved outcomes (Gamble & O'Lawrence, 2016).

Symptom management. For people with a common symptom such as anger or anxiety, symptom management groups are ideal. The focus is on sharing positive and negative experiences so that members learn coping skills from each other. A primary goal is to increase self-control or prevent relapse by helping members develop an individualized plan for action at the first appearance of symptoms.

Stress management. Often, time-limited stress management groups teach members about various relaxation techniques, including deep breathing, exercise, music, and spirituality. One such technique that is increasingly demonstrating efficacy in stress management is mindfulness (Kahnen et al., 2016). Mindfulness groups focus on developing awareness of the present moment, with the intent of inducing relaxation and promoting insight into thoughts, emotions, and physical responses.

Support and self-help groups. Support groups (often facilitated by a professional) and self-help groups (facilitated by the group itself) are structured for the purpose of providing members with the opportunity to maintain or enhance personal and social functioning through cooperation and shared understanding of life's challenges (Yalom & Leszcz, 2020). Examples include support groups for survivors of cancer, bereavement support, or support groups for families who have lost a loved one to suicide. Supportive group therapy can also benefit those with severe mental illness.

The nurse may serve as a resource for individuals and families and must be aware of the wide array of self-help groups available. One of the most important functions of such groups is to demonstrate to individuals and families that they are not alone in having a particular problem. Participants in these types of groups report feeling as though their experiences and feelings have been validated. Thus these groups provide

---

BOX 33.3 Example of Medication Education Group Protocol

Description of Group
A group for all patients, regardless of level of concentration, that prepares them for self-management of medication on discharge

Criteria for Member Selection
Open to all inpatients except those who are displaying suicidal or homicidal behaviours or the potential for assault

Visual Aids
PowerPoint slides, transparencies, flip charts, films, patient medication education sheets

Purpose
1. To educate members on the primary function of their medications
2. To provide information on adverse effects (that benefits can outweigh risks)
3. To describe a mechanism to negotiate relationships with health care workers
4. To enhance a sense of self-control over treatment

Procedure
1. Orientation and introduction to the group
2. Brief description of major symptoms in a diagnosis
3. Overview of antipsychotic drugs or antidepressants
4. Use of medication education sheets
5. Specific open question period

Behavioural Objectives
At the end of the 45-minute session, members will be able to:
1. State one of their symptoms that is treated by their medication
2. Ask at least one question about their medication
3. Identify one mechanism that helps in adhering to the medication regimen

Theoretical Justification
Even people who think they are adherent take only 80% of doses. Counselling and therapy are always adjuncts to drug therapy.

Source: Adapted from Ott, C. A. (2000). *Pediatric psychopharmacology.* South Easton: American Healthcare Institute.

Criteria	Strongly Agree	Somewhat Agree	Agree	Disagree	Strongly Disagree
1. I know the name(s) of the medication(s) I am taking.					
2. I know what symptoms the medication(s) can help me with.					
3. I know the common adverse effects of my medication(s).					
4. I feel comfortable talking to my prescriber if I am having problems with my medication(s).					
5. It is important to take my medication(s) at the same time every day.					

Fig. 33.1 Medication Group Evaluation Tool.

members with support, and their members help each other by telling their stories and providing alternative ways to view and resolve problems. Box 33.4 describes characteristics of support and self-help groups.

Advanced-Practice Nurse or Nurse Therapist
Group Psychotherapy

Group psychotherapy is a specialized treatment intervention in which a trained leader (or co-leaders) establishes a group for the purpose of treating people with psychiatric disorders. Expertise is necessary since the group is used as a tool to bring about change. Often group psychotherapy is done in conjunction with individual psychotherapy as part of an ongoing plan. The International Association for Group Psychotherapy and Group Process (https://www.iagp.com/) provides standards and training for mental health professionals, including nurses, to develop skills in this specialty.

Psychodrama groups. Psychodrama groups are specialized groups in which members are encouraged to act out life experiences or situations for the purpose of learning and insight. Leaders should have graduate-level education and training specific to this approach.

Dialectical behaviour treatment. Dialectical behavioural therapy (DBT) is a type of group psychotherapy in which people are seen each week with the goal of improving interpersonal, behavioural, cognitive, and emotional regulation skills and reducing self-destructive behaviours (Heath et al., 2021; Linehan, 1993; Rudge et al., 2020). Unlike in other types of group therapy, DBT group members are discouraged from making observations about others in the group. This treatment also requires specialized training and advanced education.

Integrative groups. An integrative group program consists of a number of sessions with a particular theme or purpose, in which individual group sessions may draw from any of the aforementioned

RESEARCH HIGHLIGHT
Benefits of an Arts-Based Mindfulness Group Intervention for Vulnerable Children

Problem
Vulnerable children, such as those who have experienced deleterious effects of abuse, neglect, loss, trauma, and family dysfunction on their physical, cognitive, emotional, social, and behavioural development face greater risks for experiencing behaviour problems that can create a myriad of difficulties in later life. It is unclear how teaching vulnerable children mindfulness-based skills and concepts would improve aspects of their resilience and self-concept such as emotion regulation and self-esteem.

Purpose of Study
To explore the effects of a 12-week arts-based mindfulness group program for vulnerable children (children who were involved with the child welfare or mental health system and experienced a variety of challenges) on their level of resiliency and self-concept.

Methods
Interpretive thematic qualitative analysis was conducted using transcribed interview data from post-group individual interviews with children or guardians. Pre- and post-intervention self-report data (using the Piers-Harris Children's Self-Concept Scale and the Resiliency Scales for Children and Adolescents) quantitative analysis was completed.

Key Findings
Qualitative analysis revealed two primary themes. The first theme had to do with the children's perceptions of Holistic Arts-Based Program (e.g., that it's a lot of fun and involves playing games, creating arts and crafts, learning mindfulness, gaining support, and making friends). Most of the children would not change anything about the group except to make it a longer duration and to conduct more activities outside. The second theme involved perceived benefits of participating in the group. Participants reported improved (1) emotion regulation, (2) mood, (3) coping and social skills, (4) confidence and self-esteem, (5) empathy, and (6) ability to pay attention and focus.

The quantitative analysis used self-report data from the participating children. There were issues with gaps in the data collected, which affected the statistical validity of the analysis. Despite these gaps, there was a significant improvement to the perceptions of self-concept. However, factors related to resiliency did not significantly differ before and after intervention.

Implications for Nursing Practice
With increased understanding of one's feelings and thoughts, a child can make better choices regarding their emotional expression, which can lead to improved functioning at school, home, and with peers. Nurses can use a group-delivered intervention to decrease the sense of isolation and improve a child's self-concept. Further research is needed regarding effective strategies to increase resilience.

Source: Coholic, D. A., & Eys, M. (2016). Benefits of an arts-based mindfulness group intervention for vulnerable children. *Child and Adolescent Social Work Journal, 33*(1), 1–13. https://doi.org/10.1007/s10560-015-0431-3

BOX 33.4 Support and Self-Help Groups

Target Population
- People who have shared the experience of a common problem, illness, crisis, or tragedy

Group Leader Activities
- May or may not be defined; may rotate among members
- Role is often more task oriented

Examples of Support Groups
- Bereavement groups for those who have experienced the loss of a loved one
- Suicide survivor groups for those who have lost a loved one to suicide
- Canadian Mental Health Association (CMHA) groups for patient or family support (or both), education, and advocacy
- Cancer support groups for families and individuals coping with the ramifications of this illness
- Internet support groups for a growing number of people, providing online, real-time interaction and support

Examples of Self-Help Groups and Resources
- Twelve-step groups that use a common model for recovery:
  - Alcoholics Anonymous (AA)—the prototype for other 12-step groups
  - Gamblers Anonymous (GA)
  - Overeaters Anonymous (OA)
  - Narcotics Anonymous (NA)
  - Co-Dependents Anonymous
  - Adult Children of Alcoholics (ACOA)
- Online listings of self-help resources in Canada:
  - eMentalHealth.ca (listing of national self-help and mutual aid groups): https://www.ementalhealth.ca/canada/en/_Selfhelp_mutual_aid_and_support_groups_a1_b44.html?filterLocalOnly=1
  - National Network for Mental Health (NNMH): https://nnmh.ca/
  - Self-Help Connection: https://selfhelpconnection.ca
  - The National Mental Health Inclusion Network (NMHIN): https://nmhin.ca/

Goals of Support and Self-Help Groups
- To provide health education and networking for resources
- To reduce anxiety and decrease feelings of isolation
- To provide support and encouragement of positive coping behaviours:
  - Decrease feelings of isolation
  - Provide mutual support
  - Provide psychoeducation and health education
  - Reduce stress
  - Help people cease self-destructive behaviours or come to terms with an overwhelming event or situation

Frequency and Duration
- Meets one or more times per week for an indefinite period of time
- Ongoing and open membership

---

approaches. An example is a group intervention for vulnerable children, which is reported in the Research Highlight box. Integrative groups may also be used to support and treat psychological symptoms that survivors of interpersonal trauma or abuse may experience. Chapter 24 further describes support and treatment approaches for people who have experienced interpersonal trauma.

Dealing With Challenging Member Behaviours

Research has identified certain behaviours of individual members that are challenging to manage within a group. Defensive behaviours interfere with people's ability to function or achieve satisfaction in their lives. Group therapy is about working through problem behaviours, but some behaviours can be especially disruptive to the group process and difficult for the leader to manage. The person who monopolizes the group, the person who complains but continues to reject help, the demoralizing person, and the silent person are examples (Yalom & Leszcz, 2020).

In dealing with any problematic behaviours in groups, members may appreciate help disclosing their own feelings and responses. The leader encourages the use of statements such as "When you speak this way, I feel …" The leader helps by noting that feelings are not right or wrong but simply exist. People tend to feel less defensive when "I feel" statements rather than "you are" statements are used. This approach helps members feel like part of the group, not alienated from it.

Monopolizing Member

The person who monopolizes the group may be attempting to deal with anxiety. As group tension grows, the person's level of anxiety rises, and the tendency to speak increases. Some people are just extremely talkative or may be hypertalkative due to hypomania or mania. In any case no one else gets a chance to be heard, and other group members eventually lose interest and begin to withdraw.

> **VIGNETTE**
> Holly is the most talkative member of the group until the nurse intervenes. Initially, Holly talks at length about her early experiences related to losing both of her parents and having to live with her grandparents. The other members of the group become bored with the same old story, and they drift off. They have heard these stories many times, not only in group therapy but also during other activities.

There are several useful strategies for dealing with an overly talkative group member. One strategy is to request a response from group members who have not had a chance to talk about the day's topic. If the behaviour continues, it may be necessary to speak directly to the monopolizing group member, either privately or in the group setting. In private you can share your observations and suggest that perhaps nervousness may be a factor causing the talkativeness. Asking for clarification may lead to a greater understanding of what the group member is experiencing. You may then ask them to limit contributions to a specific number of times (e.g., two or three). In the group setting the leader may ask the group members if they would like to share observations or feedback about other members, thereby offering a chance for growth. This strategy is probably the most challenging but potentially the most rewarding in that members feel empowered and the real therapeutic forces of groups are realized.

Complaining Member Who Rejects Help

The person who complains but continues to reject help brings problems to the group, often describing them in a manner that makes the problems seem insurmountable. In fact, the person appears to take pride in the insolubility of their problems. They come across as entirely self-centred, and the group's attempts to help are continually rejected.

The person who uses these tactics generally has highly conflicting feelings about their own dependency; any notice from the leader temporarily increases the person's self-esteem. On the other hand, the person has a pervasive mistrust of all authority figures. Most people who complain but continue to reject help have been subjected to severe deprivation early in their lives and may have experienced emotional or physical abuse or both.

> **VIGNETTE**
> Shamaila is always complaining about how horrible her relationship with her boyfriend is, and she manages to get the entire group worked up over the situation. Members tell her to leave him, not to spend all her time with him, and not to spend all her money on him, but each week she reports a new incident or crisis. In every session the group members become concerned and offer encouragement, advice, and solutions. Each time, the group becomes angry at her lack of change, and she is frustrated by her own inability to change. She asserts that the group is not helpful.

The leader should acknowledge the person's pessimism but maintain a neutral affect. If the person stays in the group long enough, and the group develops a sense of cohesion, this individual can be helped to recognize relationship patterns. The leader should encourage the person to look at the habitual "yes … but" behaviour objectively.

Demoralizing Member

Some people whose behaviour is self-centred, angry, or depressed may lack empathy or concern for other members of the group. They refuse to take any personal responsibility and can challenge the group leader and negatively affect the group process.

> **VIGNETTE**
> Dina comes to the support group on the inpatient psychiatric unit. She is very angry, stating, "I don't know why I come to these groups anyway! They don't help." Dina is to be discharged the next day to a 28-day alcohol rehabilitation program. She has a previously scheduled dental appointment before the rehabilitation intake interview, and she is being strongly encouraged by her therapist to reschedule the appointment. The therapist fears that Dina is at high risk for drinking again, because she states that she constantly has the urge to drink. When a group member who is an addictions therapist confronts Dina about not being flexible and prioritizing her need for alcohol treatment, she explodes. "I thought this group was for support. This is outrageous!" Group members are obviously uncomfortable with her anger.

In this case the group leader should listen to the comments objectively. Again, the leader may choose to speak to the group member in private and ask what is causing the anger. Sometimes this simple exchange can make the person feel a greater connection with the nurse and, more importantly, as a member of the group, which likely will decrease hostile behaviour and increase the group's benefit. In the group setting the leader can focus on positive group members, whose comments may reduce the hostility of the negative group member.

Remember that angry people may be extremely vulnerable, and devaluing or demoralizing keeps others at a distance and maintains the person's own precarious sense of safety. Leaders must empathize with the member in a matter-of-fact manner, such as "You seem angry that the group wants to support you in putting sobriety ahead of your dental needs."

Silent Member

Members who are silent in the group may be observing intently until they decide that the group is safe for them, or they may believe that they are not as competent as other, more assertive group members. Silence does not mean that the member is not engaged or involved, but it should be addressed, for several reasons. The person who does not speak cannot benefit from others' feedback, and other group members are deprived of this group member's valuable insights. Furthermore, a silent group member may make others uncomfortable and create a sense of mistrust.

> **VIGNETTE**
> Anne has attended three group sessions for survivors of childhood sexual abuse. Although she appears to be listening, she rarely makes eye contact with the leader or other group members. She responds to yes or no questions, but when it comes to open-ended questions such as "What do you think, Anne?" she tends to shrug her shoulders and respond with "I don't know." Other group members have tried to draw Anne out, as has the leader. Katia, another group member, is beginning to exhibit frustration with Anne: "Look, I have shared some of the most private and painful memories of my childhood. I feel like you think you're too good to share what happened to you."

There are several techniques that may help in this case, including allowing the person to have extra time to formulate their thoughts before responding. Saying, "I'll give you a moment to think about that" and then waiting or coming back to the group member later is often helpful. Another tactic is to make an assignment that every person in the group respond to a certain topic or question. For example, "Let's all think of a positive and assertive response to something that you generally feel helpless about. I'll give you a minute or so to think this topic over, and then I'm going to ask each of you to share."

Sometimes partnering with another group member will give the silent member the courage they need to participate. You may break the group into pairs and ask them to discuss a certain topic and then each report back to the group what they heard the other person say.

EXPECTED OUTCOMES

Expected outcomes of group participation will vary, depending on the type and purpose of the group. For education groups, such as a medication education group, the expected outcome would be demonstration of knowledge. For therapy groups, the expected outcomes will focus more on insights, behaviour changes, and reduction in symptoms. For example, in an alcohol treatment group, an expected outcome might be that the person develops insight into the connection between drinking and negative consequences. An expected behavioural outcome could be abstinence from alcohol use. In groups that focus primarily on emotional issues such as depression or anxiety standardized tests can be used to measure symptom reduction as an outcome of group participation.

KEY POINTS TO REMEMBER

- Research has identified 11 therapeutic factors that operate in groups and lead to therapeutic change for members. Yalom's therapeutic factors identify specific positive aspects of groups, such as the universality of experience, imparting information, altruism, corrective recapitulation of the primary family group, development of socializing techniques, imitative behaviour, interpersonal learning, group cohesiveness, catharsis and existential resolution, and the instillation of hope.
- When a new group is formed, similarities and differences in many dimensions, including diagnosis, age, gender, and culture, must be considered.
- A group format has advantages over individual therapy, including cost savings, increased feedback, an opportunity to practise new skills in a relatively safe environment, and the instillation of a sense of belonging.
- Groups develop through predictable phases over time.
- For a group to continue and be productive, members must fulfill specific functions known as *task* or *maintenance roles*. Individual roles are not productive and are based on individual personalities and needs.
- Clinical supervision is important so that group leaders can objectively analyze group interactions and leadership techniques.
- Nurses have opportunities to lead or co-lead therapeutic groups, some in the hospital but primarily in community settings.

- Psychoeducational groups, activity groups, task groups, and support groups are often led by nurses and provide significant treatment as part of the multi-disciplinary treatment plan.
- Advanced-practice nurses and nurse therapists may lead psychotherapy groups based on various theoretical models.
- Challenging member behaviours, such as silence, complaining, or demoralizing, can be especially difficult. A variety of interventions are recommended to minimize the disruption to the group and maximize the benefit to the person engaging in these behaviours.

CRITICAL THINKING

1. You are assigned to work with Malia, a 30-year-old woman who was admitted to the psychiatric unit with major depression after recently harming herself. Her nurse has told her she needs to attend group therapy. While lying in bed and staring at the ceiling, Malia tells you that she is a private person and that listening to other people's problems will not help and will only make her more depressed.
   a. How would you describe the benefits of group therapy to Malia?
   b. What intervention(s) might make it easier for Malia to attend group therapy?
2. Construct an outline for a medication teaching group that would cover information useful for your patients. If possible, co-lead this group with a staff member, with guidelines from your instructor.
3. Ms. Joseph is a 22-year-old Haitian-born nursing student admitted to the psychiatric unit after a nearly lethal overdose of acetaminophen (Tylenol). She admits to drinking excessively for the past 6 months. She is at risk of failing school. She complains of depressed mood, a loss of interest in her studies, decreased concentration, and social isolation. In the concurrent disorders group she has been silent for the past two sessions and sits staring at the floor.
   a. What is your evaluation of Ms. Joseph's situation?
   b. What might Ms. Joseph's nonverbal behaviour mean?
   c. What approach would you use to involve her more in the group?
   d. What criteria could you use to evaluate the effectiveness of your intervention?
   e. What cultural implications should you consider?

CHAPTER REVIEW

1. The nurse is caring for four patients. Which patient would not be appropriate to consider for group therapy?
   a. The patient with limited financial resources
   b. The patient who is acutely manic
   c. The patient who has few friends on the unit
   d. The patient who does not speak up often, yet listens to others
2. The nurse tells group members that they will be working on expressing conflicts during the current group session. Which phase of group development is represented?
   a. Formation phase
   b. Orientation phase
   c. Working phase
   d. Termination phase
3. Group members are having difficulty deciding what topic to cover in today's session. Which nurse leader response reflects autocratic leadership?
   a. "We are talking about fear of rejection today."
   b. "Let's go around the room and make suggestions for today's topic."
   c. "I will let you come to a conclusion together about what to talk about."
   d. "I'll work with you to find a suitable topic for today."
4. The nurse is planning care that includes a concurrent disorders group. A patient with which of the following disorders would be appropriate for this group?
   a. Depression and suicidal tendencies
   b. Anxiety and frequent migraine headaches
   c. Bipolar disorder and anorexia nervosa
   d. Schizophrenia and alcohol abuse
5. A member continues to dominate the group conversation despite having been asked to allow others to speak. What is the most appropriate nursing response to address this behaviour?
   a. "You are monopolizing the conversation."
   b. "When you talk constantly, it makes everyone feel angry."
   c. "You are supposed to allow others to talk also."
   d. "When you speak out of turn, I feel concerned that others cannot participate equally."

https://evolve.elsevier.com/Canada/Varcarolis/psychiatric/.

REFERENCES

Benne, K. D., & Sheats, P. (1948). Functional roles of group members. *Journal of Social Issues, 4*, 41–49. https://doi.org/10.1111/j.1540-4560.1948.tb01783.x

Burlingame, G. (2010). Small group treatments: Introduction to special section. *Psychotherapy Research: Journal of the Society for Psychotherapy Research, 20*, 1–7.

Canadian Nurses Association. (2017). *Code of ethics for registered nurses.* Ottawa: Author. Retrieved from https://hl-prod-ca-oc-download.s3-ca-central-1.amazonaws.com/CNA/2f975e7e-4a40-45ca-863c-5ebf0a138d5e/UploadedImages/documents/Code_of_Ethics_2017_Edition_Secure_Interactive.pdf

Fogger, S. A., & Lehmann, K. (2017). Recovery beyond buprenorphine: Nurse-led group therapy. *Journal of Addictions Nursing, 28*(3), 152–156. https://doi.org/10.1097/JAN.0000000000000180

Gamble, J., & O'Lawrence, H (2016). An overview of the efficacy of the 12-step group therapy for substance abuse treatment. *Journal of Health and Human Services Administration, 29*(1), 142–160.

Heath, N., Midkiff, M.F., Gerhart, J., et al. (2021). Group-based DBT skills training modules are linked to independent and additive improvements in emotion regulation in a heterogeneous outpatient sample. *Psychotherapy Research, 31*(8), 1001–1011. https://doi.org/10.1080/10503307.2021.1878306

Joyce, A. S., MacNair-Semands, R., Tasca, G. A., et al. (2011). Factor structure and validity of the Therapeutic Factors Inventory–Short Form. *Group Dynamics: Theory, Research, and Practice, 15*(3), 201.

Kahnen, D., Gerard, B., & Qin, H. (2016). How does decreasing stress impact the healthy practice environment? *Medsurg Nursing, 25*(4), S12. Retrieved from https://link.gale.com/apps/doc/A461945713/AONE?u=anon~6fb02d73&sid=googleScholar&xid=82705739

Linehan, M. M. (1993). *Cognitive behavioral treatment of borderline personality disorder.* New York: Guilford.

Niemelä, M., Marshall, C. A., Kroll, T., et al. (2016). Family-focused preventive interventions with cancers cosurvivors: A call to action. *American Journal of Public Health, 106*(8), 1381–1387. https://doi.org/10.2105/AJPH.2016.303178

Rudge, S. Feigenbaum, J. D., & Fonagy, P. (2020). Mechanisms of change in dialectical behaviour therapy and cognitive behaviour therapy for borderline personality disorder: A critical review of the literature. *Journal of Mental Health, 29*(1), 92–102. https://doi.org/10.1080/09638237.2017.1322185

Yalom, J. D. & Leszcz, M. (2020). *The theory and practice of group psychotherapy* (6th ed.). New York: Basic Books.

34

Family Interventions

Lisa-Marie Forcier
Originating US chapter by Christina Fratena, Laura G. Leahy

 https://evolve.elsevier.com/Canada/Varcarolis/psychiatric/.

OBJECTIVES

1. Define the concept of family.
2. Differentiate between functional and dysfunctional family patterns of behaviour as they relate to the five family functions.
3. Compare and contrast insight-oriented family therapy and behavioural family therapy.
4. Identify family theorists and their contributions to the family therapy movement.
5. Incorporate the family's sociocultural context when assessing and planning intervention strategies.
6. Construct a genogram using a three-generation approach.
7. Formulate outcome criteria that a nurse counsellor and family might develop together.
8. Identify strategies for family intervention in specific psychiatric clinical situations.
9. Distinguish between the nursing intervention strategies of an entry to practice nurse and those of an advanced-practice nurse with regard to counselling and psychotherapy and psychobiological issues.
10. Explain the importance of the nurse's role in psychoeducational family therapy.

KEY TERMS AND CONCEPTS

behavioural family therapy
boundaries
clear boundaries
enmeshed boundaries
family systems theory
family triangle
flexibility
genogram
insight-oriented family therapy
intergenerational issues
nuclear family
psychoeducational family therapy
rigid boundaries
sociocultural context

Although family structure and function have changed dramatically over the years, the Canadian family remains central to the fabric of Canadian society. Same-sex marriages, recognition of common-law relationships, and blended families have influenced family structure and roles. In addition, Canada is a multi-cultural society with diverse cultural expectations of family roles all of which are subject to societal influences. In the late nineteenth century the Canadian government's assimilation policies toward Indigenous peoples significantly influenced the erosion of Indigenous traditional family structure and values. The residential school system policies severely affected family structure, parenting roles, and traditions, which contributed to intergenerational trauma and cultural loss (Good2Talk, 2021). Intergenerational trauma is important to note. It occurs when trauma that is experienced by one generation is transmitted to subsequent generations, ultimately affecting their health and well-being. Historical trauma is the intentional persecution of a specific population, for example, individuals with shared ethnic, religious, cultural, or political background, by an out-group that results in a collective trauma. Historical trauma is a type of intergenerational trauma (Good2Talk, 2021).

Indigenous children were removed from their homes, forcing the loss of their culture, language, and connection to family and land. Furthermore, adoption policies during this time allowed for the removal of Indigenous children from their homes to be adopted by White families, known as the 60s scoop (Stevenson, 2021). These events have inserted patterns affected by intergenerational trauma into the lives of many families. The consequences of intergenerational trauma have impacted population mental health and inextricably changed the way people view themselves; their children, parents, and leaders; and their relationship to society (Good2Talk, 2021; Bombay et al., 2014; Gone et al., 2019). *The Truth and Reconciliation Commission of Canada* (TRC, 2015) and *The United Nations Declaration on the Rights of Indigenous Peoples* (United Nations, 2018) have established awareness and recognition of Indigenous history and culture. Expanded awareness and strength is compelling action toward healing destructive family patterns through innovative family programs such as Indigenous family court, healing programs, and Indigenous family therapy that recognize the effects of trauma and create cultural safety and growth (Ontario Centre of Excellence for Child and Youth Mental Health, 2017).

Canadian families are experiencing rapid change in these functions, and there is a growing diversity in family configurations within a rapidly changing, globalized, fast-paced society. Alongside these changing family structures, environments, and societal organization, more is being demanded of families in all facets of functioning. For example, caregiving for and support of family members who are experiencing physical illness, mental illness, and aging continue to expand, with implications for family functioning. According to Arriagada (2020), many Canadians play a central role in helping and providing care for family members or friends with a long-term condition, a physical or mental disability, or problems related to aging. In 2018 7.8 million Canadians aged 15 and older (25% of the population) were caregivers. Of these caregivers, almost 1.5 million were 65 years of age and older (Arriagada, 2020).

Family in its ideal form may provide security, kinship, a means to maintain traditions and culture, and a place of belonging. As such, family is a positive force in assisting its members through crises and the life cycle. Alternatively, family experiences may include difficulties such as all manner of crises, differences and interpersonal conflict, mental illness, poverty, or violence. It is within these diverse and challenging social and family contexts that nurses strive to provide *family-centred care*, an approach that is characterized by dignity and respect, information sharing, patient and family participation, and family–professional collaboration (Registered Nurses' Association of Ontario, 2015).

Family intervention may assist such families to gain healthy ways to adjust to change, to grow, and to gain skills for stronger ways of being. Some families may need psychotherapeutic intervention during the early years of a child's development to assist the child and family in correcting maladaptive patterns. The impact of racism, conflict, crisis, and violence on children and their longer-term mental health and functioning has been well documented (Layne et al., 2017; Willey et al., 2022), as explored in Chapters 8, 24, and 27. During times of crisis, inclusive of health crises, many families require psychological, emotional, and practical supports to restore their equilibrium. Family interventions may minimize psychological impairment and build on the strengths of the family. To facilitate non-judgemental and sensitive practice to assist families to grow with change or heal from particularly overwhelming circumstances, nurses require education in and understanding of diverse family experiences, economics, emotions, and context (Varcoe et al., 2022). This chapter explores the definitions and boundaries of families, examines sites of family conflict, and identifies specific family therapies for both entry-level and advanced practice.

FAMILY

Tam et al. (2017) suggest a "typical" family may differ between people and between cultures. For example, general definitions of a family include intact family, couple family, stepfamily, simple stepfamily, complex stepfamily, multi-generational family, and lone-parent family (Statistics Canada, 2017). These concepts are based on a range of definitions including those related to marital status, blood relations, living arrangements, and/or legal relationships. These concepts and the definitions that they are based on, however, are "monocultural" and do not embrace the complexities of other cultures, including Indigenous populations (Tam et al., 2017). It is of interest to bring forth a discussion on the complexity of conceptualizing the Indigenous family, which in Canada is often based on biological, legal, and marital relationships and household memberships (Tam et al., 2017). However, other influential factors need to be taken into consideration, such as cultural identity, kinship formation, linguistic differences, and mobility (Tam, et al., 2015).

The family is the primary system to which a person belongs. Birth, puberty, marriage, and death occur within the context of the family experience. The family can be a source of love or hate, pride or shame, and security or insecurity. Although individual family members have roles and functions, the over-riding value in families lies in the relationships among family members. It is these family relationships that provide the primary context of human development. Many family theorists consider the intergenerational connectedness of the family to be one of our greatest human resources.

> **VIGNETTE**
>
> Anna Lowen is a 54-year-old Hutterite Canadian woman who has been admitted to the acute psychiatric ward for an episode of mania. She had been diagnosed with bipolar disorder several years before and has had two previous episodes of mania. Anna lives in a Hutterite colony with her three children and her husband, Jake, and is respected for her hard work and good nature with older persons and children.
>
> Before being admitted to the hospital, she had been unable to sleep or eat for 1 week. In the mornings she was loud and irritable in the community kitchen and insisted on serving all of the children large bowls of porridge with eggs that she had collected from the henhouse. She was wandering the colony grounds, singing loudly in the middle of the night, when her family brought her to the hospital in the city. Currently, she is on a medication to stabilize her mood and help her to sleep and eat.
>
> Her husband, sisters, and several community members are visiting her at the hospital. The children have been left at the colony and do not understand what has happened to their mother. The nurse assesses the situation and adopts a family-centred nursing care approach inclusive of the community members. First, he identifies his own need to increase his understanding of the Hutterite culture, adapts psychoeducational materials to meet the family's needs, and encourages the family to bring the children to a meeting to have their questions about their mother answered.

Family Functions

Families are unique, each having its own strengths, resources, and challenges (Shajani & Snell, 2019; Varcoe et al., 2022). However, some general characteristics of a family include future obligations and caregiving functions, such as protection, nourishment, and socialization of its members (McGoldrick et al., 2016). The Vanier Institute of the Family (2021) identified the following as functions of a Canadian family:

- Provision of love and nurturance
- Socialization of children
- Social control of members
- Production and consumption of goods and services
- Addition of new family members through birth or adoption
- Physical care and maintenance of family members

These functions take place within a societal context, which also influences family members.

According to the Vanier Institute of the Family (2020), caregiving is a near-universal family experience, and at some point in our lives, most of us will provide care to a family member or friend with a long-term, physical, or mental disability or problem related to aging. In 2018 most caregivers (41%) spent 1 to 3 hours per week providing care. More than one in five (21%) spent 20 or more hours per week providing care. Further, in 2018 1 in 10 Canadians (3 million people) received care from a family member or friend for a long-term health condition, physical or mental disability or problem related to aging (Vanier Institute of the Family, 2020). Worldwide, 15% to 23% of children live with a parent with a mental illness (Leijdesdorff et al., 2017, p. 312). These children are often invisibly caregivers of their parents. Assuming too much responsibility in childhood could interfere with the attainment of children's developmental needs. These children have up to a 50% chance of developing a mental illness (Leijdesdorff et al., 2017, p. 312). Stigma also affects these children's experiences and well-being throughout their lives (Murphy et al., 2017), as it does for parents supporting adult children who are experiencing mental illness (Park & Seo, 2016; Raymond et al., 2017). Respite, education, and support are important interventions for both of these types of family members supporting other family members with mental illness experiences.

Families and Mental Illness

Historically, when mental illness occurred, health care providers often cast blame on the family. Blame was particularly predominant in the mental illness of children, especially those with autism, eating disorders, or schizophrenia. Theories charged that mothers' ways of interacting with their children were the root cause of child disturbance. Today, theories suggest holistic, complex explanations for illness (Mental Health Commission of Canada, 2015), but self-stigma and blame persist for many parents (Eaton et al., 2016). Nurses need to be aware of this history and pattern of parental blame, as remnants of these ideas linger.

An important component of nursing practice is to advise family members of appropriate support groups. Those experiencing a first episode of psychosis of a child are particularly vulnerable to being overwhelmed by the situation. Parental support groups such as the *Prevention and Early Intervention Program for Psychoses* (https://www.lhsc.on.ca/pepp-prevention-and-early-intervention-program-for-psychoses/pepp) in London, Ontario, were founded to assist such families. In addition, family support programs through the *Schizophrenia Society of Canada* and *Canadian Mental Health Association* assist all family members, parents, children, spouses, friends, and other loved ones in a number of educational, social support, and recreational program options.

CANADIAN MODELS OF FAMILY NURSING CARE AND ASSESSMENT

Three esteemed Canadian models of family care are the *McGill Model of Nursing*, developed by Dr. Moyra Allan, and the *Calgary Family Assessment Model (CFAM)* and *Calgary Family Intervention Model (CFIM)*, both based on the work of Wright and Leahey (in Shajani & Snell, 2019). These models guide both beginning and advanced-level nurses to practice from a family nursing perspective.

McGill Model of Nursing

The McGill Model of Nursing (https://www.mcgill.ca/nursing/about/model/) focuses on family health, collaboration, learning, and health promotion. It was developed in response to health care system changes that occurred when universal health care was introduced in Canada. It has been widely adopted in Canada within many diverse nursing areas. Its main assumption is that families possess strengths, motivations, and resources. These serve to assist families in moving toward health promotion, which will result in improved health outcomes. Because health behaviour is predominantly learned within the family context, it is imperative that nurses focus on working with the family by setting goals and establishing learning environments to share knowledge, build on existing knowledge, and assist in making changes in behaviours. Family members become active learners in the implementation phase of the nursing process. The processes of coping and development are dynamic (i.e., they occur in any phase). Family health is achieved by building on the strengths of the family and its individual members and using external resources, such as nurses and other health care providers. Ultimately, however, it is patients and families who are deemed experts in their own care in this model (Gottlieb, 2013).

Calgary Family Assessment Model and Calgary Family Intervention Model

The basic assumptions underlying CFAM and CFIM are derived from systems, communication, differing views of reality, and change theories. The models are multi-dimensional and consider structure, development, and function to guide a nurse's interventions with families (Shajani & Snell, 2019). The assessment and intervention approaches focus on promoting and improving family functioning in three domains: cognitive, affective, and behavioural. The CFIM recommends many relational nursing practices that promote family health and functioning, including asking interventive questions, offering commendations, providing information, validating emotional responses, encouraging illness narratives, supporting family caregivers, and encouraging respite. Within a nurturing and non-hierarchical relationship, this approach to family nursing interventions privileges family expertise and is anchored by a commitment to listen deeply to the concerns, suffering, and questions of family members.

The guidance provided by Varcoe et al. (2022) in their discussion of relational orientation and inquiry (Hartrick Doane & Varacoe, 2021) is another essential approach to relational engagement with the families encountered in a nurse's practice.

FAMILY THERAPY

Family therapy is a psychotherapeutic process that focuses on changing the interactions among the people who make up the family or marital unit. It serves to improve the family, the sub-systems within the family, and the individuals who make up the family. It focuses on evaluating these relationships and the communication patterns, structure, and rules that govern the family interactions (Boland & Verduin, 2022). Although novice nurses do not engage in family therapy, nurses may take additional educational courses to develop family therapy skills.

Every day, in every family, decisions are made regarding the functions of power, rulemaking, provision of financial support, future planning, and goods allocation. Families may address these functions in a variety of ways, but most commonly, the adults in the family determine how these functions are to be performed. In lone-parent families these functions may sometimes become overwhelming, highlighting the need for additional supports. In chaotic families a family member not well prepared to make decisions, such as a teenager, may be the decision maker. Although children learn decision-making skills as they mature and increasingly make choices about their own lives, they should not be expected to take on responsibility for the family. Cultural expectations and norms affect the allocation of roles and perspectives on how families negotiate these tasks.

Boundaries are the distinctions made between individuals in the family. Boundaries may be clear, enmeshed, rigid, or inconsistent (Box 34.1). Most families exhibit several combinations of the various boundary types (Goldenberg et al., 2017). When boundaries are functioning properly, family members work out arrangements by compromise based on an understanding of appropriate roles. Each generation is made aware of how decisions will be made and clearly understands who is in charge and when. Blurred boundary function results in family members interfering with each other's goals, creating tension and anxiety between family members. Children in these families may become confused, manipulative, and insecure.

Issues Associated With Family Therapies
Communication

Communication patterns are important in family life. Healthy communication patterns are characterized by clear and comprehensible messages (e.g., "*I would like to go now*"; "*I don't like it when you interrupt what I'm saying*"). Families with healthy communication are encouraged to ask for what they want and to express their feelings appropriately. In these families both affection and conflict are openly expressed, and members have no need to resort to manipulation. When communication is unclear, solving problems or resolving conflicts becomes difficult; therefore the cardinal rule for effective and functional communication is, "*Be clear and direct in saying what you want and need.*"

> **BOX 34.1 Types of Boundaries**
>
> - **Clear boundaries** Boundaries that are well understood by all members of the family and give family members a sense of "*I*-ness" and also "*we*-ness." They help define family members' roles and allow members to function without unnecessary interference from other members. However, they are not so rigid as to restrict contact among family members. For example, a mother tells her 14-year-old daughter, "*You don't need to worry whether your little brother eats his breakfast. Your father and I will handle that.*" This boundary may be redefined: "*I want you to make sure that your little brother gets his homework done while your father and I are at the movies.*"
> - **Enmeshed boundaries** (also called *diffuse boundaries*): Boundaries that result from a blending together of the roles, thoughts, and feelings of the individual family members so that clear distinctions fail to emerge. The members of a family that operates with enmeshed boundaries are more prone to psychological or psychosomatic symptoms. A common phenomenon within families with enmeshed boundaries is that individuals expect other members of the family to know what they are thinking (e.g., "*Why did you take that? You know I wanted it!*") and believe they know what other family members are thinking (e.g., "*I know exactly why you did that!*").
> - **Rigid boundaries** (also called *disengaged boundaries*): Boundaries in which the rules and roles are consistently adhered to no matter what; thus rigid boundaries prevent family members from trying out new roles or, in some cases, from taking on more mature functions as time goes on. In families in which rigid boundaries predominate isolation may be marked. Family members are often cut off from the community and outside influences and even from each other.

> **BOX 34.2 Examples of Dysfunctional Communication**
>
> **Manipulating:** Instead of asking directly, family members manipulate others to get what they want. A family member makes requests with "strings attached" so that the other person has a difficult time refusing the request: "*If you do this for me, I won't tell Daddy you are getting poor grades in school.*"
> **Distracting:** To avoid functional problem solving and resolve conflicts within the family, family members introduce irrelevant details into problematic issues (e.g., asking who picked up the dry cleaning when discussing communication problems).
> **Generalizing:** When dealing with problematic family issues, members use global statements like *always* and *never* instead of dealing with specific problems and areas of conflict. Family members may say "*Adem is always angry*" instead of "*Adem, what is upsetting you?*"
> **Blaming:** Family members blame other family members for failures, errors, or negative consequences of an action to keep the focus away from themselves. Blaming is a response to fear of being blamed by others.
> **Placating:** Family members pretend to be inadequate but well-meaning to keep peace in the family at any price: "*Don't yell at the children, dear. I'll put the shoes on the stairs.*"

As simple as this concept may seem, it may be difficult to activate in a family system. To be direct, individuals must first have a sense that the self is respected and loved; they then will be confident to set healthy boundaries with others. The consequences of being clear and direct may be unpleasant when boundaries are enmeshed, and confusion is the norm. Changing a family pattern will cause discomfort in the system. Explicitly stating what one wants and needs is especially difficult when one believes that family members should already know, especially if the family member is a spouse, a parent, or a close sibling. No one is able to mind-read, but emotionally undifferentiated members may believe that family members can. The following vignette describes a spousal situation that shows how easily communication can be misunderstood when clear and direct messages are not sent. See Box 34.2 for examples of unhealthy communication patterns.

> **VIGNETTE**
>
> Liz would like to spend more time on the weekends with her husband, Michael; however, Michael always seems to be busy around the house or talking with friends on the telephone. Liz feels that he does not notice her or maybe is not interested in her, so she spends a lot of time working out. Michael figures that Liz is doing what she wants to do and that it makes her happy, so he contents himself with finding things to do alone. The result is that Liz and Michael spend little time together. Liz finally confronts Michael clearly and directly about his "lack of interest" in her and tells him what she wants and needs—to spend more time together on the weekends. Michael replies that he had no idea she felt that way. He had thought she enjoyed the way things were, and he would like to have more time together too.

Emotional Support

All families encounter conflicts during their life journeys. However, in a healthy family, feelings of affection are generally uppermost, and anger and conflict do not dominate the family's pattern of interaction. Healthy families are concerned about each other and consistently meet family members' emotional and physical needs. Members feel supported and free to grow and explore new roles and facets of their personalities. A family that is dominated by conflict and anger alienates its members, leaving them isolated, fearful, and emotionally fragile. It is important for the nurse to note that patterns of family crises, including issues arising from substance use, may have underlying links to intergenerational trauma, historical oppression, and colonization.

Socialization

Within families, each member learns socialization skills. People learn coping skills and how to interact, negotiate, and plan for the future. Children learn to socialize effectively within the family and then apply their skills in society.

Family Life Cycle

The life cycle of individuals takes place within the family life cycle, the primary context of human development. Family life takes place within relationships, and changes within the relationships affect the roles of the parents. For example, as children mature and leave home, parents may renegotiate the pattern of their lives together. "Boomerang children" may unexpectedly return home, causing yet another change in family roles. Later, parents may need their adult children's help as they become less able to care for themselves. As the Canadian population ages, more family members will be providing care to older adult parents.

In the traditional Canadian family type there are six main phases of the family life cycle: (1) launching the single young adult, (2) joining families through couple formation, (3) becoming parents and caring for young children, (4) parenting adolescents, (5) launching children and moving on, and (6) experiencing later life, often encompassing the role of grandparent. Families may experience some of the phases and not others. In addition, with the increased cultural diversity of Canadian society, nurses may expect to see diverse interpretations of family tasks.

The family system moves through time, with potential for family stress at transition points (e.g., birth of a child, employment changes, children leaving home, retirement) or during an interruption in the life cycle (e.g., untoward events such as an unexpected death by suicide, first episode of psychosis of a young adult, imprisonment, divorce). At these times, therapy may be required to assist family members to proceed in the life cycle. For family members who feel trapped within a dysfunctional family system, extreme pressures can lead to distress or even suicide. Symptoms can be perceived as a response to an interruption in the family life cycle. This family life cycle assumes a traditional family organization and requires modification for increasingly non-traditional family structures (McGoldrick et al., 2016).

Working With the Family

Many concepts are used when working with families. The concepts of the *identified patient*, the *family triangle*, and the *nuclear family emotional system* are discussed here. Box 34.3 describes other concepts relevant to family work.

The Identified Patient

The *identified patient* is the individual in the family whom everyone regards as "the problem." A descriptive term for this person is the "family symptom-bearer." This family member is generally the focus of most of the family system's anxiety. They may serve to divert the attention from other more serious and debilitating problems within the family, such as a crumbling marriage, substance use, or infidelity. Furthermore, the symptoms of the identified patient may serve as a stabilizing mechanism to bring about customary behaviour in a distressed family (Goldenberg et al., 2017). The identified patient may even be aware at some level of the role they serve in "saving" the family. For example, adult children may sacrifice their autonomy by staying in the home to hold the parents together.

When a family comes for treatment, the presenting problem, which is usually related to one member of the family, must be addressed before the underlying systemic problem. The family member who is the identified patient may or may not be the one who initially seeks help from inpatient or outpatient services.

When working with families, it is important to consider not only the family as a system in a particular stage of life cycle development but also the individual developmental stage of each family member. For example, a family may present with parents in Erikson's stage of generativity versus stagnation, adolescent children dealing with identity versus role confusion issues, a school-aged child facing challenges of industry versus inferiority, and grandparents dealing with ego integrity versus despair. Thus there is more than one perspective to be considered when looking at the identified patient in terms of the family system. The focus is on the family system's anxiety.

Family Triangles

Bowen's (1985) focus was on patterns that develop in families in order to defuse anxiety. A key generator of anxiety in families is the perception of either too much closeness or too great a distance in a relationship. The degree of anxiety in any one family will be determined by the current levels of external stress and the sensitivities to particular themes that have been transmitted down the generations. If family members do not have the capacity to think through their responses to relationship dilemmas but rather react anxiously to perceived emotional demands, a state of chronic anxiety or reactivity may be set in place. Bowen described an important and common relationship process in families; it can be seen as a system of interlocking triangles. When tension in a family is low, the dyad or two-person system may interact comfortably, although some tension lies in the struggle between closeness and independence. When the tension in a close twosome builds, a third person (child, friend, or parent) may be brought in to help lower the tension. The *family triangle* (Figure 34.1) then becomes the basic building block of interpersonal relationships. All triangles contain a close side, a distant side, and a side in which conflict or tension exists between two people (Lassiter, 2019).

The intensity of the triangulation process varies among families and within the same family over time because triangles create emotional instability. The lower the level of differentiation in a family, the higher the tension is and the more important the role of triangulation is to lower tension and preserve emotional stability. As the family becomes stressed, the anxiety in the system is triggered, and the triangles become more active.

A common problem that occurs in families is the setting up of a triangle among two parents and a child; one parent is overinvolved with the child, and the other plays a more peripheral role. In this situation the child eventually becomes the means by which the parents communicate with each other about issues they cannot deal with directly. In other words, spousal conflicts may be brought into the parental arena, where they do not belong.

> **BOX 34.3 Central Concepts of Family Systems Theory**
>
> **Triangulation:** The tendency, when two-person relationships are stressful and unstable, to draw in a third person to stabilize the system through the formation of a coalition in which the two join the third. Triangles often occur with low differentiation and high anxiety and tend to draw in the third person but freeze the conflict as irresolvable.
>
> **Scapegoating:** A form of displacement in which a family member (usually the least powerful) is blamed for another family member's distress. The purpose is to keep the focus off the painful issues and problems of the blamers. In a family the blamers are often the parents, and the scapegoat is a child.
>
> **Double-bind:** A situation in which a positive command (often verbal) is followed by a negative command (often non-verbal), which leaves the recipient confused, trapped, and immobilized because there is no appropriate way to act. A double-bind is a "no win" situation in which you are "*darned if you do, darned if you don't.*"
>
> **Hierarchy:** The function of power and its structures in families, differentiating parental and sibling roles and generational boundaries.
>
> **Family life cycle:** The family's developmental process over time; refers to the family's past course, its present tasks, and its future course.
>
> **Differentiation:** The ability to develop a strong identity and sense of self while at the same time maintaining an emotional connectedness with one's family of origin.
>
> **Sociocultural context:** The broader social and ecological framework for viewing the family in terms of the influence of gender, race, ethnicity, religion, economic class, and sexual orientation.
>
> **Mino-Pimatisiwin** (an Indigenous approach to helping): In North America, Indigenous peoples belonging to the Algonquian language family use the term *mino-pimatisiwin*, which could be loosely translated as "living the good life," to describe a state of harmony, well-being, and comprehensive health based on relationships, cultural identity, and connection to the land (Landry et al., 2019).
>
> **Intergenerational issues:** The continuation and persistence from generation to generation of certain emotional interactive family patterns. Various patterns of behaviour (e.g., involving geographical distance between members, suicide, divorce, addiction, affairs, grief, triangles, historical colonization, loss) that continue to affect successive generations.

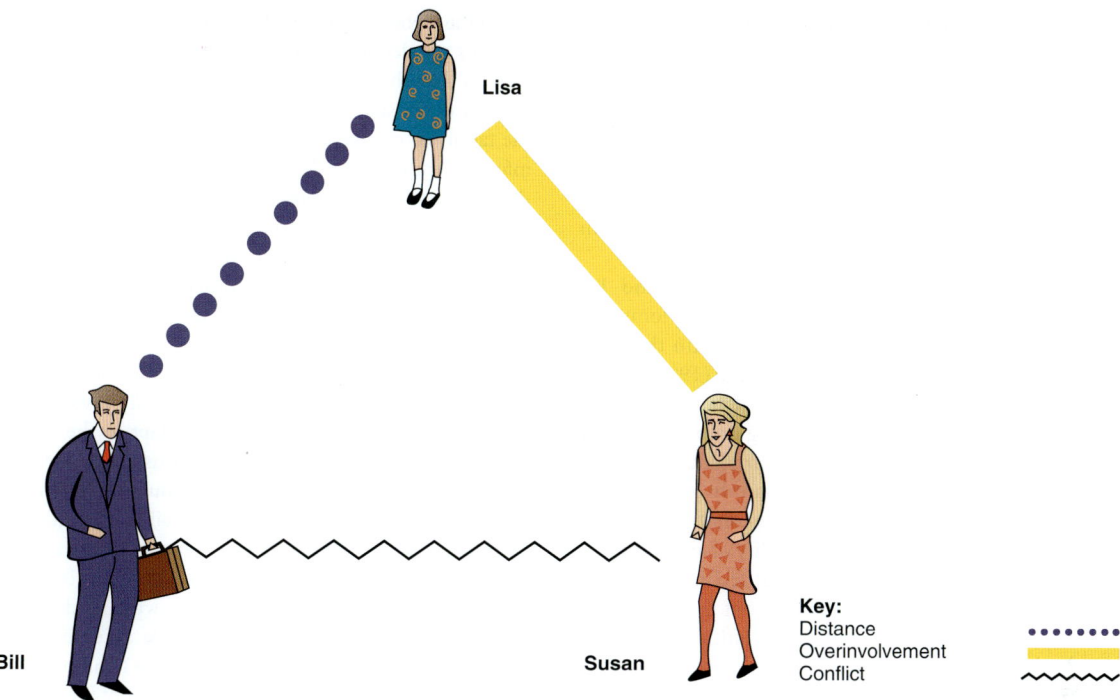

Fig. 34.1 Example of a family triangle.

VIGNETTE

Six-year-old Kami is having trouble making friends. Her mother, Makayla, has been feeling anxious and helpless as she tries to find ways to engage Kami with other youngsters. Makayla develops an overprotectiveness that further inhibits Kami from making friends. Makayla feels that her husband, Leon, is uncaring and disinterested because he thinks that she should be more relaxed about Kami's social life and let things develop naturally. Leon's job requires that he travel most of the week, so he is not involved with Makayla's daily experiences and struggles with Kami.

Makayla and Leon have been avoiding intimacy for almost a year. Makayla is angry with Leon for spending so much time with his parents, which further casts him in a peripheral role in their nuclear family, and Leon is angry with Makayla, sensing her rejection of him. Both are feeling isolated and alienated and are consequently angry with each other. Neither Leon nor Makayla addresses this issue directly. Instead, they play out their anger in the parental arena as they battle over how to handle Kami's social isolation.

The nurse's response to triangulation. The main goal of Bowenian therapy is to reduce chronic anxiety by first facilitating awareness of how the emotional system functions and then increasing levels of differentiation, where the focus is on making changes for the self rather than on trying to change others. Although entry to practice nurses do not provide family therapy, they do interact with patients and families and can assist families in awareness and insight around their patterns in relationship to one another. Nurses should also be aware of their own differentiation process and family-of-origin issues, which may affect their responses. When personal reactions interfere, the nurse may become "triangulated" into the family's system. The nurse's continued self-assessment is necessary to maintain emotional stability in the face of a chaotic family situation, in which the nurse's own issues may arise.

For advanced-practice nurses who engage in family therapy, holding family members accountable for themselves, making clear that the responsibility for change is theirs and not the nurse's, is a way of remaining clear of triangles. For example, the nurse therapist could become triangulated into a family system in any number of ways: perhaps the nurse recently experienced the loss of a family member; the nurse may belong to an enmeshed family system, in which the children are regularly drawn into spousal arguments; or perhaps stubbornness is an unresolved issue for the nurse. Any of these possibilities could allow the nurse to become triangulated into a family system, making therapeutic intervention difficult. Engaging in personal family-of-origin therapy and regular supervision is recommended when nurse therapists work with individuals, couples, or families. Supervision can be conducted with peer professionals, in groups, or privately with a more experienced clinician. One indication that a nurse is being triangulated is that their level of anxiety is greater than the situation warrants.

The Nuclear Family Emotional System

The term **nuclear family** refers to parents and the children under the parents' care. Bowen (1985) developed the concept of a *nuclear family emotional system*, defined as the flow of emotional processes within the nuclear family. This concept views symptoms as belonging to the nuclear family emotional system rather than to an individual. Bowen made a distinction between conventional medical (psychiatric) diagnosis and family diagnosis: rather than viewing a symptom as reflecting a disease that is confined to a patient, Bowen identified an emotional process that transcends the boundaries of a patient and encompasses the family relationship system. The example in the vignette of 8-year-old Luca, whom family members and others believed had attention-deficit/hyperactivity disorder (ADHD), illustrates how Luca's symptoms could be viewed as reflecting the family's conflicts and changes.

Refer to Box 34.3 for a summary of concepts central to family life.

FAMILY THERAPY THEORY

Family therapy emerged from the early child guidance clinics and marriage counselling efforts in the early twentieth century, stemming from social work movements in the United Kingdom and the United States.

Psychotherapists began to consider the effects of the social milieu on their patients and included the family in clinical observations and practice. The formal development of family therapy occurred in the 1940s and 1950s and was propelled by a focus on communication, which shifted the previous focus on individual pathology to a more systemic perspective (Becvar & Becvar, 2013). An *interactive* (interpersonal) rather than *in-dwelling* (intrapsychic Freudian) model of mental illness was becoming more widely accepted. These influences paved the way for an interest in the family system as it related to psychiatric disorders.

Leading theorists such as Virginia Satir (1972, 1983) and Jay Haley (1980, 1996) shifted the focus from the patient's symptoms *(indwelling)* to the patient's position and relationships within the family *(interactive)*. Further work by Salvador Minuchin (1996, 2012), a structural therapist, established the legitimacy of family therapy within psychiatry. Bowen (1975, 1985) was a leading proponent of the **family systems theory**, a theory that downplays problem resolution, focusing instead on the long-term awareness of family patterns and differentiation of individual family members. *Differentiation* is a term introduced by Bowen (1975) that describes the ability of an individual to make autonomous choices while separating out feelings and cognitions. Decisions are not driven by emotionality, but the individual remains emotionally connected to a significant relationship system (e.g., the family).

The aims of the family systems theory are to decrease emotional reactivity and encourage differentiation among individual family members. Parents or adults in the system are encouraged to recognize emotional patterns from their family of origin and to use resources from members of the extended family to re-engage in more mature interaction patterns. Children who are identified as the "problem" receive counselling and behavioural therapy but are not the focus of the therapy. Instead, parents are encouraged to consider system factors contributing to the child's emotional or behavioural problems.

The terms *strategic* and *structural* are used to identify the frameworks adopted by specific therapists. A *strategic model of family therapy* assumes that change in any single element in the family system will bring about change in the entire system. The aim of strategic therapy is to change the patterns, rules, and meaning of family interactions.

In the vignette about the De Santis family the family's communication patterns and decision making, partly for cultural reasons, exclude any discussion with the children. Children in such families often feel powerless and act out. Using the strategic model, the family therapist works with the family to change rigid communication patterns so that children are informed earlier in the decision-making process and so as to ease the emotional turmoil of the parents. This change provides children with an opportunity to comment or offer suggestions about how issues could be resolved. Being given a sense of control over some aspects of one's life can alleviate anxiety and reduce behavioural problems. This intervention would result in a systemic change in the way the family communicates.

The *structural model of family therapy* explains family problems from the perspective of dysfunctional boundary and role structure. These problems become evident when the family is exposed to a stressor or a transition point and is unable to adapt to the changing conditions (Goldenberg et al., 2017). A therapist using the structural model with the De Santis family in the vignette would highlight the importance of boundaries between the parental and sibling (child) subsystems rather than focus on changing a specific pattern. At the same time, the therapist would emphasize the importance of **flexibility**, which would allow for the changes inherent in normal growth and development.

In family therapy there is no single accepted model for treating families. Not all techniques are applicable to all problems, so the experienced clinician must be discerning. Most of the theoretical schools of marital and family therapy fall into two broad classifications: **insight-oriented family therapy** (a combination of behavioural therapy and education of families so that they better understand their power struggles, defense mechanisms, and other negative behaviours) and **behavioural family therapy** (a collection of psychological techniques for modifying maladaptive behaviours). Table 34.1 summarizes some of the types of therapy in each classification, describes their basic concepts and approaches, and lists the major theorists.

The Family as a System

Every family can be viewed as a unique system with its own structure, rules, and history of handling life problems and crises. Focusing on family patterns and interactions is fundamental to marital family therapy. The focus is *not* on an individual, as it is in traditional therapy, but rather on the interpersonal process of the family group (Nichols & Davis, 2022).

APPLICATION OF THE NURSING PROCESS

Assessment

Intervention is designed based on the initial assessment of family issues and adjusted with ongoing assessment throughout the nursing process. The CFAM has multiple focuses, including but not limited to (Nichols & Davis, 2022):

- Family system
- Family subsystems
- Individual members of the family
- Sociocultural context of family
- Past medical and mental health illness
- Family interactions and communication styles
- Stressors within the family system

Varcoe et al. (2022) identified a number of issues that should be assessed in family therapy, nursing practice, and counselling environments:

- Phases of the family life cycle
- Sociocultural context, beliefs
- Multi-generational concerns, intergenerational trauma, inclusive of historical oppression
- Relational practice

VIGNETTE

Eight-year-old Luca De Santis, who is hyperactive and disruptive at school and at home, is brought to the community mental health clinic to be evaluated for attention-deficit/hyperactivity disorder (ADHD). The nurse clinician performs an assessment and finds that a great deal of turmoil exists within the De Santis family. The family is composed of Luca's married parents, their other two children, and a grandmother. Luca's father has just lost his job, and his grandmother was recently diagnosed with bladder cancer. Luca's mother is considering filing for separation because of constant, unresolved arguments with her husband. She was raised a strict Roman Catholic and is unsure of this plan. Because of the family's communication patterns and cultural background, none of these issues have been discussed with Luca. Viewing this family from a strategic model, the nurse clinician sees Luca's symptoms as a function of many difficult losses and transitions that are stressing the entire family's coping mechanisms.

The nurse considers the multiple family stressors and their potential influence on Luca's symptoms of acting out and hyperactivity. Once the family issues are addressed, perhaps Luca's symptoms will subside. She refers the couple to a family therapist and, in the meantime, encourages them to focus more on their own issues and less on Luca's behaviour. An appointment is made to return to the clinic in 1 month, at which time Luca will be re-evaluated.

TABLE 34.1 Insight-Oriented and Behavioural Family Therapies

Type of Therapy	Concepts	Major Theorists
Insight-Oriented Family Therapy		
Psychodynamic therapy	Problems arise from: • Developmental arrest • Current interactions • Projections • Current stresses Improvement through insight into problematic relationships originating in the past	Nathan Ackerman James Framo Ivan Boszormenyi-Nagy
Family-of-origin therapy	Family viewed as an emotional relationship system: • Goal of fostering differentiation and decreasing emotional reactivity • Concept of triangulation • Emphasis on the family of origin	Murray Bowen
Experimental–existential therapy	Goal of therapy is to encourage the growth of family: • Symptoms express family pain • Family is responsible for its own solutions • Therapist uses nurturing and identifies dysfunctional communication patterns	Carl Whitaker Virginia Satir Leslie Greenberg Susan Johnson
Behavioural Family Therapy		
Structural therapy	Focus is on organizational patterns, boundaries, systems and subsystems, and use of scapegoating: • Restructures dysfunctional triangles • Clarifies boundaries • Looks at enmeshment and disengagement (excessive distance) issues	Salvador Minuchin
Strategic therapy	Goal is to change repetitive and maladaptive interaction patterns: • Identifies inequality of power, life cycle perspectives, and use of double-bind messages • Uses paradox • Prescribes rituals	Jay Haley Chloe Madanes Milan group (Mara Palazzoli, Gianfranco Cecchin, Giuliana Prata)
Cognitive behavioural therapy	Based on learning theory; focuses on changing cognition and behaviour: • Problem solving and solutions focused on present situations • Skills training emphasized	Gerald Patterson Richard Stuart Robert Liberman

Sociocultural Context

Rather than being viewed as an isolated unit, the family is viewed in a **sociocultural context**, wherein issues of gender, race, ethnicity, class, sexual orientation, and religion are considered equally. Each of these contextual issues affects the family's values, norms, traditions, roles, and rules. For example, the way the family relates to a terminally ill family member may be decidedly different in a first-generation Filipino Canadian Catholic family than in a long-time urban-dwelling Sikh Canadian family, a close-knit Jamaican-Canadian family, or a traditional Indigenous family. The nurse assesses how the family's cultural and religious beliefs affect acceptable care options The nurse also explicitly asks about experiences of racism and how the nurse can support anti-racism in the family's nursing care.

Gender may also be related to status and diverse cultural perspectives. In addition, beliefs about mental illness and their etiology and treatment have culturally diverse family interpretations. Cultural sensitivity prepares the nurse to provide culturally competent family intervention in all nursing practice settings (refer to Chapter 8 for further information on culture and mental health). A holistic assessment will include pertinent information on gender diversity, religious and spiritual beliefs, and trauma histories so as to provide an understanding of influencing factors on the current situation.

Intergenerational Issues

The influence of family is not restricted to the immediate family. Family is composed of the entire emotional system of at least three and sometimes four generations, meaning that the family is affected by **intergenerational issues**. Various patterns of behaviour (e.g., involving geographical distance between members, suicide, divorce, addiction, affairs, grief, triangles, historical colonization, loss) may affect successive generations. The legacy of the multi-generational family may relate to the patient's presenting problem. For example, in working with the family of an Indigenous teenager who has engaged in non-suicidal self-injurious behaviours, nurses will consider the historical and current context of the family life. A history of residential school attendance may contribute to the family's current parenting problems due to the lack of culturally appropriate role models, loss of identity, and loss of traditional way of life (Wilk et al., 2017). An astute nurse therapist will also be aware of the potential for mistrust of health care providers and authority figures related to historical oppression and incorporate this knowledge into the management of the current situation. This family may deal with grief by using silence and little outward expression of painful feelings. The nurse therapist would respect the family's way of expressing feelings. Indigenous families often bring extended family to the hospital to support the ill family member. Accommodation for this cultural expression of support is helpful for the family to resolve hospitalization issues. A trauma-informed therapy approach is a universal approach to draw on in all family therapy practice (see Chapters 8 and 21 for more on trauma-informed and anti-racist practices).

Constructing a genogram. The **genogram** is a tool for efficiently providing a clinical summary of information and relationships across generations of a family. Genograms are widely used in family therapy as a way of visually mapping out systems and recurring family patterns. Creative genograms enable families to self-define recurring personal themes and issues, thus combining both historical and experiential data on the same page (Huss & Kapulnik, 2021).

Information for the genogram should be gathered in an empathic and caring manner. Bowen (1985) provided the conceptual framework for the analysis of genogram patterns that have been further developed by McGoldrick (2016). Bowen proposed that the family is organized according to generation, age, sex, roles, functions, and interests and suggested that where each individual fits into the family structure influences the family functioning, relational patterns, and type of family formed in the next generation.

By using a genogram, nurses may map family structure and record family information inclusive of location, occupation, and educational level; functional information regarding medical, emotional, and behavioural status; and critical events such as moves, job changes, separations, abortions, imprisonment, illnesses, and deaths. Some health centres have standardized genogram forms, but genograms can also be sketched onto other forms, such as admission forms and patient care records. The genogram can be a useful tool to initiate assessment and for the family members to gain shared understanding and insight about patterns within the family.

The abilities required to do the genogram include a strong understanding of therapeutic relationships, communication, and interviewing skills. In particular, the following are needed: listening with respect, a non-judgemental attitude, empathy, capacity to reformulate and reframe responses, respect for hesitance and resistance, and ability to ask open-ended questions. Time and place are crucial considerations in the interview, and to complete this assessment and discovery intervention, a private and quiet location, ideally one with a writing surface, is selected. Since the scope of constructing a family genogram is large, it is necessary to ensure that there is sufficient time. It is acceptable, and may be practical, to complete the genogram in stages, over more than one session.

The interview may include the discussion or disclosure of difficult events, such as the death by suicide of a family member, or the experience of isolation or rejection, or specific life habits of certain family members that they would prefer not to have revealed, such as alcoholism, incest, or imprisonment. In this way it is recommended that the questions start with the more ordinary and lead later to the more delicate so that the individual or family gets used to the exploration process and gains comfort with the nurse therapist or interviewer. To put the person at ease, a simple conversational style of interview gives the best results (McGoldrick, 2016).

Practically, it is best to construct the skeleton of the genogram first, that is, to draw up the graphic representation of the various family members using the symbols of the genogram. Start systematically at first, by couples for each of the maternal and paternal ancestors, then for the descendants on both sides in chronological order by birth, for three generations, if possible. Gather the demographic information: dates of birth, death, and if helpful the place of residence, urban or rural; occupation; level of education; religion; cultural or ethnic groups; and so on.

Functional information is then explored to give information about the physical and mental health of the members of the family. Then, finally, information concerning critical events in chronological order is obtained, for example, important changes such as relationship status (separations, divorce), adoption, emigration, moves or changes in work, and finally health crises or other significant events (McGoldrick, 2016).

The specific questions required to create the genogram must be adapted to the context and the age of the person and will vary if the person is single, married, has children, and so on. The following are just some of the numerous examples of questions:

- Can you tell me about your present family situation?
- What is the occupation of each member, their dates of birth, their religious affiliation(s), and their cultures?
- How many children do you have? What are their ages? Their order of birth?
- Has your family experienced the loss of a child? How long ago?
- Has your family experienced any stillborn children, abortions, or miscarriages? Adoptions?
- Are there any development or learning concerns?
- Which family members live in the home?
- Where do the other members of the family live?
- Have any significant stressors occurred in your family recently? Can you share those with me? How have various members of the family related to the stressors?
- Has any trauma occurred in the family? Would you feel comfortable disclosing this to me?
- Have there been any changes in relationships between family members?
- What other types of changes occurred: moves, work changes?
- Are your children in relationships, partnerships, or married? Could you tell me about their partners? What are their religions, their cultures, the dates of their marriage? How many children do they have? What are their ages and order of birth? Have there been any deaths among them? When? Stillborn infants, abortions, or miscarriages? Adoptions? A child with a particular difficulty?
- Have there been any separations or divorces?
- In your extended family has there been a break in the relationship with your brothers and sisters? Parents? What might have been a part of that?

When in process or once completed, the genogram becomes part of the documentation about individual patients and family members. Figure 34.2 provides an example of a genogram derived from data about the family in the vignette.

> **VIGNETTE**
>
> Hank (of Polish Jewish descent) and Catherine Schneider (of Irish Catholic descent) are both university-educated, and each suffers from intermittent depression. Hank is an only child whose father died of a heart attack at age 55, Hank's present age. Hank's mother died by suicide at age 35. Her death is a toxic subject in Hank's family of origin. In Catherine's family of origin she is the eldest, born after three miscarriages. Much pressure and many expectations were placed on her. Catherine's brother, Mike, was born 4 years after Catherine, and their mother died during Mike's birth. Mike never finished high school. He is now 50 years old, has a serious substance use disorder, and has had three marriages that ended in divorce. One can speculate about the level of guilt Mike may feel regarding the loss of his mother.
>
> Hank and Catherine have two children, Keith and Jennifer. Keith, the identified patient, is 35 years old, has a university degree, but has not been able to hold down a job. He has problems with alcohol misuse. In 2009 Keith made a suicide attempt. In November 2010 Keith experienced an episode of psychosis for which he was hospitalized, and he was diagnosed as having schizophrenia. His younger sister, Jennifer, 31, has a university degree and is a practising pediatric nurse. She married William, a stockbroker, in 2009, the year Keith attempted suicide. Jennifer and William have two young children, Ethan and Jackson, ages 4 and 2, respectively.

Self-Awareness

Nurses frequently interact with families in hospital and community-based settings. Nurses who are aware of their personal family-of-origin issues and who practice ongoing self-awareness are most effective. Common defence mechanisms of nurses may contribute to issues in

CHAPTER 34 Family Interventions   639

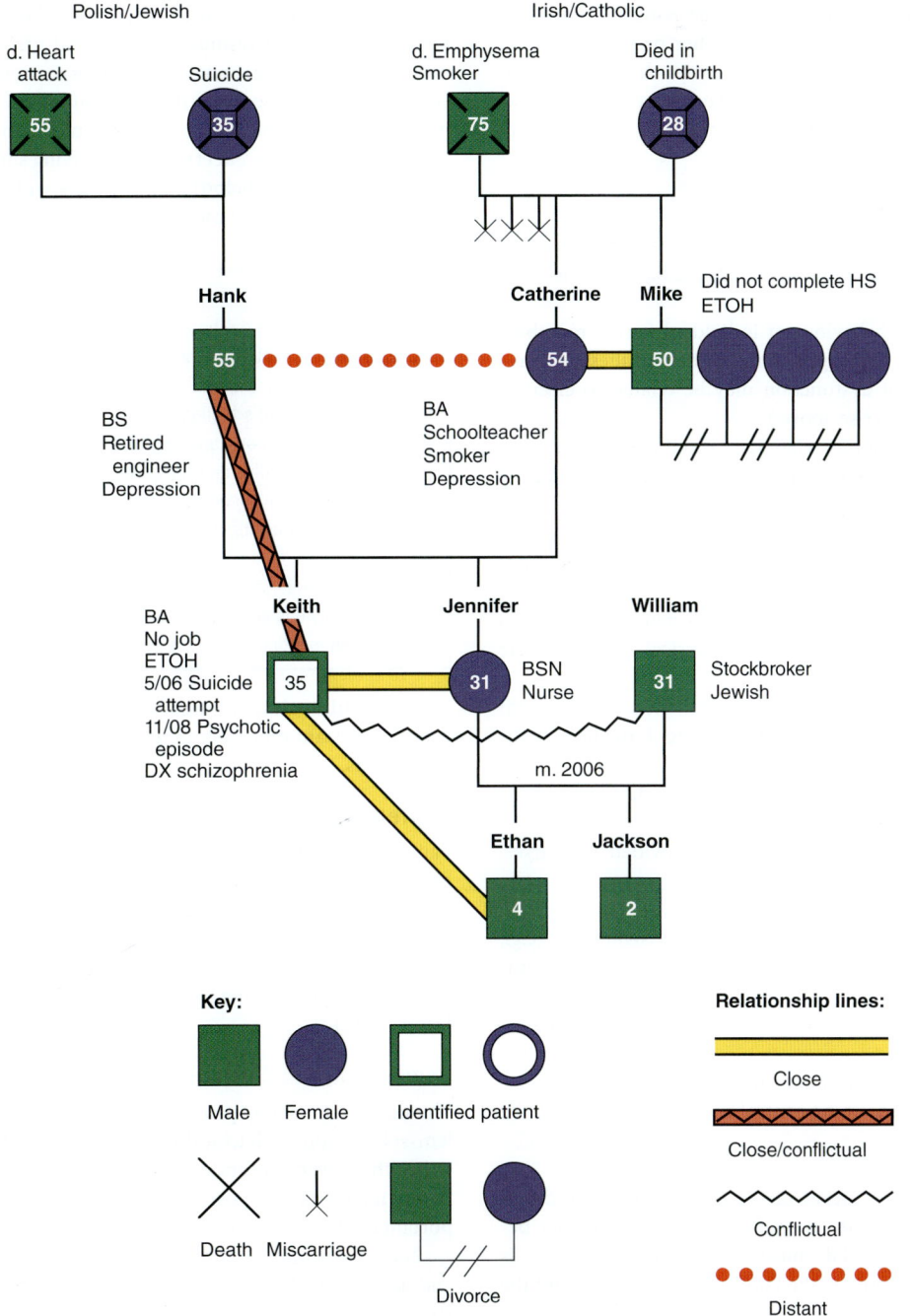

Fig. 34.2 Genogram of the Schneider family. *BA,* Bachelor of Arts; *BS,* Bachelor of Science; *BSN,* Bachelor of Science in Nursing; *d.,* deceased; *DX,* diagnosis; *ETOH,* alcohol; *HS,* high school; *m.,* married.

nurse–family relationships: the formation of triangles to reduce anxiety, defensive reactions when personal family-of-origin issues arise, and role blurring when sensitive personal issues and conflicts are triggered. Inexperienced nurses without supervision are particularly at risk for boundary violations.

An advanced-practice nurse educated at the master's level, with special training in family work, is best qualified to conduct family therapy. Nurses may experience intense reactions to alcohol or drug use, family abuse, codependency, rescue fantasies, and lifestyles choices. Clinical supervision is necessary to ensure that the nurse remains neutral and is not drawn into the patient–family dynamics.

Diagnosis

Families have unique needs at different times in their developmental stages. Family life involves new members, deaths, mental and physical illnesses, economic challenges, developmental crises, and unanticipated blows of life. Severe dysfunctional patterns (e.g., marked relational conflict, sexual misconduct, abuse, violence, suicide) exist within many families and cause significant physical or mental anguish to family members. Upon entering into a therapeutic relationship with a family to promote health and wellness, nurses need to consider the economic, social, historical, and geographical context of the family. As well, nurses must understand how their own views were formed, consider their position in society and the privilege associated with that position, and then begin to understand how other people may be in different positions (Varcoe et al., 2022). In line with the above, words such as the *dysfunctional* need to be carefully considered prior to use. Nursing diagnoses useful in working with families are identified in Box 34.4.

Outcomes Identification

Different therapists adhere to various theories and use a wide variety of methods; however, the goals of family therapy are basically the same (Nichols & Davis, 2022):

- To reduce *dysfunctional* behaviour of individual family members (Recognize the power of language and recall that families also have strengths. Root causes of dysfunction may be related to circumstances that are difficult to rise above.)
- To resolve or reduce intrafamily relationship conflicts
- To mobilize family resources and encourage adaptive family problem-solving behaviours
- To improve family communication skills
- To heighten awareness of other family members' emotional needs and help family members to meet those needs
- To strengthen the family's ability to cope with major life stressors and traumatic events, including chronic physical or psychiatric illness
- To improve integration of the family system into the societal system (i.e., especially the extended family but also school, medical facilities, workplace, and so on)
- To promote appropriate individual psychosocial development of each member of the family

Family psychoeducational teaching is often provided by nurses. Goals for the family include:

- Learning to accept a family member's illness
- Learning to deal effectively with an ill member's symptoms (e.g., hallucinations, delusions, poor hygiene, physical limitations, paranoia, aggression)
- Understanding the role of medications and when to seek medical advice
- Learning about community resources and how to access them
- Feeling less anxiety and regaining control and balance in family life

Planning

The immediate and long-term needs of the family should be determined. For example, is the family in crisis (related to a member being severely ill, homicidal, suicidal, abusive, or a victim of abuse)? Is hospitalization necessary to protect the family member? What are the family's coping mechanisms? What new skills can be used to help the family facilitate the resolution of normal life cycle crises? Is there a need for psychoeducational family interventions? Nurses are adept at educating family about the illness of one of the members (e.g., severe mental illness, dementia), providing information about medications and potential adverse effects, and identifying support groups and community resources to help the family cope with the crisis and improve quality of life for family members.

> **VIGNETTE**
>
> Doris, the head nurse on the adolescent psychiatric unit, is concerned about the negative comments staff members are making regarding the fact that none of Aaron's family has visited him for 10 days. Doris is concerned that Aaron is picking up the staff's feelings as well. After many attempts, Doris reaches Aaron's mother by phone and begins to assess the situation. She discovers that Aaron's mom is divorced and is working double shifts to meet the family's expenses. There is a 2-year-old at home and a set of twins in grade 4.
>
> Aaron's mother had been planning to visit on the weekend, but her babysitter cancelled.
>
> Once Doris understood the situation from another perspective and learned that this family has young children and is struggling to make ends meet, she called a staff meeting to address the situation.

A careful analysis of assessment data helps the nurse and other health care team members to identify the most appropriate family interventions.

Implementation

Family therapy has been applied to virtually every type of clinical disorder among children, adolescents, and adults and has demonstrated efficacy for each population studied (Nichols & Davis, 2022). Family therapy appears to be effective in the treatment of substance use disorders, child behavioural problems, marital relationship distress, and as an element of the treatment plan for schizophrenia (Nichols & Davis, 2022).

Counselling and Communication Techniques

The novice nurse may provide counselling through the use of a problem-solving approach to address an immediate-family difficulty related to health. Developing and practising strong listening skills and viewing family members in a positive, non-judgemental way are critically important qualities for nurses.

Nurses respond to family members' cues that indicate the degree and amount of stress the family system is experiencing. Indicators of stress in a family system include:

- Inability of the family or a family member to understand and act on certain recommended treatment directives
- Various somatic (physical) complaints among family members
- High degree of anxiety
- Depression
- Problems/difficulties in school
- Substance use

Promoting and monitoring a family's mental health can occur in any setting and often requires maximizing an opportune moment rather than holding a formal meeting. Sometimes an informal conversation *(therapeutic encounter)* can have a significant effect on the family.

Nurses can convey a non-judgemental approach through the way information is presented, their tone of voice, and how they ask questions. For example, the question *"Don't you think you should at least try to adhere to your medical regimen?"* would probably cause the patient

---

BOX 34.4 Possible Nursing Diagnoses for Family Interventions

- (Risk for) Caregiver role strain
- Sexual dysfunction
- Interrupted family processes
- Altered family processes
- Spiritual distress
- Risk for compromised resilience
- Ineffective denial
- Deficient knowledge
- Impaired verbal communication
- Defensive coping
- Relocation stress syndrome
- (Risk for) Impaired parenting

to become defensive, whereas the invitation statement "*Can you tell me what your medical regimen is like*" invites collaborative problem solving.

This non-judgemental approach promotes open communication among professionals and family members and respects everyone's viewpoint. Information imparted in a clear, understandable manner to all family members assists discussion and decision making regarding the patient's care. Family decision making empowers families by indicating that they are accountable and responsible for how they choose to use the information. Families also possess strengths that may be manifested in forms of resilience. Families use their skills to prevent the deterioration of their family units, oppose threats to the family, and keep their families intact (Becvar, 2013; Walsh, 2016). Refugee and immigrant families often provide examples of extraordinary efforts to keep their families together. In working with family strengths in this way to expand resilience the perspective of each family member must be elicited and heard. Often family members hear another member's view for the first time and may be surprised (e.g., "*I didn't know you felt that way*"). This approach defines the family as the central psychosocial unit of care. The vignette about Doris provides an example of maintaining neutrality, building strengths and not assigning blame, and hearing from all members.

Further possible interventions for the situation in the vignette would be to problem-solve with Aaron and his mother what is realistic for each of them regarding visiting and to organize regular telephone contact. Perhaps an extended family member or a friend can visit when the mother cannot. Long-range discharge planning for Aaron will include the identification of family supports.

Unfortunately, negative comments about family members by staff occur all too often. As a family ally and supporter, negative or discriminatory practice must be called out, and nurses should exemplify tolerance, respect, and empathy in daily practice (Willey et al., 2022). Hearing negative or discriminatory comments can present a difficult situation for the nursing student, who is entering the unit as an outsider and who realizes the negative effect this behaviour has on family members. The student should seek supervision from the instructor so that the most effective approach can be planned. One useful technique is for the student to ask questions of the head nurse and staff in such a manner that alternative ways of viewing the family are embedded in the questions. An example of this is "*Has anyone had a chance to contact Aaron's mother to see if there are any problems?*" or "*I wonder what it's like for Aaron's mother to have her son in a psychiatric unit.*"

Family Therapy

The advanced-practice nurse who has graduate or post-graduate training in family therapy may conduct private family therapy sessions. Family therapy is viewed by professionals as appropriate for most situations, although it may be contraindicated in the following circumstances (Nichols & Davis, 2022):

- The therapeutic environment is unsafe, and harm results from information, anxiety, or hostility.
- Family members demonstrate an unwillingness to be honest.
- Family members demonstrate an unwillingness to maintain confidentiality.
- A parental conflict involves issues of sexuality that are inappropriate for the children.

In most other situations traditional family therapy is useful, especially when combined with psychopharmacology in the treatment of bipolar disorder, depression, or schizophrenia. Other options that may be less costly and time consuming are psychoeducational family therapy and self-help groups.

Traditional family therapy. Family therapists use diverse theoretical philosophies and techniques to bring about change in dysfunctional behaviours and interactions. Some therapists focus on the here and now; others rely more heavily on a family's history and reports of happenings between sessions. Most family therapists use an eclectic approach, drawing on a variety of techniques to fit the particular personality and strengths of the family.

Multiple-family group therapy is used with families who have a family member in an inpatient setting. These groups can help family members gain insight into their problems, as they are reflected in the problems of other families. Several families meet in one group with one or more therapists, usually once a week until their ill family member is discharged; these groups often continue for a specific period of time after discharge.

Psychoeducational family therapy. Psychoeducational family therapy provides families with the information they need about mental illness and the coping skills that will help them best support their family member's psychiatric disorder. Psychoeducational family training has been applied successfully in the treatment of patients with schizophrenia. Family work supports families in coping with a family member with a severe mental illness.

The primary goal of psychoeducational family therapy is the sharing of mental health information. Family education groups help family members to understand their member's illness, prodromal symptoms (symptoms that may appear before a full relapse), medications, and ways to access community resources. Psychoeducational family meetings encourage the expression of feelings and identify strategies to manage problems. For example, parents may learn how to work with a child with a conduct disorder. Feelings of anger, loss, stigmatization, sadness, and helplessness can be shared and put in a perspective that the family and individual members can manage more satisfactorily.

Self-help groups. Self-help groups are led by laypeople who have the illness or a family member of someone who has the illness. They assist people with a personal problem or social deprivation and families with a member who has a specific diagnosis. Some groups focus on families with healthy members, whereas others offer assistance to families whose members are experiencing a health disorder or crisis. Nurses help patients and their families to find appropriate support groups. For many people, self-help groups provide healing and ongoing therapeutic support.

Case Management

Case managers coordinate services for patients and families and monitor the patient's condition. The patient's and family's culture, ethnicity, socioeconomic status, stage of the family life cycle, and beliefs about illness combine to affect an individual's response to case management. Case management entails teaching, giving appropriate referrals, and offering emotional support.

> **VIGNETTE**
>
> David Gilbert, aged 21 years, is leaving the hospital after experiencing his first episode of psychosis while taking his final examinations before graduation from university. David is being discharged back to his family, consisting of his mother and father; his maternal grandfather, who is bedridden; and a younger brother, Louis, who is 17 years of age. David's diagnosis is schizophrenia.
>
> While David is hospitalized and later, in post-discharge family therapy, the nurse meets with the family and takes a psychoeducational approach with them. Through reading materials and discussion, initial interventions convey information about David's mental illness and recovery. The nurse identifies psychosocial support groups and how to access them. The nurse performs ongoing assessment of the family's strengths and weaknesses, including community support. They identify areas that require discussion. Issues include:
> - Reorganizing family roles related to a newly diagnosed serious mental illness

- Managing a grandfather who is bedridden
- Attending to Louis's probable fears that he may develop this illness
- Working through potential parental guilt feelings
- Developing a care plan should David experience a relapse of psychosis
- Developing a plan for managing medication and adherence
- Reviewing any concerns about David's future, with David and family
- Formulating realistic expectations, and developing goals for the future
- Working with family to develop supports for the family, as well as how they can best support David

The nurse discusses these issues with the family and how they can best be addressed. For example, a visiting nurse will evaluate the grandfather's situation and need for home care, and a multiple-family psychoeducation group is contacted to increase the family's understanding of David's illness, help the family learn to cope with common problems, and provide a safe place for family members to share feelings of loss and grief.

Pharmacological Interventions

The nurse is often the first to explain to the family the purpose of a prescribed medication, the desired effects, and potential adverse reactions. Generally, the more information family members have, the less likely it is that anxiety will distort their observations and decision making after discharge. The nurse reviews David's medication with him and his family during his hospitalization and before discharge. The nurse monitors David to determine if adverse effects are interfering with his functioning. The nurse may consult with a physician to titrate medications based on the efficacy of the medications and David's toleration of any adverse effects.

Evaluation

Evaluation focuses on whether family members have improved functioning, reduced or resolved conflicts, improved communication skills, and strengthened coping and whether the family is more integrated into the societal system.

KEY POINTS TO REMEMBER

- Family therapy is based on a variety of theoretical concepts.
- Family therapy aims to decrease emotional reactivity and to encourage differentiation among family members.
- The primary characteristics of healthy family functioning are flexibility and clear boundaries.
- Family-oriented approaches that help family members gain insight and make behavioural changes are most successful.
- The genogram is an efficient clinical summary for providing information and defining relationships across at least three generations.
- The family's culture, ethnicity, socioeconomic status, and life cycle phase, as well as its unique beliefs about illness, affect the individual patient's progress and response to case management.
- Assessment of the family includes a focus on the family life cycle phase, multi-generational issues, the individual's developmental stage, and the family's sociocultural status.
- Nurses with basic education frequently conduct psychoeducation with families.
- Nurses with specialized education and certification provide family therapy using diverse theoretical approaches.

CRITICAL THINKING

1. Select a family with whom you've worked during your clinical experience. Evaluate this family's status in terms of functionality or dysfunctionality with reference to the family functions described in the text (i.e., provision of love and nurturance, socialization of children, social control of members, production and consumption of goods and services, addition of new family members through birth or adoption, and physical care and maintenance of family members).
2. Create your own personal genogram, including at least three generations.
   a. Be sure to include the following:
      - Location, occupation, and educational level

RESEARCH HIGHLIGHT

Problem
Often referred to as "family burden" or "carer burden," numerous problems are reported by people supporting a person with depression, including financial difficulties, feelings of isolation, reduction in social activities, relationship distress, feeling confused and overwhelmed by depressive symptoms, worry about stigma, worry about the future, and being able to access treatment. There is considerable evidence demonstrating that family interventions for mental disorders lead to improved outcomes for both patient and carer, though most of these studies have focused on caregivers of family members with schizophrenia.

Purpose of Study
The first aim of this systematic review was to evaluate the evidence for family psychoeducation (FPE) interventions for major depressive disorder (MDD). A second aim was to compare the efficacy of different modes of delivering face-to-face FPE interventions.

Methods
Ten studies (based on nine distinct samples) were identified comprising four single-family studies, four multi-family studies, one single versus multi-family comparative study, and one peer-led, mixed-diagnosis study. Seven studies measured patient functioning and six reported positive outcomes. Six studies measured carer's well-being and four reported positive outcomes. All studies examined face-to-face psychoeducation groups for people ages 14 to 85 that were specifically focused on psychoeducation for family members of people with the diagnosis of MDD.

Key Findings
Results provide preliminary evidence that FPE leads to improved outcomes for patient functioning and family-carer's well-being for persons with depression. In particular, the outcomes suggest that FPE needs to be specifically tailored to the needs of patients with MDD and their families and carers.

Findings also reveal a number of gaps in this field of study, as only 50% of trials identified (i.e., n = 5) were based on a randomized control design. Also, no studies reported level of session attendance by participants; hence it cannot be determined whether results were influenced by treatment dosage effect. Only two studies measured follow-up outcomes beyond 6 months to determine treatment retention effects. Finally, there was little consistency in the measures used across studies, limiting a more comprehensive analysis.

Implications for Nursing Practice
For those planning psychoeducation groups, the evidence shows that the more focused the topic of psychoeducational groups, the better. The value of psychoeducational groups appears promising, but longer-term follow-up studies are needed.

Source: Based on Brady, P., Kangas, M., & McGill, K. (2017). "Family matters": A systematic review of the evidence for family psychoeducation for major depressive disorder. *Journal of Marital and Family Therapy, 43*(2), 245–263. https://doi.org/10.1111/jmft.12204

- Critical events such as births, marriages, moves, job changes, separations, divorces, illnesses, and deaths
- Relationship patterns, if possible, such as emotional cutoffs, distancing, overinvolvement, and conflict

b. Analyze and reflect on patterns of behaviour that may have been transmitted through the generations within your family. These may be positive patterns or more painful patterns.

3. A family has just found out that their young son is going to die. The parents have been fighting and blaming each other for ignoring the child's ongoing symptom of leg pain, which was eventually diagnosed as advanced cancer. There are two other siblings in the family.
    a. How would you apply family concepts to help this family?
    b. What would be your outcome criterion?
4. A mother of a 6-year-old girl has recently been diagnosed with schizophrenia. How would you address her mother's diagnosis with the 6-year-old?

CHAPTER REVIEW

1. Jeff is a single, recently divorced, non-custodial parent. He will be hospitalized for several days following surgery. Which primary concern of Jeff's should the nurse anticipate during this time?
    a. Mourning the loss of his nuclear family
    b. Wondering how to deal with his spouse's extended family
    c. Attempting to restructure the relationship with his former spouse
    d. Finding ways to continue to effectively parent his child
2. While the nurse works with a family, the father, with a smirk on his face, states, *"I love my wife, and she's a good woman who would do anything for her family"* and rolls his eyes. Which behaviour should the nurse recognize?
    a. Triangulation
    b. Scapegoating
    c. Double-binding
    d. Differentiation
3. Which family member should the nurse refer to individual therapy rather than family therapy?
    a. The mother who has anxiety controlled by medication
    b. The father who is questioning his sexual orientation
    c. The brother who is verbally angry with his parents
    d. The sister who has consented to maintain confidentiality
4. The nurse is evaluating the family therapy experience. Which behaviour would indicate that further family therapy is indicated?
    a. The wife has set aside 15 minutes daily to connect with her husband.
    b. The son's grades have risen from a "D" average to a "C" average.
    c. The daughter's headaches have subsided.
    d. The mother has stopped using illicit substances, and the father's use has decreased.
5. The nurse is conducting family therapy. Which nursing intervention would be appropriate for an advanced-practice nurse?
    a. Mobilizing family resources and encouraging adaptive family problem-solving behaviours
    b. Improving family communication skills
    c. Explaining what medications can and cannot do
    d. Working with the underlying dynamics and structure of the family group

http://evolve.elsevier.com/Canada/Varcarolis/psychiatric/

REFERENCES

Arriagada, P. (2020). *The experiences and needs of older caregivers in Canada*. Retrieved from https://www12.statcan.gc.ca/census-recensement/2016/ref/guides/002/98-500-x2016002-eng.cfm

Becvar, D. S. (2013). *Handbook of family resilience*. New York: Springer.

Becvar, D. S., & Becvar, R. J. (2013). *Family therapy: A systematic integration* (8th ed.). New York: Pearson.

Boland, R., & Verduin, M. (2022). *Kaplan and Sadock's concise textbook of clinical psychiatry* (5th ed.). Philadelphia: Wolters Kluwer.

Bombay, A., Matheson, K., & Anisman, H. (2014). The intergenerational effects of Indian Residential Schools: Implications for the concept of historical trauma. *Transcultural Psychiatry, 51*(3), 320–338.

Bowen, M. (1975). Family therapy after 20 years. In S. Ariti, D. Freedman, & J. Dyrud (Eds.), *American handbook of psychiatry* (2nd ed., pp. 379–391). New York: Gardner Press.

Bowen, M. (1985). *Family therapy in clinical practice*. New York: Jason Aronson.

Eaton, K., Ohan, J. L., Stritzke, W. G. K., et al. (2016). Failing to meet the good parent ideal: Self-stigma in parents of children with mental health disorders. *Journal of Child and Family Studies, 25*(10), 3109. https://doi.org/10.1007/s10826-016-0459-9

Goldenberg, H., Stanton, M., & Goldenberg, I. (2017). *Family therapy: An overview* (9th ed.). Boston: Cengage Learning.

Gone, J. P., Hartmann, W. E., Pomerville, A., Wendt, D. C., Klem, S. H., & Burrage, R. L. (2019). The impact of historical trauma on health outcomes for Indigenous populations in the USA and Canada: A systematic review. *The American Psychologist, 74*(1), 20–35. https://doi.org/10.1037/amp0000338

Good2Talk. (2021). *Intergenerational trauma*. Retrieved from https://iknow-oce.esolutionsgroup.ca/api/ServiceItem/GetDocument?clientId=A1B5AA8F-88A1-4688-83F8-FF0A5B083EF3&documentId=0000005a-40c5-4924-b328-7e8ff3f0b0a3

Gottlieb, L. N. (2013). *Strengths-based nursing care: Health and healing for person and family*. New York: Springer.

Haley, J. (1980). *Leaving home*. New York: McGraw-Hill.

Haley, J. (1996). *Learning and teaching therapy*. New York: Guilford.

Hartrick Doane, G. H., & Varcoe, C. (2021). *How to nurse: Relational inquiry in action* (2nd ed.). Wolters Kluwer/Lippincott Williams & Wilkins.

Huss, E., & Kapulnik, E. (2021). Using creative genograms in family social work to integrate subjective and objective knowledge about the family: A participatory study. *Research on Social Work Practice, 31*(4), 390–399. https://doi.org/10.1177/1049731521992843

Landry, V., Asselin, H., & Levesque, C. (2019). Link to the land and mino-pimatisiwin (comprehensive health) of Indigenous people living in urban areas in Eastern Canada. *International Journal of Environmental Research and Public Health, 16*(23), 4782. https://doi.org/10.3390/ijerph16234782

Lassiter. L. (2019). Triangles in Bowen family therapy. In J. L. Lebow, A. L. Chambers & D. C. Breunlin (Eds.), Encyclopedia of couple and family therapy (pp. 3071–3073). Springer International Publishing. https://doi.org/10.1007/978-3-319-49425-8_363

Layne, C. M., Abramovitz, R., Stuber, M., et al. (2017). The core curriculum on childhood trauma: A tool for preparing a trauma-informed mental health workforce. *Traumatic StressPoints, 31*, 1–8. Retrieved from http://sherwood-istss.informz.net/informzdataservice/onlineversion/ind/bWFpbGluZ2luc3RhbmNlWQ9NjI1MTUwNCZzdWJzY3JpYmVyaWQ9MTA0NDYxODQ0MQ

Leijdesdorff, S., van Doesum, K., Popma, A., et al. (2017). Prevalence of psychopathology in children of parents with mental illness and/or addiction: An up to date narrative review. *Current Opinion in Psychiatry, 30*(4), 312–317.

McGoldrick, M. (2016). *The genogram casebook: A clinical companion to genograms: Assessment and intervention.* New York: W. W. Norton & Company.

McGoldrick, M., Garcia Preto, N. A., Carter, B., et al. (2016). *The expanded family life cycle: Individual, family, and social perspectives* (5th ed.). Boston: Allyn & Bacon.

Mental Health Commission of Canada. (2015). *Caregiver Mobilization Toolkit.* Retrieved from https://mentalhealthcommission.ca/resource/caregiver-mobilization-toolkit/

Minuchin, S. (1996). *Mastering family therapy.* New York: John Wiley & Sons, Inc.

Minuchin, S. (2012). *Families and family therapy.* Cambridge: New York: Routledge.

Murphy, G., Peters, K., Wilkes, L., et al. (2017). Adult children of parents with mental illness: Navigating stigma. *Child & Family Social Work, 22*(1), 330–338. https://doi.org/10.1111/cfs.12246

Nichols, M. P., & Davis, S. (2022). *Family therapy: Concepts and methods* (12th ed.). New York: Pearson.

Ontario Centre of Excellence for Child and Youth Mental Health. (2017). *Working with Indigenous families: An engagement bundle for child and youth mental health agencies.* Retrieved from http://www.excellenceforchildandyouth.ca/sites/default/files/docs/bundle_working_with_indigenous_families.pdf

Park, K., & Seo, M. (2016). Care burden of parents of adult children with mental illness: The role of associative stigma. *Comprehensive Psychiatry, 70*, 159–164. https://doi.org/10.1016/j.comppsych.2016.07.010

Raymond, K. Y., Willis, D. G., & Sullivan-Bolyai, S. (2017). Parents caring for adult children with serious mental illness. *Journal of the American Psychiatric Nurses Association, 23*(2), 119–132. https://doi.org/10.1177/1078390316685404

Registered Nurses' Association of Ontario. (2015). *Person and family centred care.* Retrieved from https://rnao.ca/bpg/guidelines/person-and-family-centred-care

Satir, V. (1972). *Peoplemaking.* Palo Alto: Science and Behaviour Books.

Satir, V. (1983). *Conjoint family therapy.* Palo Alto: Science and Behaviour Books.

Shajani, Z., & Snell, D. (2019). *Wright & Leahey's nurses and families: A guide to family assessment and intervention* (7th ed.). F. A. Davis.

Statistics Canada. (2017). *Families reference guide, census of population.* Retrieved from https://www12.statcan.gc.ca/census-recensement/2016/ref/guides/002/98-500-x2016002-eng.cfm

Stevenson, A. (2021). *Intimate integration : A history of the Sixties Scoop and the colonization of Indigenous kinship.* University of Toronto Press.

Tam, B. Y., Findlay, L. C., & Kohen, D. E. (2015). Conceptualization of family: Complexities of defining an Indigenous family. *Indigenous Policy Journal, 28*(2). Retrieved from http://www.indigenouspolicy.org/index.php/ipj/article/view/398

Tam, B. Y., Findlay, L. C., & Kohen, D. E. (2017). Indigenous families: Who do you call family? *Journal of Family Studies, 23*(3), 243–259.

Truth and Reconciliation Commission (TRC) of Canada. (2015). *Honouring the truth, reconciling for the future: Summary of the final report of the Truth and Reconciliation Commission of Canada.* Winnipeg: Author. Retrieved from https://www.trc.ca

United Nations. (2018). *United Nations declaration on the rights of Indigenous peoples.* Retrieved from https://www.un.org/development/desa/indigenouspeoples/wp-content/uploads/sites/19/2018/11/UNDRIP_E_web.pdf

Vanier Institute of the Family. (2020). *A snapshot of family caregiving and work in Canada.* Retrieved from https://vanierinstitute.ca/a-snapshot-of-family-caregiving-and-work-in-canada/

Vanier Institute of the Family. (2021). *Definition of family.* Retrieved from https://vanierinstitute.ca/definition-of-family/

Varcoe, C., Brown, H., & Cave, L. (2022). Relational nursing and family nursing in Canada. In M. Robinson, D. P. Coehlo, & P. S. Smith (Eds.), *Family health care nursing: Theory, practice, & research* (7th ed., pp. 397–416). Philadelphia: F. A. Davis.

Walsh, F. (2016). Family resilience: A developmental systems framework. *European Journal of Developmental Psychology, 13*(3), 313–324. https://doi.org/10.1080/17405629.2016.1154035

Wilk, P., Maltby, A., & Cooke, M. (2017). Residential schools and the effects on Indigenous health and well-being in Canada: A scoping review. *Public Health Reviews, 38*, 8. https://doi.org/10.1186/s40985-017-0055-6.

Willey, S., Desmyth, K., & Truong, M. (2022). Racism, healthcare access and health equity for people seeking asylum. *Nursing Inquiry, 29* (1), e12440 https://doi.org/10.1111/nin.12440

35

Integrative and Complementary Therapies

Cheryl L. Pollard
With Contributions From Karen Scott Barss

 https://evolve.elsevier.com/Canada/Varcarolis/psychiatric/.

OBJECTIVES

1. Define the terms *integrative, traditional, complementary,* and *alternative health care therapies.*
2. Identify trends in integrative health care.
3. Discuss how to help educate the public in the safe use of integrative modalities.
4. Explore information resources available through literature and online sources.
5. Explore five aspects of integrative care: whole medical systems, mind–body–spirit approaches, biologically based interventions, manipulative approaches, and energy therapies.
6. Discuss the techniques used in major traditional, complementary, and alternative modalities and potential applications to psychiatric mental health nursing practice.

KEY TERMS AND CONCEPTS

acupuncture
aromatherapy
chiropractic medicine
conventional health care
healing touch
holistic nurse
homeopathy
integrative health care
natural health products
naturopathy
reflexology
Reiki
therapeutic touch
traditional, complementary, and alternative medicine

This chapter considers *integrative care* as part of a holistic nursing philosophy. Holistic describes "whole-person care" often acknowledging body–mind–spirit. **Integrative health care** refers to practice that includes two or more disciplines or distinct approaches to care. Both terms, integrative and holistic, are associated with alternative or complementary modalities and share philosophical perspectives (Frisch & Rabinowitsch, 2019).

In Western countries **conventional health care** is also referred to as *biomedicine, allopathic medicine, Western medicine,* or *mainstream medicine* and is based largely on highly controlled systematic research that is interpreted through the lens of a Eurocentric worldview. Meanwhile, *traditional medicine* is defined by the World Health Organization (WHO, 2019) as the "sum total of the knowledge, skill and practices based on the theories, beliefs and experiences indigenous to different cultures, whether explicable or not, used in the maintenance of health as well as in the prevention, diagnosis, improvement or treatment of physical and mental illness" (p. 1). This type of therapy is of interest and used by many individuals outside of indigenous cultures. This chapter will use the WHO terminology of **traditional, complementary, and alternative medicine** (TCAM). The term *TCAM* recognizes that many of the philosophical underpinnings for the approaches presented are derived from both non-Western cultural traditions and studies in the nature of energy and reality, which have not historically been a part of conventional health care delivery. However, TCAM will be discussed in the broader context of integrative health care. With the increased use of integrative mental health therapies, it is essential that nurses have a knowledge base in this area in order to meet provincial or territorial regulatory entry-to-practice competencies (Canadian Association of Schools of Nursing & Canadian Federation of Mental Health Nurses, 2017). Refer to Table 35.1 for TCAM concurrently used as integrative therapies (not medication or supplements) for mental health.

INTEGRATIVE HEALTH CARE IN CANADA

Many Canadians seek assistance from both alternative and conventional providers and believe that using both conventional and alternative therapies is better than using either one alone. Garrett et al. (2021) report that 70% to 80% of the Canadian population use TCAM at least once, if not regularly. The rapid growth and commercialization of these products and services command the critical eye, careful assessment, and thorough communication by nurses. The four most commonly used modalities were massage, relaxation, chiropractic care, spiritual care, and yoga. Natural Health Products Regulations came into effect January 1, 2004. The term **natural health products** (NHPs) is used in Canada to refer to naturally occurring substances that are used to restore and maintain good health (Health Canada, 2016). These substances may be used in a variety of forms such as pills, tinctures, or salves. These products can be made with substances harvested from earth, air, or water. Esmail (2017) found that a majority of Canadians agreed that NHPs can be used to maintain or promote health (77%) or to treat illness (68%). Fewer (43%) agreed that NHPs were better than conventional medicine. At the same time, 81% of Canadians thought it was important to respect the role that NHPs play within cultural groups. They

TABLE 35.1 Integrative Approaches to Mental Health

Disorder	Examples of Traditional and Complementary Approaches (Not Medication/Supplements)
Anxiety	Exercise, yoga, mindfulness-based stress reduction, music, acupuncture, Reiki
Bipolar disorder	Exercise, mindfulness/meditation, yoga
Depression	Exercise, nutrition, chiropractic, bright-light therapy, music, Reiki, religious/spiritual, healing touch, qigong, massage
Post-traumatic stress disorder	Guided imagery, yoga, acupuncture
Schizophrenia/psychosis	Exercise, yoga, acupuncture
Substance use disorder	Exercise, mindfulness/meditation, yoga, qigong

Sources: Lake, J. (2015). *Integrative mental health care: A therapist's handbook.* New York: W. W. Norton; Wynn, G. H. (2015). Complementary and alternative medicine approaches in the treatment of PTSD. *Current Psychiatry Reports, 17*(8), 600. https://doi.org/10.1007/s11920-015-0600-2.

BOX 35.1 Integrative Health Care Resources

- Acupuncture Canada: https://www.acupuncturecanada.org/
- American Holistic Nurses Association: https://www.ahna.org/Home/Resources/Holistic-Mental-Health
- Canadian Association of Naturopathic Doctors: https://www.cand.ca/
- Canadian Chiropractic Association: https://www.cfacanada.com/
- Canadian Federation of Aromatherapists: https://cfacanada.com/
- Canadian Foundation for Trauma Research & Education: https://www.cftre.com/
- Canadian Holistic Nurses Association (CHNA): https://www.chna.ca/
- International Society for Complimentary Medicine Research (ISCMR): https://www.iscmr.org/
- Canadian Research Institute of Spirituality & Healing: http://www.crish.org/
- The Center for Contemplative Mind in Society: https://www.contemplativemind.org/
- Health Canada: Natural and Non-prescription Health Products: https://www.hc-sc.gc.ca/dhp-mps/prodnatur/index-eng.php
- International Network of Integrative Mental Health: https://www.inimh.org/
- Massage.ca: http://massage.ca/
- Thunderbird Partnership Foundation: https://thunderbirdpf.org/
- World Health Organization (WHO): https://www.who.int/en (Search "Traditional, Complementary, and Alternative Healing" for various guidelines and updates.)

also expressed the belief that Canadians have the right to use any NHP they choose. This attitude highlights the importance of nurses, critical awareness of the risks and benefits of these various therapies.

There is federal jurisdiction over the safety of drugs and other products used to enhance wellness or treat disease. In compliance with Canadian's Natural Health Product Regulations to address the growing trend of Canadians using NHPs, on January 4, 2004, Health Canada, recognizing its responsibility to assure all Canadians have access to a wide range of natural products that are safe, effective, and/or high quality, established the Natural Health Products Directorate. The legislation required licencing of natural products, including over-the-counter products (not needing a prescription).

However, jurisdiction over Canadian practitioners of TCAM is currently at the provincial and territorial level, resulting in a mosaic of relevant registrations, certifications, and licensures. For example, legislation requiring licensure for naturopathic doctors currently exists in British Columbia, Alberta, Saskatchewan, Manitoba, Ontario, and Nova Scotia. Many regulated health care practitioners, including those in mental health services, are integrating evidence-informed TCAM practices into their professional practice. This includes using acupuncture techniques to assist in stress reduction or pain control (Canadian Holistic Nurses Association, 2020). Further information about the current status of regulation across provinces and territories for various integrative modalities can be obtained by contacting applicable professional associations. (Box 35.1 highlights several national associations; numerous related provincial and territorial associations also exist.)

Research

There are volumes of research using conventional medicine approaches. However, research on the efficacy of TCAM is sparse by comparison. Reasons for this lack of research include (1) the relatively recent use of some of these therapies in Western countries, (2) the lack of financial incentive to support the research, and (3) the difficulties encountered when researching these modalities. These difficulties include world views, belief systems, spiritual practices, temperament of both the researcher and participants; difficulty trying to standardize modalities; and the influence of studying a phenomenon or person within a naturalistic setting.

PATIENTS AND INTEGRATIVE CARE

Patients are attracted to integrative care for a variety of reasons:
- A desire to be an active participant in their health care and to engage in holistic practices that can promote health and healing
- A desire to find therapeutic approaches that seem to carry lower risks than medications
- Dissatisfaction with the practice style of conventional medicine (e.g., rushed office visits, short hospital stays) (Esmail, 2017)

It is essential that nurses maintain up-to-date knowledge of these modalities, continue to evaluate the evidence supporting the effectiveness and safety of TCAM, and be able to help patients make safe choices about the use of these treatments for their mental health and recovery.

Safety

People who use TCAM therapies often do so without informing their conventional health care providers, which poses some risk. Approximately 12% of Canadians who used NHPs reported that they had experienced unwanted adverse effects (Health Canada, 2016). Some patients may believe that a natural substance from a health food store must be safe and effective; however, "natural" does not mean "harmless." Health Canada (2016) consumer guidelines for safe use of NHPs are listed in Box 35.2. Nurses have a professional responsibility to provide patient education that protects patients from unscrupulous practices.

Another concern regarding TCAM therapies that nurses need to address with their patients is that Western diagnosis and conventional treatment may be delayed while patients try alternative interventions, which is common with mental health disorders such as major depression and anxiety. On the other hand, many TCAM and conventional health care practitioners are aware of patients who have been injured by an uncaring conventional medical system or have suffered consequences from the use of conventional pharmaceuticals. Nurses, in consultation with all relevant practitioners, can play a key role in assisting patients to carefully and safely weigh the risks and benefits of all treatments under consideration.

CHAPTER 35 Integrative and Complementary Therapies

BOX 35.2 How Can I Use Alternative or Naturopathic Health Products Safely?

- Talk to a health care professional like a doctor, pharmacist, or naturopath before choosing a product. This is especially important for children, pregnant or breastfeeding women, older persons, and people with serious medical conditions.
- To prevent interactions, make sure your health care provider knows what other drugs and natural health products you are using.
- Use approved products. All products that have been licensed for sale in Canada have a Natural Product Number (NPN), a Drug Identification Number (DIN), or Homeopathic Medicine Number (DIN-HM) on the label. An NPN, DIN, or DIN-HM means that the product has been authorized for sale in Canada and is safe and effective when the instructions on the label are followed. Look for products with these labels only.
- Be sceptical of health-related claims that seem too good to be true. Do not rely on ads; do your own research and talk to your health care provider.
- Read and follow all instructions on the product label.
- Report unwanted side effects (adverse reactions) to your health care provider and Health Canada.

Source: Health Canada. (2016). *About natural health products: How can I use natural health products safely?* Retrieved from https://www.hc-sc.gc.ca/dhp-mps/prodnatur/about-apropos/cons-eng.php#a3. Reproduced with permission.

Efficacy

Some people make the claim that integrative therapies work through a mechanism known as the *placebo effect*. The term *placebo effect* refers to a treatment that actually does nothing, yet the condition for which it is used improves; the improvement comes about because of the power of suggestion and a belief that the treatment works. Integrative care is based on optimism. However, does any patient begin treatment for an illness or disease if there is no hope of improvement? A positive approach and the use of positive suggestion, no matter what treatment modality is being implemented, offer a greater chance of success than does communication that is negative or fosters a poor response. The placebo effect can be most powerful when the need is greatest, and a trusting relationship has been established between patient and health care provider. In fact, the literature on integrative health care increasingly refers to this positive placebo effect as "the healing response" that should intentionally be activated within holistic care to enhance healing outcomes (Mariano, 2020).

INTEGRATIVE NURSING CARE

The Canadian Holistic Nurses Association (CHNA) recognizes holistic nursing as a specialty that supports holistic health and a philosophy of holistic nursing encompassing self-care and responsibility, humanizing health care, and wellness promotion (Canadian Holistic Nurses Association, 2020). Regardless of their practice philosophy, nurses need to have a basic knowledge of treatments used in integrative care since they care for patients who increasingly use a variety of unconventional modalities to meet their health needs. Mariano (2020) defines the **holistic nurse** as one who recognizes and integrates body–mind–emotion–spirit–environment principles into practice; attends to self-awareness and personal healing; removes barriers to the healing process; facilitates growth in others; and assists illness recovery or transition to a peaceful death. To fully understand and respond to the needs of patients, nurses must ask questions about the use of TCAM as part of a holistic assessment. Such inquiry can be naturally integrated into holistic exploration of the mental, emotional, physical, spiritual, social, and cultural dimensions of the person's life and healing process.

CLASSIFICATION OF INTEGRATIVE THERAPIES

Complementary or alternative medicine is classified into five major categories of practice. These classifications include: (1) whole medical systems, (2) mind–body–spirit (MBS) approaches, (3) biologically based practices, (4) manipulative and body-based approaches, and (5) energy therapies. It is important for readers to keep in mind that these classifications are interrelated; many of the modalities discussed could fit into more than one such classification. Furthermore, many modalities are increasingly being classified as "conventional" in light of ever-expanding research and usage. It is essential for nurses to regularly revisit the literature on the effectiveness of a given modality in relation to a specific mental health issue.

Whole Medical Systems

Whole medical systems are complete systems of theory and practice. They include a defined philosophy, explanation of disease diagnosis and treatment. Whole medical systems addressed in this chapter are traditional Indigenous medicine, Ayurvedic medicine, traditional Chinese medicine (TCM), homeopathy, and naturopathy.

Traditional Indigenous Medicine

Traditional Indigenous medicine is central to integrative health care in Canada, given the large number of Canadians who are of Indigenous ancestry. In this healing system mental, emotional, spiritual, social, cultural, and physical health are inseparable (First Nations Information Governance Centre & Walker, 2020). Specific teachings vary, depending on the affiliation of Indigenous peoples. Traditional Indigenous elders and healers combine such narrative with a variety of spiritual and healing practices such as ceremonies (e.g., sweat lodges), vibrational medicine (e.g., chanting and drumming), and use of traditional medicines (e.g., native herbs) to restore balance and harmony. Physical and spiritual health must heal together. Discussed in more detail in Chapter 8, Indigenous medicine wheel teachings are increasingly being integrated into mental health treatment approaches for those of Indigenous and non-Indigenous ancestry.

Ayurvedic Medicine

Ayurvedic (pronounced i•yur•vay•dik) medicine originated in India around 5000 BC and is one of the world's oldest medical systems. *Ayurveda* means "the science of life" and is a philosophy that emphasizes individual responsibility for health. It is holistic, promotes prevention, and recognizes the uniqueness of the individual. Ayurvedic practitioners offer a variety of natural treatments such as herbs, dietary adjustments, contemplative practices, cleansing techniques, and ways of balancing the individual's *chakras*. Depending on the specific approach to ayurvedic medicine, the practitioner may work from a perspective that a patient has seven charkas (Buddhism), other schools believe there are five (Hindi). In either, a chakra is an energy pathway, a vital centre, that connects various organs and glands. The goal of treatment is to understand the energy imbalance and which chakra is being affected, and to restore the natural flow of energy, eliminate impurities, and balance the individual's unique constitution (*prakriti*) and life forces (*doshas*).

Traditional Chinese Medicine

TCM provides the basic theoretical framework for many TCAM therapies, including acupuncture, acupressure, transcendental meditation, tai chi, and qigong. TCM comes from the Eastern tradition, specifically the philosophy of Taoism, and emphasizes the promotion of harmony (health) or to bring order out of chaos (illness).

The main concept in TCM is the movement of life energy or essence, *qi*, which maintains an individual's health and wellness. If this life energy is disrupted, it can seriously affect the mind, body, and spirit (Shields & Wilson, 2016). TCM is a vast medical system based on a constellation of concepts, theories, laws, and principles of energy movement within the body. Therapy addresses the patient's illness in relation to the complex interaction of mind, body, and spirit.

Adherents of TCM say that it addresses not only physiological and psychological symptoms but also cosmological events that relate to the dynamics of the universe. These meridians become significant in the practice of acupuncture, touch therapy, and the more recent energy-based therapies used to treat emotional symptoms and promote mental health. Forms of movement such as qigong and tai chi may be used, as well as yoga. Viewed as a stressor itself, movement seems to mediate the effects of other stressors.

In TCM health is the balance between *yin* and *yang*, and illness emanates from imbalances. The TCM practitioner uses the history and physical examination to understand the imbalances of mind, body, and spirit that have caused the patient's illness. Diagnosis involves both questioning and observing body structure, skin colour, breath, body odours, nail condition, voice, gestures, mood, and pulse. Eastern goals, perspectives, and stages of healing are useful in treating mental illnesses, many of which are long term. The goals of healing in Eastern medicine include:
- Being in harmony with one's environment and with all of creation in mind, body, and spirit
- Reawakening the spirit to its possibilities
- Reconnecting with life's meaning

Homeopathy and Naturopathy

Homeopathy and naturopathy are examples of Western whole medical systems. Developed in Germany more than 200 years ago, homeopathy uses small doses (dilutions) of specially prepared plant extracts, herbs, minerals, and other materials to stimulate the body's defence mechanisms and healing processes. Infinitesimally small doses of diluted preparations that produce symptoms mimicking those of an illness are used to help the body heal itself. Homeopathy is based on the Law of Similars ("like cures like"), and dilutions are prescribed to match the patient's illness or symptom (or both) and personality profile (Shah, 2018).

Homeopathy has been difficult to study using current scientific methods because its highly diluted solutions cannot be readily measured, and homeopathic treatments are highly individualized. A systematic review found that homeopathic remedies in high dilution, taken under the supervision of trained professionals, are generally considered safe and unlikely to cause severe adverse reactions (Mathie et al., 2017). They are not known to interact with conventional drugs. Patients with addictions should be informed that some homeopathic remedies contain alcohol. The breadth of evidence does not currently support homeopathic treatments as an efficient or effective means of treatment of illness or disease.

Naturopathy emphasizes health restoration rather than disease treatment and combines nutrition, homeopathy, herbal medicine, hydrotherapy, light therapy, massage therapy, therapeutic counselling, and other treatments. It is a whole medical system that has evolved from a combination of traditional practices and health care approaches popular in Europe during the nineteenth century. Naturopathic practitioners, guided by a philosophy that emphasizes the healing power of nature, now use a variety of traditional and modern therapies. Practitioners view their role as supporting the body's inherent ability to maintain and restore health and prefer to use treatment approaches they consider the most natural and least invasive.

Mind–Body–Spirit Approaches

MBS approaches make use of the continuous interaction between mind, body, and spirit. Most of these techniques emphasize facilitating the mind and spirit's capacity to affect bodily function and symptoms; however, a reciprocal relationship is also part of the equation (i.e., physical illness affects mental and spiritual health). These approaches are based on the recent research advances in psychoneuroimmunology and psychoneuroendocrinology (Alessi & Bennett, 2020).

The MBS relationship is well accepted in conventional medicine and likely to be the domain most familiar to psychiatric mental health nurses and nurses in general. Many of the MBS interventions, such as cognitive behavioural therapy, relaxation techniques, guided imagery, hypnosis, and support groups, are now considered mainstream and have been the subject of considerable research. Research substantiates that these approaches dampen the parasympathetic responses in trauma that can lead to chronic health problems, post-traumatic stress disorder (PTSD), anxiety, and depression (Debnath et al., 2020). Meditation, prayer, spiritual healing, and therapies using creative outlets such as dance, music, and art have been researched less and often continue to be categorized as TCAM.

Guided Imagery

The use of guided imagery has been in nursing literature for at least three decades. In her seminal work Zahourek (2002) describes imagery as a holistic phenomenon that is a "multidimensional mental representation of reality and fantasy that includes not only visual pictures but also the remembrance of situations and experiences such as sound, smell, touch, movement and taste" (p. 113). As such, it can be used to promote the healing response in all dimensions of health. The clinical effectiveness of imagery has been well documented in the treatment of anxiety, depression, and a variety of stress-related illnesses (Schaub & Burt, 2013). Nurses can actively assist patients to explore what health-promoting images they can integrate into their self-care practices.

Principles of imagery have been integrated with new expressions of MBS therapy, such as somatic experiencing and self-regulation therapy, as a way of holistically processing and releasing trauma (Levine, 2010). Specialized preparation is required for the practice of these modalities.

Biofeedback

Biofeedback is the use of some form of external equipment or method of feedback that informs a person about their psychophysiological processes and state of arousal. Biofeedback equipment can include a simple handheld thermometer, cardiac monitoring equipment, and eye movement tracking tools. Almost immediate feedback is given to the individual about reactions that were previously believed to be outside of their control. Biofeedback has demonstrated a better treatment effect than placebo interventions (Tolin et al., 2020).

Meditation

Several forms of meditation have become popular self-help methods to reduce stress and promote wellness. Meditation practices include such simple behaviours as consciously breathing and focusing attention while walking, sitting, or engaging in other contemplative activity such as yoga. Other forms of meditation have arisen from scientifically based work such as that done by Benson and colleagues (Benson et al., 1974) in relation to "the relaxation response" and by Kabat-Zinn (1994) in relation to mindfulness-based stress reduction. Whatever its origins, meditation practice cultivates a contemplative state of mind that can induce an experience of deep relaxation and calm. Nurses may guide patients toward individual teachers, meditation books, audio recordings, or group classes, with religious (e.g., Hindu, Buddhist) or non-religious (e.g., mindfulness-based stress reduction) approaches, depending on patients' preferences and interests. Such meditative practices are increasingly being integrated with neuroscience by such innovators as University of Toronto psychiatrist Dr. Norman Doidge, who has pioneered their use in the promotion of brain neuroplasticity and "rewiring" in relation to anxiety, mood symptoms, and other mental health challenges (Doidge, 2016).

Hypnosis and Therapeutic Suggestion

Hypnosis is an advanced therapeutic intervention. Introductory information is provided to spark an interest in beginning practitioners to learn more about this intervention as they advance in their careers. Hypnosis is both a state of awareness (consciousness) and an intervention. As a state of consciousness, hypnosis is a natural focusing of attention that may range in susceptibility to suggestion. In stress states people are more susceptible to suggestion because their focus of attention is narrowed. People who dissociate in traumatic situations are in a trancelike state. When relaxation and imagery techniques are used, individuals frequently will enter a similarly altered state of awareness, or trancelike state, that can promote a healing response. However, there is also a risk that during these induced states, individuals may be triggered and re-experience aspects of their trauma.

> ### RESEARCH HIGHLIGHT
> *Animal-Assisted Therapy*
>
> **Problem**
> Animal-assisted interventions are not well understood within the psychiatric community. It is believed that this poses a barrier to the recognition and acceptance of this complementary therapy.
>
> **Purpose of Study**
> The purpose of the present Australian-based qualitative study was to examine equine-assisted psychotherapy (EAP) facilitators' perspectives on the biopsychosocial benefits and therapeutic outcomes of EAP for adolescents experiencing depression or anxiety.
>
> **Methods**
> A qualitative research design was used to gain an in-depth understanding of how therapists experience and create meaning in relation to EAP. Individual interviews were conducted. Themes developed from this data, and the lived experience was reported by the researchers.
>
> **Key Findings**
> The findings suggest a range of improvements within adolescent patients, including increases in confidence, self-esteem, and assertiveness, as well as a decrease in undesirable behaviours. The effectiveness of the therapy was thought to be due to the experiential nature of involving horses in therapy.
>
> **Implications for Nursing Practice**
> These results suggest that EAP is a promising intervention for treating anxiety and mood problems in adolescents experiencing depression or anxiety. Nurses are advised to be aware of the approaches and referral sources. Further research in this area is required.

Source: Wilson, K., Buultjens, M., Monfries, M., et al. (2017). Equine-assisted psychotherapy for adolescents experiencing depression and/or anxiety: A therapist's perspective. *Clinical Child Psychology and Psychiatry, 22*(1), 16–33. https://doi.org/10.1177/1359104515572379

Rhythmic Breathing

While breathing is an integral part of meditation practice, Kitko (2007) describes rhythmic breathing as an easy-to-learn and easy-to-implement MBS intervention in its own right. The nurse helps the patient focus on purposeful breath and usually breathes alongside the patient. This activity enhances the relaxation response in both nurse and patient and has implications for psychiatric mental health nurses working with agitated patients.

Spirituality

There is an increasing recognition of the importance and benefits of including spirituality in mental health care; however, nurses express barriers to integration that include lack of education and fears of exacerbating psychiatric symptoms (Neathery et al., 2020). The positive influence of spirituality on mental health has been well documented in the interdisciplinary literature in terms of enhanced coping, improved quality of life, and faster recovery (Lucchetti et al., 2019). Integration of spiritual care has been associated with fulfilled spiritual needs (such as connectedness, trust, hope, meaning, mastery, and calm), which promote enhanced overall physiologic, mental, and emotional functioning. This support, alongside opportunities to check in on distortions in spiritual thoughts, whether or not chronic psychiatric symptoms persist, is valuable for recovery (Forrester-Jones et al., 2018).

One challenge in meeting the spiritual needs of psychiatric patients is maintaining appropriate boundaries. Patients may experience difficulty in knowing where their own beliefs stop and those of the health care provider begin. Patients are in a vulnerable position of potentially being unfairly influenced by someone with strong beliefs, particularly if their functioning is compromised by psychiatric symptoms (Koenig, 2011). In meeting the spiritual needs of psychiatric patients it is imperative that nurses be continually aware and respectful of boundary issues and never impose their beliefs on patients. This awareness is particularly important in the diverse Canadian context, wherein a range of spiritual world views co-exist (Chaze et al., 2015). As such, it is important for the nurse to avoid the assumption that tending to spiritual needs involves connection to religious activity (Koduah et al., 2019).

To address the spiritual needs of patients, we nurses explore practices, concerns, beliefs, questions, and resources with patients. The assessment itself is a powerful intervention. When we ask patients about the importance of spirituality in their lives, we are helping them to mobilize their cultural and spiritual resources to promote healing (Forrester-Jones et al., 2018). In the mental health setting such inquiry must always be done in a way that does not reinforce any religious delusions that may be present.

The Canadian-based T.R.U.S.T. Model for Inclusive Spiritual Care draws on the interdisciplinary literature to offer guidelines for a non-intrusive, integrative approach to spiritual assessment and intervention in a pluralistic context (Barss, 2012) (Figure 35.1). Inclusive spiritual care is defined as relevant, non-intrusive care that tends to the spiritual dimension of health by addressing universal spiritual needs, honouring unique spiritual world views, and helping individuals to explore and mobilize factors that can help them gain or regain a sense of trust in order to promote optimal healing. The spiritual dimension of health is defined as the dimension of health associated with "matters of the spirit," as ultimately defined by each individual (Barss, 2012). The spiritual dimension may or may not involve a sense of connection to a divine presence or to religious structures or traditions, and it is associated with universal spiritual needs such as trust, hope, meaning, purpose, interconnection, reconciliation, inspiration, and creativity (Kalish, 2012). Box 35.3 includes sample questions to inform patient-centred spiritual exploration should patients wish to have it included in their holistic health care (Barss, 2012). The box highlights initial assessment questions to help nurses meet minimum standards for spiritual care that emphasize that all patients are to be invited to receive spiritual care in keeping with their individual world view (Pinto et al., 2008). The initial assessment questions are closed-ended to ensure that such inquiry is non-intrusive. They need to be accompanied by explicit statements establishing their relevance and affirming the availability of related exploration at a later time if the patient is not currently interested. Any such inquiry may need to be postponed if the patient is actively psychotic or unable to focus on such exploration (Koenig, 2011). Deep listening is essential for health care providers to be able to discern which, if any, questions are currently relevant to explore

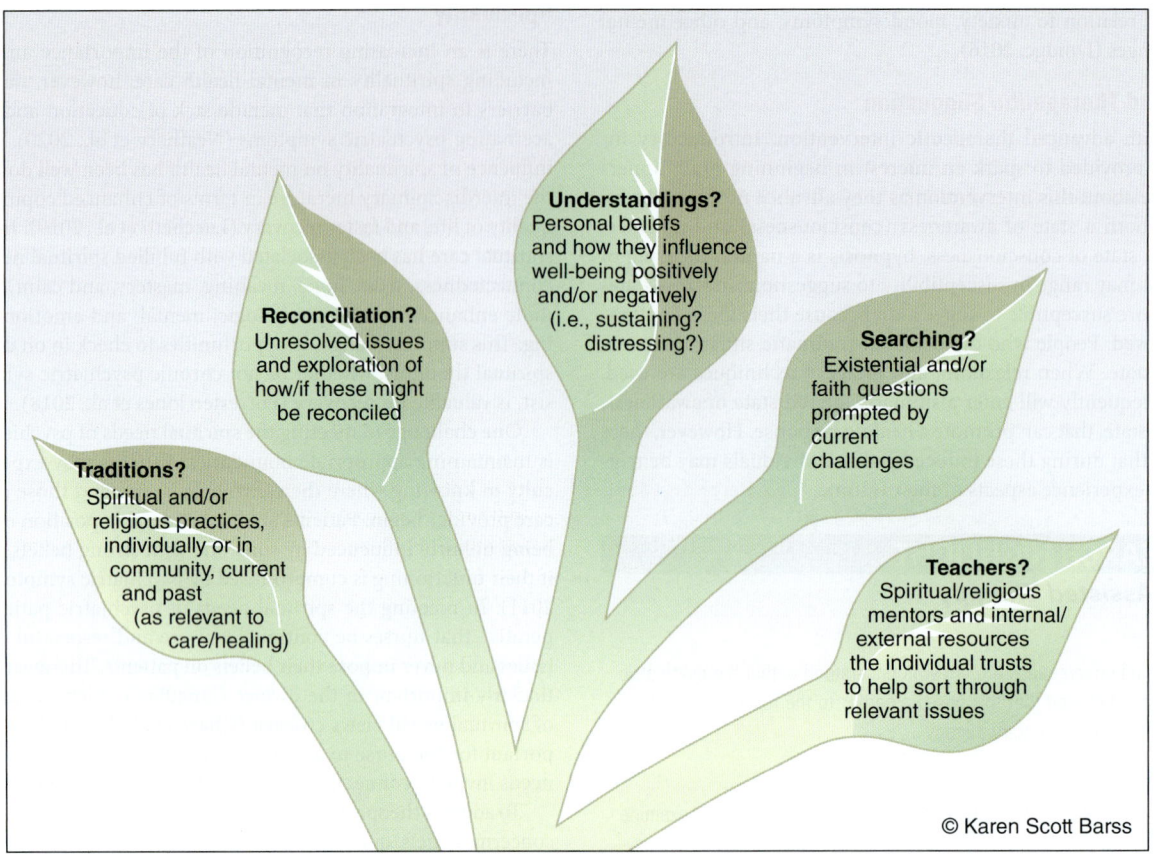

Fig. 35.1 T.R.U.S.T. Model for Inclusive Spiritual Care. (**Source:** Barss, K. S. [2008].)

with the patient; of course, such questions are just one dimension of the therapeutic dialogue (Barss, 2012). In the process patients can integrate spiritual and cultural practices and resources to support their healing. Those individuals specifically trained to offer therapy and counselling from a religious and spiritual perspective (e.g., leaders with shamanic training, Islamic imams, Christian pastors or priests, spiritual or cultural care leaders or hospital chaplains, Catholic or Buddhist nuns) may be an important resource at times of illness and crisis. Certain religious communities offer informal or formal community outreach and events that may be an important part of ongoing recovery and inclusion into community life for patients as well as families.

Biologically Based Therapies

Biologically based therapies include the use of dietary supplements such as vitamins, minerals, herbs, or other botanicals; amino acids; and substances such as enzymes, organ tissues, and metabolites. With the proliferation of literature on NHPs, many people are purchasing over-the-counter products and bypassing a visit to a health care provider. Open discussions and ongoing literature reviews on the associated risks and benefits are a must within the nurse–patient relationship. This chapter briefly introduces dietary and herbal supplements that have been used in relation to various mental health challenges and directs readers to engage in additional ongoing research in order to promote patient safety. Consultation with all relevant members of the patient's integrative health care team is also essential in accessing accurate, up-to-date information.

Diet and Nutrition

It is essential that nurses assess the patient's nutritional status and practices and address these areas in health teaching. Assess for the use of nutrients such as vitamins, protein supplements, herbal preparations, enzymes, and hormones that are considered dietary supplements. Since some nutritional supplements interact with medications, nurses should specifically ask about the use of supplements during the assessment. Nurses can review the use of the supplements and the potential interactions with foods, drugs, and other supplements to reduce risks and maximize benefits.

Nutritional therapies are used to treat a variety of mental health disorders, including depression, anxiety, attention-deficit/hyperactivity disorder (ADHD), menopausal symptoms, dementia, and addictions. The theory is that the inability to absorb nutrients from a proper diet alone may lead to the development of different illnesses. The efficacy of omega-3 fatty acids continues to be studied in the treatment of mood, impulse control, and psychotic disorders (Lange, 2020). B vitamins, especially vitamin B_6 and folic acid, appear to improve anxiety and depression (Cherak et al., 2020). According to these researchers, these vitamins often augment conventional care with antipsychotic, antidepressant, and mood-stabilizing medications.

Megavitamin therapy, also called *orthomolecular therapy*, is a specific approach to nutritional therapy used in integrative mental health care that involves taking large amounts of vitamins, minerals, and amino acids. The earliest use of megavitamin therapy was for the treatment of schizophrenia, for which a high dosage of niacin was recommended. Canadian psychiatrist Dr. Abram Hoffer pioneered this controversial approach in 1952 and continued to study and promote it throughout his career (Hoffer, 1999).

Herbal Therapy

As with dietary and nutritional supplements, health care providers need to be aware of their patients' use of herbal therapies and any potential adverse effects, interactions, and benefits. Each herbal preparation needs to be researched in the same manner as a medication in order to provide safe care. To facilitate this process, it is helpful for

BOX 35.3 T.R.U.S.T. Model for Spiritual Assessment and Care

Traditions and Practices
- **Are there things about your spiritual, religious, cultural, and/or healing traditions/practices/experiences you would like the health care team to be aware of? How might these affect how we work together?**
- What practices, activities, or issues are you inspired by/passionate about? How can these be integrated into your healing? What new practices, activities, or issues might you like to explore?
- Do you have affiliation with any particular spiritual, religious, cultural, or healing traditions? If so, do you see it/them as a current source of strength? Of distress? How so? Are there aspects of or experiences with your tradition(s) that you feel contribute to your well-being? Compromise your well-being?
- What does or do your tradition(s) say about the nature of suffering? How do you feel about that?
- What gives you hope? How can we help you connect to your sources of hope?
- How are you creative in your daily life? In your coping? How can this creativity be applied to your current challenges? To your life in general?

Reconciliation
- **Are there any unresolved issues you would like support in exploring at this time?**
- Are there situations, choices, or actions of others in your life with whom you cannot currently make peace? How does this influence your sense of well-being? What do you wish to do with this awareness?
- Do you find yourself focusing on past choices or actions that you regret? How does this focus influence your sense of well-being? What do you wish to do with this awareness?
- What does "reconciliation" mean to you? What would "reconciliation" look and feel like to you? What might be the benefits of reconciliation?
- Do your current spiritual/religious/cultural traditions play a role in finding reconciliation? What do their teachings say about "reconciliation," "forgiveness," "non-attachment," or "re-balancing"? Do they assist/interfere? How so?
- Have you found anything positive arising from your painful experiences? (e.g., development of inner strengths you didn't know you had; closer relationships; deeper trust; lessons learned; deeper appreciation for the good times; a sense of purpose or meaning, more creative coping?) If so, how does/can this enhance your daily life amidst the difficulties you face? If not, does it feel okay, for now, to grieve the losses associated with your difficulties?
- What/who can sustain you until you feel more hopeful/peaceful? Do you see yourself being able to feel more hopeful/peaceful?

Understandings
- **Are there particular personal beliefs or practices sustaining you/offering you comfort at this time? How can we help you draw upon these for strength?**
- Are you aware of any beliefs or questions that are distressing/compromising your well-being? If so, how do you wish to address these? Do you see it as possible to eventually transform them into ones that promote wellness?
- Are there particular spiritual, religious, or cultural influences that influence or inform your understandings? How do you feel about these influences?
- What do you believe about the nature of suffering? How do you think these beliefs are influencing your current healing process?
- What gives your life meaning? Is there any meaning that you make in relation to your current difficulties? If so, what? How does this influence the way you navigate your circumstances?
- Has this experience prompted you to ponder your overall life's purpose(s)? If so, what is your sense about it/them? How does this influence your well-being/your approach to life/your healing process?

Searching
- **Are there spiritually oriented questions about your current difficulties that you would like an opportunity to explore?**
- How have your current difficulties influenced your beliefs? Are there any of your previously held beliefs that you are currently questioning? How do you feel about questioning these beliefs? Does this type of questioning feel safe/unsafe? What/who contributes to this sense of safety/risk?
- What answers about life/death/spirituality are you currently seeking? How difficult is this searching?
- What/who is a source of disillusionment for you? Have you had an opportunity to grieve associated losses? If not, how might you do so?
- Has the imposition of others' beliefs added to your distress? If so, how? How can you gain protection from these intrusions?

Teachers
- **Are there people/groups/resources you find helpful in exploring spiritual questions? How can they be involved in your healing process?**
- Who do you consider to be your spiritual teachers/mentors/leaders/companions?
- What readings and activities do you find personally inspiring or comforting? How might they contribute to your healing? How can you draw these resources into your regular routine?
- What new mentors, readings, activities, and events would you like to access?
- What resources within yourself can you name and draw upon? What new internal resources would you like to develop?

Note: Bolded questions have been identified as suitable for initial assessment/trust-building.
Source: Barss, K. S. (2012). T.R.U.S.T.: An affirming model for inclusive spiritual care. *Journal of Holistic Nursing, 30*(1), 24–34. https://doi.org/10.1177/0898010111418118. Copyright © 2011 by SAGE. Reprinted with permission of SAGE Publications.

---

nurses to be aware of herbal therapies most frequently used in relation to mental health challenges. Three common herbal supplements are St. John's wort, kava, and herbal teas.

St. John's wort has been used for centuries to improve mood and alleviate pain. It has been extensively researched and generally found to be as effective as antidepressants in the treatment of mild to moderate depression. Results are inconclusive in relation to severe depression, prompting ongoing research. St. John's wort should not be taken in tandem with antidepressant pharmaceuticals due to its serotonergic effects. Caution is also warranted with bipolar disorder, as cases of mania have been reported with its use (Richardson & Brahmbhatt, 2020).

Kava is an herb from the South Pacific taken for anxiety. Kava was considered both safe and effective until 2002, when at least 25 cases of liver toxicity, including hepatitis, cirrhosis, and liver failure, were linked to its use. According to Lake (2015), the cases of liver failure, were associated with a processing error in the production of a single batch of kava. In response to this controversial information, much confusion has arisen as to its legal status in Canada. Kava is currently not legally for sale through Canadian businesses. However, private individuals may import kava-containing products from elsewhere in the world.

Herbal teas have long been used for their sedative–hypnotic effects. Common ingredients in these teas (in addition to valerian) are hops, lemon balm, chamomile, and passionflower. The most studied of these is chamomile, a tea widely used as a folk remedy. Chamomile extract has been found to bind with gamma-aminobutyric acid (GABA) receptors. These teas, along with improving sleep hygiene, may be part of a set of interventions for insomnia; they are generally safely recommended but should be used with awareness of their individual potential effects, adverse effects, and interactions. Table 35.2 provides examples of herbal and dietary supplements used with psychiatric symptoms and disorders.

Aromatherapy

Aromatherapy, the use of essential oils for enhancing physical and mental well-being and healing, is a popular therapy. Essential oils, often derived from herbs and plants, may be applied directly to the skin by carrier oil or diffused into the atmosphere through a diffuser. Essential oils are believed to stimulate the release of neurotransmitters in the brain. The sense of smell connects with the part of the brain that controls the autonomic (involuntary) nervous system. Depending on the essential oil used, the resulting effects are calming, pain reducing, stimulating, sedating, or euphoria producing (Smith & Kyle, 2008).

Smith and Kyle (2008, p. 7) provide a convenient chart on how various classifications of oils affect people:

- Rooty oils such as patchouli and valerian affect calming, grounding, and stabilizing.
- Floral oils such as ylang-ylang and jasmine create mood uplifting, relaxation, and sensuality.
- Green herbaceous oils such as lavender and chamomile create balance, regulation, and clarification.

Aromatherapy has been used to treat anxiety and mood disorders. Some individuals, particularly those with pulmonary disease, may be sensitive or allergic to essential oils when they come into contact with the skin or are inhaled. To prevent an allergic reaction, always dilute oils, administer a small amount, and perform a 24-hour skin patch test before massaging any essential oil into the skin. Ongoing consultation with a trained aromatherapist is essential, keeping in mind that the training and practice of aromatherapists currently remains unregulated (Canadian Federation of Aromatherapists, 2022).

Manipulative Practices

Manipulative practices are based on physically touching another person. (Therapeutic touch is included among the energy therapies since it technically does not involve physical touching of a patient.) The use of any physical touch in psychiatric mental health nursing practice

TABLE 35.2 Traditional, Complementary, and Alternative Medicines Used In Psychiatric Disorders

Herbal Supplement	Uses	Cautions
St. John's wort	Depression	• Interaction with other medications • Photosensitivity • Increased risk of serotonin syndrome when combined with proserotonergic medications such as antidepressants, triptans, and methadone
Kava (Kava kava)	Insomnia Fatigue Anxiety	• Warnings against use due to the link to severe liver damage
Golden root (*Rhodiola rosea*)	Anxiety Fatigue Depression	• Dizziness, dry mouth, and headaches may occur • Allergic reactions can occur
Valerian root	Insomnia Anxiety Depression	• Generally considered safe for short time periods • Mild side effects could include morning fatigue, headaches, dizziness, upset stomach
Chamomile	Sleeplessness Anxiety	• Allergic reactions can occur, particularly in those allergic to the daisy family of plants
Lavender	Anxiety Restlessness Insomnia Depression	• Topical use generally considered safe if diluted properly, although breast growth in young boys has been reported • Oil taken by mouth may be poisonous • Teas and extracts may cause side effects including GI complaints and headache • Use with medications with sedative properties may cause drowsiness to increase
Melatonin	Insomnia Jet lag Night shift	• May worsen mood in dementia • Side effects uncommon, but possibly drowsiness, dizziness, headache, nausea • Long-term use may affect the body's ability to produce melatonin on its own
SAM-e	Depression	• May interact with certain medications • Increased risk of serotonin syndrome when combined with proserotonergic medications such as antidepressants, triptans, and methadone • Side effects are uncommon
Fish oil (omega-3 fatty acids)	Depression Bipolar disorder	• Possible GI effects, like belching, indigestion • Caution with those having fish/shellfish allergies • May increase bleeding time

GI, Gastrointestinal; *SAM-e*, S-adenosylmethionine.
Source: Data from National Center for Complementary and Integrative Health (NCCIH). Retrieved from https://nccih.nih.gov.

continues to be controversial. Some believe it is not used enough, but most believe it should be used sparingly, with clear intent, recognizing that maintenance of therapeutic boundaries is extremely important, particularly with patients who have psychiatric disorders and might misinterpret touch (Cleary & Hungerford, 2021).

Chiropractic Medicine

Chiropractic medicine is one of the most widely used integrative therapies. The term *chiropractic* comes from the Greek words *praxix* and *cheir*, meaning "practice" or "treatment by hand." Chiropractic medicine focuses on the relationship between the body's structure (mainly the spine) and function and the way that relationship affects the preservation and restoration of health, using manipulative therapy as a treatment tool. Many chiropractors treat patients with depression, anxiety, and chronic pain (Kinser et al., 2021). Limited formal research is evident in regard to treatment efficacy for these illnesses.

Massage Therapy

Massage therapy includes a broad group of practices and techniques that press, rub, and manipulate muscles and soft tissues of the body. There are more than 80 different types of massage therapy (Esmail, 2017). It is intended to promote relaxation and circulation in order to promote healing. Massage has been used in the mental health context to enhance mood and reduce anxiety associated with a variety of diagnoses; as such, it is considered an appropriate adjuvant therapy for those who are so inclined (Hall et al., 2020).

Reflexology

Reflexology is a type of manipulative practice that focuses on the feet, hands, or ears. This approach is based on the understanding that zones and points on these areas of the body (most commonly the feet) correspond to other parts of the body. The purpose of treatments is to improve circulation in the feet to promote optimal function elsewhere in the body (Bahrami et al., 2020). Research on this intervention is sparse at present.

Energy Therapies

Practitioners of energy medicine believe that they are able to increase their awareness of the human energy field and enhance healing through meditation and centring (or other practice to access a sense of inner calm). Energy therapies are based on the belief that non-physical bioenergy forces pervade the universe and people. Practitioners believe that they can then detect problems in others' energy fields and adjust the quality or create balance. This detection is accomplished by placing one's hands in or through these fields to direct the energy through visualized or actual pressure or manipulation (or both). Energy is transferred between layers and eventually into the physical body through *chakras*. Disturbances of the energy field are seen as the cause of illness, and healing is understood to occur when the human energy field is balanced and energy is flowing freely (Slater, 2013).

Explanations vary as to the nature of this energy, the form of the therapies, and the rationale for how healing is believed to occur, depending on the affiliated world view. The energy is referred to as *qi* in TCM, *prana* in Indian Ayurvedic medicine, *ki* in Japanese medicine, and a variety of other names in other cultures, including *biofield energy* in contemporary Western cultures. This energy takes a particular form in each person, called the *human energy field* or *aura*.

Research on energy therapies presents particular challenges. First, determining a method to measure the success of energy therapies is difficult since their success is based on restoring balance and total healing, which are not easily quantified. Further, establishing the appropriate time for an intervention to take effect and the dosage of an energy therapy is currently impossible. Finally, establishing control groups and dealing with personality variables with individual healers and patients confound results. Therapeutic touch, healing touch, and Reiki are the most common energy therapies practised by nurses, and in many provinces and territories, the integration of such therapies into nursing practice is regulated by standards of nursing practice, alongside institutional guidelines, and always with patient consent.

Therapeutic Touch

Therapeutic touch was developed in the 1970s by Dolores Krieger, a nursing professor at New York University, and Dora Kunz, a Canadian healer. The premise for therapeutic touch is that healing is promoted by balancing the body's energies. In preparation for a treatment session practitioners focus completely on the person receiving the treatment, without any other distraction. Practitioners then assess the energy field, clear and balance it through hand movements, and direct energy in a specific region of the body. The therapist does not physically touch the patient. After undergoing a session of therapeutic touch, patients report a sense of deep relaxation (Krieger, 1993).

Healing Touch

Healing touch is a derivative of therapeutic touch developed by a registered nurse, Janet Mentgen (2001). Healing touch combines several energy therapies and is based on the belief that the body is a complex energy system that can be influenced by another through that person's intention for healing and well-being. Healing touch is related to therapeutic touch in the belief that working energetically with people to achieve their highest level of well-being, and not necessarily to relieve a specific symptom, is the goal. Healing touch involves gentle "laying of the hands" on a clothed body or moving over the body in the energy field.

Reiki

The Japanese spiritual practice of Reiki has become an increasingly popular modality for nurses to learn and practise. Reiki is an energy-based therapy in which the practitioner's energy is connected to a universal source (*chi*, *qi*, *prana*, and *ki*) and is transferred to a recipient for physical or spiritual healing. Numerous hospitals, hospices, cancer support groups, and clinics are now offering Reiki in complementary programs. Research has been conducted on such topics as reducing anxiety, depression, and pain and on promoting self-care for caregivers (Webster et al., 2020).

> ### KEY POINTS TO REMEMBER
>
> - A philosophy of holism and the promotion of a therapeutic relationship are at the heart of psychiatric mental health nursing and are important no matter what healing modality is used.
> - Traditional, complementary, alternative, and integrative approaches are in demand as patients seek a broader range of therapies than those offered by biomedical approaches.
> - With the availability of online information, patients are more likely to have researched their symptoms or conditions and identified potential TCAM treatments.
> - Nurses are in an ideal position to guide patients to reliable resources, such as National Center for Complementary and Integrative Health (NCCAM), https://www.nccih.nih.gov/ or the International Society for Traditional, Complementary and Integrative Medicine Research (ISCMR), https://www.iscmr.org/, that provide up-to-date information for health care providers and patients.
> - Nurses need to keep abreast of current research about major TCAM therapies so that they can (1) identify those that could be beneficial, affordable, and safe; (2) help patients avoid incurring unnecessary costs on ineffective therapies; (3) guide patients in discerning which therapies could be harmful; and (4) assist patients to maximize the benefits of TCAM therapies.

CRITICAL THINKING

1. As a nurse, you may have patients who use integrative therapies in conjunction with the conventional therapies prescribed by the health care provider. Identify issues that are important to assess, and discuss how you would ask about the use of these non-conventional practices.
2. Choose and research a healing modality that you would like to use for self-care. Reflect on your experience of accessing evidence-informed studies and how they improve your nursing practice.
3. Since mindfulness-based approaches demonstrate good effects for patients with anxiety and depression, consider what the nurse can do to support the patient's efforts in using these strategies.

CHAPTER REVIEW

1. A patient has questioned the nurse about the safety of an herbal supplement. Which nursing response is most appropriate?
   a. "Herbal supplements are regulated by the provinces and territories."
   b. "Since they are natural products, herbal supplements are harmless."
   c. "I know of a couple of websites and a pharmacist that can help us address your question."
   d. "If your supplement was available over the counter, it should be safe."
2. Which of the following is true of integrative health care?
   a. It is synonymous with complementary and alternative healing.
   b. It is being widely offered in the Canadian health care system.
   c. It requires nurses to focus solely on the patient.
   d. It encourages nurses to adopt an overall holistic lifestyle.
3. A patient with schizophrenia has asked the nurse about replacing prescribed antipsychotic medications with meditation and shiatsu massage. Which nursing response is most appropriate?
   a. "Both modalities may have benefits as adjuncts to your antipsychotic medication, but likely not as replacements. How can I help you find out more?"
   b. "You shouldn't even consider it. They're not safe."
   c. "I'm concerned that your illness is affecting your judgement. I think we should talk with your doctor about a medication adjustment."
   d. "I've read that they're very promising. It's worth a try."
4. In facilitating spiritual care in a mental health setting it is important for nurses to do which of the following:
   a. Avoid facilitating spiritual care with patients who are psychotic
   b. Explicitly share personal beliefs so that patients know where they stand
   c. Address spiritual needs without reinforcing any delusional thinking present
   d. Rely on referral to clergy since their expertise is needed to approach the topic
5. Contemplative practices are an important aspect of integrative mental health care because of which of the following:
   a. They have the potential to positively enhance brain structure and function.
   b. They promote a sense of calm and trust.
   c. They reduce symptoms of anxiety and depression.
   d. All of the above are important aspects of integrative mental health care.

https://evolve.elsevier.com/Canada/Varcarolis/psychiatric/.

REFERENCES

Alessi, M., & Bennett, J. (2020). Mental health is the health of the whole body: How psychoneuroimmunology & health psychology can inform & improve treatment. *Journal of Evaluation in Clinical Practice, 26*(5), 1539–1547. https://doi.org/10.1111/jep.13386

Bahrami, T., Rejeh, N., Heravi-Karimooi, M., et al. (2020). Reflexology versus aromatherapy massage for relieving anxiety and depression in hospitalized older women: A randomized clinical trial. *International Journal of Caring Sciences, 13*(1), 610–619.

Barss, K. S. (2012). T.R.U.S.T.: An affirming model for inclusive spiritual care. *Journal of Holistic Nursing, 30*(1), 24–37. https://doi.org/10.1177/0898010111418118

Benson, H., Beary, J., & Carol, M. (1974). The relaxation response. *Psychiatry, 37*(1), 37–46. https://doi.org/10.1080/00332747.1974.11023785

Canadian Association of Schools of Nursing, & Canadian Federation of Mental Health Nurses. (2017). *Entry-to-practice mental health and addiction competencies for undergraduate nursing education in Canada.* Ottawa: Canadian Association of Schools of Nursing.

Canadian Federation of Aromatherapists. (2022). *About us.* Retrieved from https://cfacanada.com/pages/about/

Canadian Holistic Nurses Association. (2020). *Specialization program in holistic nursing.* Retrieved from https://www.chna.ca/

Chaze, F., Thomson, M. S., George, U., & Guruge, S. (2015). Role of cultural beliefs, religion, and spirituality in mental health and/or service utilization among immigrants in Canada: A scoping review. *Canadian Journal of Community Mental Health, 34*(3), 87–101. https://doi.org/10.7870/cjcmh-2015-015

Cherak, S., Fiest, K., VanderSluis, L., et al. (2020). Nutrition interventions in populations with mental health conditions: A scoping review. *Applied Physiology, Nutrition, and Metabolism, 45*(7), 687–697. https://doi.org/10.1139/apnm-2019-0683

Cleary, M., & Hungerford, C. (2021). Physical touch in a changing world: Guidance for the mental health nurse. *Issues in Mental Health Nursing, 42*(2), 201–205. https://doi.org/10.1080/01612840.2020.1764679

Debnath, M., Berk, M., & Maes, M. (2020). Changing dynamics of psychoneuroimmunology during COVID-19 pandemic. *Brain, Behavior, & Immunity-Health, 5*, 100096. https://doi.org/10.1016/j.bbih.2020.100096

Doidge, N. (2016). *The brain's way of healing: Remarkable discoveries and recoveries from the frontiers of neuroplasticity.* New York: Penguin Books.

Esmail, N. (2017). *Complementary and alternative medicine: Use and public attitudes 1997, 2006, and 2016.* Fraser Institute. Retrieved from https://www.fraserinstitute.org.

First Nations Information Governance Centre, & Walker, J. D. (2020). Aging and frailty in First Nations communities. *Canadian Journal on Aging,* Retrieved from *39*(2), 133–144. Retrieved from https://muse.jhu.edu/article/756390

Forrester-Jones, R., Dietzfelbinger, L., Stedman, D., & Richmond, P. (2018). Including the "spiritual" within mental health care in the UK, from the experiences of people with mental health problems. *Journal of Religion and Health, 57*(1), 384–407. https://doi.org/10.1007/s10943-017-0502-1

Frisch, N., & Rabinowitsch, D. (2019). What's in a definition? Holistic nursing, integrative health care, and integrative nursing: Report of an integrated literature review. *Journal of Holistic Nursing, 37*(3), 260–272. https://doi.org/10.1177/0898010119860685

Garrett, B., Caulfield, T., Murdoch, B., et al. (2021). A taxonomy of risk-associated alternative health practices: A Delphi study. *Health & Social Care in the Community.* https://doi.org/10.1111/hsc.13386

Hall, G., Cant, R., Munk, N., et al. (2020). The effectiveness of massage for reducing pregnant women's anxiety and depression; systematic review and meta-analysis. *Midwifery, 90,* 102818. https://doi.org/10.1016/j.midw.2020.102818

Health Canada. (2016). *Drugs and health products: About natural health products: How can I use natural health products safely?* Retrieved from https://www.hc-sc.gc.ca/dhp-mps/prodnatur/about-apropos/cons-eng.php

Hoffer, A. (1999). *Orthomolecular treatment for schizophrenia: Megavitamin supplements and nutritional strategies for healing and recovery.* Lincolnwood: Keats.

Kabat-Zinn, J. (1994). *Wherever you go, there you are: Mindfulness meditation in everyday life* (1st ed.). New York: Hyperion.

Kalish, N. (2012). Evidence-based spiritual care: A literature review. *Current Opinions & Support in Palliative Care, 6*(2), 242–246.

Kinser, P. A., Robins, J. L. W., & Jallo, N. (2021). Complementary and integrative health approaches for women's mental health. In A. Vermeesch (Ed.), *Integrative health nursing interventions for vulnerable populations.* Cham: Springer. https://doi.org/10.1007/978-3-030-60043-3_14

Kitko, J. (2007). Rhythmic breathing as a nursing intervention. *Holistic Nursing Practice, 21,* 85–88. https://doi.org/10.1097/01.HNP.0000262023.27572.65

Koduah, A. O., Leung, A. Y. M., Leung, D. Y. L., & Liu, J.Y.W. (2019). "I sometimes ask patients to consider spiritual care": Health literacy and culture in mental health nursing practice. *International Journal of Environmental Research and Public Health, 16*(19), 3589. https://doi.org/10.3390/ijerph16193589

Koenig, H. (2011). *Spirituality & health research.* West Conshohocken: Templeton.

Krieger, D. (1993). *The personal practice of therapeutic touch.* Rochester: Bear & Company Publishing.

Lake, J. (2015). *Integrative mental health care: A therapist's handbook.* New York: W. W. Norton.

Lange, K. (2020). Omega-3 fatty acids and mental health. *Global Health Journal, 4*(1), 18–30. https://doi.org/10.1016/j.glohj.2020.01.004

Levine, P. (2010). *An unspoken voice: How the body releases trauma and restores goodness.* Berkeley: North Atlantic Books.

Lucchetti, G., Prieto Peres, M. F., & Damiano, R. F. (2019). *Spirituality, religiousness and health from research to clinical practice.* Springer International Publishing. https://doi.org/10.1007/978-3-030-21221-6

Mariano C. (2020). Holistic nursing: Scope and standards of practice. In M. Helming, et al. (Eds.), *Dossey & Keegan's holistic nursing: A handbook for practice* (8th ed., pp. 25–52). Sudbury: Jones and Bartlett.

Mathie, R. T., Ramparsad, N., Legg, L. A., et al. (2017). Randomised, double-blind, placebo-controlled trials of non-individualised homeopathic treatment: systematic review and meta-analysis. *Systematic Review, 6*(63). https://doi.org/10.1186/s13643-017-0445-3

Mentgen, J. L. (2001). Healing touch. *The Nursing Clinics of North America, 36*(1), 143–158.

Neathery, M., Taylor, E. J., & He, Z. (2020). Perceived barriers to providing spiritual care among psychiatric mental health nurses. *Archives of Psychiatric Nursing, 34*(6), 572–579. https://doi.org/10.1016/j.apnu.2020.10.004

Pinto, S., March, P., & Pravikoff, D. (2008). *Evidence-based care sheet: Spiritual needs of hospitalized patients.* Glendale: Cinahl Information Systems.

Richardson, L., & Brahmbhatt, A. (2020). Depression in primary care. *The Journal for Nurse Practitioners, 17*(2021), 37–43. https://doi.org/10.1080/15401383.2019.168821410.1016/j.nurpra.2020.09.002

Schaub, B., & Burt, M. (2013). Imagery. In B. M. Dossey, & L. Keegan (Eds.), *Holistic nursing: A handbook for practice* (6th ed., pp. 363–396). Sudbury: Jones & Bartlett.

Shah, R. (2018). Symptom similarity versus disease similarity: Revisiting the application of the Law of Similars and challenging the symptom-centric approach in homeopathy. *Homeopathy, 107*(3), 218–222. https://doi.org/10.1055/s-0038-1649499.

Shields, D. A., & Wilson, D. R. (2016). Energy healing. In B. M. Dossey, & L. Keegan (Eds.), *Holistic nursing: A handbook for practice* (7th ed., pp. 345–363). Burlington: Jones & Bartlett.

Slater, V. (2013). Energy healing. In B. M. Dossey, & L. Keegan (Eds.), *Holistic nursing: A handbook for practice* (6th ed., pp. 752–774). Sudbury: Jones & Bartlett.

Smith, M. C., & Kyle, L. (2008). Holistic foundations of aromatherapy for nursing. *Holistic Nursing Practice, 22,* 3–9. https://doi.org/10.1097/01.HNP.0000306322.03590.e9

Tolin, D. F., Davies, C. D., Moskow, D. M., et al. (2020). Biofeedback and neurofeedback for anxiety disorders: A quantitative and qualitative systematic review. In Y. K. Kim (Ed.), *Anxiety disorders. Advances in experimental medicine and biology* (Vol. 1191). Singapore: Springer https://doi.org/10.1007/978-981-32-9705-0_16.

Webster, L. C., Holden, J. M., Ray, D. C., et al. (2020). The impact of psychotherapeutic Reiki on anxiety. *Journal of Creativity in Mental Health, 15*(3), 311–326. https://doi.org/10.1080/15401383.2019.1688214

World Health Organization. (2019). *WHO global report on traditional and complementary medicine.* Geneva: Author.

Zahourek, R. P. (2002). Imagery. In M. A. Bright (Ed.), *Holistic health and healing* (pp. 113–120). Philadelphia: F. A. Davis.

APPENDIX

Standards of Practice, Code of Ethics, Beliefs, and Values

REGISTERED PSYCHIATRIC NURSES OF CANADA

Standards of Psychiatric Nursing Practice

Psychiatric nursing, as a distinct profession, provides service to individuals whose care needs are related to mental, physical, and developmental health. Registered psychiatric nurses engage in various roles providing health services to individuals, families, groups, and communities. The practice of psychiatric nursing occurs within the domains of direct practice, education, administration, and research.

Standard 1: Therapeutic Interpersonal Relationships

Registered psychiatric nurses establish professional, interpersonal, and therapeutic relationships with individuals, groups, families, and communities.

Standard 2: Application and Integration of Theory-Based Knowledge

Registered psychiatric nurses apply and integrate theory-based knowledge relevant to professional practice derived from psychiatric nursing education and continued lifelong learning.

Standard 3: Professional Responsibility

Registered psychiatric nurses are accountable to the public for safe, competent, and ethical psychiatric nursing practice.

Standard 4: Professional Ethics

Registered psychiatric nurses understand, promote, and uphold the ethical values of the profession.

The Code of Ethics

Through the *Code of Ethics*, established nationally and provincially (for example, see The College of Registered Psychiatric Nurses of Manitoba: https://crpnm.mb.ca/about-rpns/standards-and-code-of-ethics/), registered psychiatric nurses uphold the values of:
- Safe, competent, and ethical practice to ensure the protection of the public;
- Respect for the inherent worth, right of choice, and dignity of persons;
- Health, mental health, and well-being; and,
- Quality practice.

Source: Registered Psychiatric Nurses of Canada. (2010). *Code of ethics & standards of psychiatric nursing practice.* Edmonton: Author.

CANADIAN NURSES ASSOCIATION

The Canadian Nurses Association has established a code of ethics to serve as a foundation for ethical practice. It is built upon the specific values and ethical responsibilities expected of registered nurses practicing within Canada.

Values and Ethical Responsibilities

There are seven related and overlapping primary values that guide the practice of registered nurses. Listed here are the primary values are their corresponding ethical responsibilities.

1. Providing safe, compassionate, competent, and ethical care.
   - Nurses have a responsibility to conduct themselves according to the ethical responsibilities outlined in this document and in practice standards in what they do and how they interact with persons receiving care as well as with families, communities, and other members of the health care team.
   - Nurses engage in compassionate care through their speech and body language and through their efforts to understand and care about others' health care needs.
   - Nurses build trustworthy relationships with persons as the foundation of meaningful communication, recognizing that building these relationships involves a conscious effort. Such relationships are critical to understanding people's needs and concerns.
   - Nurses question, intervene, and report to address unsafe, noncompassionate, unethical or incompetent practice or conditions that interfere with their ability to provide safe, compassionate, competent, and ethical care for whom they are providing care, and they support those who do the same.
   - Nurses admit mistakes and take all necessary actions to prevent or minimize harm arising from an adverse event. They learn from near misses and work with others to reduce the potential for future risks and preventable harms.
   - When resources are not available to provide appropriate or safe care, nurses collaborate with others to adjust priorities and minimize harm. Nurses keep persons, families, and communities informed about potential and actual plans for the delivery of care. They inform employers about potential threats to safety.
   - Nurses planning to take job action or practising in environments where job action occurs take steps to safeguard the health and safety of people during the course of the job action.
   - During a natural or human-made disaster, including a communicable disease outbreak, nurses have a duty to provide care using appropriate safety precautions.
   - Nurses support, use, and engage in research and other activities that promote safe, competent, compassionate, and ethical care, and they use guidelines for ethical research that are in keeping with nursing values.
   - Nurses work to prevent and minimize all forms of violence by anticipating and assessing the risk of violent situations and by collaborating with others to establish preventative measures. When violence cannot be anticipated or prevented, nurses take action to minimize risk to protect others and themselves.
2. Promoting health and well-being.
   - Nurses provide care directed first and foremost toward the health and well-being of the person, family, or community in their care, valuing the principles of primary health care.

- When a community health intervention interferes with the individual's rights of persons receiving care, nurses use and advocate for the use of the least restrictive measures possible for those in their care.
- Nurses collaborate with other health care providers and other interested parties to maximize health benefits to persons with health care needs and concerns, recognizing and respecting the knowledge, skills, and perspectives of all.
- When experiencing moral distress, nurses take the professional responsibility to express and report on these matters.

3. Promoting and respecting informed decision-making.
   - Nurses, to the extent possible, provide persons with the information they need to make informed and autonomous decisions related to their health and well-being. They also work to ensure that health information is given to individuals, families, groups, populations, and communities in their care in an open, accurate, understandable, and transparent manner.
   - Nurses respect the wishes of capable persons to decline to receive information about their health condition.
   - Nurses recognize that capable persons may place a different weight on individualism and may choose to defer to family, cultural expectations, or community values in decision-making.
   - Nurses ensure that nursing care is provided with the person's informed consent. Nurses recognize and support a capable person's right to refuse or withdraw consent for care or treatment at any time.
   - Nurses are sensitive to the inherent actual or potential power differentials between care providers and those receiving care. They do not misuse that power to influence decision-making.
   - Nurses advocate for persons in their care if they believe that the health of those persons is being compromised by factors beyond their control, including the decision-making of others.
   - When family members disagree with the decisions made by a person with health care needs, nurses assist families in gaining an understanding of the person's decisions.
   - Nurses respect the informed decision-making of capable persons, including choice of lifestyles or treatment not conducive to good health.
   - When illness or other factors reduce a person's capacity for making choices, nurses assist or support that person's participation in making choices appropriate to their capability.
   - If a person receiving care is clearly incapable of consent, the nurse respects the law on capacity assessment and substitute decision-making in the nurse's jurisdiction.
   - Nurses, along with other health care professionals and substitute decision-makers, consider and respect the person receiving care and any previously known wishes or advance directives that apply in the situation.

4. Preserving dignity.
   - Nurses, in their professional capacity, relate to all persons with respect.
   - Nurses support persons in maintaining their dignity and integrity.
   - In health care decision-making in treatment and in care, nurses work with persons receiving care, including families, groups, populations, and communities, to take into account their unique values, customs, and spiritual beliefs, as well as their social and economic circumstances.
   - Nurses intervene, and report when necessary, when others fail to respect the dignity of a person receiving care, recognizing that to be silent and passive is to condone the behaviour.
   - Nurses respect the physical privacy of persons by providing care in a discreet manner and by minimizing intrusions as much as possible.
   - When providing care, nurses utilize practice standards, best practice guidelines, and policies concerning restraint usage.
   - Nurses maintain appropriate professional boundaries and ensure their relationships are always for the benefit of the person. They recognize the potential vulnerability of persons and do not exploit their trust and dependency in a way that might compromise the therapeutic relationship. They do not abuse their relationship for personal or financial gain and do not enter into personal relationships (romantic, sexual, or other) with persons in their care.
   - In all practice settings nurses work to relieve pain and suffering, including appropriate and effective symptom and pain management, to allow persons to live and die with dignity.
   - When a person receiving care is terminally ill or dying, nurses foster comfort, alleviate suffering, advocate for adequate relief of discomfort and pain, and support a dignified and peaceful death. This includes providing a palliative approach to care for the people they interact with, across the lifespan and across the continuum of care, and support for the family during and following the death, and care of the person's body after death.
   - Nurses understand the law so as to consider how they will respond to medical assistance in dying and their particular beliefs and values about such assistance. If they believe they would conscientiously object to being involved with persons receiving care who have requested such assistance, they discuss this with their supervisors in advance.
   - Nurses treat each other, colleagues, students, and other health care workers in a respectful manner, recognizing opportunities for sharing governance with those in formal leadership positions, staff, and students. They work with others to preserve dignity and resolve differences in a constructive way.

5. Maintaining privacy and confidentiality.
   - Nurses respect the right of persons to have control over the collection, use, access, and disclosure of their personal information.
   - When nurses are conversing with persons receiving care, they take reasonable measures to prevent confidential information in the conversation from being overheard.
   - Nurses collect, use, and disclose health information on a need-to-know basis with the highest degree of anonymity required in the circumstances and in accordance with privacy laws.
   - When nurses are required to disclose information for a particular purpose, they disclose only the amount of information necessary for that purpose and inform only those necessary. They attempt to do so in ways that minimize any potential harm to the persons, family, or community.
   - When nurses engage in any form of communication, including verbal or electronic, involving a discussion of clinical cases, they ensure that their discussion of persons is respectful and does not identify those persons unless necessary and appropriate.
   - Nurses advocate for persons to receive access to their own health care records through a timely and affordable process when such access is requested.
   - Nurses respect policies that protect and preserve persons' privacy, including security safeguards in information technology.
   - Nurses do not abuse their access to information by accessing health care records, including a family member's or any other

person's, for purposes inconsistent with their professional obligations.
- In the use of social media nurses safeguard the privacy and confidentiality of persons and other colleagues.
- Nurses intervene if others inappropriately access or disclose personal or health information of persons receiving care.

6. Promoting justice.
   - When providing care, nurses do not discriminate on the basis of a person's race, ethnicity, culture, political and spiritual beliefs, social or marital status, gender, gender identity, gender expression, sexual orientation, age, health status, place of origin, lifestyle, mental or physical ability, socioeconomic status, or any other attribute.
   - Nurses respect the special history and interests of Indigenous peoples as articulated in the Truth and Reconciliation Commission of Canada's (TRC) Calls to Action.
   - Nurses refrain from judging, labelling, stigmatizing, and humiliating behaviours toward persons receiving care, other health care professionals, or students and toward each other.
   - Nurses provide care for all persons including those seen as victims and/or abusers and refrain from any form of workplace bullying.
   - Nurses do not engage in any form of lying, punishment, or torture or any form of unusual treatment or action that is inhumane or degrading. They refuse to be complicit in such behaviours. They intervene and report such behaviours.
   - Nurses make fair decisions about the allocation of resources under their control based on the needs of persons, groups, or communities to whom they are providing care. They advocate for fair treatment and fair distribution of resources, particularly for health promotion and disease prevention.
   - Nurses support a climate of trust that sponsors openness, encourages the act of questioning the status quo, and supports those who speak out in good faith to address concerns (e.g., whistle-blowing).

7. Being accountable.
   - Nurses, as members of a self-regulating profession, practise according to the values and responsibilities in the *Code of Ethics for Registered Nurses* and in keeping with the professional standards, laws, and regulations supporting ethical practice.
   - Nurses are honest and practise with integrity in all of their professional interactions.
   - Nurses practise within the limits of their competence. When aspects of care are beyond their level of competence, they seek additional information or knowledge, report to their supervisor or a competent practitioner, and/or request a different work assignment. In the meantime nurses remain with the person receiving care until another nurse is available.
   - Nurses maintain their fitness to practise. If they are aware that they do not have the necessary physical, mental, or emotional capacity to practise safely and competently, they withdraw from the provision of care after consulting with their employer. If they are self-employed, they arrange that someone else attend to their clients' health care needs. Nurses then take the necessary steps to regain their fitness to practise.
   - Nurses are attentive to signs that a colleague is unable, for whatever reason, to perform their duties. In such a case nurses will take the necessary steps to protect the safety of persons receiving care.
   - Nurses clearly and accurately represent themselves with respect to their name, title, and role.
   - If nursing care is requested that is in conflict with the nurse's moral beliefs and values but in keeping with professional practice, the nurse provides safe, compassionate, competent, and ethical care until alternative care arrangements are in place to meet the person's needs or desires. If nurses can anticipate a conflict with their conscience, they have an obligation to notify their employers or, if the nurse is self-employed, persons receiving care, in advance so that alternative arrangements can be made.
   - Nurses identify and address conflicts of interest. They disclose actual or potential conflicts of interest that arise in their professional roles and relationships and resolve them in the interest of persons receiving care.
   - Nurses share their knowledge and provide feedback, mentorship, and guidance for the professional development of nursing students, novice nurses, and other health care team members.
   - Nurses advocate for more comprehensive and equitable mental health care services across age groups, sociocultural backgrounds, and geographic regions.

Source: Canadian Nurses Association. (2017). *Code of ethics for registered nurses* (2017 ed.). Ottawa: Canadian Nurses Association. https://www.cna-aiic.ca/en/nursing/regulated-nursing-in-canada/nursing-ethics.

GLOSSARY

A

abandonment The relinquishment of responsibilities.

abnormal motor behaviour Alterations in behaviour, including bizarre and agitated behaviours. Grossly disorganized behaviours may include mutism, stupor, or catatonic excitement.

abuse The stage of addiction when the problems resulting from misuse of a substance or behaviour become much more regular and disabling.

acculturation The process by which members of one cultural group adopt the behaviours of another cultural group, generally due to close, prolonged contact with the other group.

active listening Awareness of the patient's verbal and nonverbal communications and the monitoring of personal verbal and nonverbal communications.

acupuncture A method of traditional Chinese medicine that involves the placement of needles into the skin at meridian points to modulate the flow of energy and stimulate physical changes such as in brain activity, blood chemistry, endocrine functions, blood pressure, heart rate, and immune system response.

acute dystonia Acute sustained contraction of muscles, usually of the head and neck.

acute phase The earliest of three phases of mania, during which the person experiences poor judgement, excessive and constant motor activity, probable dehydration, and difficulty evaluating reality. The overall outcome of the acute phase is injury prevention.

acute stress disorder A short-term reaction to a highly traumatic event. Occurs within 1 month of event and resolves within 4 weeks.

addiction The persistent, compulsive dependence on or use of a substance or behaviour despite its negative consequences and the increasing frequency of those consequences.

admission criteria Factors that justify the hospitalization of an individual. Admission criteria must include evidence of one or more of the following: (1) imminent danger of harming self, (2) imminent danger of harming others, and (3) inability to care for basic needs, placing individual at imminent risk of harming self.

adult support program There are three types of adult support programs: (1) social care, (2) adult health or medical treatment programs, and (3) maintenance care. In each type, older adults are cared for during the day and stay in a home environment at night.

advance directives Documents that express patients' treatment choices.

advanced-practice nursing (APN) Includes the roles of nurse practitioner and clinical nurse specialist. Clinical nurse specialists work as consultants, educators, and clinicians in inpatient and outpatient psychiatry throughout Canada. Nurse practitioners work as consultants or collaborative team members who can diagnose, prescribe and manage medications, and provide psychotherapy.

adventitious crisis A state of imbalance that results from events not part of everyday life, such as a natural disaster, a national disaster, or the results of crime.

affect The outward representation of a person's internal state of being, manifested in facial expression, tone of voice, and body language.

affective symptoms Symptoms involving emotions and their expression.

ageism A bias against older adults based solely on age.

aggravated sexual assault A legal term used when, during a sexual assault, the life of the survivor is endangered or the assault results in injury.

aggression An emotion that results in a verbal or physical attack. Aggression is not always inappropriate.

agnosia Loss of sensory ability to recognize objects.

agonist An agent that interacts with a specific receptor and enhances the normal response for that receptor.

agoraphobia Fear of being in an open, crowded, or public place, such as a field, tunnel, bridge, congested street, or busy department store, where escape is perceived as difficult or help as not available in the case of a sudden incapacitation.

agranulocytosis An acute condition involving a severe and dangerous lowered white blood cell count, disrupting infection fighting capacity.

agraphia Inability to read or write.

akathisia Psychomotor restlessness evident as pacing or fidgeting, sometimes pronounced and very distressing.

Alcoholics Anonymous (AA) A 12-step program (the prototype for all that were subsequently developed for various types of addiction) that offers the behavioural, cognitive, and dynamic structure needed by those in recovery from alcohol addiction.

alcohol poisoning A state of toxicity that results when an individual has consumed large amounts of alcohol either quickly or over time.

alcohol withdrawal A physical reaction to the cessation or reduction of alcohol (ethanol) intake that develops within a few hours of the last intake.

alcohol withdrawal delirium An altered level of consciousness, presenting with seizures, following acute alcohol withdrawal. Alcohol withdrawal delirium is a medical emergency and can result in death even if treated.

alternate personality (alter) Also called *subpersonality*. An additional personality within a single individual that has its own pattern of perceiving, relating to, and thinking about the self and the environment.

Alzheimer's disease (AD) A form of degenerative dementia.

anergia Lack of energy or passivity.

anger A strong feeling of displeasure or hostility.

anger control assistance Facilitation of the expression of anger in an adaptive, nonviolent manner.

anhedonia The loss of ability to experience joy or pleasure in living.

anorexia nervosa An eating disorder characterized by a refusal to maintain a minimally normal weight for height and by an intense fear of gaining weight.

anosognosia An inability to recognize illness in oneself, which is caused by the illness itself.

antagonist An agent that interacts with a specific receptor site and blocks or depresses the normal response for that receptor.

antianxiety (anxiolytic) drugs Drugs that enhance $GABA_A$ receptors or increase 5-HT, norepinephrine, or both.

anticholinergic-induced delirium A potentially life-threatening medical emergency secondary to use of anticholinergic drugs and characterized by dry mucous membranes; reduced or absent peristalsis; mydriasis; nonreactive pupils; hot, dry, red skin; hyperpyrexia without diaphoresis; tachycardia; agitation; unstable vital signs; worsening of psychotic symptoms; delirium; urinary retention; seizure; and repetitive motor movements.

anticholinesterase drugs Drugs that interfere with the action of acetylcholinesterase with the result of elevated levels of the neurotransmitter acetylcholine.

anticipatory grief A patient's or loved one's experience of grief ahead of time, after a life-limiting diagnosis or when threatened with loss of ability to function independently, loss of identity, or changes in role definition.

anticonvulsant drugs A group of drugs (e.g., carbamazepine, valproic acid) used especially in treating people with mania that has been refractory to lithium therapy. These drugs are also useful in treating people who need rapid de-escalation and do not respond to other treatment approaches.

anxiety A feeling of apprehension, uneasiness, uncertainty, or dread resulting from a real or perceived threat.

aphasia Loss of language ability.

apraxia Loss of purposeful movement in the absence of motor or sensory impairment.

aromatherapy The use of essential oils for enhancing physical and mental well-being and healing.

assault Reasonable belief that a person means to cause one harm.

assent Expressed agreement to participate in health care or research.

assertive community treatment (ACT) An intensive type of case management developed in response to the community-living needs of people with serious, persistent psychiatric symptoms.

assimilation The process by which different cultural groups come to share a culture; generally, when a minority group adapts to the dominant culture and loses its uniqueness.

associative looseness Disorganized thinking, manifested as jumbled and illogical speech and impaired reasoning (also known as *looseness of association*).

asylums Retreats from society designed with the hope that, with early intervention and several months of rest, people with mental illness could be cured.

attention-deficit/hyperactivity disorder (ADHD) A disorder that causes an inappropriate degree of inattention, impulsiveness, and hyperactivity, all of which interfere with functioning or development.

automatic obedience An exaggerated attempt to cooperate with a request or a command made by another person.

automatic thoughts Rapid, unthinking, often irrational responses based on schemata. These responses are particularly intense and frequent in psychiatric disorders such as depression and anxiety. Also called *cognitive distortions*.

autonomy The rights of others to make their own decisions.

B

barriers to treatment Factors that impede access to psychiatric care, including stigma, geographic challenges, financial limitations, policy issues, and system shortcomings.

battery Harmful or offensive touching.

Beck's cognitive triad Three thoughts that perpetuate depression: (1) a negative, self-deprecating view of self; (2) a pessimistic view of the world; and (3) the belief that negative reinforcement (or no validation for the self) will continue in the future.

behavioural family therapy A collection of psychological techniques for modifying maladaptive behaviours.

behavioural therapy A treatment method that is concerned with patterns of behaviour rather than inner motivations. Behavioural therapy is effective in treating people with phobias, alcoholism, schizophrenia, and many other conditions.

beneficence The duty to act to benefit or promote the good of others.

Benson's relaxation technique A method, influenced by Eastern practices, for switching from the fight-or-flight response to a state of relaxation; achieved by adopting a calm and passive attitude and focusing on a pleasant mental image in a calm and peaceful environment.

bereavement The period of grieving following a death.

bibliotherapy The use of literature for children or adolescents to help the individual express feelings in a supportive environment, gain insight into feelings and behaviour, and learn new ways to cope with difficult situations.

binge eating disorder An eating disorder characterized by repeated episodes of binge eating, after which patients experience significant distress but, in most cases, do not use compensatory behaviours.

bioethics Deontological principles that are irreducible and must be balanced in clinical situations.

biofeedback A form of behavioural therapy, especially effective in stress management, which uses sensitive instrumentation to provide immediate and exact information about physiological responses.

biopsychiatry A theoretical approach to understanding mental health disorders as biological malfunctions of the nervous system.

biopsychosocial model A model that takes a holistic view of the client, including the person's biology, social environment and skills, and psychological characteristics.

bipolar I disorder A chronic, recurrent illness marked by shifts in mood, energy, and ability to function and in which at least one episode of mania alternates with major depression. Psychosis may accompany the manic episode.

bipolar II disorder A chronic, recurrent illness marked by shifts in mood, energy, and ability to function and in which hypomanic episodes alternate with major depression. Psychosis is not present. Hypomania tends to be euphoric and often increases functioning; depression in this disorder tends to put people at particular risk for suicide.

bisexual A term to describe people who are attracted to both men and women when describing their sexual orientation.

blame Attachment of personal responsibility for the assault onto the victim.

blood alcohol level (BAL) A measure (by urinalysis or Breathalyzer) of the level of alcohol in the blood.

boundaries Distinctions made between individuals in the family. Boundaries may be clear, enmeshed, rigid, or inconsistent.

boundary impairment An impaired ability to sense where one's self ends and others' selves begin.

bulimia nervosa An eating disorder characterized by repeated episodes of binge eating followed by compensatory behaviours, such as self-induced vomiting; misuse of laxatives, diuretics, or other medications; fasting; or excessive exercise.

bullying A repetitive behaviour that sustains an imbalance of power.

C

callousness A lack of concern about the feelings of others; the absence of remorse or guilt except when facing punishment; and a disregard for meeting school, family, and other obligations.

Canadian Federation of Mental Health Nurses An organization of registered nurses across Canada who specialize in psychiatric mental health nursing. Under the umbrella of the Canadian Nurses Association and with consumer input, this organization set the standards of practice for psychiatric mental health nursing for registered nurses.

Cannabis sativa Marijuana (*Cannabis sativa*) is a member of the hemp family of plants with one major distinction: it contains delta 9-tetrahydrocannabinol (THC). This is the psychoactive ingredient found in the resin secreted from the flowering tops and leaves of the female cannabis plant.

caregiver burden The physical, psychological, emotional, social, and financial stresses that individuals experience as a result of providing care.

case management Care coordination activities the nurse does with or for the patient; includes referrals, assistance with paperwork applications, connection to resources, and overall navigation of the health care system.

catastrophic reactions Over-reactions to a seemingly normal, nonthreatening situation, commonly experienced in Alzheimer's disease.

catatonia A psychomotor disorder usually involving a lack of movement and communication, but may also altered movements and expression include agitation, confusion, and restlessness.

chiropractic medicine A system of medicine based on the relationship between the body's structure (mainly the spine) and function and its relationship to the preservation and restoration of health, using manipulative therapy as a treatment tool.

circadian rhythms The fluctuation of various physiological and behavioural parameters over a 24-hour cycle.

circumstantiality The inclusion of unnecessary and often tedious details in one's conversation.

cisgender A term that refers to one's gender identity being aligned with the gender assigned at birth.

clang associations The stringing together of words because of their rhyming sounds, without regard to their meaning.

classical conditioning Bringing about involuntary behaviour or reflexes through conditioned responses to stimuli.

clear boundaries Boundaries that are well understood by all members of the family and that give family members a sense of both "I-ness" and "we-ness."

clinical epidemiology A broad field that addresses what happens after people with illnesses are seen by clinical care providers.

clinical pathway A guideline that is used to describe and implement clinical standards. It helps to provide quality and efficient patient care.

clinical supervision A mentoring relationship characterized by evaluation and feedback and a gradual increase in autonomy and responsibility.

closed-ended questions Questions that elicit a "yes" or "no" response. They are useful for getting information efficiently, as in an assessment, but do little to encourage the sharing of feelings.

cluster suicide A term that describes deaths by suicide that follow a highly publicized suicide of a public figure, an idol, or a peer in the community.

CMHA Canadian Mental Health Association. (cmha.ca)

cognitive behavioural therapy (CBT) A commonly employed, effective, and well-researched therapeutic tool based on both cognitive psychology and behavioural theory that is used to treat a variety of psychiatric disorders (e.g., depression, anxiety, phobias, pain problems).

cognitive distortions Rapid, unthinking, often irrational responses based on schemata. Prevalent in many forms of mental illness. Also called *automatic thoughts*.

cognitive reframing The changing of an individual's perceptions of stress through the reassessment of a situation and the replacing of irrational beliefs ("I can't pass this course") with more positive self-statements ("If I choose to study for this course, I will increase my chances of success").

cognitive symptoms Difficulty with attention, memory, information processing, cognitive flexibility, and executive functions (e.g., decision making, judgement, planning, problem solving).

collaboration Formal links between mental health and addiction service personnel who work together to develop and implement a recovery plan.

collectivist (collectivism) The value, principle or practice of giving priority to the collective group over individuals.

colonization The process whereby a people are overcome by a more powerful group and the views, philosophies, values, and beliefs of the powerful group are imposed on the original inhabitants of the land.

command hallucinations "Voices" that direct the person to take an action.

community treatment orders (CTOs) Mandatory treatment provided in a less restrictive community setting.

comorbid condition Having more than one mental disorder at a time.

competency The capacity to understand the consequences of one's decisions.

complicated grief Grief that is prolonged, maladaptive, and dysfunctional, experienced after the loss of a loved one.

compulsions Ritualistic behaviours or thoughts an individual feels compelled to perform in an attempt to reduce anxiety.

compulsive behaviour Behaviour that does not have a biological element but only psychological and social elements. Some examples are exercising, gaming, gambling, Internet use, pornography viewing, shopping, smartphone use, studying, and work.

concrete thinking An impaired ability to think abstractly. The person interprets statements literally.

concurrent disorder The complex combination of a diagnosis of mental illness and a substance abuse disorder or addiction.

conditioning The pairing of a behaviour with a condition that reinforces or diminishes the behaviour's occurrence.

conduct disorder A disorder characterized by a persistent pattern of behaviour in which the rights of others are violated and age-appropriate societal norms or rules are disregarded.

confabulation The creation of stories or answers in place of actual memories to maintain self-esteem.

confidentiality A person's right to privacy of information.

conflict Open disagreement among members. Positive conflict resolution within a group is key to successful outcomes.

confusional arousal disorders Recurrent episodes of incomplete waking from sleep with or without terror or movement, usually occurring during the first third of the major sleep episode and contributing to impaired nighttime and daytime safety or functioning.

conscious One of Freud's levels of awareness. It contains all of the material a person is aware of at any one time, including perceptions, memories, thoughts, fantasies, and feelings.

consent A person's capacity to understand information and voluntarily to act on this information.

consequentialist theory The belief that every person in society has the right to be happy and that we have an obligation to make sure happiness results from our actions.

consultation A process that involves informal links between mental health and addiction service personnel along with additional human services as may be needed for the client.

contemplation The process through which patients become aware that they are stuck in a situation and must decide whether they wish to change or remain where they are.

conscientious objection An individual refuses to perform a legal or professional responsibility because of moral or other personal beliefs.

continuation phase Lasts for 4 to 9 months. Although the overall outcome of this phase is relapse prevention, many other outcomes must be accomplished to achieve relapse prevention.

contract An agreement, either stated or written, that contains the place, time, date, and duration of the meetings between nurse and patient.

controlled style of coping A contained response to an event that may be ambiguous in appearance and reactions and exhibited by a lack of affective response or even calm or subdued behaviours.

conventional health care A system of medicine based largely on highly controlled, evidence-informed scientific research. Also known as *biomedical*, *allopathic*, or *mainstream medicine*.

conversion disorder Also called *functional neurological disorder*. An illness in the absence of a neurological diagnosis that presents with neurological symptoms such as deficits in voluntary motor or sensory functions, including paralysis, blindness, movement disorder, gait disorder, numbness, paresthesia (tingling or burning sensations), loss of vision or hearing, or episodes resembling epilepsy.

coping Navigating through challenges using skills, either learned or natural, to meet goals.

coping methods The thinking, behavioural, and emotional processes individuals use to support functioning in the face of stressors.

coping skills Healthier ways of looking at and dealing with illness (e.g., assertiveness training, cognitive reframing, problem-solving skills, social supports).

coping styles Personal attributes people develop to help manage stress.

correctional nursing Nursing practice organized by the location of the work or the legal status of the patient, rather than by the role or functions being performed. The role involves all aspects of nursing practice.

counter-transference The health care worker's unconscious personal response to the patient.

crisis An acute state of psychological imbalance resulting in poor coping with evidence of distress and functional impairment.

crisis intervention A process focused on resolution of the immediate problem through personal, social, and environmental resources.

crisis situation A situation that puts stress on a family that includes a violent member.

critical incident stress debriefing (CISD) A group-level crisis intervention carried out very soon after a traumatic event.

cultural competence The ability of nurses to apply knowledge and skill appropriately in cross-cultural situations and to adapt care delivery to meet the patient's cultural needs and preferences.

cultural concepts of distress Sets of signs and symptoms that are common in a limited number of cultures but virtually nonexistent in most other cultural groups.

cultural diversity The existence of a number of cultures in one space.

cultural filters Filters through which each of us interprets ourselves, others, and the world.

cultural humility A process of self-reflection and humbly recognizing oneself as a learner about the experience of another, with the responsibility to grow and awareness that therapeutic relationships are reciprocal and formed, over time, with mutual respect.

cultural safety An awareness of power relations between health care professionals and clients; it is of particular importance in light of Indigenous peoples' experiences of colonization.

cultural sensitivity reflects the idea that people have culturally-based understandings, practices, and customs and that health care providers need to be aware of those understandings.

cultural violence When an individual is harmed as a result of practices that are part of her or his culture, religion, or tradition.

culture The shared beliefs, values, and practices of a group that shape members' thinking and behaviour in patterned ways. Culture can also be viewed as a blueprint for guiding actions that affect care, health, and well-being.

custodial care Assistance in performing the basic daily necessities of life, such as dressing, eating, using a toilet, walking, and so on.

cyclothymia Hypomanic episodes that alternate with minor depressive episodes of at least 2 years' duration. Individuals with cyclothymia tend to have irritable hypomanic episodes.

cyclothymic disorder Symptoms of hypomania alternate with symptoms of mild to moderate depression for at least 2 years in adults and 1 year in children.

D

death by suicide The act of taking one's own life. Also called *suicide*.

decompensation Deterioration of mental health.

de-escalation Reduction in the intensity or potential for violence of an interaction.

de-escalation techniques Methods and tools, including advanced communication skills, used to defuse any incident of acting out, anger, aggression, or violence.

defence mechanisms Innate, unconscious means of preventing conscious awareness of threatening feelings or of denying or distorting reality to ward off anxiety.

deinstitutionalization The shift from caring for people with mental illness in institutions to caring for them in communities.

delirium A neurocognitive disturbance characterized by inattention, disorganized thinking, altered consciousness, and fluctuations in mental status.

delusions Alterations in *thought content* (what a person thinks about). Delusions are false fixed beliefs that cannot be corrected by reasoning.

dementia Global deterioration of cognitive functioning (e.g., memory, judgement, ability to think abstractly, orientation). Often progressive and irreversible, depending on the underlying cause.

deontology Duty-based ethics with the central concepts of reason and duty.

depersonalization A nonspecific feeling that a person has lost their identity, that the self is different or unreal, or that the person is an observer of their own body or mental processes. An aspect of depersonalization/derealization disorder.

depressive disorder due to another medical condition May be caused by disorders that affect the body's systems or from long-term illnesses that cause ongoing pain.

derealization An aspect of depersonalization/derealization disorder that results in individuals experiencing a recurring feeling that their surroundings are unreal or distant—an external or outside feeling of disconnect.

Diagnostic and Statistical Manual of Mental Disorders, fifth edition (DSM-5) The official guideline for diagnosing psychiatric disorders.

dialectical behaviour therapy (DBT) Evidence-informed therapy used to treat chronically suicidal people with borderline personality disorder.

diaspora This refers to any group dispersed outside of their original geographic homeland. dominant culture.

diathesis–stress model A general theory that explains psychopathology using a systems approach. This theory helps us understand how personality disorders emerge from the multifaceted factors of biology and environment.

diathesis–stress model of depression A theory that depression results from a dynamic interplay of biology and the environment.

disaster risk reduction (DRR) A systematic approach to identifying, assessing and reducing the risks of disaster.

disasters Events that threaten the well-being of citizens.

disenfranchised grief Grief that can promote a sense of isolation and occurs when losses are not always openly acknowledged, supported, or recognized as significant, such as a loss through a suicide, the loss of a friend, the loss of a pet, or the grief of someone thought incapable of grieving (e.g., a child, a person with dementia).

disorganized thinking The loosening of associations, manifested as jumbled and illogical speech and impaired reasoning.

disruptive mood dysregulation disorder Characterized by severe and recurrent temper outbursts that are inconsistent with developmental level.

dissent Expressed refusal to participate in health care or research.

dissociative amnesia An inability to recall important autobiographical information, often of a traumatic or stressful nature, that is too pervasive to be explained by ordinary forgetfulness.

dissociative disorders A group of illnesses in which mind–body connections are unconsciously altered.

dissociative fugue A subtype of *dissociative amnesia*, characterized by sudden, unexpected travel away from the customary location and an inability to recall one's identity and information about some or all of the past.

dissociative identity disorder (DID) An illness in which a person experiences two or more distinct personality states that alternately and recurrently take control of the person's behaviour.

distress A negative, draining energy that results in anxiety, depression, confusion, helplessness, hopelessness, and fatigue.

dominant culture refers to those deeply rooted understandings that tend to be taken up as "truths" about individuals, society, and social relationships.

Dorothea Dix A passionate social reformer, she advocated for improved treatment and public care of people with mental illness and was influential in lobbying for the first public mental hospital in the United States and for reform in institutions in Britain and Canada.

double-bind messages Communication that contains two contradictory messages given by the same person at the same time, to which the receiver is expected to respond, putting the receiver in "a bind," or an impossible conflict. Constant double-bind situations result in feelings of helplessness, fear, and anxiety in the recipient of such messages.

double messages Conflicting messages (also known as *mixed messages*).

drug misuse A stage where people experience problems as a result of their drug use (see also: misuse).

duty to protect Responsibility of the nurse when the nurse determines—or, pursuant to professional standards, should have determined—that the patient presents a serious danger to another.

duty to warn Responsibility to notify a potential victim of a threat to their well-being or to notify authorities of such a threat.

dyssomnias Sleep disturbances associated with the initiation and maintenance of sleep or with excessive sleepiness.

dysthymic disorder (DD) A chronic depressive syndrome that is usually present for most of the day, more days than not, for at least 2 years.

E

echolalia The pathological repeating of another's words, often seen in catatonia.

echopraxia The mimicking of the movements of another.

ecological model An analytical tool that identifies personal (victim or perpetrator) characteristics, family members, the immediate social context (often referred to as *community factors*), and the characteristics of the larger society to help understand the multilevel, multifaceted nature of violence.

ego One of three psychological processes that make up the Freudian system of personality (id, ego, superego). The ego is one's sense of self and provides such functions as problem solving, mobilization of defence mechanisms, reality testing, and the capability of functioning independently. The ego is said to be the mediator between one's primitive drives (the id) and internalized parental and social prohibitions (the superego).

electroconvulsive therapy (ECT) A procedure in which electric currents are passed through the brain, intentionally triggering a brief seizure.

electronic health care Health care services provided from a distance through the Internet.

elopement Absence from the unit without leave.

emergency response Strategic, coordinated and systematic actions taken in crisis situations.

emotional dysregulation A term that describes poorly modulated mood characterized by mood swings.

emotional intelligence The capacity to perceive, use, understand, manage, and handle emotions and to handle interpersonal relationships with awareness and empathy of the emotions of others.

emotional lability Moods that alternate rapidly from one emotional extreme to another.

emotional violence When someone says or does something to make a person feel belittled or worthless.

empathy The ability of one person to imagine him- or herself inside another's world and see things from the other person's perspective and to communicate this understanding to the other person.

enculturation The learning, usually passed from parents, about which behaviours, beliefs, values, and actions are "right" and which are "wrong."

engagement The connection between the self and another. It is through this connection that nurses can develop a meaningful understanding of another person's experience, perspective, and vulnerability.

enmeshed boundaries A blending together of the roles, thoughts, and feelings of the individual family members so that clear distinctions fail to emerge. Also called *diffuse boundaries*.

epidemiology The quantitative study of the distribution of mental disorders in human populations.

equity-oriented health care is comprised of three *intersecting* key dimensions – cultural safety, trauma- and violence-informed care (TVIC) and harm reduction.

ethics An expression of the values and beliefs that guide practice.

ethnicity The sharing of common traits, customs, and race. Ethnic groups have a common heritage, history, and world view.

ethnocentrism A perception that one's own values, beliefs, and behaviours are superior.

euphoric mood When associated with mania, unstable mood during which the patient may describe an intense feeling of well-being. The overly joyous mood may seem out of proportion to the situation, and cheerfulness may be inappropriate for the circumstances, considering that the person is full of energy but has had little or no sleep.

eustress A positive, beneficial energy that motivates and results in feelings of happiness, hopefulness, and purposeful movement.

euthanasia A deliberate act undertaken by a person with the intention of ending the life of another person in order to relieve that person's suffering and where that act is the cause of death.

evidence-informed decision making Promoted by the Canadian Nurses Association in nursing practice as a model for decision making that incorporates the best available research evidence, with professional clinical judgement, client preference, and collaboration with other key health stakeholders.

evidence-informed practice Care based on the collection, interpretation, and integration of valid, important, and applicable patient-reported, clinician-observed, and research-derived evidence.

excessive sleepiness (ES) At least 1 month of prolonged sleep episodes or daytime sleep episodes that occur almost daily and cause significant distress and social and vocational impairment.

expressed style of coping An outwardly expressed behavioural response to an event (e.g., crying, withdrawing, smoking, abusing alcohol and drugs, talking about the traumatic event).

extinction The absence of reinforcement through the withholding of a reward that has become habitual.

extrapyramidal side effects (EPS) Adverse effects, including akathisia, acute dystonias, pseudoparkinsonism, and tardive dyskinesia, caused by blockage of D_2 dopamine receptor sites in the motor areas.

F

false imprisonment Detention of a voluntarily admitted patient, with no agency or legal policies to support detaining the patient.

family systems theory A theory of family therapy that downplays problem resolution, focusing instead on the long-term ability of family members to make autonomous choices. Its goals are to decrease emotional reactivity and encourage differentiation among individual family members.

family triangle A basic building block of interpersonal relationships; a third person is brought into a dyad to lower tensions once they build. All triangles contain a close side, a distant side, and a side in which conflict or tension exists between two people.

fear A reaction to a specific danger.

feedback Communication of one person's impressions of and reactions to another person's actions or verbalizations.

feeding disorder An inability or difficulty in eating or drinking sufficient quantities to maintain optimal nutritional status.

fight-or-flight response The body's way of preparing for a situation perceived as a threat to survival; this response results in increased blood pressure, heart rate, and cardiac output.

financial abuse The withholding of financial support or the illegal or improper exploitation of funds or other resources for one's personal gain.

first-generation antipsychotic drugs Also referred to as typical, traditional, or conventional antipsychotics developed in the 1950s to treat psychosis.

flashbacks Dissociative experiences during which the event is relived and the person behaves as though they is experiencing the event in the present.

flexibility Allowance for the changes inherent in normal growth and development.

flight of ideas A nearly continuous flow of accelerated speech, with abrupt changes from topic to topic that are usually based on understandable associations or plays on words.

forensics The utilization of scientific processes to support legal investigation.

forensic nursing The application of nursing science to public or legal proceedings. The practice combines the forensic and biopsychosocial aspects of health care in the scientific investigation of trauma or death of victims and perpetrators of abuse, violence, criminal activity, and traumatic accidents.

forensic psychiatric mental health nurse A nurse who integrates nursing philosophy and theory with knowledge of and skill in mental health care and legal proceedings in the investigation or treatment of the trauma of victims and perpetrators of criminal activity.

Four Gifts of Resolving Relationships A predictable sequence of communications about four processes that can be shared with a person who is dying (forgiveness, love, gratitude, farewell).

frotteurism Rubbing or touching a nonconsenting person.

G

gay A term that refers to a man being attracted to another man. Also called *homosexual*.

gender A person's identity and social classifications, often based on masculine or feminine qualities and traits.

gender dysphoria Feelings of unease about one's maleness or femaleness.

gender identity A person's sense of maleness or femaleness. Gender identity is not inborn but is usually established by the age of 3 years.

gender non-conforming Individuals who have a gender expression that does not conform to traditional gender norms of male and female.

general adaptation syndrome (GAS) A three-stage theory of stress proposed by Hans Selye: (1) the *alarm* stage, the initial, brief, and adaptive response (fight or flight) to the stressor; (2) the *resistance* stage, during which sustained and optimal resistance to the stressor occurs; (3) the *exhaustion* stage (occurring only when attempts to resist the stressor prove futile)—resources are depleted, and the stress may become chronic, producing a wide array of psychological and physiological responses and even death.

generalized anxiety disorder (GAD) An anxiety reaction characterized by persistent and exaggerated apprehension and tension.

genogram A tool for efficiently providing a clinical summary of information and relationships across generations of a family.

genuineness Self-awareness of one's feelings as they arise within the nurse–patient relationship and the ability to communicate them when appropriate.

grandiosity A state in which people with mania may exaggerate their achievements or importance, say that they know famous people, or believe that they have great powers. Grandiosity is also apparent in behaviour. Boasts of exceptional powers and status can take delusional proportions. Also called *inflated self-regard*.

grief All of an individual's reactions to loss (e.g., depressed mood, insomnia, anxiety, poor appetite, shock, denial, guilt); sorrow experienced in anticipation of, during, and after a loss.

grounding techniques Promote awareness of in-the-moment physical reality and help to counter dissociative episodes.

group Two or more people who come together for the purpose of pursuing common goals, interests, or both.

group content All that is said in the group.
group norms Expectations for behaviour in the group that develop over time and provide structure for members (e.g., starting on time, not interrupting).
group process The dynamics of interaction among the members (e.g., who talks to whom, facial expressions, body language).
group psychotherapy A specialized treatment intervention in which a trained leader (or co-leaders) establishes a group for the purpose of treating people with psychiatric disorders.
group themes Members' expressed ideas or feelings that recur and have a common thread. The leader can clarify a theme to help members recognize it more fully.
group work A method whereby individuals with a common purpose come together and benefit by giving and receiving feedback within the context of group life.
guardianship An involuntary trust relationship in which one party, the guardian, acts on behalf of an individual, the ward.
guided imagery A process whereby a person is led to envision images that are both calming and health enhancing; can be used in conjunction with Benson's relaxation technique.

H

hallucinations The perception of a sensory experience for which no external stimulus exists (e.g., hearing a voice when no one is speaking).
hallucinogen A distinct psychoactive agent, in that it does not primarily produce euphoria but rather disrupts the central and peripheral nervous systems, producing a disconnect between the physical world and the user's perception of the physical world.
harm reduction A range of programs, policies, and interventions designed to reduce or minimize the adverse consequences, such as overdose, infections, and spread of communicable diseases, associated with drug use.
healing touch A therapeutic modality related to therapeutic touch that combines several energy therapies and is based on the belief that the body is a complex energy system that can be influenced by another, through that person's intention for healing and well-being.
health equity Can be understood as a social justice goal focused on pursuing the highest possible standard of health and health care for all people, with particular attention paid to those at greatest risk of poor health, and taking into account broader socio-political and economic influences on health and access to care.
health inequity Can be understood as socially constructed, unjust, and avoidable differences in health and well-being between and within groups of people.
health teaching Includes identifying the health education needs of the patient and teaching basic principles of physical and mental health, such as giving information about coping, interpersonal relationships, social skills, mental health disorders, the treatments for such illnesses and their effects on daily living, relapse prevention, problem-solving skills, stress management, crisis intervention, and self-care activities.
heterosexual A term that means to be sexually attracted to the opposite sex.
holistic approach An approach to care that addresses both the psychological and the physiological needs of the patient.
holistic nurse A nurse who recognizes and integrates body–mind–emotion–spirit–environment principles and modalities in daily life and clinical practice.
homeopathy A system of treatment of disease that uses small doses (dilutions) of specially prepared plant extracts, herbs, minerals, and other materials to stimulate the body's defence mechanisms and healing processes.
homosexual A term that means to be sexually attracted to the same sex.
hospice palliative care (HPC) Whole-person health care aimed at relieving suffering and improving quality of life rather than at a cure; grounded in the belief that each of us has the right to die pain-free and with dignity.
hypermetamorphosis A compulsion to touch everything in sight.
hyperorality The need to taste and chew, resulting in putting everything in one's mouth.
hypersomnia Excessive daytime sleep.
hypersomnia disorder Excessive sleepiness that occurs three or more times per week for 3 or more months despite a main sleep lasting 7 hours or longer.
hypnotic An effect, produced by drugs, of blunting the degree to which a person feels alert and focused, often resulting in drowsiness.
hypomania State in which people have voracious appetites for social engagement, spending, activity, and even indiscriminate sex. During hypomania, constant activity and a reduced need for sleep prevent proper rest.

I

id One of three psychological processes that make up the Freudian system of personality (id, ego, and superego). The id is the source of all primitive drives and instincts.
ideal body weight A weight that is believed to be maximally healthful for a person, based chiefly on height but modified by factors such as gender, age, build, and degree of muscular development.
ideas of reference The giving of personal significance to trivial events; the perception that events relate to one when they do not.
illness anxiety disorder An illness that results in the misinterpretation of physical sensations as evidence of a serious illness.
illusions Misperceptions or misinterpretations of a real experience.
immigrants are those persons born outside of Canada who have been granted the right to live in Canada permanently.
impaired impulse control A state or condition in which a person has trouble controlling emotions or behaviors.
implied consent Nonwritten consent.
impulse-control training Assisting the person to mediate impulsive behaviour through application of problem-solving strategies to social and interpersonal situations.
impulsivity Manifests in acting quickly in response to emotions without considering the consequences.
incidence The number of new cases of mental disorders in a healthy population within a given period of time.
index offence A reference to highly acute and serious types of offences, including murder, homicides, aggravated assaults and arson.
Indigenous A term referencing a historical community with an extensive and long habitation of a geographic region. Typically, this precedes Western settlements in countries like Canada, the USA, Australia, and New Zealand.
Indigenous peoples A collective term used in this text to identify original peoples and their descendants living in Canada.
individualism Values, principles and practices that favour the individual over the collective.
informed consent A patient's approval of recommended treatment with the knowledge of the potential positive and adverse effects of treatment; based on a person's right to self-determination and the ethical principle of *autonomy*.
inhalants Include volatile gases, substances that exist in a gaseous form at body temperature, refrigerants, solvents, general anaesthetics, and propellants.
insight-oriented family therapy A combination of behavioural therapy and education of families in better understanding their power struggles, defence mechanisms, and other negative behaviours.
insomnia disorder A state of constant hyperarousal, involving biological, psychological, and social factors, that disrupts sleep and impairs daytime functioning for three or more nights per week for 3 or more months.
institutionalized Dependent on the services and structure of institutions and therefore unable to function independently outside such institutions.
integrated use Refers to when a substance is used to enhance an already pleasurable and ongoing experience (e.g., a social occasion)
integration The provision of addiction and mental health services in a single treatment setting to meet the often multiple and high needs of the client.
integrative health care An interdisciplinary, nonhierarchical blending of both conventional health care and traditional, complementary, or alternative health care, with the intent to synergistically blend the best of all evidence-informed healing practices to provide relationship-based, holistic care.
intentional torts Voluntary acts intended to bring about a physical or mental consequence.
interdisciplinary A team approach that integrates separate discipline approaches. A common understanding of the patient issues is

developed, and team members move beyond the silo of their discipline to work toward the best possible patient outcome.

intergenerational issues Various patterns of behaviour (e.g., involving geographical distance between members, suicide, divorce, addiction, affairs, grief, triangles, historical colonization, loss) that affect successive generations.

internalized homophobia A concept that refers to a set of negative beliefs and attitudes toward homosexuality and one's own homosexuality.

interpersonal psychotherapy An effective short-term therapy that is predicated on the notion that disturbances in interpersonal relationships can play a role in initiating or maintaining clinical depression. The goal of interpersonal psychotherapy is to reduce or eliminate psychiatric symptoms (particularly depression) by improving interpersonal functioning and satisfaction with social relationships.

interpersonal violence Includes child abuse, intimate partner violence, and older adult abuse and can involve all nine types of violence: physical, sexual, psychological, emotional, spiritual, cultural, verbal abuse, financial abuse, and neglect.

intersex A set of medical conditions that features a congenital anomaly of the reproductive system or genitals.

intrapsychic conflict A mental struggle, often unconscious, between the id, ego, and superego; it is no longer widely thought to be valid, and such therapy requires a lengthy period of treatment, making it prohibitively expensive for most.

intrusive thoughts Thoughts about a sexual assault that break into the survivor's conscious mind during the day and during sleep. May include flashbacks (re-experiencing of the traumatic event) or dreams with violent content.

ISx PATH WARM scale A mnemonic device used to help assess individuals at immediate risk for suicide. Each letter corresponds with a risk factor frequently experienced within the last few months before suicide. Suicide Ideation, Substance Abuse, Purposelessness, Anger, Trapped, Hopelessness, Withdrawing, Anxiety, Recklessness, Mood Change.

J

journaling The keeping of an informal diary of daily events and activities; journalling is an extremely useful therapeutic means used to reduce depression, anxiety, and distress as well as improve overall well-being.

justice The duty to distribute resources or care equally, regardless of personal attributes.

L

la belle indifférence Lack of emotional concern about the symptoms.

learned helplessness Martin Seligman's theory of depression in which individuals perceive a lack of control over a situation.

lesbian A term that refers to a woman being attracted to another woman. Also called *homosexual*.

lethality The degree of suicidal risk.

light therapy A treatment used in seasonal affective disorder (SAD) consisting of 30 to 45 minutes of exposure daily to a 10 000-lux light source.

limbic system Complex set of brain structures, including the hypothalamus, the amygdala, and the hippocampus, that plays a crucial role in emotional status and psychological function.

limit setting Establishing the parameters of desirable and acceptable personal behaviour.

lithium carbonate Mood stabilizer drug used in patients with bipolar disorder.

locus of control (LOC) An inherent factor in our experience and expression of mood.

M

maintenance/adaption Focuses on supporting and consolidating the gains made during the action stage and continued focus on avoiding lapse or more significant relapse.

maintenance phase A stage of change during which the patient focuses on actively working to maintain changes made and prevent relapse. Also, the final phase of bipolar disorder, the focus of which is prevention of relapse and limitation of the severity and duration of future episodes.

major depressive disorder (MDD) A history of one or more major depressive episodes without a history of manic or hypomanic episodes.

major neurocognitive disorders Commonly referred to as *dementia*, which is progressive and irreversible.

malpractice An act or omission of an act that breaches the duty of due care and results in or is responsible for a person's injuries.

mania An exaggerated euphoria or irritability.

manic episode Individuals experiencing a *manic episode* feel euphoric and energized, do not sleep or eat, and are in perpetual motion. They often take significant risks and engage in hazardous activities.

maturational crisis A critical period of increased vulnerability and heightened potential—a turning point.

medical assistance in dying (MAiD) The situation where a person seeks and obtains medical help to end their life.

medically assisted death Providing another with the knowledge or means to intentionally end their own life through medicine (e.g., a physician prescribes medication to a patient with advanced terminal illness, who uses the drugs to end their life).

medication reconciliation The process of developing the most accurate list possible of all medication a patient is taking.

medicine wheel An ancient symbol that can be interpreted in many ways—the four directions, the four grandfathers, the four components of human nature (physical, mental, spiritual, and emotional)—and that represents the interrelatedness of all aspects of the person, a holistic world view of health and illness based on deep personal connections to the natural world and the tribe.

meditation A discipline for training the mind to develop greater calm and then using that calm to bring penetrative insight into one's experience.

melatonin A naturally occurring hormone; although it is a popular over-the-counter nutraceutical, there are few data to support its use in the management of insomnia.

mental health A state of well-being in which the individual is able to realize their potential, cope with the normal stresses of life, work productively and fruitfully, and make a contribution to the community. Psychiatry's definition is continually evolving since it is shaped by the prevailing culture, societal values, and political climate.

mental health emergency A state of overwhelming anxiety that can lead to serious personality disorganization, depression, confusion, and behavioural disturbances.

mental health first aid (MHFA) The help provided to a person who is developing a mental health problem or experiencing a mental health crisis.

mental illness Alterations in cognition, mood, or behaviour that are coupled with significant distress and impaired functioning.

mental status examination (MSE) Analogous to the physical examination in general medicine. The purpose is to evaluate an individual's current cognitive, affective (emotional), and behavioural functioning.

metabolites The products that result from the body's breaking down a drug.

mild anxiety The level of anxiety that occurs in the normal experience of everyday living and that allows an individual to perceive reality in sharp focus. A person experiencing a mild level of anxiety sees, hears, and grasps more information, and problem solving becomes more effective.

mild neurocognitive disorders Result from changes in the brain that produce less pronounced deficits than do major neurocognitive disorders.

milieu therapy The use of a living, learning, or working environment, including people, setting, structure, and emotional climate, to treat psychiatric patients. Milieu therapy uses naturally occurring events in the environment as rich learning opportunities for patients.

mindfulness A centuries-old form of meditation that is based on the premise that we are not aware of ourselves moment to moment but operate on a sort of mental autopilot. Being mindful requires observing and monitoring the content of our consciousness and recognizing that thoughts are just thoughts and that negative interpretations can become positive.

misuse The stage of addiction when people begin to experience problems associated with their use of alcohol, other drugs, or other behaviours.

moderate anxiety A level of anxiety that interferes with what a person sees, hears, and grasps—the perceptual field narrows, and some details are excluded from observation.

monoamine oxidase inhibitors (MAOIs) Group of antidepressant drugs that prevent the destruction of monoamines by inhibiting the action of monoamine oxidase.

mood disorders A group of diagnoses related to disturbances in mood.

mood stabilizer Drug used to treat mood disorders by balancing brain neurotransmitters.

moral agent A person who has the power and capacity to do what is good and right.

moral distress A response to one's values and commitments being compromised.

moral residue Feelings that are carried forward from situations that resulted in moral distress or uncertainty.

moral resilience The ability and willingness to speak and take the most fitting action in the presence of moral and ethical dilemmas.

moral treatment Social and psychological approaches to treatment that included retreats from society, calm environments, and several months of rest.

moral uncertainty An uneasy feeling that results from a person's being unable to make an ethical decision.

motivational interviewing An approach to both assessment and treatment whereby nurses and other practitioners work with patients to facilitate movement through fluctuations between the stages of change.

mourning Things people do to cope with their grief, including shared, social expressions of grief, such as attending funerals and participating in bereavement groups.

multiculturalism The presence of diverse racial and ethnic minorities who identify themselves as different and wish to remain so; a set of ideals celebrating the cultural diversity of Canada adopted at the federal, provincial, and municipal levels.

multidisciplinary A team approach that consists of individuals from distinct disciplines approaching the patient from their own perspectives.

mutual aid Community-based (face-to-face or online) support that usually involves peer-to-peer support groups where people recovering from problematic substance use meet to share their challenges and successes in an effort to assist one another to achieve and maintain sobriety (e.g., Alcoholics Anonymous, Narcotics Anonymous). Mutual aid is also used by people to gain understanding and coping skills in the face of living with someone with problematic substance use (e.g., AlAnon or Alateen family groups).

mutual storytelling A psychodramatic technique developed to help young children express themselves verbally.

N

natural health products (NHPs) Substances such as vitamins and minerals, herbal medicines, homeopathic preparations, energy drinks, probiotics, and many alternative and traditional medicines.

naturopathy A system guided by a philosophy emphasizing the healing power of nature and restoring the body's natural ability to maintain and restore health using a variety of traditional and modern therapies.

negative reinforcement The removal of an unpleasant consequence of a behaviour; it is not the same as *punishment*. This concept is related to *positive reinforcement*.

negative symptoms The absence of something that should be present but is not (e.g., apathy, lack of motivation, anhedonia, poor thought processes).

negativism The trait of being negative, pessimistic or overly critical to the suggestions of others or as a general attitude.

neglect Failure to provide basic needs for a dependant. Includes physical neglect (failure to provide for basic needs or to protect from harm), emotional neglect (failure to attend to basic emotional needs and nurturing), educational neglect (failure to provide a child with experiences, including formal education necessary for intellectual growth and development), and medical neglect (failure to provide basic medical, dental, or psychiatric care).

negligence Carelessness.

neologisms Made-up words (or idiosyncratic uses of existing words) that have meaning for the person but a different or nonexistent meaning to others. This eccentric use of words represents disorganized thinking and interferes with communication.

neurocognitive disorders Result from changes in the brain and are marked by disturbances in orientation, memory, intellect, judgement, and affect.

neurodevelopmental disorders Disorders characterized by developmental deficits in the young (i.e., preschool-aged) child that produce impairments in social skills, intelligence, academic and occupational functioning, and communication skills.

neuroleptic malignant syndrome (NMS) A potentially fatal reaction to antipsychotic medications. Symptoms include muscular rigidity, hyperpyrexia, and sometimes oculogyric crises.

neurons Specialized nerve cells that process and transmit information through electrical and chemical signals.

neurotransmitters Chemicals that transmit signals from one neuron to the next across synapses.

non-binary A term for gender identities that are neither male nor female—identities that are outside the gender binary.

nonmaleficence The duty to minimize harm and do no wrong to the patient.

nonsuicidal self-injury Characterized by self-harming behaviour with no intent to die.

nontherapeutic communication techniques Any method of communication that detracts from the therapeutic relationship.

nonverbal behaviours Behaviours such as body language, the crossing of arms or tapping of the foot or fingers on a surface, tone of voice, and other expressions other than the content of speech.

nonverbal communication Interpersonal communication conveyed through such nonverbal behaviours as body language, eye contact, facial expressions, tone of voice, or gestures.

normal anxiety A healthy reaction necessary for survival, providing the energy needed to carry out everyday tasks and strive toward goals.

not criminally responsible (NCR) A circumstance where a criminal act has taken place, however the accused is deemed not responsible due to a serious and significant mental health impairment.

nuclear family Parents and the children under their care.

Nursing Interventions Classification (NIC) A tool used to standardize, define, and measure nursing care.

Nursing Outcomes Classification (NOC) A reference that provides a comprehensive list of standardized outcomes, definitions, and measures to describe client outcomes influenced by nursing practice.

O

obsessions Thoughts, impulses, or images that persist and recur and cannot be dismissed from the mind. Obsessions often seem senseless to the individual who experiences them (*ego-dystonic*), and their presence causes severe anxiety.

open-ended questions Questions that encourage lengthy responses and information about experiences, perceptions, or responses to a situation and cannot be answered by a simple "yes" or "no" response.

operant conditioning A type of behaviour modification in which voluntary behaviours are increased or decreased through reinforcement or punishment.

opioid A drug that acts on endorphin receptors with a secondary effect on dopamine.

oppositional defiant disorder A recurrent pattern of negativistic, disobedient, hostile, defiant behaviour toward authority figures without going so far as to seriously violate the basic rights of others.

orientation phase The phase during which the nurse conducts the initial interview; can last for a few meetings or extend over a longer period.

outcome criteria The hoped-for outcomes that reflect the maximal level of patient health that can realistically be achieved through nursing interventions.

P

palliative care An interdisciplinary and collaborative approach to care for the treatment of pain and suffering of chronically and terminally ill patients.

pandemic A disease process prevalent over a whole country, multiple countries or globally.

panic The most extreme level of anxiety, marked by an inability to process the meaning of activity in the environment, noticeably disturbed behaviour, and, sometimes, a lost sense of reality.

panic attack The sudden onset of extreme apprehension or fear, usually associated with feelings of impending doom. The feelings of terror present during a panic attack are so severe that normal function is suspended, the perceptual field is severely limited, and misinterpretation of reality may occur.

panic disorder (PD) An anxiety disorder characterized by recurring severe panic attacks. It may also effect significant behavioural changes lasting at least a month and ongoing worry about having other attacks.

paranoia Any intense and strongly defended irrational suspicion.

perpetrators Those who initiate violence. Perpetrators often consider their own needs to be more important than anyone else's and look to others to meet their needs.

perseveration The repetition of phrases or behaviour.

persistent depressive disorder Diagnosed when feelings of depression occur for most of the day, for the majority of days.

persona Latin word meaning *mask* and the origin of the word *personality*. May refer to the person as other people see them.

personality The combination of qualities or characteristics that makes a person a distinct individual. Personality determines the quality of experiences among people and serves as a guide for one-to-one interaction and in social groups.

personality disorders Disorders that cause significant challenges in self-identity or self-direction and problems with empathy or intimacy within relationships.

personality trait A stable characteristic of a person, such as neuroticism, extraversion, openness to experience, agreeableness, and conscientiousness.

personality type A way to describe a cluster of traits.

pharmacodynamics Biochemical and physiological effects of drugs on the body, which include the mechanisms of drug action and its effect.

pharmacogenetics An approach to treatment that takes into consideration individual genetic differences when determining which and how much medication to prescribe.

pharmacokinetics The study of the action of drugs within the body; used to determine the blood level of a drug and to guide the dosage schedule.

phases of crisis Four distinct phases of physical and psychological experiences in response to a crisis as identified by Caplan.

Philippe Pinel Eighteenth-century reformer who, along with William Tuke, introduced the moral treatment era of psychiatry, which attempted to focus on providing peaceful, nurturing environments for people with mental illness.

physical dependency A physiological state of cellular adaptation that arises when the central and peripheral nervous systems become habituated to a psychoactive agent such that the person physically needs the drug to function or to avoid the physical pain of withdrawal.

physical stressors Negative changes to our environment (e.g., trauma, excessive cold or heat) or physical beings (e.g., infection, hemorrhage, hunger, pain).

physical violence The infliction of physical pain or bodily harm (e.g., slapping, punching, hitting, choking, pushing, restraining, biting, throwing, burning).

pica The persistent eating of non-nutritive substances without an aversion to eating food. Infants and toddlers may eat paint, plaster, string, or cloth.

play therapy Usually, a one-to-one session the therapist has with a child in a playroom. The therapist offers a choice of play materials to the child to aid self-expression, assess developmental and emotional status, determine diagnosis, and institute therapeutic interventions.

polysomnography (PSG) The most common sleep test; used to diagnose and evaluate people with sleep disorders related to breathing, nocturnal seizure disorders, and various parasomnias or with unusual sleep patterns that interrupt functioning.

population health approaches Actions and strategies taken at the community and systems level of intervention for the purposes of strengthening mental health at all levels of prevention.

population mental health The state of psychological and emotional wellbeing at the population level and among different groups of people.

positive reinforcement The presentation of a reward immediately following a behaviour, making the behaviour more likely to occur in the future.

positive symptoms The presence of something that is not normally present (e.g., hallucinations, delusions, bizarre behaviour, paranoia).

post-traumatic stress disorder (PTSD) An acute emotional response to a traumatic event or situation involving severe environmental stress.

postvention Interventions with the family and friends of a person who has died by suicide. Postvention aims to both reduce the traumatic aftereffects and explore effective means of addressing survivor problems using primary and secondary interventions.

preconscious One of Freud's levels of awareness. Just below the surface of awareness, it contains material that can be retrieved rather easily through conscious effort.

precontemplation The first stage of the Transtheoretical Model of Change (TTM), it recognizes that an individual will be resistant to change and typically has no intention of altering behaviour in the near future.

premenstrual dysphoric disorder A cluster of symptoms that occur in the last week before the onset of a woman's menstrual period.

preorientation phase The phase of the therapeutic relationship during which the nurse prepares for the orientation phase—for instance, by familiarizing himself or herself with the patient's background or engaging in self-reflection.

preparation Also known as the determination stage, it involves some commitment from the patient that changing their drug-using behaviour is being considered along with the anticipation of what this future action may look like.

prevalence The total number of cases, new and existing, in a given population during a specific period of time, regardless of when the subjects became ill.

primary care In terms of mental health care, care that promotes mental health and reduces mental illness to decrease the incidence of crisis.

primary dementia An irreversible, progressive dementia that is not secondary to any other disorder.

primary intervention In relation to suicide, activities that provide support, information, and education to prevent suicide.

primary prevention In regard to abuse, measures taken to prevent the occurrence of abuse.

principle of least restrictive intervention This principle requires that more restrictive interventions be used only after less restrictive interventions to manage the behaviour have been attempted.

prolonged grief Severe and disabling chronic grief.

progressive muscle relaxation (PMR) A stress relaxation technique performed by tensing groups of muscles (beginning with feet and ending with face) as tightly as possible for 8 seconds and suddenly releasing them.

pseudodementia A disorder that mimics dementia.

pseudoparkinsonism A medication-induced, temporary constellation of symptoms associated with Parkinson's disease: tremor, reduced accessory movements, impaired gait, and stiffening of muscles.

psychiatric consultation liaison nurse (PCLN) A nurse who functions as a consultant to other nurses in managing psychological concerns and symptoms of psychiatric disorders and who works directly with patients as a clinician to help them deal more effectively with physical and emotional problems.

psychodynamic therapy A therapy focused on the present that uses many of the tools of psychoanalysis, such as free association, dream analysis, transference, and counter-transference, but in which the therapist has increased involvement and interacts with the patient more freely.

psychoeducation An approach to care that emphasizes helping a person gain knowledge necessary to manage the illness.

psychoeducational family therapy Therapy that provides families with the information they need about mental illness and the coping skills that will help them deal with their loved one's psychiatric disorder.

psychoeducational groups Groups that aim to increase knowledge or skills about a specific subject and allow members to communicate emotional concerns.

psychological dependency When a drug becomes so important to an individual's thoughts and actions that the person believes she or he cannot manage without the substance.

psychological stressors Changes that are cognitive- or emotion-based (e.g., divorce, loss of a job, unmanageable debt, the death of a loved one, retirement, fear of a terrorist attack); psychological stressors also include changes we might consider positive (e.g., marriage, the arrival of a new baby, unexpected success).

psychological violence When someone uses threats and causes fear in an individual to gain control.

psychomotor agitation The need to fidget (e.g., constant pacing and wringing hands).

psychomotor retardation The slowing of physical movements and, often, of thoughts.

psychoneuroimmunology An area of study focused on the relationship between the mind, the nervous system, and the immune system.

psychosis Altered cognition, altered perception, or an impaired ability to determine what is or is not real (an ability known as reality testing).

psychosocial assessment An evaluation of the person's social functioning and the systems in which the person operates.

public health emergency Crisis situations occurring impacting wider societal and population level health circumstances.

punishment An unpleasant consequence of a behaviour.

Q

queer A term often used as an umbrella term for individuals who do not identify as heterosexual.

R

race A *socially constructed* category of "difference" without biological meaning. Although the concept of distinct "races" has generally been rejected, the notion of racism remains important.

racism A set of attitudes and behaviours in which social groups are identified, separated, treated as inferior or superior, and given differential access to power and other valued resources.

racialization A process of differentiation underpinned by the assumption that "race" is the primary, natural, and neutral means of categorization. From this perspective, behavioral characteristics are also linked with "race." Power is exerted through everyday actions and attitudes and from institutionalized polices and practice that disadvantage individuals and groups on the basis of presumed biological, physical, or genetic differences.

rage An uncontrollable, violent state of anger that prevents a person from thinking clearly or logically, impeding psychosocial or cognitive behavioural interventions.

rape-trauma syndrome A variant of post-traumatic stress disorder that consists of an acute phase and a long-term reorganization process that occurs after an actual or attempted sexual assault.

rapid cycling Four or more mood episodes in a 12-month period. The term is used to indicate more severe symptoms, such as poorer global functioning, high recurrence risk, and resistance to conventional somatic treatments.

rapport A relationship characterized by trust, support, and understanding.

reality testing The ability to determine accurately whether or not an experience is based in reality.

receptors Protein molecules, embedded in a cell, to which one or more specific kinds of signalling molecules may attach.

recidivism The return, or repeat of criminal behaviours typically resulting in re-incarceration.

recovery The ability of a patient to work, live, and participate in the community after an illness.

recovery model A patient-centred approach that stresses hope, living a full and productive life, and eventual recovery. Patients partner with health care providers and aim to extend their improvement beyond stability.

recovery-oriented Approaches and strategies that are centred on recovery and the recovery model.

reflexology A form of manipulative therapy based on the understanding that zones and points of the body relate to one another. Focuses primarily on the feet to improve circulation and promote optimum function elsewhere in the body.

refugee A person who is seeking asylum in a new country due to threat of trauma or actual trauma and violation of human rights.

Registered Psychiatric Nurses of Canada An organization representing the four Western provincial associations for registered psychiatric nurses.

rehabilitation A program focused on managing patients' deficits and helping patients learn to live with their illnesses.

Reiki An energy-based therapy in which the practitioner's energy is connected to a universal source and is transferred to a recipient for physical or spiritual healing.

reinforcement An outcome that causes a behaviour to occur more frequently.

relapse prevention The process that occurs after formal treatment.

relational ethics A developing ethical theory with the core elements of mutual respect, engagement, embodied knowledge, interdependent environment, and uncertainty.

resilience A characteristic of mental health that aids people to recognize stressors and negative emotions, deal with them, and learn from the experience.

respect for autonomy Respecting the rights of others to make their own decisions (e.g., acknowledging the patient's right to refuse medication promotes autonomy).

reticular activating system (RAS) Part of the brain that helps to control sleep, motivation, and breathing.

reuptake Reabsorption of a neurotransmitter by a neuron following impulse transmission across a synapse.

right to privacy The assurance that only people with a right to know will have access to privileged information.

right to refuse treatment A person's ability to understand and appreciate their condition and determine if they will accept treatment.

rigid boundaries Boundaries in which the rules and roles are consistently adhered to no matter what. Rigid boundaries prevent family members from trying out new roles or, in some cases, from taking on more mature functions as time goes on. Also called *disengaged boundaries*.

rumination disorder The repeated regurgitation and rechewing of food without apparent nausea, retching, or gastrointestinal problems.

S

SAD PERSONS scale A simple and practical guide for triaging potentially suicidal patients.

safety plan A plan for a rapid escape when abuse recurs.

seclusion protocol An outline of the proper reporting procedure, through the appropriate channels, to be used when seclusion is used as a treatment.

secondary care In terms of mental health, care that includes intervention during an acute crisis to prevent prolonged anxiety from diminishing personal effectiveness and personality organization.

secondary dementia A form of dementia that occurs as a result of some other pathological process (e.g., metabolic, nutritional, or neurological).

secondary gains Benefits derived from the symptoms alone.

secondary intervention In relation to suicide, a treatment of the actual suicidal crisis. It is practised in clinics, hospitals, and jails and on telephone hotlines.

secondary prevention In regard to abuse, early intervention in abusive situations to minimize their disabling or long-term effects.

secondary victimization The sexual assault survivor's experiencing further stress or trauma when seeking help.

second-generation antipsychotic drugs Drugs used to treat psychosis that target both the positive and possibly the negative symptoms of schizophrenia and may produce fewer extrapyramidal side effects.

selective inattention An impairment in the ability to see or hear everything in the environment.

selective serotonin reuptake inhibitors (SSRIs) Medications that increase both serotonin and norepinephrine.

self-care activities Personal responsibility for activities of daily living (ADL).

self-help groups Groups (often run by the members themselves) that are structured for the purpose of providing members with the opportunity to maintain or enhance personal and social functioning through cooperation and shared understanding of life's challenges. Also called *support groups*.

serotonin syndrome A potentially life-threatening reaction caused by concurrently taking two medications that increase the level of serotonin.

serotonin–norepinephrine reuptake inhibitor (SNRI) A drug used to treat generalized anxiety disorder (GAD), social anxiety disorder (SAD), and panic disorder (PD).

severe anxiety A level of anxiety that seriously impairs the person's ability to notice their environment, even when it is pointed out by another. A person with severe anxiety may instead focus on one particular detail or many scattered details.

sexual assault Any sexual activity for which consent is not obtained or freely given. Also called *sexual violence*.

sexual assault nurse examiners (SANEs) Nurses who are specially trained in the care and assessment (including of psychological and emotional trauma) of adult and pediatric victims of sexual assault (*SANE-A* and *SANE-P*, respectively).

sexual orientation A person's sexual identity in relation to the gender to which they are attracted. Sexual orientation is biological; people are born heterosexual, homosexual, or bisexual.

sexual violence When a person is forced to unwillingly take part in sexual activity. Sexual violence against adults may be referred to as *rape*, or in legal terms as *sexual assault*.

sexuality The ways in which people experience and express themselves as sexual beings.

situational crisis Acute imbalance that arises from events that are extraordinary, external rather than internal, and unanticipated.

sleep architecture The structural organization of non–rapid eye movement (NREM) and rapid eye movement (REM) sleep.

sleep continuity The distribution of sleep and wakefulness across the sleep period.

sleep deprivation The discrepancy between hours of sleep obtained and hours of sleep required for optimal functioning.

sleep efficiency Ratio of sleep duration to time spent in bed.

sleep fragmentation Disruption of sleep stages as indicated by excessive amounts of stage 1 sleep, multiple brief arousals, and frequent shifts in sleep staging.

sleep hygiene Conditions and practices that promote continuous and effective sleep.

sleep latency The time it takes to go to sleep.

sleep restriction Limiting the total sleep time to create a temporary, mild state of sleep deprivation and strengthen the sleep homeostatic drive.

social determinants of health Elements of one's lifestyle that affect health, including economic status, genetics, job security, employment opportunities, access to safe and affordable housing, child care availability, food security, and inclusion and exclusion from society.

social phobia Also called *social anxiety disorder (SAD)*. Severe anxiety or fear provoked by exposure to a social or performance situation (e.g., fear of being scrutinized, saying something that sounds foolish in public, not being able to answer questions in a classroom, eating in public, performing on stage).

social relationship A relationship that is initiated primarily for the purpose of friendship, socialization, enjoyment, or accomplishment of a task. Mutual needs are met during social interaction (e.g., participants share ideas, feelings, and experiences).

social skills training The teaching of a wide variety of social and activities of daily living (ADL) skills.

sociocultural context The equal consideration of issues of gender, race, ethnicity, class, sexual orientation, and religion.

somatic symptom disorders Thoughts, feelings, and behaviours caused by excessive worry about physical signs and symptoms.

somatic therapies Also known as *sensorimotor psychotherapy*. These therapies combine talk therapy with body-centred interventions and movement to address dissociative symptoms.

somatization Emotional or psychological distress expressed as physical pain.

specific phobias High levels of anxiety or fear in response to specific objects or situations (e.g., an animal, dirt), activities (e.g., meeting strangers, leaving the familiar setting of a home), or physical situations (e.g., heights, open or closed spaces).

spiritual (religious) violence When someone uses an individual's spiritual beliefs to manipulate, dominate, or control that person.

splitting A primary defence or coping style used by people with borderline personality disorder. Splitting makes the person unable to incorporate positive and negative aspects of people (self or others) into a whole image.

standard drink 1.5 ounces of 40% alcohol comprises a standard drink.

standards of nursing practice Authoritative statements that promote, guide, direct, and regulate professional nursing practice.

stereotyped behaviours Repeated motor behaviours that do not presently serve a logical purpose.

stereotyping A generalized conscious or unconscious conceptualization of a group of people that does not allow for individual differences with the group.

stigma Negative attitudes or behaviours toward a person or group based on a belief that they possess negative traits.

stigmatized persons with medical conditions Patients assumed by health care workers to be bad, disgusting, or even just unusual; often include those who have mental illnesses, those who are HIV positive, and those who have undergone transgender surgeries or treatments.

stimulus control A strategy of adherence to five basic principles that decrease negative associations with the bed and bedroom and strengthen the stimulus for sleep.

stressors Psychological or physical stimuli that are incompatible with current functioning and require adaptation.

structural violence The existence of unequal power, restricted access to resources, and systematic oppression resulting in the denial of basic needs.

subpersonality Also called *alternate personality (alter)*. An additional personality within a single individual that has its own pattern of perceiving, relating to, and thinking about the self and the environment.

substance-induced anxiety disorder The onset of symptoms of anxiety, panic attacks, obsessions, or compulsions that develop with the use of a substance or within a month of discontinuing use of the substance.

substance/medication-induced depressive disorder A depressive disorder, such as major depressive disorder, that is a result of prolonged use of or withdrawal from drugs and alcohol.

suicidal behaviour Actions that cause self-harm (also referred to as self-injury) initiated with a clear intent to cause bodily harm or death by suicide.

suicidal ideation Also known as *suicidal thoughts*. These thoughts can range from a fleeting idea about one's own death (or about not being here) that does not include the act of killing oneself to a detailed plan, including the final act of killing oneself.

suicide The act of taking one's own life. Also called *death by suicide*.

sundowning Also known as *sundown syndrome*. Symptoms become more pronounced in the evening. This symptom-exacerbation pattern may occur in people who have either delirium or dementia.

superego One of three psychological processes that make up the Freudian system of personality (id, ego, superego). The superego consists of the conscience and the ego ideal. The superego represents the ideal rather than the real and seeks perfection rather than pleasure or reason.

support groups Groups (usually facilitated by a professional) that are structured for the purpose of providing members with the opportunity to maintain or enhance personal and social functioning through cooperation and shared understanding of life's challenges. Also called *self-help groups*.

supported-employment model A model of care that includes rapid job placement, on-the-job support, and provision of a job coach who is linked to the mental health team.

supportive psychotherapy An approach that stresses empathic understanding, a nonjudgemental attitude, and the development of a therapeutic alliance.

survivor A person who has endured abuse and recovered. This term recognizes the recovery and healing process that follows victimization.

survivors of suicide Family and friends of a person who has died by suicide.

survivorship A movement referencing a survival experience, not of an illness, but of the psychiatric system of care and treatment.

synapse Structure that permits a neuron (or nerve cell) to pass an electrical or chemical signal to another cell.

T

tangentiality A departure from the main topic to talk about less important information; going off on tangents in a way that takes the conversation off topic.

tardive dyskinesia (TD or TDK) A persistent extrapyramidal side effect that usually appears after prolonged treatment and persists even after the medication has been discontinued. TD consists of involuntary tonic muscular contractions that typically involve the tongue, fingers, toes, neck, trunk, or pelvis.

temperament The style of behaviour habitually used to adapt to the demands and expectations of the environment. This style is present in the infant, is modified by maturation, and develops in the context of the social environment.

termination phase The final, integral phase of the nurse–patient relationship, during which the patient and nurse summarize the achievement of goals and discuss the continued implementation by the patient of strategies learned.

tertiary care In terms of mental health care, provision of support for those who have experienced a severe crisis and are now recovering from a disabling mental state.

tertiary intervention In relation to suicide, interventions with the family and friends of a person who has died by suicide. Tertiary interventions aim to both reduce the traumatic aftereffects and explore effective means of addressing survivor problems using primary and secondary interventions.

tertiary prevention In regard to abuse, the facilitating of the healing and rehabilitative process through counselling of individuals and families, provision of support for groups of survivors, and provision of assistance to survivors of violence to achieve their optimal level of safety, health, and well-being.

therapeutic communication skills and strategies Communication that reflects the use of skills such as warmth, respect, and empathy and strategies such as using silence, recognizing strengths, and making observations.

therapeutic encounter A brief, informal meeting between nurse and patient that is useful and important for the patient.

therapeutic factors Aspects of the group experience that facilitate therapeutic change.

therapeutic games Specific games played with children that elicit children's fears and fantasies and help with assessment and treatment.

therapeutic index The ratio of the lethal dose to the effective dose; a measure of overall drug safety regarding the possibility of overdose or toxicity.

therapeutic relationship A relationship in which the nurse maximizes their communication skills, understanding of human behaviours, and personal strengths to enhance the patient's growth.

therapeutic touch A healing modality based on the premise that healing is promoted by balancing the body's energies through hand movements and direct energy (but no physical touch) to the energy field of the body.

therapeutic use of self One's individual, genuine ways of being with another person based on one's personal values and beliefs of humanity and enhanced by the application of microcommunication skills to guide the process of developing, maintaining, and terminating a therapeutic relationship.

tidal model A model that focuses on the interpersonal relationships as the context for recovery.

tolerance A physiological experience that occurs when a person's reaction to a substance decreases with repeated administrations of the same dose.

tort law Law developed from obligations to another.

traditional, complementary, and alternative medicine (TCAM) A system of medicine that recognizes that many of the philosophical underpinnings for different approaches are derived from both non-Western cultural traditions and newer concepts from quantum physics and studies in the nature of energy and reality, which have not historically been a part of conventional health care delivery.

transcranial magnetic stimulation (TMS) A noninvasive treatment modality that uses magnetic resonance imaging (MRI)-strength magnetic pulses to stimulate focal areas of the cerebral cortex.

transference The patient's experience of feelings toward the nurse or therapist that were originally held toward significant others in their life.

transgender An incongruence between a person's gender identity and the gender assigned at birth.

Transtheoretical Model of Change A behaviour change model that is the basis for developing effective interventions to promote health behaviour change in addictions services.

trauma Experiencing or witnessing events that threaten an individual's very survival (physical or psychological).

trauma-informed care Care focused on patients' past experiences of violence or trauma and the role this violence or trauma currently plays in their lives.

trauma-informed practice An approach that recognizes the impacts of previous traumatic events on current health and mental health situations.

tricyclic antidepressants (TCAs) Drugs that block the reuptake of norepinephrine for the secondary amines and both norepinephrine and serotonin for the tertiary amines.

two-spirit A term used by some Indigenous people to describe their gender, sexual, or spiritual identity; it refers to a person who embodies both a male and a female spirit.

typology of interpersonal violence Four modes in which the abuse of power may be inflicted: physical abuse, sexual abuse, psychological or emotional abuse, and deprivation or neglect. (Economic abuse is another mode in which violence can be inflicted.)

U

unconscious One of Freud's levels of awareness. The unconscious includes all repressed memories, passions, and unacceptable urges lying deep below the surface. The unconscious exerts a powerful yet unseen effect on the conscious thoughts and feelings of the individual.

unintentional torts Unintentional acts that produce injury or harm to another person.

utilitarianism Bringing about the greatest good and the least harm for the greatest number of people.

V

vagus nerve stimulation (VNS) Electrical stimulation of the vagus nerve to increase the level of neurotransmitters and improve mood.

values Abstract standards that represent an ideal, either positive or negative.

vegetative signs of depression Alterations in those activities necessary to support physical life and growth (e.g., change in bowel movements and eating habits, sleep disturbances, disinterest in sex).

verbal abuse When someone uses language, whether spoken or written, to cause harm to an individual.

verbal communication All the words a person speaks.

vicarious trauma A term used to describe the disruptions in thinking and perspectives of those who are exposed to the stories of people who are traumatized; it is of concern for nurses and others working with sexual assault victims.

violence Any action that has the intent to harm. It can be directed at self, others, or objects.

violence in the workplace Aggression, violence or harms that occur within the work environment.

violence-informed practice Recognition of the impact of prior violent or traumatic events on current experiences. See also trauma informed care.

virtual care A broad term that encompasses all the ways healthcare providers remotely interact with their patients.

virtue ethics An ethical theory that espouses that good people will make good decisions.

virtues Attitudes, dispositions, or character traits that enable us to be and to act in ways that develop ethical potential and ensure ethical outcomes.

vocational rehabilitation A program providing vocational training, financial support for attaining employment, or supported-employment services.

vulnerable person An adult or child who, as a result of illness, physical condition, or experiences, is at greater risk than the general population for being harmed.

W

waxy flexibility A condition in which a person remains in a position for an unusually long time after someone else places him or her in a position.

Weir Report A report released in 1932 by the Canadian Medical Association and the Canadian Nurses Association. It concluded that drastic changes to nursing education programs were needed, including the standardization of curriculum, work hours, and instructor training, and that the care of people with mental illnesses needed to be integrated into all generalist programs.

Western tradition A world view based on the scientific biomedical model and aligned with values of autonomy, individualization, and independence.

William Tuke Eighteenth-century reformer who, along with Philippe Pinel, introduced the moral treatment era of psychiatry, which attempted to focus on providing peaceful, nurturing environments for people with mental illness.

withdrawal The experiences and physiological changes that occur when blood and tissue concentrations of a drug decrease in individuals who have maintained heavy and prolonged use of a substance.

word salad A jumble of words that is meaningless to the listener—and perhaps to the speaker as well—because of an extreme level of disorganization.

working phase The phase of the nurse–patient relationship during which the nurse and patient identify and explore areas that are causing problems in the patient's life.

workplace violence Acts of aggression or violence by patients directed at staff or others.

world view A major paradigm that is used to explain the world and its mysteries, including beliefs about health, illness, and the hereafter. The major world views used to explain health and illness phenomena are attributed to the paradigms of magic and religion, empirical science, and holistic health.

2SLGBTQQIA (two-spirit, lesbian, gay, bisexual, transgender, queer, questioning, intersex, and asexual.

INDEX

Page numbers followed by "*f*" indicate figures, "*t*" indicate tables, and "*b*" indicate boxes.

A

AA. *See* Alcoholics Anonymous
Abandonment, 101
ABCD-ER mnemonic tool, for abuse screening, 491, 493*b*
Abilify. *See* Aripiprazole
Abnormal Involuntary Movement Scale (AIMS), 172, 290, 293*f*
Abnormal motor behaviour, with schizophrenia, 272
Aboriginal peoples
   alcoholism prevalence statistics in, 354
   federal government funding mental health care for, 25
Abstraction, 79*b*–80*b*
Abuse
   as adventitious crisis, 434
   case study and nursing care plan in, 502*b*–504*b*
   comorbidity of, 487*b*, 487
   define, 482
   epidemiology of, 485
   myth vs. fact in, 494*t*
   nursing process application in, 489
      assessment in, 489, 490*b*
      diagnosis in, 495
      evaluation in, 502
      implementation in, 496
      outcomes identification in, 496, 496*t*
      planning in, 496
   power and control in, 488, 489*f*
   prevention of, 499
   reporting, 496
   screening tools in, 491, 492*f*
Abuse Assessment Screen, 491, 492*f*
Acamprosate (Campral), 374
Accepting, as therapeutic communication technique, 143*t*–144*t*
Access to care
   as key strategy area for Canadian mental health care, 7, 8*b*
   of older adults, 559
Accidents
   concurrent with substance abuse disorders, 354
   due to sleep deprivation, 414
Accountability, of health care workers, 126
Acetylcholine (ACh), 156, 157*t*
   in anger and aggression, 468
   depression and, 225
   first-generation antipsychotic drugs and, 171
   reduction of, 158*b*
   tricyclic drugs and, 168
Acetylcholinesterase, 156, 341
Acrophobia, 188*t*
Actigraphy, 418
Action phase, of Transtheoretical Model of Change, 370–371

Action potential, 156
Active listening, as therapeutic communication technique, 140
Active negativism, 279
Acupuncture, 646, 648
Acute care, 311
   for anorexia nervosa, 311
   for bulimia nervosa, 315
Acute chemical impairment, 359*b*
Acute confusion
   with dementia, 329
   NOC outcomes related to, 330*t*
Acute confusional state, 326
Acute dystonia, from conventional antipsychotics, 290, 291*t*–292*t*
Acute intoxication, assessment of, 358*b*, 358
Acute phase
   of bipolar disorders
      implementation for, 258, 259*t*
      outcomes identification in, 257
      planning in, 258
   of depression, 232
   of manic episodes, 258
   of rape-trauma syndrome, 510, 511*b*
   of schizophrenia, 275, 283, 284, 284*t*
      interventions, 284
      setting, 284
Acute stress disorder, description of, 185, 196*b*, 196
AD. *See* Alzheimer's disease
Adapting, resilience and, 5
Adaptive servo-ventilation (ASV), 418
Adaptive uses, of defences, 186*t*–187*t*
Addiction, 351
   comprehensive conceptualization of, 351, 352*f*
   definition of, 352
   development, process of, 351, 353*f*
      excessive use, 352
      experimentation, 352
      integrated use, 352
      no contact, 351
   helping patients change and, 369
   psychological changes due to, 369
   self-assessment and self-awareness due to, 369
   services, funding of, 25
Addiction supportive housing (ASH), 382
Adenosine, 417
ADHD. *See* Attention deficit-hyperactivity disorder
Adherence
   to medication, 37
   as treatment issues, in serious mental illness, 576*b*
Admission assessment, by psychiatric nurse, 36
Admission criteria, for hospitalization, 30
Adolescent-onset conduct disorder, 547
Adolescents, 533

Adolescents (Continued)
   anxiety disorders in, 550
      assessment guidelines for, 550*b*
      generalized anxiety disorder (GAD), 550
      Nursing Outcomes Classification (*NOC*) for, 551*t*
      separation anxiety disorder, 543*b*, 550
   assessment of, 77*b*, 77
   bipolar and related disorders in, 551
   bipolar disorders in, 251*t*, 252
   characteristics of mentally healthy, 537*b*
   depression in, 223
      assessment of, 229–230
   depressive disorders in, 551
   disorders of, 533
      brain development and biochemicals in, 536
      comorbidity of, 534
      cultural factors, 536
      environmental factors, 536
      epidemiology of, 534
      genetic factors in, 535
      resilience factors, 536
      temperament in, 536
   disruptive, impulse control, and conduct disorders in, 546
      adolescent-onset conduct disorder, 547
      bullying, 547
      childhood-onset conduct disorder, 547
      conduct disorders, 547, 548*b*
      nursing process application to, 548*b*, 548, 548*t*
      oppositional defiant disorder, 546, 548*b*
      techniques for managing, 549*b*
   feeding and eating disorders, 551
   gender dysphoria in, 526*b*
   hostility toward lesbian, gay, bisexual and transgender, and queer, 537*b*
   mood disorders in, 551
   neurodevelopmental disorders in, 542
      attention deficit-hyperactivity disorder (ADHD), 543*b*, 543, 545*b*, 547*b*
      autism spectrum disorders, 542
      communication disorders, 542
      intellectual disabilities, 542
      motor disorders, 544
      Nursing Outcomes Classification (*NOC*) for, 546*t*
      nursing process application to, 544, 545*b*, 545*t*
      specific learning disorder (SLD), 544
      stereotypic movement disorder, 544
      Tourette's disorder, 544
   post-traumatic stress disorder (PTSD) in, 543*b*, 551
   psychiatric mental health nursing, 536
      assessment data in, 538*b*, 538
      behavioural therapy, 539
      bibliotherapy, 541–542

Adolescents *(Continued)*
    cognitive behavioural therapy, 539
    cultural factors in, 539
    data collection in, 537
    developmental assessment in, 538
    family therapy, 539
    group therapy, 539
    medication treatment of, 543*b*
    mental status examination in, 538
    milieu management, 540*b*, 540
    mind-body therapies, 540
    mutual storytelling, 541*b*, 541
    play therapy, 541
    principle of least restrictive intervention, 539
    psychopharmacology, 542
    quiet room, 540
    risk assessment in, 539
    seclusion and restraint in, 540
    therapeutic drawing, 542
    therapeutic games, 541, 542*b*
    time out, 540
  risk factors for mental illness in, 534, 535*b*
  use of antidepressant drugs by, 241
  yoga for, 541*b*
Adrenal cortex, stress response and, 61
Adrenal glands, role of, in mental function, 155
α_1-adrenergic receptors, 171
α_2-adrenergic receptors, 168–169
Adults, gender dysphoria in, 526*b*
Adult support programs, 568–569
Advance directives, 97
  in Canadian hospice palliative care treatment model, 594
  nursing responsibilities with, 97
Advanced-practice interventions, 418*b*, 427
  for anorexia nervosa, 312
  for bulimia nervosa, 315
  in sexual assault, 518
  in violence and abuse, 500
Advanced-practice nursing (APN), 21, 626
Advanced-practice psychiatric mental health nurses, as members of psychiatric mental health treatment teams, 34*b*
Advanced-practice psychiatric mental health nurses interventions, 11*t*
Adverse childhood experiences (ACEs), 64
Adverse effects, of lithium carbonate, 170
Advice, giving, 142, 145*t*
Affect
  assessment of, during mental status examination, 79*b*–80*b*
  depression assessment of, 229
Affection, for managing disruptive behaviours, in children and adolescents, 549*b*
Affective blunting, in schizophrenia, 279*t*
Affective disorders, 220
Affective symptoms, of schizophrenia, 276, 280
Age, considerations for, during assessments, 76
Ageism
  and drug testing, 560

Ageism *(Continued)*
  older adult, 559
  and public policy, 560
Aggravated sexual assault, definition of, 508
Aggression, 465
  behavioural theories, 469
  biological factors, 468
  case management, 472
  cognitive and cognitive behavioural theories, 469
  comorbidity, 467
  de-escalation techniques for, 472*b*, 472
  defining, 465, 482
  engaging patient, 473
  health teaching and health promotion, 471
  implementation, 471
  inpatient psychiatric settings, 476
  nursing diagnosis, 471
  nursing outcomes, 471
  nursing process application to, 470, 471*b*, 473*b*, 475*b*, 476*b*–477*b*
  patients with neurocognitive disorders, 477
  personality theory, 469
  pharmacological interventions, 473
  physical interventions, 474
  planning interventions, 471
  quiet rooms, 472
  safety and, 32
  social learning theories, 470
  sociocultural factors, 470
  words describing different types of, 465
Aggressive behaviour
  goals with personality disorders, 404*t*
  with personality disorders, 402, 404*t*, 406*b*, 407*t*
Aging. *See also* Older adults
  as challenge to psychiatric mental health nurses, 11
  facts and myths about, 556*b*
  and frailty in first nations communities, 556*b*
  major theories of, 555, 556*b*
  mental health issues related to, 556
    anxiety disorders, 557
    depression in, 557
    late-life mental illness in, 556
    substance use disorders, 557
    suicide risk, 557
  normal, major neurocognitive disorder vs., 332*t*
  of population, 555
Agitation
  with delirium, 328
  with dementia, 336–337
Agnosia, 335
Agonist, 164–165
  buspirone as, 166
Agoraphobia, 185–188, 188*b*, 188*t*
Agranulocytosis, 290
  from conventional antipsychotic, 291*t*–292*t*
Agreement, element of LEAP approach, 271
Aguilera, Donna, 433
Akathisia
  from conventional antipsychotics, 290, 291*t*–292*t*
  suicide and, 455
Al-Anon, 380–381, 383*b*–384*b*

Alateen, 380–381
Alcohol abuse
  CAGE-AID screening tool, 557
  Michigan Alcoholism Screening Test-Geriatric Version (MAST-G), 558*b*
  as most prevalent substance abuse disorder, 354
  by older adults, 557, 558*b*
  pharmacological interventions during, 374
Alcohol dependence, with depression, case study on, 383*b*–384*b*
Alcohol intoxication, effects in non-tolerant individuals, 360–361, 362*t*
Alcohol poisoning
  prevalence statistics in Canada, 360
  signs and symptoms of, 360
Alcohol-related neurodevelopmental disorder (ARND), 355
Alcohol use
  in LGBTQ, 529
  in violence and abuse, 495
Alcohol withdrawal
  alcohol withdrawal delirium, 362–363
  benzodiazepines for, 166
  signs and symptoms of, 360, 360*t*–361*t*
Alcoholics Anonymous (AA), 380, 381*b*, 558
  by older adults, 557, 558*b*
Alcoholism
  Michigan Alcoholism Screening Test-Geriatric Version (MAST-G), 558*b*
  prevalence statistics in Canada, 354
All-or-nothing thinking, 51*t*
  in cognitive distortions, 311*b*
Allies, 525
Allopathic medicine, 645
Alogia, in schizophrenia, 279*t*
Alprazolam (Xanax), 165, 166*f*, 212*b*–214*b*
Alterations
  in behaviour, 279
  in perception, 278
  in speech, 276–278
  in thinking, 276
Alternate personality (alter), 199
Altruism, 621*b*
  as defence mechanism, 186*t*–187*t*
Alzheimer's disease (AD), 332, 332*t*
  brain injury and, 334
  in Canada, 334
  drugs for, 174
  environmental factors in, 334
  epidemiology of, 334
  genetic factors in, 334
  genetics in, 334
  as most common cause of dementia, 332
  positron emission tomography scan of brain with, 161, 163*f*
  progression of, 333
  stages of, 333, 333*t*
  symptoms of, 335
Alzheimer Society of Canada, 338
Amino acids, 157*t*
Amitriptyline hydrochloride (Elavil), 212*b*–214*b*, 236*b*–237*b*, 238
Amphetamines, 174, 417
  description and medical uses for, 366

Amygdala, emotions and psychological function and, 158–159
β-amyloid, 161
Anergia
  in schizophrenia, 279t
  with seasonal affective disorder, 221
Anger, 465, 481–482
  behavioural theories, 469
  during bereavement, 603t
  biological factors, 468
  case management, 472
  cognitive and cognitive behavioural theories, 469
  comorbidity, 467
  as counter-transference, 127t
  de-escalation techniques for, 472b, 472
  depression and, 229
  engaging patient, 473
  escalates, safety when, 128–130, 130t
  etiology of, 468
  health teaching and health promotion, 471
  implementation, 471
  inpatient psychiatric settings, 476
  nursing diagnosis, 471
  nursing outcomes, 471
  nursing process application to, 470, 471b, 473b, 475b–477b
  patients with neurocognitive disorders, 477
  personality theory, 469
  pharmacological interventions, 473
  physical interventions, 474
  planning interventions, 471
  psychological factors and, 468
  quiet rooms, 472
  social learning theories, 470
  sociocultural factors, 470
Anger control assistance, interventions for, 406b
Anhedonia
  depression and, 228
  in schizophrenia, 279t
Animal-assisted therapy, 649b
Animistic charms, 17
Anorexia nervosa, 305, 308
  acute care in, 311
  advanced-practice interventions for, 312
  assessment of, 308, 310b
  case study and nursing care plan for, 317
  characteristics of, 305b
  clinical picture of, 304
  cognitive distortions in, 311b
  comorbidity of, 307
  criteria for hospital admission of, 309b
  culture and, 5–6
  depression co-occurring with, 234t
  diagnosis of, 310
  epidemiology of, 305
  etiology of, 307
  evaluation of, 313
  general assessment for, 309
  health teaching and health promotion for, 311
  implementation in, 311
  medical complications of, 309b
  milieu management of, 311
  NOC outcomes related to, 310t

Anorexia nervosa (Continued)
  nursing process, application of, 308
  outcomes identification of, 310
  pharmacological interventions for, 311
  planning of, 310
  psychosocial interventions for, 311b, 311
  psychotherapy for, 312
  self-assessment of, 310
  signs and symptoms of, 309t
  state of treatment for, 312t
  thoughts and behaviours associated with, 308b
  vignette in, 311b–312b
Anosognosia, 280, 573, 576
Antagonism, vs. compliance, 401, 402t
Antagonist, 164–165
  buspirone as, 166
Anthony, Dr. William, on recovery model for depression, 232
Antiandrogens, in gender dysphoria, 527
Anti-anxiety (anxiolytic) drugs, 164
  for anxiety disorders, 212b–214b, 214–215
  for bipolar disorders, 262
  gamma-aminobutyric acid as, 164–165
Anticholinergic-induced delirium, from antipsychotics, 290, 291t–292t
Anticholinesterase drugs, for Alzheimer's disease, 174
Anticipatory grief
  dementia and, 336
  signs of, 599b, 599
Anticonvulsants, 262
  for anxiety disorders, 212b–214b, 215
  for bipolar disorders, 262, 263b
Antidepressant drugs, 234
  for anxiety disorders, 166, 167f, 212b–214b, 214
  for bulimia nervosa, 315
  monoamine oxidase inhibitors (MAOIs) as, 167, 169, 236b–237b, 239, 240b
  selective serotonin reuptake inhibitors (SSRIs) as, 166, 168, 236b–237b, 237
  serotonin and norepinephrine disinhibitors (SNDIs) as, 168
  serotonin-norepinephrine reuptake inhibitors (SNRIs) as, 166, 168, 236b–237b, 237
  for sleep disorders, 426t
  suicide risk and, 170
  tricyclic antidepressants, 167, 168f, 236b–237b, 238, 239b
  use by children and adolescents, 241
  use by older adults, 241
  use by pregnant women, 240
Antidepressants, 166
Antidipsotropics, 374
Antihistamines
  for anxiety disorders, 212b–214b, 215
  for sleep disorders, 426t
Anti-manic agents, 290
Antipsychotics
  first-generation, 171, 172f
  for schizophrenia, 288
    adjuncts to, 290

Antipsychotics (Continued)
  atypical, 288, 289t
  conventional, 289, 289t, 291t–292t
  issues in, 288
  potentially dangerous responses to, 290b, 290
  when to change, 290
  second-generation, 172f, 173
  aripiprazole (Abilify), 173
  clozapine (Clozaril) as, 173
  olanzapine (Zyprexa) as, 173
  paliperidone (Invega) as, 173
  quetiapine, 173
  risperidone (Risperdal) as, 173
  ziprasidone (Zeldox) as, 173
Anti-seizure drugs, for bipolar disorder, 171
Anti-social personality disorder (ASPD)
  characteristics and behaviours associated with, 391, 397, 398b
  nursing and therapy guidelines for, 398, 405t
  treatment of, 398
Anti-stigma practice, 110–111
Anxiety, 181, 199
  clinical picture on, 185
  defences against, 184, 186t–187t
  defined by Sullivan, 46
    application of, by Peplau, 47
  definition of, 181
  depression assessment of, 228
  disorders, 185
  drugs for, 165
    antidepressants as, 166
    selective serotonin reuptake inhibitors (SSRIs), for, 166
  due to non-psychiatric medical conditions, 189, 190t
  in eating and feeding disorder, 307
  fear vs., 181
  flowchart illustrating, 185f
  levels of, 182, 184t
    case study and nursing care plan for, 182b–183b
    mild, 182, 184t, 208, 208t
    moderate, 182, 184t, 208, 208t
  NANDA-I classifications of, 437
  normal, 182
  operationally defined, 64f
  panic, 182, 184t, 208, 209t
  reduction techniques in crisis situation, 439
  related to hospitalization, 475
  schizophrenia and, 273
  self-control, in anorexia nervosa, 310t
  with serious medical illness, 588b, 588
  severe, 182, 184t, 208, 209t
  in Sigmund Freud's psychoanalytic theory, 42
  in violence, 494
Anxiety disorders, 180
  applying nursing process to, 201
  assessment of, 201, 202b, 202t, 203f, 204t–205t
  evaluation for, 216
  implementation for, 207, 208t–209t
  nursing diagnosis of, 205, 206t–207t
  outcomes of, 205, 207t

Anxiety disorders *(Continued)*
    planning for, 205
    behavioural therapy for, 215–216
    case study and nursing care plan for, 182b–183b
    in children and adolescents, 550
        assessment guidelines for, 550b
        generalized anxiety disorder (GAD), 550
        Nursing Outcomes Classification (NOC) for, 551t
        separation anxiety disorder, 543b, 550
    cognitive therapy for, 216
    comorbidity of, 190
    counselling for, 210
    culture-bound syndromes, 201
    drug treatment for, 212b–214b
    epidemiology of, 190
    etiology of, 199
        biological factors in, 199
        environmental factors in, 200
        psychological factors in, 200
        sociocultural factors in, 200, 201b
    health teaching and health promotion for, 210
    integrative therapy for, 215, 215b
    milieu therapy for, 212
    pharmacological interventions for, 212
        anti-anxiety drugs, 212b–214b, 212
        antidepressants, 212b–214b, 214
    psychosocial interventions for, 210, 211b
    selective serotonin-norepinephrine reuptake inhibitors for, 212b–214b
    selective serotonin reuptake inhibitors for, 212b–214b, 214
    self-care promotion for, 212
        elimination, 212
        nutrition and fluid intake, 212
        personal hygiene and grooming, 212
        sleep, 212
    suicide risk in, 450
    types of
        acute stress disorder, 196b, 196
        agoraphobia, 185–188, 188b
        generalized anxiety disorder, 188, 189b, 189t
        obsessive-compulsive disorders, 193b, 193, 195t
        panic attack, 185b, 185
        panic disorder, 185b, 185
        phobias, 188b, 188, 188t
        post-traumatic stress disorder, 196
        substance-induced anxiety disorder, 189
Anxiolytics, 214–215
Apathy, in dementia, 337t
Aphasia, 335
Apiphobia, 188t
APN. *See* Advanced-practice nursing
Appearance, assessment of, during mental status examination, 79b–80b
Appetite
    changes with depression, 229
    serotonin regulating, 224–225
Approachability, in abuse screening, 493b
Approval, giving, 142, 145t
Apraxia, 335

Aripiprazole (Abilify), 173
    for bipolar disorders, 263b
    for schizophrenia, 288–289, 289t
ARND. *See* Alcohol-related neurodevelopmental disorder
Aromatherapy, 652
Art therapists, as members of psychiatric mental health treatment teams, 34b
Asenapine (Saphris), 174
ASH. *See* Addiction supportive housing
ASPD. *See* Anti-social personality disorder
Assault, 100, 100t
    define, 482
    violence and, 466
Assent, in child health care decision making, 535
Assertive communication, 146
Assertive community treatment, 31b–32b, 31
    for serious mental illness, 578
Assessment
    of adolescents, 77b, 77
    age considerations in, 76
    of anorexia nervosa, 308, 310b
    of bulimia nervosa, 313, 314b
    of children, 76
    cultural and social, 81
    language barriers and, 77
    of older adults, 77
    in psychiatric mental health, purpose of, 77
    psychosocial, 80, 81b
    rating scales for, 82, 83t
    religious, 80
    of schizophrenia, 275, 277f
    spiritual, 80
    standards of practice and, 75
    validation of, 82
Assimilation, 107
Association of Registered Nurses of Newfoundland and Labrador, 21
Associative looseness, 276–278
    counselling and communication techniques for, 286
Astraphobia, 188t
Asylums, 16–17
    Canadian, early, 17
    introduction of nurses to, 18
Ataque de nervios, 115
Atenolol (Tenormin), 212b–214b
Atlantic Canada, history of psychiatric nursing licensing in, 19
Atomoxetine (Strattera), 174
Atonia
    muscle during REM sleep, 416
    rapid eye movement behaviour disorder and, 420
Attending behaviour, for patient's growth, 133–134
Attention, 79b–80b
    norepinephrine modulating, 224–225
Attention deficit-hyperactivity disorder (ADHD), 418–419
    assessment guidelines in, 545b
    as comorbid condition, 534
    description of, 543
    drugs for, 174, 543b, 547b
    prevalence statistics of, in Canada, 9t

Attitude
    in abuse screening, 493b
    behaviours in personality and, 402t
Atypical antipsychotics, 273
    for anorexia nervosa, 311
    aripiprazole (Abilify), 263b
    for bipolar disorders, 262, 263b
    olanzapine (Zyprexa), 263b
    quetiapine fumarate (Seroquel), 263b
    risperidone (Risperdal), 263b
    for schizophrenia, 288, 289t
    ziprasidone (Zeldox), 263b
Atypical features, with major depressive disorder, 221
Atypicals, 173
Auditory functions, area of brain responsible for, 159f
Auditory hallucinations, 278, 278t
    coping with, 286b–287b
    with major depressive disorder, 221
Aura, 653
Authorization of treatment, 95
Autism spectrum disorders, 542, 543b
Autocratic leader, 623
Automatic obedience, 279
Automatic thoughts, 50
Autonomic dysfunction, from conventional antipsychotics, 291t–292t
Autonomic nervous system, regulation of, 154, 155f
Autonomic physiological responses, as non-verbal behaviour, 139t
Autonomy
    defined, 91–92
    principle of, 96
    respect for, 90
Autoreceptors, 158
Aversion therapy, 49
Avoidance training, 49
Avoidant personality disorder
    characteristics and behaviours associated with, 391, 400b, 400
    nursing and therapy guidelines for, 400, 405t
    treatment of, 400
Avoidant/restrictive food intake disorder, 305
Avolition, in schizophrenia, 279t
Awareness, levels of, in Sigmund Freud's psychoanalytic theory, 42, 42f
Ayurvedic medicine, 647

B

Baby boomers, 555
Bachelor of science degrees in nursing (BScN), 20
Baclofen, 374
Bad medicine, 115
BALs. *See* Blood alcohol levels
Bandura, Albert, 55t–56t
Bariatric surgery, for binge eating disorder, 316, 317b
Barriers
    to accurate pain assessment, in older adults, 560
    to treatment, as future issue in psychiatric mental health care, 37

INDEX

Barry, Pat, 21
Basal ganglia, 160
Bath salts, description and medical uses for, 366
Bathing, in guidelines for self-care for individuals with cognitive impairment, 340b–341b
Battery
 in cycle of violence, 485
 liability issues with, 100, 100t
 signs of, 483
Battlefords and District Co-operative Ltd. v. Gibbs, 93
BDNF. *See* Brain-derived neurotrophic factor
Beauport asylum, 17
Beck, Aaron T., 50, 50f
Beck's cognitive triad, 226
Beers, Clifford W., 7
Behavioural contract, for managing disruptive behaviours, in children and adolescents, 549b
Behavioural crises, management of, 37
Behavioural family therapy, 636, 637t
Behavioural health home care, 569
Behavioural theories, 48, 469
 of anxiety disorders, 200
 behaviourism theory as, 48
 classical conditioning theory as, 48, 48f
 implications of, in nursing practice, 49
 operant conditioning theory as, 48, 48f
Behavioural therapy, 48
 for anxiety disorders, 215–216
 aversion therapy as, 49
 biofeedback as, 49
 for children and adolescents, 539
 modelling, 49
 operant conditioning, 49, 49t
 systematic desensitization as, 49
Behaviours
 assessment of, during mental status examination, 79b–80b
 attitudes in personality and, 401, 402t
 bipolar disorders and, 255b, 255
 with delirium, 328
 with dementia, 336–337, 337t
  medications for, 342
 non-verbal, 139, 139t
 norepinephrine modulating, 224–225
Behaviourism theory, 48
Beliefs
 in abuse screening, 493b
 in therapeutic relationships, 126
Belongingness, need for, 54
Beneficence, 90, 97
Benner, Patricia, 47t
Benson, Herbert, 67
Benson's relaxation technique, 67, 68b
Benzodiazepines (sedative-hypnotics), 165, 166f, 375–376
 for anxiety disorders, 212b–214b
 for schizophrenia, 290
 for sleep disorders, 426t
Bereavement, 601
 communication and, 604b
 depression with, 222–223
 exclusion, 222–223

Bereavement *(Continued)*
 guidelines for dealing with, 605b
 phenomena experienced during, 603t
Best action principle, 91
Best practice
 establishing, 94
 standards of practice, 94
Beta-blockers, for anxiety disorders, 212b–214b, 215
Bettelheim, Bruno, 54
Bias, cultural, 146
Bibliotherapy, 541–542
Biigajiiskaan, 108, 110b
Bilevel positive airway pressure (BPAP), 418
Binet, Alfred, 44
Binet Intelligence Test, 44
Binge eating disorder, 305, 316
 bariatric surgery for, 316, 317b
 characteristics of, 305b
 clinical picture of, 304
 comorbidity of, 307
 epidemiology of, 305
 etiology of, 307
 state of treatment for, 312t
Biochemical factors, with depression, 224, 225f
Bioethics, 90–91
Biofeedback, 648
 as behavioural therapy, 49
 as relaxation technique, 69
Biofield energy, 653
Biologic endowment, as key social determinant of health, 12
Biological approach, 153
Biological factors
 in aggression and violence, 468
 with depression, 224
 in eating and feeding disorders, 307
 in non-suicidal self-injury, 459
 with substance use disorders, 355, 356f
 in suicide, 452
Biological interventions, during psychiatric mental health nursing process, 85
Biological model, 54
 implications of, for nursing practice, 54
Biological theories, 54
 advent of psychopharmacology and, 54
 biological model and, 54
Biological therapy, as basic-level psychiatric mental health nursing intervention, 11t
Biologically based integrative therapies, 650
 aromatherapy as, 652
 diet and nutrition as, 650
 herbal therapy as, 650
 megavitamin therapy as, 650
Biologically based mental illness, 572
Biopsychiatry
 as biological approach to nervous system malfunctions, 153
 and psychotropic drugs, 153
Biopsychosocial assessment, 33, 34b
Biopsychosocial care manager, 35
Biopsychosocial model, 33
Bipolar disorders, 171, 249
 acute phase of

Bipolar disorders *(Continued)*
  implementation for, 258, 259t
  outcomes identification in, 257
  planning in, 258
 advanced-practice interventions, 264
 anti-seizure drugs for, 171
 behavioural symptoms of, 255
 biological factors of, 252
 carbamazepine for, 171
 in children and adolescents, 551
 clinical picture on, 249
  bipolar I disorder, 249, 251b
  bipolar II disorder, 250
  cyclothymic disorder, 251
 cognitive symptoms of, 256
 comorbidity of, 252
 continuation phase of
  implementation for, 258
  outcomes identification in, 258
  planning in, 258
 continuum symptoms of, 250f
 cultural considerations for, 253b
 drug treatment for, 170
 electroconvulsive therapy for, 262
 environmental factors of, 253
 epidemiology of, 251, 251t
 etiology of, 252
 euphoric mood associated with, 255
 flight of ideas and, 256
 genetics and, 252
 health teaching and health promotion for, 264b, 264
 hypomania in
  behaviour symptoms of, 255
  with bipolar II disorder, 250
  transition to mania, 255
 lamotrigine for, 171
 lithium carbonate, 170
 maintenance phase of
  implementation for, 260
  outcomes identification in, 258
  planning in, 258
 milieu management for, 262
 Mood Disorder Questionnaire for, 254f, 254
 nursing process application to, 254
  assessment in, 254, 254f, 257b
  case study and nursing care plan for, 265b
  evaluation for, 265
  implementation for, 258
  nursing diagnosis of, 256, 257t
  outcomes identification in, 257
  planning in, 258
 pharmacological interventions for, 260, 263b
  anti-anxiety drugs, 262
  anticonvulsant drugs, 262, 263b
  atypical antipsychotics, 262
  lithium carbonate, 260, 261b, 261t, 263b
  omega-3 fatty acids, 263b
 prevalence statistics of, in Canada, 9t
 psychological factors of, 253
 psychotherapy for, 264
 suicide risk in, 450

Bipolar disorders *(Continued)*
    support groups for, 264
    thought and speech symptoms of, 256
    valproate for, 171
Bipolar I disorder, 249
    comorbidity of, 252
    diagnostic criteria for, 251b
Bipolar II disorder, 250
    comorbidity of, 252
Bisexual, 525
    hostility toward, 537b
Black Lives Matter movement, 12
Bladder function, in guidelines for self-care for individuals with cognitive impairment, 340b–341b
Blame
    during family therapy, 633b
    in sexual assault, 515
Bleuler, Eugen, coined the term schizophrenia, 272
Blood alcohol content (BAC), 362t
Blood alcohol levels (BALs), testing of, 358
Blurred boundaries, 125, 125t
Blurred vision, from conventional antipsychotics, 291t–292t
Body language
    during clinical interview, 149
    as non-verbal behaviour, 139t
Borderline personality disorder (BPD)
    case study and nursing care plan on, 408b–410b
    characteristics and behaviours associated with, 391, 394, 397b
    nursing and therapy guidelines for, 396, 405t
    pathological personality traits seen in, 395, 396
    treatment of, 397
Boredom, as counter-transference, 127t
Boundaries
    blurred, 125, 125t
    establishing, 124
    in family therapies, 632, 633b
    relationship, 124
    self-check on, 126, 128f
Boundary impairment, 278
Bowel function, in guidelines for self-care for individuals with cognitive impairment, 340b–341b
Brain
    activities of, 154
    biopsychiatry and, 153
    cellular composition of, 156, 156f
    control of biological drives and behaviour in, 155
    development and biochemicals, in child and adolescent disorders, 536
    functions of, 154b, 154
    homeostasis in, maintenance of, 154
    lobes and associated functions of, 159, 160f
    organization of, 158
        brainstem in, 158, 159f
        cerebellum, 159, 159f–160f
        cerebrum, 159, 160f
    structure of, 154

Brain *(Continued)*
    visualization of, 160, 161t, 162f–163f
Brain-derived neurotrophic factor (BDNF), monoamines and, 170
Brain imaging, 335
Brain injury
    delirium, major neurocognitive disorders, depression, comparison of, 325t
    traumatic, in Alzheimer's disease, 334
Brain structure abnormalities, 273
Brain structure and function, bipolar disorders and, 253
Brainstem, 158, 159f
Breach of duty, 101
Breathing exercises, 68b, 68
Breathing-related disorders, 420
    affecting sleep, 420
Brexpiprazole, for schizophrenia, 288–289
Brief psychotic disorder, 272b
Brief therapies, 52–53, 53b
BScN. *See* Bachelor of science degrees in nursing
Bulimia nervosa, 305, 313
    acute care for, 315
    advanced-practice interventions for, 315
    assessment of, 313, 314b
    case study and nursing care plan for, 319b–320b
    characteristics of, 305b
    clinical picture of, 304
    comorbidity of, 307
    counselling for, 315
    diagnosis of, 314
    epidemiology of, 305
    etiology of, 307
    evaluation of, 316
    general assessment of, 313
    health teaching and health promotion for, 315
    implementation in, 315
    medical complications of, 313b
    NOC outcomes related to, 315t
    nursing process, application of, 313
    outcomes identification of, 314
    pharmacological interventions for, 315
    planning for, 315
    psychotherapy for, 315
    self-assessment of, 314
    signs and symptoms of, 314t
    state of treatment for, 312t
    thoughts and behaviours associated with, 314b
    vignette in, 313b, 315b
Bullycide, 450
    suicide and, 450
Bullying, 466
    in children and adolescents, 547
    culture in schools, 466
Buprenorphine (Suboxone), 375
Bupropion (Wellbutrin), 236b–237b
    for bulimia nervosa, 315
    for depression, 169
Burden on family, in dementia, 337t
Buspirone (BuSpar), 166, 166f
    as alternative to addictive benzodiazepines, 215

Buspirone hydrochloride (Bustab), 212b–214b

C

Caffeine
    addiction to, 367
    physical complications related to abuse of, 355t
    reduction/cessation of intake of, as stress buster, 64b
CAGE-AID Screening Tool, for substance abuse, 557
Calgary Family Assessment Model (CFAM), 632, 639f
Calgary Family Intervention Model (CFIM), 632
Callousness, 397–398
CAM. *See* Confusion Assessment Method
Canada
    correctional nursing in, 614
    cultural landscape of, 111
    forensic mental health system in, 613
Canada Health Act, 25, 89
Canada's Fentanyl public health crisis, 364b
Canadian Association for Suicide Prevention, 456b
Canadian Association of Schools of Nursing (CASN), 20–21
Canadian Community Health Survey (CCHS), 24
Canadian Council of Psychiatric Nurses (CCPN), 20
Canadian Federation of Mental Health Nurses (CFMHN), 20–21, 95
    standards of practice, 10, 20–21
Canadian Gerontological Nursing Association, 563
Canadian Holistic Nurses Association (CHNA), 647
Canadian Hospice Palliative Care Association (CHPCA), 594
Canadian Human Rights Tribunal (CHRT), 107
Canadian Index of Wellbeing (CIW), 63–64
Canadian Medical Association, 18–19
Canadian Mental Health Association (CMHA), 7
    housing and support established by, 27
Canadian National Association of Trained Nurses, 18
Canadian Network for Mood and Anxiety Treatments (CANMAT), 262
Canadian Nurses Association (CNA), 18
    on addiction in the workplace, 385
    certification by, 21
    code of ethics, 90b, 90–91
    confidentiality and, 98
    culture and, 105–106
    history of, 18–19
    standards of practice set by, 10
Canadian Nurses Protective Society (CNPS), 101–102
Canadian Perspectives Survey Series (CPSS), 24

Cancer
    anxiety caused by, 194*t*
    pain, visual analogue scale for, 563*f*
CANMAT. *See* Canadian Network for Mood and Anxiety Treatments
Cannabis sativa, 367
Cannon, Walter, 59
Cannon's theory, 59–61
Carbamazepine (Tegretol), 171, 212*b*–214*b*
    for bipolar disorders, 262, 263*b*
Cardiovascular diseases
    anxiety caused by, 194*t*
    in dementia, 334
    depression co-occurring with, 223*t*
    that may mimic psychiatric illness, 78*b*
Care theory, ethics of, 45
Caregiver
    families as, 631
    role strain, in dementia, 336
    service, for dementia, 341*t*
Caregiver burden
    for older adults, 559
    serious mental illness and, 575
Caring, during end-of-life (EOL) care, 596
Cariprazine, for schizophrenia, 288–289
Case management, 36
    as basic-level nursing intervention, 27
CASN. *See* Canadian Association of Schools of Nursing
Catastrophic reactions, 336*b*
    aggression and, 477
Catastrophizing, 51*t*
    in cognitive distortions, 311*b*
Catatonia, 279
    associated with another medical condition, 272*b*
    excited phase, 295
    withdrawn phase, 294
Catatonic features, with major depressive disorder, 221
Catharsis, 621*b*
Cathartic method, 42
Cause in fact, 101
CBT. *See* Cognitive behavioural therapy
CCPN. *See* Canadian Council of Psychiatric Nurses
Cellular composition, of brain, 156, 156*f*
Cellular reuptake, 156, 156*f*
Central nervous system (CNS)
    alcohol affecting, 354
    depressants, 223*t*, 359, 359*t*
    gamma-aminobutyric acid (GABA) and, 165
    stimulants, intoxication, overdose and withdrawal, 364, 366*t*
Cerebellum, 159, 159*f*–160*f*
Cerebral hypoxia, 329
Cerebrum, 159, 160*f*
CFAM. *See* Calgary Family Assessment Model
CFIM. *See* Calgary Family Intervention Model
CFMHN. *See* Canadian Federation of Mental Health Nurses
Chakras, 647, 653
Chamomile extract, 652, 652*t*

Changing Directions, Changing Lives: The Mental Health Strategy for Canada, 27
Chemical dependence and marginal coping, 476
Child abuse, 481
    as adventitious crisis, 434
    in Canada, 485
    characteristics of abusive parents, 488*b*
    Duluth "Abuse of Children" wheel, 490*f*
    Duluth "Nurturing Children" wheel in, 501*f*
    epidemiology of, 485
    factors to assess in home visits in, 495*b*, 495
    interventions for, 498*b*
    neglect and, 485
    nursing process application in, 489
        assessment in, 489, 490*b*
        diagnosis in, 495, 496*t*
        evaluation in, 502
        implementation in, 496
        outcomes identification in, 496, 496*t*
        planning in, 496
    reporting suspected, 99*b*, 99
    risk factors for mental illness in, 535*b*, 535
    sexual, 484
    vulnerability in, 488, 490*f*
Childhood experiences, as key social determinant of health, 12
Childhood-onset conduct disorder, 547
Children
    anxiety disorders in, 550
        assessment guidelines for, 550*b*
        generalized anxiety disorder (GAD), 550
        Nursing Outcomes Classification (*NOC*) for, 551*t*
        separation anxiety disorder, 550
    assessment of, 76
    bipolar disorders in, 252, 551
    characteristics of mentally healthy, 537*b*
    depression in
        assessment of, 229–230
        stress leading to, 223
    depressive disorders in, 551
    disorders of, 533
        brain development and biochemicals in, 536
        comorbidity of, 534
        cultural factors, 536
        environmental factors, 536
        epidemiology of, 534
        genetic factors in, 535
        medication treatment of, 543*b*
        resilience factors, 536
        temperament in, 536
    disruptive, impulse control, and conduct disorders in, 546
        adolescent-onset conduct disorder, 547
        bullying, 547
        childhood-onset conduct disorder, 547
        conduct disorders, 547, 548*b*
        nursing process application to, 548*b*, 548, 548*t*
        oppositional defiant disorder, 546, 548*b*
        techniques for managing, 549*b*
    Duluth "Nurturing Children" wheel in, 501*f*

Children (*Continued*)
    feeding and eating disorders, 551
    mood disorders in, 551
    neurodevelopmental disorders in, 542
        attention deficit-hyperactivity disorder (ADHD), 543, 545*b*, 547*b*
        autism spectrum disorders, 542
        communication disorders, 542
        intellectual disabilities, 542
        motor disorders, 544
        Nursing Outcomes Classification (*NOC*) for, 546*t*
        nursing process application to, 544, 545*b*, 545*t*
        specific learning disorder (SLD), 544
        stereotypic movement disorder, 544
        Tourette's disorder, 544
    post-traumatic stress disorder (PTSD) in, 551
    psychiatric mental health nursing, 536, 537*b*
        assessment data in, 538*b*, 538
        behavioural therapy, 539
        bibliotherapy, 541–542
        cognitive behavioural therapy, 539
        cultural factors in, 539
        data collection in, 537
        developmental assessment in, 538
        family therapy, 539
        group therapy, 539
        mental status examination in, 538
        milieu management, 540*b*, 540
        mind-body therapies, 540
        mutual storytelling, 541*b*, 541
        play therapy, 541
        principle of least restrictive intervention, 539
        psychopharmacology, 542
        quiet room, 540
        risk assessment in, 539
        seclusion and restraint in, 540
        therapeutic drawing, 542
        therapeutic games, 541, 542*b*
        time out, 540
    risk factors for mental illness in, 535*b*, 535
    use of antidepressant drugs by, 241
    vulnerable to abuse, 488, 490*f*
Chiropractic medicine, 653
Chlordiazepoxide hydrochloride (Librax), 212*b*–214*b*
Chlorpromazine (Largactil, Thorazine), 6, 54, 473*b*
    for anorexia nervosa, 311
    for schizophrenia, 289*t*
CHNA. *See* Canadian Holistic Nurses Association
Cholestatic jaundice, from conventional antipsychotics, 291*t*–292*t*
Cholinergics, 157*t*
Cholinesterase inhibitors, for Alzheimer's disease, 174, 341
CHPCA. *See* Canadian Hospice Palliative Care Association
Chronic fatigue syndrome, 422
Chronic sorrow, 601
Chronological age, 555

Circadian drive, 417
Circadian process, 417
Circadian rhythm sleep disorder, 420
Circadian rhythms, 156, 414
   circadian rhythm sleep disorder, 420
Circumstantiality, in communication, 278
Cirrhosis, concurrent with substance abuse disorders, 354
CISD. *See* Critical incident stress debriefing
Cisgender, 525
Citalopram (Celexa), 168, 212*b*–214*b*, 236*b*–237*b*
Civil obligations, 99, 100*t*
CIW. *See* Canadian Index of Wellbeing
Clang associations, 256
   in communication, 278
Clarification, for managing disruptive behaviours, in children and adolescents, 549*b*
Clarifying techniques, as therapeutic communication technique, 141, 143*t*–144*t*
Classical conditioning theory, 48
   vs. operant conditioning, 48*f*
Classical psychoanalysis, 43
   counter-transference in, 43–44
   transference in, 43–44
Claustrophobia, 188*t*
Clear boundaries, 633*b*
Cleverley, Kristin, 20–21
Clinical competence, of health care workers, 126
Clinical consultation, 623
Clinical epidemiology, 9
Clinical Institute Withdrawal Assessment for Alcohol (CIWA-Ar), 360, 360*t*–361*t*
Clinical interview, 136
   attending behaviours during, 148
   clinical supervision during, 149
   helpful guidelines for, 148
   initiating, 148
   introductions during, 148
   pace of, 147
   preparation, 147
   process recordings during, 149, 150*t*
   seating in, 148
   setting of, 147
   tactics to avoid during, 148, 148*t*
Clinical nurse specialist, province licensing regulations for, 21
Clinical Opiate Withdrawal Scale (COWS), 364, 365*t*
Clinical pathway, discharge planning and, 30–31
Clinical supervision, 126
Clomipramine hydrochloride (Anafranil), 212*b*–214*b*, 236*b*–237*b*
Clonazepam (Rivotril), 165, 166*f*, 212*b*–214*b*
Closed-ended questions, 142
Closed group, 621*b*
Clozapine (Clozaril), 173
   for schizophrenia, 288, 289*t*
Clozaril. *See* Clozapine
Cluster A personality disorders, 391, 393
Cluster B personality disorders, 391, 394

Cluster C personality disorders, 391, 400
Cluster suicide, 453
CMHA. *See* Canadian Mental Health Association
CNA. *See* Canadian Nurses Association
Cocaine, 365
   vs. methamphetamine, 367*t*
   physical complications related to abuse of, 355*t*
Code of ethics
   Canadian Nurses Association, 90*b*, 90–91
   Registered Psychiatric Nurses of Canada, 90*b*, 90–91
Code White responders, 473
Codeine, intoxication, overdose and withdrawal from, 364*t*
Cognition, 324
   assessment of, during mental status examination, 79*b*–80*b*
Cognitive and cognitive behavioural theories, 469
Cognitive behaviorism, 469–470
Cognitive behavioural therapy (CBT), 50, 52*b*, 622, 623*t*
   for anxiety disorders, 216
   for binge eating disorder, 316
   for bipolar disorders, 265
   for bulimia nervosa, 315
   for children and adolescents, 539
   for depression, 242–243
   for insomnia, 425, 427*b*
   internet-delivered, for obsessive-compulsive disorder, 195*b*
   for serious mental illness, 578
Cognitive changes, 229
Cognitive development, 44, 55*t*–56*t*
Cognitive distortions, 50, 51*t*, 69
   in anorexia nervosa, 311*b*, 311
Cognitive disturbances, in delirium, 328
Cognitive function, 324
   bipolar disorders and, 256
Cognitive impairment
   case study and nursing care plan, 344*b*–347*b*
   self-care for individuals with, guidelines for, 340*b*–341*b*
   with substance abuse or behavioural addictions, 373*t*
Cognitive reframing, 69, 69*t*
Cognitive restructuring process, 216
Cognitive symptoms, of schizophrenia, 276, 279–280
Cognitive theories, 50
   of anxiety disorders, 200
   cognitive behavioural therapy and, 50, 52*b*
   of depression, 226
   dialectic behavioural therapy as, 51
   implications of, in nursing practice, 52, 53*b*
   rational emotive behaviour therapy and, 50
Cognitive therapy, for anxiety disorders, 216
Cogwheel rigidity, from conventional antipsychotics, 291*t*–292*t*
Collaboration
   as key strategy area for Canadian mental health care, 7, 8*b*

Collaboration *(Continued)*
   of primary health care and mental health care, 586, 587*b*
Collagen vascular diseases, that may mimic psychiatric illness, 78*b*
Collective violence, 467
Collectivist (collectivism), 108
Colonization, 107
Command hallucinations, 279*b*, 279
Communicable diseases, confidentiality and, 99
Communication, 136
   for associative looseness, 287
   for catatonia, 294, 295
   for delusions, 286*b*, 286
   in dementia, 337, 339*b*–340*b*
   depression and, 229
   disorders, in children and adolescents, 542
   for disorganization, 295
   dysfunctional, in family therapy, 632, 633*b*
   factors affecting, 137
   in group therapy, 623*t*
   for hallucinations, 286*b*–287*b*, 286
   importance of effective, during end-of-life (EOL) care, 597, 598*b*
   non-verbal, 139
   operational definition of, 138*f*
   for paranoia, 294
   process of, 137, 138*f*
   for schizophrenia, 285
   skills for nurses, 140
      assertive communication in, 146
      evaluation of, 147, 147*f*
      therapeutic communication strategies in, 140
   style, 146
   techniques
      of group leader, 623*t*
      with substance abuse patients, 371, 371*t*, 372*t*
   therapeutic strategies, 140, 143*t*–144*t*
      active listening as, 140
      asking questions and eliciting patient responses as, 142
      clarifying techniques as, 141, 143*t*–144*t*
      exploring as, 142
      listening with empathy as, 141
      paraphrasing as, 141
      reflecting as, 141
      restating as, 141
      silence as, 140
      summarizing as, 143*t*–144*t*
   verbal, 139
Community-based groups, 337–338
Community-based programs, for older adults, 569
Community-based treatment, 381
Community mental health centres, 27, 28*b*
   deinstitutionalization and, 27
   interprofessional team model in, 27
   psychiatric mental health nurse in, 27
   recovery and, 27
Community mental health workers, as members of psychiatric mental health treatment teams, 34*b*

Community psychiatric mental health nursing, 32
Community supports, for Alzheimer's disease, 338, 341t
Community treatment orders (CTOs), 96–97, 581
Community violence, 112–113
Comorbid condition, defined, 8
Comparison, encouraging, as therapeutic communication technique, 143t–144t
Compensation defence mechanism, 186t–187t
Competency, 96
   early defining of, in psychiatric mental health nurse, 21
   in older adult abuse, 497
   in relationship building, 124
Complaining member, 627, 628b
Complementary therapies, 645
Complete suicide, 449
Complicated grief, 601
Compulsions, 193, 195t, 201
Compulsive behaviours, 351
Computed tomography (CT scans), description and psychiatric uses for, 161t
Concentration, 79b–80b
   difficulties with depression, 229
Concordance
   depression in identical twins and, 224
   in identical twin brain image research, 162f, 164
Concrete operational stage, of cognitive development, 44
Concrete thinking, 276
   in schizophrenia, 280
Concreteness, 280
Concurrent disorder programs, 381
Concurrent disorders, 354, 574
   groups, 625
   programs, 26, 381, 382b
Conditioning
   classical, 48f, 48
   defined, 48
   operant, 48f, 48
Conduct disorders, in children and adolescents, 543b, 547, 548b
Confabulation, 335
Confidentiality
   in abuse screening, 493b
   adolescents and, 77
   after death, 99
   communicable diseases and, 99
   in nurse-patient relationship, 131
   rights regarding, 98
Confinement, 16
Conflict
   in groups, 621b
   nurse responses to, 129t–130t
Confusion Assessment Method (CAM), 326
Confusional arousal disorders, 419
   types of, 418
Connecting, during end-of-life (EOL) care, 596
Conscientious objection, 92

Conscious mental activity, brain function and, 156
Conscious mind, 42
Consensual validation, seeking, as therapeutic communication technique, 143t–144t
Consent
   in child health care decision making, 535
   informed, 96
Consequentialist theory, 91
Consistency, in nurse-patient relationship, 132
Constipation
   from conventional antipsychotics, 291t–292t
   depression co-occurring with, 234t
Constraint, vs. impulsivity, 401, 402t
Consultation, 385
   by advanced-practice psychiatric mental health nurses, 11t
Contemplation, 370
Contemplation phase, of Transtheoretical Model of Change, 370
Content, of message, 139
Continuation phase
   of bipolar disorders
     implementation for, 258
     outcomes identification in, 258
     planning in, 258
   of depression, 232
   of manic episodes, 258
Continuum of psychiatric mental health treatment, 26f, 26
Contract, for nurse-patient relationship, 131
Contraindications, 261
Control
   in nurse-patient relationships, 132
   of perpetrators, 488
Controlled drinking, 377
Controlled style, of coping, 511b, 513
Conventional antipsychotics, 171
   for anorexia nervosa, 311
   medication, 273
   for schizophrenia, 289, 289t, 291t–292t
Conventional health care, 645
Conversion defence mechanism, 186t–187t
Conversion disorder, 190, 192, 193b
Coordination of care
   as basic-level psychiatric mental health nursing intervention, 11t
   in psychiatric mental health nursing, 85
Coping
   definition of, 432
   "ineffective" diagnosis in crisis situations, 437, 439t
   styles, assessment of, 65
Coping mechanisms
   four phases of crisis, 435
   in sexual assault, 512
   with stress and crisis, 433
   in violence, 494, 494t, 495b
Coping skills
   anger and aggression and
     healthy, overwhelmed, 475
     marginal, 475–476
   anxiety disorders and, 204
   factors compromising, 433

Coping skills *(Continued)*
   as key social determinant of health, 12
   mental illness and, 586, 590, 591t, 592b
Copycat suicide, 453
Coronavirus disease 2019 (COVID-19) pandemic. *See* COVID-19 pandemic
Correctional nursing, 614, 615b
Corrections and Conditional Release Act (1992), 615
Corticosteroids, stress response and, 61
Corticotropin, nerve cells of brain influenced by, 155
Corticotropin-releasing factor (CRF), depression and, 225
Corticotropin-releasing hormone (CRH), nerve cells of brain influenced by, 155
Cortisol
   depression and, 225
   nerve cells of brain influenced by, 155
Counselling
   for anxiety disorders, 210
   as basic-level nursing intervention, 26
   for bulimia nervosa, 315
   communication techniques with depression, 232, 233b
   for dementia, 337
   for managing disruptive behaviours, in children and adolescents, 549b
   for schizophrenia, 285
   for sexual assault, 515
   for sleep disorders, 425
   techniques in crisis situation, 440
   for violence and abuse, 497
Counsellors, as members of psychiatric mental health treatment teams, 34b
Counter-transference, 125–126, 127t, 280
   in classical psychoanalysis, 43–44
COVID-19 pandemic, 432, 448–449, 451, 453, 458–459, 485, 578b
   maternal psychological distress and mental health service use during, 30b–31b
   mental health service and, 26
   social isolation in, 110
COWS. *See* Clinical Opiate Withdrawal Scale
Crack, 365
Crash, 364–365
CRF. *See* Corticotropin-releasing factor
CRH. *See* Corticotropin-releasing hormone
Crime, Canada's National Crime Prevention Strategy, 611b, 611
Criminal Code, 613
   in reporting abuse, 497
   in sexual assault, 509
Criminal responsibility, 614
Criminalization
   decreased, mobile crisis intervention team and, 28
   of mentally ill, 613
Crisis, 432
   Aguilera's paradigm on outcomes of, 433f, 433
   coping and coping methods, 432
   defining, 432
   "ineffective" diagnosis in crisis situations, 437

Crisis (Continued)
  NANDA-I classifications of anxiety associated with, 437
  nursing process application to
    diagnosis of, 437b, 437, 438t
    outcomes identification of, 437, 438b, 439t
    phases of, 435
      phase 1, 435
      phase 2, 435
      phase 3, 435
      phase 4, 435
    resolution from the state of, 433, 433f
    situation, abuse and, 488
    theory, 433, 434f
    two necessary conditions (Roberts) for, 432
    types of, 434
      adventitious, 434
      maturational, 434
      situational, 434
Crisis intervention
  cultural considerations, 436b
  definition of, 433
  five elements of, 433
  foundation for, 435b
  guidelines for, 439–440, 440t
  nursing process application to
    assessment of, 433f, 435, 435b–436b
    case study and nursing care plan on, 442b–445b
    evaluation of, 441, 442b
    implementation of, 439, 441b
    planning of, 439
  process of, 433
  Roberts's seven-stage model of, 433, 434f
  self-assessment in, 437
Crisis intervention teams, mobile, 28, 29b
Crisis management, 37
  behavioural, 37
  medical, 37
Crisis theory, nursing process application to, 435
Critical incident stress debriefing (CISD), phases of, 441b, 441
Cross-language facilitation, 114–115
Crying, nurse responses to, 129t–130t
CTOs. See Community treatment orders
Cues, non-verbal, 139, 139t
Cultural competence, 105–106
Cultural concepts of distress, 115
Cultural considerations
  for bipolar disorders, 253b
  crisis resolution, 434f, 434
  eye contact, 146
  on gender bias in diagnosing personality disorders, 398b
  non-verbal communication, 146
  regarding sexual orientation and gender identity, 525b
  regarding sleep in Canadian culture, 417b
  touch, 146
  weight bias/weight stigma, 308b
Cultural contexts, on end-of-life (EOL) care, 596
Cultural diversity, 105–106

Cultural encounters, 110
Cultural filters, 146
Cultural humility, 106–107
Cultural norms, 108
Cultural safety, 106, 107b
  awareness of, 107
Cultural sensitivity, 105–106
Cultural violence, 483t, 484
Culturally safe practice, 110
Culture
  assessment of, 81
  beliefs of, regarding mental illness, 5
  defined, 105
  as key social determinant of health, 12
  as mediator of stress response, 63
  mental health and, 105
  pharmacogenetics and, 165b, 165
  world view of, 108
Culture-bound syndromes, 5–6
  anxiety disorders and, 201b, 201
Custodial care, 17
Cutting, as self-harm, 454
Cyberbullying, 466
Cycle of violence, 485, 486f
Cyclic stage, in cycle of violence, 485
Cyclothymic disorder, 251
  comorbidity of, 252
  epidemiology of, 252
Cytokines
  depression and, 62
  stress response and, 62

D

Damages, 101
Dance therapists, as members of psychiatric mental health treatment teams, 34b
Data collection
  definition of, 74
  primary source for, 76
Date rape, 509, 510t
Day treatment programs, 568
Daytox programs, 381
  for drug abuse, 381
  for schizophrenia, 284
DBT. See Dialectical behaviour therapy
D-Cycloserine, for anxiety disorders, 215
Death
  Canadian hospice palliative care treatment model and, 595
  confidentiality after, 99
  in eating disorders, 308–309
  guidelines when caring for the dying, 599b
  by suicide, 449
  Woodruff's Total Suffering Model, 597f, 597
Debriefing, 149
"Decade of the brain", 7
Decision making
  in crisis situations, 439t
  in dementia, 337t
  evidence-informed, 83, 84b
Decompensation, 26
Deep-breathing exercise, 68b
De-escalation techniques, 472b, 472
Defamation, of character, 100

Defence mechanisms
  in Alzheimer's disease, 335
  in Sigmund Freud's psychoanalytic theory, 42
Defences
  adaptive and maladaptive uses of, 186t–187t
  against anxiety, 184, 185f, 186t–187t
Deficient fluid volume, in delirium, 329
Deinstitutionalization, 20, 611
  consequences of, 29
  lack of funding for, 27
  trend of, 27
Delirium, 326b, 326
  alcohol withdrawal, 362–363
  assessment of, 326, 329b
  clinical picture of, 326
  common causes of, 327b
  comorbidity and etiology of, 326
  diagnosis of, 329, 330t
  diagnostic criteria for, 326b
  epidemiology of, 326
  evaluation of, 329
  implementation in, 329, 331b
  major neurocognitive disorders, depression, and brain injury, comparison of, 325t
  outcomes identification in, 329, 330t
  planning for, 329
  vignette in, 328b
Delirium tremens (DTs), 362–363
Delusional disorder, 272b
Delusions, 271
  coping with, 286b–287b
  counselling and communication techniques for, 286
  with dementia, 336–337
  with major depressive disorder, 221
  people experiencing, 286b
  with schizophrenia, 271
  summary of, 277t
Dementia, 325, 330
  from Alzheimer's disease, 332
  care at home, guidelines for, 342b
  as challenge to psychiatric mental health nurses, 11–12
  clinical picture of, 332
  communication, guidelines for, 337, 339b–340b
  counselling and communication techniques for, 337
  delirium, depression, and brain injury, comparison of, 325t
  diagnostic criteria for, 331b
  epidemiology of, 334
  etiology of, 334
    biological factors in, 334
    environmental factors in, 334
  evaluation for, 344
  Functional Dementia Scale in, 338f
  health teaching and health promotion in, 337
  within Indigenous peoples in Canada, 333b
  normal aging vs., 332t
  nursing process, application of, 335
    assessment of, 335b, 335

Dementia (Continued)
  case study and nursing care plan in, 344b–347b
  diagnosis of, 335
  implementation in, 336, 339b
  outcomes identification in, 336, 337t, 338b
  planning for, 336
  palliative care for patients with, 605
  pharmacological interventions for, 338
  self-care for individuals with cognitive impairment, guidelines for, 340b–341b
  services that may be available to people with, 341t
  types of, 332t
  vignette in, 334b
Democratic leader, 623
Demoralizing member, 628b, 628
Denial, 370
  with Alzheimer's disease, 335
  as defence mechanism, 186t–187t
  with serious medical illness, 588, 589b
Deontology, 90–91
Dependent personality disorder
  characteristics and behaviours associated with, 391, 400b, 400
  nursing and therapy guidelines for, 400, 405t
  treatment of, 400
Depersonalization/derealization disorder, 198, 199b, 278, 515
  sexual assault and, 515
Depot medications, 288
Depression, 169
  advanced practice interventions for
    group therapy, 243
    psychotherapy, 242–243
  affecting basic sex and hunger drives, 155
  alcohol dependence with, case study on, 383b–384b
  antidepressant drugs for, 234
    by children and adolescents, 241
    choosing, 236
    monoamine oxidase inhibitors, 236b–237b, 239, 240b
    by older adults, 241
    by pregnant women, 240
    selective serotonin reuptake inhibitors (SSRIs), 236b–237b, 237
    serotonin-norepinephrine reuptake inhibitors (SNRIs), 236b–237b, 237
    tricyclic antidepressants, 236b–237b, 238, 239b
  assessment of, 226, 231b, 280
    age considerations in, 229
    areas to assess, 229
    in children and adolescents, 229–230
    guidelines in, 231b
    key findings in, 228
    in older adults, 230
    screening tools in, 226, 228f
    self-assessment in, 230
    suicidal ideation in, 227
  Beck's cognitive triad and, 226
  during bereavement, 603t

Depression (Continued)
  case study and nursing care plan for, 244b–246b
  clinical picture, 220
  comorbidity of, 224
  cytokines and, 62
  delirium, major neurocognitive disorders, and brain injury, comparison of, 325t
  with dementia, 336–337
  diagnosis of, 231, 231t
  drug treatment for, 167, 167f
    potential receptor interactions of, 167f
  in eating and feeding disorder, 307
  epidemiology of, 223, 224f
    in children and adolescents, 223
    in older adults, 223
  etiology of, 224
    biochemical factors in, 224, 225f
    biological factors in, 224
    cognitive theory in, 226
    diathesis-stress model in, 225
    genetic factors in, 224
    hormones in, 225
    inflammation in, 225
    learned helplessness and, 226
    neurotransmitters and, 224–225
    psychological factors in, 226
    risk factors in, 224b
    stress factors in, 225
  evaluation for, 243
  Geriatric Depression Scale, 565b, 565
  vs. grief, 601
  and grieving, 222
  implementation for, 232
    acute phase, 232
    continuation phase, 232
    counselling and communication techniques in, 232, 233b
    electroconvulsive therapy in, 241, 241f
    health teaching and health promotion, 232
    maintenance phase, 232
    milieu management in, 233
    pharmacological interventions in, 234, 235f
    promotion of self-care activities in, 233
    transcranial magnetic stimulation in, 242, 242f
    vagus nerve stimulation in, 242f, 242
    for vegetative signs, 234t
  integrative therapy for, 243b
    exercise, 243b
    light therapy, 243b
    St. John's wort, 243b
  in LGBTQ, 529
  monoamine theory of, 167f, 167, 170
  NOC outcomes related to, 232, 232t
  nursing process, application of, 226
  in older adults, 557
  PET scan images, before and after medication, 225f, 225
  planning in, 232
  positron emission tomography scan of brain with, 161, 163f
  recovery model for, 232, 232t
  schizophrenia and, 273

Depression (Continued)
  serious medical illness and, 587, 588b
  spirituality and religious beliefs influencing, 229
  sub-types and specifiers of, 221
    atypical features, 221
    catatonic features, 221
    melancholic features, 221
    postpartum onset, 221
    psychotic features, 221
    seasonal features, 221
  suicide risk in, 450
  symptoms of, 231t
    anger, 229
    anhedonia, 228
    communication difficulties, 229, 232, 233b
    grooming lapses, 229
    mood and feelings, 229, 231t
    physical behaviour, 229
    psychomotor agitation, 229
    psychomotor retardation, 229
    sleep issues, 229, 234t
    vegetative signs, 228, 231t, 234t
Depressive disorders, 220
  in children and adolescents, 551
  disruptive mood dysregulation disorder, 221
  due to another medical condition, 222, 223t
  major depressive disorder, 220–221
  persistent depressive disorder, 222
  pre-menstrual dysphoric disorder, 222
  substance/medication-induced depressive disorder, 222
Depressive episodes, 258
  treatment during bipolar, 258
Derealization, 278, 515
Desensitization, systematic, as behavioural therapy, 49
Desipramine hydrochloride (Norpramin), 212b–214b, 238
Destigmatizing Practices and Mental Illness, 110–111
Desvenlafaxine (Pristiq), 168
Determination stage, 370
Detox, 381
Development, stages of
  Erikson's, 45t
  moral, 44
  psychosexual, 43, 43t
Developmental theories, 44
  cognitive development as, 44
  ethics of care theory and, 45
  implications of, for nursing practice, 46
  moral development stages, 44
  theory of psychosocial development and, 45t, 46
Dexamethasone, 225
Diagnostic and Statistics Manual of Mental Disorders, fifth edition *(DSM-5)*, 4–5, 9, 111, 193
  in gender dysphoria, 526b, 526
  and nursing diagnoses, 11
  organizational structure of, 9
  for schizophrenia, 272

INDEX

Dialectical behaviour therapy (DBT), 51, 626
    for binge eating disorder, 316
    for personality disorders, 406, 408f
    for violence, 501
Diarrhea, 373t
Diaspora, 113b–114b
Diathesis, defining, 392
Diathesis-stress model, 6
    of depression, 225
    of personality disorders, 392
    of schizophrenia, 273
Diazepam (Valium), 165, 166f, 212b–214b, 473b
DID. *See* Dissociative identity disorder
Diet
    for integrative health care, 650
    as mediator of stress response, 63
Differentiation, 396, 634b, 636
Diffuse boundaries, 633b
Dignity, to the dying, 594
Diphenhydramine (Benadryl, Nytol), 426t
Disability Assessment Schedule 2.0, 10
Disability, mental health-related, 24
Disapproval, giving, 142
Disaster response teams, 28
Disasters, 432
    as adventitious crisis, 434
    critical incident stress debriefing (CISD), 441b, 441
    five elements of intervention, 433
    resilience and, 5
Discrimination
    advocacy groups to fight Canadian mental health care, 7
    against mentally ill persons, 93
Disenfranchised grief, 601
Disengaged boundaries, 633b
Disinhibitor, 168–169
Disorganization, 295
Disorganized thinking, with schizophrenia, 272
Disorientation
    with delirium, 327–328
    with dementia, 336, 337t
Disparities, reduction of, as key strategy for Canadian mental health care, 7, 8b
Displacement, 186t–187t
Disqualifying the positive, 51t
Disruptive, impulse control, and conduct disorders, in children and adolescents, 546
    adolescent-onset conduct disorder, 547
    bullying, 547
    childhood-onset conduct disorder, 547
    conduct disorders, 543b, 547, 548b
    nursing process application to, 548b, 548, 548t
    oppositional defiant disorder, 546, 548b
    techniques for managing, 549b
Disruptive mood dysregulation disorder, 221
Dissent, in child health care decision making, 535
Dissociation, 79b–80b
    as defence mechanism, 186t–187t
Dissociative amnesia, 196, 199

Dissociative disorders, 180, 198
    assessment guidelines for, 203b–204b
    comorbidity of, 199
    depersonalization/derealization disorder, 198, 199b
    dissociative amnesia, 199
    dissociative identity disorder, 199
    epidemiology of, 199
    nursing diagnoses for, 207t
    nursing interventions for, 211t
    sexual assault and, 514b, 514
Dissociative fugue, 199
Dissociative identity disorder (DID), 198–199
Distortions, cognitive, 50, 51t, 69
    in anorexia nervosa, 311b, 311
Distracting, during family therapy, 633b
Distress, 61, 207
    cultural concepts of, 115
Disturbed thought processes, with delirium, 329
Diuretics, use of, 315b
Divalproex sodium (Epival), for bipolar disorders, 262, 263b
Diversion
    of drugs, 95
    signs with nurses, 385b, 385
Diversity
    increasing, as challenge for psychiatric mental health nurses, 11
    as key strategy for Canadian mental health care, 8b
Dix, Dorothea, 17
Documentation, 37
    in abuse screening, 493b
    of care, 98
    importance in seclusion protocol, 263
    legal considerations for, 85b–86b
    in nursing process, 85
    of suicide risk assessment, 454b
Dominant culture, 105
Donepezil (Aricept), 174
    for Alzheimer's disease, 341, 343f
Dopamine, 157t
    in anger and aggression, 468
    reduction of, 158b
    substance use disorders and, 355–356
    theory, of schizophrenia, 273
    use of, by neuronal circuitry, 164
    wakefulness and, 417
Dopamine system stabilizer, aripiprazole as, 173
Double-bind messages, 140
Double messages, 140
Doubt, voicing, as therapeutic communication technique, 143t–144t
Doxepin hydrochloride (Adapin, Sinequan), 212b–214b, 238
Dressing, in guidelines for self-care for individuals with cognitive impairment, 340b–341b
Drug-facilitated sexual assault, 510, 510t
Drug misuse, 373
Drugs
    effects that may mimic psychiatric illness, 78b
    mental health dysfunction and, 164

Drug therapy, 344
Drug use
    in LGBTQ, 529
    in violence and abuse, 495
Dry eyes, from conventional antipsychotics, 291t–292t
Dry mouth, from conventional antipsychotics, 291t–292t
Dual Process Model, of coping with bereavement, 602
Duloxetine (Cymbalta), 168
Duloxetine hydrochloride (Cymbalta), 212b–214b
    for major depressive disorder, 236b–237b
Duluth "Abuse of Children" wheel, 490f
Duluth "Equality" wheel, 500f
Duluth "Nurturing Children" wheel, 501f
Duluth "Power and Control" wheel, 489f
Dutton, Dr. Donald, 485
Duty, 101
    breach of, 101
    to protect, 98
    vignette regarding, 101b
    to warn, 98
Dyssomnia, 413
Dysthymia, drug treatment for, 543b

E

Early detection, 275
Early-onset Alzheimer's disease, 334
Eastern Canada, history of psychiatric nursing licensing in, 19
Eating and feeding disorders, 304, 306b–307b
    anorexia nervosa as, 308
        acute care in, 311
        advanced-practice interventions for, 312
        assessment of, 308, 310b
        case study and nursing care plan for, 317
        characteristics of, 305b
        clinical picture of, 304
        cognitive distortions in, 311b
        comorbidity of, 307
        criteria for hospital admission of, 309b
        diagnosis of, 310
        epidemiology of, 305
        etiology of, 307
        evaluation of, 313
        general assessment for, 309
        health teaching and health promotion for, 311
        implementation in, 311
        medical complications of, 309b
        milieu management of, 311
        NOC outcomes related to, 310t
        outcomes identification of, 310
        pharmacological interventions for, 311
        planning of, 310
        psychosocial interventions for, 311b, 311
        psychotherapy for, 312
        self-assessment of, 310
        signs and symptoms of, 309t
        thoughts and behaviours associated with, 308b
        vignette in, 311b–312b
    avoidant/restrictive food intake disorder as, 305

Eating and feeding disorders *(Continued)*
  binge eating disorder as, 316
    bariatric surgery for, 316, 317*b*
    characteristics of, 305*b*
    clinical picture of, 304
    comorbidity of, 307
    epidemiology of, 305
    etiology of, 307
  bulimia nervosa as, 313
    acute care for, 315
    advanced-practice interventions for, 315
    assessment of, 313, 314*b*
    case study and nursing care plan for, 319*b*–320*b*
    characteristics of, 305*b*
    clinical picture of, 304
    comorbidity of, 307
    counselling for, 315
    diagnosis of, 314
    epidemiology of, 305
    etiology of, 307
    evaluation of, 316
    general assessment of, 313
    health teaching and health promotion for, 315
    implementation in, 315
    medical complications of, 313*b*
    NOC outcomes related to, 315*t*
    outcomes identification of, 314
    pharmacological interventions for, 315
    planning for, 315
    psychotherapy for, 315
    self-assessment of, 314
    signs and symptoms of, 314*t*
    thoughts and behaviours associated with, 314*b*
    vignette in, 313*b*, 315*b*
  in children and adolescents, 551
  coping with a family member who has, 313*b*
  NIC interventions for, 315, 316*b*
  not otherwise specified, 304
  pica as, 305
  prevalence statistics of, in Canada, 9*t*
  rumination disorder as, 305
  screening, 314*b*
  state of treatment for, 312*t*
Echolalia, in communication, 278
Echopraxia, 279
E-cigarettes, 375
Economic abuse, 489*f*–490*f*
Ecstasy, 368
Education
  in abuse screening, 493*b*
  clinical levels of, in psychiatric mental health nursing, 11
  early university-based nursing curriculum and, 20
  as key social determinant of health, 12
  medication, 625
  shifts in control over nursing and, 18
  Weir Report and, 18–19
Effective emergency response, 440*b*
Ego, 42*f*, 42
Electrical conductivity, adverse effect of lithium on, 170–171, 171*t*

Electrical impulses, conducted by neurons, 156
Electroconvulsive therapy (ECT), 17–18
  adverse reactions, 241
  for bipolar disorders, 262
  for depression, 241, 241*f*
  indications, 241
  procedure, 241
  risk factors, 241
Electroencephalograms (EEGs), measuring sleep, 414
Electrolyte imbalance
  with anorexia nervosa, 309
  with delirium, 329
Electronic documentation, guidelines for, 98
Elimination, anxiety disorders and, 212
Ellis, Albert, 50*f*, 50, 55*t*–56*t*, 469–470
Ellis, Kathryn, 19–20
Elopement, safety and, 32
Embodied knowledge, as relational ethics principle, 91
EMDR therapy. *See* Eye movement desensitization and reprocessing (EMDR) therapy
Emergency care, mental health first aid (MHFA), 442*b*
Emotional aggression, 465
Emotional dysregulation
  defining, 392
  emotional stability vs., 401, 402*t*
Emotional intelligence, 468
Emotional lability, 396
Emotional reactions
  in coping, 511*b*
  in dementia, 337*t*
Emotional reasoning, 51*t*
  in cognitive distortions, 311*b*
Emotional stability, vs. emotional dysregulation, 401, 402*t*
Emotional trauma
  long-lasting, 510
  signs and symptoms of, 511*b*, 513
Emotional violence
  definition of, 483*t*, 484
  devastating consequences in children, 484
  in "Power and Control" wheel, 489*f*
Emotions
  control and regulation of, 468
  resilience and, 5
Empathy
  element of LEAP approach, 271
  listening with, 141
  for patients' growth, 133
  sympathy vs., 133
Employee assistance programs, for substance use disorders, 385
Employment, as key social determinant of health, 12
Employment Equity Act, 89
Empowering, during end-of-life (EOL) care, 596
Endocrine disorders
  depression co-occurring with, 223*t*
  that may mimic psychiatric illness, 78*b*
Endocrine system, regulation of, 154, 155*f*
End-of-life care
  art, presence, and caring of nursing in, 596

End-of-life care *(Continued)*
  assessment for spiritual issues during, 596
  hospice palliative care nursing, 596
  importance of effective communication during, 597, 598*b*
  nursing care at, 596
Endorphins, stress response and, 61
Energy therapies, 653
  healing touch as, 653
  Reiki as, 653
  therapeutic touch as, 653
Engagement, as relational ethics principle, 91
Enmeshed boundaries, 633*b*
Environmental factors
  affecting communication, 137
  in eating and feeding disorders, 308
  in violence and abuse, 487
Environmental stressors, in schizophrenia, 274
Enzymes, that destroy neurotransmitter, 156
Epidemiology, defined, in mental health, 7
Epilepsy, 6
  in aggression and violence, 468
"Epp Report," *Mental Health for Canadians: Striking a Balance*, 3, 4*f*
EPSs. *See* Extrapyramidal side effects
Equality, in Canadian mental health care, 7
Equity-oriented health care (EOHC), 106
Erikson, Erik, 44
  stages of development, 44, 45*t*
Erotomanic delusion, 277*t*
Escitalopram oxalate (Cipralex), 168, 212*b*–214*b*, 236*b*–237*b*
Essential hypertension, anxiety caused by, 194*t*
Esteem, need for, 54
Estrogen, in gender dysphoria, 527
Ethical concepts, 89, 90*f*
Ethical dilemma, 91–92
Ethics
  defined, 89
  relational, 90–91
  virtue, 91
Ethnic groups, pharmacogenetics and, 165*b*, 165
Ethnicity, 106
Ethnocentrism, defined, 106
Etiology, diagnostic titles and, 82
Etuaptmumk, 108
Euphoric mood, associated with mania, 255
Eustress, 61
Euthanasia, 453
Evaluation
  definition of, 74
  in nursing process, 85
Evidence-informed decision making, 83, 84*b*
Evidence-informed practice, 11
Excessive questioning, 142, 145*t*
Excessive sleepiness (ES), due to sleep deprivation, 414
Excessive use, 352
Excitotoxicity, 174
Exercises
  for depression, 243*b*
  physical, as relaxation technique, 68
  for relaxation, 65

Exercises *(Continued)*
 as stress buster, 64*b*
Existential resolution, 621*b*
Existentialism, 55*t*–56*t*
Expert witnesses, forensic psychiatric mental health nurses as, 613
Exploring, as therapeutic communication technique, 142, 143*t*–144*t*
Expressed style, of coping, 511*b*, 512
Extinction, 48
Extrapyramidal side effects (EPSs), in conventional antipsychotics, 289
Extraversion, vs. introversion, 401, 402*t*
Eye cast, 139, 139*t*
Eye contact
 during clinical interview, 148
 cultural considerations to, 146
Eye movement desensitization and reprocessing (EMDR) therapy, for sexual assaults, 518

F

Facial expressions, as non-verbal behaviour, 139, 139*t*
Facilitative skills checklist, 147*f*, 147
False imprisonment, 100, 100*t*
Falsely reassuring, 145*t*
Family, 631*b*, 631
 application of the nursing process, 636
  assessment, 636
  case management, 641
  counselling and communication techniques, 640
  diagnosis, 639
  evaluation, 642
  implementation, 640, 641*b*–642*b*
  interventions, 640*b*
  outcomes identification, 640
  pharmacological interventions, 642
  planning, 640
  self-awareness, 638
 Canadian models of nursing care, 632
  Calgary Family Assessment Model (CFAM), 632, 639*f*
  Calgary Family Intervention Model (CFIM), 632
  McGill Model of Nursing, 632
 as caregivers, 631
 diversity, Canadian, 630–631
 emotional support from, 633
 functions, 631
 ideal form, 631
 identified patient, 634
 life cycle, 633
 and mental illness, 632
 socialization and, 633
 as system, 636
 triangles, 634, 635*f*
 working with, 634*b*, 634
Family assessment
 Calgary Family Assessment Model (CFAM), 632
 Calgary Family Intervention Model (CFIM), 632
 McGill Model of Nursing, 632
Family-centred care, 631

Family coping patterns, in violence, 495*b*, 495
Family education, therapeutic groups and, 625
Family-focused therapy, for bipolar disorders, 265
Family interventions, 630
Family psychotherapy, in violence and abuse, 501*f*, 501
Family service, for dementia, 341*t*
Family systems theory, 634*b*, 636
Family therapy, 632, 641
 boundaries, 632, 633*b*
 for children and adolescents, 539
 dysfunctional communication during, 632, 633*b*
 psychoeducational, 641
 for schizophrenia, 295, 296*b*
 theory, 635
 traditional, 641
Family triangles, 634, 635*f*
Family violence, 112
 case study and nursing care plan in, 502*b*–504*b*
 coping responses in, 494, 494*t*
 diagnosis of, 495, 496*t*
 long-term effects of, 487*b*
 maintaining accurate records in, 491, 493*b*
 myth vs. fact in, 494*t*
 nursing process application in, 489
  assessment in, 489, 490*b*
  diagnosis in, 495, 496*t*
  evaluation in, 502
  implementation in, 496
  outcomes identification in, 496, 496*t*
  planning in, 496
Farewell, in death and dying situations, 600
FAS. *See* Fetal alcohol syndrome
FASD. *See* Fetal alcohol spectrum disorder
Fear, 180
 anxiety vs., 181
 in delirium, 329
 of dependency, with serious medical conditions, 589*b*, 589
 phobias, 188*b*, 188, 188*t*
 systematic desensitization of, 49
Federal government, role of, in psychiatric mental health care funding, 25
Feedback, in communication process, 137, 138*f*
Feeding disorders, 305
Feelings, 230, 231*b*
 depression and, 229
 minimizing, 145*t*
Fentanyl, 364*t*
Fetal alcohol spectrum disorder (FASD), 355
Fetal alcohol syndrome (FAS), 355
Fiddler, Nettie, 19
Fidelity, principle of, 91
Fight-or-flight response, 59
 with anger and aggression, 468
Financial abuse, 483*t*, 484–485
First aid, psychological, 28
First-generation antipsychotic medications, 171, 273, 288
First Nations
 federal government role in funding mental health care for, 25

First Nations *(Continued)*
 as key strategy area for Canadian mental health care, 8*b*
First Nations Mental Wellness Continuum (FNMWC) framework, 108, 110*b*
Fish oil, 652*t*
5-Hydroxytryptamine (5-HT), 167
Flashbacks, 196
Flight of ideas, with bipolar disorders, 256
Flooding, for anxiety disorders, 216
Fluid intake issues, with substance abuse or behavioural addictions, 373*t*
Flunitrazepam (Rohypnol, "roofies"), 360
Fluoxetine hydrochloride (Prozac), 168
 for anorexia nervosa, 311
 for anxiety disorders, 212*b*–214*b*
 for bulimia nervosa, 315
 for depression, 236*b*–237*b*
Flupentixol, for schizophrenia, 289*t*
Fluphenazine, for schizophrenia, 289*t*
Flurazepam (Dalmane, Som Pam), 166, 426*t*
Fluvoxamine maleate (Luvox), 168, 212*b*–214*b*, 236*b*–237*b*
Focusing, as therapeutic communication technique, 143*t*–144*t*
Follicle-stimulating hormone, 155
Follow-up care, in sexual assault, 516
Forced treatment, advocacy groups to fight Canadian mental health care, 7
Forchuk, Cheryl, 20–21
Forensic correctional nurses, 611
Forensic geriatric or pediatric nurses, 611
Forensic nurse examiners, 611
Forensic nursing, 611
 education of, 612
 nurse coroner or death investigator, 613
 roles and functions of, 612
 sexual assault nurse examiner (SANE), 612
Forensic psychiatric mental health nurses, 613
 competencies associated with, 614*b*
 as expert witnesses, 613
 roles and functions of, 613
Forensic psychiatric nursing, 613
Forensics, 611
Foreseeability, of harm, 101
Forest bathing, 68
Forget-me pill, 510*t*
Forgiveness, in death and dying situations, 599–600
Formal contract, for nurse-patient relationship, 131
Formal operational stage, of cognitive development, 44
Fortune-telling error, 51*t*
Four Gifts of Resolving Relationships, 599, 600*b*
Frankl, Viktor, 55*t*–56*t*
Free association, 42
Freud, Sigmund, 42, 452
 psychoanalytic theory by, 42
  defence mechanisms and anxiety, 42, 184, 186*t*–187*t*
  levels of awareness in, 42, 42*f*
  personality structure in, 42
  psychosexual stages of development in, 43, 43*t*

Frontotemporal dementia, 332*t*
Functional Dementia Scale, 338*f*
Functional magnetic resonance imaging (fMRI), 160
   description and psychiatric uses for, 161*t*
Functional neurological symptom disorder, 190, 192
Funding, for psychiatric mental health care, 24*b*–25*b*, 25

G

GABA. *See* Gamma-aminobutyric acid
Gabapentin (Neurontin), 171, 212*b*–214*b*, 263*b*
GAD. *See* Generalized anxiety disorder
Galantamine (Reminyl), 174
   for Alzheimer's disease, 343*f*
Gamma-aminobutyric acid (GABA), 157*t*
   in anger and aggression, 468
   anti-anxiety actions of, 164
   associated with substance abuse, 356
   types of receptors for, 165
Gamma-hydroxybutyrate (GHB), 510*t*
Gang involvement, 535
GAS. *See* General adaptation syndrome
Gastritis, concurrent with substance abuse disorders, 354
Gastrointestinal disorders, that may mimic psychiatric illness, 78*b*
Gay, 525
   hostility toward, 537*b*
Gender, 525
   bias in diagnosing personality disorders, 398*b*
   definition of, 525, 526*b*
   incongruence, 526
      of adolescents or adults, 527*b*
      of childhood, 527*b*
      criteria for, 527*b*
   as key social determinant of health, 12
   nursing process application in, 527
      assessment, 527, 528*b*
      evaluation, 530
      implementation, 528, 529*b*
      mental health issues, 529
      planning, 528
      providing safe and inclusive nursing care, 529
Gender-affirming surgery, in gender dysphoria, 527
Gender dysphoria, 526
   advanced interventions in, 527
   clinical picture of, 527
   criteria for, 526*b*
   epidemiology of, 527
   nursing care for, 527
Gender identity
   cultural considerations, 525*b*
   definition of, 525
Gender non-conforming, 525
General adaptation syndrome (GAS), 61, 468, 586
Generalized anxiety disorder (GAD)
   in children and adolescents, 550
   description of, 188, 189*b*, 189*t*
   prevalence statistics of, in Canada, 9*t*

Generalized anxiety disorder (GAD) (*Continued*)
   selective serotonin reuptake inhibitors for, 166
Generalizing, during family therapy, 633*b*
Genes, mapping of, neurological illness and, 7
Genetic endowment, as key social determinant of health, 12
Genetics
   anxiety disorders and, 199
   bipolar disorders and, 252
   in dementia, 334
   depression and, 224
   in eating and feeding disorders, 307
   Human Genome Project, 6, 12
   in identical twin brain image research, 162*f*, 164
   personality disorders and, 392
   substance use disorders and, 356
Genogram, 637–638, 638*b*, 639*f*
Genuineness
   element of LEAP approach, 271
   for patients' growth, 133
Geriatric Depression Scale, 230
Germ theory, 6
Gestures
   non-verbal communication through, 139, 139*t*
   use of, for managing disruptive behaviours, in children and adolescents, 549*b*
GHB. *See* Gamma-hydroxybutyrate
Ghost sickness, 116
Gilligan, Carol, 45–46
Ginkgo biloba, 174
Glossophobia, 188*t*
Glutamate, 157*t*
   in anger and aggression, 468
   depression and, 225
Glycogen synthase kinase 3ß (GSK3ß), 170
Golden root, 652*t*
Goldie, Katie, 110
Graduate nursing programs, CFMHN recommendations for, 20–21
Grandeur delusion, 277*t*
Grandiosity, with mania, 256
Gratitude, in death and dying situations, 600
Grey matter, 159, 160*f*
Grey Nuns, 17
Grief
   anticipatory grief, 599*b*, 599
   defined, 601*b*, 601
   guidelines for, 604*t*
   normal, 601
   nursing care for, 601
   psychoanalytic model of, 602
   with serious medical illness, 588*b*, 588
   theories of, 602
   types of, 601
Grieving, depression and, 222
Grooming
   anxiety disorders and, 212
   depression and, 229
   non-verbal communication through, 139*t*
Grounding techniques, for sexual assaults, 518

Group, 620
   cohesiveness, 621*b*
   development, phases of, 621
   observation, 624
   planning, 620
   psychoeducational, 625
   therapeutic factors in, 620, 621*b*
Group content, 621*b*
Group discussion, nurse-patient relationship and, 128
Group homes, in schizophrenia, 284
Group norms, 621*b*
Group process, 621*b*, 623*t*
Group psychotherapy, 626
   in violence and abuse, 501–502
Group themes, 621*b*
Group therapy, 36–37
   for children and adolescents, 539
   for depression, 243
   ethical issues in, 624
   modalities, for older adults, 567*t*
   theoretical foundations for, 623*t*
Group work, 620, 621*b*
   terms describing, 621*b*
Growth, patients'
   attending behaviour, 133–134
   develop resources for, 134
   empathy for, 133
   factors that encourage and promote, 133
   genuineness for, 133
   positive regard for, 133
Guardianship, 97
Guided imagery, 68*b*, 68, 540, 648
Guilt
   during bereavement, 603*t*
   depression assessment of, 229
   with major depressive disorder, 221
Gustatory hallucination, 278*t*

H

Haldol. *See* Haloperidol
Hallucinations, 271, 278, 285
   assessment of, during mental status examination, 79*b*–80*b*
   auditory, 278, 278*t*
   causes of, 278
   command, 279
   counselling and communication techniques for, 285*b*, 285
   with delirium, 329, 336–337
   with dementia, 332
   gustatory, 278*t*
   hypnagogic, 419
   illusions and, 278
   with major depressive disorder, 221
   olfactory, 278*t*
   with schizophrenia, 271
   with substance abuse or behavioural addictions, 373*t*
   summary of, 278, 278*t*
   tactile, 278*t*
   visual, 278*t*, 279
Hallucinogens, intoxication, overdose and withdrawal, 368, 369*t*
Haloperidol, 473*b*
   for schizophrenia, 289*t*

Hamilton Anxiety Rating Scale, 201–202, 202t
Hamilton Depression Rating Scale, 226b–227b, 226
Hamilton Psychiatric Hospital, 20–21
Harm Command Safety Protocol, 280, 281f–282f
Harm reduction approaches, for drug abuse programs, 376
HAT. See Heroin assisted treatment
Head injury, in dementia, 334
HEADSSS psychosocial interview technique, 77b
Healing touch, 653
Health
    culture and, 105
    equity, 106–107
    inequity, 106–107
Health Canada
    approved drug treatment
        for anxiety, 212b–214b, 212
        for bipolar disorders, 262, 263b
    on natural health products, 175
Health care aides, as members of psychiatric mental health treatment teams, 34b
Health determinants, used in psychiatric mental health nursing, 12
Health indicators, 63
Health information acts, provincial and territorial, 76t, 82
Health maintenance, pharmacological interventions during, 373
Health Professions Act (HPA), 94
Health promotion
    for anorexia nervosa, 311
    for bulimia nervosa, 315
    for dementia, 337
    interventions in psychiatric mental health nursing and, 85
    regarding sleep hygiene, 419b, 425
    for schizophrenia, 287
    in violence and abuse, 498
Health services, as key social determinant of health, 12
Health teaching
    for anorexia nervosa, 311
    as basic-level nursing intervention, 27
    as basic-level psychiatric mental health nursing intervention, 11t
    for bulimia nervosa, 315
    for dementia, 337
    interventions in psychiatric mental health nursing and, 85
    regarding sleep hygiene, 419b, 425
    for schizophrenia, 287
    in violence and abuse, 498
Hearing
    area of brain responsible for, 159, 160f
    in communication, 137
    issues when assessing older adults, 77
Helplessness
    as counter-transference, 127t
    depression assessment of, 229, 231t
Hematophobia, 188t
Herbal teas, 651–652
Herbal therapy, 650

Heroin
    intoxication, overdose and withdrawal from, 364t
    physical complications related to abuse of, 355t
Heroin-assisted treatment (HAT), 377
Heterogeneous group, 621b
Heterosexual, 525
Hierarchy, in families, 634b
High-quality emotional support, 63
Hincks, Clarence M., 7
Hippocampus, emotions and psychological function and, 158–159
Histamine, 157t
Historical trauma, 112, 470b
History
    of early Canadian asylums, 17
    of early psychiatric treatments, 17–18
    Rockwood Asylum Nursing School, 18
Histrionic personality disorder
    characteristics and behaviours associated with, 391, 398, 399b
    nursing and therapy guidelines for, 399, 405t
    treatment of, 399
Holistic approach, 586
Holistic medicine, from indigenous peoples in Canada, 17
Holistic nurse, 647
Holmes, David, 20–21
Home care
    for dementia, 341t
    guidelines for, 342b
Homeless, increase of individuals with mental illness in, deinstitutionalization and, 29
Homeopathy, 648
Homeostasis
    cycle of sleep and wakefulness and, 155
    maintenance of, brain and, 154
Homeostatic processes, for sleep drive, 417
Homicide
    in Canada, 610–611
    concurrent with substance abuse disorders, 354
    potential, in violence and abuse, 495
Homogeneous group, 621b
Homosexual, 525
Honesty, misuse of, as counter-transference, 127t
Honeymoon stage, in cycle of violence, 485
Hope
    bulimia nervosa and, 315t
    inspiration for anxiety disorders, 209b
    instillation, in therapeutic groups, 621b
Hope and Healing: A Practical Guide for Survivors, 458–459
Hopelessness, 112
    as counter-transference, 127t
    depression assessment of, 229, 231t
    with substance abuse or behavioural addictions, 373t
Hormones, 468
    depression and, 225
    in gender transition, 527
    mental health dysfunction and, 164
    regulation of, 155

Hospice palliative care, 594, 595b
Hospital admission, of patients with eating disorders, 308–309, 309b
Hospital policies and procedures, 95
Housing instability, serious mental illness and, 575
How a Nurse Helped Me, in LEAP approach, for schizophrenia, 271b, 271
HPA. See Health Professions Act
Human energy field, 653
Human Genome Project, 6, 12
Human immunodeficiency virus (HIV) infection, with dementia, 332t
Human rights abuses, of stigmatized persons with medical conditions, 589
Humanism, 55t–56t
Humanistic psychology theory, 53
    hierarchy of needs, 53, 53f, 54b
Humanistic theories, 53
    Abraham Maslow's humanistic psychology theory as, 53
Humour, 70
    for managing disruptive behaviours, in children and adolescents, 549b
Huntington's disease, with dementia, 332t
Hwa-Byung, 115
Hydromorphone (Dilaudid), intoxication, overdose and withdrawal from, 364t
Hydrophobia, 188t
Hydrotherapy, 18
Hydroxyzine hydrochloride (Atarax), 212b–214b
Hydroxyzine pamoate (Vistaril), 212b–214b
Hygiene
    anxiety disorders and, 212
    with substance abuse or behavioural addictions, 373t
Hyperpyrexia, from conventional anti-psychotics, 291t–292t
Hypersomnia disorders
    description and types of, 419
    with seasonal affective disorder, 221
Hypertension, sleep disorders and, 421
Hypnosis, 649
Hypnotics
    benzodiazepines used in Canada for, 166
    short-acting sedative, 166
Hypochondriasis, 192
Hypocretin, 419
    wakefulness and, 417
Hypomania
    behaviour symptoms of, 255
    with bipolar II disorder, 250
    transition to mania, 255
Hypotension, from conventional anti-psychotics, 291t–292t
Hypothalamic–pituitary–thyroid–adrenal (HPTA) axis, associated with mood disorders, 253
Hypothalamus, 158–159
    emotions and psychological function and, 158–159
    role in mental function, 155
    stress response and, 61

Hypothyroidism
    associated with hypersomnia, 422
    depression and, 253
    mimicking depression, 79
Hypoxia, 329
Hysteria, 5, 42

I
IAFN. *See* International Association of Forensic Nurses
Id, 42*f*, 42
Ideal body weight, 310
    definition of, 311
Ideas of harming self or others, assessment of, during
    mental status examination, 79*b*–80*b*
Ideas of influence, in delusions, 277*t*
Ideas of reference, 294
    in delusions, 277*t*
Identical twins
    autism concordance rate for, 542
    brain image research on, 162*f*, 164
    depression concordance in, 224
Identification, as defence mechanism, 186*t*–187*t*
Identified patient, 634
Illness anxiety disorder, 190, 192
Illusions, 278
    assessment of, during mental status examination, 79*b*–80*b*
    with delirium, 329
Imaging, of brain, in anorexia nervosa, 307
Imipramine hydrochloride (Tofranil), 212*b*–214*b*
Immigrants
    definition of, 111
    mental health concerns of, 113
Immune stress response, 61
Impaired executive functioning, 280
Impaired impulse control, 279
Impaired information processing, 280
Impaired memory, 280
Impaired social interaction, with delirium, 329
Impaired verbal communication, in delirium, 329
Implementation
    definition of, 74
    within psychiatric mental health nursing process, 84
Implied consent, 96
Impossibility, principle of, 91
Impotence, from conventional anti-psychotics, 291*t*–292*t*
Impulse control
    goals with personality disorders, 404*t*
    training, interventions for, 406*b*
Impulse self-control, in bulimia nervosa, 315*t*
Impulsivity
    constraint vs., 401, 402*t*
    manifestation of, 396
Incest, 510
Incidence, defined, in mental health epidemiology, 7–8
Income, as key social determinant of health, 12

Incontinence, in dementia, 337*t*
Indian Act, 112
Indian Residential Schools (IRSs), 112
Indigenous people
    defined, 106
    end-of-life care and, 596–597
    family structure of, 630
    mental health concerns of, 111
    mental wellness needs of, 56*b*
    residential school system, 630
Indigenous Services Canada, 449–450
Indigenous Wellness Framework, 109*f*
Indigenous world view, 108
Individual psychotherapy, in violence and abuse, 500*f*, 500
Individualism, 108
Infections
    depression co-occurring with, 223*t*
    mental health dysfunction and, 164
    that may mimic psychiatric illness, 78*b*
Inflammation, depression and, 225
Inflammatory disorders, depression co-occurring with, 223*t*
Informal contract, for nurse-patient relationship, 131
Information
    giving, as therapeutic communication technique, 143*t*–144*t*
    imparting of, in groups, 621*b*
    Personal Information Protection and Electronic Documents Act, 76
    privacy of, right to, 98
Informed consent, 96
In-group workplace violence, 466–467
Inhalants, intoxication, overdose and withdrawal of, 363, 363*t*
Initial impressions, in nurse-patient relationship, 132
Inpatient psychiatric mental health programs, 29
    entry to, 29, 30*b*
    preparation for discharge to the community in, 30, 31*b*
Insight, 79*b*–80*b*
Insight-oriented family therapy, 636, 637*t*
Insomnia
    with delirium, 329
    with dementia, 336–337
    depression co-occurring with, 234*t*
    disorders
        description and types of, 418
        sleep hygiene and, 419*b*, 419
    drugs for, 165, 426*t*, 543*b*
    melatonin for, 419, 426*b*
    NANDA definition of, 424
    three factors contribute to, 418
Institutionalization, 27
Instrumental aggression, 465
Insulin shock treatment, 17–18
Integrated use, 352
Integrative groups, 626–627
Integrative health care
    biologically based integrative therapies for, 650
    aromatherapy as, 652
    diet and nutrition as, 650

Integrative health care *(Continued)*
    herbal therapy as, 650
    megavitamin therapy as, 650
    in Canada, 645
    definition of, 645
    manipulative practices for, 652
        chiropractic medicine, 653
        massage therapy, 653
        reflexology, 653
    patients and, 646
    resources, 646*b*
    whole medical systems of, 647
        acupuncture, 646
        Ayurvedic medicine, 647
        homeopathy and naturopathy, 648
        traditional Chinese medicine, 647
        traditional Indigenous medicine, 647
Integrative nursing care, 647
Integrative therapy, 645
    for anxiety disorders, 215, 215*b*
    as basic-level psychiatric mental health nursing intervention, 11*t*
    classification of, 647
    for depression, 243*b*
        exercise, 243*b*
        light therapy, 243*b*
        St. John's wort, 243*b*
    ma huang, 310*b*
    melatonin for insomnia, 426*b*
    during psychiatric mental health nursing process, 85
Intellectual disabilities, in children and adolescents, 542
Intellectualization, as defence mechanism, 186*t*–187*t*
Intelligence, fund of, 79*b*–80*b*
Intentional torts, 100, 100*t*
Interdependent environment, as relational ethics principle, 91
Interdisciplinary team, care plans and, 35
Intergenerational issues, with families, 634*b*, 637
Intergenerational trauma, 111–112, 630
Interleukins, depression and, 62
International Association of Forensic Nurses (IAFN), 612
International Classification of Diseases (ICD), 10
    ICD-10-CA, 10
    ICD-11, 10
Interpersonal and social rhythm therapy, for bipolar disorders, 265
Interpersonal and structural violence, 112
Interpersonal psychotherapy, 46
Interpersonal Relations in Nursing, 46, 126
Interpersonal relations, Peplau's theory of, 46
Interpersonal theories, 46
    implications of, for nursing practice, 48
    interpersonal psychotherapy in, 46
    Peplau's theory of interpersonal relations, 46
    by Sullivan, 46
    theory of object relations in, 46
Interpersonal therapy
    for binge eating disorder, 316
    in groups, 623*t*

Interpersonal violence, 481
  case study and nursing care plan in, 502b–504b
  clinical picture of, 481
  comorbidity of, 487b, 487
  define, 482f
  effective nursing intervention in, 482b, 482
  epidemiology of, 486
  etiology of, 487
  myth vs. fact in, 494t
  nursing process application in, 489
    assessment in, 489, 490b
    diagnosis in, 495, 496t
    evaluation in, 502
    implementation in, 496
    outcomes identification in, 496, 496t
    planning in, 496
  typology of, 481, 482f
Interprofessional team model
  in community mental health centres, 27
  members of, 35
Intersex, 525
Interventions
  advanced-practice, 85
  basic-level, 85
  basic-level and advanced-practice psychiatric, 11t
  for nicotine replacement therapy, 375
  Nursing Interventions Classification (NIC), 11
  for opioid, 375
  pharmacological, biological and integrative, 85
  substance misuse, for those resisting treatment, 374
  pharmacologic, 374
Interviewing techniques
  abuse and, 491, 492f, 493b
  HEADSSS psychosocial interview, 77b
  motivational, in substance abuse cases, 371, 372b
  for older adults, 565b
Intimate partner abuse, 481
  in Canada, 486
  epidemiology of, 486
  interventions for, 498b
  nursing process application in, 489
    assessment in, 489, 490b
    diagnosis in, 495, 496t
    evaluation in, 502
    implementation in, 496
    outcomes identification in, 496, 496t
    planning in, 496
Intimate relationships, between patients, 32
Intoxication
  assessment of acute, 358b, 358
  signs of, 359
Intrapsychic conflict, 43
Intravenous drugs, comorbid conditions in users, 355
Introjection, as defence mechanism, 186t–187t
Introversion, vs. extraversion, 401, 402t
Intrusive thoughts, of sexual assaults, 511

Inuit people
  federal government role in funding mental health care for, 25
  as key strategy area for Canadian mental health care, 8b
Inventory of Voice Experiences, 283
Involuntary admission, 30
  criteria, 97
Isolation, with serious mental illness, 575

J
Jacobson, Edmund, 65–67
Jealousy delusion, 277t
Jet lag, 426b
Jordan's Principle, 107
Journaling, 69
Judgement, 79b–80b
  delaying, of health care workers, 126
Jumping to conclusions, 51t
Justice, 91
Justice view, of morality, 46

K
Kava kava, 174, 215b, 651, 652t
Keon, Wilbert, 27
Ketamine, 368, 369t, 510t
Kinesics, 149
Kirby, Michael, 27
Kleine-Levin Syndrome, 420
Knowledge, fund of, 79b–80b
Kohlberg, Lawrence, 44, 55t–56t
Korsakoff's syndrome, 354
Kraepelin, Emil, coined the term schizophrenia, 272
Kübler-Ross, Dr. Elisabeth, 594–595
  Four Gifts of Resolving Relationships, 599

L
La belle indifférence, 192–193
Labelling, 51t
Laboratory data, during psychiatric mental health nursing assessments, 79
Laissez-faire leader, 623
Lamotrigine (Lamictal), 171
  for bipolar disorders, 262, 263b
  for schizophrenia, 290
Language, 79b–80b
  area of brain responsible for, 159–160, 160f
  barriers to, assessments and, 77
Laryngeal dystonia, from conventional anti-psychotics, 291t–292t
Lateral workplace violence, 466b, 466, 470b
Latuda. *See* Lurasidone
Laughing gas, 363
Lavender, 652t
Leadership, 622
  clinical supervision for, 623
  as key strategy area for Canadian mental health care, 7, 8b
  nurse as group leader, 622
  styles of, 623, 624t
  in therapeutic groups, 623
LEAP approach, to schizophrenia, 271b, 271

Learned helplessness, depression and, 226
Learning theory, of anxiety disorders, 200
Least restrictive type, of mental health care, 97b, 97
Leeching, 17–18
Legal issues, documentation guidelines and importance, 85b–86b, 85
Legislation, mental health, 89, 93b, 93
Leininger, Madeleine, 105–106
Lesbian, 525
  hostility toward, 537b
Lethality, of suicide plan, 455
Letourneau, Nicole, 20–21
Level of consciousness, assessment of, during mental status examination, 79b–80b
Levels of awareness, in Sigmund Freud's psychoanalytic theory, 42, 42f
Levels of prevention, for substance use disorders, 376
  primary, 376
  secondary, 376
    controlled drinking in, 377
    harm reduction in, 376
    heroin assisted treatment in, 377
    managed alcohol programs in, 378
    methadone treatment and methadone maintenance in, 376
    needle exchange programs in, 376
    relapse, 378, 379b
    self-help groups in, 380–381
    supervised consumption sites, 377
  tertiary, 381
    addiction supportive housing in, 382
    alternative living environment in, 382
    assessment and referral in, 381
    community-based (outpatient), 381
    day, 381
    nurses and addiction in the workplace, 385
    Onen'tó:kon Healing Lodge in, 382
    recovery homes in, 382
    short-term residential, 381–382
    withdrawal management services in, 381
Lewy bodies, dementia with, 332t
LGBT (lesbian, gay, bisexual, and transgender), 525
LGBTQ (lesbian, gay, bisexual, transgender, and queer), 525
LGBTTIQQ2SA (lesbian, gay, bisexual, transsexual, transgender, intersex, queer, questioning, two-spirited, and allies), 525
Liability issues, 100t
Libel, 100, 100t
Libido, serotonin regulating, 224–225
Licensed Natural Health Products Database, 175
Licensed practical nurses, as members of psychiatric mental health treatment teams, 34b, 35
Licensure
  province regulations regarding APN, 21
  for psychiatric nurse, history of, 19
Life After Service Studies, 449
Life changes, depression and, 225
Light therapy, for depression, 243b

Limbic system
　benzodiazepines and, 165
　roles and neurotransmitters associated with, 158–159
Limit setting
　for managing disruptive behaviours, in children and adolescents, 549b
　with manipulative behaviour, 406b
Lindemann, Erich, 433
Linehan, Marsha, 51
Listening
　active, 140
　element of LEAP approach, 271
　in nurse-patient relationship, 132
Lithium carbonate, 170, 171t
　for bipolar disorders, 260, 261b, 261t, 263b
　contraindications to, 261
　indications for bipolar disorders, 260
　maintenance therapy for, 260
　therapeutic and toxic levels of, 260, 261t
Little Albert, 48
Live Life, 456
Liver
　disorders concurrent with substance abuse disorders, 354
　drug metabolism and, 164–165
Lobotomies, 17–18
LOC. *See* Locus of control
Locus of control (LOC), 469
Loneliness, with serious mental illness, 575
Lone-parent families, 632
Long-term reorganization phase, of rape-trauma syndrome, 511
Loose ego boundaries, 278
Looseness of association, with schizophrenia, 156
Lorazepam (Ativan), 166, 212b–214b, 473b
Loss
　helping people cope with, 603
　with serious medical illness, 588b, 588
Loss-oriented stressors, 602–603
Love
　in death and dying situations, 600
　need for, 54
Low-quality support relationships, 63
Loxapac. *See* Loxapine
Loxapine, 473b
　for schizophrenia, 289t
LSD. *See* Lysergic acid diethylamide
Lurasidone (Latuda), 174
　for schizophrenia, 288
Luteinizing hormone, 155
Lysergic acid diethylamide (LSD), 164, 368, 369t

M

Ma huang, 310b
Madness, 16
Magnetic resonance imaging (MRI), description and psychiatric uses for, 161t
Magnification, 51t
Mahler, Margaret, 46
Maintenance of wakefulness test (MWT), 418
Maintenance phase
　of bipolar disorders
　　implementation for, 260

Maintenance phase *(Continued)*
　　outcomes identification in, 258
　　planning in, 258
　of depression, 232
　of schizophrenia, 275, 283–285
　of Transtheoretical Model of Change, 371
Major depressive disorder (MDD), 220–221
　case study on, 220b
　diagnostic criteria for, 221b
　drug treatment for, 543b
　epidemiology of, 223
　medical conditions and substances or medications associated with, 223t
　prevalence statistics of, in Canada, 9t
　sub-types and specifiers of, 221
　　atypical features, 221
　　catatonic features, 221
　　melancholic features, 221
　　postpartum onset, 221
　　psychotic features, 221
　　seasonal features, 221
Major neurocognitive disorder. *See* Dementia
Maladaptive uses, of defences, 186t–187t
Malpractice, 100–101, 100t
Managed alcohol programs (MAPs), 378
Mania, 249
　with bipolar disorder, 249–250, 251b
　case study and nursing care plan for, 265b–267b
　euphoric mood associated with, 255
　spectrum of symptoms of, 255
Manic depression, 249
Manic episodes
　with bipolar disorder, 249
　treatment during bipolar, 258, 259t
Manipulative behaviour
　during family therapy, 633b
　with personality disorders, 402, 404t, 406b, 407t
Manipulative practices, 652
　chiropractic medicine, 653
　massage therapy, 653
　reflexology, 653
MAO. *See* Monoamine oxidase
MAOIs. *See* Monoamine oxidase inhibitors
MAPs. *See* Managed alcohol programs
Maslow, Abraham, humanistic psychology theory by, 53
Mass disasters, five elements of intervention, 433–434
Massage, 653
　as stress buster, 64b
Master biological clock, 417
MAST-G. *See* Michigan Alcoholism Screening Test-Geriatric Version
McGill Model of Nursing, 632
MDD. *See* Major depressive disorder
MDQ. *See* Mood Disorder Questionnaire
Media, in communication process, 137
Medical Assistance in Dying (MAiD), 338, 453
Medical comorbidity, 354
Medical conditions
　anxiety caused by, 194t
　application of nursing process, 590
　　assessment, 590b, 590, 591t
　　diagnosis, 591

Medical conditions *(Continued)*
　　evaluation, 592
　　implementation, 591
　　outcomes identification, 591
　　planning, 591
　depression co-occurring with, 223t, 224
　human rights abuses of stigmatized persons with, 589
　psychiatric consultation liaison nurse (PCLN), 592
　psychological factors affecting, 586
　psychological responses to serious, 587
　psychosis associated with, 272b
　psychosocial assessment, 590b, 590
　　coping skills, 590, 591t, 592b
　　quality of life assessment, 590
　　social and spiritual support, 590
　that may mimic psychiatric illness, 78b, 78
Medical crises, management of, 37
Medical physicians, as members of psychiatric mental health treatment teams, 34b
Medical records
　as evidence, 99
　organizational use of, 99
Medicare Act, 25
Medication adherence, 577b
Medication-induced dementia, 332t
Medication-induced psychotic disorder, 272b
Medication prescriptive authority, of advanced-practice psychiatric mental health nurses, 11t
Medications
　for anxiety disorders, 212, 215
　　anti-anxiety drugs, 212b–215b, 212, 215
　　antidepressants, 212b–214b, 214
　for behavioural symptoms, 342
　delirium from, 328
　for depression, 234, 235f, 236b–237b
　depression co-occurring with, 223t
　education group protocol, 625b, 625, 626f
Medicine wheel, 108, 109f
Meditation, 67, 648
Medulla oblongata, 159f
Megavitamin therapy, 650
Melancholic features, with major depressive disorder, 221
Melatonin, 652t
　for insomnia, 419, 426b
Memantine (Ebixa, Namenda), 174
　for Alzheimer's disease, 342, 343f
Memory
　assessment of, during mental status examination, 79b–80b
　brain and, 156
　impairment, in dementia, 337t
Memory deficits
　normal aging vs. major neurocognitive disorder, 332t
　with substance abuse or behavioural addictions, 373t
Menstrual periods, pre-menstrual dysphoric disorder, 222
Mental Disorder Continuum, 3–4
Mental disorders
　classification of, 9
　epidemiology of, 7, 8b

Mental filter, 51*t*
Mental function, disturbances of, 164, 164*f*
Mental health, 2*b*, 2
   contributing factors to, 4, 4*f*
   culture in, 105
   Mental Health for Canadians: Striking a Balance, defining three major challenges, 7
   outcomes of, 4
   positive, attributes of, 2–3, 3*f*
   psychiatric nursing, 10
   recovery of, 5*b*, 5
   two conceptualizations of, 3
   WHO definition of, 2–3
Mental Health Act, 469
Mental health care
   barriers and pathways to, in multi-cultural context, 114
      communication, 114
      misdiagnosis as, 115
   continuum of, 25
      evolving venues of practice in, 25, 26*b*
   least restrictive type of, 97*b*, 97
   primary health care and, 586, 587*b*
Mental Health Care Law: Ten Basic Principles, 93*b*, 93
Mental Health Commission of Canada (MHCC), 458
   Changing Directions, Changing Lives: The Mental Health Strategy for Canada, 7
   cultural diversity identified by, 12
   defining strategies for mental health, 7, 8*b*
   on mental illness, recovery from, 573–574
Mental Health Commission of Canada (MHCC) Changing Directions, Changing Lives: The Mental Health Strategy for Canada, 533
   on mental health issues related to aging, 556
Mental health concerns
   of immigrants, 113
   of Indigenous people, 111
   of refugees, 113
Mental health emergency, defining in phase four of crisis coping, 435
Mental health first aid (MHFA), 437
Mental Health for Canadians: Striking a Balance, "Epp Report," 3, 4*f*
   challenges/goals identified by, 7
Mental health nursing practice, psychiatric, ethical responsibilities and legal obligations for, 89
Mental health-related disability, 24
Mental illness, 2*b*, 2, 421*b*, 421
   definition of, 3
   early care for, 16
   families and, 632
   vs. physical illness, 6
   psychiatric definitions of, 3
   stigma, 110
   stigma of, 37
Mental status examination, 79*b*–80*b*, 79
   of children and adolescents, 538
Meperidine (Demerol), addiction effects of, 364*t*
Mephedrone, 366
Mescaline (peyote), 368, 369*t*

Mesnick, Janice, 433
Mesocortical pathways, 158–159
Mesolimbic pathways, 158–159
Messages
   in communication process, 137, 138*f*
   double, 140
   double-bind, 140, 634*b*
   process of, 139
Metabolic disorders, that may mimic psychiatric illness, 78*b*
Metabolites, 164–165
Methadone (Metadol), 364*t*, 375
Methadone maintenance (MM), 376
Methadone treatment (MT), 376
Methamphetamine, description and medical uses for, 366, 367*t*
Methylenedioxypyrovalerone (MDPV), 366
Methylphenidate (Biphentin, Concerta, Ritalin), 174, 546
Métis
   federal government role in funding mental health care for, 25
   as key strategy area for Canadian mental health care, 8*b*
Meyer, Adolph, 46
MHCC. *See* Mental Health Commission of Canada
MHFA. *See* Mental health first aid
Michigan Alcoholism Screening Test-Geriatric Version (MAST-G), 558*b*
Midbrain, 159*f*
Mild Alzheimer's disease, 333*t*
Mild anxiety, 182, 184*t*
   interventions for, 208, 208*t*
Mild brain injury, 468
Mild neurocognitive disorders, 325, 330, 331*b*
Milieu
   for children and adolescents, 540*b*, 540
   defined, 54–55
   management, 36
      for anorexia nervosa, 311
      for bipolar disorders, 262
      for catatonia, 295
      for depression, 233
      for disorganization, 295
      in older adults, 568
      for paranoia, 294
      for schizophrenia, 285
      as suicide precautions, 457, 457*t*
   needs, 294–295, 295*b*
   therapeutic factors in, 540*b*
Milieu management, of schizophrenia, 285*b*, 285
Milieu therapy, 54
   for anxiety disorders, 212
   as basic-level psychiatric mental health nursing intervention, 11*t*
   implications of, for nursing practice, 55
   as part of psychiatric mental health nursing process, 85
Mind-body-spirit approaches, to integrative health care, 648
   biofeedback, 648
   guided imagery, 648
   hypnosis, 649

Mind-body-spirit approaches, to integrative health care *(Continued)*
   meditation, 648
   rhythmic breathing, 649
   spirituality, 649
   therapeutic suggestion, 649
   T.R.U.S.T. model, 649–650, 650*f*, 651*b*
Mind-body therapies, 65
   for children and adolescents, 540
Mindfulness, 69
   for schizophrenia, 288*b*
Mindfulness-based therapy, 648–649
Mind-reading, 51*t*
Minimization, 51*t*
Mino-Pimatisiwin, 634*b*
Mirtazapine (Remeron), 168–169, 236*b*–237*b*
Misdiagnosis, of mental illness, 115
Misperceptions, with delirium, 329
Mistaken beliefs, in dementia, 337*t*
Misuse, 352
Mixed messages, 140
Miyo-mahcihoyān, 123*b*
MM. *See* Methadone maintenance
Mnemonic tool ABCD-ER, 491, 493*b*
Mobile crisis intervention teams, 28, 29*b*
Mobile crisis outreach, 442*b*
Mobile mental health units, 26
MoCA. *See* Montreal Cognitive Assessment
Moclobemide (Aurorix, Manerix), 236*b*–237*b*
Modecate. *See* Fluphenazine
Model of care, for mental illness, 573
Modelling
   for anxiety disorders, 215
   as behavioural therapy, 49
   for managing disruptive behaviours, in children and adolescents, 549*b*
Moderate Alzheimer's disease, 333*t*
Moderate anxiety, 182, 184*t*
   interventions for, 208, 208*t*
Monoamine oxidase (MAO), 156
   definition of, 169*f*, 169
   as destructive enzyme, 156
Monoamine oxidase inhibitors (MAOIs), 167, 169
   actions and effects of, 236*b*–237*b*
   adverse reactions and toxic effects of, 240, 240*t*
   for anxiety disorders, 212*b*–214*b*, 214
   common adverse reactions, 240
   contraindications, 240
   definition of, 169
   for depression, 236*b*–237*b*, 239, 240*b*
   drugs that can interact with, 238, 239*b*
   foods that can interact with, 239, 239*t*
   indications, 240
   potential toxic effects, 240
Monoamine theory, of depression, 167, 170
Monoamines, 157*t*
   definitions, 169
   normal release, reuptake, and degradation of, 167*f*, 167
Monophobia, 188*t*
Monopolizing member, 627*b*, 627
Montreal Cognitive Assessment (MoCA), in delirium, 328

Mood
    assessment of, during mental status examination, 79b–80b
    bipolar disorders and, 255
    in delirium, 328
    depression assessment of, 229
Mood Disorder Questionnaire (MDQ), 254f, 254
Mood disorders, 220
    in children and adolescents, 551
    in eating and feeding disorder, 307
    Mood Disorder Questionnaire for, 254f, 254
    prevalence statistics of, in Canada, 9t
Mood stabilizers, 170, 290
    for bipolar disorders, 260
Moral agent, 91–92
Moral development, stages of, 44, 55t–56t
    conventional level of, 45
    post-conventional level of, 45
    pre-conventional level of, 44
Moral distress, 92b–93b, 92
Moral residue, 92
Moral resilience, 92b–93b, 92
Moral treatment, 16–17
Moral uncertainty, 92
Morphine, intoxication, overdose and withdrawal from, 364t
Motivation theory, implications of, for nursing practice, 54
Motivational interviewing (MI), 577b
    in substance abuse cases, 371, 372b
    supplementing goal setting for families using, 137b
Motor disorders, in children and adolescents, 544
Motor functions, area of brain responsible for, 159–160, 160f
Mount, Balfour, 595
Mourning, 601
    four tasks of, 603
    goals of, 602
MT. *See* Methadone treatment
Multi-culturalism, 111
Multi-disciplinary teams, care plans and, 35
Multiple sleep latency test (MSLT), 418
Muscarinic receptors, 168, 172
Muscle atonia, rapid eye movement behaviour disorder, 420
Music, as stress buster, 64b
Music therapists, as members of psychiatric mental health treatment teams, 34b
Must statements, 51t
Mutual aid, 380
Mutual avoidance, defined, 133
Mutual storytelling, 541, 542b
MWT. *See* Maintenance of wakefulness test
Mysophobia, 188t

N

NA. *See* Narcotics Anonymous
Naltrexone (ReVia), 374
NANDA-I. *See* North American Nursing Diagnosis Association International
Narcissistic personality disorder
    characteristics and behaviours associated with, 391, 399b, 399
    nursing and therapy guidelines for, 399, 405t
    treatment of, 399
Narcolepsy, 419
Narcotics Anonymous (NA), 380
National Crime Prevention Strategy (NCPS), 611b, 611
National Eating Disorder Information Centre (NEDIC), 315
National Inuit Suicide Prevention Strategy, 450
National Native Alcohol and Drug Abuse Program (NNADAP), 113
National Network for Mental Health, 627b
National Sleep Foundation, recommended hours of sleep per night, 414
Native Wellness Assessment Tool, 115
Natural disasters, critical incident stress debriefing (CISD), 441, 442b
Natural health products (NHPs), 174, 175b
    in Canada, 645–646
Natural Health Products Directorate (NHPD), 646
Natural Health Products Regulations (NHPR), 645–646
Nature vs. nurture, 6
Naturopathy, 648
Navane. *See* Thiothixene
Nav-CARE, 559b
Navigation, resilience and, 5
NCPS. *See* National Crime Prevention Strategy
NDRIs. *See* Norepinephrine-dopamine reuptake inhibitors
NEDIC. *See* National Eating Disorder Information Centre
Needle exchange programs, 376
Needs
    for belongingness, 54
    for esteem, 54
    hierarchy of, 53, 53f, 54b
    for love, 54
    physiological, 53
    safety, 54
Negative reinforcement, 48
Negative symptoms, of schizophrenia, 272, 276, 279, 279t
Negativism, 279
Neglect, 483t, 485
    as risk factor for mental illness, 535
Negligence, 100–101
    as liability issue, 100t
    by peers, 95
Negotiation, resilience and, 5
Neologisms, in communication, 278
Neoplastic disorders, depression co-occurring with, 223t
Nerve stimulation, 242
Nervous system, 154, 155f
Neuman, Betty, 47t
Neurasthenia, 115
Neurobiological factors, 334
    anxiety disorders and, 200
    bipolar disorders and, 252
    in eating and feeding disorders, 307
Neurobiology, 392
Neurochemical factors, in aggression and violence, 468
Neurochemical hypotheses, of schizophrenia, 273
Neurochemistry, 392
Neurocognitive disorders, 324–325
    case study and nursing care plan in, 344b–347b
    delirium as, 326
        assessment of, 326, 329b
        clinical picture of, 326
        common causes of, 327b
        comorbidity and etiology of, 326
        diagnosis of, 329, 330t
        diagnostic criteria for, 326b
        epidemiology of, 326
        evaluation of, 329
        implementation in, 329, 331b
        major neurocognitive disorders, depression, and brain injury, comparison of, 325t
        outcomes identification in, 329, 330t
        planning for, 329
        vignette in, 328b
    dementia as, 330
    major, 325, 330, 331b
    mild, 325, 330, 331b
    nursing process, application of, 326
    types of, 332t
Neurodevelopmental disorders
    in children and adolescents, 542
        attention deficit-hyperactivity disorder (ADHD), 543b, 543, 545b, 547b
        autism spectrum disorders, 542
        communication disorders, 542
        intellectual disabilities, 542
        motor disorders, 544
        Nursing Outcomes Classification (NOC) for, 546t
        specific learning disorder (SLD), 544
        stereotypic movement disorder, 544
        Tourette's disorder, 544
        nursing process application to, 544, 545b, 545t
Neurodevelopmental factors, in aggression and violence, 468
Neuroendocrine, 253
Neuroimaging techniques, 253
    refinement of, 7
Neuroleptic malignant syndrome (NMS), from conventional antipsychotics, 290, 291t–292t
Neurological disorders, 468
    anger, aggression and violence, 468
    depression co-occurring with, 223t
    that may mimic psychiatric illness, 78b, 78
Neurological factors, in aggression and violence, 468
Neuromodulators, receptors and mental disorders associated with, 157t

Neurons, 156
 activity of, 156f
 as psychotropic drug targets, 165
Neuropathic pain, antidepressant drugs for, 168
Neuropeptides, 158
Neurotensin (NT), 157t
Neurotransmitters
 associated with bipolar disorder, 252–253
 associated with depression, 224
 circadian rhythms and, 156
 destruction of, 156
 excess transmission of, 164f
 of limbic system, 158–159
 normal transmission of, 164f
 as psychotropic drug targets, 165
 reduction of, in the synapse, 158b
 release of, 156
 stress response and, 61
 substance use disorders and, 356
Neurotrophic factors, 158
NHPD. *See* Natural Health Products Directorate
NHPR. *See* Natural Health Products Regulations
NHPs. *See* Natural health products
NIC. *See* Nursing Interventions Classification
Nicotine, 367, 375
 dependence, in schizophrenia, 273
 description and medical uses for, 367
 physical complications related to abuse of, 355t
Nicotine replacement therapy (NRT), 375
 options, 376t
Nightingale, Florence, 20, 81
Nightmare disorder, 419
Nitrazepam (Mogadon), 166, 426t
N-methyl-D-aspartate (NMDA) receptor antagonist, for Alzheimer's disease, 342
NMS. *See* Neuroleptic malignant syndrome
NNADAP. *See* National Native Alcohol and Drug Abuse Program
NOC. *See* Nursing Outcomes Classification
Non-adherence, as treatment issues, in serious mental illness, 575
Non-benzodiazepines, for anxiety disorders, 212b–214b
Non-binary, 525
Non-maleficence, 90, 97
Non-rapid eye movement (NREM) sleep
 description and EEG illustration of, 414
 patterns and efficiency of, 418
Non-specific bruising, in abuse, 483
Non-steroidal anti-inflammatory drugs (NSAIDs), for Alzheimer's disease, 342
Non-suicidal self-injury, 448
 assessment of, 460
 biological factors, 459
 clinical picture of, 459
 comorbidity of, 459
 diagnosis of, 460
 epidemiology of, 459
 evaluation of, 460

Non-suicidal self-injury *(Continued)*
 interventions for, 460
 outcomes criteria of, 460
 plan of care for, 460
 psychosocial factors, 459
 risk factors for, 459
 societal factors, 459
Non-therapeutic communication techniques, 142, 145t
 asking "why" questions as, 144, 145t
 excessive questioning as, 142, 145t
 giving advice as, 142, 145t
 giving approval/disapproval as, 142
Non-therapeutic relationships, 132f, 132–133
Non-verbal clues, suicide and, 454
Non-verbal communication, 139
 cultural considerations for, 146
 interaction with verbal communication, 139, 140b
Noradrenaline, 157t
Norepinephrine (NE), 157t
 circadian rhythms and, 156
 depression and, 224–225
 reduction of, 158b
 selective serotonin reuptake inhibitors (SSRIs), 167, 168
 substance use disorders and, 356
 wakefulness and, 417
Norepinephrine-dopamine reuptake inhibitors (NDRIs), for depression, 236b–237b
Norepinephrine reuptake inhibitors (NRIs), for depression, 236b–237b
Normal anxiety, 181–182
Normal autism, 396
Normal sleep cycle, 414
North American Nursing Diagnosis Association International (NANDA-I), 10
 crisis-related anxiety issues, 437
 Nursing Diagnoses: Definitions and Classification 2012–2014, 10
 sleep disorders, 424
Nortriptyline hydrochloride (Aventyl, Norventyl), 167–168, 212b–214b, 236b–237b
NRIs. *See* Norepinephrine reuptake inhibitors
NSAIDs. *See* Non-steroidal anti-inflammatory drugs
Nuclear family, 635
 emotional system, 635
Nurse
 addiction in the workplace and, 385b, 385
 as group leader, 622
Nurse coroner or death investigator, 613
Nurse-patient relationship, 123
 boundaries of, 124
 confidentiality in, 131
 counter-transference in, 125–126, 127t
 establishing rapport in, 131
 factors that enhance, 132–133
 factors that hinder, 132
 formal/informal contract in, 131
 parameters of, 131
 Peplau's model of, 126

Nurse-patient relationship *(Continued)*
 orientation phase of, 130
 pre-orientation phase of, 128, 129t–130t
 termination phase of, 131
 working phase of, 131
 Registered Psychiatric Nurses of Canada (RPNC) on, 84
 social relationship, 123
 therapeutic relationship, 124
Nurse practitioners, province licensing regulations for, 21
Nurse therapist, 626
Nursing
 care for those who grieve, 601
 end-of-life (EOL) care, 596
 self-care and, 600
 shifts in control over, 18
Nursing care, 36b, 36
 crisis management and, 37
  behavioural crises, 37
  medical crises, 37
 documentation and, 37
 establishing a therapeutic relationship in, 36
 medication administration in, 37
  adherence to, 37
  for pain management, 37
 mental and physical health assessment in, 36
 milieu management and, 36
 structured group activities and, 36
Nursing diagnosis
 definition of, 74
 DSM-5 and, 11
 North American Nursing Diagnosis Association International (NANDA-I), 10
 Nursing Diagnoses: Definitions and Classification 2012–2014, 10
 within psychiatric mental health nursing process, 82
 structural components of, 82
Nursing help boxes
 on anxiety disorders, 181b
 on bipolar disorders, 250b
 on co-worker abuse reporting, 351b
 on critical incident stress debriefing, 441b
 on dementia, 324b–325b
 on eating and feeding disorders, 304b
 on major depressive disorder, 220b
 on personality disorders, 390b–391b
 on worrying and insomnia, 413b–414b
Nursing Interventions Classification (NIC), 11
 for aggressive, manipulative and impulsive behaviours, 402, 406b
 for anxiety disorders, 208, 209b
 for delirium, 329, 331b
 for eating disorders, 315, 316b
 within psychiatric mental health nursing process, 84
 for sexual assault, 515
Nursing Outcomes Classification (NOC), 11, 82–83
 for aggressive, manipulative and impulsive behaviours, 404t

Nursing Outcomes Classification (NOC) (Continued)
  for anorexia nervosa, 310, 310t
  for anxiety disorders, 205, 207t
  for bipolar disorders, 257
  for bulimia nervosa, 315t
  for crisis-related anxiety issues, 437, 439t
  for delirium, 329, 330t
  for depression, 232, 232t
  related to neurocognitive disorders, 338b
  for sexual assault, 515
  for sleep disorders, 424, 425t
Nursing practice, relevant theories and therapies for, 41
Nursing process, standards of care for psychiatric mental health nursing and, 74, 75f, 76b
  advanced-practice interventions in, 85
  assessment and, 75
  basic-level interventions, 85
  documentation of, 85
  evaluation in, 85
  implementation, 84
  nursing diagnosis in, 82
  outcomes identification in, 82, 84t
  planning for, 83
Nursing shortage, in mental hospitals, 19–20
Nutrition
  anxiety disorders and, 212
  in guidelines for self-care for individuals with cognitive impairment, 340b–341b
  for integrative health care, 650
Nutritional disorders, that may mimic psychiatric illness, 78b, 78
Nutritional status, in anorexia nervosa, 310t
Nyctophobia, 188t

O

Obesity
  in Canada, 308
  sleep disorders and, 421
Object constancy, 396
Object, defined, 46
Object relations, theory of, 46
Obsessions, 189, 193, 195t
Obsessive-compulsive disorder (OCD)
  with anorexia nervosa, 307
  characteristics and behaviours associated with, 391, 400, 401b
  comorbidity of, 194
  description of, 193b, 193, 195t
  drug treatment for, 543b
  epidemiology of, 194
  medications for, 212b–214b
  nursing and therapy guidelines for, 401, 405t
  positron emission tomography scan of brain with, 161, 162f
  prevalence statistics of, in Canada, 9t
  selective serotonin reuptake inhibitors for, 166
  treatment of, 401
  Yale-Brown Obsessive Compulsive Scale (YBOCS) for, 202
Obstructive sleep apnea hypopnea syndrome, description and types of, 420

Occupational therapists, as members of psychiatric mental health treatment teams, 34b
OCD. See Obsessive-compulsive disorder
Oculogyric crisis, from conventional antipsychotics, 291t–292t
Olanzapine (Zyprexa), 173, 473b
  for anorexia nervosa, 311
  for bipolar disorders, 263b
  for schizophrenia, 288, 289t
Older adult abuse, 481
  competency in, 497
  epidemiology of, 487
  factors to assess in home visits in, 495b, 495
  interventions for, 498b
  neglect and, 487
  nursing process application in, 489
    assessment in, 489, 490b
    diagnosis in, 495, 496t
    evaluation in, 502
    implementation in, 496
    outcomes identification in, 496, 496t
    planning in, 496
  vulnerability in, 488
Older adults
  access to care in, 559
  ageism, 559
  aging of the population, 555
  assessment of, 77
  care giver burden and, 559
  care settings in, 568
    behavioural health home care, 569
    community-based programs, 569
    day treatment programs, 568
    long-term care facilities, 568
    partial hospitalization, 568
    respite care, 569
  depression in, 557
    assessment of, 230, 565b, 565
    Geriatric Depression Scale, 565b, 565
    and suicide risk, 557
  factors to assess in home visits in, 495b, 495
  facts and myths regarding, 556b
  group therapy modalities for, 567t
  late-life mental illness in, 556
  milieu management, 568
  nursing care of, 563
    assessment strategies for, 564, 564f, 565b
    health teaching and health promotion, 567b, 567, 567t
    intervention strategies, 566
    interview and, 565b
    pharmacological interventions, 567
    promotion of self-care activities in, 567
    psychosocial interventions in, 566b, 566, 567t
    standards of care, six categories of, 563
  pain in, 560, 560f–561f, 562b, 563f
  pharmacological pain management in, 563b
  psychosocial needs of, 555
  serious mental illness in, 572, 573b
  sleep hypnogram vs. young adults, 415f, 416
  suicide rate among, 557
  trauma in, 558

Older persons, 223
  suicide among, 450
    interventions, 451
    risk factors, 451
    warning signs, 451
Olfactory hallucination, 278t
Omega-3 fatty acids, 652t
  for bipolar disorders, 263b
Onen'tó:kon Healing Lodge, 382
Open-ended questions, 142
Open group, 621b
Operant conditioning, 48, 539
  as behavioural therapy, 49, 49t
Operant conditioning theory, 48
  vs. classical conditioning, 48f
Operation, defined, 44
Operational Stress Injury Social Support (OSISS) programs, 25
Opioid substitution therapy, 376
Opioids, 356, 375
  addiction to, 363, 364b
    case example, 351b
  intoxication, overdose and withdrawal, 364t
  physical complications related to abuse of, 355t
  withdrawal, 364, 365t
Opisthotonos, from conventional antipsychotics, 291t–292t
Opium (paregoric), intoxication, overdose and withdrawal from, 364t
Oppositional defiant disorder, in children and adolescents, 546, 548b
Orap. See Pimozide
Orem, Dorothea, 47t
Orientation phase
  of Peplau's model of nurse-patient relationship, 130
  in therapeutic group, 621
Orientation, to reality, 79b–80b
Orthomolecular therapy, 650
OSISS programs. See Operational Stress Injury Social Support (OSISS) programs
Out of the Shadows at Last, 27, 38, 534
Outcome criteria, 82–83, 84t
Outcome identification, definition of, 74
Outcomes, seven domains of, 11
Outpatient treatment, 381
Overeating, with seasonal affective disorder, 221
Overgeneralization, 51t
  in cognitive distortions, 311b
Overidentification, as counter-transference, 127t
Overinvolvement, as counter-transference, 127t
Oxazepam (Serax), 166, 212b–214b
Oxcarbazepine (Trileptal), 171

P

Pacing, 132
Pain
  barriers to accurate pain assessment, in older adults, 560
  in older adults, 560

Pain (Continued)
  Pain Assessment in Advanced Dementia (PAINAD) scale, 560, 561f, 562b
  pharmacological pain management in older adults, 563b
  visual analogue scale, for cancer pain, 563f
  Wong-Baker FACES Pain Rating Scale, 560f, 560
Pain Assessment in Advanced Dementia (PAINAD) scale, 560, 561f, 562b
Pain management
  medication administration for, 37
  in older adults, 563b
PAINAD scale. See Pain Assessment in Advanced Dementia (PAINAD) scale
Paliperidone (Invega), 173
  for schizophrenia, 289t
Palliative care, 595
  cultural contexts of, 596, 597b
  guidelines when caring for the dying, 599b
  patient-centred, 594
  for patients with dementia, 605
  symptom management, 597
Pancreatitis, concurrent with substance abuse disorders, 354
Panic, 182, 184t
  interventions for, 208, 209t
  and school phobia, drug treatment for, 543b
Panic attack, description of, 185b, 185
Panic disorder (PD), 185b, 185
  generic care plan for, 187t
  Panic Disorder Severity Scale (PDSS) for, 202
  prevalence statistics of, in Canada, 9t
  selective serotonin reuptake inhibitors for, 166
Panic Disorder Severity Scale (PDSS), 202
Paranoia, 290
  communication guidelines for, 294
  milieu needs for, 294
  in schizophrenia, 296b–298b
  self-care needs for, 294
Paranoid personality disorder
  characteristics and behaviours associated with, 392–393, 393b
  nursing and therapy guidelines for, 393, 405t
  treatment of, 393
Paraphrasing, as therapeutic communication technique, 141
Parasympathetic nervous system, regulation of, 155f, 155
Parents, characteristics of abusive, 488b
Parkinson's disease, with dementia, 332t
Paroxetine (Paxil), 168, 212b–214b, 236b–237b
Partial hospitalization
  in older adults, 568
  programs, 29b–30b, 29
    criteria for referral to, 29
  in schizophrenia, 284
Participant observer, 48

Partnership
  element of LEAP approach, 271
  and family support, for serious mental illness, 578
Passive negativism, 279
Paternalism, 95
Patient and family teaching
  on bipolar disorder, 264b
  coping with a major medical illness, 592b
  coping with auditory hallucinations or delusions, 286b–287b
  guidelines for care at home, 342b
  guidelines for self-care for individuals with cognitive impairment, 340b–341b
  on lithium therapy, 261b
  regarding selective serotonin reuptake inhibitors, 238b
  regarding tricyclic antidepressants, 238, 239b
  in schizophrenia, 287b
Patient Health Questionnaire-9 (PHQ-9), 226, 228f
Patient Health Questionnaire-15 (PHQ), 202–203, 203f
Patient safety, as liability issue, 100t
Patients
  intimate relationships between, 32
  tracking whereabouts and activities of, 32
Patient's rights, under law, 95
Pauly, Bernie, 20–21
Pavlov, Ivan, 48
PCLN. See Psychiatric consultation liaison nurse
PCP. See Phenylcyclohexyl piperidine
PDSS. See Panic Disorder Severity Scale
Peer supervision, 623
Penitentiary system, increase of individuals with mental illness in, deinstitutionalization and, 29
Peplau, Hildegard, 20, 46, 47f, 126
  theory of interpersonal relations by, 46
Peplau's model of nurse-patient relationship, 126
  orientation phase of, 130
  pre-orientation phase of, 128, 129t–130t
  termination phase of, 131
  working phase of, 131
Peptic ulcer, anxiety caused by, 194t
Peptides, receptors and mental disorders associated with, 157t
Perceived Stress Scale, 64, 67f
Perception, 50
  assessment of, during mental status examination, 79b–80b
  encouraging description of, as therapeutic communication technique, 143t–144t
  as mediator of stress response, 62
Perceptual disturbances
  assessment of, during mental status examination, 79b–80b
  in delirium, 328
Perceptual disturbances, in delirium, 328
Peripheral nerves, 154
Perpetrators
  sexual assault, 509, 518
  of violence, 488, 490f

Perpetuating factors, of insomnia, 418
Perphenazine, for schizophrenia, 289t
Persecution, in delusions, 277t
Perseveration, 335
Persistent depressive disorder, 222
Persona, as origin of term "personality", 390
Personal appearance, as non-verbal behaviour, 139t
Personal factors, affecting communication, 137
Personal hygiene and grooming, 212
Personal Information Protection and Electronic Documents Act, 76
Personal power, 469
Personal question, nurse responses to, 129t–130t
Personal space, in nurse-patient relationships, 125
Personality
  defined by Sullivan, 46
  defining, 390
  five dimensions of, 401, 402t
  from Latin word persona, 390
  as mediator of stress response, 62
  structure of, in Sigmund Freud's psychoanalytic theory, 42
Personality disorders, 390–391
  advanced-practice interventions for, 406
  aggressive behaviour with, 402, 404t, 406b, 407t
  case management of, 404
  clinical picture of, 391b, 391
  cluster A, 393
    paranoid personality disorder, 392, 393b, 393
    schizoid personality disorder, 391, 393, 394b
    schizotypal personality disorder (STPD), 391, 394b, 394
  cluster B, 394
    anti-social personality disorder (ASPD), 391, 397
    borderline personality disorder, 391, 394, 397b
    histrionic personality disorder, 391, 398, 399b
    narcissistic personality disorder, 391, 399b, 399
  cluster C, 400
    avoidant personality disorder, 391, 400b, 400
    dependent personality disorder, 391, 400b, 400
    obsessive-compulsive personality disorder, 391, 400, 401b
  comorbidity of, 392
  dialectical behaviour therapy treatment for, 406, 408f
  in eating and feeding disorder, 307
  epidemiology of, 391
  etiology of, 392
    biological factors in, 392
    environmental factors in, 392
    genetics in, 392
    neurobiology and neurochemistry in, 392

Personality disorders *(Continued)*
   impulsive behaviour with, 402, 404*t*, 406*b*, 407*t*
   manipulative behaviour with, 402–403, 404*t*, 406*b*, 407*t*
   nursing process application to, 401
      assessment of, 401, 403*b*
      case study and nursing care plan on, 408*b*–410*b*
      diagnosis of, 402, 403*t*
      evaluation of, 408
      implementation of, 402, 406*b*, 407*t*
      outcomes identification of, 402, 404*t*
      patient history in, 401
      planning of, 402
      self-assessment in, 402
   pharmacological interventions of, 404
   psychological factors in, 392
   psychotherapy for, 406
   safety and teamwork for, 403, 407*t*
   system factors in, 392
Personality trait, defining, 390
Personality type, defining, 390
Personalization, 51*t*
   in cognitive distortions, 311*b*
Pets, as stress buster, 64*b*
Pharmacists, as members of psychiatric mental health treatment teams, 34*b*
Pharmacodynamics, 164–165
   ethnic variation in, 114
   interactions, 356
Pharmacogenetics, 165*b*, 165
Pharmacokinetics, 164–165
Pharmacological interventions, 374
   for Alzheimer's disease, 338, 343*f*
   for anorexia nervosa, 311
   as basic-level psychiatric mental health nursing intervention, 11*t*
   for bulimia nervosa, 315
   for older adults, 567
   during psychiatric mental health nursing process, 85
   for schizophrenia, 288
Phases of crisis, 435
   phase 1, 435
   phase 2, 435
   phase 3, 435
   phase 4, 435
Phenelzine sulphate (Nardil), 212*b*–214*b*, 236*b*–237*b*
Phenylcyclohexyl piperidine (PCP), 368, 369*t*
Phobias, 188*b*, 188
   common types of, 188*t*
   social, 188
   specific, 188
Photosensitivity, from conventional antipsychotics, 291*t*–292*t*
PHQ. *See* Patient Health Questionnaire-15
PHQ-9. *See* Patient Health Questionnaire-9
Physical activities, for anxiety disorders, 209*b*
Physical behaviours
   in delirium, 328
   depression and, 229
Physical characteristics, as non-verbal behaviour, 139*t*
Physical dependency, 351

Physical distance, for managing disruptive behaviours, in children and adolescents, 549*b*
Physical environments, as key social determinant of health, 12
Physical exercise, 68
Physical illness
   vs. mental illness, 6
   psychological factors affecting, 586
   schizophrenia and, 273
Physical needs
   in delirium, 328
   in dementia, 337*t*
Physical restraint, for managing disruptive behaviours, in children and adolescents, 549*b*
Physical stressors, 62
Physical trauma
   mental health dysfunction and, 164
   signs and symptoms of, 513
Physical violence, 467
   common presenting problems in, 483*b*
   definition of, 483*b*, 483, 483*t*
Physiological needs, 53
Piaget, Jean, 44, 55*t*–56*t*
Pibloktoq, 5–6
Pica, 305
Pimozide, for schizophrenia, 289*t*
Pinel, Philippe, 16–17
Pituitary glands, role of, in mental function, 155
Placating, during family therapy, 633*b*
Placebo effect, 647
Planned ignoring, for managing disruptive behaviours, in children and adolescents, 549*b*
Planning
   definition of, 74
   within psychiatric mental health nursing process, 83, 84*b*
   for terms of termination, in nurse-patient relationship, 131
Play therapy, 541
Police Service Mobile Crisis Intervention Team, Toronto's, 26, 26*b*
Pollard, Cheryl L., 20–21
Polypharmacy, aging and, 555
Polysomnography (PSG), 418
Pons, 159*f*
Population mental health, 581
Positive regard, for patients' growth, 133
Positive reinforcement, 48
Positive symptoms, 276
   of schizophrenia, 276
Positron emission tomography (PET) scan
   for depression, before and after medication, 225*f*, 225
   description and psychiatric uses for, 161*t*
   in Alzheimer's disease, 161, 163*f*
   in depression, 161, 163*f*
   in obsessive-compulsive disorder, 161, 162*f*
   in schizophrenia, 161, 162*f*
Postpartum onset, with major depressive disorder, 221
Postsynaptic neuron, 156

Post-traumatic stress disorder (PTSD)
   with adventitious crisis, 434
   case study and nursing care plan for, 196*b*–198*b*
   in children and adolescents, 543*b*
   description of, 196
   flashbacks and, 196
   prevalence statistics of, in Canada, 9*t*
Postural hypotension, from conventional antipsychotics, 291*t*–292*t*
Posture, non-verbal communication through, 139, 139*t*
Post-vention, for survivors of suicide, 458, 458*b*
Potlatch, 17
Poverty
   of content of speech, in schizophrenia, 279*t*
   serious mental illness and, 575
   of speech, in schizophrenia, 279*t*
"Power and Control" wheel, 489*f*
Power, of perpetrators, 488
Practising, 396
Prayer, 63
Precipitating factors, of insomnia, 418–419
Preconscious mind, 42
Precontemplation phase, of Transtheoretical Model of Change, 370
Predisposing factors, of insomnia, 418–419
Prednisone, mental health dysfunction and, 164
Pregnancy, violence and, 488
Prejudice, cultural, 146
Pre-menstrual dysphoric disorder, 222
Pre-natal stressors, in schizophrenia, 274
Pre-operational stage, of cognitive development, 44
Pre-orientation phase, of Peplau's model of nurse-patient relationship, 128, 129*t*–130*t*
Preparation, 370
Preparation phase, of Transtheoretical Model of Change, 370
Pre-psychotic phase, of schizophrenia, 276
Prescription medications, for suicide, 455
Present, giving, nurse responses to, 129*t*–130*t*
Presenting reality, as therapeutic communication technique, 143*t*–144*t*
Presynaptic neuron, 156
Prevalence, defined, in mental health epidemiology, 7–8
Prevention, as key strategy area for Canadian mental health care, 7, 8*b*
Primary alveolar hypoventilation, 420
Primary care, for crisis intervention, 440
Primary central sleep apnea, 420
Primary prevention, 376
   of abuse, 499
Principle of least restrictive intervention, 539
Prion, 332*t*
Prison, in Canada, 610
Privacy, right to, 98
Problem, in nursing diagnoses, 82
Process, of message, 139
Process recordings, 46–47, 149, 150*t*
Profile, of sexual perpetrators, 509
Progressive muscle relaxation, 65–67

Projection, as defence mechanism, 186t–187t
Prolonged grief disorder, 605
Promotion, as key strategy area for Canadian mental health care, 7, 8b
Propranolol (Inderal), 212b–214b
Protective factors, for suicide, 452b
Protein kinase A (PKA), suicide and, 452
Provincial governments
　health professions acts in, 94t
　mental health acts in, 93–94, 94t
Proxemics, 149
Proximate cause, 101
Pseudodementia, 223–224, 335
Pseudoparkinsonism, in conventional antipsychotics, 290, 291t–292t
Psilocybin (mushrooms), 368, 369t
Psychiatric comorbidity, 354
Psychiatric consultation liaison nurse (PCLN), 592
Psychiatric mental health advanced-practice nurses, as members of psychiatric mental health treatment teams, 34b
Psychiatric mental health care
　barriers to treatment as, 37
　funding for, 25
　future issues in, 37
　meeting changing demands as, 38
　roles and responsibilities in, 32
　　biopsychosocial assessment as, 33, 34b
　　biopsychosocial care manager as, 35
　　community psychiatric mental health nursing as, 32
　　interprofessional team member as, 35
　　nursing care as, 36
　　relevant to educational preparation, 33t
　　treatment goals and interventions as, 34
　　treatment team as, 35
　settings of, 26
　　assertive community treatment as, 31b–32b, 31
　　characteristics, treatment outcomes, and interventions by, 33t
　　community mental health centres as, 27, 28b
　　disaster response teams as, 28
　　ensuring safety in, 31
　　inpatient psychiatric mental health programs as, 29
　　mobile crisis intervention teams as, 28, 29b
　　partial hospitalization programs as, 29b–30b, 29
Psychiatric mental health nurse, roles and responsibilities of, 32
　biopsychosocial assessment as, 33, 34b
　biopsychosocial care manager as, 35
　community psychiatric mental health nursing as, 32
　in community setting, 27
　interprofessional team member as, 35
　nursing care as, 36
　relevant to educational preparation, 33t
　treatment goals and interventions as, 34
　treatment team as, 35
Psychiatric mental health nursing, 10
　assessment in, 77
　of children and adolescents, 536, 538b

Psychiatric mental health nursing (Continued)
　assessment data in, 538
　behavioural therapy, 539
　bibliotherapy, 541–542
　cognitive behavioural therapy, 539
　cultural factors in, 539
　data collection in, 537
　developmental assessment in, 538
　family therapy, 539
　group therapy, 539
　mental status examination in, 538
　milieu management, 540b, 540
　mind-body therapies, 540
　mutual storytelling, 541b, 541
　play therapy, 541
　principle of least restrictive intervention, 539
　psychopharmacology, 542
　quiet room, 540
　risk assessment in, 539
　seclusion and restraint in, 540
　therapeutic drawing, 542
　therapeutic games, 541, 542b
　time out, 540
　clinical practice of, levels of, 11
　cultural implications for, 105
　defined, 10
　future challenges and roles in, 11
　future of, 21
　historical overview of, 16
　national organizations for, 21
　shifts in control over, 18, 19b
　twelve key social determinants of health used in, 12
Psychiatric mental health programs, for inpatients, 29
　entry to, 29, 30b
　preparation for discharge to the community in, 30, 31b
Psychiatric mental health treatment, continuum of, 26f, 26
Psychiatrists, as members of psychiatric mental health treatment teams, 34b
Psychiatry, early treatments in, 17
Psychic secretion, 48
Psychoactive substance use and treatment, 350–351, 357, 386
　addiction and
　　compulsive behaviour vs., 351
　　development, process of, 351
　　withdrawal stage, 352
　comorbidity and, 354
　　medical, 354, 355t
　　psychiatric, 354
　concurrent disorders and, 354
　definitions associated with
　　addiction definition, 352
　　tolerance, 352
　epidemiology of, 352
　etiology of, 355
　　biological factors in, 355, 356f
　　psychological factors in, 356
　　sociocultural factors in, 357
　initial and active, 373
　nursing process application to, 357
　　assessment of, 357, 358b

Psychoactive substance use and treatment (Continued)
　　case study and nursing care plan on, 380b, 383b–384b
　　diagnosis of, 373, 373t
　　evaluation of, 385, 386f
　　helping patients change in, 369
　　implementation of, 373
　　interventions of, 374
　　outcomes identification of, 373
　　planning of, 373, 383b–384b
Psychoanalysis, classical, 43
　counter-transference in, 43–44
　transference in, 43–44
Psychoanalytic theories, 42
　implications of, for nursing practice, 44
　psychodynamic therapy and, 44
　Sigmund Freud's, 42
　　defence mechanisms and anxiety, 42
　　as foundation for group therapy, 623t
　　levels of awareness in, 42, 42f
　　personality structure in, 42
　　psychosexual stages of development in, 43, 43t
Psychobiological intervention, as basic-level nursing intervention, 27
Psychodrama groups, 626
Psychodynamic theories, of anxiety disorders, 200
Psychodynamic therapy, 44
　in groups, 623t
Psychoeducation, adherence to treatment and, 576b
Psychoeducational family therapy, 641
Psychoeducational groups, 625
Psychological dependency, 351
Psychological effects, of sexual assault, 510
Psychological factors
　anger and, 468
　anxiety disorders and, 200
　with depression, 226
　in eating and feeding disorders, 307
　with substance use disorders, 356
Psychological first aid, 28
Psychological stressors, 62
　in schizophrenia, 274
Psychological violence, 483t, 484
Psychologists, as members of psychiatric mental health treatment teams, 34b
Psychomotor agitation, 228, 279
　depression and, 229
Psychomotor retardation, 228, 279
　depression and, 229
Psychoneuroimmunology, 61–62
　mind-body therapies and, 65
Psychopharmacology
　advent of, 54
　for children and adolescents, 542
Psychosexual stages of development, 43, 43t
Psychosis, 270
　associated with another medical condition, 272b
　drugs for, 171
　family psychoeducation interventions for, 296b
　prevalence statistics of, in Canada, 9t

Psychosocial assessment, 80, 81b
Psychosocial factors, 204
  of suicide, 452
Psychosocial interventions
  for anorexia nervosa, 311b, 311
  in older adults, 566b, 566, 567t
Psychostimulants, depression co-occurring with, 223t
Psychotherapy, 406
  by advanced-practice psychiatric mental health nurses, 11t
  for anorexia nervosa, 312
  for bipolar disorders, 264
  for bulimia nervosa, 315
  for depression, 242–243
  for serious mental illness, 579b, 579
Psychotic disorders
  aggression and violence and, 476
  other than schizophrenia, 272b
Psychotic features, with major depressive disorder, 221
Psychotic symptoms, drug treatment for, 543b
Psychotropic drugs, 153, 154b, 165b
  adverse effects of, serious mental illness and, 576
  for Alzheimer's disease, 174
  for anxiety and insomnia, 165
  for attention-deficit/hyperactivity disorder, 174
  biopsychiatry and, 153
  for bipolar disorders, 170
  for depression, 167, 167f
  non-adherence to, 165
  for psychosis, 171
  use of, 164
PTSD. See Post-traumatic stress disorder
Punishment, 48
Pyrophobia, 188t

Q

Qi, 647–648
Quality of life, psychosocial assessment of, 590
Quality palliative care, 595
Queer, 525
  hostility toward, 537b
Questions, avoidance of, in Alzheimer's disease, 335
Quetiapine, 173
  for schizophrenia, 288, 289t
Quetiapine fumarate (Seroquel), for bipolar disorders, 263b
Quiet room, 472, 540

R

Race, mental health and, 105
Racialization, 106
Racism, 106
Rage, defining, 465
Rape. See also Sexual assault
  date, 509, 510t
  myth vs. fact in, 514t
  sexual violence and, 509
Rape-trauma syndrome, 510
  acute phase of, 510, 511b

Rape-trauma syndrome (Continued)
  diagnosis of, 513
  interventions for, 515b, 515
  long-term reorganization phase of, 511
Rapid cycling, with bipolar disorder, 251
Rapid eye movement (REM), sleep
  description and EEG illustration of, 414
  patterns and efficiency of, 414
Rapid eye movement behaviour disorder (RBD), 420
Rapport, in nurse-patient relationship, 131
Rapprochement, 396
RAS. See Reticular activating system
Rating scales, for assessment, 82, 83t
Rational emotive behaviour therapy (REBT), 50
Rationalization, as defence mechanism, 186t–187t
RBD. See Rapid eye movement behaviour disorder
Reaction formation, as defence mechanism, 186t–187t
Reactive aggression, 466
Readiness for enhanced sleep, NANDA definition of, 424
Reality testing, 42
  in schizophrenia, 270, 276
Reattribution treatment, for anxiety disorders, 210, 211b
REBT. See Rational Emotive Behaviour Therapy
Receiver, in communication process, 137, 138f
Recent Life Changes Questionnaire, 64, 66t
Receptor desensitization, 170
Receptors, 156, 157t
  as psychotropic drug targets, 165
Recognition
  in abuse screening, 493b
  as therapeutic communication technique, 143t–144t
Recovery
  as critical aspect to improving well-being, 27
  importance with bipolar disorder, 264
  as key strategy area for Canadian mental health care, 7, 8b
Recovery homes, 382
Recovery model, 283
  for depression, 232, 232t
Recovery-oriented approaches, 110–111
Recreational therapists, as members of psychiatric mental health treatment teams, 34b
Redirection, for managing disruptive behaviours, in children and adolescents, 549b
Refeeding syndrome, 310
Reflection, as therapeutic communication technique, 141, 143t–144t
Reflexes, role of medulla oblongata in, 159f
Reflexology, 653
Refugees
  defined, 111
  mental health concerns of, 113

Registered nurses, as members of psychiatric mental health treatment teams, 34b, 35
Registered Nurses' Association of Ontario (RNAO), history of psychiatric nursing licensing and, 19
Registered practical nurses, as members of psychiatric mental health treatment teams, 34b, 35
Registered Psychiatric Nurse Regulators of Canada (RPNRC), 20
Registered Psychiatric Nurses Act, 19–20
Registered psychiatric nurses, as members of psychiatric mental health treatment teams, 34b, 35
Registered Psychiatric Nurses of Canada (RPNC)
  baccalaureate and graduate programs for, 21
  code of ethics, 21, 90b, 90–91
  on nurse-patient relationships, 84
  standards of practice, 21, 90–91, 91b
Regression, as defence mechanism, 186t–187t
Rehabilitation, concept of, for serious mental illness, 573
Reiki, 653
Reinforcement, 48
Reis Typology, 381, 382b
Rejection, giving, nurse responses to, 129t–130t
Relapse, prevention strategies, 378f, 378, 379b
Relational aggression, 466
Relational ethics, 90–91
Relational violence, 467
Relationship, 123
  social, 123
  therapeutic, 124
Relationship factors, affecting communication, 137
Relaxation techniques
  for anxiety disorders, 209b
  Benson's, 67, 68b
  biofeedback as, 69
  cognitive reframing as, 69, 69t
  humour as, 70
  journaling as, 69
  meditation as, 67
  mindfulness as, 69
  physical exercise as, 68
  progressive muscle relaxation as, 65–67
  for stress, 65
Religion, 81
  anxiety disorders and, 204
  assessment of, 80
  medical conditions and, 590
Religious beliefs
  depression and, 229
  as mediator of stress response, 63
Reminiscence therapy, 567t
Remotivation therapy, 567t
Repetitiveness, in dementia, 337t
Repression, as defence mechanism, 186t–187t
Rescue, as counter-transference, 127t
Research, evidence-informed practice and, 11

Research highlight boxes
  adolescents' experiences of internet-delivered cognitive behavioural therapy for obsessive-compulsive disorder, 195*b*
  animal-assisted therapy, 649*b*
  on borderline personality disorder, 403*b*
  on crisis interventions in rural vs. urban settings, 442*b*
  DSM-5 classifications of, 418
  family interventions, 642*b*
  family psychoeducation interventions for psychosis and schizophrenia, 296*b*
  on fear of cancer recurrence, 587*b*
  First Nations communities and palliative care, 597*b*
  group intervention for vulnerable children, 626*b*
  in intimate partner violence, 491*b*
  on mental health first aid (MHFA), 438*b*
  nursing students' knowledge, attitude, and cultural competence, 529*b*
  population health burden of depression, 230*b*
  post-traumatic stress disorder (PTSD) for sexual assault, 519*b*
  recognition, prevention, and treatment of delirium in emergency department, 327*b*
  recovery communities for people with serious mental illness, 574*b*
  screening eating disorders, 314*b*
  self-harm and suicidal behaviour, 451*b*
  sleep in nursing education programs, 416*b*
  smoking cessation via mobile texting, 368*b*
  supplementing goal setting for families using motivational interviewing, 137*b*
  survivors' satisfaction with nurse-led sexual assault and domestic violence care, 612*b*
  in violence, 469*b*
  on youth with bipolar disorder seeking health information online, 255*b*
Residential crisis centres, in schizophrenia, 284
Resilience
  assessment of, 5*b*
  of children and adolescents, 536
  definition of, 5
  goals with personality disorders, 404*t*
Resources, helping patients develop, 134
Respect
  in abuse screening, 493*b*
  for autonomy, as principle of bioethics, 90
  as relational ethics principle, 91
Respiratory disorders, that may mimic psychiatric illness, 78*b*, 78
Respiratory retraining, 68
Response prevention, for anxiety disorders, 216
Restating, as therapeutic communication technique, 141, 143*t*–144*t*

Restitution, for managing disruptive behaviours, in children and adolescents, 549*b*
Restless leg syndrome (RLS), 420*b*, 420
Restlessness, with delirium, 329
Restoration-oriented stressors, 602
Restraint
  abuse, 483
  for children and adolescents, 540
  contraindications to, 97*b*
  least restrictive, 97
  liability issues with, 100
  with violence, 474*b*, 474
Restrictive food intake disorder, 305
Restructuring, for managing disruptive behaviours, in children and adolescents, 549*b*
Reticular activating system (RAS), 158
Retrograde amnesia, 241
Reuptake, 156
  cellular, 156, 158*b*
Revenge porn, 466
Rexulti. *See* Brexpiprazole
Rhodiola, 652*t*
Rhythmic breathing, 649
Rights
  as key strategy area for Canadian mental health care, 7, 8*b*
  to privacy, 98
  to refuse treatment, 96*b*, 96
  regarding confidentiality, 98
Rigid boundaries, 633*b*
Risk
  in home, 337*t*
  for injury, with delirium, 329
  outside the home, 337*t*
  for self-mutilation, 460
Risk factors, with depression, 224*b*
Risperdal. *See* Risperidone
Risperidone (Risperdal), 173
  for bipolar disorders, 263*b*
  for schizophrenia, 288, 289*t*
  for violent behaviour, 473*b*
Ritalin, 376
Rivastigmine (Exelon), 174
  for Alzheimer's disease, 342, 343*f*
RLS. *See* Restless leg syndrome
RNAO. *See* Registered Nurses' Association of Ontario
Road rage, 465
Rockwood Asylum Nursing School, 18
Rogers, Carl, 55*t*–56*t*
Rohypnol, 510*t*
Role performance, in crisis situations, 439*t*
Role-playing, for managing disruptive behaviours, in children and adolescents, 549*b*
"Roofies," 510*t*
Royal Commission on Aboriginal Peoples, 111
Roy, Sister Callista, 47*t*
RPNC. *See* Registered Psychiatric Nurses of Canada
RPNRC. *See* Registered Psychiatric Nurse Regulators of Canada
Rumination disorder, 305

Running amok, 5–6
Russell, E. Kathleen, 20
Ryan-Nicholls, Kimberley, 20–21

S
SAD. *See* Seasonal affective disorder; Social anxiety disorder
SAD PERSONS scale, 455, 455*t*
Safe environment, in guidelines for care at home, 342*b*
Safety
  Accreditation Canada, patient safety practices required by, 32
  cultural, 106, 107*b*
  in delirium, 329
  needs, 54
  plan, in violence and abuse, 497
  during planning, 83
  in psychiatric mental health care settings, 31
    goals for, 32*b*
  of staff, violence and, 472
  of traditional, complementary, and alternative medicine, 646, 647*b*
SAMe, 652*t*
SANE. *See* Sexual assault nurse examiner
SARI. *See* Serotonin antagonist and reuptake inhibitor
SARTs. *See* Sexual assault response teams
Saunders, Dame Cicely, 595
Scapegoating, 634*b*
Schizoaffective disorder, 272*b*
Schizoid personality disorder
  characteristics and behaviours associated with, 391, 393, 394*b*
  nursing and therapy guidelines for, 393, 405*t*
  treatment of, 394
Schizophrenia
  advanced-practice interventions for, 295, 296*b*
    family therapy in, 295, 296*b*
  assessment of, 275
    affective symptoms, 280
    cognitive symptoms, 276, 279–280
    general, 276, 277*f*
    guidelines for, 282*b*
    interventions for overcoming obstacles to, 281*t*
    negative symptoms, 272, 279, 279*t*
    positive symptoms, 276
    during pre-psychotic phase, 276
    self-assessment, 280, 281*f*–282*f*, 281*t*
  case study and nursing care plan in, 296*b*–298*b*
  catatonia in, 294
  clinical picture of, 271
    abnormal motor behaviour, 272
    delusions, 271
    disorganized thinking, 272
    hallucinations, 271
    negative symptoms, 272
  comorbidity of, 272
  counselling and communication techniques in, 285*b*, 285, 286*b*
  course of, 275

Schizophrenia *(Continued)*
   delusions, summary of, 276, 277t
   diagnosis of, 283, 283t
   epidemiology of, 272
   etiology of, 273
      biological factors, 273
      brain structure abnormalities, 273
      environmental stressors, 274
      genetic factors, 273
      neurobiological factors, 273
      pre-natal stressors, 274
      psychological, social, and environmental factors, 274
      psychological stressors, 274
   evaluation of, 296
   hallucinations, summary of, 278, 278t
   health teaching and health promotion in, 287b, 287
   implementation of, 284
   interventions of, 284
   LEAP approach in, 271b, 271
   maintenance of, 285
   milieu management of, 285
   nursing process, application of, 275
   outcomes identification in, 283, 284t
   paranoia in, 290
   pharmacological interventions for, 288
      additional medication administration issues, 288
      adjuncts to, 290
      atypical antipsychotics, 288, 289t
      conventional antipsychotics, 289, 291t–292t, 293f
      potentially dangerous responses to, 290
   phases of, 275
   planning for, 283
   positron emission tomography scan of brain with, 161, 162f
   prevalence statistics of, in Canada, 9t
   prognosis of, 275
   psychotic disorders other than, 272b, 272
   reality testing in, 276
   settings in, 284
   stabilization of, 285
   stigma of, 274b
   suicide risk in, 450
   word salad with, 156
Schizophrenia spectrum and other psychotic disorders, 270, 271b
   LEAP approach in, 271b, 271
Schizophreniform disorder, 272b
Schizotypal personality disorder (STPD)
   characteristics and behaviours associated with, 391, 394b, 394
   nursing and therapy guidelines for, 394, 405t
   treatment of, 394
Seasonal affective disorder (SAD)
   depressive features of, 221
   light therapy for, 221, 243b
Seasonal features, with major depressive disorder, 221
Seclusion
   for children and adolescents, 540
   contraindications to, 97b

Seclusion *(Continued)*
   history of, 97
   liability issues with, 100
   protocol, careful documentation of bipolar, 262–263
   with violence, 474b, 474
Second-generation antipsychotic medication, 173, 273, 288
Secondary care, for crisis intervention, 440–441
Secondary gains, 200, 204
Secondary prevention, 376
   of abuse, 499
Secondary traumatic stress, 437
Secondary victimization, 509
Secret, keeping, nurse responses to, 129t–130t
Security operations, defined by Sullivan, 46
Sedation, benzodiazepines causing, 166
Seeing, in communication, 137
Selective inattention, 182
Selective serotonin-norepinephrine reuptake inhibitors (SSNRIs), for anxiety disorders, 212b–214b
Selective serotonin reuptake inhibitors (SSRIs), 166, 168
   actions and side effects of, 236b–237b
   for anorexia nervosa, 311
   for anxiety disorders, 212b–214b, 214
   for binge eating disorder, 316
   for bulimia nervosa, 315
   common adverse reactions, 237
   for depression, 236b–237b, 237
   disorders treated by, 166
   indications, 237
   patient and family teaching regarding, 238b
   potential toxic effects, 237
   serotonin syndrome, 237, 238b
Self-actualization, 54
   characteristics of persons who have, 54b
Self-assessment, 369
   in abuse, 494, 494t
   in non-suicidal self-injury, 460
   in sexual assault, 513
   in suicide, 455
Self-awareness, 369
   in therapeutic relationships, 126
Self-care
   guidelines for, when caring for the dying, 600
   promotion of
      for anxiety patients, 212
      elimination, 212
      nutrition and fluid intake, 212
      in older adults, 567
      personal hygiene and grooming, 212
      sleep, 212
Self-care activities
   for anorexia nervosa, 311
   promotion of
      as basic-level nursing intervention, 27
      in psychiatric mental health nursing, 85
      in violence and abuse, 498
   in sexual assault, 516
Self-care deficits
   with delirium, 329
   depression co-occurring with, 234t

Self-care deficits *(Continued)*
   with substance abuse or behavioural addictions, 373t
Self-care needs
   for catatonia, 294–295
   for disorganization, 295
   for paranoia, 294
Self-check, on boundaries, 126, 128f
Self-determination, right to, 96
Self-esteem
   in anorexia nervosa, 311
   enhancement, for anxiety disorders, 209b
Self-harm, 450, 451b
   in LGBTQ, 530
   risk factors associated with, 450
   suicidal behaviour and, research highlight on, 451b
Self-help groups, 63, 625, 627b, 641b–642b, 641
   for patient and family/friends, 380–381
Self-injurious behaviours, in eating and feeding disorder, 306
Self-injury, non-suicidal, 448
   assessment of, 460
   biological factors, 459
   clinical picture of, 459
   comorbidity of, 459
   diagnosis of, 460
   epidemiology of, 459
   evaluation of, 460
   interventions for, 460
   outcomes criteria of, 460
   plan of care for, 460
   psychosocial factors, 459
   risk factors for, 459
   societal factors, 459
Self-mutilation, 460
   with borderline personality disorder (BPD), case study and nursing care plan, 408b–410b
Selye, Hans, 61
   on general adaptation syndrome, 586
Sender, in communication process, 137, 138f
Sensorimotor stage, of cognitive development, 44
Sensory functions, area of brain responsible for, 159–160, 160f
Separation anxiety disorder, in children and adolescents, 543b, 550
Serious mental illness
   across the lifespan, 572
      in older adults, 572, 573b
      in younger adults, 573b, 573
   adherence, treatment issues, 576b
   anosognosia, 573, 576
   chronic or recurrent, 572
   comorbid conditions and, 574
   current issues on, 581
      criminal offences and incarceration, 581
      involuntary treatment, 581
      population health & social justice approaches, 581
   definition of, in Canada, 572
   depression and suicide, 574
   development of, 573
   economic challenges, 575

Serious mental illness *(Continued)*
  establishing a meaningful life and, 574
  evidence-informed treatment approaches with, 578
    assertive community treatment, 578
    cognitive behavioural therapy, 578
    family support and partnership, 578
    social skills training, 578
    supportive psychotherapy, 579b, 579
    vocational rehabilitation and related services, 579
  exercise for, 579
  impairments associated with, 572
  isolation and loneliness, 575
  non-adherence, treatment issues, 575
  nursing care of patients with, 579, 580b, 580t
  rehabilitation vs. recovery for, 573
  resources for, 577
    comprehensive community treatment, 577
    consumer-run programs, 579
    exercise, 579
    substance abuse treatment, 578b, 578
    wellness and recovery action plans, 579
  social problems with, 575
  stigma of, 575
  substance abuse, 574
  victimization, 575
Seroquel. *See* Quetiapine
Serotonin
  in anger and aggression, 468
  circadian rhythms and, 156
  depression and, 166, 224–225
  in eating disorders, 307
  reduction of, 158b
  stress response and, 61
  substance use disorders and, 356
Serotonin (5-HT), 157t
Serotonin and norepinephrine disinhibitors (SNDIs), 168
  for depression, 236b–237b
Serotonin antagonist and reuptake inhibitor (SARI), 169
Serotonin modulator and stimulator, 168
Serotonin-norepinephrine reuptake inhibitors (SNRIs), 166, 168
  for depression, 236b–237b, 237
Serotonin syndrome, 174–175, 237, 238b
Sertraline hydrochloride (Zoloft), 168, 212b–214b, 236b–237b
Severe Alzheimer's disease, 333t
Severe anxiety, 182, 184t
  case study and nursing care plan for, 182b–183b
  interventions for, 208, 209t
Sex offenders, defining, 508
Sexual abuse, as risk factor for mental illness, 535
Sexual advances, nurse responses to, 129t–130t
Sexual assault, 508
  clinical picture of, 509
  date rape and, 509, 510t
  definition of, 508
  epidemiology of, 509

Sexual assault *(Continued)*
  myth vs. fact in, 514t
  nursing process application to, 511
    assessment, 512, 512b–514b
    case study and nursing care plan, 516b–518b
    diagnosis of, 513, 514b
    evaluation, 519
    implementation, 515b, 515
    outcomes identification, 515
    planning, 515
    trauma-informed approach, 511, 512b
  secondary victimization in, 509
  sexual assault nurse examiner (SANE) and, 513
Sexual assault nurse examiner (SANE), 513, 518, 612
  adults, 612
  pediatric, 612
Sexual assault response teams (SARTs), 613
Sexual exploitation, 508
Sexual history, algorithm for taking, 528b, 528
Sexual interest, depression and, 229
Sexual orientation
  considering culture in, 525b
  definition of, 525
Sexual violence, 508
  in Canada, 487
  definition of, 483–484, 483t
Sexuality, 524
  definition of, 525, 526b
  nursing process application in, 527
    assessment, 527, 528b
    evaluation, 530
    implementation, 528, 529b
    mental health issues, 529
    planning, 528
Shaken baby syndrome, 483
Shea, Shawn, 139
Shelters, for abused person, 497
Shift-work disorder, 426b
Short-Acting Sedative-Hypnotic Sleep Drugs, 166
Short-term residential treatment, 381–382
Should statements, 51t
Signals, use of, for managing disruptive behaviours, in children and adolescents, 549b
Signs and symptoms
  of anxiety disorders, 206t
  of bipolar disorders, 257t
  of depression, 231t
  within nursing diagnoses, 82
Silence, as therapeutic communication technique, 140, 143t–144t
Silent member, 628b, 628
Similarities test, 276
SISs. *See* Supervised injection sites
SKA2 gene expression, suicide and, 452
Skinner, B. F., 48
Slander, 100t
SLD. *See* Specific learning disorder
Sleep, 414 *See also* Sleep-wake disorders
  anxiety disorders and, 212

Sleep *(Continued)*
  circadian process or drive, 417
  dyssomnia, 413
  efficiency, 418
  functions of, 417
  general health and, 422b, 422
  in guidelines for self-care for individuals with cognitive impairment, 340b–341b
  hypnogram illustrating young vs. older adult, 415f, 416
  loss, consequences of, 414
  normal cycle and stages of, 414
  patterns and efficiency, 418, 422
  readiness for enhanced, 424
  regulation of, 417
  requirements, 417
  serotonin regulating, 224–225
  as stress buster, 64b
  studies, 418, 424
Sleep and wakefulness, cycle of, 155
Sleep architecture, hypnogram illustrating young adult vs. older adult, 415f, 416
Sleep continuity, definition of, 416
Sleep deprivation
  consequences of
    accidents, 414, 419
    excessive sleepiness, 414
    hypersomnia, 414, 419
    medical disorders associated with, 421b, 421
    psychiatric disorders associated with, 421b, 421
  definition of, 414
  in delirium, 329
  NANDA definition of, 424
  pharmacological interventions for, 425
Sleep diary, 416f, 425–426
Sleep disturbances, 425t
Sleep efficiency, 418
Sleep fragmentation, definition of, 416
Sleep hygiene, 419
  health teaching and health promotion regarding, 419b, 425
  importance for bipolar patients, 264
Sleep latency, 414–416
Sleep paralysis, 420
Sleep reactivity, 418
Sleep restriction, to strengthen homeostatic drive, 425–426
Sleep terrors, 419
Sleep–wake cycles, 414
  with substance abuse or behavioural addictions, 373t
Sleep–wake disorders, 413, 418
  advanced-practice intervention of, 418b, 427
  anxiety and, 427
  Canadian Sleep Society research on, 413
  clinical picture of, 418
  cognitive behavioural therapy for, 425
  comorbidity of, 421
  epidemiology of, 421
  functioning and safety for, 422–424
  identifying, 422, 424b
  medications to treat, 424–425, 425t
  mental illness and, 421b, 421

Sleep–wake disorders (Continued)
 non-pharmacological methods for, 426
 nursing process application to, 422
  assessment, 422
  diagnosis, 424
  evaluation, 427
  implementation, 425
  outcomes identification, 424
  planning, 424
 self-assessment of, 424
 types of
  breathing-related disorders, 420
  circadian rhythm sleep disorder, 420
  confusional arousal disorders, 419
  hypersomnia disorders, 419
  insomnia disorders, 418
  Kleine-Levin Syndrome, 420
  narcolepsy, 419
  nightmare disorder, 419
  obstructive sleep apnea hypopnea syndrome, 420
  primary alveolar hypoventilation, 420
  primary central sleep apnea, 420
  rapid eye movement behaviour disorder, 420
  restless legs syndrome, 420b, 420
  sleep paralysis, 420
  sleep terrors, 419
  sleepwalking, 419
  substance-induced sleep, 422
Sleepwalking, 419
Smoking
 cessation
  bupropion for, 168
  research via mobile texting, 368b
 in LGBTQ, 530
 in schizophrenia, 273
SNDIs. See Serotonin and norepinephrine disinhibitors
SNRIs. See Serotonin-norepinephrine reuptake inhibitors
Social anxiety disorder (SAD)
 description of, 188, 188t
 selective serotonin reuptake inhibitors for, 166
Social assessment, 81
Social determinants of health, 105
 in psychiatric mental health nursing, 12
Social interaction
 impaired, with delirium, 329
 skills, goals with personality disorders, 404t
Social learning theory, 55t–56t, 470
Social phobia
 anxiety symptoms with, 188b, 188, 188t
 drug treatment for, 543b
Social relationship, 123
Social skills
 brain functioning and, 156
 training, for serious mental illness, 578
Social status, as key social determinant of health, 12
Social support
 as key social determinant of health, 12
 as mediator of stress response, 63
 medical conditions and, 590

Social workers, as members of psychiatric mental health treatment teams, 34b, 35
Societal factors, of non-suicidal self-injury, 459
Sociocultural context, of family, 637
Sociocultural factors
 anger and, 470
 with substance use disorders, 357
Sociopaths, 397
Somatic delusion, 277t
Somatic reaction, in coping, 511b
Somatic symptom disorders, 190
 assessment guidelines for, 203b
 case study and nursing care plan for, 191b–192b
 clinical picture on, 190
 comorbidity of, 193, 194t
 conversion disorder, 192, 193b
 epidemiology of, 193
 illness anxiety disorder, 192
 interventions for, 210t
 nursing diagnoses for, 206t
 somatic symptom disorder, 190
Somatic therapy
 for dissociative disorders, 216
 for sexual assaults, 518
Somatization, 115, 190
Somatostatin (SRIF), 157t
Somnambulism, 419
Soporific drugs, benzodiazepines as, 166
Spatial processing, 79b–80b
Specific learning disorder (SLD), in children and adolescents, 544
Specific phobias, anxiety and, 188
Speech
 area of brain responsible for, 159–160, 160f
 assessment of, during mental status examination, 79b–80b
 patterns, bipolar disorders and, 256
Spinning, 17–18
Spiritual carers, as members of psychiatric mental health treatment teams, 34b, 35
Spiritual issues, assessment for, during end-of-life (EOL) care, 596
Spiritual support, medical conditions and, 590
Spiritual violence, 483t, 484
Spirituality, 80–81
 anxiety disorders and, 204
 assessment of, 80
 depression and, 229
 as integrative health care, 649
 as mediator of stress response, 63
Splitting
 characteristics and behaviours associated with, 396
 as defence mechanism, 186t–187t
SSNRIs. See Selective serotonin-norepinephrine reuptake inhibitors
SSRIs. See Selective serotonin reuptake inhibitors
St. John's wort, 651, 652t
 for depression, 243b
 interactions of, with conventional medications, 174–175

Stabilization phase, of schizophrenia, 275, 283–285
Standard drink, 352, 361–362, 377
Standards of care, 95
 guidelines for ensuring adherence to, 95
 nursing process and, for psychiatric mental health nursing, 74, 76b
  assessment, 75
  documentation, 85
  evaluation, 85
  implementation, 84
  nursing diagnosis, 82
  outcomes identification, 82, 84t
  planning, 83
Standards of nursing practice, 74
Standards of practice, 95
 Registered Psychiatric Nurses of Canada (RPNC), 90–91, 91b
Starson v. Swayze, 96b, 96
Stereotyped behaviours, 279
Stereotypic movement disorder, in children and adolescents, 544
Stereotyping, culture and, 106
Stevens-Johnson syndrome, 171
Stigma
 advocacy groups to fight Canadian mental health care, 7
 human rights abuses of stigmatized persons with medical conditions, 589
 mental illness and, 110
 of schizophrenia, 274b
 of serious mental illness, 575
Stigmatized persons with medical conditions, 589
Stimulants, 376
Stimulus
 in communication process, 137, 138f
 control, in CBT sleep-improvement techniques, 426
STPD. See Schizotypal personality disorder
Strategic model of family therapy, 636b, 636
Stress
 acute, reactions to, 61t
 adverse childhood experiences (ACEs), 64
 anxiety flowchart and, 185f
 coping mechanisms during crisis and, 439t
 defined, 59
 depression and, 225
 diathesis-stress model and, 6, 392
 effective busters of, 64b
 effects of, 59
 management groups, 625
 measurement of, 63, 65f, 66t
 mental health and, 586
 operationally defined, 64f
 prolonged, reactions to, 61t
 recovery, 62b
 reduction, benefits of, 65
 relaxation techniques for, 65
  Benson's, 67, 68b
  biofeedback as, 69
  breathing exercises and, 68b, 68
  cognitive reframing as, 69, 69t
  exercises, 65
  guided imagery as, 68b, 68
  humour as, 70

Stress *(Continued)*
  journaling as, 69
  meditation, 67
  mindfulness as, 69
  physical exercise as, 68
  progressive muscle relaxation as, 65–67
  responses to, 59, 60f
    early theories in, 59, 60f
    immune, 61
    mediators of, 62
    neurotransmitters and, 61
    nursing management of, 63
    positive and negative, 67t
    understanding of, 59
  substance use disorders and, 356
Stress system, 61
Stressors, 62
  defined, 59
  physical, 62
  psychological, 62
  in schizophrenia, 274
Structural model of family therapy, 636
Structural violence, 107, 112
Structured group activities, 36
Sub-group, 621b
Subject, changing, 145t
Sublimation, as defence mechanism, 186t–187t
Suboxone maintenance, 376
Suboxone treatment, 376
Subpersonality, 199
Substance abuse
  depression co-occurring with, 223t
  in LGBTQ, 530
  in peers, 95
  substance-induced anxiety disorder, 189
Substance-induced anxiety disorder, 185, 189
Substance-induced dementia, 332t
Substance-induced disorders, assessment of, 357
Substance-induced psychotic disorder, 272b
Substance-induced sleep disorder, 422
Substance/medication-induced depressive disorder, 222
Substance misuse interventions, 374
Substance P (SP), 157t
Substance use, 113
  assessment of, 357
  serious medical illness and, 588
Substance use disorders
  in eating and feeding disorder, 307
  etiology of, 355
    biological factors in, 355, 356f
    psychological factors in, 356
    sociocultural factors in, 357
  motivational interviewing for, 371, 372b
  nursing process application to, 357
    assessment, 357, 358b
    case study and nursing care plan, 380b, 383b–384b
    diagnosis, 373, 373t
    evaluation, 385, 386f
    helping patients change, 369
    implementation, 373
    interventions, 374
    outcomes identification, 373
    planning, 373, 383b–384b

Substance use disorders *(Continued)*
  in older adults, 557
  prevalence statistics of, in Canada, 9t
  psychological changes due to, 369
  schizophrenia and, 272
  self-assessment and self-awareness due to, 369
  suicide risk in, 450
Subsyndromal depression, 223–224
Suicidal behaviour, 448, 453–454
  self-harm and, research highlight on, 451b
Suicidal ideation
  among Inuit in Canada, 223b
  with anger, helplessness and hopelessness, 229
  assessment in depressed patients, 227
  definition of, 450
  verbal and non-verbal clues of, 454
Suicidal patients, long and short-term goals for, 84t
Suicide, 448
  among older persons, 450
    interventions, 451
    risk factors, 451
    warning signs, 451
  assessment of, 454, 454b
    guidelines for, 455b
    tools for, 455, 455t
    in young child, 539
  biological factors, 452
  in Canada, 610
  cultural beliefs regarding, 5
  in eating and feeding disorder, 306
  epidemiology of, 449
  etiology of, 452
  in Indigenous peoples, 112
  Indigenous peoples statistics of, 449
  in LGBTQ, 530
  interventions for
    case management for, 458
    counselling for, 458
    health teaching and health promotion for, 458
    implementation of, 455
    milieu management for, 457
    pharmacological, 458
    precautions, 457b
    primary, 456, 456b
    secondary, 457
    tertiary, 457
  medical assistance in dying (MAiD), 453
  nurse responses to, 129t–130t
  nursing process application to, 453
    assessment, 454
    evaluation, 459
    implementation, 455
  potential, in violence and abuse, 495
  precautions, 457, 457t
  prevalence statistics of, in Canada, 9t
  protective factors, 452b
  psychosocial factors, 452
  risk
    antidepressant drugs and, 170
    in older adults, 557, 566
  risk factors for, 450, 452b
  in schizophrenia, 273

Suicide *(Continued)*
  self-assessment of, 455
  societal factors, 453
  warning signs of, 453b
Suicide Risk Assessment Guide: A Resource for Health Care Organizations, 454
Sullivan, Harry Stack, 46, 200
Summarizing, in therapeutic communication, 143t–144t
Sundance, 17
Sundown syndrome, 327–328
Sundowning, 327–328
Superego, 42f, 42
Supervised consumption sites (SCS), 377
Supervised injection sites (SISs), 377
Supervision, clinical, 149
Supervision, of health care workers, 126
Supervisory liability, 100t
Support groups, 625, 627b
  for bipolar disorders, 264
Support system
  in abuse, 495
  available, in sexual assault, 512
Supported-employment model, for serious mental illness, 579
Supported play, 77
Supporting data, within nursing diagnoses, 82
Supportive psychotherapy, for serious mental illness, 579b, 579
Supportive therapies, 44
Suppressed anger, 465
Suppression, as defence mechanism, 186t–187t
Survivor
  of abuse, 488
  of sexual assaults, 508–509, 518
  of suicide, 448
Susto, 115
Sweat lodge, 17
Symbiosis, 36
Sympathy, empathy vs., 133
Synapse, 156
  reduction of neurotransmitters in, 158b
Systematic desensitization
  for anxiety disorders, 215–216
  as behavioural therapy, 49
Systemic medications, depression co-occurring with, 223t

T

Tachycardia, from conventional antipsychotics, 291t–292t
Tacrine (Cognex), for Alzheimer's disease, 341
Tactile hallucination, 278t
Talk therapy, Freud's use of, 42
Tangentiality, in communication, 278
Tarasoff v. Regents of University of California, 98
Tardive dyskinesia (TD/TDK), from conventional antipsychotics, 290, 291t–292t
TCAM. *See* Traditional, complementary, and alternative medicine
TCAs. *See* Tricyclic antidepressants

Technology, expanding, mental health and, 12
Tegretol. *See* Carbamazepine
Telemedicine, 12
Telepsychiatry, 12
Temazepam (Restoril), 166, 426*t*
Temperament
    in child and adolescent disorders, 536
    defining, 392
Temporal lobe dysfunction, 468
Tension-building stage, in cycle of violence, 485
Tension headache, anxiety caused by, 194*t*
Terminal illness
    assessment for spiritual issues, 596
    caring for patients with, 594, 595*b*, 599*b*
    Kübler-Ross, Dr. Elisabeth, 594–595
Termination phase
    of Peplau's model of nurse-patient relationship, 131
    of therapeutic group, 621
Territorial governments
    health professions acts in, 94*t*
    mental health acts in, 93–94, 94*t*
Terrorism, 434
Tertiary care, for crisis intervention, 441
Tertiary prevention, 381
    of abuse, 499–500
Testosterone, in gender dysphoria, 527
Theories
    behavioural, 48
        behaviourism theory as, 48
        classical conditioning theory as, 48, 48*f*
        implications of, in nursing practice, 49
        operant conditioning theory as, 48, 48*f*
    biological, 54
        advent of psychopharmacology and, 54
        biological model and, 54
    cognitive, 50
        cognitive behavioural therapy and, 50, 52*b*
        dialectic behavioural therapy as, 51
        implications of, in nursing practice, 52, 53*b*
        rational emotive behaviour therapy and, 50
    comparison of, 52*t*
    developmental, 44
        cognitive development as, 44
        ethics of care theory and, 45
        implications of, for nursing practice, 46
        moral development stages, 44
        theory of psychosocial development and, 45*t*, 46
    humanistic, 53
        Abraham Maslow's humanistic psychology theory as, 53
    interpersonal, 46
        implications of, for nursing practice, 48
        interpersonal psychotherapy in, 46
        Peplau's theory of interpersonal relations, 46
        by Sullivan, 46
        theory of object relations in, 46
    psychoanalytic, 42
        classical psychoanalysis, 43

Theories *(Continued)*
        implications of, for nursing practice, 44
        psychodynamic therapy and, 44
        Sigmund Freud's, 42
    selected nursing theorists in, 47*t*
Therapeutic communication
    basic vs., 136
    skills and strategies, 140
    strategies, 140, 143*t*–144*t*
        accepting as, 143*t*–144*t*
        active listening as, 140
        asking questions and eliciting patient responses as, 142
        clarifying techniques as, 141, 143*t*–144*t*
        exploring as, 142
        listening with empathy as, 141
        paraphrasing as, 141
        reflecting as, 141
        restating as, 141
        silence as, 140
        summarizing as, 143*t*–144*t*
Therapeutic drawing, 542
Therapeutic encounter, 124
Therapeutic factors, in groups, 620, 621*b*
    terms central to, 621*b*
Therapeutic games, 541, 542*b*
Therapeutic groups, 620
    member roles, 621, 622*t*
    support and self-help groups, 625
Therapeutic index, 170–171, 171*t*
Therapeutic relationships, 36, 122*b*–123*b*, 122
    beliefs in, 126
    blurred boundaries in, 125, 125*t*
    Peplau's model of, 126
        orientation phase of, 130
        pre-orientation phase of, 128, 129*t*–130*t*
        termination phase of, 131
        working phase of, 131
    phases of, 132*f*
    self-awareness in, 126
    values in, 126
Therapeutic suggestion, 649
Therapeutic touch, 653
Therapeutic use of self, 123
Thiothixene, for schizophrenia, 289*t*
Third generation antipsychotic medications, 288–289
Thought broadcasting, in delusions, 277*t*
Thought insertion, in delusions, 277*t*
Thought processes
    area of brain responsible for, 159, 160*f*
    bipolar disorders and, 256
    depression assessment of, 229
    disturbed, with delirium, 329
Thought stopping, for anxiety disorders, 216
Thought withdrawal, in delusions, 277*t*
Thoughts
    assessment of, during mental status examination, 79*b*–80*b*
    automatic, 50
Tidal model, 47
Time out, 540

Token economy, 49
Tolerance, definition of substance, 352
Tonic factors, 378–379
Topiramate (Topamax), 171, 374–375
    for bipolar disorders, 263*b*
Toronto's Police Service Mobile Crisis Intervention Team, 26, 26*b*
Tort law, 100
Touch
    in communication process, 137
    control, for managing disruptive behaviours, in children and adolescents, 549*b*
    cultural considerations to, 146
Tourette's disorder, in children and adolescents, 544
Toxicity, of lithium carbonate, 260, 261*t*
Traditional Chinese medicine, 647
Traditional, complementary, and alternative medicine (TCAM), 645, 646*t*
    biologically based integrative therapies for, 650
        aromatherapy as, 652
        diet and nutrition as, 650
        herbal therapy as, 650
        megavitamin therapy as, 650
    in Canada, 650
    definition of, 645
    jurisdiction over, 646
    manipulative practices for, 652
        chiropractic medicine, 653
        massage therapy, 653
        reflexology, 653
    patients and, 646
    research on, 646
    resources, 646*b*
    safety of, 646, 647*b*
    whole medical systems of, 647
        acupuncture, 646
        Ayurvedic medicine, 647
        homeopathy and naturopathy, 648
        traditional Chinese medicine, 647
        traditional Indigenous medicine, 647
Traditional Indigenous medicine, 647
Traditional medicine, definition of, 645
Traditional practice knowledge, 95
Trait aggression, 469
Transcranial magnetic stimulation (TMS), for depression, 242, 242*f*
Transference, 125
    in classical psychoanalysis, 43–44
Transgender, 525
    hostility toward, 537*b*
Translators, professional health care, 77
Transmitters, 157*t*
Transtheoretical model of Change (TTM), 370
    stages of, 370, 370*f*
        action, 370–371
        contemplation, 370
        evaluation/termination, 371
        maintenance/adaption, 371
        pre-contemplation, 370
        preparation, 370
Tranylcypromine sulphate (Parnate), 212*b*–214*b*, 236*b*–237*b*

Trauma
    as adventitious crisis, 434
    historical, 112
    on older adults, 558
    physical, mental health dysfunction and, 164
    resilience and, 5
    as risk factor for mental illness, 535
Trauma and stressor disorders, 196
Trauma- and violence-informed care (TVIC), 106, 107b
Trauma-informed approach, to sexual assault, 511, 512b
Trauma-informed care, 470–471
Trauma-informed practice, 107–108
Traumatic brain injury, 332t, 468
    in dementia, 334
Travelbee, Joyce, 47t
Trazodone (Oleptro, Trazodone, Trazorel), 426t
    for depression, 169
TRD. See Treatment-resistant depression
Treatment
    authorization of, 95
    Nursing Interventions Classification (NIC), 11
Treatment plans, clinical pathway and, 30–31
Treatment-resistant depression (TRD), 242
Treatment team, 35
    collaboration of, 98
Triangulation, 634b, 635f, 635
Triazolam (Halcion), 166, 426t
Tri-Council Policy Statement: Ethical Conduct for Research Involving Humans,, 92
Tricyclic antidepressants (TCAs), 167, 168f
    actions of, 236b–237b, 238
    adverse drug interactions, 238
    adverse reactions and toxic effects of, 238
    for anxiety disorders, 212b–214b
    for bulimia nervosa, 315
    common adverse reactions, 238
    contraindications, 238
    for depression, 236b–237b, 238
    indications, 238
    patient and family teaching, 238
    patient and family teaching regarding, 238, 239b
    potential toxic effects, 238
Triskaidekaphobia, 188t
T.R.U.S.T. Model for Inclusive Spiritual Care, 649–650, 650f, 651b
Truth and Reconciliation Commission of Canada, 111
Tryptophan, 307
Tuberculosis, with long term alcohol abuse, 354
Tuke, William, 16–17
Two-Eyed Seeing, 108
Two-spirit, 525
Typical antipsychotic medications, 288
Typology of interpersonal violence, 481, 482f
Tyramine, 169, 239, 239t

U

UBC. See University of British Columbia
Ultra-metabolizers, 165
Uncertainty, as relational ethics principle, 91
Unconscious mind, 42
Unconventionality, 390, 402t
Undoing, as defence mechanism, 186t–187t
Unemployment, with serious mental illness, 575
Unintentional torts, 100
United Nations Declaration on the Rights of Indigenous Peoples (UNDRIP), 111
Universality, 621b
University-based nursing curriculum, 20
University of Alberta, 20
University of British Columbia (UBC), 20
University of Saskatchewan, 20
University of Toronto, 20
University of Western Ontario, 20
Unpleasant Voices Scale, 280, 281f–282f
Unrealistic expectations of self, 230b, 230
Urban tree canopy, 62b
Urinary retention, from conventional antipsychotics, 291t–292t
Useful activities, in guidelines for care at home, 342b
Utilitarianism, 91
Utility, principle of, 91

V

Vagus nerve stimulation (VNS), for depression, 242f, 242
Valerian root, 651–652, 652t
Valproate, 171, 262
Valproate (Depakote, Depakene), 171
Valproic acid (Depakote, Depakene), 212b–214b
    for bipolar disorders, 262, 263b
    for schizophrenia, 290
Value judgements
    making, 145t
    suspending, for patient's growth, 134
Values, in therapeutic relationships, 126
Valuing, during end-of-life (EOL) care, 596
Vascular dementia, 332t
Vegetative signs, of depression, 229, 231t, 234t
Venlafaxine hydrochloride (Effexor), 168, 212b–214b, 236b–237b
Ventral tegmental pathway, 158–159
Verbal abuse, 483t, 484
Verbal clues, suicide and, 454
Verbal communication, 139
    interaction with non-verbal communication, 139, 140b
Verbal tracking, during clinical interview, 149
Vicarious liability, 100t
Vicarious trauma, 437, 513
Victimization
    in inmates with a mental illness, 611
    with serious mental illness, 575
    in sexual assault, 510t
        perpetrators and, 509
Vignette, 311
Violence, 465, 482, 611
    behavioural theories, 469
    biological factors, 468
    case management, 472
    cognitive and cognitive behavioural theories, 469
    comorbidity, 467

Violence *(Continued)*
    coping responses in, 494, 494t
    cycle of, 485, 486f
    de-escalation techniques for, 472b, 472
    defining, 466, 481
    drugs treatments for emergency management of, 473b
    ecological model of, 487
    epidemiology of, 467
    health teaching and health promotion, 471
    implementation, 471
    inpatient psychiatric settings, 476
    milieu characteristics conducive to, 467b, 467
    nursing diagnosis, 471
    nursing outcomes, 471
    nursing process application in, 489
        assessment in, 489, 490b
        diagnosis in, 495, 496t
        evaluation in, 502
        implementation in, 496
        outcomes identification in, 496, 496t
        planning in, 496
    nursing process application to, 470, 471b, 473b, 475b–477b
    patients with neurocognitive disorders, 477
    personality theory, 469
    pharmacological interventions, 473
    physical interventions, 474
    planning interventions, 471
    quiet rooms, 472
    restraints or seclusion use with, 474b, 474
    as risk factor for mental illness, 535
    safety and, 32
    social learning theories, 470
    sociocultural factors, 470
    types of, 482, 483t
Violence-informed practice, 107–108
Virtual health care, 12
Virtue ethics, 91
Virtues, defined, 91
Vision, area of brain responsible for, 159, 160f
Visitors, safety and, 32
Visual hallucinations, 278t, 279
Visual processing, 79b–80b
Vital signs, in bulimia nervosa, 315t
Vocal quality, during clinical interview, 149
Vocational rehabilitation, for serious mental illness, 579
Voice-related behaviours, as non-verbal behaviour, 139t
Voices, in hallucinations, 278–279
Vomiting
    with anorexia nervosa, 312
    with bulimia nervosa, 305, 313b, 313, 315
    with substance abuse or behavioural addictions, 373t
Vortioxetine (Trintellix), 168
Vraylar. See Cariprazine
Vulnerability
    coping with crisis and, 434–435
    ethical dilemma and, 92
    as relational ethics principle, 91
Vulnerable population, as target of abuse
    children, 488, 490f
    older adult, 488
    women, 488

W

Wakefulness, neurotransmitters responsible for, 417
Wandering
　with dementia, 336–337
　in guidelines for care at home, 342b
War, as adventitious crisis, 434
Watson, John B., 48
Waxy flexibility, 279
Weight bias, 308b
Weight gain behaviour, in anorexia nervosa, 310t
Weight maintenance behaviour, in bulimia nervosa, 315t
Weight stigma, 308b
Weir Report, 18–19
Wernicke's encephalopathy, 354
Western Canada, history of psychiatric nursing licensing in, 19
Western worldview, 108
White matter, 159, 160f
Whole medical systems, of integrative health care, 647
　acupuncture, 646
　Ayurvedic medicine, 647
　homeopathy and naturopathy, 648
　traditional Chinese medicine, 647
　traditional Indigenous medicine, 647
"Why" questions, asking, 144, 145t
Willis-Ekbom disease, 420b, 420
Withdrawal, signs of, 359

Withdrawal stage
　definition of addiction, 352
　management services, 381
　pharmacological interventions during, 373
Women
　sexual assault of, 485
　vulnerability of, in abuse, 488
Wong-Baker FACES Pain Rating Scale, 560f
Woodruff's Total Suffering Model, 597f, 597
Word salad, 278
　with schizophrenia, 156
Working conditions, as key social determinant of health, 12
Working phase
　of Peplau's model of nurse-patient relationship, 131
　of therapeutic groups, 621
Workplace
　addiction in nurses, 385b, 385
　violence, 466
Workplace harassment, 466
Workplace violence, 466
World Health Organization (WHO), 375
　defining traditional medicine, 645
　Disability Assessment Schedule 2.0, 10
　in ecological model of violence, 487f, 487
　in interpersonal violence, 481
　Mental Health Care Law: Ten Basic Principles, 93b
　mental health defined by, 2–3

Worldview
　culture and, 108
　indigenous, 108
　Western, 108

Y

Yale-Brown Obsessive Compulsive Scale (YBOCS), 202
YBOCS. *See* Yale-Brown Obsessive Compulsive Scale
Yin and *yang*, 648
Yoga, 648–649
　for adolescents, 541b
Young
　serious mental illness in, 573b, 573
　sleep hypnogram vs. older adults, 415f, 416

Z

Z-drugs, 166
Zeitgebers, 417
Zeldox. *See* Ziprasidone
Ziprasidone (Zeldox), 173
　for bipolar disorders, 263b
　for schizophrenia, 288, 289t
Zoophobia, 188t
Zopiclone (Imovane, Rhovane), 166, 426t
Zuclopenthixol, 473b
　for schizophrenia, 289t
Zung Self-Rating Depression Scale, 226
Zyprexa. *See* Olanzapine